QUICK INDEX OF CONDITIONS AND REGIONS

Note: Page numbers in italics denote figures and exhibits, entries followed by "t" denote tables.

(continues)

Differential Diagnosis and Management for the Chiropractor

PROTOCOLS AND ALGORITHMS

FIFTH EDITION

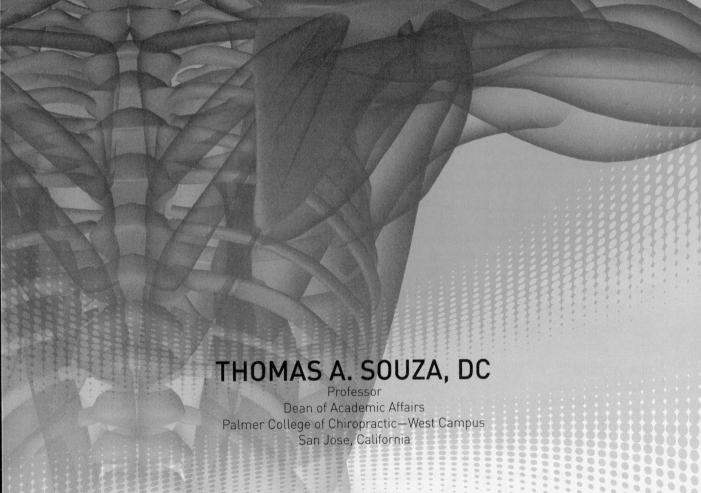

THOMAS A. SOUZA, DC

Professor
Dean of Academic Affairs
Palmer College of Chiropractic—West Campus
San Jose, California

JONES & BARTLETT
LEARNING

World Headquarters
Jones & Bartlett Learning
5 Wall Street
Burlington, MA 01803
978-443-5000
info@jblearning.com
www.jblearning.com

Jones & Bartlett Learning books and products are available through most bookstores and online booksellers. To contact Jones & Bartlett Learning directly, call 800-832-0034, fax 978-443-8000, or visit our website, www.jblearning.com.

Substantial discounts on bulk quantities of Jones & Bartlett Learning publications are available to corporations, professional associations, and other qualified organizations. For details and specific discount information, contact the special sales department at Jones & Bartlett Learning via the above contact information or send an email to specialsales@jblearning.com.

Production Credits

Publisher: Cathy L. Esperti
Acquisitions Editor: Ryan Angel
Associate Editor: Kayla Dos Santos
Editorial Assistant: Raven Heroux
Associate Director of Production: Julie C. Bolduc
Production Manager: Tina Chen
Marketing Manager: Grace Richards

Manager of Photo Research, Rights & Permissions: Amy Rathburn
VP, Manufacturing and Inventory Control: Therese Connell
Cover Design: Kristin Parker
Cover Image: Skeleton: © Medioimages/Photodisc/Digital Vision /Thinkstock; background: © Hemera/Thinkstock
Composition: Cenveo® Publisher Services
Printing and Binding: Edwards Brothers Malloy
Cover Printing: Edwards Brothers Malloy

Library of Congress Cataloging-in-Publication Data
Souza, Thomas A., author.
  Differential diagnosis and management for the chiropractor : protocols and algorithms / Thomas A. Souza. — Fifth edition.
     p. ; cm.
  Includes bibliographical references and index.
  ISBN 978-1-284-02230-8
  I. Title.
  [DNLM: 1. Chiropractic—methods. 2. Algorithms. 3. Clinical Protocols. 4. Diagnosis, Differential. WB 905]
  RZ250
  615.5'34—dc23
                          2014029050
6048

Printed in the United States of America
19 18 17 16   10 9 8 7 6 5 4 3

To Aaron.

CONTENTS

ACKNOWLEDGMENTS

I would like to express my appreciation to those who have contributed to editing the *Fifth Edition*. This includes many of the academic deans and department chairs at various chiropractic colleges and suggestions from practitioners and students. As usual, a task this size is not possible without the dedication and hard work of the editorial and production staff at Jones & Bartlett. Special thanks to Kayla Dos Santos, Joanna Lundeen, Ryan Angel, Vastavikta Sharma, Julie Searls, and everyone else who assisted in this project.

INTRODUCTION

In the five years since the previous edition of this book, there have been dramatic changes to the U.S. healthcare system that, in concept and evolution, will be placing more demand on evidence and outcomes. The literature has been exponentially growing, providing more evidence not only in the area of diagnostic accuracy but also outcomes. With that carries a larger responsibility for the average practitioner who has little time to keep up with these advances. The intention, always, with this text is to provide a predigested and critiqued summary of what is known and is likely to be relevant to the practicing chiropractor as well as to students who will need to understand processes of critical thinking and also have a quick option for evaluating complaints.

Chiropractors are finally positioned to become part of what is coined the Patient-Centered Medical Home (PCMH) or whatever future evolution this may involve. As part of a healthcare team, chiropractors can not only participate as spine specialists but also apply their broader knowledge to be participants in a well-integrated support group for patients.

In 2013, the North American Spine Society, in its guidelines for lumbar disc-related radiculopathy, listed manipulation as a viable option.[1] This is a monumental advance when one considers that not long ago, chiropractors were often accused of causing disc herniation and were considered off-limits by most MDs for the management of "complicated" low back pain with radiation below the knee. The literature in the last two years has in fact demonstrated that for both cervical and lumbar radiculopathy, manipulation may be a safe and effective alternative.[2, 3] In addition, other approaches such as directional-preference exercise approaches are good adjunctive and safe procedures.

In the field of physiotherapy and rehabilitation, some new approaches, or older approaches with new evidence, are dominating the discussion, including the use of shockwave therapy, low-level laser treatment, injections such as plasma rich protein (PRP), and vibration therapy, among others. The literature is growing and indicates that these alternatives are possible options to surgical management.

At the same time, gene-related approaches in both medication selection and surgical options are growing. In the case of stem-cell research, with advances in the use of adipose-derived cells, new opportunities for replacing worn-out or damaged tissues have become a potential reality in the near future.

New to this Edition

As usual, there have been a number of major revisions and additions to this new edition. These include but are not exclusive to the following:

- An additional 500 references
- Clinical summaries of the diagnostic literature for orthopaedic areas (see Translations Into Clinical Practice [TIPS]) at the end of orthopaedic-related chapters.
- For select chapters, a new graphical representation of likelihood ratios for tests involving the cervical and lumbar spine, the shoulder, and the knee.
- A widely expanded Pharmacology for the Chiropractor appendix. This expansion focuses on the mechanisms of common categories of medications prescribed for common complaints encountered in clinical practice by most chiropractors.
- A new appendix on how to incorporate literature evidence into practice and how to interpret the literature. There is a special emphasis on how practitioners can measure in their own practices; the scientist-clinician.
- Updated algorithms
- Expanded sections on:
  1. Pain
  2. Weakness
  3. Stroke
  4. Concussion

The reader is also directed to the list of websites that follows, which provides valuable resources for chiropractic-related sites, evidence-based sites, practice guideline sites, and links to databases and search engines for keeping up with our ever-expanding knowledge base.

Instructor Resources

As a benefit and an incentive for using this textbook, and to save the instructor valuable time in the preparation and instruction of this course, the publisher is pleased to provide for the first time the following resources to accompany *Differential Diagnosis and Management for the Chiropractor: Protocols and Algorithms, Fifth Edition*:

- Learning Objectives
- Lecture Outlines in PowerPoint format

- Sample Syllabus
- Test Bank
- Image Bank
- Transition Guide

Video Updates

Readers are encouraged to subscribe to Dr. Souza's update videos at **http://www.coffeebreaku.com**. These concise, timely video presentations will keep you current between editions with short, informative reviews of the most significant articles relevant to chiropractic practice. Subscribers will receive new video summaries each month and have access to a growing video library archive.

Students are directed to **http://www.jblearning.com /catalog/9781284022308/** for an access code to be redeemed on http://www.coffeebreaku.com and a discounted subscription.

References

1. Kreiner DS, Hwang SW, Easa JE, et al. An evidence-based clinical guideline for the diagnosis and treatment of lumbar disc herniation with radiculopathy. *Spine J.* 2014;14(1):180–191.
2. Peterson CK, Leemann S, Lechmann M, Pfirrmann CW, Hodler J, Humphreys BK. Symptomatic magnetic resonance imaging-confirmed lumbar disk herniation patients: a comparative effectiveness prospective observational study of 2 age- and sex-matched cohorts treated with either high-velocity, low-amplitude spinal manipulative therapy or imaging-guided lumbar nerve root injections. *J Manipulative Physiol Ther.* 2013;36(4):218–225.
3. Peterson CK, Schmid C, Leemann S, Anklin B, Humphreys BK. Outcomes from magnetic resonance imaging-confirmed symptomatic cervical disk herniation patients treated with high-velocity, low-amplitude spinal manipulative therapy: a prospective cohort study with 3-month follow-up. *J Manipulative Physiol Ther.* 2013;36(8):461–467.

Websites

Chiropractic Websites

American Chiropractic Association
http://www.acatoday.org/

International Chiropractors Association
http://www.chiropractic.org/

Evidence-Based Websites

Agency for Healthcare Research and Quality
http://www.ahrq.gov/

Cochrane Collaboration
http://www.cochrane.org/

Centre for Evidence-Based Medicine
http://www.cebm.net/

Evidence-Based Medicine
http://ebm.bmjjournals.com/

Practice Guideline Websites

CCGPP—Council on Chiropractic Guidelines and Practice Parameters
http://www.ccgpp.org/

National Guidelines Clearinghouse: Guidelines from the Agency for Healthcare Research and Quality, the U.S. Preventive Services Task Force, and other agencies
http://www.guidelines.gov

New Zealand Guidelines Group
http://www.nzgg.org.nz

National Institute for Health and Care Evidence (NICE)
http://cks.nice.org.uk/

Scottish Intercollegiate Guidelines Network (SIGN): How the literature is rated.
http://www.sign.ac.uk/

Database Search Sources

PubMed
http://**www.pubmed.org**

CINAHL (Cumulative Index to Nursing and Allied Health Literature)
http://www.ebscohost.com/cinahl/

MANTIS (chiropractic literature not on PubMed)
http://www.healthindex.com/

Cochrane Library
http://www.thecochranelibrary.com/view/0/index. html

Clinical Evidence
http://**www.clinicalevidence.com**

PEDro (Physiotherapy Evidence Database)
http://www.pedro.fhs.usyd.edu.au/

Part

1

Musculoskeletal Complaints

General Approach to Musculoskeletal Complaints

Context

The approach to a patient's musculoskeletal complaint is a standardized, often sequential search for what can and what cannot be managed by the examining doctor. There is always an ultimate decision: rule in or rule out referable conditions.

- The crucial decision with acute traumatic pain is to rule out fracture (and its complications such as neural or vascular damage), dislocation, and gross instability.
- The crucial decision with nontraumatic pain is to rule out tumors, inflammatory arthritides, infections, or visceral referral.

There appears to be a misinterpretation regarding the amount of information necessary to make diagnostic or management decisions. One error is to think of all joints as distinctly different because the names of structures, disorders, or orthopaedic tests are different for each joint. Another error is to make the assumption that the joint operates as an independent contractor without accountability to other joints. The first error leads to an overspecialization effort that often leaves the doctor unwilling to attack the vast amount of individual information for each joint. The second error leads the examiner to an approach that excludes important information that may contribute to the diagnosis of a patient's complaint. Each is an error in extremes: the first is that too much knowledge is assumed necessary; the second assumes that too little baseline information is needed for making diagnostic and treatment decisions.

A general approach to evaluation of any joint (and surrounding structures) utilizes the perspective that a joint is a joint. Although a specific joint may function differently because of its bony configuration, structurally,

it is composed generally of the same tissues. Most joint regions have bone, ligaments, a capsule, cartilage and synovium, surrounding tendons and muscles, associated bursae, blood vessels, nerves, fat, and skin. All of these structures may be injured by compression or stretch. Compression may lead to fracture in bones or neural dysfunction in nerves. Stretch leads to varying degrees of tendon/muscle, ligament/capsule, neural/vascular, or bone/epiphyseal damage ranging from minor disruption to full rupture. Joints can be further divided into weight-bearing and non-weight-bearing. Non-weight-bearing joints may be transformed into weight-bearing joints through various positions such as handstands or falls with the upper extremity, hyperextension of the spine, or any axial compression force to the joint. Weight-bearing joints are generally more susceptible to chronic degeneration and osteoarthritis.

Bones and joints are also susceptible to nonmechanical processes that involve seeding of infection or cancer as well as the development of primary cancer and the immunologically based rheumatoid and connective tissue disorders. Clues to rheumatoid and seronegative arthritides include a pattern of involvement with a specific predilection to a joint or groups of joints coupled with laboratory investigation.

The approach to evaluation of a neuromusculoskeletal complaint is also directed by a knowledge of common conditions affecting specific structures (regardless of the specific names). Following is a list of these structures and the disorders or conditions most often encountered with each:

- Bone
  1. tumor, primary or metastatic
  2. osteochondrosis/apophysitis
  3. fracture
  4. osteopenia (osteoporosis)
  5. osteomyelitis

- Soft tissue
  1. muscle
     - strain or rupture
     - trigger points
     - atrophy
     - myositis ossificans
     - muscular dystrophy
  2. rhabdomyolysis tendon
     - tendinitis
     - tendinosis paratenonitis
     - rupture
  3. ligament
     - sprain or rupture
  4. bursa
     - bursitis
  5. fascia
     - myofascitis
- Joint
  1. arthritis
  2. subluxation/fixation (chiropractic)
  3. synovitis
  4. infection
  5. joint mice
  6. dislocation/subluxation (medical)

General Strategy

History

Clarify the onset.

- Is the complaint traumatic?
- Is there a history of overuse?
- Is the onset insidious?

Clarify the type of complaint.

- Is the complaint one of pain, numbness or tingling, stiffness, looseness, crepitus, locking, or a combination of complaints?
- Localize the complaint to anterior, posterior, medial, or lateral if applicable.

Clarify the mechanism if traumatic (for extremities see **Table 1–1**).

- If there was a fall onto a specific region or structure within that region, consider fracture, dislocation, or contusion.
- Determine whether there was an excessive valgus or varus force, internal or external rotation, or

Table 1–1 Joint-Specific Injury Mechanism

Mechanism	Possible Structure(s) Damaged
Shoulder	
Fall on an outstretched arm (extended elbow)	Rotator cuff tear
	Glenoid labrum tear
	Posterior dislocation
	Clavicular fracture
Arm forced into abduction/external rotation	Anterior dislocation
	Anterior musculature strain
Blow to the shoulder area	Fracture
	Acromioclavicular separation
	Dislocation
Fall onto top of shoulder	Shoulder pointer
	Acromioclavicular separation
	Distal clavicular fracture
Traction injury to arm	Plexus injury
	Medical subluxation
Elbow	
Direct fall on tip of elbow or fall on hand with elbow flexed	Olecranon fracture
Fall on hand with extended elbow	Radial head fracture
Hyperextension injury to elbow	Elbow dislocation
	Supracondylar fracture in children

Table 1–1 Joint-Specific Injury Mechanism (continued)

Mechanism	Possible Structure(s) Damaged
Severe valgus stress	Capitellum fracture
	Avulsion of medial epicondyle
	Medial collateral ligament sprain or rupture
Sudden traction of forearm	Radial head subluxation
Wrist/hand	
Fall on dorsiflexed hand	Navicular fracture
	Epiphyseal and torus fractures in children
	Carpal dislocation, or instability
Hyperextension or abduction of thumb	Gamekeeper's thumb (ulnar collateral ligament damage)
Axial compression of thumb	Bennett's fracture
	Dislocation
Hyperextension of finger	Volar plate injury
	Jersey finger (rupture of flexor digitorum profundus)
	Dislocation
Hyperflexion of finger	Avulsion of central slip
	Mallet finger (rupture of extensor tendon)
Valgus/varus stress injury to finger	Collateral ligament or volar plate injury
Axial compression	Capsular irritation
	Fracture
Hip	
Fall on hip	Fracture
	Synovitis
	Hip pointer
	Trochanteric bursitis
Blow to flexed, abducted hip	Posterior dislocation
Knee	
Hyperextension	Anterior cruciate ligament tear
Sudden deceleration	Anterior cruciate ligament tear
Blow to a flexed knee at proximal tibia or hyperflexion	Posterior cruciate ligament tear
Blow to anterior knee/patella	Irritation of plica
	Patellar fracture
	Bursitis
	Infrapatellar fat pad irritation
Valgus force	Medial collateral ligament tear
	Pes anserine strain
Rotational injury with foot fixed on ground	Meniscus
Rotational injury with a valgus force	Anterior cruciate ligament, meniscus, medial collateral ligament
Foot/ankle	
Plantarflexion, inversion of ankle	Ankle sprain with possible associated bifurcate ligament damage, fracture, or peroneal tendon snapping from torn retinaculum
Eversion injury to ankle	Deltoid ligament sprain or rupture
	Fracture
	Dislocation
Hyperextension of great toe	Turf-toe injury to capsular ligaments
Landing on heels	Fat pad irritation
	Ankle or tibial fracture

flexion or extension. Consider ligament/capsule or muscle/tendon.

- If there was sudden axial traction to the joint, consider sprain or subluxation.
- If there was axial compression to the joint, consider fracture or synovitis.

Determine whether the mechanism is one of overuse.

- In what position does the patient work?
- Does the patient perform a repetitive movement at work or during sports activities? Consider muscle strain, tendinitis, trigger points, or peripheral nerve entrapment.

If insidious, determine the following:

- Are there associated systemic signs of fever, malaise/fatigue, lymphadenopathy, multiple affected areas, etc.?
- Are there local signs of inflammation including swelling, heat, or redness?
- Is there local deformity?
- Is there associated weakness, numbness, tingling, or other associated neurologic dysfunction?

Determine whether the patient has a current or past history or diagnosis of his or her complaint or other related disorders.

- Are there associated spinal complaints or radiation from the spine? Consider subluxation, nerve root entrapment, or compression.
- Does the patient have a diagnosis of another arthritide, systemic disorder such as diabetes, or past history of cancer?

- Does the patient have "visceral" complaints such as abdominal or chest pain, fever, weight loss, or other complaints?

Evaluation

- With trauma, palpate for points of tenderness and test for neurovascular status distal to the site of injury; obtain plain films to rule out the possibility of fracture/dislocation.
- Palpate for swelling, masses, and warmth.
- Determine whether swelling is present and if so, whether it is intra- or extra-articular. If extra-articular, attempt to differentiate between bursal versus vascular inflammation.
- If deformity or mass is evident, attempt to differentiate between soft versus bony tissue. The most common soft tissue causes would include lipomas, neuromas, and ganglions (or other cysts), or fascial herniation.
- With no history of trauma or overuse, consider the use of special imaging, including MRI or CT; bone scan for cancer seeding screen or for stress fracture; electrodiagnostic studies if persistent neurological findings are present; laboratory if systemic findings are present; or synovial fluid analysis if swelling is present or if an arthritide is suspected but in need of differentiation (see **Table 1–2**).
- Palpate and challenge the ligaments and capsule of the joint.
- Challenge the musculotendinous attachments with stretch, contraction, and a combination of contraction in a stretched position.

Table 1–2 Synovial Fluid Examination

Type	Examples	Color	Clarity	WBC (per μL)	PMNs	Culture	Glucose	Volume
Normal		Clear	Transparent	<200	<25%	Negative	Nearly = to serum	<3.5
Group I (Noninflammatory)	DJD Trauma Osteochondritis dissecans PVS Osteochondromatosis Neuropathic arthropathy	Yellow	Transparent	200–300	<25%	Negative	Nearly = to serum	Often >3.5

Table 1–2 Synovial Fluid Examination (continued)

Type	Examples	Color	Clarity	WBC (per μL)	PMNs	Culture	Glucose	Volume
Group II (Inflammatory)	RA Active crystal-induced (gout, pseudogout) Seronegatives (AS, Reiter's psoriatic) Enteropathic (IBD) Rheumatic fever SLE Scleroderma Tuberculosis Mycotic infection	Yellow to opalescent	Transparent to opaque	3,000–50,000	50% or more	Negative	>25; lower than serum	Often >3.5
Group III (Purulent)	Pyogenic bacterial infection	Yellow to green	Opaque	>50,000	75% or more	Usually positive	<25; much lower than serum	Often >3.5

Note: Joint aspiration findings for hemorrhagic causes, including hemophilia, trauma (with or without fracture), neuropathic arthropathy, PVS, and benign neoplasms (e.g., hemangioma) are dominated by blood in the joint. *Legend:* WBC = white blood cell; PMN = polymorphonuclear leukocytes; PVS = pigmented villonodular synovitis; IBD = inflammatory bowel disease (includes ulcerative colitis and regional enteritis)

- Measure the functional capacities of the region involved; determine any associated biomechanical faults that may be contributing to the problem.

Management

- Refer fracture/dislocation, infection, and tumors for orthopaedic management.
- Refer or comanage rheumatoid and connective tissue disorders.
- If the problem is one of instability without ligament rupture, stabilize the joint through an appropriate exercise program using a brace initially, if necessary, to assist.
- If the problem is weakness, strengthen the associated muscle.
- Functionally retrain the individual for a return to daily activities and occupational or sport requirements.
- Use manipulation/mobilization for articular dysfunction.

History

A mnemonic approach to the patient's complaints may be helpful in organizing the vast number of possibilities. Beginning with a description of the patient's complaint, a list of common causes may be attached. WIRS Pain is a mnemonic for **weakness**, **instability**, **restricted movement**, **surface complaints**, and **pain**.

Weakness

Weakness may be due to pain inhibition, muscle strain, or neurologic interruption at the myoneural junction, peripheral nerve, nerve root, or spinal cord and above. Weakness may be a misinterpretation by the patient when instability or a "loose" joint is present or the patient has stiffness that must be overcome by increased muscular activity.

Instability

Instability is due to either traumatic damage to ligamentous or muscular support or due to the inherent looseness found in some individuals' joints. This inherent looseness is usually global and can be identified in other joints or acquired as a result of repetitive overstretch positioning. Instability is most apparent when the joint is positioned so that muscles have less mechanical advantage (e.g., overhead shoulder positions) or when a quick movement demand is faster than the reaction time for the corresponding muscles (e.g., cutting or rotating knee movements).

Restricted Movement

Restricted movement may be due to pain, muscle spasm, stretching of soft tissue contracture, or mechanical blockage by osteophytes, joint mice, fracture, or effusion.

Surface Complaints

Superficial complaints include skin lesions, cuts/abrasions, swelling, and a patient's subjective sense of numbness or paresthesias.

Pain

Pain is nonspecific; however, the cause usually will be revealed by combining a history of trauma, overuse, or insidious onset with associated complaints and significant examination findings. It is important to determine local pain versus referred pain. Following are some guidelines:

- Referred pain from scleratogenous sources: Scleratogenous pain presents as a nondermatomal pattern with no hard neurologic findings such as significant decrease in myotomal strength or deep tendon reflex changes. Although the term is used broadly, here we are referring mainly to facet- and disc-generated pain.
- Referred pain from visceral sources: In most cases a historical screening of patients will reveal primary or secondary visceral complaints. It is important to know the classic referral zones, such as scapular/shoulder pain with cholelithiasis and medial arm pain with cardiac ischemia.
- Bone pain: Bone pain is deep pain, commonly worse in the evening. Trauma may indicate an underlying fracture requiring radiographic evaluation. An overuse history may be suggestive of a stress fracture requiring a radiographic evaluation. If results of the radiograph are negative, but a stress fracture is still suspected, a bone scan is warranted.

A careful history will usually indicate the diagnosis or, at the very least, narrow down the possibilities to two or three. Physical examination and imaging studies more often are used as a confirmation of one's suspicion(s). Generalizing a history approach allows the doctor to address any complaint regardless of region. Generally speaking, damage to structures locally is due to (1) exceeding the tensile stress of ligaments, capsule, muscles, and tendons; (2) compression of bone; (3) demineralization of bone; or (4) intrinsic destructive processes involving arthritides (e.g., pannus formation with rheumatoid arthritis [RA], crystal deposition with gout or pseudogout), infections, or cancer). Although the first two categories are almost always the result of trauma or overuse, the latter two are more commonly insidious. Traumatic and overuse disorders are classically local with regard to signs and symptoms, whereas arthritides and cancer are often either generalized or stereotypical based on the type.

Suspicion of specific structures is based on a basic knowledge of what causes damage to any similar structure regardless of which region or joint is involved. Ligament or capsular injury is often the result of excessive force on the opposite side of the ligament/capsule. For example, a valgus stress (outside to inside force) to the knee will cause an injury to the medial collateral ligament; a varus force, the lateral collateral ligament. Although more dramatically evident in an acute injury, it must be remembered that low-level, chronic stresses are often the cause of ligamentous or capsular sprain. Muscle injury can be divided into stretch injury and contraction injury. Often when ligaments are damaged, muscle/tendon groups are also involved. Muscles/tendons often act as static stabilizers simply because when they cross the joint, they are in the way when outside forces stretch that joint. Additionally, muscles will often contract in an attempt to protect the joint and either incur damage or impose more damage to the joint. This occurs especially when a joint is in extension (such as the knee and elbow) or in neutral (such as the wrist and ankle). Contraction injury is divided into concentric and eccentric. Usually an overexertion problem, concentric injury often occurs when too heavy a weight is lifted or a sudden explosive muscle activity is required. Concentric injury occurs as the muscle is shortening. Eccentric injury occurs while the muscle is lengthening. Although eccentric injury may occur with lifting, this pattern is frequently seen with overuse or repetitive activity and/or injuries that challenge the decelerator or stabilizer role of the muscle.

Tendons are susceptible primarily to overstrain from a sudden, forceful muscle contraction or from overuse. Occasionally, direct trauma may damage or inflame the tendon or its sheath. Rheumatoid and connective tissue disorders can also affect the synovial lining or paratenon. Sometimes the use of various terminologies in the description of tendon disorders is confusing. Newer terminology replacing older nomenclature causes some of this difficulty, coupled with new theories as to the types of tendon pathology that occur related to its structure and function.[1] Following is an updated list:

- Paratenonitis—This term is replacing tenosynovitis, tenovaginitis, and peritendinitis. It is characterized by inflammation of only the paratenon (lined by synovium or not). Clinical signs are swelling, pain, crepitation along the tendon, local tenderness, and warmth.
- Tendinitis—Now used in place of strain or tear of a tendon. This term refers to symptomatic degeneration of a tendon with vascular disruption and an inflammatory repair response. Stages include: acute, < 2 weeks; subacute, 4–6 weeks; and chronic, > 6 weeks. Three subgroups include: (1) purely inflammatory with acute hemorrhage and tearing, (2) inflammation that is in addition to preexisting degeneration, and (3) calcification and tendinosis that is chronic.
- Tendinosis—The newer term used to indicate intratendinous degeneration due to atrophy (due to aging, microtrauma, vascular compromise, etc.). This is considered noninflammatory with hypocellularity, variable vascular ingrowth, local necrosis, and/or calcification, with accompanying fiber disorientation. Palpable nodules can be found, such as in the Achilles, with or without tenderness.
- Paratenonitis with tendinosis—This describes a paratenon inflammation associated with intratendinous degeneration. Unlike tendinosis, this combination of pathologies presents clinically with a possible palpable tendon nodule, with accompanying signs of swelling and inflammation.

Bursae are protective cushions placed strategically at points of friction, particularly between muscle/tendon and bone. Although there are standard bursae in most individuals, adventitious bursae may develop at sites of repetitive friction in individuals performing specific activities. Bursae may be deep or superficial. Superficial bursae are susceptible to direct traumatic forces. Deep bursae are more susceptible to compression by bone or soft tissue structures. Compression is often position-specific, such as during overhead movements with the shoulder. Bursitis may be secondary to other soft tissue involvement such as calcific tendinitis.

When musculoskeletal pain does not have an obvious mechanical or traumatic cause, a search is initiated for myofascial disorders, arthritides, psychological factors, connective tissue disorders, cancer, and infection (see **Table 1–3**).

Arthritis has a "geriatric" connotation, yet it may affect any age group. The term simply means that the joint is affected. Generally, arthritis is due to degeneration or destruction that is age-related or trauma-related, infectious, inflammatory, and/or autoimmune. Based on the cause, arthritis may present as a monoarthropathy (i.e., single joint), an oligoarthropathy (2–4 joints), or a polyarthropathy (≥ 5 joints). When a single joint is involved, gout (first toe), infectious (direct infection or indirect spreading from another source such as gonococcal), or trauma should be considered. When multiple joints are involved a distinction in thinking occurs differentiating degenerative, inflammatory (primarily rheumatoid and rheumatoid variants), and crystalline induced (primarily gout, pseudogout, amyloidosis, etc.). Seronegatives and enteropathic arthropathies tend to be oligoarticular, whereas RA and LE tend to involve more joints.

When considering arthritis as a cause of joint pain, there are several other general factors that when considered separately and then clustered together provide a good tool for narrowing the large list of possibilities. The sequence of how these factors are considered may change given the presentation of the patient, yet the discussion will begin with age. There are very few arthritides that affect the young. Primarily, juvenile rheumatoid arthritis or arthritis secondary to other diseases would be considered. For the young to middle-aged adult, primarily inflammatory and/or autoimmune arthritides are considered, including:

- Seronegative arthritides (i.e., negative for rheumatoid factor) including ankylosing spondylitis (AS), Reiter's, and psoriatic
- Rheumatoid arthritis (RA)
- Scleroderma
- Lupus erythematosus (LE)
- Osteitis condensins illi
- Synoviochondrometaplasia

For onset in the senior, the primary considerations include:

- Degenerative joint disease; osteoarthritis (OA)
- Diffuse idiopathic skeletal hyperostosis (DISH)
- Hypertrophic osteoarthropathy
- Gout
- Pseudogout; calcium pyrophosphate dihydrate (CPPD) deposition disease

Considering gender, males are more prone toward AS, Reiter's, gout, hypertrophic osteoarthropathy, and secondary OA. Females are more prone toward juvenile

Table 1–3 Selected Arthritic Disorders

Type	Features	Management Issues
Degenerative		
Primary osteoarthritis	**Age of Onset**—Generally > 45 y/o **Gender Predominance**—Ratio of female to male = 10:1 **Common Joints Involved**—Hips, knees, SI joint, AC joint, first MCP, first MC trapezium, DIP joints of hands Often initially asymptomatic; gradual increase in joint stiffness and pain. Deformity may be apparent (e.g., Heberden's nodes in hands). May eventually lead to joint subluxation and instability. Radiographically: The distribution is asymmetric, with nonuniform loss of joint space, osteophyte formation, subchondral sclerosis (eburnation), subchondral cysts.	Management in early and middle stages should include strengthening around involved joints. If weight-bearing joint, begin with non-weight-bearing and progress cautiously to weight-bearing if possible. Maintenance of normal joint motion and function may be facilitated by adjusting/manipulation or mobilization. Dietary approaches include glucosamine and chondroitin sulfate. Medical management may include recommendations for NSAIDs, in particular, COX-2 inhibitors. Some medical specialists may recommend viscosupplementation (injection of hyaluronic acid into the degenerative joint). This is of questionable value. In some joints, joint replacement is necessary.
Secondary osteoarthritis	**Age of Onset**— > 25 years **Gender Predominance**—Equal **Common Joints Involved**—GH, AC, SI, hip, elbow, knee, foot, hand Cause is secondary to other disorders or diseases/injuries such as trauma, septic or inflammatory arthritis, slipped epiphyses, dysplasias, fracture/dislocation, avascular necrosis, ochronosis, and acromegaly. Similar radiographic presentation.	Management in early and middle stages should include strengthening around involved joints. If weight-bearing, begin with non-weight-bearing and progress cautiously to weight-bearing if possible. Maintenance of normal joint motion and function may be facilitated by adjusting/manipulation or mobilization. Dietary approaches include glucosamine and chondroitin sulfate. Medical management may include recommendations for NSAIDs, in particular, COX-2 inhibitors. Some medical specialists may recommend viscosupplementation (injection of hyaluronic acid into the degenerative joint). This is of questionable value. In some joints, joint replacement is necessary.
Erosive osteoarthritis	**Gender Predominance**—Female **Common Joints Involved**—Interphalangeal joints of hand **Age of Onset**—40–50 y/o Inflammatory variant of DJD characterized by cartilage degeneration and synovial proliferation. Acute episodes that appear similar to inflammatory/synovial arthritis; chronically may evolve to subluxation and development of Heberden's nodes. Radiologically similar to OA with additional finding of central erosions.	Management in early and middle stages should include strengthening around involved joints. If weight-bearing, begin with non-weight-bearing and progress cautiously to weight-bearing if possible. Dietary approaches include glucosamine and chondroitin sulfate. Medical management may include recommendations for NSAIDs, in particular, COX-2 inhibitors. In addition, the following anti-inflammatory medications may be suggested: • DMARDs—Disease-modifying antirheumatic drugs (e.g., methotrexate [Rheumatrex and Trexall], hydroxychloroquine [Plaquenil], and leflunomide [Arava]). These are toxic and may take weeks to months to work, yet are highly effective. • Biologic agents—reduce the production of tissue necrosis factor (TNF) (e.g., Enbrel and Remicade sometimes given together with methotrexate).

Degenerative spine disease	**Age of Onset**— > 30 y/o **Gender Predominance**—Equal **Common Joints Involved**—Specific spinal involvement at C5-C7, T2-T5, T10-T12, L4-S1 with additional involvement of uncovertebral, costovertebral, discovertebral, and apophyseal (facet) joint involvement. Range from asymptomatic to severely symptomatic with pain and stiffness. Radiographic to clinical correlation is poor. May contribute to IVF narrowing and spinal stenosis. Common radiographic findings include disc space narrowing, hypertrophy of smaller joints such as facets and costovertebral, synovial cysts, Schmorl's nodes, and intradiscal vacuum phenomena. In middle stages, joint and capsular laxity may lead to subluxation and listhesis.	Management in early and middle stages should include strengthening of the spinal muscles with a focus on abdominal strengthening and extensor strengthening and stretching. The three-joint complex model stresses the need to consider the interrelationship of facets joint and intervertebral disc joints in the progression of DJD of the spine. Maintenance of normal joint motion and function may be facilitated by adjusting or manipulation or mobilization. Dietary approaches include an anti-inflammatory dietary regimen and use of glucosamine and chondroitin sulfate. Medical management may include recommendations for NSAIDs, in particular, COX-2 inhibitors for pain management.
Diffuse idiopathic skeletal hyperostosis (DISH) (synonyms: ankylosing hyperostosis, Forestier's disease)	**Age of Onset**—50 y/o and older **Gender Predominance**—Male **Common Joints Involved**—Spine; predominantly T7-T11 (calcification of anterior longitudinal ligament) with 30% peripheral joint involvement. Found in 25% of men and 15% of women >50 y/o (common). May be asymptomatic; when symptomatic, similar complaints associated with DJD such as stiffness and pain; 20% of patients report dysphagia; occasional complaints involving the Achilles tendon, extensor wad of wrist/forearm, plantar fascia, and quadriceps tendon (may find enthesophytes at corresponding sites); about a quarter of patients have diabetes. Radiographically: Diffuse, thick, hyperostosis primarily along the anterolateral aspect of spine ("flowing wax" appearance); 50% of patients also have ossification of the PLL, especially in the cervical spine.	Management in early and middle stages should include strengthening of the spinal muscles with a focus on abdominal strengthening and extensor strengthening and stretching. Dietary approaches include an anti-inflammatory dietary regimen and use of glucosamine and chondroitin sulfate, yet DISH appears to follow its own course of progression specific to the individual but generally always progressive. Medical management may include recommendations for NSAIDs, in particular, COX-2 inhibitors for pain management.
Neuropathic (neurotrophic) arthropathy	**Age of Onset**—Variable **Gender Predominance**—Variable **Common Joints Involved**—Knee, hip, ankle, spine, shoulder, elbow, wrist, foot. Variable upper motor and lower motor lesions cause a combination of loss of proprioception and pain perception leading to joint destruction. Conditions include syringomyelia, diabetes, tabes dorsalis, multiple sclerosis, Charcot-Marie-Tooth disease, prolonged used of intra-articular corticosteroids, pernicious anemia, and leprosy, among others. A somewhat separate but related cause is spinal cord damage resulting in paraplegia or quadriplegia, which results in usually asymptomatic bony ankylosis. Radiographically neuropathic arthropathy is seen as joint collapse, pseudarthrosis, fragmentation, and deformity.	Treatment is directed toward the primary disease. If in weight-bearing joints, mechanical assistance is often required. In severe cases, amputation is necessary.

(continues)

Table 1–3 Selected Arthritic Disorders (continued)

Type	Features	Management Issues
Synoviochondrometaplasia (idiopathic synovial osteochondromatosis)	**Age of Onset**—30–50 y/o **Gender Predominance**—Ratio of male to female = 3:1 **Common Joints Involved**—Knee, hip, ankle, elbow, wrist. Synoviochondrometaplasia, as the name implies, is a synovial metaplasia that results in the formation of cartilage that then forms loose bodies in the joint. This process is usually idiopathic but may be the result of trauma. The patient will report increasing pain, swelling, crepitus, and locking due to the loose bodies. Radiographically the loose bodies can be seen if radiopaque. Sometimes erosion may occur as in the "apple-core" deformity of the hip.	Synovectomy for most patients. Joint replacement may be recommended for older patients.
Inflammatory		
Positive for Rheumatoid Factor (Seropositive)		
Rheumatoid arthritis (RA)	**Age of Onset**—25–55 y/o **Gender Predominance**—Female to male ratio = 2:1 to 3:1 **Common Joints Involved**—Hand, foot, wrist, knee, elbow, GH joint, AC joint, and cervical spine (atlantoaxial). A symmetric, bilateral, polyarticular disorder of the synovial membrane resulting in joint pain, swelling, and destruction. Also involved are ligaments, tendons, and bursae. The diagnostic criteria includes: Deformities such as Boutonniere, swan-neck, phalangeal deviation, and arthritis mutilans; morning stiffness that lasts longer than 1 hour, specific swelling of several joints (including the PIP joints, MCP joint, and wrist), rheumatoid nodules, positive for rheumatoid factor, and radiographic evidence that includes erosions or periarticular osteopenia or both in hands or wrists or both. Need four or more of the above for at least 6 weeks. Additional symptoms may include fatigue, anorexia, weight loss, and muscular pain/stiffness. Special concern is for atlantoaxial instability due to ligament erosion and a resulting risk of excessive movement leading to spinal cord compression.	Caution with rheumatoid conditions is unpredictable flare-ups. Given that some of the therapies employed by chiropractic are mechanical, including adjusting, soft tissue therapy, and physiotherapy, it is important to keep in mind that this is an inflammatory condition and can be exacerbated by these therapies. Incorporate an anti-inflammatory diet regimen (see Table 1–9). Medical management includes: • NSAIDs—COX-1 inhibitors (e.g., ibuprofen, naproxen) or COX-2 inhibitors (e.g., Celebrex). • Corticosteroids • DMARDs—disease-modifying antirheumatic drugs (e.g., methotrexate [Rheumatrex and Trexall], hydroxychloroquine [Plaquenil], and leflunomide [Arava]). These are toxic and may take weeks to months to work, yet are highly effective. • Biologic agents—Reduce the production of tissue necrosis factor (TNF) (e.g., Enbrel and Remicade sometimes given together with methotrexate). May be administered as infusion therapy.

Juvenile chronic arthritis	**Age of Onset**—5–10 y/o **Gender Predominance**—Variable based on specific disorder **Common Joints Involved**—Hand, foot, wrist, knee, elbow, heel, hip, and cervical spine. Several types including: • Juvenile-onset adult RA—same findings as RA • Still's disease—more of a systemic disease • Juvenile onset of seronegative arthropathies—see each disorder Radiographically similar with the possible addition of growth disturbances of bone and epiphyseal compression fractures.	Caution with rheumatoid conditions is unpredictable flare-ups. Given that some of the therapies employed by chiropractic are mechanical, including adjusting, soft tissue therapy, and physiotherapy, it is important to keep in mind that this is an inflammatory condition and can be exacerbated by these therapies. Medical management includes: • NSAIDs—COX-1 inhibitors (e.g., ibuprofen, naproxen) or COX-2 inhibitors (e.g., Celebrex). • DMARDs—disease-modifying antirheumatic drugs (e.g., methotrexate [Rheumatrex and Trexall], hydroxychloroquine [Plaquenil], and leflunomide [Arava]). These are toxic and may take weeks to months to work, yet are highly effective. • Biologic agents—Reduce the production of tissue necrosis factor (TNF) (e.g., Enbrel and Remicade are sometimes given together with methotrexate). May be administered as infusion therapy. • Corticosteroids—Rarely needed.
Negative for Rheumatoid Factor (Seronegative)		
Ankylosing spondylitis (AS)	**Age of Onset**—15–35 y/o **Gender Predominance**—Male to female ratio = 4:1 to 10:1 **Common Joints Involved**—SI joint, thoracolumbar spine, cervical spine, symphysis pubis, hip, shoulder, and heel. Complaints often begin with SI pain and progress to low back and thoracic stiffness. Eventually there may be a decrease in chest expansion. Peripheral joint involvement occurs in approximately 50% as does radiating pain to the lower extremity. Areas of concern include iritis (20% of cases), aortic insufficiency, aneurysms, pulmonary fibrosis, pleuritis, IBD, and amyloidosis. Laboratory findings include an increased ESR during active phases, negative for RA and LE factors; HLA B-27, positive in 80% (positive in 6–8% of general population). Radiographically there are classic signs, including symmetrical involvement of the SI joints, ligament calcification, and marginal syndesmophytes, eventually leading to "trolley-track" sign, and bamboo spine.	Caution with rheumatoid conditions is unpredictable flare-ups. Given that some of the therapies employed by chiropractic are mechanical, including adjusting, soft tissue therapy, and physiotherapy, it is important to keep in mind that this is an inflammatory condition and can be exacerbated by these therapies. Medical management includes: • NSAIDs—COX-1 inhibitors (e.g., ibuprofen, naproxen) or COX-2 inhibitors (e.g., Celebrex). • DMARDs—disease-modifying antirheumatic drugs (e.g., methotrexate [Rheumatrex and Trexall], hydroxychloroquine [Plaquenil], and leflunomide [Arava]). These are toxic and may take weeks to months to work, yet are highly effective. • Biologic agents—Reduce the production of tissue necrosis factor (TNF) (e.g., Enbrel and Remicade are sometimes given together with methotrexate). May be administered as infusion therapy. • Corticosteroids—Rarely needed.

(continues)

Table 1-3 Selected Arthritic Disorders (continued)

Type	Features	Management Issues
Reiter's syndrome	**Age of Onset**—15–35 y/o **Gender Predominance**—Male to female ratio = 5:1 to 50:1 depending upon study **Common Joints Involved**—SI joint, foot, heel, ankle, knee, hip, spine; more rarely the upper extremity. Urethritis and other eye complaints often following a STD or gastrointestinal infection. Keratitis, keratoderma, and keratosis of nails may be found. Systemic findings may include fever, weight loss, thrombophlebitis, or amyloidosis. Lab findings may include positive HLAB27 (75%), leukocytosis, anemia, and elevated ESR. Radiographically SI joint is prominent, atlantoaxial instability, nonmarginal syndesmophytes. Similar to psoriatic arthritis, a single digit may be involved (sausage finger) and enthesopathies are common as in AS. Monitor for aortic regurgitation in chronic cases.	Caution with rheumatoid conditions is unpredictable flare-ups. Given that some of the therapies employed by chiropractic are mechanical, including adjusting, soft tissue therapy, and physiotherapy, it is important to keep in mind that this is an inflammatory condition and can be exacerbated by these therapies. Medical management includes: • NSAIDs—COX-1 inhibitors (e.g., ibuprofen, naproxen) or COX-2 inhibitors (e.g., Celebrex). • DMARDs—disease-modifying antirheumatic drugs (e.g., methotrexate [Rheumatrex and Trexall], hydroxychloroquine [Plaquenil], and leflunomide [Arava]). These are toxic and may take weeks to months to work, yet are highly effective. • Biologic agents—Reduce the production of tissue necrosis factor (TNF) (e.g., Enbrel and Remicade are sometimes given together with methotrexate). May be administered as infusion therapy. • Corticosteroids—Rarely needed.
Psoriatic	**Age of Onset**—20–50 y/o **Gender Predominance**—Generally equal **Common Joints Involved**—Hand, foot, SI joint, thoracolumbar spine, and cervical spine. Only about 5% of those with skin disease have the joint involvement. There are various patterns, yet many times the proximal and distal IP joints are involved. A deforming type may lead to arthritis mutilans. In addition to possibly having scaly patches of skin (psoriasis) on the extensor surfaces of the knees and elbows, patients may also have nail changes, including pitting, discoloration, and splintering. In some cases hyperostosis occurs at the SC joint. Other skin lesions may occur in the hands and feet. Lab includes HLA-B27 antigen (60% of cases), mild anemia, elevated ESR during active periods, occasionally elevated uric acid levels. Radiographically the involvement of the hands is similar to RA. In addition, one digit is often affected (sausage finger) and tuft resorption and proliferation (ivory phalanx) occur. In the spine, nonmarginal syndesmophytes may be seen.	Caution with rheumatoid conditions is unpredictable flare-ups. Given that some of the therapies employed by chiropractic are mechanical, including adjusting, soft tissue therapy, and physiotherapy, it is important to keep in mind that this is an inflammatory condition and can be exacerbated by these therapies. When arthritis is present, cyclosporine, methotrexate, and acitretin are used. Methotrexate is associated with hepatic toxicity; cyclosporine associated with hypertension and nephrotoxicity; and acitretin is associated with elevated serum lipids, mucocutaneous toxicity, and teratogenicity. New drugs are being marketed that, although highly promising, are extremely expensive. These drugs are part of a new class of medications called immune modulators (also known as biological response modifiers or "biologics"). The mechanism for these new drugs is either to block and reduce abnormal T-lymphocyte activity or the inflammatory response. Examples are alefacept and etanercept. (The "-cept" ending is an indication of the drug's effect, which is fusion of a receptor to the Fc portion of human IgGI.)

Condition	Details	Management
Enteropathic (associated with inflammatory bowel disease [IBD])	**Age of Onset**—Variable **Gender Predominance**—Variable **Common Joints Involved**—SI joint and spine; occasionally peripheral joint involvement. Many inflammatory disorders affecting the GI tract may result in an arthritis similar to the seronegative arthritides. Disorders include Crohn's, ulcerative colitis, Whipple's disease, and infections, including Salmonella, Shigella, and Yersinia. Intestinal bypass surgery may also be related. The frequency of IBD and AS is about 15%. Laboratory reveals HLA-B27 in 90% of those with IBD and arthritis. Radiographic findings are similar to AS, including SI involvement and the spine.	Caution with rheumatoid conditions is unpredictable flare-ups. Given that some of the therapies employed by chiropractic are mechanical, including adjusting, soft tissue therapy, and physiotherapy; it is important to keep in mind that this is an inflammatory condition and can be exacerbated by these therapies. Use anti-inflammatory approaches in diet and supplement recommendations and physiotherapy management. Medical management includes: • NSAIDs—COX-1 inhibitors (e.g., ibuprofen, naproxen) or COX-2 inhibitors (e.g., Celebrex). • DMARDs—disease-modifying antirheumatic drugs (e.g., methotrexate [Rheumatrex and Trexall], hydroxychloroquine [Plaquenil], and leflunomide [Arava]). These are toxic and may take weeks to months to work, yet are highly effective. • Biologic agents—Reduce the production of tissue necrosis factor (TNF) (e.g., Enbrel and Remicade are sometimes given together with methotrexate). • Corticosteroids.
Systemic lupus erythematosus (SLE)	**Age of Onset**—20–45 y/o **Gender Predominance**—Female more than male **Common Joints Involved**—Hand and osteonecrosis, specifically of femur (head and condyles) and sometimes shoulder (humeral head). A systemic autoimmune disorder characterized by multisystem involvement resulting in generalized findings such as fever, anorexia, weight loss, malaise, and weakness. Visceral inflammation occurs. Skin affects include rashes (e.g., butterfly malar rash). Polyarthritis is common. Like many patients with autoimmune rheumatoid conditions, tendons are weakened and may rupture. Laboratory reveals anemia with leucopenia and plasma protein abnormalities (protein electrophoresis usually ordered due to globulin increase). Antinuclear antibody and LE cells present. A false-positive syphilis test may occur. Radiographically a symmetric, nonerosive yet deforming arthropathy is seen. Osteonecrosis may be seen due to the disease or due to treatment (corticosteroids).	Given that some of the therapies employed by chiropractic are mechanical, including adjusting, soft tissue therapy, and physiotherapy; it is important to keep in mind that this is an inflammatory condition and can be exacerbated by these therapies. Protection of the skin includes avoiding sunlight, and it is important when exposed to use a sunblock with SPF 15 or higher. Primary treatment is prednisone for joint pain, cutaneous lesions, and renal and CNS involvement. Other medical therapies include antimalarials (hydroxychloroquine) and NSAIDs. Infection is common due to immunosuppression and is the cause of death in one-third of cases. Blacks and Hispanics fare worse. Pericarditis is found in 25% of patients. Also, screening for renal function is important to determine disease activity.
Scleroderma (progressive systemic sclerosis)	**Age of Onset**—20–30 y/o **Gender Predominance**—Female more than male **Common Joints Involved**—Hand, wrist, foot, ribs, and, more rarely, the spine. There are two types of this collagen-vascular disease: one with systemic involvement (progressive) and one without (localized). Scleroderma is characterized by involvement of multiple organs including skin, heart,	Management is for various aspects of the disease. Following are combinations of medical and conservative approaches: *Raynaud's* • Calcium channel blockers • Peripheral adrenergic blockers • Protective measures against cold, cessation of smoking, and decreased use of caffeine and other sympathomimetics

(continues)

Table 1–3 Selected Arthritic Disorders (continued)

Type	Features	Management Issues
	lungs, kidneys, GI tract, and musculoskeletal system; therefore, signs and symptoms are quite variable. Muscle weakness, including dysphagia; Raynaud's phenomenon; hyperpigmentation; vitiligo and telangiectasias; and thickening and tightening of the skin of the face, hands, and feet. Laboratory findings include an elevated ESR (60–70%), positive RF (20–40%), positive ANA (35–96%), and a high protein level in synovial fluid. Radiographically there are periarticular and subcutaneous calcifications including paraspinal, phalangeal tuft, and superior rib erosions.	*Renal* • Initially ACE inhibitors; may lead to dialysis or kidney transplant *Pulmonary hypertension* • May require oxygen or lung transplant in serious cases *Esophageal reflux* • Avoid large meals and a recumbent position after meals • Avoid sympathomimetic substances and certain foods • H2 inhibitors and/or proton-pump inhibitors *Arthralgias* • NSAIDs Given that some of the therapies employed by chiropractic are mechanical, including adjusting, soft tissue therapy, and physiotherapy, it is important to keep in mind that this is an inflammatory condition and can be exacerbated by these therapies.
Dermatomyositis and poly-myositis	**Age of Onset**—5–10 y/o and again at 20–50 y/o **Gender Predominance**—Female to male ratio = 2:1 **Common Joints Involved**—Soft tissues primarily of the thigh, leg, and arm. Dermatomyositis affects skin and muscle, whereas polymyositis affects primarily muscle. The affect is inflammation and degeneration of striated muscle with a laying down of sheet-like calcifications in soft tissue. About half of patients have arthritis while one-third have Raynaud's phenomenon. Disability occurs due to progressive symmetric, proximal muscle weakness. Laboratory findings include CPK elevations and elevations in urinary creatinine levels. EMG reveals a proximal myopathy as does muscle biopsy. Radiographically, there is soft tissue atrophy coupled with sheet-like soft tissue calcifications and sometimes ossification. Like other inflammatory conditions, there is phalangeal tuft resorption.	Given that some of the therapies employed by chiropractic are mechanical, including adjusting, soft tissue therapy, and physiotherapy, it is important to keep in mind that this is an inflammatory condition and can be exacerbated by these therapies. Protection of the skin with sunblock of SPF 15 or higher is important; provide physical therapy to keep muscle stretch and strength. If dysphagia is present, speech therapy should be employed. Inflammatory aspect may be managed medically with prednisone, immunosuppressive therapy such as methotrexate or azathioprine. Approximately 50% go into remission in 5 years, with an approximate 75% 8-year survival. Those who do not remiss remain on therapy.
Mixed connective tissue disease	**Age of Onset**—20–50 y/o **Gender Predominance**—Female more than male **Common Joints Involved**—Hand, wrist, and foot. This group of conditions is an overlap of several specific diseases such as RA, SLE, dermatomyositis, and scleroderma. Laboratory findings include specific findings for each disorder and presence of ribonuclease-sensitive extractable nuclear antigen. Radiographic findings are those for each disorder and include joint destruction with marginal erosions and soft tissue calcification.	Caution with rheumatoid conditions is unpredictable flare-ups. Given that some of the therapies employed by chiropractic are mechanical, including adjusting, soft tissue therapy, and physiotherapy, it is important to keep in mind that this is an inflammatory condition and can be exacerbated by these therapies. The medical management approach would include those for the underlying disorders. See management under each.

Hypertrophic osteoarthropathy (Marie-Bamberger syndrome or pulmonary osteoarthropathy)	**Age of Onset**—40–60 y/o **Gender Predominance**—Primarily male **Common Joints Involved**—Fingers (clubbing); periostitis in tibia, fibula, radius, and ulna. There is a triad of peripheral arthritis with clubbing of the fingers and periostitis of the distal long bones. This process appears to be secondary to processes in thorax or abdomen, most commonly, bronchogenic carcinoma, and seems to be neurovascular due to vagus nerve dysfunction. Patients often have signs only of the underlying disorder. Radiographic findings include the digital clubbing and long bone symmetrical periostitis.	Identification of the underlying disorder directs appropriate treatment measures. In some cases the hypertrophic osteoarthropathy may improve or disappear with effective care. This may include chemotherapy for tumors or antibiotic therapy for chronic pulmonary infection. In some cases vagotomy or percutaneous vagal blockade is necessary for symptomatic relief. NSAIDs and similar agents are used initially for symptom control.
Osteitis condensins illi	**Age of Onset**—20–40 y/o **Gender Predominance**—Female to male ratio = 9:1 **Common Joints Involved**—Sacroiliac. This bilateral disorder affects females probably through a combination of ligament laxity (hormonally induced) and mechanical stresses that lead to sclerotic changes in the iliac subchondral bone. The process is often asymptomatic. When symptomatic, may present as low back pain with or without leg pain; however, caution must be taken when attempting to relate the radiographic changes to symptoms. The condition, if symptomatic, appears to be primarily self-limiting.	When symptomatic, management includes anti-inflammatory approaches. Generally self-resolving.
Osteitis pubis	**Age of Onset**—Varies, but with females during the reproductive years **Gender Predominance**—Female predominant **Common Joints Involved**—Symphysis pubis. An inflammatory process secondary to trauma, pelvic surgery, or childbirth. This is particularly true if complicated by infection. Possibly due to intraosseous venous congestion and/or infection. Radiographically appears as joint space widening, subchondral sclerosis, localized osteoporosis, and joint erosions.	Initial management may be with NSAIDs and rest. More severe cases may require oral or locally injected corticosteroids. In rare cases, arthrodesis is necessary.

Metabolic

Crystal Deposition

Gout	**Age of Onset**—> 30 y/o (in females, postmenopausal) **Gender Predominance**—Male **Common Joints Involved**—First MTP joint of foot, feet, ankle, and knees	For those with single attack, lifestyle modification first. Diet—attention to hydration, low-purine diet (avoid meat, yeasts including beer/alcohol, beans, legumes), alcohol avoidance, lose weight. Medication avoidance—hyperuricemic meds such as thiazide and loop diuretics; also avoid low-dose aspirin and niacin.

(continues)

Table 1–3 Selected Arthritic Disorders (continued)

Type	Features	Management Issues
	First attack is often sudden and nocturnal, affecting the first MCP joint of foot. This may follow excess alcohol or meat intake. Fever is common during the acute attack. The joint is red and swollen. Desquamation and pruritus after the acute attack are common. Tophi (calcium urate deposits) appear after several attacks of gout and are found behind the ears, olecranon, prepatellar bursae, hands, and feet. There is a dramatic response to NSAIDs or colchicines during the acute attack. Those with gout should be evaluated for associated conditions including alcoholism, various nephropathies, myeloproliferative disorders, hypertension, and insulin resistance.

Occurrence in 2nd and 3rd decade indicates hereditary disorders such as hypoxanthine guanine phosphoribosyltransferase deficiency. Hyperuricemia is common, especially during acute attacks; joint aspiration reveals calcium urate crystals. Radiographically, joint destruction with soft tissue swelling and radiolucent spots (urate crystals) are evident. | Medical approach—acute attacks; NSAIDs or corticosteroids, or colchicines (for inflammation); long-term approach incorporates drugs to reduce serum uric acid and decrease tophi deposits; primarily allopurinol (xanthine-oxidase inhibitor) and probenecid. Low-dose colchicines are acceptable as a prophylaxis for first 6 months. |
| Calcium pyrophosphate deposition disease (CPDD) | **Age of Onset**—> 50 y/o
Gender Predominance—Generally equal dependent on cause
Common Joints Involved—Knee, symphysis pubis, hand, wrist, hip, shoulder, elbow, spine.

CPDD crystal deposition in soft tissue occurs due to trauma, several metabolic diseases, and other causes. The general term *chondrocalcinosis* is associated with metabolic disorders that include hemochromatosis, hyperparathyroidism, ochronosis, diabetes, hypothyroidism, Wilson's disease, among others. There are various subtypes such as pseudogout, pseudorheumatoid arthritis, and pseudodegenerative joint disease. The most common, pseudogout, may appear similar to gout; however, it occurs at a later age in most instances. May be asymptomatic or symptomatic. When symptomatic, pain and swelling occur. Joint aspiration reveals pyrophosphate crystals in synovial fluid. ESR is elevated during acute attacks.

Calcification of intra- and extra-articular structures with eventual articular destruction and fragmentation. | Management may include joint aspiration, short-term use of NSAIDs or colchicines, or corticosteroid injection during acute attacks. For recurrent attacks, low-dose colchicines have been used as have corticosteroids. Antimalarial medications have also been used in some cases. Radioactive synovectomy has also been performed on some patients. |

Hydroxyapatite deposition disease	**Age of Onset**—40–70 y/o **Gender Predominance**—Equal **Common Joints Involved**—Shoulder, hip, cervical spine. This idiopathic process results in calcium (hydroxyapatite) deposition in tendons, bursae, and other periarticular soft tissue. In the spine this may include nucleus pulposus calcification. Technically not an arthritis, pain is felt around joints. It is believed that symptoms develop as the process resolves (inflammation) rather than during the deposition process. Radiographically, soft tissue opacities are seen around the joint.	Management may include joint aspiration, short-term use of NSAIDs or colchicines, or corticosteroid injection during acute attacks. For recurrent attacks, low-dose colchicine has been used as has corticosteroids. Pulsed ultrasound using iontophoresis may be of benefit.
Other		
Sarcoidosis	**Age of Onset**—20–40 y/o **Gender Predominance**—Equal **Common Joints Involved**—Hands, wrists, and feet. This is a systemic disease that produces noncaseating granulomas. It is more common in Scandinavian and Black populations. Generalized symptoms/signs predominate with low-grade fever, rash, lymphadenopathy, malaise, fatigue, arthralgias, and iritis. A subgroup of patients has Lofgren's syndrome. Laboratory findings include a reverse A/G ratio, elevated ESR, hypercalcemia, and a positive Kveim test. Skeletal involvement occurs in 15% of patients. Radiographically, granulomas are seen in the perihilar region of the lungs with infiltrates and fibrosis. In joints there may be circumscribed, lytic, intraosseous lesions.	Arthritis is managed similar to rheumatoid arthritis, incorporating corticosteroids in severe cases or colchicine as is used with gout. Unknown whether an anti-inflammatory diet is helpful.
Hemochromatosis	**Age of Onset**—40–60 y/o **Gender Predominance**—Male to female ratio = 10:1 to 20:1 **Common Joints Involved**—Hip, knee, shoulder, wrist, hand. Rare disorder involving deposition of iron into various tissues. Triad includes bronze skin, liver cirrhosis, and diabetes mellitus. When joints are affected there may be pain, stiffness, and swelling; usually bilaterally; however, may begin in a single joint. Laboratory includes elevated ESR and serum iron, increased saturation of plasma iron binding protein transferring, and liver biopsy findings. Radiographically, usually bilateral involvement with osteoporosis, CPDD crystal deposition (50% of patients), and involvement of MCP joints.	Weekly phlebotomy is the treatment approach to prolong lives.

(continues)

Table 1–3 Selected Arthritic Disorders (continued)

Type	Features	Management Issues
Alkaptonuria (ochronosis)	**Age of Onset**—30–40 y/o (present at birth though) **Gender Predominance**—Equal **Common Joints Involved**—Spine, hip, and knee. A hereditary disorder of tyrosine characterized by absence of homogentisic acid oxidase leading to deposition in tissues throughout the body. The accumulation of homogentisic acid oxidizes to form a black pigment. Ochronosis (brown-black pigmentation in connective tissue not usually seen until age 20), discoloration of urine and ochronotic arthropathy that includes acute exacerbations of arthritic pain in the spine. Cartilage of nose and ears may appear brown but blue on transillumination. Renal and prostate stones are common. Laboratory findings include urine that turns black on standing, homogentisic acid in urine. Radiographically, there is accelerated DJD of the spine with eventual bamboo spine, often beginning with calcification of the interspinous ligament.	Homogentisic acid accumulation could theoretically be controlled through dietary restrictions of phenylalanine and tyrosine, yet the long-term results have not proven this to be an effective treatment. Similarly, theoretically ascorbic acid supplementation could block oxidation of homogentisic acid, but the effectiveness of this approach has not been confirmed.
Pigmented villonodular synovitis (PVNS)	**Age of Onset**—20–40 y/o **Gender Predominance**—Male (slight) **Common Joints Involved**—Knee, hip, elbow, ankle. A synovial proliferative disorder of unknown origin, although 50% of individuals report a history of trauma; usually occurs in one joint. In the hand or foot, a tendon involvement is termed giant cell tumor. Slowly developing joint pain with associated swelling, tenderness, and warmth. Aspiration may reveal hemorrhage. Radiographically, a "popcorn" appearance is seen with initial preservation of joint space. Cystic erosions with hemorrhagic joint effusion can be seen. MRI is diagnostic.	Treatment is complete synovectomy. Irradiation has also been used in some patients.
Hemophillic arthropathy	**Age of Onset**—2–3 y/o **Gender Predominance**—Male **Common Joints Involved**—Knee and elbow commonly affected, although most other appendicular joints can be affected. Hemophilia is a group of disorders that share a problem with clotting factors and result in dysfunctional blood coagulation. The result is bleeding throughout the body, manifested externally as bruising, and prolonged bleeding, such as nose bleeds. Within joints, bleeding occurs and gradually causes changes that include swelling, contractures, fibrosis, and joint destruction. Due to the age of onset, radiographic findings include epiphyseal overgrowth, accelerated skeletal maturation, and radiolucent joint effusions. At some point the joint has a similar appearance radiographically to juvenile rheumatoid arthritis.	At the first sign of hemarthrosis, infusion of factor VIII or IX is initiated. The involved joint is kept in as much extension as possible while NSAIDs and local icing are used for pain control. COX-2 inhibitors are preferred. For chronic scenarios associated with hypertrophied synovium, synovectomy, either open or arthroscopic, may be recommended.

Infectious	Arthritis may be secondary to bacterial, fungal, or viral infections, causing infiltration of synovial or periarticular tissues.	
	There are a number of risk factors for joint infections including: older age (over half of cases in patients over 60 years of age); joint surgery; intravenous drug use; alcoholism; diabetes; immunosuppressive illnesses or use of immunosuppressive medications; malignancy; chronic disease of the liver, lung, or kidney; or skin infections. For acute arthritis, the most common bacterial cause in adults is *Neisseria gonorrhoeae*. Others include *Staphylococcus aureus*, streptococci, and some gram-negative such as Enterobacter, *Pseudomonas aeruginosa*, and *Serratia marcescens*. For chronic arthritis, primary causes include mycobacterium and fungi. Early clinical signs are pain, swelling, and warmth. Radiographic changes with bacterial causes include early soft tissue and synovial swelling. After about 2 weeks, joint space narrowing and erosions begin to appear. With chronic causes, joint space is preserved longer. Synovial fluid analysis will reveal a high WBC count with a decrease in viscosity and glucose. Gram staining and culture will usually reveal the causative organism.	Antibiotic therapy is often given parenterally, and joint aspiration is performed as well as lavage and debridement dependent on degree of involvement. For fungal infections, amphotericin B and similar medications are needed.
Hyperlipidemia	Recurrent, migratory joint pain involving the knee and other large joints is seen in patients with familial hypercholesterolemia. The appearance is that of inflammatory process with fever, swelling, tenderness, and warmth. The onset is generally acute. The joint pain may not be in the joint itself but represent periarthritis or peritendinitis given that there is usually no joint damage. Xanthomas have been reported in the Achilles tendon, patellar tendon, and extensor tendons of the hands and feet. Diagnostic suspicion is high with a finding of familial hypercholesterolemia on laboratory evaluation coupled with the onset of recurrent migratory arthritis. Radiographs may show osteopenia and bone cysts.	Acute management is with NSAIDs or similar approaches. Long-term management may involve the use of HMG CoA reductase inhibitors; however, these may cause myalgias or polymyositis

and adult RA, LE, scleroderma, and osteitis condensins illi, as examples. Further distinction can be made from a pattern of joint involvement. For example, OA tends to affect large joints such as the knee and hip, with eventual involvement in the hands (specifically first metacarpal phalangeal and distal interphalangeal joints), whereas RA tends to affect the metacarpal and proximal interphalangeal joints of the hand first and then larger joints. Gout tends to affect the first toe and knees primarily. The seronegatives tend to affect the sacroiliac joint or spine with possible affect in peripheral joints. Finally, associated systemic signs may help relate the arthritis to disorders such as LE, scleroderma, enteropathic arthritides (i.e., arthritis associated with inflammatory bowel disease), and so on.

Assembling and applying this information, if a middle-aged female presented with a polyarthropathy that included the hands but not the spine, without other systemic involvement, RA would be high on the list of differentials. If a young to middle-aged male presented with sacroiliac pain, no spinal pain, and involvement of a finger, Reiter's or AS would be high on the list of differentials.

A review article by Margaretten et al.[2] evaluated the ability of a clinician to determine whether their adult patient has septic arthritis. The history indicators would be whether the patient is diabetic, has rheumatoid arthritis, HIV infection, skin infection, has had joint surgery, or a hip or knee prosthesis. Joint pain, a history of joint swelling, and fever were the only findings that occurred in more than 50% of patients. Other findings such as night sweats and rigors were inconsistent and often not found with septic arthritis. However, the addition of synovial fluid analysis for WBCs and percentage of polymorphonuclear cells from arthrocentesis were needed to confirm the likelihood prior to Gram stain and culture test results.

Examination

Acute Traumatic Injury

An approach to acute injury evaluation initially focuses on neurovascular status distal to and local to the injury site. These neurovascular injuries often are secondary to fracture. Motor assessments with active and active resisted attempts evaluate both muscle and neural integrity. Sensory testing incorporates the use of a pin in an attempt to test pain perception and a paper clip for testing two-point discrimination in the fingers. Palpation

of pulses is useful in determining major vascular injury. Although these tests are more applicable to extremity injury, injury to the spine requires the same diligent search for an intact neurovascular system. With these conditions reasonably eliminated, the specific sequence one uses is less important than the fact that the approach is comprehensive.

General Approach

However complex the orthopaedic evaluation may become, the basics remain the same regardless of which joints and/or surrounding structures are involved (**Table 1–4**). Generally, orthopaedic testing attempts to (1) reproduce a patient's complaint (i.e., elicit pain, provoke numbness/tingling, or reproduce popping or clicking); (2) reveal laxity; (3) demonstrate weakness; or (4) demonstrate restriction (orthopaedic evaluation, in the context of a chiropractor, also includes accessory motion evaluation at a joint). The possible caveats to these attempts are that pain may be due to many factors and is therefore nonspecific (localization and injury pattern help better define); laxity may be normal for an individual (especially if bilateral) or pathologic; weakness may be due to reflex inhibition caused by pain (relatively nonspecific), laxity, muscle injury, or neurologic damage; and restriction to movement may be due to soft tissue or bony blockage.

The mechanics of orthopaedic tests have similarities regardless of any assigned name. Testing involves one of three approaches: (1) stretch, (2) compress, or (3) contract. When performing a named orthopaedic test, reflection on what is the intended use coupled with the understanding of what other structures may be challenged is imperative to appreciate and interpret fully the variety of patient responses possible. Although a test is designed to stretch a ligament, also stretched are muscles, tendons, and nerves. The same maneuver may elicit a positive response through compression of tissues. For example, a valgus force stretches the medial knee yet compresses the lateral knee. Although not the intended response, any pain response to a maneuver may provide important information if simple biomechanics are kept in mind.

Another general principle is that similar structures are tested similarly (**Table 1–5**).

- Ligaments/capsules—Use direct palpation (if possible) and perform a stress test that usually involves stabilizing one bone while moving the neighboring bone on it (for example, drawer

Table 1–4 Selective Tension Approach

Condition	Active ROM	Passive ROM	Resisted Movement	Key Points
Arthritis/capsulitis	Painful at limit of range	Painful at limit of range	Usually painless within range of motion	Often specific capsular pattern of one or two restricted movement patterns
Tendinitis Tendinosis	Variable	Pain on stretch	Painful, especially if contracted in stretched position	Insertion of tendon is often tender or slightly proximal to insertion
Tendon rupture	None	Full; painless	Weak; painless	Note displaced muscle belly
Ligament sprain	Decreased; limited by pain	Pain on stability challenge	Painless if full rupture, painful if partial	Overpressure laxity may indicate degree of damage
Muscle strain	Painful, often midrange	Passive stretch may increase pain	If resistance is sufficient, pain is produced	Check with resistance throughout full range of movement
Intra-articular body	Sudden onset of pain in a specific range of motion	Sudden onset of pain in a specific range of motion is also possible	Usually painless	An "arc" of pain with a "catching" or blockage is highly suggestive
Acute bursitis (deep)	Painful in most directions	Empty end-feel is often present	Isometric testing is often painful	Positional relief is less common than with muscle/tendon injury

Table 1–5 General Approach Based on Structure

Structure	Initial Evaluation	Specific Imaging Evaluation
Bone		
Tumor—primary or metastatic	Radiograph	MRI or CT, bone scan for metastasis (nonspecific)
Osteochondrosis/apophysitis	Local tenderness and radiograph	Possible bone scan
Fracture	Palpation, percussion, tuning fork, radiograph	CT or possibly MRI
Stress fracture	Palpation, percussion, radiograph	Bone scan, SPECT scan; quantified CT, dual-energy absorptiometry
Osteopenia (osteoporosis)	Radiograph	Quantified CT, dual-energy absorptiometry
Osteomyelitis	Radiograph	MRI
Soft Tissue		
Muscle		
Strain or rupture	Active resistance	For rupture, sonography, or MRI
Trigger points	Palpation	None
Atrophy	Observation	Electrodiagnostic studies
Myositis ossificans	Palpation, radiograph	CT
Muscular dystrophy	Muscle testing, creatine kinase (CK) on lab	Electrodiagnostic studies
Tendon		
Tendinitis/tendinosis	Stretch and contraction	Sonography
Paratenonitis	Stretch	Sonography or MRI
Rupture	Lack of passive tension effect	Sonography or MRI

(continues)

Table 1–5 General Approach Based on Structure (continued)

Structure	Initial Evaluation	Specific Imaging Evaluation
Ligament		
Sprain or rupture	Stability testing	MRI
Bursa		
Bursitis	Palpation	MRI or bursography
Fascia		
Myofascitis	Palpation	None
Joint		
Arthritis	Characteristic joint involvement, laboratory findings including rheumatoid factor, HLA-B27, ANA, and radiographic characteristics	CT for bone, MRI for soft tissue involvement
Subluxation/fixation (chiropractic)	Palpation, indirect radiographic findings	CT for facet joints (research only)
Synovitis	Capsular pattern of restriction	MRI, joint aspiration
Joint mice	Restricted ROM, radiograph	CT or MRI
Dislocation/subluxation (medical)	Observation and radiograph	CT

testing of the shoulder, knee, and ankle). In essence, motion palpation of a joint is the same as many ligament stability tests, yet the intent is different; locate restrictions, not instability.

- Tendons—Use direct palpation and stretch into end-range (contraction at end-range stretch may also be used).
- Muscles—Use direct palpation and contraction. Although traditionally used to detect weakness, the main focus is to determine reproduction of a patient's complaint.
- Nerves—Tapping (i.e., Tinel's) and compression are direct tests for superficial nerves; indirect tests include motor and sensory evaluation of specific peripheral nerves, nerve plexus, nerve root, or central nervous system (CNS) involvement including muscle tests, deep tendon reflex testing, and sensory testing with a pin/brush or pinwheel.

Palpation is a valuable tool when accessing superficial tissues. Accessibility is limited, based on the joint and its location. The fingers and toes are thin accessible structures, whereas the hip and shoulder are not. Direct palpation of ligaments and tendons may reveal tenderness. Muscles may also be palpated for tenderness and possible associated referred patterns of pain. These trigger points have been mapped by Travell and Simons.[3] Their work serves as a road map for investigation.

New studies help clarify the etiology and diagnosis of trigger points. In two studies Shah et al.[4,5] evaluated the biochemical environment of a trigger point as compared to a normal control match. Using a microdialysis needle and sampling B21 (an acupuncture point and myofascial trigger point) they were able to measure pH, bradykinin, substance P, calcitonin gene-related peptide, tumor necrosis factor, and inflammatory fractions of interleukin, serotonin, and norepinephrine. All levels were higher in the active trigger points than in the controls. Another study of promise was conducted by Chen et al.[6] These researchers attempted to investigate the presence of taut bands of myofascial trigger points (MTP) using magnetic resonance elastography (MRE). There are some concerns regarding this study, but preliminary interpretation suggests that this technology may be able to identify and distinguish these MTP bands.

The reliability of soft tissue palpation has been evaluated for the spine and the extremities. In general, it is evident that soft tissue palpation findings are not as reliable as bony palpation among examiners. When specific sites in the extremities are exposed through specific positioning, however, the reliability may increase.[7]

Although orthopaedic testing is the standard for orthopaedists, more involved investigations are usually added by the chiropractor and/or manual therapist. The first is based on the work of Cyriax,[8] which emphasizes the "feel" of soft tissue palpation, especially at end-range.

Combined with this end-range determination, a selective tension approach is incorporated using the responses to active, active resisted, and passive movements to differentiate between contractile (muscle/tendon) and noncontractile (ligament/capsule and bursa) tissue. Another approach is to challenge specifically each joint to determine fixation or hypermobility. Finally, a functional approach to movement as proposed by Janda[9] and Lewit[10] is often used. This approach addresses the quality of movement and the "postural" tendencies toward imbalance of strength and flexibility of muscles.

Selective Tension Approach

Cyriax[8] divided the quality of passive end-range at a joint into normal and abnormal. Some normal end-feels include the following:

- Soft tissue approximation—This is a soft end-feel that occurs when a muscle opposes another muscle; for example, when the calf muscles hit the hamstrings or the forearm hits the biceps on flexion.
- Muscular—This is an elastic end-feel that occurs when a muscle is stretched to its end-range. This occurs with straight leg raising with the hamstrings.
- Bone-on-bone or cartilaginous—This occurs when the joint anatomically stops, as occurs with elbow extension.
- Capsular—This occurs with a tight, slightly elastic feel such as occurs with full hip rotation. It is due to the elastic tension that develops in the joint capsule when stretched.

Abnormal end-feels include the following:

- Spasm—When muscle spasm is present, pain will prevent full range of motion.
- Springy block or rebound—This occurs when there is a mechanical blockage such as a torn meniscus in the knee or labrum in the shoulder. The end-range occurs before a full range of motion is attained.
- Empty—This occurs when there is an acute painful process such as a bursitis. The patient prevents movement to end-range.
- Loose—This end-feel is indicative of capsular or ligamentous damage and is in essence the end-feel that is found with a positive ligament stability test.

Many examiners probably sense these different end-range palpation findings. They have not categorized them, yet interpret them intuitively.

Some examiners will equate timing of the onset of pain on passive testing with staging of injury as follows:

- Pain felt before end-range is considered an acute process that would obviate the application of vigorous therapy.
- Pain felt at the same time as end-range is indicative of a subacute process and would be amenable to gentle stretching and mobilization.
- Pain felt after end-range is indicative of a chronic process that may respond to aggressive stretching and manipulation.

By taking the patient through passive range of motion (PROM) and active range of motion (AROM) and testing resisted motion, a clearer idea of contractile versus noncontractile tissue involvement may be appreciated (**Figure 1–1** and Table 1–5). It should be evident that contractile tissue may be painful with either stretch or midrange contraction. If both findings are present, they should be present in opposite directions (e.g., contraction into flexion hurts anteriorly while passive extension does also). If end-range stretch is not painful but contraction at end-range is, the tendon of the involved muscle is likely involved. If pain is not found with active movement but passive movement into end-range causes pain, noncontractile tissue is probably involved. Active movement should not affect most noncontractile tissue unless it is compressed. This is more likely to occur at end-range. Cyriax's selective tension approach is a logical attempt to localize the involved tissue, yet until recently it has remained unchallenged. One study demonstrated a high interexaminer reliability using these methods. The interexaminer agreement was 90.5% with a kappa statistic of 0.875.[13]

An extension of the selective tension approach is to determine the effect of mild isometric contractions on restricted range of motion. If a patient provides a mild resistance for several seconds to the agonist and antagonist pattern of restriction (e.g., flexion/extension) and repeats this several times followed by an attempt at stretch by the examiner, a distinction between soft tissue or bony blockage to movement may be determined. For example, if a patient presented with a restriction to abduction of the shoulder, repetitive, reciprocal contraction (minimal contraction for 5 to 6 seconds) into abduction and adduction several times will increase the available range if soft

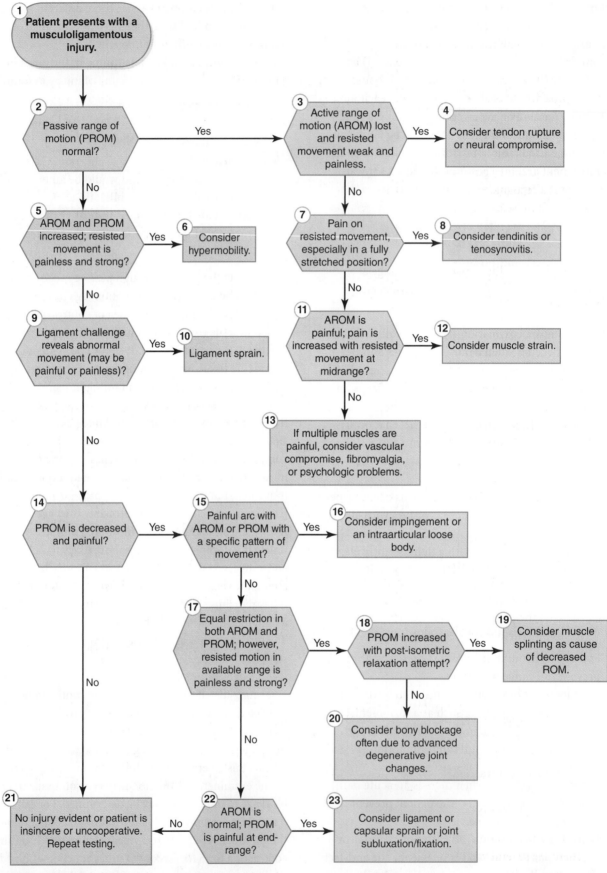

Figure 1–1 Assessment of Musculoligamentous Injury—Algorithm

tissue is the cause (**Exhibit 1–1**). Bony blockage from OA, fracture, or a torn labrum will result in little or no increase in motion with the same procedure.

Functional Approach

Traditional muscle evaluation involves a test of muscle strength only. Janda[9] and Lewit[10] and others[14] advocate an approach that takes into account not only the quantity of contraction (strength) but also the quality of movement. There is a recognized natural imbalance in muscle strength. Not all muscles are created equal. It is known that small muscles are often phasic, required to react quickly to changes in the environment, whereas larger muscles are often tonic, posturally assigned. Certain movement patterns are biased. For example, supination is stronger than pronation and internal rotation of the shoulder is stronger than external rotation. This bias is in large part due to the size or number (or both) of muscles used in the movement pattern. Strength is also positionally dependent. Certain positions place at a disadvantage some muscles of a synergistic group.

There is another perspective with regard to muscle weakness and tightness that may affect evaluation and eventually management. An observation by Janda[9] and Lewit[10] is that there are crossed and layered patterns of weakness and tightness. For example, in the low back it is not uncommon to find a pattern of anterior weakness in the abdominal muscles associated with posterior tightness of the erector spinae (sagittal pattern). A vertical pattern is illustrated by the association of the tight erector spinae's being sandwiched between weak gluteal muscles inferiorly and weak lower trapezius muscles superiorly. These two planes create a "crossed" pattern whereby tightness of the erector spinae is associated with tightness of the iliopsoas, and weakness of the abdominal muscles is associated with weakness of the gluteal muscles. This pattern is relatively consistent throughout the body and is a reflection of two concepts: (1) muscles that function to resist the effects of gravity (postural muscles) have a tendency to become tight in sedentary people, and (2) muscles that function more dynamically are underused and become weak and prone to injury. Additionally, muscles that cross more than one joint are prone toward tightness. For example, the rectus femoris, which crosses the hip and knee, is prone toward tightness, whereas the medialis obliquus, which does not cross a joint and is primarily a "dynamic" muscle, is often weak.

Exhibit 1–1 Postisometric Relaxation, Proprioceptive Neuromuscular Facilitation (PNF) Hold-Relax, and PNF Contract-Relax

Postisometric Relaxation

- Stretch the affected muscle to patient tolerance.
- Maintain the stretch position while the patient isometrically contracts the muscle for 6 to 10 seconds at a 25% effort against doctor's resistance.
- Instruct the patient to relax fully (taking in a deep breath and letting it out may help).
- Attempt a further stretch of the muscle with the patient relaxed.
- Repeat this procedure five or six times or until no further stretch seems possible (whichever comes first).

PNF Hold-Relax

- This technique is very similar to a postisometric relaxation approach; however, classically the patient attempts a maximum contraction of either the agonist or antagonist.
- Caution must be used with maximal contractions. The author prefers to start with a postisometric approach using a 25% contraction before proceeding to more forceful resistance.

PNF Contract-Relax

- This is a full isotonic contraction followed by a stretch into a new position.
- There are several variations of this technique. A popular one is called CRAC (contract-relax-antagonist-contract).

With the above concepts in mind, Lewit and Janda have focused on an observation of quality of movement with an emphasis on the timing and recruitment during a movement pattern. Often these two concepts overlap when the timing of the movement is a reflection of recruitment. For example, hip extension in a lying position requires a timing of contraction beginning with the hamstrings. This is followed by gluteal contraction, then erector spinae contraction. If the hamstrings or gluteals do not participate, the erector spinae contract, causing a weak contraction and a lordotic/compressive load to the low back. In the neck, flexion may reveal an imbalance in movement. If the patient's jaw juts forward at the beginning of the pattern, weak neck flexors with associated "strong" sternocleidomastoids are indicated.

Functional Movement Approach to Assessment

An approach to asymptomatic individuals as well as symptomatic individuals is to examine, rate, and rank, patterns to discover and correct limitations to specific movement patterns or asymmetries in specific movement patterns. One such approach by Cook[11] is divided into two sequences. One is devoted to the asymptomatic individual and is called a Functional Movement Screen (FMS). This approach is not diagnostic. The second approach for symptomatic individuals is called Selective Functional Movement Assessments (SFMA). This uses patterns broken down into component elements (**Table 1–6**). A key concept is to find the pattern with the most limitation or most asymmetry and remediate this "weakest" link. The reason may be joint restriction, muscle tightness, poor segmental stability, or a combination of these. The core components of the FMS include primitive movement patterns, progressing through transitional movement patterns that have a requirement for more stability and coordination, and then to higher level movement patterns. There is caution expressed in the literature that demonstrates that the intraexaminer reliability of this method is good, but the interreliability is not causing the authors of one study to suggest that this approach should not be used "indiscriminately" to screen the athlete at greatest risk for injury.[12]

Table 1–6 Functional Movement Patterns of Assessment

Approach	Rating System	Movements or Evaluation		Purpose of Assessment
FMS	3 = complete movement (no issues)	Deep squat		Mobility and stability
		Hurdle step	The Big Three	Both the SLR and shoulder
	2 = complete movement with compensation, deviation from standard, or both	Inline lunge	(Functional)	mobility tests for mobility;
		Shoulder mobility reaching		the stability pushup and
		Active SLR		rotary stability for stability
	1 = incomplete	Trunk stability pushup	The Little Four	
	0 = pain on any test (nullifies test)	Rotary Stability	(Fundamental)	
		In general focus is on Little Four first		
		Asymmetrical split-side tests are more important than symmetrical tests such as the squat, trunk stability pushup		
SFMA		*All of the following have "breakout" movement assessments (largely regional)*		
		Cervical spine		
		Upper extremity		
		Multisegmental flexion		
		Multisegmental extension		
		Multisegmental rotation		
		Single leg stance		
		Overhead deep squat		
		Rolling patterns		

Legend: Functional Movement Screen (FMS), Selective Functional Movement Assessments (SFMA), Straight Leg Raise (SLR)

Accessory Motion

One of the indicators for manipulation or adjusting is blockage of accessory motion.[15] Accessory motion is that subtle amount of bone-on-bone movement that is not under voluntary control. For example, although the humerus moves on the glenoid during abduction, there is a degree of movement measured in millimeters that is necessary yet not under the control of the shoulder abductor muscles. Determining whether accessory motion is available involves placing the joint in a specific position and attempting passively to move one bone on another. If the end-feel is springy, then joint play is available. If there is a perceived restriction, however, movement at the joint may be restricted. It is important to distinguish between the end-range descriptions of Cyriax[8] and the end-feel of accessory motion. Cyriax is referring to the end-range of an extremity or spinal movement such as flexion, extension, abduction, or adduction. Accessory motion is palpated at the joint both with the joint in a neutral or open-packed position and also with a coupled movement pattern taken to end-range actively and passively. The joint would not be restricted by the tension of the capsule or muscle with the neutral position method. The active and passive techniques take advantage of the end-range position to determine whether the accompanying accessory motion is, in fact, occurring. There are specific guidelines for both assessment and application of treatment to accessory motion barriers.

Specific patterns of extremity and spinal movement are coupled with specific accessory motion so that restrictions in active movement may be indirectly an indicator of dysfunction of the accompanying accessory motion.[16]

Radiography and Special Imaging

When making choices regarding the need for radiographs or special imaging, it is important to keep one major question in mind: Is there a reasonably high expectation that the information provided by the study will dictate or alter the type of treatment or dictate whether medical referral is needed? If the answer is no, it is important to delay ordering expensive, unnecessary studies at that given time. As time passes, the answer to the question may change. Some secondary issues with regard to further testing are as follows:

- What are the risks to the patient?
- What is the cost? Are there less expensive methods of arriving at the same diagnosis?
- What are the legal ramifications if the study or studies are or are not performed?

The decision for the use of radiographs is based on relative risk. Patients often can be categorized into high- and low-risk groups by combining history and examination data. Many groups have developed similar standards for absolute or relative indications for the need for radiographs.[17–19] Generally, for patients with joint pain, the following are some suggested indicators:

- Significant trauma
- Suspicion of cancer (unexplained weight loss, prior history of cancer, patients over age 50 years)
- Suspicion of infection (fever of unknown origin above 100°F and/or chills, use of intravenous drugs, recent urinary tract infection)
- Chronic corticosteroid use
- Drug or alcohol abuse
- Neuromotor deficits
- Scoliosis
- History of surgery to the involved region
- Laboratory indicators such as significantly elevated erythrocyte sedimentation rate, alkaline phosphatase, positive rheumatoid factor, monoclonal spiking on electrophoresis
- Dermopathy suggestive of psoriasis, Reiter's syndrome, melanoma, and the like
- Lymphadenopathy
- Patients unresponsive to 1 month of conservative care
- Medicolegal requirements or concerns

Choice of imaging is based on the sensitivity and specificity of a given imaging tool, the cost, and the availability (see Table 1–6). In general:

- Radiography—Signs of many conditions, including cancer, fracture, infection, osteoporosis, and degeneration, often are visible. The degree of sensitivity is quite low with early disease, however.
- Magnetic resonance imaging (MRI) is extremely valuable in evaluating soft tissue such as tendons, ligaments, and discs. In evaluating the volume of tumor or infection involvement, MRI is also valuable. Spinal cord processes such as multiple sclerosis or syringomyelia are well visualized on MRI (**Table 1–7**).
- When attempting further to clarify the degree of bony spinal stenosis, the extent of fracture, or other bony processes, computed tomography (CT) is often a sensitive tool—better than MRI in many

Table 1–7 Magnetic Resonance Imaging for the Chiropractor

MRI Better Than CT	MRI Equal to CT	CT Better Than MRI
MRI of the Head		
Severe headaches	Hydrocephalus	Fracture of the calvaria
Visual disturbance	Brain atrophy	Fracture of the skull base
Sensory-neural hearing loss		Cholesteatoma of inner ear
Primary brain tumor		Intracranial hemorrhage 1–3 days old
Metastatic brain tumor		Cerebral infarction 1–3 days old
Intracranial infection		Intracranial calcifications
Age-related CNS disease		
Multiple sclerosis		
Dementia		
Chronic subdural hematoma		
Posttraumatic evaluation of the brain		
Intracranial hemorrhage older than 3 days		
Cerebral infarction older than 3 days		
MRI of the Cervical and Thoracic Spines		
Tumors or masses at the level of the foramen magnum	Spinal stenosis	Occult fracture of a vertebra
Chiari I malformation		Complex fracture of a vertebra
Cervical or thoracic herniated disc		Bony foraminal encroachment
Posttraumatic syrinx		
Core or conus tumor		
Acquired immunodeficiency syndrome-related myelopathy		
Multiple sclerosis of the spinal cord		
Posttraumatic epidural hematoma		
Epidural metastatic disease		
Epidural abscess		
MRI of the Lumbar Spine		
Small lumbar herniation	Large lumbar herniation	Occult fracture
Foraminal herniation	Spinal stenosis	Hypertrophic bony overgrowth or spurring
Interruption of the posterior longitudinal ligament		Bony foraminal encroachment
Root sleeve compression		Spondylolysis
Postoperative scar versus recurrent lumbar herniation (with gadolinium)		Evaluation of posterior element fusion
MRI of the Shoulder		
Posttraumatic bone bruise	Rotator cuff tear	Subtle glenoid labrum tear
Avascular necrosis of humeral head		Evaluation of the glenohumeral ligaments
Impingement syndrome		
Lipoma (or soft tissue mass)		
Tumor		
Brachial plexus tumor		

Table 1–7 Magnetic Resonance Imaging for the Chiropractor (continued)

MRI Better Than CT	MRI Equal to CT	CT Better Than MRI
MRI of the Knee		
Posttraumatic bone bruise	Meniscal tear	Evaluation of the meniscus following previous meniscectomy
Osteochondritis dissecans		Evaluation of the articular cartilage
Anterior cruciate ligament tear		
Posterior cruciate ligament tear		
Collateral ligament tear		
Patellar tendon abnormalities		
Infection		
Tumor		
Osteochondritis dissecans		

Courtesy of Murray Solomon, M.D., Redwood City, California.

cases. Recent cerebrovascular events and some tumors are well visualized with CT.

- When the search is for stress fracture, metastasis to bone, or avascular necrosis, bone scans often provide valuable information.
- When determining the degree of osteoporosis in a patient, dual x-ray radiographic absorptiometry is more sensitive than standard radiography.

In late 2007, a set of diagnostic imaging practice guidelines for musculoskeletal complaints in adults was released.[20] The guidelines were the result of years of research including an extensive literature search, an external review by 12 chiropractic specialists for external review, and finally, a two-round modified Delphi process involving 149 international experts. The agreement on recommendations was quite high (approximately 85%). Generally, these guidelines are intended to inform clinicians as to the best scientific evidence currently available, and are intended to be used in conjunction with sound clinical judgment and experience. The hope is that in addition to identifying patients in need of further diagnostic workup, unnecessary use of radiographs, and therefore the time and cost for health care will be reduced, while maintaining or improving patient care.

A new approach being studied and utilized by physical therapists internationally is rehabilitative ultrasound imaging (RUSI).[21–28] The concept is to use diagnostic ultrasonography (US) to evaluate morphological changes while therapy is being applied. By determining the best position for stretch or for the effects of care, RUSI is

being advocated as an important adjunct to musculoskeletal management. For example, RUSI would be used to measure the cross-sectional area of a muscle or tendon.

Management

Recently, a growing focus for many practitioners involved in a manual therapy, physical medicine/therapy approach is a basic science explanation for why these approaches are effective and may be necessary alternatives to the often short-term goal effects of various surgical solutions to common musculoskeletal problems. The concept is an old one but is resurfacing as a generalized concept of approach called mechanotherapy. The premise of this general and broad concept is mechanotransduction where a mechanical stimulus or loading is converted into cellular responses. As a result of this mechanical input, processes are set into play to promote structural change. In an article by Khan and Scott[29] in 2009 published in the *British Journal of Sports Medicine*, the authors review and categorize the main steps in this transduction of mechanical stimulus to cellular response. They break down the process into three steps: (1) mechanocoupling, which involves the mechanical trigger; (2) cell–cell communication throughout the tissue to communicate the loading message; and (3) the effector response at a cellular level to set into play the production of necessary materials in the correct alignment of that tissue. For the communication via cell signaling to occur, an "information network" of messenger proteins, ion channels, and lipids must be present. The signaling substances include calcium and inositol triphosphate. Specific changes have been demonstrated, including in tendons there is an up-regulation of insulin-like growth factor (IGF-I) associated with cellular proliferation and matrix remodeling within the tendon. Other growth factors and cytokines in addition to IGF-I also are likely to play a role.[30] In a study[31] involving rehabilitation of Achilles tendinosis, after a follow-up of almost four years many of the tendons exposed to an eccentric loading approach to rehabilitation demonstrated normal structure. Taken together, these illustrate that the body's normal response to stimulus is to adapt and make an attempt at recreating normal structure.

Conservative management of a musculoskeletal problem is based on several broad principles.

- Initial management involves a greater degree of passive care with a transition into active care dominance over time.
- The goals for patient management vary based on the acuteness of the problem.
- Rehabilitation progresses in a sequence: passive motion to active motion to active resisted motion (begins with isometrics and progresses to isotonics) to functional training.

Although traditionally it was the doctor's role to be active and the patient's to be passive with treatment, it is becoming clear that there is a point at which role switching is necessary. When a patient has acute pain, the goal is to reduce the pain and assist healing. Many of the treatment methods used with acute pain employ procedures that are doctor-dependent. As the patient progressively improves, there should be a focus on the patient's active participation in restoring normal function. Nelson[32] has outlined some criteria for passive care (**Figure 1–2**). These include a history of recent trauma, acute condition or flare-up, inflammation, or dependency behavior. There are generally four types of care that may overlap, as follows:

1. Care for inflammation might include the traditional approach of protection, rest, ice, and, if appropriate, compression and elevation. Modalities that are available include high-voltage galvanic stimulation, ultrasound, therapeutic heat, contrast baths, and nonsteroidal anti-inflammatory drugs (NSAIDs), or enzyme alternatives.
2. Options for care for pain include manipulation, mobilization, trigger-point therapy, transcutaneous electrical nerve stimulation (TENS), interferential stimulation, (**Table 1–8**), ice, cryotherapy, acupuncture, and NSAIDs.
3. Care for hypomobility includes various forms of stretch, manipulation, mobilization, and soft tissue approaches such as myofascial release techniques.
4. Care for hypermobility includes protection with taping, casts, splints, or various braces.

Low-Level Laser Therapy (LLLT)

There are many types of lasers. Those used therapeutically can be divided into several subtypes. Those without a strong thermal effect are often referred to as *cold lasers*. These are divided into two types based on wavelength. Far-red to infrared wavelengths (longer than 800nm) penetrate deeper and are therefore indicated for treatment of deep acupuncture points, trigger points, and large muscles. The second type, visible red wavelengths (shorter than 800nm) are more appropriate for more superficial tissue because they do not penetrate as far.

There are a number of proposed effects of LLLT, which include:

- Reduction of pain through inhibition of fast axonal transmission in small- and medium-diameter $A\delta$ and C fibers
- Potentially reduces peripheral nociceptive afferent input to the dorsal horn and possible reorganization of synaptic connections in the CNS that modulate pain
- Improve oxidative metabolism
- Increase production of endogenous opioids, reduce swelling, reduce prostaglandin E_2 levels, and inhibition of cyclooxygenase 2

If the output power (mW) and beam area (cm²) are known, one can calculate the remaining parameters that determine dosage. The output refers to the number of photons emitted at the particular wavelength of the laser diode. The thermal effect of photons at the treatment area is measured as the Power Density. Energy Densities in the range 0.5 to 4 J/cm² are most effective in producing a photobiological stimulating response. Dosages of 8 to 12 J/cm² and higher are proposed to cause bioinhibition, and may be effective with pain management. To change dosages it is recommended to maintain a fixed output power and alter the emission time.

In a Cochrane Review[33] published in 2008 the reviewers cautioned that there was insufficient evidence to draw firm conclusions about LLLT for nonspecific low back pain. They state that although three small studies

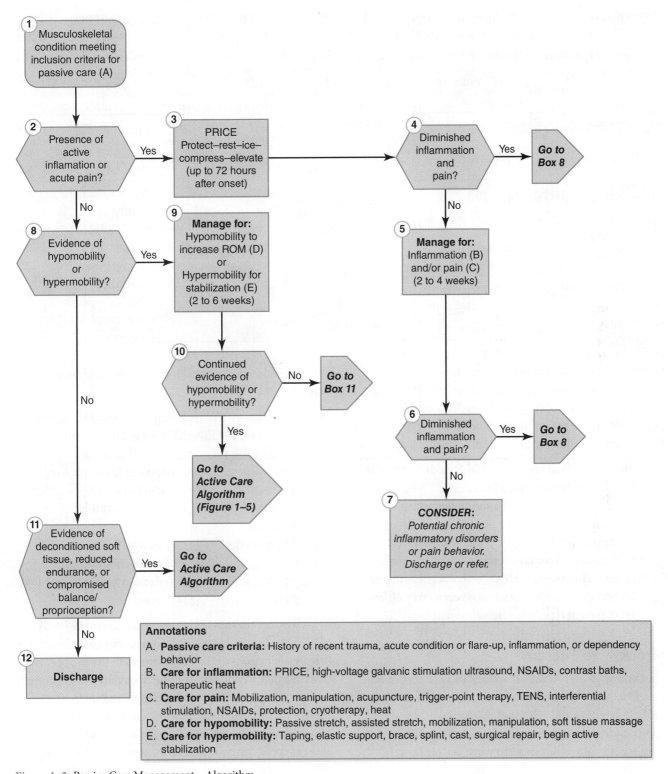

Figure 1–2 Passive Care Management—Algorithm
Reproduced from D.L. Nelson, *Topics in Clinical Chiropractic*, Vol. 1, No. 4, p. 75, © 1994, Aspen Publishers, Inc.

showed statistically significant differences, they did not show clinically important differences. They did conclude though that real LLLT is perhaps better than sham LLLT but not better than exercise for pain and disability in the short term. They indicate that two small studies

demonstrated that the relapse rate was significantly lower for patients treated with LLLT at six months compared to the control group.

Although a review[34] in *Lancet* in 2009 concluded that LLLT reduces pain immediately after treatment for acute

Table 1–8 Physiotherapy Approaches for Musculoskeletal Complaints

Various Transcutaneous Electrical Nerve Stimulation (TENS) Approaches

Type	Pulse Width (pps)	Pulse Rate	Amplitude	Treatment Time
High frequency	High: 75–100	< 200	Increase to discomfort	20 min.–24 hrs
Low frequency	Low: < 10	200–300	Increase to elicit strong rhythmic contractions	30–60 min.
Brief and intense	TENS—150	150	Increase to strong but comfortable contraction	20–60 min.

Pulsed High-Volt Galvanic

Treatment Effect	Mode	Frequency (pps)	Type of Stimulation	Time (min.)
Reduce edema	Continuous	High: 80–100	Sensory	20
Reduce muscle spasm	Continuous	High: 80–120	Sensory/motor	20–30
Autonomic response	Uninterrupted/pulse	High: 80–100	Sensory	20–30
Neuro/hormonal	Uninterrupted/pulse	Low: 2–5	Motor (twitch)	30–60
Muscle pumping	Surged 1:3	Low: 30–50	Motor	20–30

neck pain and for patients with chronic pain up to 32 weeks after treatment with LLLT, there were limitations to strength of these conclusions. Three of the studies quoted and utilized in the review that had the largest reported mean differences in favor of LLLT had limitations or errors:

- Two studies had significant baseline differences in favor of the active treatment.
- A typing error indicated a significant mean difference when in the original study, there was no significant difference.
- Pooling of data for nonspecific neck pain, myofascial pain syndrome, and cervical osteoarthritis may be inappropriate because each may represent a different set of patient types and clinical responses.

Shockwave Therapy

Shockwave therapy (SWT) is utilized in a number of musculoskeletal as well as visceral disorders. Commonly used for kidney stones and gallstones management, a similar approach to tendon, muscle, and ligament problems has been successfully utilized over the last decade or so.

By definition, shock waves involve a sequence of single sonic pulses with the following characteristics:

- High peak pressure (100 mPa)
- A fast rise in pressure (< 10 nanoseconds)
- A short life cycle (10 microseconds)

Therapeutically, SWT is applied based on energy output and frequency of impulses. SWT is

generally classified according to two energy levels with different effects:

- Low-energy SWT—defined as having an energy flux density (EFD) of less than 0.12 mJ/mm^2. Shock-wave therapy at an EFD lower than 0.09 mJ/mm^2 is reported to produce a neoangiogenic effect by increasing expression of vascular endothelial growth factor (VEFG) and its receptor.
- High-energy SWT—defined as having an EFD between 0.12 and 0.38 mJ/mm^2. At the higher ends of high-energy SWT, local anesthesia is often necessary.

A distinction must be made between two types of SWT. The first is called focused SWT and may be generated via electrohydraulic, electromagnetic, or piezoelectric mechanisms. Based on how the energy is generated, the focal area and tissue penetration and their effects on tissue vary. Focused shockwaves are concentrated through focusing reflectors to the target site. The other type is termed radial shockwave therapy or radial pulse therapy (RPT). Radial "shock" waves are not actually shockwaves being generated by a ballistic source and so therefore, do not have the characteristics of real medical shockwaves. Their effect is superficial; they do not have a penetrating effect on tissue.

Short-term effects of real SWT include analgesic and anti-inflammatory results likely due to removal of inflammatory mediators coupled with nociceptive inhibition through a gate-control mechanism. Longer term healing-effects may be related to acute vessel rupture and subsequent angiogenesis in soft tissues. EFD between 0.04 and 0.22 mJ/mm^2 have very few side effects as reported in the literature including pain, erythema, local soft tissue swelling, and local subcutaneous hematomas among others. High-energy SWT is quite uncomfortable without local anesthetic.

At the current time, based on literature evidence, treatment parameters appear empirical. The clinician weighs the advantage of high-energy treatment with the comfort level of low-energy treatment. It does appear that both high- and low-energy protocol procedures are equally effective if the total energy applied is approximately the same. The compensation then is to utilize a low-energy protocol but use more impulses over more treatment sessions to achieve a similar result to high-energy treatment protocols, especially when administered by chiropractors who are not able to utilize local anesthetic in-office.

Common uses for SWT include calcific tendinitis, lateral epicondylitis, patellar tendinitis, and plantar fasciitis.[27c, 27d, 27e]

Platelet-Rich Plasma (PRP) and Other Injections for Soft Tissue

A relatively new therapy has gained popular attention due to its use with well-known athletes. However, until recently, there has been little data to support the myriad claims. The approach is sometimes classified as a form of prolotherapy involving injection into a joint, muscle, tendon, or ligament. Although there is a heterogeneous group of injectables, the most popular is an injection that contains platelet-rich plasma (PRP). It is autogenic, meaning it is created by taking a patient's own blood and spinning it down into a platelet concentrate. The theory is that PRP is rich in growth factors and will help in healing and repair. Although this approach has been used for the conditions listed below, most studies are small and without randomization.

- acute ligament injury involving medial collateral ligament rupture of knee and elbow, lateral collateral ligament rupture of ankle, etc.
- chronic tendon problems such as rotator cuff tear, lateral epicondylitis of elbow, patellar tendinosis, Achilles tendinitis, plantar fasciitis, etc.
- chondromalacia or osteoarthritis of the knee, shoulder, and SI joint

Concerns about the underlying principle and theory of PRP injection include:

- For chronic processes, most of the growth factors are expressed within one hour after intra-articular PRP injection, so it is unlikely that it has a significant effect on the existing damage from chronic diseases.
- The pain relief seems consistent across studies but comparison to control groups is rarely utilized in the study design.[38]
- The basic science support is largely based in rat research that has demonstrated that PRP increased the number of collagen fibers and fibroblasts in the early phase of the healing process after damage to tendons.
- PRP has also been shown to stimulate the synthesis of hepatocyte growth factor (HGF) and vascular endothelial growth factor (VEGF) found within tendon cells, which increases cellular proliferation and vascular regeneration. However, only demonstrated in in-vitro studies, PRP affected human osteoarthritic chondrocytes by inhibiting the action of inflammatory cytokines such as IL-1 and NF-kB.[39]

There are mixed results that may be based on a balance of formulation of PRP. One study[39] suggests that rather than a focus on increasing platelets in an effort to maximize anabolic signaling, reducing leukocytes to minimize catabolic signaling may be more important. Although increasing the platelet concentration within lrPRP preparations results in the more anabolic growth factor delivery and less proinflammatory cytokines, the biological tradeoff is an effect on tendons of diminished metabolism indicated by a decrease in the synthesis of both COL1A1 and COL3A1. Therefore a balance must be accomplished where minimizing leukocytes in PRP becomes more important than maximizing platelet numbers with an overemphasis on concentration. This refocus should result in decreasing inflammation while enhancing matrix gene synthesis.

Following is a list of conclusions from recent reviews:

- In a systematic review of studies comparing PRP to a control group none of them showed any benefit of an autologous growth factor injection when compared with a control group.[40]
- Another systematic review of a number of injection therapies including corticosteroid, sclerosing agents, glycosaminoglycans, botulinum toxins, and PRP concluded that corticosteroid injection is beneficial in the short term for the treatment of tendinopathies

(potentially worse than other treatments in the intermediate and long terms). There was no clear evidence of benefit of other injections including PRP, except for sodium hyaluronate in the short and long term in overall improvement and pain reduction of lateral epicondylalgia.[41]

Another claim is a change in osteoarthritis progression with an injection of PRP. In a 2012 study,[42] investigators utilized MRI to detect whether PRP therapy for early knee osteoarthritis altered or stalled osteoarthritic changes as seen on MRI. They also measured clinical outcomes such as pain and function. Qualitative MRIs demonstrated no change in at least 73% of cases at one year. This is in contrast to some longitudinal studies that suggest annual decreases of up to 4 to 6% of cartilage

volume in knee osteoarthritis. This suggests a benefit at prevention but more studies are necessary given there was no control group. Noteworthy is that the American Academy of Orthopaedic Surgeons (AAOS) have approved PRP protocols only for use in research, and that PRP is not recommended for treatment purposes.[43] Also, some countries, including Korea, state that the use of PRP is illegal. Their concern is that there is not enough science to back up claims, yet hospitals and other groups are using this procedure as a major revenue source.[44]

Stretching of Soft Tissue

Numerous techniques for stretching and soft tissue pain control are used. **Exhibits 1–2** through **1–4** outline many

---

Exhibit 1–2 Rhythmic Stabilization

A variation of hold-relax, this technique uses a reciprocal contraction of the agonist and the antagonist following the approach outlined below:

- Stretch the involved muscle to patient tolerance.
- Use a physician's contact on both sides of a joint.
- Ask the patient to contract with a 25% contraction in the direction of agonist contraction for 5 to 8 seconds.
- Without resting, ask the patient to contract into the opposite direction for 5 to 8 seconds.
- Repeat this procedure five or six times.
- Ask the patient to relax.
- Stretch into new position.
- Repeat the above five or six times or until no more stretch appears available (whichever comes first).

Exhibit 1–3 Cross-Friction Massage and Spray and Stretch

Cross-Friction Massage

Cross-friction massage is a technique popularized by Cyriax.[8] The rationale behind its use is somewhat dependent on the patient's presenting phase of injury. For example, in subacute injury the intent is to align collagen for stronger scar formation. With chronic conditions the cross-friction approach is used to break up adhesions and increase blood supply. A secondary effect of cross-friction massage is a pressure anesthesia, which occurs after a couple minutes of application. There are several suggestions for the proper use of cross-friction massage:

- It appears to be most effective with tendons and ligaments.
- The tendon or ligament should be placed under slight tension (by stretching the involved structure) while cross-friction is performed.
- The contact is skin on skin with no lotion.
- The pressure is applied as a transverse motion (90° to the involved structure).
- Monitoring the patient every 2 minutes for a total of 6 to 9 minutes is recommended.
- Prior to application, some practitioners recommended ice; others recommend moist heat for approximately 5 minutes.
- Treatment is given every other day for 1 to 2 weeks (up to 4 weeks maximum).

Spray (Cold) and Stretch

Although the technique of using fluoromethane spray for stretching muscles was popularized by Travell and Simons,[3] concerns over damage to the ozone layer and increasing unavailability of the spray have led to a return to the use of ice. With the use of either tool, the technique of application has several common protocol components:

- The muscle being stretched is placed in a position of mild to moderate stretch. Maintain this stretch while applying the cold stimulus.
- The cold stimulus is applied in a series of linear strokes to the skin overlying the muscle and its associated pain referral zone. This is applied in the direction of pain referral.
- Gradually increase the stretch while applying the cold.
- Following the stretch, the skin should be briefly rewarmed with a moist heat pack.
- The muscle should then be put through a full range of motion, passively and then actively (this is an attempt to avoid posttreatment soreness).

Exhibit 1–4 Myofascial Release Techniques (MRTs)

Several techniques have been developed and popularized under different technique names. Most techniques involve a stripping motion of a muscle. A combination of these techniques is found with MRT (or ART) as proposed by Leahy and Mock.[45] These techniques are best used when a muscle is determined to be dysfunctional. This is accomplished through a combination of palpation, range of motion (ROM) findings, and muscle testing. This technique is not intended for acute injury (within 24 to 36 hours) or for ligaments and tendons that respond better to cross-friction massage. In essence, this is an extension of other myofascial or trigger-point approaches. Skin lotion should be used when possible. Following is a summary of this approach. There are four levels. Use the highest level that patient tolerance permits.

Level 4
- Place the muscle in its shortest position.
- Apply a firm contact to the muscle just distal to the site of palpable adhesion.
- Ask the patient to move the limb actively through an antagonist pattern (if the joint is in extension, the patient flexes), elongating the muscle.
- Always maintain a fixed contact on the patient so that the adhesions are forced under the contact point.

Level 3
- Place the muscle in its shortest position.
- Apply a firm contact to the muscle just distal to the site of palpable adhesion.
- Passively move the limb through an antagonist pattern, elongating the muscle.
- Always maintain a fixed contact on the patient so that the adhesions are forced under the contact point.

Level 2
- Place the muscle in a stretched position (creating tension).
- Apply muscle-stripping massage (along the direction of muscle fibers) using a broad contact, concentrating on areas of adhesion.

Level 1
- Place the muscle in a neutral position (no tension).
- Apply muscle-stripping massage, concentrating on areas of adhesion.

Treatment usually involves several passes over the muscle, treatment every other day, and resolution within the first few treatments.

Adjunctive care involves prescription of exercises for the involved muscle, starting with facilitation.

of these approaches, including rhythmic stabilization, postisometric relaxation, proprioceptive neuromuscular facilitation (PNF) hold-relax and contract-relax techniques, cross-friction massage, spray and stretch, myofascial release techniques (MRT or active resistive technique [ART][45]), and Graston technique. These are further discussed below.

Recommendations for the frequency of manual therapy generally have been outlined by the Mercy Guidelines (**Figures 1–3** and **1–4**).[50] A brief summary follows:

- If the condition is acute (<6 weeks) and uncomplicated (no red flags indicating referral), there may be an initial trial treatment phase of 2 weeks at a frequency of three to five times per week.
- At 2 weeks the case is reevaluated (unless there is progressive worsening); if improving, the patient is given an education program regarding activities of daily living (ADL) and a graduated program of exercise and stretching, with treatment continuing for up to 8 weeks depending on the patient's progress; if not improved, a 2-week trial with a different treatment plan is suggested.
- If after the second 2-week trial, the patient has not improved, consultation or referral is suggested.
- Cases that will likely have a prolonged recovery include those with symptoms lasting longer than 8 days, severe pain, more than four previous episodes, or preexisting structural or pathologic conditions.

Active care criteria include decreasing pain and inflammation and an improvement in range of motion and joint mobility (**Figures 1–5** and **1–6**). There is a phase where passive and active care coexist. During this stage, isometrics performed in limited arcs are helpful initiators and facilitators for a progressive exercise program. Progressing through a graded program involves setting criteria for passing each stage. The most common criteria are range of motion, strength levels, and performance without pain.

Active care elements include training to increase range of motion, strengthening primary and secondary stabilizers of a given joint or region, increasing the endurance capabilities of the muscles, proprioceptively training for balance and reaction time, and finally, functionally training for a specific sport or occupational task. Each element involves different training strategies (**Table 1–9** and **Exhibits 1–5** through **1–7**).

Strength and Endurance

Strengthening begins with facilitation. This is accomplished either through isometrics performed at every 20° to 30° or rhythmic stabilization using elastic tubing, performing very fast, short-arc movements for 60 seconds or until fatigue or pain limits further performance. Strengthening may then progress to holding end-range isometrics with elastic tubing for several seconds, and slowly releasing through the eccentric (negative) contraction. In some cases, these end-range isometrics may be performed initially against only gravity. If these elements are strong and pain free, progressing to full-arc isotonics using weights or elastic tubing may be introduced. It is best to begin with three to five sets of high repetitions (12 to 20) using 50% to 70% of maximum weight. After 1 to 3 weeks of this training, progression through a more vigorous strengthening program may be determined by the daily adjustable progressive resistance exercise (DAPRE) approach[48] (although the exercises are performed every other day). This is a pyramid approach using lower weight with more repetitions and progressing through sets to higher weight and fewer repetitions. The last number of repetitions performed determines the working weight for the next workout.

Proprioceptive Training

Proprioceptive training incorporates various balance devices such as wobble boards, giant exercise balls, and mini trampolines. The intention is to have the body part react to changing support as quickly as possible and to integrate the rest of the body in this attempt.

Functional Training (also see Functional Movement Evaluation earlier in this chapter)

Functional training is based on the requirements of a given sport or occupational activity and requires a knowledge of the biomechanics involved. Various PNF techniques may be employed. Simulated task performance is another approach for occupational retraining.

Whole-Body Vibration Therapy

Whole body vibration (WBV) has become a popular approach in the physiotherapy and rehabilitation arena. It is applied through a broad contact area that involves a sitting or standing platform. The vibration is in the range of 0.5 to 80 Hz. Aliases include *biomechanical stimulation* (BMS), *vibration therapy*, and *biomechanical oscillation* (BMO).

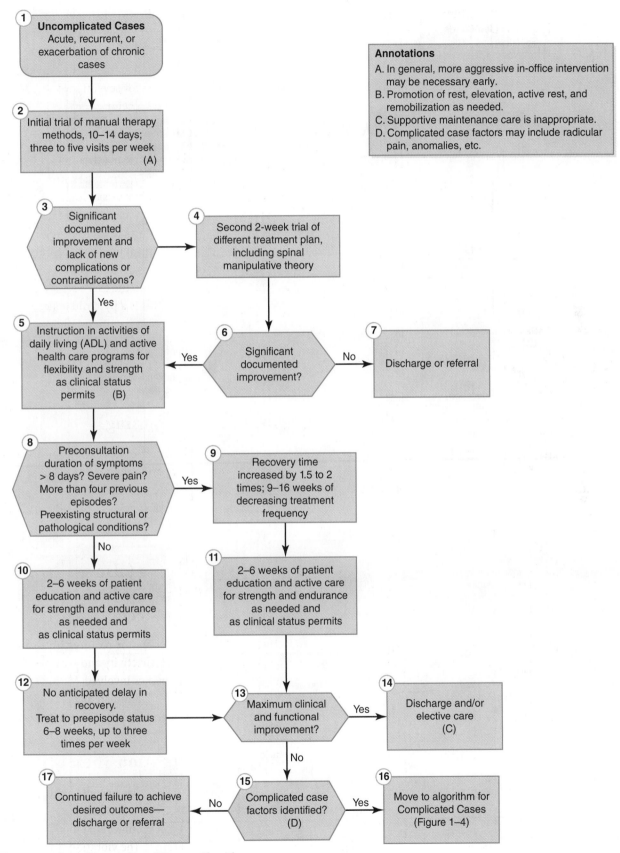

Figure 1–3 Acute/Uncomplicated Cases—Algorithm

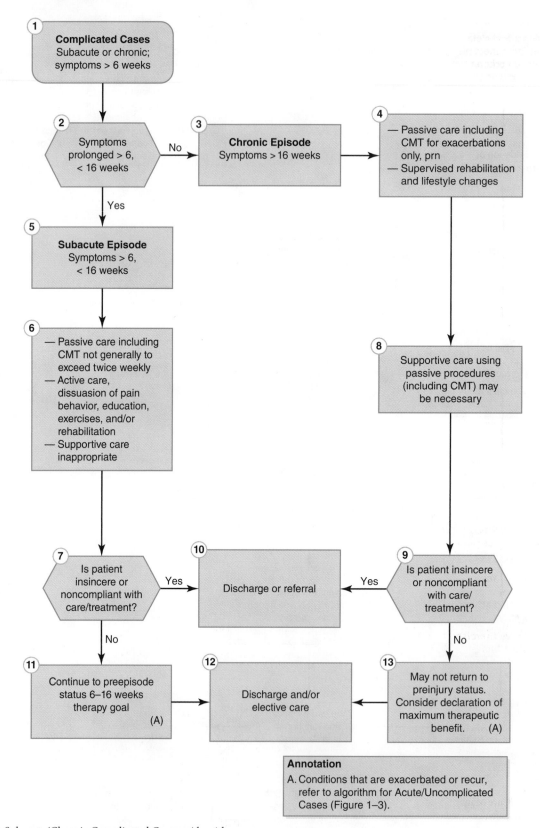

Figure 1–4 Subacute/Chronic Complicated Cases—Algorithm

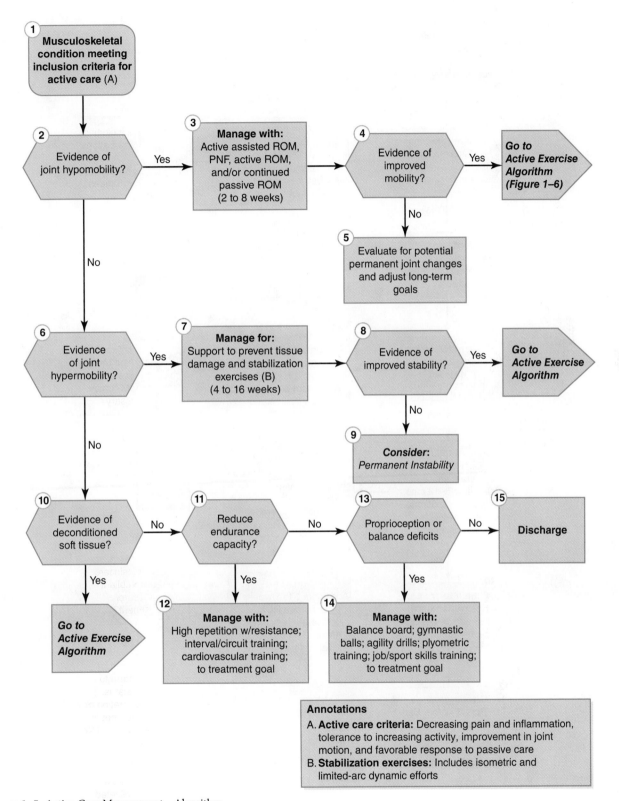

Figure 1–5 Active Care Management—Algorithm

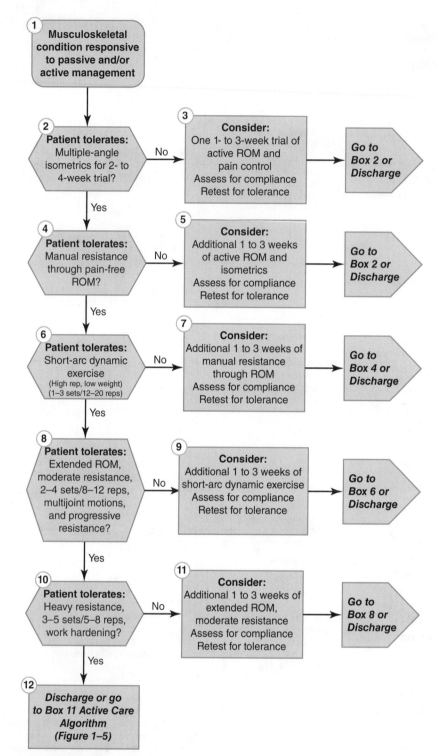

Figure 1–6 Active Care: Exercise—Algorithm

Reproduced from D.L. Nelson, *Topics in Clinical Chiropractic*, Vol. 1, No. 4, p. 77, © 1994, Aspen Publishers, Inc.

Table 1–9 The Daily Adjustable Progressive Resistance Exercise (DAPRE) Approach

Set	Weight	Repetitions
1	½ working weight	10
2	¾ working weight	6
3	Full working weight	Maximum
4	Adjusted working weight (based on Set 3)	Maximum

- Use the following table to determine working weight for Set 4 (based on number of repetitions in Set 3).
- Full working weight (Set 3) of the next training session is based on number of repetitions performed in the Set 4.

No. of Repetitions	For Set 4	Next Session Full Working Weight
0–2	Decrease 5–10 lb	Decrease 5–10 lb
3–4	Decrease 0–5 lb	The same
5–6	The same	Increase 5–10 lb
7–10	Increase 5–10 lb	Increase 5–15 lb
11 or more	Increase 10–15 lb	Increase 10–20 lb

As with most therapies, it is not as simple as one therapy—there are a multitude of types, brands, protocols, and claims. General parameters include the direction and force of vibration matched to the intention. Machines may vibrate in one or more than one direction: sideways (x), front and back (y), and up and down (z). The z-axis has the largest amplitude and is the most defining component in generating and inducing muscle contractions. Machines that offer side alternation (x-axis) usually can provide a larger amplitude of oscillation and a frequency range of about 5 to 35 Hz.

Following are some standard divisions based on type and use:

- High Energy Lineal (HVL), commonly found in gyms and vibration training centers. HVL machines focus on the vertical or upward movement of the platform, which is intended to increase gravity's effect eliciting a strong stretch-reflex contraction in muscles. Linear/upright systems deliver lower amplitudes but higher frequencies in the range of 20 to 50 Hz.
- Premium Speed Pivotal, basically a teeter-totter movement, often used for exercise workouts at speeds up to 30 Hz.
- Other types include Medium Energy Lineal, which accounts for the majority of lineal platforms produced. Often made of plastic, their construction may be less durable.
- Low Energy/Low Amplitude Lineal and Low Energy/High Amplitude Lineal, used primarily for

the older population with the intended outcomes of improved circulation, osteoporosis prevention, and minimal fitness maintenance.

Although WBV has been proposed for a multitude of disorders ranging from musculoskeletal disorders (including tendinosis, osteoporosis, strength training), stroke, neurological disorders (including multiple sclerosis, cerebral palsy, Parkinson's, spinocerebellar ataxia), and even the metabolic profile of metabolic syndrome and diabetes, there appears to be no clear evidence at this time that it leads to any clinically significant changes. Many studies either show no difference between groups randomized to placebo or WBV or only statistically significant changes; not clinically significant. An example would be for a 10-m or Timed Up and Go Test, the differences amount to 1 second or less and, although passing the test of statistical significance, are unlikely to make any difference to a patient. Secondly, there are no indications of what protocol to use. There are differences that include standard WBV, nonrandom rotational, or vertical higher frequency (20–50 Hz) vibration (used in most WBV research), and stochastic meaning random, low-frequency vibration (2.0–6 Hz).

A commonly tested claim of WBV proponents that it is effective in improving balance through a process whereby vibration stimulates nerves that stimulate alpha-motor neurons that cause muscle contraction at an increased rate and more effectively when compared to other approaches, there is little evidence to support such a claim.

Exhibit 1–5 Eccentric Exercise Protocols

General Comments

- Eccentrics are usually begun in the subacute phase of healing.
- Although there is some disagreement, the initial phase begins somewhere between 3 and 7 days after injury depending on severity.
- The superiority of eccentrics over concentrics occurs only during the first 19 days postinjury.
- A load of up to 20% above a one-repetition maximum is considered safe.
- It is suggested by the literature to perform between 3 and 20 repetitions with a three-set maximum; two to three times per week. Two times per week will probably prevent delayed-onset muscle soreness (DOMS).
- Rest periods are not as important due to the low oxygen demand. Somewhere between 30 seconds to 1 minute is sufficient.
- Training begins with slow progressing to faster repetitions.
- Two concerns are chance of overload injury and DOMS.
- Generally, there are three phases of training. An example for the lower extremity follows:
  1. Two-leg concentric/eccentric training is followed by two-leg concentric/injured leg eccentric work.
  2. Slow, submaximal, single-leg eccentrics are performed. The first two phases are usually completed in 3 weeks or less.
  3. Functional eccentrics are performed in preparation for plyometrics. This phase usually takes 2 to 3 weeks to complete.

Functional Eccentrics for the Lower Extremity

A sample of a functional eccentric program would include the following:

1. One-leg step-up onto 12-inch stool; noninvolved leg steps up first, down last.
2. One-leg step-up; involved leg steps up first, down last.
3. Repeat with 18-inch step height.
4. Slow quarter squats.
5. Rapid quarter squats.
6. Slow parallel squats.
7. Rapid parallel squats.

Curwin and Stanish[47] Eccentric Protocol for Tendinitis/Tendinosis

1. Static stretching for 15–30 seconds is repeated three to five times.
2. Eccentric exercise is begun with gravity or light weights. For the first 2 days they are performed slowly. During days 3–5 they are performed at moderate speed. On days 6 and 7 the exercises are performed quickly. Three sets of 10 are performed.
3. After the eccentric phase, a repeat of the static stretching phase is performed.
4. Follow with 5–10 minutes of icing.

Curwin and Stanish suggest that there should be some pain felt in the third set. If not, the resistance should be increased slightly. If pain is felt in the first two sets, weight should be decreased slightly.

Based on the literature, there is a limit to the strength of conclusions for most studies regarding effect. What is fairly clear at this point is that:

- Used for the purpose of weight loss, there is no support for this proposed effect.[50]
- Reduction or prevention of chronic low back pain is not evident from current studies.[51, 52]
- There is insufficient evidence of the effect of WBV training on functional performance of neurodegenerative disease patients.[53]

Exhibit 1–6 Advanced Training Approaches

Russian Stimulation Protocol

- Place one electrode over the muscle and one over the associated nerve root.
- Use a 2500-Hz carrier wave; modulate at 50 pulses per second.
- Increase intensity to patient tolerance.
- Use 10-second maximum contraction with 50-second rest periods equaling 10 contractions in 10 minutes.
- Use three to five treatments per week for 5 to 7 weeks for a total of 23 to 35 treatments (2-day rest period per week).
- Protocol is used one time per year, best at night and not before or after strenuous exercise.

Plyometrics for the Lower Extremity

- Plyometrics are advanced exercises used only under the following conditions:
    1. Strength and flexibility are preinjury.
    2. Static stability is demonstrated with the following:
       —single-leg stance
       —single-leg quarter squat
       —single-leg half squat

All can be performed for 30 seconds with eyes open and closed.

- A plyometric workout should be sport-specific and include the following (general conditioning):
    1. Warm-up for 10 to 20 minutes.
    2. Low-intensity drills: 3 to 5 exercises; 10 to 20 repetitions.
    3. Moderate-intensity drills: 3 to 4 exercises; 5 to 8 repetitions.
    4. High-intensity drills: 2 to 3 exercises; 10 to 20 repetitions.

- A plyometric protocol begins with horizontal and progresses to vertical movements.
- Horizontal progression is as follows:
    1. Double-leg forward hopping in a straight line.
    2. Side-to-side hopping, double leg.
    3. Combination of side-to-side and forward hopping.
    4. Follow with single-leg progression following the above sequence.
- Vertical progression is as follows:
    1. Jump from the floor to a box and back down, starting with 6-inch box and progressing to 12-inch, then 18-inch, then 20-inch.
    2. Jump in a line using boxes of variable height.

Never use plyometrics for an athlete with quadriceps or patellar tendinitis.

Most promising are the use of WBV for the following:

- Neuropathy—some improvements with diabetic neuropathy associated with increases in blood flow.[54]
- Adjunct to management of type 2 diabetes—including some limited information about metabolic improvement, increased blood flow, and adiposity.[54, 55]
- Osteoarthritis of the knee—decreases in knee pain.[56]
- Mild increases in osteogenic activity with variable indicators of increased bone mineral density.[57]

Exhibit 1–7 Classic Elastic Tubing Protocol

Facilitation

A fast midrange movement is performed for 30 to 60 seconds or until painful. The number of sets is determined by the overall status of the patient. When this can be performed pain free for 2 or 3 days, move on to the next phase.

Strength

A slow full-range movement is performed and held for an isometric contraction of up to 30 seconds at end-range. This is followed by a slow eccentric phase (at least twice as long as the concentric). Rest for 10 seconds and perform again for up to 10 repetitions (pain or fatigue dependent). When performed for 2 or 3 days pain free, move to the next phase.

Endurance

A fast full-range movement is performed at the rate of one per second. This may be performed for 50 to 60 seconds or until pain or fatigue is felt. Several sets may be performed with resting phases of 30 seconds. When this is possible for 2 or 3 days pain free, the patient has the option of progressing to pulley or free-weight exercise.

- The thickness and length of the tubing determine the resistance.
- Thicker, shorter tubing is more resistant and requires more patient effort.
- Resistance increases throughout the concentric contraction and decreases through the eccentric phase.

Variations of Elastic Tubing Exercise Protocols

- Currently, short-arc, fast repetitions are used for stabilization. May be used every 20° or so or may focus on position of instability (e.g., 20° to 30° knee flexion for anterior cruciate ligament tears).
- Eccentric focus only for tendinitis. For example, place knee in final position of flexion or extension and resist tubing while lengthening the muscle. For example, extend knee, apply tubing behind, and gradually allow tubing to overcome resistance; end position of knee flexion.
- Sports cord training.
- Closed-chain exercise: squats or seated foot dragging.
- Functional PNF diagonal pattern training.

Note: Always ice after any of the above exercises.

- Postural control in the elderly, potentially preventing falls.[58]
- Improved blood flow in the elderly—works as a pump on the blood vessels through rapid contraction and relaxation of muscles at 20 to 50 times per second. Patients often feel a tingling sensation as a result of the increased vasodilation.[59]
- Benefit for the management of tendinopathy, in particular as an alternative to Achilles rehab if eccentric exercise is unsuccessful.[60]
- Benefits in avoiding muscle atrophy with bed rest or post-surgery for ACL reconstruction.[61, 62]

Taping

There are a number of different taping approaches based on the texture and structure of the tape and its intended purpose. All taping has the potential of providing, beyond the structural support, several neurological advantages including decreased pain due to large-fiber mechanoreceptor stimulation of the skin, increased proprioception through increased stimulation to cutaneous mechanoreceptors, and changes in muscle recruitment patterns due to this stimulation.[63, 64]

Standard white (Zonas) taping is structurally unforgiving and is more often used for stability with ankle sprains and AC separations, yet the time frame upon which the support is provided has been shown to be rather limited. Even more rigid is Leukotape (McConnell taping) or "brown" tape, which is more supportive. This approach has been used for patellar stability among others. Yet, again the effect seems less on the stability, which does not appear to last long, but more likely based on the same neurological reflex responses seen with all tape.

Most recently there has been an interest and increased use of several types of taping that have some similar qualities. The first to gain widespread attention is Kinesio tape. This approach is less focused on support and more on the following unique characteristics and proposed mechanisms of effect in addition to standard taping:[65]

- It has elasticity in one direction and can be stretched to 140% of its original length. As a result there is a constant pulling (shear) force to the skin.
- It is air-permeable and water-resistant and can be worn for several days.
- There may be improved circulation of blood and lymph by eliminating tissue fluid or bleeding beneath the skin through constant compression and pumping effect.
- It may affect the function of fascia and muscle.

Instrument-Assisted Soft Tissue Mobilization

As the original approach to instrument-assisted soft tissue mobilization (IASTM), Graston Technique utilizes a set of metal instruments to deliver a directional massage. As part of an even larger concept of tissue therapy called provocation therapy, its goal is to break down scar tissue and fascial restrictions. The practitioner performs a "scan" of the involved area and through the metal is able to perceive areas of adhesion that then direct application. Often the beveled side of the tool is used for broader areas of application and, in addition, a lotion is applied prior to treatment. Rules governing directional application are similar to standard massage (in the direction of lymphatic flow) and with caution regarding a temporary skin reaction of small petechiae, practitioners deliver a treatment session that is generally quite short. The general rule of thumb is that a response should be felt almost immediately and sustained for at least several hours. This is a prime indicator of potential long-term effectiveness. Many practitioners combine the treatment concept of IASTM with other techniques such as myofascial release

or functional movement to create an approach that uses movement coupled with application of Graston or Graston-like instrument massage. Although these techniques are now quite widespread with the development of a number of modifications of the original Graston tools, other than a handful of case studies, there is still little evidence in the literature at this time to support this approach.[66, 67] It is hoped that new research will emerge on this new resurfacing of an age-old approach (i.e., coin therapy in Asia).

Nutritional Support

The nutritional support needed for musculoskeletal healing is based on recommendations made by Gerber.[49]

- In the inflammatory phase of healing, proteolytic enzymes, bioflavonoids, and vitamins C and E are recommended. Bromelain in doses of 1200 mg/d of 2400μ potency taken between meals for several days may be beneficial.
- In the proliferative phase, arginine, glycine, proline, vitamins A and C, pantothenic acid, and zinc may be of benefit. Connective tissue repair may be aided with glycosaminoglycans, manganese, and chondroitin sulfate.
- Fracture healing may be enhanced with adequate dietary calcium, vitamin D, phosphorus, and magnesium; microcrystalline hydroxyapatite may also be of benefit (6 to 8 g/d).

The Anti-Inflammatory Diet

Linoleic acid from n-6 fatty acids is converted to arachidonic acid and through several steps into prostaglandin-E2 (PGE2) and other pro-inflammatory eicosanoids. It may be that many chronic diseases and cancers are in part maintained or supported by this pro-inflammatory environment. Breast cancer is one example. One study indicates that women with high n6 fatty acid intake and a low n3 fatty acid intake were more prone to develop breast cancer.[69] N-6 fatty acids are found in high amounts in most seeds (and their oils) as well as in grains and their manufactured varieties (e.g., flours, pasta, cereal, chips, desserts). Meats, dairy fats, and shellfish are also converted to arachidonic acid, which is converted to PGE2. There is a belief that a ratio of n6 to n3 fatty acids should be close to 1:1 for humans to maintain an anti-inflammatory internal environment. Ratios in the modern diet can be as high as 10:1 to 30:1. If a diet consisted of less grain and seed and more vegetables, fruit, and fish, the proper balance of n6 to n3 would be maintained. It is possible to buy eggs and beef that have a higher n3 content. Ω-3 fatty acids may also be supplemented in the form of fish oil (obtainable from eicosapentaenoic acid and docosahexaenoic acid (EPA/DHA) and alpha-linolenic acid (ALA) from flaxseed oil. Typical doses for EPA/DHA are 1 to 2 grams per day and for ALA, 2 grams per day.

A popular theory regarding the cause of many diseases that appear autoimmune is that both molecular mimicry and a "leaky gut" are factors in establishing an autoimmune response in the body. According to the proposed model of molecular mimicry, microbial antigens resemble self-antigens when exposed to the mucosal immune system and an auto-immune process is triggered. The process is set in play and perpetuated by the body's own immune response and then becomes independent of exposure to the environmental trigger and is therefore self-perpetuating and irreversible.

The leaky gut theory is based on a model that proposes that the normal macromolecule trafficking dictated mainly by intestinal paracellular permeability involves alterations in intestinal permeability due to changes in the competency of barriers called tight junctions.[70]

The molecular mimicry theory is an extrapolation of the viral mimicry theory that is believed to be the mechanism by which some diseases such as multiple sclerosis are activated. The dietary version suggests that, in genetically susceptible individuals, certain undigested food particles can mimic human protein, such as collagen, and elicit an autoimmune response. For example, bovine serum albumin (BSA) found in cow's milk may be considered by the body as an antigen, and given that it is similar in sequence to human collagen may cause an autoimmune reaction.[71] Another example is glycine-rich protein found in grains and legumes, which has a similar protein sequence to connective tissue. Other suspected agents include wheat germ agglutinin (WGA) found in wheat, phytohemagglutinin (PHA) found in kidney beans, and peanut lection (PNA) found in peanuts.

In addition to digestion, the gastrointestinal system, specifically the intestinal lining, provides an immune defense for the body. Immune defense is accomplished partly by the intestinal mucosa that acts as a physical barrier, by intestinal secretions (e.g., secretory IgA

antibodies), and via intramural lymphocytes. One suggested test for the leaky gut syndrome is the lactulose-mannitol test.

Dietary support for providing an intact and functioning intestinal lining (see **Table 1–10**) includes:

- Glutamine—acts as a fuel source for intestinal cell maintenance and repair.
- Vitamins C and E, lipoic acid, zinc, and ginkgo biloba—act as antioxidants, protecting the mucosal lining from free-radical damage.
- Deglycyrrhizinated licorice (DGL)—thought to increase cell wall integrity of mucosal cells.
- N-acetylglucosamine (NAG)—helps to heal extracellular tissue and may decrease binding of some lectins.
- Probiotics—believed to counteract harmful bacteria.
- Hydrochloric acid and digestive enzymes—believed by some that if food particles are digested with the assistance of supplemental HCL and digestive enzymes, the less likely it will be that antigenic responses will occur.

Modification of the Inflammatory Response

Aspirin, nonsteroid anti-inflammatories (NSAIDs), and cyclooxygenase inhibitors (COX) block the cyclooxygenase enzyme that converts arachidonic acid to prostaglandin E-2, decreasing or blocking inflammation. Also, corticosteroids inhibit phospholipase A2, which inhibits arachidonic acid release from phospholipids in the cell membrane. Cell-signaling molecules, which stimulate genes, induce the expression of the COX enzyme. Aspirin, NSAIDs, and corticosteroids inhibit binding of cell-signaling molecules such as NFκ-B, which reduces inflammation (see **Exhibit 1–8**). Conversely, NFκ-B activation induces COX-2 activation, which leads to inflammation. The expression of the coding gene for COX-2 for the production of prostaglandins is transcriptionally regulated by NFκ-B. It is in the cytoplasm and is bound to its inhibitor. Free radicals release NFκ-B from the inhibitor, which then moves into the nucleus to activate genes responsible for COX-2 activation.

Green tea polyphenols, resveratrol from red wine, vitamins C and E, curcumin, and glutathione reduce the activation of NFκ-B. It is possible that carotenoids

Table 1–10 Nutritional Support for Osteoarthritis

Substance	How Might It Work?	Dosage	Special Instructions	Contraindications and Possible Side Effects
Glucosamine sulfate	Stimulates the rebuilding of damaged cartilage	500 mg three times per day	Take with meals. Take 6–8 weeks to determine effect	No contraindications. May cause some gastrointestinal upset. Does not interfere with other anti-inflammatory drugs. Some products processed with sodium chloride; use caution with patients who are hypertensive
Boswellia	Decreases inflammation	150 mg three times per day (for example, if extract contains 37.5% boswellic acids, need 400 mg of extract taken three times/day)	Take for 8 to 12 weeks	None at recommended dosage
Horsetail	Decreases inflammation	Taken as a tea at 1–4 g/day; tincture would be taken as 2–6 ml three times per day	Take for 8 to 12 weeks	None at recommended dosage
SAM (S-adenosylmethionine)	Possibly raises levels of dopamine	1600 mg/day	None	Occasional gastrointestinal upset. Some caution about patients with manic-depression switching from depression to a manic episode. Apparently safe in pregnancy
Vitamin E	Antioxidant	100–300 IU/day	None	None at recommended dosage
Niacinamide	Form of vitamin B3; may relieve symptoms and increase mobility	250 mg of niacinamide or nicotinamide 4–16 times/day	Improvement may take 3–4 months of supplementation	None at recommended dosage. Rare liver problems at several thousand milligrams per day
Vitamin C, iron (glycinate), and alpha-ketoglutaric acid	Required for hydroxylation of L-proline to L-hydroxyproline needed for quality collagen production	Vitamin C—3000–6000 mg/day in divided dosages. Iron (glycinate)—8–12 mg/day in divided dosages. Alpha-ketoglutaric acid—15 mg/day in divided dosages	Improvement may take 3–4 months of supplementation	Use caution with high dosages of vitamin C; it may lead to diarrhea or urinary tract irritation in some people

Note: These substances have not been approved by the Food and Drug Administration for the treatment of this disorder.

Exhibit 1–8 Contributors and Mediators of Inflammation: A Simplified Presentation

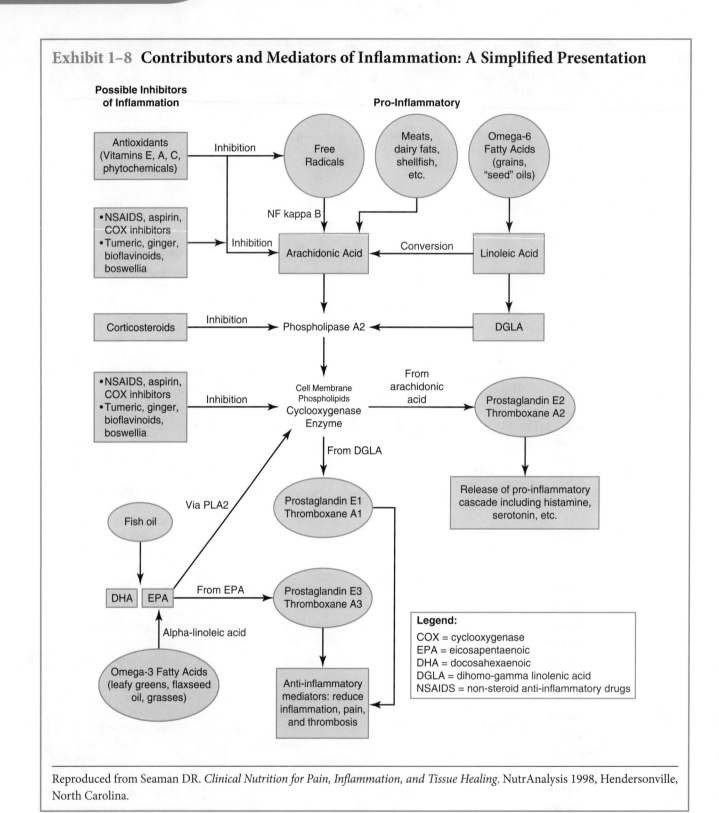

Reproduced from Seaman DR. *Clinical Nutrition for Pain, Inflammation, and Tissue Healing.* NutrAnalysis 1998, Hendersonville, North Carolina.

and flavonoids also have similar actions. Also, the anti-inflammatory omega-3 fatty acids are found in green vegetables, most fish, wild game, grass-fed meat, and EPA/DHA fish oil.

Table 1–11 presents a general nutritional approach to tendinosis and other soft tissue injury.

Tables 1–12, 1–13, and **1–14** outline common medications used in the management of musculoskeletal pain and inflammation.

Chondroitin sulfate is occasionally suggested for OA. Probably same effect or less than glucosamine sulfate. If taken, typical level is 400 mg three times per day.

Table 1–11 General Nutritional Approach to Tendinitis/Tendinosis and Other Soft Tissue Injury

Substance(s)	Recommended Amount
Proteolytic enzymes (trypsin, chymotrypsin, bromelain)	Bromelain at 1200 mg/day of 2400 mcu (milk clotting units) in divided doses in between meals is at the high end of recommended dose. This is for acute inflammatory phase only (for several days only). Contraindicated in patients with bleeding tendencies (or peptic ulcer); systemic infection; or allergy to source product such as pineapple, pork, beef, or papaya.
Bioflavonoids (quercetin, hesperidin, rutin, etc.)	600–1800 mg/day. Often taken at 200 mg every 2 waking hours. Taken before peak of inflammatory phase.
Herbs (boswellia, ginger, turmeric, cayenne)	Boswellia—400 mg, ginger—300 mg, turmeric—200 mg, cayenne—50 mg taken every 2 waking hours during inflammatory phase.

Table 1–12 Pain Medications

Drug Class	Examples	General Mechanism	Interactions/Side Effects
NSAIDs	Aspirin (acetylsalicylic acid) Alka-Seltzer A.S.A. Aspergum Bayer Cosprin Easprin Ecotrin Empirin Entrophen Novasen St. Joseph's Triaphen-10 ZORprin	Inhibits the formation of pro-inflammatory prostaglandins. Acts as an anti-inflammatory, antipyretic, and analgesic. Also has an antiplatelet effect. Used in the management of pain, fever, and prophylactically for its anticlotting action for prevention of stroke (transient ischemic attack), recurrence of MI, and thrombus formation (such as deep vein thrombosis).	Some individuals are allergic to aspirin and may have a hypersensitivity reaction including an asthma-like response. Heartburn and stomach upset may be due to irritation leading to peptic ulcer formation. Anemia may be due to blood loss or hemolytic anemia. Ototoxic effects include tinnitus and hearing loss. High doses may impair renal function.
	Naproxen Naproxen sodium Aleve Anaprox Apo-Naproxen Naprolen Naprosyn	NSAID. Similar to ibuprofen, ketoprofen, etc. Inhibits inflammatory prostaglandin synthesis. Actions include analgesic, anti-inflammatory, and antipyretic. Inhibits platelet aggregation and prolongs bleeding time but does not affect clotting.	May cause headache, drowsiness, dizziness, anorexia, heartburn, nausea, GI bleeding, and rarely agranulocytosis.
	Indomethacin Indameth Indocid Indocin Indocin SR	NSAID used to reduce pain and fever. May reduce activity of PMNs, development of cellular exudates, and vascular permeability when tissue is damaged.	Hypersensitivity possible with rash, dyspnea, asthma syndrome if patient is an aspirin-sensitive asthmatic, edema, hypotension. Also, concern of GI bleeding and rarely an aplastic anemia affect or renal function impairment.

(continues)

Table 1–12 Pain Medications (continued)

Drug Class	Examples	General Mechanism	Interactions/Side Effects
COX-2 inhibitors	Celecoxib Celebrex	NSAID: cyclooxygenase (COX) 2 inhibitor (does not inhibit COX-1) used primarily for arthritis (osteo, rheumatoid, and rheumatoid variants), acute pain, and menstrual cramps. Reduces fever. Also approved to prevent and reduce the size of polyps in patients with genetic disease.	May cause back pain, peripheral edema, GI problems, dizziness, headache, pharyngitis, and rash.
Opioids	Codeine Methylmorphine Paverol	An opiate derivative from morphine. Antihistamine effect stronger than morphine. Effective for pain relief and cough suppression.	May cause constipation, dizziness, urticaria, anaphylactic reaction, or urinary retention.
	Meperidine Demerol Pethadol Pethidine HCL	An opiate receptor agonist having the effects of analgesia, respiratory depression, and sedation.	May cause dizziness, sedation, nausea, constipation, allergic reaction, respiratory depression, convulsions, cardiovascular collapse.
	Pentazocine Talwin Talwin Nx	A synthetic analgesic, narcotic, CNS depressant used in the management of moderate to severe pain and preoperative sedation.	Not to be used with head injury. Will cause drowsiness, lightheadedness, and sedation. May cause dizziness, nausea/vomiting, constipation, urinary retention, rash, respiratory depression, or shock.
	Propoxyphene Darvon Novopropoxyn	Related to methadone; a strong opioid. Used for mild to moderate pain. Also used to manage narcotic withdrawal.	Caution that use with alcohol or high doses may cause death. Also more commonly causes drowsiness, constipation, skin reactions, GI upset, and rarely circulatory collapse or coma.
	Tramadol Ultram	Tramadol and its main metabolite bind to opioid receptors. Also reduces uptake of norepinephrine and serotonin. A pain reliever that is similar in action to narcotics with less of a risk for addiction or abuse.	May cause constipation, dizziness, nausea/vomiting, headache, and pruritus.
Opioid combinations with NSAIDs or acetaminophen	Hydrocodone/ acetaminophen Anexsia Lorcet Lorcet Plus Norco Vicodin Vicodin ES	Narcotic pain reliever and cough suppressant similar to codeine (CNS depression). The acetaminophen component is a non-narcotic pain reliever and fever reducer.	May cause dry mouth, nausea, vomiting, lightheadedness, dizziness, euphoria, dysphoria, some respiratory depression, and rash.
	Hydromorphone hydrochloride Dilaudid Dilaudid–HP	Similar to morphine but much stronger analgesic effect. Used for mild to moderate pain and cough suppression.	May cause drowsiness, respiratory depression, euphoria, dizziness, and various GI symptoms.

Table 1–12 Pain Medications (continued)

Drug Class	Examples	General Mechanism	Interactions/Side Effects
	Oxycodone Oxycontin Oxyfast Percolone Roxicodone	Binds to stereo-specific receptors in the CNS having the effects of a potent analgesic; ten times more potent than codeine. Used in the management of pain with fractures, bursitis, dislocations, postsurgery, and postpartum.	May cause sedation, constipation, respiratory depression, or hepatotoxicity.
Non-benzodiazepine muscle relaxants	**Cyclobenzaprine** Cycloflex Flexeril	Similar in structure to tricyclic antidepressants, these medications are used as muscle relaxants acting primarily on the CNS specifically at the brainstem. Increases circulating norepinephrine by blocking reuptake. Also has sedative effects and anticholinergic effects.	Drowsiness, dizziness, dry mouth, edema of the tongue, palpitations, chest pain, pruritus, and similar side effects of tricyclic antidepressants. Contraindicated for patients with heart problems.
	Chlorzoxazone Paraflex Parafon Forte	Used as a "muscle relaxant" due to action of depression of nerve transmission. Has slight sedative action. Used in combination with other medications in the treatment of low back and neck pain associated with muscle spasm.	May cause drowsiness, dizziness, nausea, vomiting, constipation, rash, or jaundice.

Table 1–13 Rheumatic Drugs Including DMARDs (Biologics and Nonbiologics)

Drug Class	Examples	General Mechanism	Interactions/Side Effects
Disease modifying antirheumatic drugs (DMARD) a.k.a.-Biologics	**Abatacept** Orencia	A disease-modifying antirheumatic drug (DMARD) inhibits T-cell proliferation and inhibits tumor necrosis factor alpha, gamma-interferon and interleukin-2, and decreases anticollagen antibody production. Used in the management of rheumatoid arthritis in patients who have inadequate response to other DMARDs. Used as mono therapy or in combination. Given as IV infusion.	Hypersensitivity reactions, headache, dizziness, hypertension, upper respiratory infection, malignancies, urinary tract infections.
	Etanercept Enbrel	A recombinant DNA substance that binds to tissue necrosis factor–alpha (TNF) receptors. TNF is a cytokine that induces an inflammatory action through interleukins. Affective in the management of Crohn's disease and inflammatory arthritic disorders such as RA and psoriatic arthritis.	May cause the usual GI disturbances, headache, dizziness, fatigue, loss of hair, pruritus. Rarely cause MI, serious infections, or pancytopenia.
	Adalimumab Humira	A disease-modifying antirheumatic drug (DMARD) is used alone or with methotrexate for the treatment of rheumatoid arthritis and similar disorders. A human monoclonal antibody, it works by blocking tissue necrosis factor (TNF)–alpha, a major protein involved in inflammation.	May cause a local injection response, rash, or increase the risk of serious infection such as tuberculosis, neurologic events, or malignancies. Very expensive.

(continues)

Table 1–13 Rheumatic Drugs Including DMARDs (Biologics and Nonbiologics) (continued)

Drug Class	Examples	General Mechanism	Interactions/Side Effects
	Infliximab Remicade	An IgG1-K monoclonal antibody that binds to tissue necrosis factor–alpha (TNF). TNF is a cytokine that induces an inflammatory action through interleukins. Affective in the management of Crohn's disease and inflammatory arthritic disorders such as RA and psoriatic arthritis.	May cause the usual GI disturbances, headache, dizziness, fatigue, lupus-like syndrome, loss of hair, pruritus, and increased liver enzymes.
Anti-inflammatory	**Prednisone** Dethasone Liquid Pred Medrol Oral Liquid Pediapred Prednisolone	Synthetic oral corticosteroid used to suppress immune system reaction including inflammation. These medications mimic actions of cortisol (hydrocortisone) produced by the adrenal gland. Used in the treatment of inflammatory arthritis, colitis such as Crohn's and ulcerative colitis, asthma, bronchitis, some skin rashes, allergic or inflammatory conditions affecting the nose and eyes.	Long-term use may cause suppression of bone growth, osteopenia and resultant fractures, Cushing's syndrome (osteoporosis, skin atrophy, abnormal glucose tolerance, anemia, behavioral abnormalities, etc.). Increased risk of candida (yeast) infection.
	Sulfasalazine Azulfidine Sulfasalazine Salazopyrin S.A.S.-500	A long-acting sulfonamide used in the management of clostridium and *E. coli* infections, inflammatory bowel disease, and RA. Anti-inflammatory effect may be due to inhibition of prostaglandins, and may have antibacterial effect due to conversion to sulfapyridine and 5-ASA.	May cause nausea, vomiting, bloody diarrhea, anorexia, rash, and allergic reactions.
	Methotrexate Rheumatrex Trexall	An antimetabolite that blocks the metabolism of fast-growing cells. Blocks folate reduction through inhibitory effect on dihydrofolate reductase. Used in the treatment of cancer and rheumatoid-like conditions such as psoriatic arthritis and RA. Cancers include acute lymphocytic leukemia; osteogenic sarcoma; Burkitt's lymphoma; non-Hodgkin's lymphoma; cancers of the brain, head, or neck; and small-cell lung choriocarcinoma. Also used to induce miscarriage (e.g., in ectopic pregnancy).	May cause bone marrow suppression, GI ulcers, nephrotoxicity, hepatotoxicity, nausea, diarrhea, or pulmonary infiltrates.
	Sulindac Clinoril	An indole, prostaglandin inhibitor (similar to indomethacin) used similar to aspirin with fewer GI effects than aspirin. Primarily used for inflammatory arthritis such as RA, ankylosing spondylitis, acute attacks of gout, acute bursitis of the shoulder.	May cause dizziness, headache, abdominal pain, prolonged bleeding time, aplastic anemia, anaphylaxis, toxic epidermal necrosis syndrome.
Combination effect	**Gold sodium thiomalate** Myochrysine	An injectable water-soluble gold compound used in the treatment of rheumatoid arthritis. Appears to have immunosuppressant and anti-inflammatory properties possibly through inhibition of inflammatory prostaglandins.	May cause photosensitivity, dizziness, syncope, proteinuria, stomatitis, GI symptoms, grey to blue discoloration of skin, hypersensitivity and erythema dermatitis.
	Gout Medications **Allopurinol** Alloprin Lopurin Novopurinol Zyloprim	A xanthine oxidase inhibitor used in the treatment of gout. It decreases endogenous uric acid. Inhibiting xanthine oxidase prevents conversion of hypo-xanthine to xanthine and then xanthine to uric acid. Not used for anti-inflammatory effect.	May cause nausea, vomiting, diarrhea, abdominal pain. Concerns over possible hepatotoxicity, renal insufficiency, aplastic anemia, and thrombocytopenia. Check with CBC and liver function tests.

Table 1–13 Rheumatic Drugs Including DMARDs (Biologics and Nonbiologics) (continued)

Drug Class	Examples	General Mechanism	Interactions/Side Effects
	Colchicine Novocolchine	Used as an anti-inflammatory agent in the treatment of gout. Sometimes used for sarcoid arthritis and pseudogout.	May cause nausea, vomiting, diarrhea, abdominal pain, steatorrhea, and pancreatitis. Also, a syndrome of muscle weakness may occur with accompanying elevation of serum creatine kinase.
	Probenecid Benemid Benuryl Probalan	A renal tubular blocking agent that prevents the reabsorption of uric acid, thereby, promoting its excretion. Used in the management of chronic hyperuricemia associated with gout.	May cause headache, GI complaints, hemolytic anemia, respiratory depression, and rarely hepatic necrosis.

Table 1–14 Neuralgia Drugs

Drug Class	Examples	General Mechanism	Interactions/Side Effects
Calcium channel blocker	**Pregabalin** Lyrica	Used in the management of the following: neuropathic pain (diabetic peripheral neuropathy), postherpetic neuralgia, adjunctive therapy for partial seizures, and fibromyalgia. Blocks calcium dependent of pronociceptive neurotransmitter's release.	Dizziness, sleepiness, edema, blurred vision, weight gain, and difficulty with concentration.
Glutamate antagonist	**Carbamazepine** Carbatrol Tegretol Tegretol-XR	Sodium, potassium, and calcium currents are reduced across neuronal membranes decreasing neuronal transmission. Has an antidiuretic effect. Used in the treatment of seizures and facial neuralgias, also sometimes schizophrenia.	CNS toxicity including sedation, dizziness, imbalance, and nausea/vomiting. Agranulocytosis or aplastic anemia. Also possible cause of birth defects.
GABA agonist	**Gabapentin** Neurontin	Related to gamma aminobutyric acid (GABA). Used as an adjunctive treatment of seizures; also used for herpetic neuropathy.	May cause tiredness, ataxia, dizziness, or other CNS effects.

Appendix 1–1

Web Resources

General Orthopaedics and Arthritis

National Institute of Arthritis and Musculoskeletal and Skin Diseases
(877) 220-4267; **www.niams.nih.gov**
The Arthritis Society
(800) 321-1433; **www.arthritis.ca**
American Academy of Orthopaedic Surgeons
(800) 824-BONES (26637); **www.aaos.org**

Autoimmune Disorders

American Autoimmune Related Disease Association
(800) 598-4668; http://**www.aarda.org**

Appendix 1–2

References

1. Clancy WG. Tendon trauma and overuse injuries. In: Leadbetter WB, Buckwalter JA, Gordon SL, eds. *Sports-Induced Inflammation*. Park Ridge, IL: AAOS; 1990.

2. Margaretten ME, Kohlwes J, Moore D, Bent S. Does this adult patient have septic arthritis? *JAMA.* 2007;297(13):1478–1488.

3. Travell J, Simons DG. *Myofascial Dysfunction: The Trigger Point Manual.* Baltimore: Williams & Wilkins; 1993.

4. Shah JP, Phillips TM, Danoff JV, Gerber LH. An in vivo microanalytical technique for measuring the local biochemical milieu of human skeletal muscle. *J Appl Physiol.* 2005;99(5):1977–1984.

5. Shah JP, Danoff JV, Desai MJ, et al. Biochemicals associated with pain and inflammation are elevated in sites near to and remote from active myofascial trigger points. *Arch Phys Med Rehabil.* 2008;89(1):16–23.

6. Chen Q, Bensamoun S, Basford JR, Thompson JM, An KN. Identification and quantification of myofascial taut bands with magnetic resonance elastography. *Arch Phys Med Rehabil.* 2007;88(12):1658–1661.

7. Mattingly GE, Mackarey PJ. Optimal methods for shoulder tendon palpation: a cadaver study. *Phys Ther.* 1996;2:166–174.

8. Cyriax J. *Textbook of Orthopaedic Medicine.* London: Ballière Tindall; 1982.

9. Janda V. Evaluation of muscular imbalance. In: Liebenson C, ed. *Rehabilitation of the Spine: A Practitioner's Manual.* Baltimore: Williams & Wilkins; 1996:97.

10. Lewit K, ed. *Manipulative Therapy in Rehabilitation of the Locomotor System.* 2nd ed. Oxford, England: Butterworth-Heinemann; 1991.

11. Cook G. *Movement: Functional Movement Systems. Screening, Assessment, and Corrective Strategies.* Santa Cruz: On Target Publications; 2010.

12. Shultz R, Anderson SC, Matheson GO, Marcello B, Besier T. Test-retest and interrater reliability of the functional movement screen. *J Athl Train.* 2013;48(3):331–336.

13. Pellechia GL, Paolino J, Connell J. Intertester reliability of the Cyriax evaluation in assessing patients with shoulder pain. *J Orthop Sports Phys Ther.* 1996;23:34–38.

14. Liebenson C, ed. *Rehabilitation of the Spine: A Practitioner's Manual.* Baltimore: Williams & Wilkins; 1996.

15. Schafer RC, Faye LJ. *Motion Palpation and Chiropractic Technique: Principles of Dynamic Chiropractic.* Huntington Beach, CA: Motion Palpation Institute; 1989.

16. Greenman PE. *Principles of Manual Medicine.* Baltimore: Williams & Wilkins; 1990.

17. Deyo RA, Diehl AK. Lumbar spine films in primary care: current use and effects of selective ordering criteria. *J Gen Intern Med.* 1986;1:20.

18. Howard BA, Rowe LJ. Spinal X-rays. In: Haldeman S, ed. *Principles and Practice of Chiropractic.* 2nd ed. Norwalk, CT: Appleton & Lange; 1992:361–364.

19. Schultz G, Philips RB, Cooley J, et al. Diagnostic imaging of the spine in chiropractic practice: recommendations for utilisation. *Chiro J Aust.* 1992;22:141–152.

20. Bussieres AE, Peterson C, Taylor JA. Diagnostic imaging practice guidelines for musculoskeletal complaints in adults—an evidence-based approach: introduction. *J Manipulative Physiol Ther.* 2007;30(9):617–683.

21. Raney NH, Teyhen DS, Childs JD. Observed changes in lateral abdominal muscle thickness after spinal manipulation: a case series using rehabilitative ultrasound imaging. *J Orthop Sports Phys Ther.* 2007;37(8):472–479.

22. Henry SM, Teyhen DS. Ultrasound imaging as a feedback tool in the rehabilitation of trunk muscle dysfunction for people with low back pain. *J Orthop Sports Phys Ther.* 2007;37(10):627–634.

23. Painter EE, Ogle MD, Teyhen DS. Lumbopelvic dysfunction and stress urinary incontinence: a case report applying rehabilitative ultrasound imaging. *J Orthop Sports Phys Ther.* 2007;37(8):499–504.

24. Teyhen D. Rehabilitative Ultrasound Imaging Symposium San Antonio, TX, May 8-10, 2006. *J Orthop Sports Phys Ther.* 2006;36(8):A1–3.

25. Teyhen DS, Childs JD, Flynn TW. Rehabilitative ultrasound imaging: when is a picture necessary. *J Orthop Sports Phys Ther.* 2007;37(10):579–580.

26. Teyhen DS, Gill NW, Whittaker JL, Henry SM, Hides JA, Hodges P. Rehabilitative ultrasound imaging of the abdominal muscles. *J Orthop Sports Phys Ther.* 2007;37(8): 450–466.

27. Whittaker JL, Teyhen DS, Elliott JM, et al. Rehabilitative ultrasound imaging: understanding the technology and its applications. *J Orthop Sports Phys Ther.* 2007;37(8):434–449.

28. Whittaker JL, Thompson JA, Teyhen DS, Hodges P. Rehabilitative ultrasound imaging of pelvic floor muscle function. *J Orthop Sports Phys Ther.* 2007;37(8):487–498.

29. Khan KM, Scott A. Mechanotherapy: how physical therapists' prescription of exercise promotes tissue repair. *Br J Sports Med.* 2009;43(4):247–252.

30. Olesen JL, Heinemeier KM, Gemmer C, et al. Exercise-dependent IGF-I, IGFBPS, and type I

collagen changes in human peritendinous connective tissue determined by microdialysis. *J Appl Physiol.* 2007;102:214–220.

31. Ohberg L, Lorentzon R, Alfredson H. Eccentric training in patients with chronic Achilles tendinosis: normalised tendon structure and decreased thickness at follow-up. *Br J Sports Med.* 2004;38:8–11.

32. Nelson DL. Assuring quality in the delivery of passive and active care. *Top Clin Chiro.* 1994;1(4):20–29.

33. Yousefi-Nooraie R, Schonstein E, Heidari K, et al. Low level laser therapy for nonspecific low-back pain. *Cochrane Database Syst Rev.* 2008(2):CD005107.

34. Chow RT, Johnson MI, Lopes-Martins RA, Bjordal JM. Efficacy of low-level laser therapy in the management of neck pain: a systematic review and meta-analysis of randomised placebo or active-treatment controlled trials. *Lancet.* 2009;374(9705):1897–1908.

35. Galasso O, Amelio E, Riccelli DA, Gasparini G. Short-term outcomes of extracorporeal shock wave therapy for the treatment of chronic non-calcific tendinopathy of the supraspinatus: a double-blind, randomized, placebo-controlled trial. *BMC Musculoskelet Disord.* 2012;13:86.

36. Lee SS, Kang S, Park NK, et al. Effectiveness of initial extracorporeal shock wave therapy on the newly diagnosed lateral or medial epicondylitis. *Ann Rehabil Med.* 2012;36(5):681–687.

37. Speed C. A systematic review of shockwave therapies in soft tissue conditions: focusing on the evidence. *Br J Sports Med.* 2013. doi: 10.1136/bjsports-2012-091961.

38. van Buul GM, Koevoet WL, Kops N, et al. Platelet-rich plasma releasate inhibits inflammatory processes in osteoarthritic chondrocytes. *Am J Sports Med.* 2011;39(11):2362–2370.

39. de Vos RJ, van Veldhoven PL, Moen MH, Weir A, Tol JL, Maffulli N. Autologous growth factor injections in chronic tendinopathy: a systematic review. *Br Med Bull.* 2010;95:63–77.

40. Boswell SG, Schnabel LV, Mohammed HO, Sundman EA, Minas T, Fortier LA. Increasing platelet concentrations in leukocyte-reduced platelet-rich plasma decrease collagen gene synthesis in tendons. *Am J Sports Med.* 2014;42(1):42–49.

41. Hart L. Corticosteroid and other injections in the management of tendinopathies: a review. *Clin J Sport Med.* 2011;21(6):540–541.

42. Halpern B, Chaudhury S, Rodeo SA, et al. Clinical and MRI outcomes after platelet-rich plasma treatment for knee osteoarthritis. *Clin J Sport Med.* 2013;23(3):238–239.

43. Martinez S. Practical guidelines for using PRP in the orthopaedic office [Internet]. Rosemont: American Academy of Orthopaedic Surgeons; c2012 [cited 2012 Apr 15]. Available from: http://www.aaos.org/news /aaosnow/sep10/clinica3.asp

44. Park YG, Han SB, Song SJ, Kim TJ, Ha CW. Platelet-rich plasma therapy for knee joint problems: review of the literature, current practice and legal perspectives in Korea. *Knee Surg Relat Res.* 2012;24(2):70–78.

45. Leahy PM, Mock LE III. Myofascial release technique and mechanical compromise of peripheral nerves of the upper extremity. *Chiro Sports Med.* 1992;6:139–150.

46. Haldeman S, Chapman-Smith D, Petersen DM, Jr., eds. *Guidelines for Quality Assurance and Practice Parameters.* Gaithersburg, MD: Aspen Publishers, Inc.; 1992.

47. Curwin S, Stanish WD. *Tendinitis: Its Etiology and Treatment.* Lexington, MA: Collamore Press; 1984.

48. Knight K. Knee rehabilitation by the daily adjustable progressive resistance technique. *Am J Sports Med.* 1979;7:336–337.

49. Gerber JM. *Handbook of Preventive and Therapeutic Nutrition.* Gaithersburg, MD: Aspen Publishers, Inc.; 1993.

50. Roelants M, Delecluse C, Goris M, Verschueren S. Effects of 24 weeks of whole body vibration training on body composition and muscle strength in untrained females. *Int J Sports Med.* 2004;25(1):1–5.

51. del Pozo-Cruz B, Hernandez Mocholi MA, Adsuar JC, Parraca JA, Muro I, Gusi N. Effects of whole body vibration therapy on main outcome measures for chronic non-specific low back pain: a single-blind randomized controlled trial. *J Rehabil Med.* 2011;43(8):689–694.

52. Rittweger J, Just K, Kautzsch K, Reeg P, Felsenberg D. Treatment of chronic lower back pain with lumbar extension and whole-body vibration exercise: a randomized controlled trial. *Spine (Phila Pa 1976).* 2002;27(17):1829–1834.

53. Sitjà Rabert M, Rigau Comas D, Fort Vanmeerhaeghe A, Santoyo Medina C, Roqué i Figuls M, Romero-Rodríguez D, Bonfill Cosp X. Whole-body vibration training for patients with neurodegenerative disease. *Cochrane Database of Systematic Reviews* 2012, Issue 2. Art. No.: CD009097. DOI: 10.1002/14651858. CD009097.pub2.

54. Kessler NJ, Hong J. Whole body vibration therapy for painful diabetic peripheral neuropathy: a pilot study. *J Bodyw Mov Ther.* 2013;17(4):518–522.

55. Del Pozo-Cruz B, Alfonso-Rosa RM, Del Pozo-Cruz J, Sanudo B, Rogers ME. Effects of a 12-week whole-body vibration based intervention to improve type 2 diabetes. *Maturitas*. 2013:(1):52–58.

56. Park YG, Kwon BS, Park JW, et al. Therapeutic effect of whole body vibration on chronic knee osteoarthritis. *Ann Rehabil Med*. 2013;37(4):505–515.

57. Ligouri GC, Shoepe TC, Almstedt HC. Whole body vibration training is osteogenic at the spine in college-age men and women. *J Hum Kinet*. 2012;31:55–68.

58. Verschueren SM, Roelants M, Delecluse C, Swinnen S, Vanderschueren D, Boonen S. Effect of 6-month whole body vibration training on hip density, muscle strength, and postural control in postmenopausal women: a randomized controlled pilot study. *J Bone Miner Res*. 2004;19(3):352–359.

59. Sanudo B, Alfonso-Rosa R, Del Pozo-Cruz B, Del Pozo-Cruz J, Galiano D, Figueroa A. Whole body vibration training improves leg blood flow and adiposity in patients with type 2 diabetes mellitus. *Eur J Appl Physiol*. 2013;113(9):2245–2252.

60. Horstmann T, Jud HM, Frohlich V, Mundermann A, Grau S. Whole-body vibration versus eccentric training or a wait-and-see approach for chronic Achilles tendinopathy: a randomized clinical trial. *J Orthop Sports Phys Ther*. 2013;43(11):794–803.

61. Fu CL, Yung SH, Law KY, et al. The effect of early whole-body vibration therapy on neuromuscular control after anterior cruciate ligament reconstruction: a randomized controlled trial. *Am J Sports Med*. 2013;41(4):804–814.

62. Belavy DL, Hides JA, Wilson SJ, et al. Resistive simulated weightbearing exercise with whole body vibration reduces lumbar spine deconditioning in bed-rest. *Spine (Phila Pa 1976)*. 2008;33(5): E121–131.

63. Murray H, Husk L. Effect of kinesiotaping on proprioception in the ankle. *J Orthop Sports Phys Ther*. 2001;31:A-37.

64. Halseth T, McChesney JW, DeBeliso M, et al. The effects of kinesiotaping on proprioception at the ankle. *J Sports Sci Med*. 2004;3:1–7.

65. Kase K, Tatsuyuki H, Tomoki O. Development of Kinesio Tape. Kinesio Taping Perfect Manual. 1996.

66. Hammer WI. The effect of mechanical load on degenerated soft tissue. *J Bodyw Mov Ther*. 2008;12(3):246–256.

67. Schaefer JL, Sandrey MA. Effects of a 4-week dynamic-balance-training program supplemented with Graston instrument-assisted soft-tissue mobilization for chronic ankle instability. *J Sport Rehabil*. 2012;21(4):313–326.

68. Burke J, Buchberger DJ, Carey-Loghmani MT, Dougherty PE, Greco DS, Dishman JD. A pilot study comparing two manual therapy interventions for carpal tunnel syndrome. *J Manipulative Physiol Ther*. 2007;30(1):50–61.

69. Capone SL, Bagga D, Glaspy JA. The relationship between omega-3 and omega-6 fatty acid ratios and breast cancer. *Nutrition*. 1997;13:822–824.

70. Fasano A. Leaky gut and autoimmune diseases. *Clin Rev Allergy Immunol*. Feb 2011;42(1):71–78.

71. Cordain L, Toohey L, Smith MJ, Hickey MS. Modulation of immune function by dietary lectins in rheumatoid arthritis. *Br J Nutr*. 2000;83:207–217.

Neck and Neck/Arm Complaints

Context

The cervical spine serves a unique function as a positioner of the head in space. This function requires a proprioceptive integration that results in optimization of head position through reflex setting of muscle tone. Although having the head perched atop the cervical spine allows better appreciation of the surrounding environment, this arrangement creates a potentially damaging lever arm in acute injury events that force the head to move quickly into extremes of flexion, extension, or lateral flexion. In addition to the cervical spine itself, soft tissue and neural structures may be damaged in the extremes of these movements. The lever effect also is operative in a more insidious manner when a forward head position is maintained for prolonged periods, as in a computer work environment. The demands on posterior musculature are dramatically increased by the weight of the head as it moves forward of the body.

The cervical spine is a focus for investigation of complaints that involve the head and upper extremities. The unique association between the upper cervical spinal nerves and the trigeminal nerve is postulated to have effects that result in complaints of headache, facial pain, or ear pain. Upper extremity complaints may be caused or augmented by cervical spine pathology that affects the spine, nerve roots, or brachial plexus.

Common patient presentations include the following:

- Acute injury neck and/or arm pain (e.g., whiplash, cervical "stingers")
- Acute, pseudotorticollis (not a true torticollis but a painful limitation of all neck movement)
- Postural pain or stiffness due to poor ergonomics in the work environment

- Osteoarthritis associated stiffness or pain
- Headaches

When arm complaints accompany neck pain, it is essential to make the determination of whether nerve root irritation or a referred phenomenon is the source. Chiropractors are often faced with patients who, upon examination, demonstrate no objectifiable neurologic deficit in the arm(s) even though numbness/tingling or weakness is part of their complaint. Many of these patients appear to obtain relief from chiropractic procedures, suggesting a referral connection between what is manipulated and what causes the "phantom" symptoms. This is most likely the facet joint. Whether the complaint is local to the neck or referred to the arm, Bogduk[1] states that facet joint pain accounts for the majority of patient complaints. Neck and arm complaints also require a consideration of brachial plexus or peripheral nerve involvement.

The National Board of Chiropractic Examiners (NBCE) Job Analysis 2005[2] estimates that neck pain accounts for approximately 18.7% of all chiropractic visits. In a Canadian study, Cote et al.[3] found that the age-adjusted lifetime prevalence for neck pain was 66.7% and the point prevalence was 22.2%. According to the National Health Interview Survey (NHIS) 13.8% of the population in the United States reported having neck pain in 2004.[4] Data reported in the Task Force on Neck Pain and Its Associated Disorders provides a range for the 12-month prevalence of 12.1% to 71.5% in the general population and 27.1% to 47.8% in workers (Haldeman). However, the one-year prevalence of disability due to neck pain was between 1.7% and 11.5% in the general population. A more narrow range of only 11% to 14.1% of workers report being limited in their activities during a one-year time frame. Only about 25% of individuals with neck pain seek conventional medical care. However, one to five years after the initial episode of neck pain, 50% to 85% of individuals will again report neck pain. Data from three national surveys indicates that 64% of ambulatory visits for neck pain resulted in a pain diagnosis rather than a pathology diagnosis. In hospitals, 94% of patients with neck pain received a pathology diagnosis with 79% of those patients requiring surgery.

The appropriateness of chiropractic manipulation of the cervical spine for various conditions has been addressed in two major publications: the 1995 scientific monograph of the Quebec Task Force on Whiplash-Associated Disorders[5] entitled "Redefining 'Whiplash' and Its Management," and the 1996 Rand Corporation report[6] entitled *The Appropriateness of Manipulation and Mobilization of the Cervical Spine.* More recently the Bone and Joint Decade 2000–2010 Task Force on Neck Pain and Its Associated Disorders[7] has reviewed the literature and made recommendations regarding evaluation and management. Manipulation is one of the approaches recommended for mechanical neck pain. Although the literature support is not as strong as for the low back, both studies recognize the potential value of manipulation in the management of some cervical spine complaints.

General Strategy

History

- Screen the patient for "red flags" that indicate the need for either immediate radiographs/special studies or referral to or consultation with a specialist, including severe trauma, direct head trauma with loss of consciousness, nuchal rigidity, bladder dysfunction associated with onset of neck pain, associated dysphasia, associated cranial nerve or central nervous system (CNS) signs/symptoms, onset of a "new" headache, and preexisting conditions such as rheumatoid arthritis, cancer, Down syndrome, alcoholism, drug abuse, or an immunocompromised state.
- If there is a history of trauma, determine the mechanism and severity.
- For patients involved in a motor vehicle accident (MVA), take a thorough history with regard to angle of collision; speed; use of brakes, seat belt, shoulder harness, and air bag; position of the patient in the car; subsequent legal concerns with regard to police reports; and so forth (**Exhibit 2–1**).

- Determine whether the complaint is one of pain, stiffness, weakness, or a combination of complaints.
- Determine whether the complaint is limited to the neck or is radiating to the head or upper extremity unilaterally or bilaterally.
- Determine the level of pain and functional capacity with a questionnaire such as the Neck Disability Index (**Exhibit 2–2**) with a pain scale (e.g., Visual Analog Scale [VAS]).

Examination

- For patients with nuchal rigidity and/or a positive Brudzinski's or Kernig's sign, refer for medical management.
- For patients with suspected fracture or dislocation (e.g., MVA, compressive or distractive injury to the neck), infection, or cancer, obtain radiographs of the cervical spine.
- For patients with neck pain only, perform a thorough examination of the neck, including inspection, observation of the patient's movements, palpation of soft and bony tissues, motion palpation of the spine, passive and active range of motion (using a goniometer or inclinometer), a functional assessment (e.g., according to Janda[8]), and a brief orthopaedic screening.
- For patients with neck and arm pain, add a thorough orthopaedic/neurologic examination, including compressive and neural stretch maneuvers to the neck in various positions, nerve stretch maneuvers, deep tendon reflex testing, sensation testing (include pain, temperature, light touch, and vibration), and myotome testing.
- Radiographs should be obtained for patients who have radicular findings, including an anteroposterior (AP), AP-open mouth, lateral, and oblique. Flexion-extension views may be added when searching for instability.
- Special imaging, including computed tomography (CT) or magnetic resonance (MR), should be reserved for the differential of radicular or myelopathic cases where there is a need for further distinction among stenosis, tumor, herniated disc, or multiple sclerosis. Electrodiagnostic studies should be reserved for cases where the cause of radicular complaints remains unclear.

Exhibit 2–1

Automotive Crash Form

Billing Information

Patient name:

Date of injury: _____ Time of injury: _____ ☐ AM ☐ PM

City and street where crash occurred: _____

What is the estimated damage to your vehicle? $ _____

☐ Yes ☐ No   Do you have automobile medical insurance coverage?_____

_____

Name/address/phone _____

_____

What is your car insurance medical coverage limit? $_____

What is the claim number? _____

☐ Yes ☐ No   Do you know the claims adjuster's name? _____

☐ Yes ☐ No   Have you reported this injury to your car insurance company? _____

☐ Yes ☐ No   Did the police come to the accident scene and make a report? _____

☐ Yes ☐ No   Is an attorney representing you? Name/address/phone: _____

Auto Accident Description

Describe how the crash happened _____

_____

_____

_____

_____

_____

_____

_____

_____

_____

Collision Description

Check all that apply to you:

☐ Single-car crash   ☐ Two-vehicle crash   ☐ More than thee vehicles
☐ Rear-end crash   ☐ Side crash   ☐ Rollover
☐ Head-on crash   ☐ Hit guardrail/tree   ☐ Ran off road

You were the

☐ Driver   ☐ Front passenger   ☐ Rear passenger

Describe the vehicle you were in

Model year and make: _____

☐ Subcompact car   ☐ Compact car   ☐ Mid-sized car
☐ Full-sized car   ☐ Pickup truck   ☐ Larger than 1-ton vehicle

Describe the other vehicle

☐ Subcompact car   ☐ Compact car   ☐ Mid-sized car
☐ Full-sized car   ☐ Pickup truck   ☐ Larger than 1-ton vehicle

Estimated crash speeds

Estimate how fast your vehicle was moving at time of crash.   _____ mph
Estimate how fast the other vehicle was moving at time of crash   _____ mph

(continues)

Exhibit 2–1 (continued)

At the time of impact your vehicle was
☐ Slowing down   ☐ Stopped   ☐ Gaining speed   ☐ Moving at steady speed

At the time of impact the other vehicle was
☐ Slowing down   ☐ Stopped   ☐ Gaining speed   ☐ Moving at steady speed

During and after the crash, your vehicle
☐ Kept going straight, not hitting anything   ☐ Spun around, not hitting anything
☐ Kept going straight, hitting car in front   ☐ Spun around, hitting car in front
☐ Was hit by another vehicle   ☐ Spun around, hitting object other than car

Describe yourself during the crash
Check only the areas that apply to you:
☐ You were unaware of the impending collision.
☐ You were aware of the impending crash and braced yourself.
☐ Your body, torso, and head were facing straight ahead.
☐ You had your head and/or torso turned at the time of collision:
     ☐ Turned to left   ☐ Turned to right
☐ You were intoxicated (alcohol) at the time of crash.
☐ You were wearing a seat belt.
     If yes, does your seat belt have a shoulder harness?   ☐ Yes   ☐ No
☐ You were holding onto the steering wheel at the time of impact.

Indicate if your body hit something or was hit by any of the following:
Please draw lines and match the left side to the right side.

Head	Windshield
Face	Steering wheel
Shoulder	Side door
Neck	Dashboard
Chest	Car frame
Hip	Another occupant
Knee	Seat
Foot	Seat belt

Check if any of the following vehicle parts broke, bent, or were damaged in your car
☐ Windshield   ☐ Seat frame   ☐ Knee bolster
☐ Steering wheel   ☐ Side/rear window   ☐ Other _____
☐ Dashboard   ☐ Mirror   ☐ Other _____

Rear-end collisions only
Answer this section only if you were hit from the rear.
Does your vehicle have
☐ Movable head restraints
☐ Fixed, nonmovable head restraints
☐ No head restraints

Please indicate how your head restraint was positioned at the time of crash.*
☐ At the top of the back of your head
☐ Midway height of the back of your head
☐ Lower height of the back of your head
☐ Located at the level of your neck
☐ Located at the level of your shoulder blades (upper back) below neck

*Estimate the distance between the back of your head and the front of the head restraints. _____ inches

Exhibit 2–1 (continued)

All types of collisions
Answer this section regardless of the type of crash, indicating those relevant to your case.

Yes   No

☐   ☐   Did any of the front or side structures, such as the side door, dashboard, or floor board of your car, dent inward during the crash?

☐   ☐   Did the side door touch your body during the crash?

☐   ☐   Were your hands on the steering wheel or dashboard during the crash?

☐   ☐   Did your body slide under the seat belt?

☐   ☐   Was a door of your vehicle damaged to the point where you could not open the door?

Emergency department

Yes   No

☐   ☐   Did you go to the emergency department after the accident?
        What is name of the emergency department? _____
        When did you go (date and time)? _____

☐   ☐   Did you go to the emergency department in an ambulance?

☐   ☐   Did you or another person drive you to the emergency department?

☐   ☐   Where you hospitalized overnight?

☐   ☐   Did the emergency department doctor take X-rays? Check what was taken:
        ☐ Skull
        ☐ Neck
        ☐ Low back
        ☐ Arm or leg

☐   ☐   Did the emergency department doctor give you pain medications?

☐   ☐   Did the emergency department doctor give you muscle relaxants?

☐   ☐   Did you have any cuts or lacerations?

☐   ☐   Did you require any stitching for cuts?

☐   ☐   Were you given a neck collar or back brace to wear?

When did you first notice any pain after injury?
☐ Immediately   ☐ ____ Hours after injury   ☐ ____ Days after injury

If you did not see a doctor for the first time within the first week, indicate why
Check all that apply
☐ No pain was noticed   ☐ No appointment schedule available
☐ No transportation   ☐ Work/home schedule conflicts

If you did not see a doctor for the first time within the first month after injury, indicate why
Check all that apply
☐ No pain was noticed   ☐ No appointment schedule available
☐ No transportation   ☐ Work/home schedule conflicts
☐ I thought pain would go away   ☐ I had no insurance or money
☐ I self-treated with over-the-counter drugs   ☐ I took hot showers, used ice, heat

Have you been unable to work since injury?
☐ Yes   ☐ No If yes, you were off work   ☐ partially or   ☐ completely
Please list date off work: _____ to _____.

Management

- Patients with clinical, radiographic, or laboratory evidence of tumor, infection, fracture, or dislocation should be sent for medical evaluation and possible management.
- Patients who appear to have a mechanical cause of pain should be managed conservatively for one month; if unresponsive, further testing or referral for a second opinion is suggested.

Relevant Anatomy and Biomechanics

The cervical spine is often discussed as two separate yet interdependent sections: the upper cervical spine (the occiput and C1-C2) and the lower cervical spine (C2-C7/T1). This is due in part to a functional distinction based on the great degree of rotation available at the upper cervical spine, allowed by the unique articulation between the C2 and C1 vertebrae. The dens of C2 acts as a pivotal point for rotation. The intricate musculature support and control in this region are important in substituting for a generally more lax ligamentous system, compared with the thoracic and lumbar regions. Another important difference in the upper cervical region is the lack of intervertebral foramina and discs between the occiput (C0), C1, and C2. From a neurologic perspective, the upper cervical spinal cord has a unique connection with the CNS through the trigeminocervical nucleus, an intermingling of the spinal nucleus of the trigeminal nerve and the dorsal horn of the upper cervical spinal nerves.[9] This connection allows for interactions and misinterpretations postulated to be the cause of headaches, dizziness, and facial pain.

The vertebral arteries enter the transverse foramen at C6 and ascend through the other transverse foramina. At C2 they take sharp turns to run more laterally and horizontally to reach the transverse foramen of C1. At the transverse foramen of C1 and C2, the vertebral arteries are anchored with fibrous tissue restricting their movement. Continuing upward, the vertebral arteries travel posteromedial to run around the lateral mass of C1. Running through a groove in the posterior arch of C1, the vertebral arteries pass between the atlantooccipital membrane and capsule before entering the dura mater at the foramen magnum. These two sites—C6 and the upper cervical region—are proposed to be tethering or

compressive sites leading to occlusion or intimal tearing resulting in vertebrobasilar events (vascular accidents) although studies that evaluate these effects in cadavers have not demonstrated this as likely with maneuvers that simulate cervical manipulation. Vertebrobasilar events are extremely rare and although they have been associated not only with cervical spine adjustments they also occur with common daily activities such as turning the head while driving and extending the head for a shampoo at the hairstylist as well.[10] When damage does occur it is usually due to trauma to the arterial wall leading to either vasospasm or intimal tearing. Intimal tears may occur in isolation or be complicated by embolic formation or dissection of the arterial wall.[11] The dorsolateral medullary syndrome (Wallenberg's) and the locked-in syndrome or cerebromedullospinal disconnection syndrome are two possible consequences of vertebrobasilar injury. Wallenberg's syndrome usually involves occlusion of the posterior inferior cerebellar artery with resulting problems of vertigo, diplopia, and dysarthria. Most patients regain a significant degree of neurologic function. The locked-in syndrome is much more serious, leaving the patient conscious but paralyzed.

The Discs

Like all intervertebral discs, the cervical disc is composed of a central nucleus pulposus and an outer annulus. However, by age 40 years the nucleus pulposus is essentially nonexistent, having changed to a ligamentous-like, dry material.[12] Herniation is therefore theoretically not possible in the older patient unless small hyaline pieces become free. The cervical discs have much less weight to bear than the lumbar discs for two reasons: (1) only the head plus gravity is borne and (2) the distribution of load is approximately equal among the disc and the two facet joints (i.e., each bears one-third the load). Like the other regions of the spine, the outer annulus fibrosus is innervated by the sinuvertebral nerves as are the vertebral bodies. **Exhibit 2–3** illustrates the innervations of deep spinal structures.

In a recent study[13] examining the discs of rats, researchers demonstrated that the C5/C6 disc was innervated multisegmentally from the dorsal root ganglions of C2-C8. In addition, there was innervation sympathetically from the stellate ganglion and parasympathetically from the nodose ganglion (vagus). Seventy-nine percent of the nerve fibers innervating the IVD were sensory nerves and 20.4% were autonomic nerves. Specifically,

Exhibit 2–2 Neck Disability Index

This questionnaire has been designed to give the doctor information as to how your neck pain has affected your ability to manage in everyday life. Please answer every section and mark in each section only the *one* box that applies to you. We realize you may consider that two of the statements in any one section relate to you, but please just mark the box that most closely describes your problem.

Section 1—Pain Intensity
☐ I have no pain at the moment.
☐ The pain is very mild at the moment.
☐ The pain is moderate at the moment.
☐ The pain is fairly severe at the moment.
☐ The pain is the worst imaginable at the moment.

Section 2—Pesonal Care (Washing, Dressing, etc.)
☐ I can look after myself normally without causing extra pain.
☐ I can look after myself normally but it causes extra pain.
☐ It is painful to look after myself and I am slow and careful.
☐ I need some help but manage most of my personal care.
☐ I do not get dressed, I wash with difficulty and stay in bed.

Section 3—Lifting
☐ I can lift heavy weights without extra pain.
☐ I can lift heavy weights but it gives extra pain.
☐ Pain prevents me from lifting heavy weights off the floor, but I can manage if they are conveniently positioned, for example, on a table.
☐ Pain prevents me from lifting heavy weights, but I can manage light to medium weights if they are conveniently positioned. I can lift very light weights.
☐ I cannot lift or carry anything at all.

Section 4—Reading
☐ I can read as much as I want to with no pain in my neck.
☐ I can read as much as I want to with slight pain in my neck.
☐ I can read as much as I want with moderate pain in my neck.
☐ I can't read as much as I want because of moderate pain in my neck.
☐ I can hardly read at all because of severe pain in my neck.
☐ I cannot read at all.

Section 5—Headaches
☐ I have no headaches at all.
☐ I have slight headaches that come infrequently.
☐ I have moderate headaches that come infrequently.
☐ I have moderate headaches that come frequently.
☐ I have severe headaches that come frequently.
☐ I have headaches almost all the time.

Section 6—Concentration
☐ I can concentrate fully when I want to with no difficulty.
☐ I can concentrate fully when I want to with slight difficulty.
☐ I have a fair degree of difficulty in concentrating when I want to.
☐ I have a lot of difficulty in concentrating when I want to.
☐ I have a great deal of difficulty in concentrating when I want to.
☐ I cannot concentrate at all.

Section 7—Work
☐ I can do as much work as I want to.
☐ I can only do my usual work, but no more.
☐ I can do most of my usual work, but no more.
☐ I cannot do my usual work.
☐ I can hardly do any work at all.
☐ I can't do any work at all.

Section 8—Driving
☐ I can drive my car without any neck pain.
☐ I can drive my car as long as I want with slight pain in my neck.
☐ I can drive my car as long as I want with moderate pain in my neck.
☐ I can't drive my car as long as I want because of moderate pain in my neck.
☐ I can hardly drive at all because of severe pain in my neck.
☐ I can't drive my car at all.

Section 9—Sleeping
☐ I have no trouble sleeping.
☐ My sleep is slightly disturbed (less than 1 hr. sleepless).
☐ My sleep is mildly disturbed (1–2 hrs. sleepless).
☐ My sleep is moderately disturbed (2–3 hrs. sleepless).
☐ My sleep is greatly disturbed (3–5 hrs. sleepless).
☐ My sleep is completely distubed (5–7 hrs. sleepless.)

Section 10—Recreation
☐ I am able to engage in all my recreation activities with no neck pain at all.
☐ I am able to engage in all my recreation activities with some pain in my neck.
☐ I am able to engage in most, but not all, of my usual recreation activities because of pain in my neck.
☐ I can hardly do any recreation activities because of pain in my neck.
☐ I can't do any recreation activities at all.

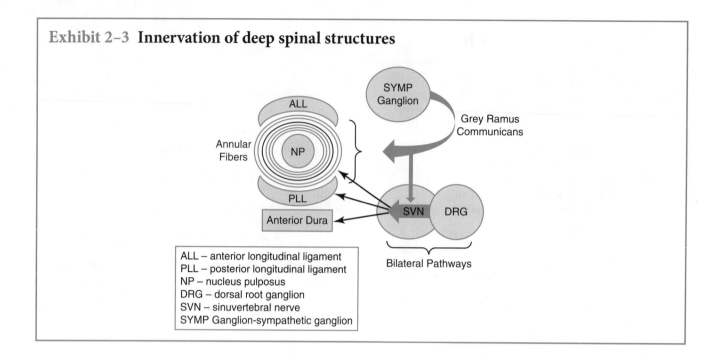

Exhibit 2–3 Innervation of deep spinal structures

ALL – anterior longitudinal ligament
PLL – posterior longitudinal ligament
NP – nucleus pulposus
DRG – dorsal root ganglion
SVN – sinuvertebral nerve
SYMP Ganglion-sympathetic ganglion

23.9% of the nerve fibers innervating the IVD were afferent sensory pain-related nerves, 8.9% were efferent sympathetic nerves, and 11.5% were efferent parasympathetic nerves. Given the varied and unusual clinical signs and symptoms related to cervical disc injury, this finding of autonomic innervation may partially explain why. Potentiating the effect and extent of sympathetically mediated pain is a structure named "Terminal Dogiel's nests," described as bundles of sprouting sympathetic axons in the dorsal root ganglia that seem to form after injury.[14]

The Facets

The facets of the upper cervical spine are angled approximately 35° to the horizontal plane, whereas the lower cervical spine facets are oriented at approximately a 65° angle.[15] The facets (zygapophyseal) joints are surrounded by a joint capsule that is generally looser in the cervical region than in the thoracic and lumbar regions, allowing for more range of motion. The capsule is lined with synovium on the upper and lower aspects. There are often inclusions of fat-filled synovial folds and meniscoids that extend between the facets. Although they are believed primarily to be shock absorbers, these inclusions can become trapped, causing a mechanical lock.[16, 17] It is unlikely, however, that they are the primary cause of vertebral fixation given that meniscoids are not always present in fixed joints and that patients with rheumatoid arthritis have a

higher incidence of meniscoids yet no higher incidence of fixation.[18] However, in children and in those who develop sudden neck pain without significant trauma that is relieved with manipulation, a synovial entrapment or extrapment (caught outside the joint) is likely the cause.

Histological studies of facet joints demonstrate the existence of substance P reactive fibers suggesting a potential role in mediating pain.[19] Facet-joint capsules contain low-threshold mechanoreceptors, mechanically sensitive nociceptors, and silent nociceptors. The speed at which mechanoreceptors are stimulated may affect their role in pain. Low stretch levels activate proprioceptors in the facet-joint capsule whereas sudden severe capsular stretch activates nociceptors, which may lead to prolonged discharge and damage to the capsule and to axons in the capsule.[20]

The facet joints are innervated by the medial branch of the posterior primary rami. Recent evidence from rat research[21] indicates that sensory nerve fibers of cervical C5-C6 facet joints are derived from the dorsal root ganglia (DRG) of multisegmental levels, from C3 to T3. This likely explains common referral patterns from the facets including neck and head pain from the C2-C3 joints and neck and shoulder pain from the C5-C6 joints. Also, this multisegmental innervation may determine more global neurological reactions to pain generated at a local segment.

The DRG themselves are at risk due to a peculiar vascular structure.[22] Primarily internal arterialization coupled with a superficial venous drainage places the DRG at risk for ischemic damage from external pressure (e.g., degenerative osteophytes) or from internal edematous pressure leading to a form of "compartment syndrome."

Although it might be assumed that all spinal levels have contributions to the DRG, a study by Tubbs et al.[23] indicates that at the C1 level there is substantial variation with potential clinical results. The researchers found that in all specimens there were C1 and C2 spinal nerves, but only 46.6% of specimens had C1 dorsal rootlets and of these, only 28.5% had an associated dorsal root ganglion. In 50% of specimens, the spinal accessory nerve joined with dorsal rootlets of C1. When the spinal accessory nerve combined with the dorsal rootlets of C1, there was no C1 DRG.

Calcitonin gene-related peptide (CGRP) immunoreactive dorsal root ganglion neurons innervate the cervical facets and are affected by trauma. One study[24] indicated that although the number of CGRP cells decreased after trauma, there was a phenotypical switch to larger cells.

Ligaments and Muscles

The upper cervical spine has an intricate system of ligaments and muscles to stabilize and control fine head movements. In addition, the muscles serve a function of providing important proprioceptive input integrated into the reflex control of the head and neck and posture in general. Studies have demonstrated that injections into the upper cervical spine area result in various symptoms, including vertigo.[25]

Three ligaments help stabilize the dens of C2 to the anterior arch of C1. These include the alar ligament, cruciform (cruciate) ligament, and tectorial membrane. These continue down as the posterior longitudinal ligament. A prominent section of the cruciate ligament is the transverse ligament. This ligament is the primary stabilizer of the dens. Deterioration of the transverse ligament, usually through rheumatoid processes, will allow abnormal movement between C2 and C1. The posterior longitudinal ligament (PLL) is broad in the cervical spine, providing more protection against lateral disc herniation than found in the lumbar region. Also, the joints of Luschka provide some bony protection to nerve root impingement from disc herniation. The ligamentum flavum is posterior to the PLL, attaching to the laminae forming the anterior support for the facet joint capsules and protecting the spinal cord. A recent study indicates

that contrary to accepted knowledge, the ligamentum flavum does not connect the posterior arch of the atlas to the laminae of the axis 15a. Bogduk[1] emphasizes that the interspinous ligament is nonexistent in the cervical region and that the sagittal and superficial component of the ligamentum nuchae are simply extensions of other structures.

The muscles of the cervical spine are often divided into posterior and anterior with subdivisions of superficial and deep sections. The more superficial muscles are involved with upper extremity movement and respiration. The deeper muscles are involved more with posture and head/neck movement. The posterior muscles, including the semispinalis, spinalis, and splenius, are essential as antigravity/postural muscles, often being called upon to fire eccentrically during flexion of the neck/head, and are chronically strained during forward head positions. The four suboccipital muscles (obliquus capitis inferior and superior and the rectus capitis posterior major and minor) plus the deep "shunt" muscles of the middle and lower cervical spine, such as the interspinales, multifidus, rotatores, intertransversarii, and longus cervicis, are important for intersegmental movement. In addition, they play a major role in providing afferent proprioceptive input to the spinal cord used both for gross postural control and spinal segmental (involuntary) positioning. This is due to the high density of muscle spindles in this region.[26]

Thoracic Outlet

The thoracic outlet is the path taken by the brachial plexus and associated vasculature into the arm from the neck. Thoracic outlet syndrome (TOS) is an over-diagnosed condition. It is purported to be caused by neurologic or neurovascular compromise of the brachial plexus and/or subclavian-axillary vessels. The potential sites of entrapment or compression include: at the cervical ribs (elongated C7 transverse processes), the scalene muscles, the costoclavicular interval, and the subcoracoid loop involving the pectoralis minor. When TOS is present it is most common to have involvement of the lower brachial plexus (C7-T1) with related medial arm and hand complaints. Factors that have been suggested as causes include trauma, posture (rounded shoulders), tight scalenes or pectoralis minor, and cervical ribs. Leffert[27] states, however, that patients who have had stabilizing surgery for the shoulder have had accompanying TOS symptoms resolved.

Biomechanics

The various motion patterns available to the cervical spine are determined by both active and passive elements. The passive elements include the facets, discs, ligaments, and bone. The various components of functional patterns that may be affected include range of motion (ROM), coupling patterns, the instantaneous axis of rotation (IAR), and the neutral zone. Many of the biomechanical studies have focused on how the various static components contribute to movement and ROM, and therefore must be considered cautiously when extrapolated to patients. Many of the manipulative maneuvers used by chiropractors and others, however, require elimination of muscular participation; therefore, the studies may have some clinical validity.

The cervical spine flexes, extends, rotates, and bends laterally. Flexion and extension occur mainly at three areas: (1) the atlantooccipital joint, (2) the C1-C2 level, and (3) between C4 and C6. Each accounts for about 20° of flexion/extension. The other segments contribute between 10° and 20°. Flexion at the atlantooccipital joint is accompanied by a coupled movement of slight anterior translation of the occiput relative to C1.

The facet orientation in the cervical spine allows for a large degree of motion. Approximately 50% to 60% of axial rotation occurs between C1 and C2.[28] It is in large part due to the pivot-shaped articulation between these segments. On the other hand, axial rotation is minimal (0° to 5°) at the atlantooccipital articulation. Lateral bending between segments increases from the upper to the lower cervical spine. In the upper cervical spine only about 5° is available; in the middle and lower cervical spine 5° to 10° is available. With lateral bending in the middle and lower cervical regions, the spinous processes rotate to the opposite side (i.e., left lateral bending causes the spinous processes to move to the right). This coupling occurs most at C2-C3 and decreases in the lower segments. With rotation, C2-C3 and segments above bend laterally in the opposite direction of rotation (i.e., right rotation causes left lateral bending). Below this level, however, the cervical spine generally bends to the same side as head rotation. Another coupled pattern with rotation is flexion and extension. Above the C4-C5 level, extension accompanies rotation; below this level, flexion occurs with rotation. These coupling patterns change with the beginning head position.[29] For example, if the head rotates while in full flexion, lateral flexion coupled with axial rotation decreases compared to neutral.

These coupled patterns may be important factors for planning positioning and force application with manipulative procedures.

Because acceleration/deceleration injury to the cervical spine is a common mechanism of injury in patients seeking chiropractic care, a brief overview of the biomechanics of whiplash is presented. There is considerable research to indicate a "typical" sequence of events following a rear-end collision. They are divided into phases by Croft:[30]

- *Phase One*—When a vehicle is rear-ended, the patient's torso is forced back into the seat and at the same time moves upward. This upward movement is accompanied by straightening of the cervical spine as it is being compressed axially. The head and neck then begin to extend.
- *Phase Two*—As the head and neck are extending, the vehicle has reached its peak acceleration. Energy stored in the seat from the backward movement of the body into the seat may add more acceleration to the torso as a "diving board" effect. The upward (vertical) movement of the torso may allow ramping over the headrest, adding an element of extension. If the driver's foot is taken off the brake, acceleration may be prolonged.
- *Phase Three*—Acceleration diminishes while the head and torso are thrown forward. It may be accentuated if the driver's foot is reapplied to the brakes.
- *Phase Four*—As the body moves forward, a seat belt and shoulder harness (if applicable) will restrain the torso, allowing the head to decelerate forward.

The older model of hyperextension/hyperflexion injury associated with a "whiplash" or rear-end collision is not always the case. In fact, in recent studies the global neck motion did not extend beyond the normal range of motion.[31] Although global hyperextension does not always occur, intersegmental hyperextension does appear to occur and may be the most prominent injury mechanism. Recent evidence suggests that low-speed rear-impact collisions (LOSRIC) result in a distinct s-shaped curvature with the lower cervical segments hyperextending and the upper cervical segments flexing.[32] As a result of the injury sequence, the instantaneous axis of rotation changes in the lower cervical segments placing more compressive forces on the facet joints and discs in a rapid manner (within 100 msec), particularly at C5-C6.

Evaluation

History

The first line of business is to attempt to rule out "serious" causes of neck or neck and arm pain. It is important to consider the possibility of meningitis when there is accompanying fever and a complaint of neck stiffness. Although neck stiffness may be a common complaint with the flu, the severity of pain and the response to passive flexion of the head are usually less remarkable. When neck pain is associated with a severe headache that is "new" or worse than any headache previously experienced, a red flag should be raised for infection, tumor, or vascular causes.

When patients have a complaint of neck and arm pain, clues to the cause may be evident from the history (**Table 2–1**). If the complaint is of a strip of pain connecting the neck or shoulder to the hand and this strip overlaps several dermatomes or in the hand is rather diffuse, nerve root compression is unlikely. Patients with this presentation often have a referred pain that is unrelated to nerve root compression. These patients rarely complain of weakness in the arm (or if they do it is usually not objectifiable). Patients with nerve root compression will have complaints not only of pain (often localized to a dermatome) but also of eventual motor weakness that can be objectified on the physical examination.

Traumatic/Overuse Injury

When there is direct trauma to the head or neck, it is important to gauge the degree of injury, the mechanism of injury, and whether there was loss of consciousness. There are some classic patterns of injury with respect to specific types of fractures (**Table 2–2**). When these mechanisms are evident from the history, radiographic evaluation can be more focused. In addition to the well-known Ottawa Knee and Ankle Rules, Canadian Cervical Spine Rules[33] have been developed in an attempt to determine who does or does not need radiographic examination following trauma to rule out fracture. Developed a number of years ago, these rules have stood the test of time and comparison to other approaches, and have proven very sensitive for detecting patients in need of radiographic evaluation following trauma.[34, 35] The rules are a set of questions:

- Are there any high-risk factors involved (i.e., age greater than or equal to 65 years, work with dangerous mechanisms, or paresthesias in extremities)? If the answer is yes, then x-rays are indicated.
- Are there any low-risk factors that allow safe assessment of range of motion (i.e., simple rear-end collision, sitting in emergency department or ambulatory since injury, delayed onset neck pain, or absence of midline cervical spine tenderness)? If not, x-rays are indicated. If so, move on to the next question.
- Is the patient able to actively rotate neck 45° right and left? X-rays are indicated if the answer is no.

These rules are intended only to detect those individuals who might have a cervical spine fracture.

Similarly the National Emergency X-Radiography Utilization Study (NEXUS)[36] rules state that, for patients with neck trauma no radiographs are needed if all of the following are true:

- No posterior or central cervical spine tenderness
- No evidence of intoxication
- A normal level of alertness
- No focal neurologic deficit
- No painful distracting injuries

If the patient was involved in an MVA, it is important to acquire detail such as type of vehicle, angle of collision, and damage to the vehicle(s) (see Exhibit 2–1). Information to be elicited from the patient includes his or her position in the car, whether a seat belt and shoulder harness were worn, whether an air bag was triggered, and whether the head or other body parts made contact with the windshield, steering wheel, or dashboard.

Lateral flexion injury to the neck is common in sports and MVAs. When a patient reports having his or her neck snapped to the side, compression injury on the side of head/neck movement and stretch injury on the side opposite are likely. When the brachial plexus is stretched, the upper section is most often involved. The patient will report a sudden onset of weakness in the arm, often with a burning or tingling pain down the outside of the arm to the hand. This type of injury is often referred to in sports as a "burner" or a "stinger." Most injuries are transient; however, some cases may need further evaluation with electrodiagnostic studies. When a lateral flexion injury is reported, it is a caution to the chiropractor not to take the head/neck into the position of injury when adjusting the neck.

When forced flexion is the mechanism, in addition to fractures of the vertebral bodies, myelopathy from a stenotic spinal canal must be considered when the patient has arm or leg complaints. If the patient

Table 2–1 History Questions for Cervical Spine Injuries

Primary Question	What Are you Thinking?	Secondary Questions	What Are You Thinking?
Were you involved in an accident?	Sprain/strain, subluxation, dislocation, fracture, disc lesion	Was your head forced forward?	Sprain/strain of posterior neck muscles/ligaments, fracture of vertebral body, facet dislocation, disc lesion
		Was your head forced back?	Sprain/strain of anterior neck muscles/ligaments, facet compression, hangman's or teardrop fracture at C2-C3
		Was your head turned and flexed?	Facet subluxation or dislocation, sprain/strain
		Was your head stretched to the side?	Brachial plexus stretch lesion, facet fracture, nerve root compression on side of head flexion
		Was your head turned and extended?	Facet compression, articular pillar fracture, sprain/strain
		Did you hit the top of your head?	Possible Jefferson fracture
Does the pain radiate to your arm(s)?	Disc lesion, nerve root entrapment, referred pain, myelopathy, brachial plexus damage, double crush	Is there isolated weakness or numbness?	Nerve root involvement
		Was there associated numbness/tingling or weakness that resolved over a few minutes?	Burner or stinger if involved with a lateral flexion injury
		Is there associated difficulty with walking or urinary dysfunction?	Myelopathy possible
		Is there more numbness and tingling in a diffuse or ill-defined pattern?	Referred pain from facet or trigger points
Are you unable to move your head in a specific direction?	"Torticollis," osteoarthritis, fracture/dislocation, meningitis	Did you simply wake up with this?	Acute "pseudotorticollis" due to global muscle spasm
		Is there associated fever? Is it worse with flexion?	Possible meningitis if flexion pain is severe
		Was there a gradual onset? (in an older patient)	Likely osteoarthritis
		Did this occur after head or neck trauma?	Consider fracture or dislocation
Do you have chronic pain or stiffness?	Osteoarthritis, postural syndrome, subluxation	Does work involve a forward head posture or lateral flexion while on the phone?	Postural syndrome
		Is there local pain with specific movement?	Subluxation

has accompanying complaints of urinary dysfunction, myelopathy must be suspected and investigated further via physical examination and radiographs.

Overuse injury is in most instances postural "injury." A line of questioning regarding occupational mechanical stresses is particularly important for patients with chronic neck pain. Questions should be asked regarding workstations (i.e., height of chair, desk, and computer monitor) and how the telephone is answered and for how long during a one-day period. For those patients whose

Table 2–2 Fractures of the Cervical Spine

Mechanism	Fracture	Best Radiographic View	Stable/Unstable?
Hyperflexion	Wedge fracture of vertebral body	AP and lateral views; loss of anterior body height	Generally stable; based on neurologic signs or potential risk
	Clay shoveler's [C6-T1 spinous process]	Lateral; may need swimmer's view	Generally stable; however, may require several weeks in a hard collar or in rare cases surgical excision
	Teardrop	Lateral view	Unstable; may be associated with anterior cord injury
	Burst fracture	Lateral view	Generally stable; however, requires close monitoring for neurologic compromise
	Bilateral facet dislocation	Lateral view demonstrates instability	Unstable
Flexion/rotation	Unilateral facet dislocation	Lateral view may demonstrate anterior body translation or a dysrelationship of the normal overlap of facets	May be unstable
Hyperextension	Extension teardrop fracture of anteroinferior body of C2	Lateral view	Relatively stable in flexion; unstable in extension
	Hangman's: bilateral pedicle fracture of C2	Lateral view	Highly unstable, requiring halo traction immobilization
Hyperextension/rotation	Articular pillar	Lateral view may show a double outline; AP may show a disruption of the smooth cortical line; oblique or pillar views may be necessary; if found, CT is suggested	Generally stable; however, swelling may produce some radicular signs
Hyperextension/lateral flexion	Facet fracture	Obliques	Usually neurologically stable; however, must be assessed for stability after healing
Compression	Jefferson burst fracture of C1	Visible on AP open mouth; on lateral view increase in retropharyngeal space	Highly unstable, requiring halo traction immobilization

Key: AP, anteroposterior; CT, computed tomography.

Reproduced with permission from S.M. Foreman, Long-Term Prognosis, in *Whiplash Injuries: The Cervical Acceleration/Deceleration Syndrome*, 2nd ed., S.M. Foreman and A.C. Croft, eds., ©1995, Lippincott Williams & Wilkins.

employment requires less sitting and more lifting, it is important to determine the degree of overhead lifting, which often requires a degree of hyperextension of the neck. Dentists, mechanics, plumbers, electricians, and others represent a unique population who often work in awkward positions. It is important to have the patient give a detailed explanation of common prolonged positions or any single position that causes pain. From this description, a relationship regarding which anatomic structures are stretched and which are compressed can be appreciated.

Stiffness/Restricted Motion

For many patients, the biggest concern is stiffness or restricted ROM; they complain that looking over the shoulder is not possible. In an acute setting, the patient often will present with an insidious onset that began upon waking. He or she will complain of difficulty moving the head in any direction with accompanying pain. Often this acute "torticollis" is not a torticollis at all, because all ranges are affected and the patient's head is held in neutral and not cocked to one side. Although there is no known cause, the global muscle-splinting effect makes this a painful but benign condition in the majority of cases.

Instability

Instability is a concern with trauma to the head or neck. The type of fracture often suggests the mechanism of injury (Table 2–2). Fracture should always be considered with compressive or distractive injury to the neck. Instability is always a concern with patients who have signs or symptoms or a previous diagnosis of rheumatoid arthritis, seronegative arthritides (i.e., ankylosis spondylitis, Reiter's syndrome, or psoriatic arthritis), or Down syndrome.

Examination

Inspection, palpation, and ROM testing are the clinical approach taken when neck pain or stiffness is the primary complaint. A recent study evaluated the intrarater and interrater reliability of visual assessment of cervical and lumbar lordosis (without the use of a measurement instrument).[37] This study included chiropractors, physical therapists, physiatrists, rheumatologists, and orthopaedic surgeons. Subjects were divided into those with back pain and those without. Raters were asked to rate photographs placed in a PowerPoint presentation. Lateral views of relaxed individuals' cervical and lumbar curves were rated as normal, increased, or decreased. Interestingly, there was no difference in rating between those with or without back pain. The intrarater reliability was statistically fair ($\kappa = 0.50$) and the interrater reliability was poor ($\kappa = 0.16$). When the

complaint involves radiation into the back or extremities, specific orthopaedic and neurologic tests are added. The primary intention of orthopaedic tests is to compress or stretch pain-producing structures such as facets and nerve roots. The standard battery of orthopaedic tests includes various forms of cervical compression, cervical distraction, shoulder depression, the brachial plexus stretch test, Soto-Hall test, and Lhermitte's test. Cervical compression also referred to as Spurling's test (**Figure 2–1**) is usually axially applied with the patient's head in neutral and then in all positions of lateral flexion, flexion, extension, and rotation. Local pain felt more on extension and/or rotation indicates facet involvement, while radiating pain down the arm indicates nerve root involvement. Cervical distraction is an attempt to reduce local or radiating complaints. If the maneuver is more painful, muscle splinting is likely. There are very few orthopaedic tests for the cervical spine. Most of these tests are provocative or relief tests for cervical radiculopathy. Recently, a study evaluating the sensitivity and specificity of Spurling's test determined that although not very sensitive, Spurling's test is a specific test for cervical radiculopathy.[38] Therefore, the test is not useful in screening, but is useful in confirming a cervical radiculopathy diagnosis. Shoulder depression can cause nerve root or brachial plexus stretching on the side opposite head deviation, or nerve root compression on the side of lateral flexion; however, there is no evidence for the value of this test. Shoulder depression, in fact, is imbedded in the upper limb tension test and does not need to be performed separately. Cervical distraction too is part of the upper limb tension group of testing maneuvers and will be discussed later (**Figure 2–2**). Soto-Hall and

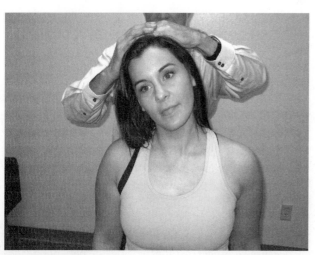

Figure 2–1 Spurling's test.

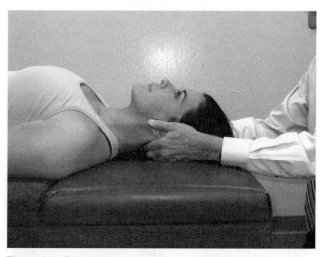

Figure 2–2 Distraction.

Lhermitte's tests involve passive flexion of the patient's neck. Electric shock sensations down the arm or arms is a positive Lhermitte's response and is occasionally found with multiple sclerosis or cervical myelopathy.

Vikari-Juntura and colleagues[39, 40] evaluated the interexaminer reliability and validity of some common clinical evaluation procedures for the cervical spine. Inspection of atrophy of small muscles of the hand, sensitivity tests for touch and pain, and the cervical compression and distraction tests were considered reliable. Muscle strength testing and an estimation of ROM were considered fairly reliable. Palpation for trigger points, the brachial plexus stretch test, and the shoulder abduction relief test (relief of arm pain when holding the arm above shoulder level), however, were considered poor. When 43 patients with known cervical disc disease were tested with cervical compression, distraction, and shoulder depression the specificity was high; however, the sensitivity was low (25% to 50%). Therefore, patients with cervical disc disease did not consistently have pain provoked or relieved by these maneuvers. When the test was positive, however, it was fairly specific to a disc lesion. Adding neurologic and radiographic information raised the sensitivity to between 40% and 64%. A recent study[41] suggests that the addition of cervical nonorganic signs to assess abnormal illness behavior may be helpful.

A more recent and high-level review by Wainner et al.[42] on the diagnostic accuracy of the clinical examination and patient self-report for cervical radiculopathy indicates that there may be some value in clusters of findings. The upper limb tension test (ULTT), sometimes referred to as the brachial plexus stretch test, was found to be a very good screening to rule out cervical radiculopathy. As with the lumbar spine examination, the neurological examination for dermatome, myotome, and deep-tendon reflex abnormalities is relatively specific but not sensitive (i.e., the patient may have nerve-root involvement and not have neurological evidence upon examination). The recommended cluster of test findings was:

- The ULTT
- Cervical rotation of less than 60°
- The distraction test (i.e., relief of radicular symptoms)
- Spurling's "A" test

Exhibit 2–4 provides a graphical example of how the likelihood of cervical radiculopathy is estimated using this approach. It was estimated that if three out of

these four tests were positive, the probability of having cervical radiculopathy increased to 65%. If all four were positive, the probability increased to 90%. (For a description of how to perform these tests see **Table 2–3** and **Figure 2–3**.) The authors caution the clinician in applying the cluster in practice. They indicate that the 95% confidence intervals (CI) for diagnostic accuracy for individual examination tests, and the test cluster, were wide due to the limited sample size and low prevalence of radiculopathy in their study. Another review by Rubinstein et al.[43] concurs with this caution stating that more high-quality studies are needed.

Nordin et al.[44] have made recommendations as the Task Force on Neck Pain and Its Associated Disorders committee addressing assessment. The committee came to similar conclusions in other studies. Specifically, they found that the interexaminer reliability was quite variable for muscle strength testing and sensitivity to touch. There was better reliability for increased versus decreased sensation. For radiculopathy, they concluded that a specific portion of the ULTT was highly sensitive and potentially specific. This position was a contralateral rotation of the head and extension of the arm and fingers. For nonemergency neck pain, the evidence does not support the diagnostic validity of provocation discography, anesthetic facet or medial branch blocks, surface electromyography, dermatomal somatosensory evoked responses, or quantitative sensory testing for radiculopathy. It is important to note that facet or medial branch blocks are also used as treatment, and this group did not address this use given that their focus was on diagnosis.

Other tests with acceptable diagnostic accuracy included cervical flexion less than 55°, a decrease in biceps reflex and muscle strength, the Valsalva test, a variation of Spurling's (test A), shoulder abduction weakness, C5 dermatome involvement, and two history questions: "Where are your symptoms most bothersome?" and "Do your symptoms improve with moving or positioning of your neck?"

The standard neurologic examination attempts to differentiate the cause of associated arm pain, numbness and tingling, or weakness. This process attempts to rule in or rule out nerve root compression, peripheral nerve entrapment, referred pain, brachial plexus injury, and spinal cord injury. This is accomplished by determining whether regions specific to a nerve root or peripheral nerve have sensory or motor deficits (see **Figure 2–4**). Larger, more diffuse patterns of sensory or motor loss require a search for brachial plexus or spinal cord involvement. Bilateral patterns suggest systemic polyneuropathies or spinal cord involvement.

It is important to note that weakness found on physical examination is actually more common than subjective weakness. Of patients with radiculopathy, 64% to 75% demonstrate weakness upon examination while only 15% to 34% complain of weakness. Deep tendon reflex involvement is found in 84% of patients with radiculopathy and dermatome sensory changes in only 33%.

The most commonly involved nerve root is C7 followed by C6. The standard muscle test for C7 is elbow extension. For C6, the standard muscle test used is wrist extension. A recent study[45] evaluated the value of adding forearm pronation to these muscle tests. Their results

Exhibit 2–4 Likelihood Patient Has a Cervical Radiculopathy

Approximating Probability: The likelihood ratios (LRs) in this graphical representation represent estimates of probability based on the aggregate of multiple reviews of each test finding. They are only approximations and only reliable indicators of a change in the context of a patient having an intermediate pre-test probability of between 20% to 80%. If the pre-test probability is very high or very low, the LR has little effect on changing the probability.

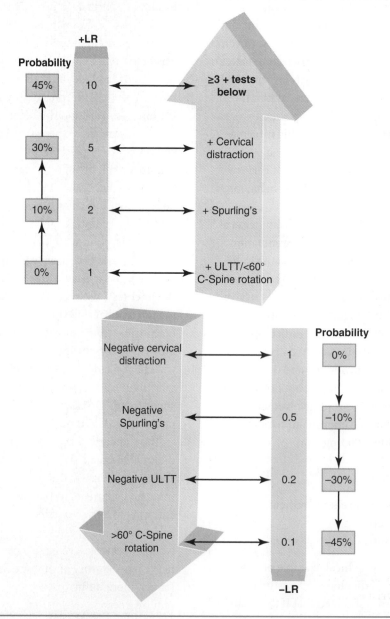

TABLE 2–3 Tests as Described and Performed in the Wainner et al.[1] Study

Name of Test	How to Perform	Positive Test Finding
Spurling's test A	With the patient seated, the neck is passively laterally bent toward the symptomatic side and the examiner applies over-pressure.	Symptom reproduction
Spurling's test B	With the patient seated, the neck is passively placed in a combination of laterally bending, coupled with rotation and extension toward the symptomatic side and the examiner applies over-pressure.	Symptom reproduction
Neck distraction	The patient is tested supine. The examiner's contact is under the chin and occiput. The patient's neck is then flexed to a position of comfort. Gradual distraction is then applied up to 14 kg.	Symptom decrease or elimination
Upper limb tension (Part A)	The patient is supine. The patient is positioned sequentially through six positions. The first five gradually increase stretch to the nerves and therefore may create a positive reproduction of arm symptoms. Scapular depression is followed by shoulder abduction (with scapular stabilization), then forearm supination coupled with wrist and finger extension. Next, shoulder external rotation, then elbow extension is added followed by contralateral cervical side-bending. The final position is movement of the head to ipsilateral cervical side-bending. This final position should provide relief of arm symptoms if positive.	In addition to reproduction of the patient's complaints with any of the first five maneuvers, or relief of symptoms with ipsilateral side-bending of the neck, side-to-side differences of >10° in elbow extension are also considered a positive.
Cervical rotation	The patient is seated and asked to perform two repetitions in each direction and then a single measure with a long-arm goniometer is performed.	Cervical rotation <60°
Cervical flexion	The patient is seated and asked to perform two repetitions. A single inclinometer is used to measure.	Cervical flexion <55°

1. Data from Wainner RS, Fritz JM, Irrgang JJ, Boninger ML, Delitto A, Alison S. Reliability and diagnostic accuracy of the clinical examination and patient self-report measures for cervical radiculopathy. *Spine*. 2003;28(1):52–62.

indicated that with C6 radiculopathies, forearm pronation was weak in 72% of patients, twice the number of patients demonstrating weak wrist extension. For C7, elbow extension and forearm pronation were weak in 23% of patients but in 10% of patients the only weakness found was in the forearm.

The basic approach to detecting nerve root involvement is a search for corresponding deficits in sensory, motor, and reflex function. Following is a basic pattern for spinal levels C5-T1 (patterns may vary depending on the source due to root overlap):

- C5—motor supply to the deltoid (shoulder abduction) and biceps (elbow flexion/supination), biceps reflex, and sensory supply to outer shoulder (axillary nerve)
- C6—motor supply to the biceps (elbow flexion/supination) and wrist extension, brachioradialis reflex, and sensory supply to the outer forearm

- C7—motor supply to the triceps (elbow extension), finger extensors and wrist flexors, triceps reflex, and sensory supply to the middle finger
- C8—motor supply to the finger flexors, no reflex, and sensory supply to the little and ring fingers
- T1—motor supply to the interosseous muscles of the hand (abduction/adduction of fingers), no reflex, and sensory supply to the medial arm

It is interesting to note though that in a study by Murphy et al.[46] patients with radiculopathy do not seem to indicate a dermatomal pattern to their radiating pain. Only 30.3% of patients with cervical radiculopathy reported a dermatomal pattern to their radiating pain (69.7% reported a nondermatomal pattern) with the exception of C4 where 60% of patients reported a dermatomal pattern. Given C4 is not often involved in radiculopathy, the majority of patients then describe a nondermatomal pattern.

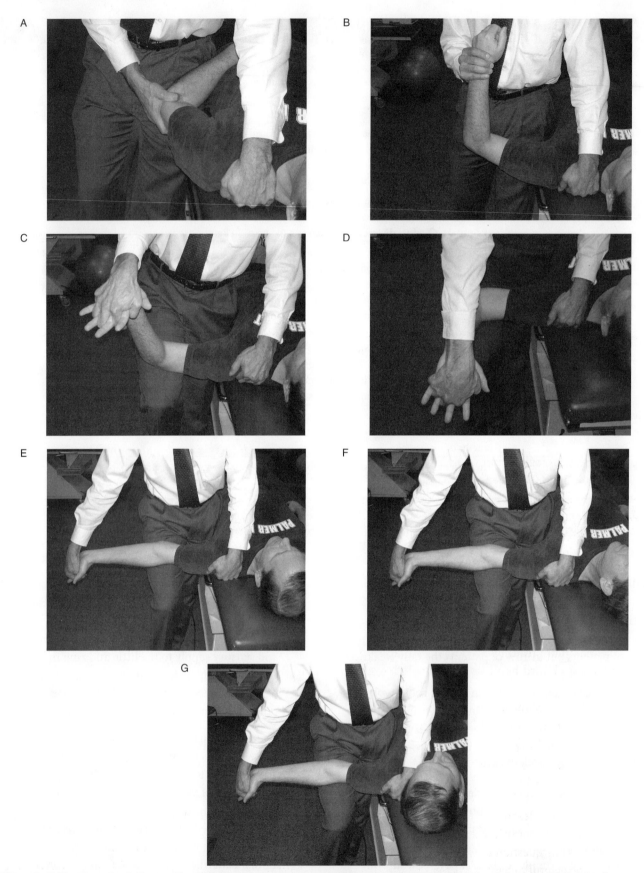

Figure 2–3 The Upper Limb Tension Test (ULTT): (A) Step 1—scapular depression; (B) Step 2—shoulder abduction; (C) Step 3—forearm supination, wrist and finger extension; (D) Step 4—shoulder external rotation; (E) Step 5—elbow extension; (F) Step 6—contra lateral cervical side-bending (lateral bending); (G) Step 7—ipsilateral cervical side-bending (lateral).

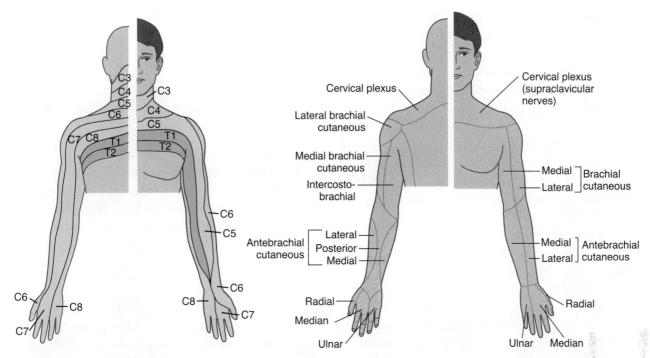

Figure 2–4 Neck complaints. Dermatomes of the upper extremity and the cutaneous innervation of the arm by the peripheral sensory nerves.

Part of the neurologic examination includes evaluation of grip strength. The most common device used is a Jamar dynamometer (Bissell Healthcare Corporation, Bolingbrook, Illinois). This device has been shown to be accurate, and the interrater reliability is high. There are, however, positional and postural effects on readings:[47]

- The wrist can be between 15° of palmar flexion and 30° of extension without an effect on strength; grip is stronger in supination, weaker in pronation; use neutral as the standard forearm position.
- The maximum readings are found with the second- and third-handle positions of a Jamar dynamometer.
- The first and second attempts are the strongest.
- Hand dominance may cause a 10% to 15% higher reading on that side.
- Test and retest reliability is best with the mean of three trials (attempts) (0.80).
- The patient should be tested in a seated position with the elbow flexed 90° at the patient's side.
- Patients test stronger in the standing position.
- If there is any question as to patient participation, it may be helpful to have the patient test with each handle position; a bell curve should appear even with neurologic weakness (i.e., strongest in the middle handle positions, weakest in the shortened and lengthened positions).

Common muscle imbalances at or affecting the cervical spine include tightness of the sternocleidomastoids (SCMs); short, deep neck extensors; upper trapezius; levator scapulae; and the pectoralis major and minor. Muscles that tend to be inhibited include the deep neck flexors and the lower stabilizers of the scapulae, including the lower and middle trapezius and the rhomboids. Taken together, these imbalances often lead to a rounded shoulder, forward head position. Functional testing as described by Janda[8] includes the spine-chin tuck test. The supine patient is instructed to tuck the chin in as much as possible and then raise the head 1 cm off the table. If the chin pokes or juts forward or if the head shifts up or down, Janda considers this an indication of substitution by the SCMs for the deep neck flexors.

TOS is often considered in the differential diagnosis of patients with arm complaints. Unfortunately, much of this testing is associated with a high level of false-positive and false-negative responses. These maneuvers are designed to compress the brachial plexus by specific structures in the hope of reproducing the patient's arm complaint. If a diminished pulse is used as a positive, however, a false-positive rate of 50% occurs.[48] Tests include Adson's, Halstead's, Wright's, and Roos' hyper-abduction test. Adson's and Halstead's tests attempt to isolate the anterior or middle scalenes, respectively, as compression sites. The patient's arm is passively abducted while the patient turns his or her head to one side and then the other. The examiner palpates the radial pulse for a decrease; however, a true positive is reproduction of the patient's arm complaints. Wright's hyperabduction test is similar; however, the arm is abducted and extended back. The Roos' test is a functional assessment. The patient is asked to hold the hand up above the head and repeatedly grip and release for 20 to 60 seconds in an attempt to reproduce the arm complaint(s).

Although numerous factors have been implicated as potential predispositions to vascular injury, none has been demonstrated to be significant for vertebrobasilar risk.[49] Analysis of the literature published before 1993 that reported vertebrobasilar artery dissection and occlusion leading to brainstem and cerebellar ischemia and infarction totaled 367 case reports.[51] Of these, 160 cases were of spontaneous onset with no association to manipulation, whereas 115 cases were of onset after spinal manipulation, 58 cases were associated with trivial trauma, and 37 cases were caused by major trauma. An analysis of possible causative head positions or specific manipulative procedures failed to identify any consistent pattern. In a review article by Haldeman et al., data from 64 cases of CVA associated with cervical spine manipulation did not reveal any inherent predictors in the history or physical examination that would assist in determining which patients are at risk.[52]

Routine radiography of the cervical spine is considered unnecessary unless it can potentially change the management of a case. Conditions that might warrant routine radiography include trauma, infection, gross instability, fracture/dislocation, and cancer. Another possible indication is radiating pain or numbness/tingling into the arm/hand. The decision is based on a thorough history and examination, however. Routine radiographs to evaluate degenerative changes are considered of limited value.[53] Radiographic examination of the cervical spine begins with a standard three-shot series including an AP, an AP open-mouth, and a lateral. Based on what is viewed on these basic films, a decision to complement the evaluation with oblique, flexion/extension, swimmer's, or pillar view can be made. Oblique views are valuable for visualizing the intervertebral foraminae (IVF) in search of foraminal encroachment due to osteophytes or dislocation. A bilateral or unilateral pillar view may be helpful when concerned about a possible hidden fracture

of the posterior elements.[54] The unilateral view is safest with the patient's head turned 45° and slightly flexed. There is a 30° to 35° caudad tube tilt based on the degree of cervical lordosis. When segmental instability is suspected, the lateral view will provide sufficient evidence for the middle and lower cervical spine. The criteria that are used include the following:

- fanning of adjacent spinouses
- a kyphotic angulation greater than 11°
- greater than 3 mm anterior displacement between the inferior posterior border of the superior vertebra and the superior posterior border of the adjacent inferior vertebra

Medical evaluation of instability may involve a radiographic traction stretch test.[55]

For the upper cervical spine, instability is often the result of rheumatoid or congenital disorders, although trauma is a possible cause. In patients with rheumatoid arthritis, the seronegative arthropathies, or Down syndrome, an evaluation of the atlantodental interspace is warranted. It is measured on a lateral view; most evident in flexion on a flexion/extension series. A measurement of the distance between the posterior margin of the anterior tubercle of C1 and the anterior surface of the odontoid is referred to as the atlantodental interspace (ADI), and it is an indirect measure of the integrity of the transverse ligament of the atlas. For adults the normal ADI measurement is between 1 and 3 mm; in children, it is between 1 and 5 mm.

Intersegmental hypermobility has been suggested as a biomechanical factor worth investigating; however, examiners have not been able to establish either the criteria or the ability to detect this entity.[56] The standard approach is to use flexion/extension lateral views to observe or to mark intersegmental movement not visible on a neutral lateral view.

A measure of the spaciousness of the spinal canal can be estimated on the lateral cervical view. The distance is measured with a line drawn from the posterior surface of the vertebral body extending to the same-level spinolaminar junction. The diameter varies based on the segmental level and the age of the patient (i.e., adults versus children); however, a canal less than 12 mm is considered stenotic. Another approach is to take the ratio of the sagittal diameter (same as above) to the vertebral body sagittal diameter. A ratio of less than 0.82 is considered evidence of stenosis (Pavlov or Torg ratio).[57]

With regard to TOS, many doctors will assume that the presence of cervical ribs is diagnostic. Yet less than

1% of the population have cervical ribs; of these individuals, less than 10% will have symptoms. Also, the more common cause of TOS is fibrous bands not visible on a radiograph.[58] Three spaces can be measured if a soft tissue mass is believed to be anterior to the cervical vertebrae: the retropharyngeal (at C2-C3), retrolaryngeal (at C4-C5), and retrotracheal (at C5-C7) spaces. Normal values on the neutral are 5 mm at C2, 7 mm at C3-C4, and 20 mm at C5-C7.[59]

When ordering special studies, it is always important to consider which imaging tool best evaluates what type of tissue. It also is extremely important to correlate clinical findings with special study findings due to the significant number of abnormal findings in asymptomatic patients. CT scans and MR imaging are valuable only when radiographs fail to determine the exact cause of a complaint of radiation of symptoms into the arms or back. Even then, it is probably worth a conservative trial prior to using these expensive tools. If stenosis is suspected, a CT scan is quite valuable. If disc herniation, multiple sclerosis, tumor, infection, or cancer is suspected, MR imaging is probably more valuable in most cases.

Electrodiagnostic studies occasionally are needed in the differentiation of neck and arm pain. Electromyography (EMG) and nerve conduction velocity (NCV) tests are valuable in differentiating nerve root compression from peripheral neuropathies. Somatosensory-evoked potentials (SEPs) and dermatomal somatosensory-evoked potentials (DSEPs) may be helpful in evaluating the patient suspected of having cervical myelopathy and determining the degree of involvement.

Management

The Neck Pain Task Force (Guzman et al.[60]) recommends a triage approach. They have devised four grades with associated recommendations:

- Grade I—Neck pain with no signs of serious pathology and little or no difference with daily activities. No further work-up is necessary; reassurance and self-care should be emphasized.
- Grade II—Neck pain with no signs of serious pathology but interference with daily activities. Assess factors and advise about methods that may help decrease interference in daily activities; discuss options for short-term relief.
- Grade III—Neck pain with neurologic signs of nerve compression. Monitor if deficits are stable

and minor; consider MRI and referral if deficits are major or progress; an EMG might be needed.
- Grade IV—Neck pain with signs of major structural pathology. Investigate according to the suspected condition.

Recommendations regarding options for short-term relief include exercise training and mobilization for those with neck pain after a traffic collision. For those with no trauma the task force recommends exercise training, manipulation, mobilization, acupuncture, analgesics, and low-level laser treatment. **Table 2–4** is a summary of all of the conclusions and recommendations of The Bone and Joint Decade 2000–2010 Task Force on Neck Pain and Its Associated Disorders.

The Mercy Guidelines[61] and other sources suggest that approximately six weeks of care is usually all that is needed in most "uncomplicated" cases. Initial high-frequency treatment ranging from three to five treatments for one to two weeks is considered appropriate. Treatment past this point is gradually decreased if the patient is responding; if not, a second two-week trial using a different form of treatment is suggested. If unsuccessful, then special studies or referrals for medical consultation are suggested. It is suggested that a questionnaire such as the Neck Disability Index (Exhibit 2–2) be used as a baseline measurement of patient status. This tool has been demonstrated to be a reliable indicator of the patient's functional improvement.[62]

The Bone and Joint Decade 2000–2010 Task Force on Neck Pain and Its Associated Disorders (Haldeman et al.[63]) provides a list of modifiable risk and protective factors, which include smoking, exposure to environmental tobacco, and participation in physical activity. Although they found insufficient evidence of the effectiveness of workplace interventions, they did find that high quantitative work demand, low social support at work, repetitive work, precision work, and sedentary work position all increased the risk of neck pain. Poor prognosis was associated with:

- poor health
- prior neck pain episodes
- poor psychological health
- worrying
- becoming angry or frustrated in response to neck pain

Indicators of a good prognosis included a coping style that involved self-assurance, optimism, and less need to socialize. Recovery appeared to be unrelated to a

Table 2–4 Conclusions and Recommendations from the Task Force on Neck Pain and Its Associated Disorders

Intervention	Recommendations
Nonsurgical Intervention[1] Whiplash-Associated Disorders	
Education or advice	• Evidence that an educational pamphlet was not associated with recovery in patients with acute WAD.
	• Some evidence that an educational video in combination with usual urgent or emergency care is associated with lower pain ratings at six months with acute WAD compared to usual care alone.
Exercise	• Some evidence that using an exercise component was positively associated with more favorable results in short- and long-term outcomes with acute or subacute WAD when compared to passive interventions including education.
	• Supervised and home exercise have marginal effects over advice but not in the long term.
Medications	• Cervical facet injections were not associated with greater pain reduction at three months.
	• Infusion of methylprednisolone was not associated with greater pain relief in the short term for acute WAD.
Manual therapies	• Mobilization was associated with greater pain relief in the short term for acute WAD as compared to passive modalities or general advice.
	• No advantage for a rigid collar for two weeks and mobilization over usual care at 12 months follow-up.
Physical modalities	• No advantage for passive modalities (TENS, ultrasound, diathermy) alone or in combination with mobilization in the short term compared to exercise and manual therapy for acute or subacute WAD.
Collars	• No advantage for soft or rigid collars compared to other approaches for acute WAD.
Combined approaches	• Evidence that multidisciplinary management was associated with quicker claim closure for WAD compared to usual care.
	• Evidence that fitness training or in- or outpatient rehabilitation plus usual care may increase recovery time for acute WAD.
"Nonspecific" Neck Pain	
Education or advice	• No evidence of advantage in education or advice over other interventions.
Exercise	• Evidence that a neck exercise program alone or in combination with spinal manipulation decreases pain and disability in the short term when compared to manipulation alone, TENS, or usual GP care.
	• Evidence that manual therapy or pulsed diathermy with neck exercise and coping advice were not associated with improvement compared to exercise and advice alone.
	• Compared to endurance exercise, strengthening exercise was not associated with a better outcome in the short and long term with female workers.
Medications	• No advantage to botulinum toxin A.
	• No advantage of piroxicam over indomethacin in the short term.
	• Some evidence that orphenadrine and paracetamol are associated with greater pain relief in the short term.
	• Some evidence that manipulation with advice and salicylates is more effective in the short term compared to salicylates with advice, massage electrical stimulation, or traction.

Table 2–4 Conclusions and Recommendations from the Task Force on Neck Pain and Its Associated Disorders (continued)

Intervention	Recommendations
Manual therapies	• Evidence that cervical spine manipulation along or with advice and home exercise was not associated with either pain or disability outcomes in the short or long term compared to mobilization with or without exercise, strengthening exercise, or instrumental manipulation. • Mobilization or exercise alone or in combination with medications was associated with better pain and functional outcomes in the short term compared with usual CP care, pain medication, or advice to stay active. • Evidence that manipulation or mobilization was not associated with better pain or disability outcome for subacute or chronic neck pain as compared to exercise alone or to exercise with massage or passive modalities.
Physical modalities	• Consistent evidence that passive modalities alone or in combination with other passive treatments or modalities have no advantage in the short or long term compared to usual CP, other modalities, or sham interventions. • Percutaneous neuromodulation therapy was associated with better intermediate post-treatment measure of pain, improved sleep, and more physical activity after three weeks with cervical disc disease causing chronic pain.
Acupuncture	• Inconsistent evidence of effectiveness. • Some evidence that acupuncture was better in the short term when compared to massage in the short term for patients with chronic pain. • Evidence that acupuncture was not better than mobilization or traction in the short term.
Laser therapy and magnetic therapy	• Evidence that low-level laser therapy was associated with improvements in pain and function in the short term for patients with subacute or chronic neck or shoulder pain. • Evidence that magnetic stimulation had better pain and disability outcome in the short term for myofascial pain compared to TENS or placebo.
Combined approaches	• Combinations of exercise, manual therapy, and advice were positively associated with decreased pain and disability and decreased time for sick leave compared to usual PCP care, surgery, cervical collar, or advice to stay active.
Workplace or employee interventions	• Evidence that any of the following were not associated with better outcomes: ergonomic interventions, relaxation or behavioral support, software-simulated work breaks which included rest or exercise, and physical training and stress management programs. • Evidence that endurance or strength training in combination with dynamic exercise involving the upper and lower extremities was associated with better one-year pain and disability outcomes in female office workers with chronic or recurrent neck pain compared to advice to perform exercises.
Invasive Interventions[2]	
Cervical injections for neck pain and radiculopathy	• There is evidence that treatment using a short course of epidural or selective root injections with corticosteroids gives short-term relief for radicular symptoms in patients involved in litigation. No evidence that multiple injections offer a benefit beyond one to three injections. • No evidence that cervical root or epidural injections in seriously symptomatic individuals reduce the need for surgery.

(continues)

Table 2–4 Conclusions and Recommendations from the Task Force on Neck Pain and Its Associated Disorders (continued)

Intervention	Recommendations
Cervical injection or radiofrequency neurotomy for neck pain without radiculopathy	• Evidence that intra-articular steroid injection is not effective for facet joint pain as compared to other anesthetic blockage protocols. • No evidence to support the use of radiofrequency neurotomy for facet pain.
Open surgical treatment of cervical radiculopathy	• No evidence for long-term benefit of surgery for radiculopathy; however, evidence for substantial short-term decrease of pain and impairment. • Evidence that anterior plating in one- and two-level fusions reduces kyphosis progression after surgery. • No evidence that complex approaches (fusion, case, plates, or fusion augmentation with bone) have an advantage over cervical decompression alone.
Open surgical treatment for neck pain without radiculopathy	• No support for the use of anterior cervical fusion or cervical disc arthroplasty for neck pain without radiculopathy. • No evidence to support surgical intervention for suspected upper cervical ligamentous injury following whiplash as determined by spinal change within these ligaments on MRI.
Complications with surgery	• With cervical foraminal or epidural injections—minor adverse effects in 15% to 20% of patients; serious events in < 1%. • Cervical open surgical procedures—serious complications in 4% of patients (higher in older patients and those with surgery for myelopathy); minor complications such as dysphagia, hoarseness, and donor site pain are frequently reported but resolved in most cases.

WAD = whiplash-associated disorder.
Data from: 1. Hurwitz EL, Carragee EJ, van der Velde G, et al. Treatment of neck pain: noninvasive interventions: results of the Bone and Joint Decade 2000–2010 Task Force on Neck Pain and Its Associated Disorders. *Spine.* 2008;33(4 Suppl):S123–152; 2. Carragee EJ, Hurwitz EL, Cheng I, et al. Treatment of neck pain: injections and surgical interventions: results of the Bone and Joint Decade 2000–2010 Task Force on Neck Pain and Its Associated Disorders. *Spine.* 2008;33(4 Suppl):S153–169.

specific workplace or physical work demands with those patients who included general exercise or sports as part of their lifestyle.

Following are a list of some of the side effects or complications with various treatment approaches (Guzman et al.[63]):

• Anti-inflammatory medication—dyspepsia (heartburn), GI bleeding in up to 2% of individuals with chronic use, heart attacks, hypertension
• Muscle relaxants or narcotics—drowsiness in one out of three individuals
• Exercise—transitory increases in pain
• Manipulation or manual medicine—transitory increase in pain in up to 30% of individuals; less common with mobilization

• Injections—transient increases in pain, numbness, and dizziness in up to 16% of individuals; major complications in less than 1%
• Surgery—transitory hoarseness and difficulty swallowing, rarely permanent hoarseness, nerve or spinal cord injury, or stroke

The recent Thiel et al.[64] prospective national survey involved more than 28,000 treatment consultations and over 50,000 cervical spine manipulations. There were no serious adverse events reported. Minor side effects with possible neurologic involvement were most common, with the highest risk occurring immediately after treatment for fainting, dizziness, or light-headedness (approximately 16 per 1,000 treatment consultations). For up to seven days post-treatment, the risks were headache (at most approximately 4 per 100), numbness or tingling in the upper limbs (approximately 15 per 1,000), and fainting, dizziness, or light-headedness (approximately 13 per 1,000).

Rubinstein et al.,[65] in a prospective, multicenter, cohort study, have also demonstrated that although adverse effects are relatively common (56%), they are short-lived and rarely severe in intensity (13%). Patients were initially treated three times. Symptoms such as tiredness, dizziness, nausea, or ringing in the ears were uncommon (less than 8%). At 12 months, 1% of patients reported being worse. Of patients who returned for a fourth visit, about 50% reported recovery.

Ernst[66, 67] is commonly critical of cervical manipulation and its associated risk (as evident in several publications). Bronfort et al.[68] clearly point out the methodological flaws in Ernst's arguments.

The strongest study to date by Cassidy et al.[69] evaluated vertebrobasilar (VBA) stroke and chiropractic care. This very large population-based, case-control, and case-crossover study evaluated over 100 million person-years and found there were 818 VBA stroke patients who were hospitalized. Individuals younger than 45 years were three times more likely to see a chiropractor or a primary care practitioner (PCP) before their stroke as compared to controls. There was no increased association between VBA stroke and chiropractic visits in those older than 45 years. However, there was an association between VBA stroke and patients of all ages visiting a PCP prior to stroke. Those billed for headache or neck complaints were highly associated with subsequent VBA stroke. The conclusions that are drawn are:

- A VBA stroke is extremely rare.
- Given there is at least an equal association between chiropractic visits and PCP visits and stroke, it is unlikely that there is something unique to the chiropractic treatment that would contribute as a cause of the stroke.
- Given that patients who subsequently had a stroke had complaints of headache and/or neck complaints, it is likely that dissection (intimal tearing) was occurring at the time of presentation and not due to an intervention in the PCP's or chiropractor's office.

Another revealing report by Boyle et al.[70] reviewed the statistics for VBA stroke in Saskatchewan (over eleven years) and Ontario (over nine years) covering more than 100,000 person-years in each province. It appears that the incidence for VBA in Saskatchewan was 0.855 per 100,000 person-years and 0.750 per 100,000 person-years in Ontario. The study revealed that there was an increase of 300% of cases in Saskatchewan in 2000 and only a 38% increase in Ontario in the same year. Correspondingly, there was only a small increase in chiropractic utilization in Saskatchewan and an actual decrease in chiropractic utilization in Ontario during this year. This data would seem to suggest that there is no association between the increase in VBA stroke and chiropractic utilization.

Finally, a number of basic science investigations into the effect on vertebral artery blood flow by manipulation or positioning for manipulation have been conducted on cadavers and live participants. A 2014 publication[71] confirmed what other studies have found. In this study using phase-contrast magnetic resonance imaging on asymptomatic volunteers, physiologic measures of VA blood flow and velocity at the C1-C2 spinal level were obtained after three different head positions and a chiropractic upper cervical spinal manipulation. There were no significant changes in blood flow or velocity in the vertebral arteries with any positions or with manipulation.

Prior to the use of manipulation for the cervical spine, it has often been suggested that the patient be informed of the very rare yet potential risk of a vertebrobasilar accident. As mentioned earlier, there is no sensitive or reliable screening test, and it is not enough to rely on a past history of uncomplicated manipulation treatment.[49] It must be accepted that the risk is small but real, and there is no known clinical test to identify those who will have an accident. The patient should be informed of this rare complication, given the potential for neurologic compromise.

Postural advice regarding work and everyday posture is considered an important adjunct by many chiropractors. The focus should be to maintain a neutral head position. This often involves a focus on stretching of the short spinal extensors with strengthening of the deep neck flexors. Supportive to this attempt is correction of the factors contributing to a hyperlordotic lumbar spine or hyperkyphotic thoracic spine when possible. Exercises should include stretching of the upper trapezius/levator scapulae, pectorals, lumbar extensors, and hip flexors, followed by strengthening of the middle/lower trapezius, abdominals, and gluteals. Ergonomically, workstations should be oriented to provide a straight-ahead view of a computer screen, shoulder support or a headpiece for long-term telephone usage, and arm supports on the chair.

The sequence of prescribed exercises usually begins with mild isometrics, progressing to a more functional approach. Minimal contractions into all six movement patterns of flexion, extension, lateral bending, and rotation are initiated as soon as pain restriction permits.

Mechanical Traction

Although traction is often utilized for neck pain, there are few studies to substantiate effect. One study[50] in 2009 attempted to predict improvement with mechanical traction for mechanical neck pain by evaluating the effect of several variables. A clinical prediction rule utilizing five variables was created based on patient response which included: (1) patient reported peripheralization with lower cervical spine (C4-7) mobility testing; (2) positive shoulder abduction test; (3) age > or =55; (4) positive upper limb tension test A; and (5) positive neck distraction test. The prediction for success with mechanical traction when three out of five predictors were present resulted in a +LR equal to 4.81 (95% CI = 2.17-11.4). This increased the likelihood of success with cervical traction from 44% to 79.2%. But dramatically increasing the effect was if four out of five variables were present. Then the LR was equal to 23.1 (2.5-227.9), increasing the post-test probability of having improvement with cervical traction to 94.8%. The protocol for application included:

- Intermittent traction was applied to a supine patient with 24° flexion.
- If full flexion was not possible, the angle was reduced to 15°.
- The application was one minute on; 20 seconds off. During the off-phase, 50% of the traction pull was maintained.
- Starting pull was 10–12 pounds and was increased in an attempt to reduce symptoms.
- Traction time was 15 minutes.
- There were a total of six sessions at two to three per week for three weeks.

Exercise

Most systematic reviews (including Cochrane) have concluded that exercise is an integral part of management for neck pain patients.[72-74] There is strong evidence for the incorporation of deep neck flexor strengthening either alone or in combination with mobilization or manipulation. There are several approaches to strengthening the neck flexors, yet it appears that the most commonly used are generally equal in effect.[75] The most common approaches are:

- Instruct the supine patient to lift the head and tuck the chin while maintaining the craniocervical area in neutral for a goal of three sets of 12 repetitions. The patient initially uses head weight against gravity. If unable to perform the 12 repetitions, the table is tilted to reduce the effect of gravity until the patient reaches the 12 repetitions goal. After three sets of 12 repetitions is reached, 0.5 kg are added with the goal of 12 repetitions always as the target. Eventually, over a four-week program, the goal is three sets of 20 repetitions.
- Using a pressure biofeedback device, patients are instructed to focus on the craniocervical junction to deemphasize the superficial neck flexors. The patient's head rests on a pressure-sensitive device to a level of 22–30 mm/hg and holds for 10 seconds. The goal is 10 repetitions with small rest periods in between.

An interesting study by Chiu et al.[76] randomized patients with chronic neck pain into either an infrared irradiation and neck care advice group, or a group that added an active exercise program that strengthened deep neck flexors for six weeks. There was a benefit at six weeks for those in the active exercise group; however, this appears to be lost at six-month follow-up when compared to the infrared irradiation plus neck care advice only group.

Two studies published in 2012 compared manipulation with exercise. The first study by Evans et al.[77] compared three groups: (1) supervised exercise with manipulation, (2) supervised exercise alone, and (3) home exercise. Both supervised exercise groups demonstrated similar success; better than the home exercise group. The second study by Bronfort et al.[78] was designed to compare manipulation, medication, and home exercise as a treatment approach for acute, and subacute neck pain. This randomized controlled trial compared these groups for benefit at three, six, and twelve months. There was no real difference between the manipulation and home exercise groups, although there was a significant advantage for manipulation compared with medication, especially at the one-year follow-up.

Fitz-Ritson[79] suggests exercises that are based on reflex mechanisms similar to the work of Feldenkrais and Alexander. His study indicated a marked improvement in pain and in disability index rating compared with a group using standard (stretching/isometric/isokinetic) exercises. This approach is based on influencing the vestibulo-ocular reflex (VOR), which involves a quick (phasic) coordination of the eye, head, and neck through integration and processing of vestibular, visual, and proprioceptive input.

Manipulation

The effectiveness of chiropractic manipulation for chronic neck pain is supported in the recent literature;[80-84] however, more randomized trials must be performed. In the study by Giles and Muller,[80] a comparison of manipulation to acupuncture and a nonsteroidal anti-inflammatory drug indicated a significant improvement in pain and disability for the manipulated patients as compared with patients undergoing other treatment approaches. Hurwitz et al.[83] published a study as part of the clinical outcomes section of the UCLA Neck-Pain study. The researchers randomized patients with neck pain who were part of a health maintenance organization (HMO) into manipulation with or without heat, manipulation with or without electrical muscle stimulation, mobilization with or without heat, and mobilization with or without electrical muscle stimulation. Cervical spine manipulation and mobilization provided similar clinical outcomes with neither demonstrating an advantage at six months. Giles and Muller[84] conducted a randomized clinical trial on patients with chronic spinal pain presenting to a sports clinic in Australia. They compared treatment results using data from patients randomized to medication, acupuncture, or spinal manipulation. The results indicate greater short-term improvement with manipulation. The largest number of patients who were asymptomatic the earliest were those who were treated with manipulation (27.3%), followed next by acupuncture (9.4%), and then medication (5%). A systematic review[85] published in 2014 concluded that after review of 51 randomized controlled trials, manipulation or mobilization and exercise in combination were effective for management of adults with chronic neck pain.

The management of cervical disc herniation is controversial. An interesting study by Croft[86] demonstrated a "standard" of adjusting (manipulating) patients with known cervical disc herniation among the doctors polled. This finding is interesting given that chiropractors can be accused of causing disc herniation. The majority of chiropractors, however, would not adjust the affected level. There are published case studies[82-88] indicating that chiropractic management of cervical disc herniation may be successful.

Although controversial, manipulation under anesthesia (MUA) for chronic spinal pain has some published support. An early study by West et al.[89] for cervical spine pain indicated good results. Almost all patients were back to work after six months and use of medication dropped significantly. Since then, there have been no large studies using a control group.

Whiplash

A recent report by the Task Force on Neck Pain and Its Associated Disorders (Carroll et al.[90]) noted that approximately 50% of those with whiplash associated disorder (WAD) report neck pain symptoms one year following the initial injury. Some predictors for prolonged recovery appear to be more symptoms, greater initial pain, and greater initial disability. Also prognostic for prolonged recovery were depressed mood, fear of movement, and a passive coping style. Interestingly, factors related to the actual collision such as direction, position, headrest type, and so on, were not found to be prognostic. It is proposed, though, that the number of WAD patients has been decreased by a seat design that has been changed over the last decade. Softer seats that absorb the body's backward movement prevent some ramping, while also bringing the head/neck to the head restraint sooner.

In a study by Cassidy et al.[91] patients who were involved in a whiplash injury were divided into four groups determined by their follow-up care:

1. Fitness training at a health club
2. Outpatient rehabilitation
3. Inpatient rehabilitation
4. Standard care

Those receiving fitness training or outpatient rehabilitation had slower recovery times than patients in the other two groups. Patients in the inpatient rehabilitation group did not differ in outcome as compared to those assigned to standard care. Another study by Cassidy et al. reflects a similar finding when a patient is returned to work too quickly following a WAD.

For massage, a systematic review published in 2007 by Ezzo et al.[92] concluded that no recommendations could be made based on the existing literature regarding the contribution, type, frequency, multimodal application, or effect on patients with mechanical neck disorders. They recommend better research designed to determine the role of massage therapy.

There have been some small studies[93, 94] with patients suffering from myofascial chronic neck pain that suggest that low-level laser treatment (830 nm or 904 nm) may be effective alone or in combination with other treatment as compared to a sham laser treatment. Although a 2009 review[95] in Lancet concluded that LLLT reduces pain immediately after treatment for acute neck pain and for patients with chronic pain up to 32 weeks after treatment with LLLT, there were limitations to the strength of these conclusions. Three of the studies quoted and utilized in the review that had the largest reported mean differences in favor of LLLT had limitations or errors.

- Two studies had significant baseline differences in favor of the active treatment
- A typing error indicated a significant mean difference when in the original study, there was no significant difference
- Pooling of data for nonspecific neck pain, myofascial pain syndrome, and cervical osteoarthritis may be inappropriate because each may represent a different set of patient types and clinical responses

A more recent study[96] published in 2011 was a small RCT that compared patients randomized to CMT, CMT with LLLT, or a group with both therapies combined concluded that the combination therapy demonstrated better results. However, this was a small group and the effect differences were minimal. More studies need to be conducted with a larger group of participants.

The Quebec Task Force on Whiplash-Associated Disorders[5] concluded that there is little or no evidence for the efficacy of soft cervical collars, corticosteroid injections of the facet joints, pulsed electromagnetic treatment, magnetic necklace, and subcutaneous sterile water injection. Use of soft collars beyond the initial 72 hours postinjury will probably prolong disability. The task force also found that the literature did not support the use of cervical pillows, postural alignment training, acupuncture, spray and stretch, heat, ice, massage,

muscle relaxation techniques, epidural or intrathecal injections, psychological interventions, ultrasound, laser, or short-wave diathermy. It is important to note that lack of literature support often means that no significant research has been performed to evaluate efficacy, even though many of these approaches are commonly used. In other words, it does not mean that they are ineffective; more often they are simply untested. Often this is due to the complacent attitude of, "if it works, why question it?"

The contribution of zygapophyseal joint pain to chronic neck pain following whiplash injury was evaluated in a study by Barnsley et al.[97] Fifty consecutive patients with chronic neck pain following whiplash were studied using a double-blind controlled approach incorporating local anesthetic blocks of cervical zygapophyseal joints. Joint blockade injections provided relief to 54% of patients.

In addition to pain, it appears that other reflex abnormalities may occur and persist as a result of cervical spine afferent activation. The question is whether these "late effects" are the result of damage at the time of injury, chronic pain, or cervical afferent activation. These effects include:

- abnormal neuropsychological test results[98]
- vestibular hyperreactivity and abnormalities of the vestibulo-ocular reflex[99]
- cervicocephalic kinesthetic sensibility decreases (ability to return to a neutral cervical position after movement)[100]
- reduction of smooth pursuit ability with neck torsion (ability to smoothly track a moving object)[101]

Results from another study[102] implied a possible positive association between a history of neck injury in an MVA and headaches, disabling neck pain, and a perception of lower general health compared to those with no history of neck injury. Although interesting, it is important to realize that these results do not imply a cause-and-effect relationship between the injury and these subsequent complaints. Low-speed rear-impact collisions (LOSRIC) account for as many as 80% of rear-impact collisions. The range of speed in these LOSRICs is between 6 and 12 mph.

Recent, encouraging research[103, 104] indicates that patients with symptoms of chronic whiplash injury respond well to chiropractic management. Interestingly, one of these studies[103] identified a subgroup of patients who did not respond well to most therapies. These patients include those with severe neck pain, yet with a full range of motion and no neurologic symptoms/signs specific to a myotome or dermatome. These patients often complained of other symptoms and signs such as blackouts, visual disturbances, nausea and vomiting, chest pain, and a nondermatomal pattern of pain.

Algorithms

Algorithms for traumatic neck pain, nontraumatic neck and arm pain, nontraumatic neck pain with no radiation, and annotations are presented in **Figures 2–5** through **2–8**.

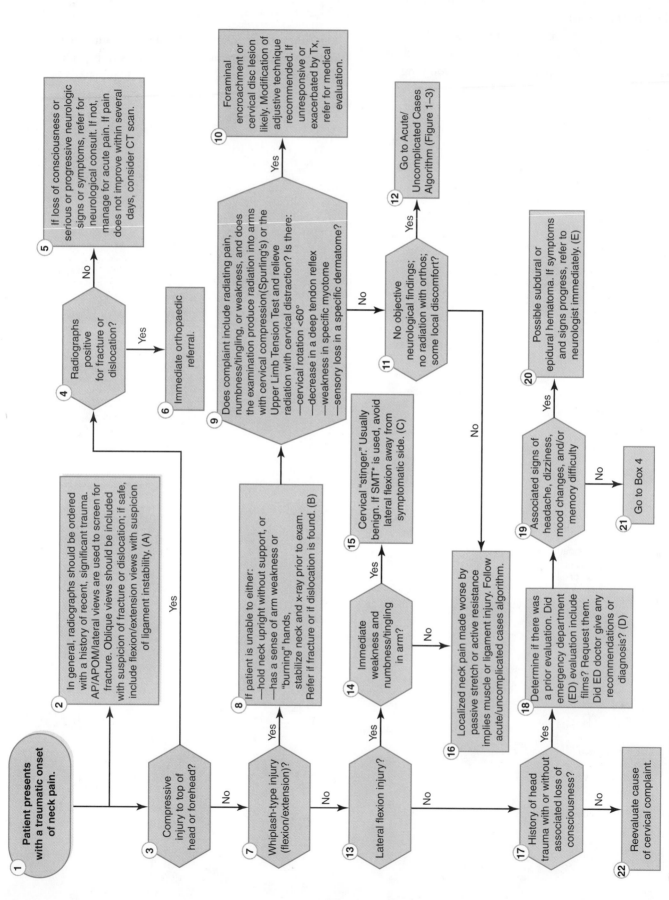

Figure 2–5 Traumatic Neck Pain—Algorithm

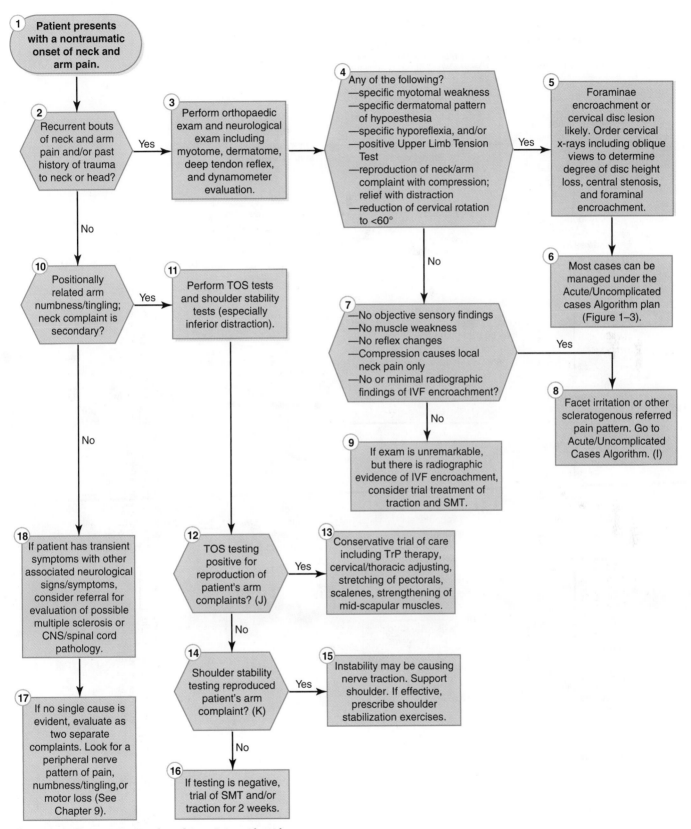

Figure 2–6 Nontraumatic Neck and Arm Pain—Algorithm

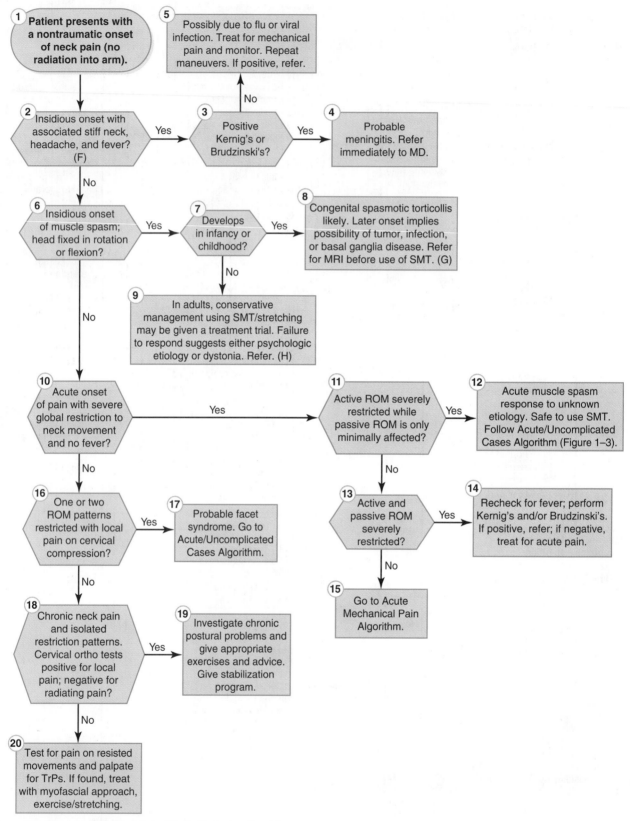

Figure 2–7 Nontraumatic Neck Pain (No Radiation)—Algorithm

A. If trauma is significant or patient is unable to move their neck without significant discomfort, stabilize neck and shoot x-rays prior to orthopaedic examination.

B. Burning-hands syndrome represents spinal cord injury due to stenosis or fracture. Radiographs to determine fracture and degree of stenosis should also include lateral flexion/extension views to determine any contributory instability. Most cases of burning-hands syndrome are self-resolving; however, prolonged recovery is not uncommon.

C. A "stinger" usually involves a traction injury of either the nerve root or plexus. Most are brief occurrences representing a neuropraxia, however, with more severe trauma an axonotmesis can occur requiring referral to a neurologist.

D. It is extremely important to get information regarding any evaluation at another facility. Often films are available and a previous diagnosis and/or patient instructions have been given including some contraindications to manipulation.

E. Any patient with a Hx of head trauma should be monitored for several weeks. Usually due to a torn vein, pressure may develop slowly resulting in very subtle neuro signs/symptoms. With patients who do not seem "quite right," referral to neurologist is warranted. Epidural hematomas usually involve a temporal bone fracture and bleeding from an artery usually resulting in a more rapid onset of neuro signs.

F. Subarachnoid hemorrhage is essentially a brain bruise. It may result from trauma or a ruptured aneurysm or AVM. With vessel rupture, the onset is sudden and there is no associated fever. This may help distinguish the presentation from meningitis. Immediate referral is necessary.

G. Spastic torticollis (wryneck) may be congenital and is self-resolving or is correctable within the first few months. Other causes may include basal ganglion disorders, infection, tumors, and psychiatric disorders. A thorough evaluation is needed prior to application of CMT. Note that the restriction is limited to one side.

H. Dystonia may first present with torticollis and an accompanying distortion of another body part such as the feet. It is rare yet progressive resulting in sustained abnormal postures.

I. Sclerotogenous pain patterns are less distinct than dermatomal or peripheral nerve patterns. Additionally, reflexes, sensory testing, and muscle strength are normal.

J. TOS tests may produce frequent false positives. It is not enough to obtain a diminished pulse. The test must reproduce the patient's complaint of arm pain/numbness/tingling.

K. Shoulder instability has been shown to produce similar symptoms as TOS due to tractioning of the plexus.

Figure 2–8 Annotations for neck pain—Algorithm

Selected Causes of Cervical Spine Pain

Cervical Radiculopathy

Classic Presentation

The patient complains of neck and arm pain. Onset often follows neck injury; however, it may be insidious. There is often a past history of multiple bouts of neck pain following minor injuries. The patient also complains of some weakness in the hand. The pain is described as a deep ache. Some patients report some relief with the hand held behind the head.

Cause

Unlike the lumbar spine, herniation of the nucleus pulposus accounts for only 20% to 25% of cases in the cervical spine. The clear difference is the natural history of the intervertebral disc of the cervical spine, which dehydrates to the point of almost a ligamentous structure by the age of 40 to 50 years. In fact, the peak incidence occurs at approximately 50 to 54 years old when the disc can no longer herniate, and a history of trauma is found in only about 15% of cases. The prevalence is quite low compared to the lumbar spine: only 0.8 to 3.5 per 100,000 patients.[105] Seventy percent to seventy-five percent of cases are due to foraminal encroachment due to degeneration, including decreased disc height, uncovertebral joint arthrosis, and facet joint arthrosis.

Evaluation

The patient often will have a painful restriction in active and passive ROM, often more on one side. Orthopaedic testing with cervical compression (Figure 2–1) may reproduce the neck and arm pain. Radiation into the medial scapular area also is possible. Cervical distraction (Figure 2–2) may relieve the arm pain. All of these orthopaedic tests are relatively insensitive but moderately specific.[106] Some patients report some relief of the arm pain by putting the hand behind the head, thereby decreasing any traction effect. Neurologic testing should reveal a decreased corresponding deep tendon reflex, weakness in a related myotome, and sensory abnormality in a related dermatome. Radiographic evaluation of the neck should include oblique views to determine the degree of bony foraminal encroachment. MR imaging or CT scans are reserved for patients with severe pain or those unresponsive to nonsurgical management. Electrodiagnostic studies may be helpful three to four weeks after the onset of symptoms if a specific cause has not yet been identified or the patient is unresponsive to care.

Management

The natural history appears favorable.[107] Conservative treatment is used for approximately 74% of cases. Ninety percent of patients fully recover or have only mild residual dysfunction. A small prospective study[108] published in 2013 evaluated the short-term effectiveness of manipulation for patients with MRI-confirmed radiculopathy caused by disc herniation. There was no comparative group for natural history or other treatment approach, yet, the improvement rates were, at two weeks 55.3%, at one month 68.9%, and at three months 85.7%. Given there was no comparative control group, it is important to note that for subacute and chronic patients, 76.2% were improved at three months. No adverse events related to manipulation were reported in this previously-assumed high-risk group of patients.

A prospective study[109] published in *Spine* in 2013 compared the results of a structured physiotherapy approach versus anterior decompression surgery and physiotherapy for patients with cervical radiculopathy and followed patients over two years. At a one-year follow-up, 87% of the patients in the surgical group rated their symptoms as "better/much better" versus 62% in the nonsurgical group. At two years, the percentage for improvement using the above rating was 81% in the surgical group versus 69% in the structured physiotherapy group. Improvement was more rapid in the surgical group; however, at two years, there were significant reductions in the Neck Disability Index, in neck pain, and with arm pain compared with baseline in both groups.

Cervical manipulation at sites other than the herniation is used by many chiropractors.[86] If osseous adjusting is to be used, it should be applied with a trial of mild mobilization impulses at the involved level to determine patient response. The degree of force application should be the least possible. It should always be kept in mind that if the patient has hard neurologic evidence of nerve root compression, the chiropractor is at risk of irritating the nerve and being accused of causing the herniation. Nonosseous techniques may be attempted for a short course to determine therapeutic effect.

A first-time randomized controlled trial[87] examined the management of cervical radiculopathy with either a semihard cervical collar or physiotherapist-direct exercise versus rest during the first six weeks of onset. Although the use of a cervical collar for neck pain has decreased significantly based on evidence that it does not seem to make a difference for whiplash patients, there was no evidence for or against the use of a cervical collar for patients with cervical radiculopathy.

Reduction in arm pain at six weeks in the wait-and-see group was approximately 19 points on a 100-point scale. Comparatively, the semirigid collar group experienced on average a reduction of 31 points on a 100-point scale at six weeks. Reduction in neck pain at six weeks in the wait-and-see group was only 5 points, whereas the reduction in the semirigid collar group was an additional 9–12 points.

Consider using a semihard cervical collar for patients with recent onset cervical radiculopathy, in particular, if there is concern by you or the patient regarding manipulation. Instruct the patient to wear the brace during the day. To avoid complications, wean the patient off of the brace over a period of six weeks. The results of this study also support the opposite approach; have patients perform mild exercising and stretching of the neck during the first six weeks of onset with caution if symptoms are increased by the exercise.

Cervical traction and physical therapy may also be incorporated. Home traction for 15 minutes twice a day will be of benefit to some patients. The response is usually evident within a few days.[110] Patients who are unresponsive or are simply in too much pain should be referred for medical comanagement.

Myelopathy

Classic Presentation

Patient presentation may differ depending on the type and degree of compression. Classically, a patient presents with complaints of bilateral symptoms of clumsiness of the hands, difficulty walking, possible urinary dysfunction, and possible shooting pains into the arms.

Cause

Cervical spine myelopathy is present in 90% of individuals older than 70 years of age and is the most common cause of spinal cord dysfunction in individuals older than 55 years of age. It is more common in males and in Asians.

There are numerous causes of spinal cord compression (myelopathy), including tumor, herniated disc, and spondylotic sources. Depending on which portion of the spinal cord or whether nerve roots are also involved, the signs and symptoms will vary. Direct pressure on the posterior columns often occurs with spondylotic myelopathy, causing disturbances in vibration perception and proprioception. If compression of nerve roots also occurs, signs of a lower motor neuron problem will surface.

Evaluation

If the anterior cord is involved, then pain, pathological reflexes and/or hyperactive deep tendon reflexes or motor weakness may be evident. If the posterior cord is involved, then loss of dexterity, gait abnormalities, poor coordination, clumsiness, or sensory loss may the dominant signs and symptoms. Overlap may occur so that headache, neck stiffness, shoulder pain, paresthesia in one or both arms or hands, or other radiculopathic signs may also be present.

Long tract signs, such as Hoffmann's, Babinski sign, clonus, the crossed-abductor sign, the inverted supinator sign, or hand withdrawal reflex testing, reflect the disinhibition of the primitive afferent or efferent (pyramidal) spinal cord pathways that are normally suppressed or modulated in the adult. Mixed findings of UMNL and LMNL signs may occur. At the level of involvement, LMNL signs may be present and below the level of involvement, UMNL signs. Mixed findings may be found including LMNL signs in the upper extremity with UMNL signs in the lower extremity. Sensory loss may include both numbness and vibration loss bilaterally, or if unilateral involvement is present it may cause contralateral numbness with unilateral vibration loss. There is a dynamic component where extension of the cervical spine may add compression through buckling of the ligamentum flavum or with flexion compression from the posterior longitudinal ligament, especially if calcified.

Cook et al.[111] conducted a systematic review and through classifying exam findings into gait abnormalities, pathological signs, and deep tendon reflex changes, they determined the following:

- Gait or balance—Both abnormal gait (ataxia, wide-based gait, or spastic gait) and a positive static or dynamic Romberg sign were very specific but not sensitive for cervical spine myelopathy.
- Pathological signs—Hoffmann sign, Babinski sign, and clonus were very specific but not very sensitive for cervical spine myelopathy.
- DTR changes—Hyperreflexia was very specific but not very sensitive for cervical myelopathy.

In other words, most tests for cervical myelopathy are specific but not sensitive, meaning that finding a positive is relatively good at ruling-in myelopathy but not finding positive tests is not very good at ruling-out myelopathy. The inverted supinator sign is probably the most sensitive test. It is similar to the brachioradialis reflex test with the patient's forearm placed in slight pronation on the examiner's knee. A few quick strikes with a percussion hammer near the radial styloid process with a pathological response of slight finger flexion or elbow extension.

The researchers combined the following to develop a clinical prediction rule.[112] The Babinski sign, inverted supinator sign, Hoffmann sign, and gait dysfunction (spastic, wide-based gait, or ataxia) and age older than 45 years. If only 1 of 5 tests was positive (4 tests are negative) the sensitivity was 0.94 with a −LR of 0.18 (rule-out). If there were 3 of 5 positive tests, the +LR was 30.9 (rule-in) (95% CI = 5.5-181.8) with a posttest probability of 94%.

The most common finding in patients with myelopathy identified on MRI is gait abnormality found in 91% of patients. Babinski's was found positive in only about 44% of myelopathic patients.[113] Hyperreflexia was more common in the lower extremity (81%) compared to the upper extremity (67%). Eighty-four percent of patients had a positive clinical examination.

Radiographic measurement of spinal canal diameter may be accomplished on the lateral view of the cervical spine. The width is measured from the posterior vertebral body to the lamina-pedicle junction. Anything less than 13 mm should warrant concern. Anything less than 10 to 11 mm is an indication of absolute stenosis. The Torg (or Pavlov) ratio uses the spinal canal width over the anterior to posterior width of the vertebral body. A ratio less than 0.82 is considered stenotic.[114] If there are myelopathic findings on exam or absolute stenosis evident on radiographs, order MRI (or CT). Evidence of myelopathy is primarily seen on sagittal images. Evidence of spinal cord compression on MRI is indicated by an indentation on the spinal cord parenchyma. More significant involvement is indicated by a T2 signal abnormality in the spinal cord, which is indicated by the presence of a hyperintense signal within the spinal cord parenchyma.[115] This finding should be confirmed on axial images to avoid an artifact effect causing a false positive.

MRI has been shown to be 79–95% sensitive and 82–88% specific with a positive likelihood ratio (LR) of 4.39–7.92 and a negative likelihood ratio (LR) of 0.06–0.27 for identifying selected abnormalities such as space-occupying tumors, disk herniation, and ligamentous ossification. Although special imaging is the "gold standard," in some individuals the presence of radiographic spinal cord compression is seen without clinical symptoms or physical signs of cervical myelopathy. Findings are seen in 16% of asymptomatic patients younger than 64 years of age, increasing to 26% of those older than 64 years of age.

Electrodiagnostic studies may be helpful in estimating the degree of involvement and perhaps the level. The most valuable tests are SEPs and DSEPs because they may determine latency of signal transmission through the spinal cord.[116]

Management

Surgery is often recommended in cases where there are "hard" lesions such as spondylosis or ossification of the posterior longitudinal ligament because of the possibility of permanent neurologic damage. "Soft" lesions such as disc lesions may resolve over time. Decompression surgery for spondylotic myelopathy has variable results between 33% and 74%.[117] In 2002, a Cochrane review of surgery for cervical spondylotic radiculomyelopathy determined that although the short-term effects of surgery were superior to conservative management for pain, weakness, or sensory loss, the effect was lost at one year where there was no significant difference between the two groups.[118] For those with a mild functional deficit associated with cervical myelopathy, there were no significant differences two years following treatment. A follow-up Cochrane review[119] in 2010 still maintained that there was lack of evidence for surgery's having a superior long-term effect. Recommendations should be based on the severity of functional impairment and failure of conservative management.

Murphy et al.[120] published a case-series report on patients with early and mild myelopathy managed chiropractically. Seventy percent of patients, on average, improved although there was a wide range of 0–100%. No neurological signs developed and no major complications occurred. A management approach to the patient with cervical myelopathy based on this study is:

- If there are mild myelopathic signs/symptoms or MRI evidence of compression with *no* T2 changes, consider an initial trial of HVLA adjusting using premanipulative positioning (i.e., setting up without thrusting) to determine if peripheralization occurs or not. It is important to find a position that does not peripheralize prior to adjusting. Make this clinical decision for treatment with patient education, input, and approval.
- If there are advanced or severe clinical findings of myelopathy or T2 hyperintense signal changes on MRI, surgical consult or a trial of nonmanipulative approaches is suggested.

Comanagement is recommended for patients who show no improvement after one to two weeks.

Burner/Stinger

Classic Presentation

The patient reports a sudden onset of burning pain and/or numbness along the lateral arm with associated arm weakness following a lateral flexion injury of the neck/head (e.g., lateral "whiplash"). The symptoms usually last only a couple of minutes.

Cause

"Burner" or "stinger" are the names given to injury of the brachial plexus or nerve roots caused by a lateral flexion injury. This is a common injury in sports and has a high percentage of underreporting (70%) because of the transient symptoms.[121] In general, lateral flexion of the head away from the involved side with accompanying shoulder distraction (depression) on the involved side causes a brachial plexopathy. Compression on the side with lateral flexion is more likely to result in nerve root compression. When the brachial plexus is involved, the upper trunk (C5-C6) is most often affected. Varying degrees of injury may occur; however, the majority of injuries are mild, with transient symptoms.

Evaluation

The most common physical finding is weakness of shoulder abduction, external rotation, and arm flexion. Both muscle weakness and sensory findings may be delayed; therefore, it is important to reexamine patients within about one week postinjury. Persistent symptoms require a radiographic evaluation for instability, including flexion and extension views. If arm weakness is persistent after three weeks, an EMG study may be helpful.[122] If a nerve root problem is suspected, an MRI may be of help. Otherwise, most cases require no special testing evaluation.

Management

It is important to avoid reproduction of the injury with a lateral-flexion type of adjustment. Given that recurrence of the injury is common in sports, athletes are encouraged to strengthen their neck muscles and wear protective gear when appropriate. Repeated episodes may lead to more damage requiring neurologic consultation.

Thoracic Outlet Syndrome

Classic Presentation

The patient presents with diffuse arm symptoms, including numbness and tingling. Often the patient will describe a path down the inside of his or her arm to the little and ring fingers. This is often made worse by overhead activity.

Cause

The brachial plexus and/or subclavian/axillary arteries can be compressed at various sites as they travel downward into the arm. Several common sites are possible, including an elongated C7 transverse process (cervical rib), the scalene muscles, the costoclavicular area, and the subcoracoid area (between the coracoid and the pectoralis minor). Muscular compression at the scalenes or with the pectoralis minor is believed to be due to tight muscles and/or posturally induced (forward head and rounded shoulder habit). Leffert[123] reports that in 40% of cases there is a report of inciting trauma. It is important to recognize that only 1% of the population has cervical ribs, and only 10% of those individuals have symptoms.[124] A fibrous band connecting the cervical rib to the first rib also may be the culprit in some cases.

Evaluation

Although a number of provocative tests are used, there are often false positives and false negatives. The intent of the tests is to reproduce symptoms in the arm. If the positive is based on simply a reduction of the radial pulse, many false positives will be found. When the scalenes are being tested, the patient is asked to look either toward (Adson's test) or away (Halstead's test) from the involved side with the arm held in slight abduction. When the pectoralis minor is tested, the arm is lifted into abduction and horizontal abduction (Wright's test). A functional test is to have the patient raise the arms above head level and repeatedly grip and release the hands for 20 to 60 seconds (Roos' test) in an attempt to reproduce arm symptoms or weakness. It is always important to perform a neurologic evaluation in an attempt to differentiate TOS from lower brachial plexus, nerve root, or peripheral entrapment problems.

Management

Generally, management is conservative with an approach based on postural correction, stretching of tightened muscles, and strengthening of weakened muscles. This includes strengthening of the middle and lower trapezius and rhomboids, and stretching of the pectorals and scalenes. Trigger-point therapy is also advocated by Travell and Simons.[125] Taping or bracing may help with a proprioceptive training program for postural correction. There is also a belief that a first rib subluxation may cause the signs and symptoms of TOS. Several investigators have suggested manipulation of the first rib in an attempt to correct this problem.[126-128] Surgery is suggested for a minority of patients (approximately 24%) who do not respond to conservative management.[129]

Facet/Referred

Classic Presentation

The patient often will report a minor (e.g., sudden turning of the head) to moderate (e.g., motor vehicle accident) traumatic onset of neck and arm pain. In some patients the onset can be insidious with no recent trauma. The patient often will draw a line of pain down the outer arm to the hand. The arm and hand pain do not often fit a specific dermatome.

Cause

Irritation of the facet joints or deep cervical muscles causes a referred pain down the arm. The most common location is down the outer arm to the hand. This location often implicates segmentally related facet joints of C5-C7.

Evaluation

It is assumed that what chiropractors affect are facet joints, yet there have been no studies to correlate findings of facet involvement with facet injections for pain relief. A recent study by King et al.[130] evaluated patients who were diagnosed by physical therapists as having facet joint dysfunction. The patients who were willing to participate then had controlled diagnostic blocks performed to determine which facets, in fact, were involved. The manual examination was sensitive, but not specific, for facet involvement.

A standard orthopaedic and neurologic examination of the neck and upper extremity should be performed. With referred pain, there is rarely any hard neurologic evidence. Deep tendon reflexes are normal, muscle strength is normal or weakness does not fit a specific myotome, and numbness is often subjective with no objective sensory findings. Local pain may be reproduced with cervical compression (Figure 2–1) with the neck in extension and rotation to the involved side. A search for trigger-point referral should be made, including supraspinatus or infraspinatus involvement. Radiographic evaluation may be performed to detect any foraminal encroachment on the oblique views. Patients with mild foraminal encroachment, however, may still have referred pain as opposed to nerve root impingement if the neurologic examination is normal.

Management

Manipulation of the neck is the treatment of choice. If unsuccessful, cervical traction may be of benefit. Any myofascial contribution may be addressed with stretch-and-spray techniques, trigger-point therapy, or myofascial release.

Torticollis

Classic Presentation

There may be several presentations of torticollis based on age and cause. In congenital torticollis, the infant will have a fixed asymmetry of the head that is seen within hours (or sometimes weeks) of delivery. In the adult version, a patient presents with painful spasm of the SCM, causing the head to be held in rotation and sometimes slight flexion. In pseudotorticollis, the patient presents with the inability to move the head in any direction without pain. The patient reports having awakened with the condition; there is no trauma or obvious cause. The head is held in neutral.

Cause

The congenital cause of torticollis is probably birth trauma, often breech delivery. Damage to the SCM causes it to become fibrous. The adult version may be due to a number of causes, including CNS infection, tumor, basal ganglion disease, or psychiatric disease. Pseudotorticollis has no known cause. It differs from classic torticollis in that all movements are painful and there is no deviation of the head.

Evaluation

It is important to determine whether there is a moderate to high fever, which would be suggestive of meningitis. Kernig's or Brudzinski's signs would be positive, causing severe pain and/or flexion of the lower limbs on passive flexion of the neck. Palpation of the SCMs and the anterior neck for masses is important. Patients with pseudotorticollis often have markedly increased passive ROM when examined carefully in the supine position. The amount of passive ROM is used as the gauge as to whether or not manipulation is appropriate. A neurologic check for upper motor and lower motor neuron dysfunction will reveal any medically referable causes. Radiographs are usually not necessary. MR imaging or CT scans may be needed when CNS disease is suspected.

Management

The congenital type of torticollis may respond to physical therapy attempts to lengthen the SCM; however, the therapy must be consistent and often takes up to one year. For the adult who has no known cause, attempts at neck manipulation and physical therapy may help, or the condition may self-resolve. With pseudotorticollis, manipulation should be applied cautiously as soon as possible in an attempt to decrease the global muscle spasm. Failure to resolve warrants a referral for medical evaluation.

The Evidence—Cervical Spine

Translation into Practice Summary (TIPS)

Directed by the patient presentation, the evaluation for cervical spine fracture, instability, and radiculopathy are important specific focuses of the examination. The history and examination together are good at determining the need for radiography in the evaluation of fracture and instability. The history is poor but the examination good at ruling-in cervical radiculopathy. There is no evidence for the value of the clinical examination to screen for risk of vertebrobasilar accidents.

The Literature-Based Clinical Core

- The clinical examination together with specific historical indicators is sensitive for cervical spine fracture. Both the NEXUS and Canadian Spine Rule are very good at ruling-out (but not ruling-in) fracture of the cervical spine.
- The Sharp-Purser test may be valuable in ruling-in cervical spine instability.
- The patient history is not helpful in ruling-in or ruling-out cervical radiculopathy.
- The biceps and brachioradialis DTRs are good at ruling-in (but not ruling-out) C5 and C6 nerve root involvement. However, the triceps DTR is only fair at ruling-in, but bad at ruling-out C7 nerve root involvement.
- Although the specificity for myotome and dermatome testing for radiculopathy is good, the overall performance based on LRs is poor. Adding resisted pronation testing may increase the sensitivity of detecting a C6 or C7 nerve root involvement.
- Patients are less likely to report weakness compared to the finding of weakness by the examiner so that strength testing should always be performed with patients complaining of radiating pain.
- It is less common for patients to describe a dermatomal pattern when a radiculopathy is present; therefore, any radiation warrants the application of the clinical prediction rule stated below.
- The combination of the upper limb tension test (ULTT), Spurling's, cervical distraction, and ROM less than 60° together are very good at ruling-in cervical radiculopathy

- The ICCs are good for ROM testing and cervical strength and endurance testing.
- The kappa values are poor for assessing pain with palpation and intervertebral motion testing. Palpation of cervical facets posteriorly has a good −LR and a fair +LR.
- With the exception of a forward flexed head, the kappa values for postural assessment and muscle length assessment of the cervical spine area are good.
- There is no evidence for the reliability or validity of any tests for thoracic outlet syndrome (TOS) when evaluating for the medically defined entity of TOS.

The Expert-Opinion-Based Clinical Core

- When all neurological findings are negative including the upper limb tension test, it is likely that a patient's radiating pain is not, in fact, radicular and more likely scleratogenous with the main sources coming from internal disc disruption and cervical facet joints.
- Mapping of a patient's description of radiation should always include a scleratogenous and trigger point comparison.
- Use of TOS testing may have some value when determining a myofascial component of radiating complaints of numbness, tingling, or pain.
- Screening tests for vertebrobasilar accidents (ischemia) are of no value and may introduce false positives that compromise clinical decision making. None of the tests from George's or deKleyn's are of value in screening for VBA.
- Older patients should always be screened for myelopathy especially with gait problems or with neurological symptoms or radiating complaints (especially bilaterally).
- Older patients with diffuse symptoms in both arms/hands should also be evaluated for T4 syndrome.

APPENDIX 2–1

References

1. Bogduk N. The anatomical basis for spinal pain syndromes. Conference proceedings of the Chiropractic Centennial Foundation. Presented at the Chiropractic Centennial; July 6–8, 1995; Washington, DC.

2. National Board of Chiropractic Examiners. *Job Analysis of Chiropractic: A Project Report, Survey Analysis, and Summary of the Practice of Chiropractic Within the United States.* Greeley, CO: National Board of Chiropractic Examiners (NBCE); 2010.

3. Cote P, Cassidy JD, Carroll L. The Saskatchewan Health and Back Pain Survey. The prevalence of neck pain and related disability in Saskatchewan adults. *Spine.* 1998;23(15):1689–1698.

4. Riddle DL, Schappert SM. Volume and characteristics of inpatient and ambulatory medical care for neck pain in the United States: data from three national surveys. *Spine.* 2007;32(1):132–140;discussion 141.

5. Spitzer WO, Skovron ML, Salmi LR, et al. Redefining "whiplash" and its management. Scientific monograph of the Quebec Task Force on Whiplash-Associated Disorders. *Spine.* 1995;20(85):1S–73S.

6. Coulter ID, Hurwitz EL, Adams AH, et al. *The Appropriateness of Manipulation and Mobilization of the Cervical Spine.* Santa Monica, CA: Rand Corporation; 1996.

7. Haldeman S, Carroll L, Cassidy JD, Schubert J, Nygren A. The Bone and Joint Decade 2000–2010 Task Force on Neck Pain and Its Associated Disorders: executive summary. *Spine.* 2008;33(4 Suppl):S5–7.

8. Janda V. Muscles and cervicogenic pain syndromes. In: Grant R, ed. *Physical Therapy of the Cervical and Thoracic Spine.* New York: Churchill Livingstone; 1988:153–166.

9. Bogduk N. A neurological approach to neck pain. In: Glasgow EF, Twomey IV, Seall ER, et al., eds. *Aspects of Manipulative Therapy.* New York: Churchill Livingstone; 1985.

10. Weintraub M. Beauty parlor stroke syndrome: a report of 5 cases. *JAMA.* 1993;269(16):2085–2086.

11. Terrett AGJ, Kleynhans AM. Cerebrovascular complications of manipulation. In: Haldeman S, ed. *Modern Developments in the Principles and Practice of Chiropractic.* New York: Appleton-Century-Crofts; 1994:579–598.

12. Bland JH. Cervical and thoracic pain. *Curr Opin Rheumatol.* 1991;3:218–225.

13. Fujimoto K, Miyagi M, Ishikawa T, et al. Sensory and autonomic innervation of the cervical intervertebral disc in rats: the pathomechanics of chronic discogenic neck pain. *Spine (Phila Pa 1976).* 2012;37(16):1357–1362.

14. Garcia-Poblete E, Fernandez-Garcia H, Moro-Rodriguez E, et al. Sympathetic sprouting in dorsal root ganglia (DRG): a recent histological finding? *Histol Histopathol.* 2003;18(2):575–586.

15. Panjabi M, Oxland T, Parks E. Quantitative anatomy of cervical spine ligaments, part II: middle and lower cervical spine. *J Spinal Disord.* 1991;4:277–285.

16. Webb AL, Collins P, Rassoulian H, Mitchell BS. Synovial folds—a pain in the neck? *Man Ther.* 2011;16(2):118–124.

17. Webb AL, Rassoulian H, Mitchell BS. Morphometry of the synovial folds of the lateral atlanto-axial joints: the anatomical basis for understanding their potential role in neck pain. *Surg Radiol Anat.* 2012;34(2):115–124.

18. Mootz RD. Theoretic models of chiropractic subluxation. In: Gatterman MI, ed. *Foundations of Chiropractic: Subluxation.* St. Louis, MO: Mosby-Year Book; 1995:176–189.

19. Kallakuri S, Li Y, Chen C, Cavanaugh JM. Innervation of cervical ventral facet joint capsule: Histological evidence. *World J Orthop.* 2012;3(2):10–14.

20. Cavanaugh JM, Lu Y, Chen C, Kallakuri S. Pain generation in lumbar and cervical facet joints. *J Bone Joint Surg Am.* 2006;88 Suppl 2:63–67.

21. Ohtori S, Takahashi K, Chiba T, Yamagata M, Sameda H, Moriya H. Sensory innervation of the cervical facet joints in rats. *Spine (Phila Pa 1976).* 2001;26(2):147–150.

22. Parke WW, Whalen JL. The vascular pattern of the human dorsal root ganglion and its probable bearing on a compartment syndrome. *Spine (Phila Pa 1976).* 2002;27(4):347–352.

23. Tubbs RS, Loukas M, Slappey JB, Shoja MM, Oakes WJ, Salter EG. Clinical anatomy of the C1 dorsal root, ganglion, and ramus: a review and anatomical study. *Clin Anat.* 2007;20(6):624–627.

24. Ohtori S, Takahashi K, Moriya H. Calcitonin gene-related peptide immunoreactive DRG neurons innervating the cervical facet joints show phenotypic switch in cervical facet injury in rats. *Eur Spine J.* 2003;12(2):211–215.

25. DeJong PTVN, DeJong JMBV, Cohen B, Jongkees LBV. Ataxia and nystagmus induced by injection of local anesthesia in the neck. *Ann Neurol.* 1977;1:240–246.

26. Richmond FJR, Vidal PP. The motor system: joints and muscles of the neck. In: Peterson BW, Richmond F, eds. *Control of Head Movement.* New York: Oxford University Press; 1988.

27. Leffert RD. Thoracic outlet syndrome and the shoulder. *Clin Sports Med.* 1983;2:439.

28. Panjabi MM, Vasavada A, White AA III. Cervical spine biomechanics. *Semin Spine Surg.* 1993;5:10–16.

29. Panjabi MM, Oda T, Crisco J J III, et al. Posture affects motion coupling patterns of the upper cervical spine. *J Orthop Res.* 1993;11:525–536.

30. Croft AC. Advances in the clinical understanding of acceleration/deceleration injuries to the cervical spine. In: Lawrence DJ, Cassidy JD, McGregor M, et al., eds. *Advances in Chiropractic.* St. Louis, MO: Mosby-Year Book; 1995;2:1–37.

31. Otto K, Kaneoka K, Wittek A, Kajzer J. Cervical injury mechanism based on the analysis of human cervical vertebral motion and head-neck torso kinematics during low speed rear impacts. 41st Stapp Car Crash Conference Proceedings. SAE paper 973340, 1997; 339–356.

32. Grauer JN, Panjabi MM, Chelewicki J, et al. Whiplash produces an s-shaped curvature of the neck with hyperextension at lower levels. *Spine* 1997;22:2489–2494.

33. Stiell IG, Wells GA, Vandemheen KL, et al. The Canadian C-spine rule for radiography in alert and stable trauma patients. *JAMA.* 2001;286(15):1841–1848.

34. Bandiera G, Stiell IG, Wells GA, et al. The Canadian C-spine rule performs better than unstructured physician judgment. *Ann Emerg Med.* 2003;42(3):395–402.

35. Stiell IG, Clement CM, McKnight RD, et al. The Canadian C-spine rule versus the NEXUS low-risk criteria in patients with trauma. *N Engl J Med.* 2003;349(26):2510–2518.

36. Panacek EA, Mower WR, Holmes JF, Hoffman JR. Test performance of the individual NEXUS low-risk clinical screening criteria for cervical spine injury. *Ann Emerg Med.* 2001;38(1):22–25.

37. Fedorak C, Ashworth N, Marshall J, Paul H. Reliability of the visual assessment of cervical and lumbar lordosis: how good are we? *Spine.* 2003;28(16):1857–1859.

38. Torg HC, Haig AJ, Yamakawa K. The Spurling test and cervical radiculopathy. *Spine.* 2002;27(2):156–159.

39. Vikari-Juntura E. Interexaminer reliability of observations in physical examinations of the neck. *Phys Ther.* 1987; 67:1526–1532.

40. Vikari-Juntura E, Porros M, Lassomen EM. Validity of clinical tests in the diagnosis of root compression in cervical disc disease. *Spine.* 1989;14:253–257.

41. Sobel JB, Sollenberger P, Robinson R, et al., Cervical Nonorganic Signs: A New Clinical Tool to Assess Abnormal Illness Behavior in Neck Pain Patients: A Pilot Study. *Arch Phys Med Rehabil.* 2000;81:170–175.

42. Wainner RS, Fritz JM, Irrgang JJ, Boninger ML, Delitto A, Allison S. Reliability and diagnostic accuracy of the clinical examination and patient self-report measures for cervical radiculopathy. *Spine.* 2003;28(1):52–62.

43. Rubinstein SM, Pool JJ, van Tulder MW, Riphagen, II, de Vet HC. A systematic review of the diagnostic accuracy of provocative tests of the neck for diagnosing cervical radiculopathy. *Eur Spine J.* 2007;16(3):307–319.

44. Nordin M, Carragee EJ, Hogg-Johnson S, et al. Assessment of neck pain and its associated disorders: results of the Bone and Joint Decade 2000–2010 Task Force on Neck Pain and Its Associated Disorders. *Spine.* 2008;33(4 Suppl):S101–122.

45. Rainville J, Noto DJ, Jouve C, Jenis L. Assessment of forearm pronation strength in C6 and C7 radiculopathies. *Spine.* 2007;32(1):72–75.

46. Murphy DR, Hurwitz EL, Gerrard JK, Clary R. Pain patterns and descriptions in patients with radicular pain: does the pain necessarily follow a specific dermatome? *Chiropr Osteopat.* 2009;17:9.

47. Souza TA. Which orthopedic tests are really necessary? In: Lawrence DJ, Cassidy JD, McGregor M, et al., eds. *Advances in Chiropractic.* St. Louis, MO: Mosby-Year Book; 1994;1:101–158.

48. Sieke FW, Kelly TR. Thoracic outlet syndrome. *Am J Surg.* 1988;156:54–57.

49. Ferezy JS. Neurovascular assessment for risk management in chiropractic practice. In: Lawrence DJ, Cassidy JD, McGregor M, et al., eds. *Advances in Chiropractic.* St. Louis, MO: Mosby-Year Book; 1994:455–475.

50. Raney NH, Petersen EJ, Smith TA, et al. Development of a clinical prediction rule to identify patients with neck pain likely to benefit from cervical traction and exercise. *Eur Spine J.* 2009;18(3):382–391.

51. Haldeman S, Kohlbeck FJ, McGregor M. Risk factors and precipitating neck movements causing vertebrobasilar artery dissection after cervical trauma and spinal manipulation. *Spine.* 1999;24(8):785–794.

52. Haldeman S, Kohlbeck FJ, McGregor M. Unpredictability of cerebrovascular ischemia associated with cervical spine manipulation therapy: a review of sixty-four cases after cervical spine manipulation. *Spine.* 2002;27(1):49–55.

53. Helfet CA, Stanley P, Lewis Jones B, Heller RF. Value of X-ray examinations of the cervical spine. *Br Med J.* 1983;287:1276–1278.

54. Jaeger SA, Baum CA, Linquist GR. The many faces of the facets. In: Lawrence DJ, Cassidy JD, McGregor

M, et al., eds. *Advances in Chiropractic*. St. Louis, MO: Mosby-Year Book; 1995;2:331–372.

55. White AA, Panjabi MM, eds. *Clinical Biomechanics of the Spine*. Philadelphia: J B Lippincott; 1978:229.

56. McGregor M, Mior S, Shannon H, Hagino C, Schut B. The clinical usefulness of flexion-extension radiographs in the cervical spine. *Top Clin Chiro*. 1995;2(3):19–28.

57. Torg JS. Cervical spine stenosis with cord neuropraxia and transient quadriplegia. *Curr Opin Orthop*. 1994;5(11):97.

58. Karas SE. Thoracic outlet syndrome. *Clin Sports Med*. 1990;9:297–310.

59. Sistrom CL, Southall EP, Peddada SD, et al. Factors affecting the thickness of the cervical prevertebral soft tissues. *Skeletal Radiol*. 1993;22:167.

60. Guzman J, Hurwitz EL, Carroll LJ, et al. A new conceptual model of neck pain: linking onset, course, and care; the Bone and Joint Decade 2000–2010 Task Force on Neck Pain and Its Associated Disorders. *Spine*. 2008;33(4 Suppl):S14–23.

61. Haldeman S, Chapman-Smith D, Petersen DM, Jr. *Guidelines for Chiropractic Quality Assurance and Practice Parameters: Proceedings of the Mercy Center Consensus Conference*. Gaithersburg, MD: Aspen Publishers, Inc; 1993.

62. Vernon H, Mior S. The neck disability index: a study of reliability and validity. *J Manipulative Physiol Ther*. 1991; 14:409–415.

63. Guzman J, Haldeman S, Carroll LJ, et al. Clinical practice implications of the Bone and Joint Decade 2000–2010 Task Force on Neck Pain and Its Associated Disorders: from concepts and findings to recommendations. *Spine*. 2008;33(4 Suppl):S199–213.

64. Thiel HW, Bolton JE, Docherty S, Portlock JC. Safety of chiropractic manipulation of the cervical spine: a prospective national survey. *Spine*. 2007;32(21):2375–2378; discussion 2379.

65. Rubinstein SM, Leboeuf-Yde C, Knol DL, de Koekkoek TE, Pfeifle CE, van Tulder MW. The benefits outweigh the risks for patients undergoing chiropractic care for neck pain: a prospective, multicenter, cohort study. *J Manipulative Physiol Ther*. 2007;30(6):408–418.

66. Ernst E. Adverse effects of spinal manipulation: a systematic review. *J R Soc Med*. 2007;100(7):330–338.

67. Ernst E, Canter PH. A systematic review of systematic reviews of spinal manipulation. *J R Soc Med*. 2006; 99(4):192–196.

68. Bronfort G, Haas M, Moher D, et al. Review conclusions by Ernst and Canter regarding spinal manipulation refuted. *Chiropr Osteopat*. 2006;14:14.

69. Cassidy JD, Boyle E, Cote P, et al. Risk of vertebrobasilar stroke and chiropractic care: results of a population-based, case-control, and case-crossover study. *Spine*. 2008;33(4 Suppl):S176–183.

70. Boyle E, Cote P, Grier AR, Cassidy JD. Examining vertebrobasilar artery stroke in two Canadian provinces. *Spine*. 2008;33(4 Suppl):S170–175.

71. Quesnele JJ, Triano JJ, Noseworthy MD, Wells GD. Changes in vertebral artery blood flow following various head positions and cervical spine manipulation. *J Manipulative Physiol Ther*. 2014;37(1):22–31.

72. Gross AR, Goldsmith C, Hoving JL, et al. Conservative management of mechanical neck disorders: a systematic review. *J Rheumatol*. 2007;34(5):1083–1102.

73. Gross AR, Hoving JL, Haines TA, et al. A Cochrane review of manipulation and mobilization for mechanical neck disorders. *Spine*. 2004;29(14):1541–1548.

74. Kay TM, Gross A, Goldsmith C, Santaguida PL, Hoving J, Bronfort G. Exercises for mechanical neck disorders. *Cochrane Database Syst Rev*. 2005(3):CD004250.

75. O'Leary S, Jull G, Kim M, Vicenzino B. Specificity in retraining craniocervical flexor muscle performance. *J Orthop Sports Phys Ther*. 2007;37(1):3–9.

76. Chiu TT, Lam TH, Hedley AJ. A randomized controlled trial on the efficacy of exercise for patients with chronic neck pain. *Spine*. 2005;30(1):E1–7.

77. Evans R, Bronfort G, Schulz C, et al. Supervised exercise with and without spinal manipulation performs similarly and better than home exercise for chronic neck pain: a randomized controlled trial. *Spine (Phila Pa 1976)*. May 15, 2012;37(11):903–914.

78. Bronfort G, Evans R, Anderson AV, Svendsen KH, Bracha Y, Grimm RH. Spinal manipulation, medication, or home exercise with advice for acute and subacute neck pain: a randomized trial. *Ann Intern Med*. 2012;156(1 Pt 1):1–10.

79. Fitz-Ritson D. Phasic exercises for cervical rehabilitation after "whiplash" trauma. *J Manipulative Physiol Ther*. 1995;18:21–24.

80. Giles LG, Muller R. Chronic spinal pain syndromes: a clinical pilot trial comparing acupuncture, a nonsteroidal anti-inflammatory drug, and spinal manipulation. *J Manipulative Physiol Ther*. 1999;22(6):376–381.

81. Aker PD, Gross AR, Goldsmith CH, Peloso RS. Conservative management of mechanical neck pain: systematic overview and metaanalysis. *Br Med J.* 1996;313:1291–1296.

82. Hurwitz EL, Aker PD. Manipulation and mobilization of the cervical spine. *Spine.* 1996;21(15):1746–1760.

83. Hurwitz EL, Morgenstern H, Harber P, et al. A randomized trial of chiropractic manipulation and mobilization for patients with neck pain: clinical outcomes from the UCLA Neck Pain study. *Am J Public Health* 2002; 92:1634–1641.

84. Giles LG, Muller R. Chronic spinal pain: a randomized clinical trial comparing medication, acupuncture, and spinal manipulation. *Spine.* 2003;28(14):1490–1503.

85. Bryans R, Decina P, Descarreaux M, et al. Evidence-based guidelines for the chiropractic treatment of adults with neck pain. *J Manipulative Physiol Ther.* 2014;37(1):42–63.

86. Croft AC. Standards of care in cervical disk herniation: results from our nationwide survey of 3500 DCs. *SRISD Fact Sheet.* 1995;3:1–2.

87. Kuijper B, Tans JT, Beelen A, Nollet F, de Visser M. Cervical collar or physiotherapy versus wait and see policy for recent onset cervical radiculopathy: randomised trial. *BMJ.* 2009;339:b3883.

88. Ben-Eliyahu D. Magnetic resonance imaging follow-up study of 27 patients receiving chiropractic treatment for cervical and lumbar disc herniations. Conference proceedings of the Chiropractic Centennial Foundation. Presented at the Chiropractic Centennial; July 6–8, 1995; Washington, DC.

89. West DT, Mathews RS, Miller MR, Kent GM. Effective management of spinal pain in one hundred seventy-seven patients evaluated for manipulation under anesthesia. *J Manipulative Physiol Ther.* 1999;22(5):299–308.

90. Carroll LJ, Holm LW, Hogg-Johnson S, et al. Course and prognostic factors for neck pain in whiplash-associated disorders (WAD): results of the Bone and Joint Decade 2000–2010 Task Force on Neck Pain and Its Associated Disorders. *Spine.* 2008;33(4 Suppl):S83–92.

91. Cassidy JD, Carroll LJ, Cote P, Frank J. Does multidisciplinary rehabilitation benefit whiplash recovery? Results of a population-based incidence cohort study. *Spine.* 2007;32(1):126–131.

92. Ezzo J, Haraldsson BG, Gross AR, et al. Massage for mechanical neck disorders: a systematic review. *Spine.* 2007;32(3):353–362.

93. Gur A, Sarac AJ, Cevik R, Altindag O, Sarac S. Efficacy of 904 nm gallium arsenide low-level laser therapy in the management of chronic myofascial pain in the neck: a double-blind and randomized-controlled trial. *Lasers Surg Med.* 2004;35(3):229–235.

94. Chow RT, Heller GZ, Barnsley L. The effect of 300 mW, 830 nm laser on chronic neck pain: a double-blind, randomized, placebo-controlled study. *Pain.* 2006;124(1–2): 201–210.

95. Chow RT, Johnson MI, Lopes-Martins RA, Bjordal JM. Efficacy of low-level laser therapy in the management of neck pain: a systematic review and meta-analysis of randomised placebo or active-treatment controlled trials. *Lancet.* 2009;374(9705):1897–1908.

96. Saayman L, Hay C, Abrahamse H. Chiropractic manipulative therapy and low-level laser therapy in the management of cervical facet dysfunction: a randomized controlled study. *J Manipulative Physiol Ther.* 2011;34(3):153–163.

97. Barnsley L, Lord SM, Wallis BJ, Bogduk N. The prevalence of chronic cervical zygapophyseal joint pain after whiplash. *Spine.* 1995;20(1):20–26.

98. Otte A, Ettlin TM, Mitsche EU, et al. PET and SPECT in whiplash syndrome: a new approach to a forgotten brain? *J Neuro Neurosurg Psychiat.* 1997;63:368–372.

99. Fischer AJEM, Verhagen WIM, Huygen PLM. Whiplash injury. A clinical review with emphasis on neurotological aspects. *Clin Otolaryngol* 1997;22:192–201.

100. Heikkila HV, Wenngren BI. Cervicocephalic kinesthetic sensibility, active range of cervical motion, and occulo-motor function in patients with whiplash injury. *Arch Phys Med Rehab* 1998;79:1089–1094.

101. Tjell C, Rosenhall U. Smooth pursuit neck torsion test—a specific test for cervical dizziness. *Am J Otol.* 1988; 19:76–81.

102. Cote P, Cassidy JD, Carroll L. Is a lifetime history of neck injury in a traffic collision associated with prevalent neck pain, headache, and depressive symptomatology? *Accident Analysis and Prevention.* 2000;32:151–159.

103. Khan S, Cook JCH, Gargan M, Bannister GC. A symptomatic classification of whiplash injury and the implications for treatment. *J Orthop Med.* 1999;21(1):22–25.

104. Woodward MN, Cook JCH, Gargan ME, Bannister GC. Chiropractic treatment of chronic whiplash injury. *Injury.* 1996;27:643–645.

105. Radhakrishnan K, Litchy WJ, O'Fallon WM, Kurland LT. Epidemiology of cervical radiculopathy. A

population-based study from Rochester, Minnesota, 1976 through 1990. *Brain.* 1994;117(Pt 2):325–335.

106. Vikari-Juntura E, Porros M, Lassomen EM. Validity of clinical tests in the diagnosis of root compression in cervical disc disease. *Spine.* 1989;14:253–257.

107. Carette S, Fehlings MG. Clinical practice. Cervical radiculopathy. *N Engl J Med.* 2005;353(4):392–399.

108. Peterson CK, Schmid C, Leemann S, Anklin B, Humphreys BK. Outcomes From Magnetic Resonance Imaging-Confirmed Symptomatic Cervical Disk Herniation Patients Treated With High-Velocity, Low-Amplitude Spinal Manipulative Therapy: A Prospective Cohort Study With 3-Month Follow-Up. *J Manipulative Physiol Ther.* 2013;36:461–467.

109. Engquist M, Lofgren H, Oberg B, et al. Surgery Versus Nonsurgical Treatment of Cervical Radiculopathy: A Prospective, Randomized Study Comparing Surgery Plus Physiotherapy With Physiotherapy Alone With a 2-Year Follow-up. *Spine. (Phila Pa 1976).* 2013;38(20):1715–1722.

110. Venditti PP, Rosner AL, Kettner N, Sanders G. Cervical traction device study: a basic evaluation of home-use supine cervical traction devices. *J Neuromusculoskeletal Sys.* 1995;3:82–91.

111. Cook CE, Wilhelm M, Cook AE, Petrosino C, Isaacs R. Clinical tests for screening and diagnosis of cervical spine myelopathy: a systematic review. *J Manipulative Physiol Ther.* 2011;34(8):539–546.

112. Cook C, Brown C, Isaacs R, Roman M, Davis S, Richardson W. Clustered clinical findings for diagnosis of cervical spine myelopathy. *J Man Manip Ther.* 2010;18(4):175–180.

113. Harrop JS, Naroji S, Maltenfort M, et al. Cervical Myelopathy: A Clinical and Radiographic Evaluation and Correlation to Cervical Spondylotic Myelopathy. *Spine (Phila Pa 1976).* 2010. Feb 10. [Epub ahead of print].

114. Torg JS, Pavlov H, Genuario S, et al. Neuropraxia of the cervical spine cord with transient quadriplegia. *J Bone Joint Surg Am.* 1986;68:1354–1370.

115. Bell GR, Ross J. Diagnosis of nerve root compression. *Orthop Clin North Am.* 1992;23:405–415.

116. Swenson R. Dermatomal somatosensory evoked potentials: a review of literature. *J Neuromusculoskeletal Sys.* 1994;2(2):45–51.

117. Yone K, Sakov T, Yanese M, Ijuri K. Preoperative and postoperative magnetic resonance image evaluation of the spinal cord in cervical myelopathy. *Spine.* 1994;17(10S):390–392.

118. Fouyas IP, Statham FX, Sandercock P A G. Cochrane review on the role of surgery in cervical spondylotic radiculomyelopathy. *Spine.* 2002;27:736–747.

119. Nikolaidis I, Fouyas IP, Sandercock PA, Statham PF. Surgery for cervical radiculopathy or myelopathy. *Cochrane Database Syst Rev.* 2010(1):CD001466.

120. Murphy DR, Hurwitz EL, Gregory AA. Manipulation in the presence of cervical spinal cord compression: a case series. *J Manipulative Physiol Ther.* 2006;29(3):236–244.

121. Hershman EB. Brachial plexus injuries. *Clin Sports Med.* 1990;9(2):311–329.

122. Sallis RE, Jones K, Knopp W. Burners: offensive strategy for an underreported injury. *Physician Sportsmed.* 1992; 20:47–55.

123. Leffert RD. Thoracic outlet syndrome: a correspondence newsletter to the American Society of Surgery of the Hand, December 12, 1988.

124. Brown SCW, Charlesworth D. Results of excision of a cervical rib in patients with thoracic outlet syndrome. *Br J Surg.* 1988;75:431.

125. Travell J, Simons DG. *Myofascial Dysfunction: The Trigger Point Manual.* Baltimore: Williams & Wilkins; 1983.

126. Grice AC. Scalenus anticus syndrome: diagnosis and chiropractic adjustive procedure. *J Canad Chiro Ass.* 1977; 5:35–37.

127. Lee R, Farquarson T, Domleo S. Subluxation and blockierung der ersten rippe: eine ursache fur das "thoracic outlet syndrome." *Manuelle Medizin.* 1993;31:126–127.

128. Lindgren KA, Leino E. Subluxation of the first rib: a possible thoracic outlet syndrome mechanism. *Arch Phys Med Rehabil.* 1988;69:692–695.

129. Swaraz ZT. The thoracic outlet syndrome: first rib subluxation syndrome. In: Gatterman MI, ed. *Foundations of Chiropractic: Subluxation.* St. Louis, MO: Mosby-Year Book; 1995:360–377.

130. King W, Lau P, Lees R, Bogduk N. The validity of manual examination in assessing patients with neck pain. *Spine J.* 2007;7(1):22–26.

APPENDIX 2–2

Neck Diagnosis Table

Diagnosis	Comments	History Findings	Positive Examination Findings	Radiography/Special Studies	Treatment Options
Segmental Dysfunction of Cervical Spine Joints	• Should be used when chiropractic manipulation is used as Tx for any cervical spine problem/Dx. • Can be primary Dx if patient is asymptomatic or patient has tenderness and no pain. • Must indicate chiropractic exam findings to support Dx.	*Nonspecific*	*Palpation*—Local tenderness or other signs of subluxation *Ortho*—None *Neuro*—None *Active ROM*—Variable restriction *Passive ROM*—Endrange restriction *Motion palpation*—Specific vertebral segmental restriction or symptoms produced on endrange	• Radiography not required for the diagnosis of subluxation. • Radiographic biomechanical analysis may assist in treatment decisions. • For specifics see radiographic guidelines.	• Chiropractic adjustive technique. • Decisions regarding specifically which technique(s) is/are applied and modifications to the given approach will be directed by the primary Dx and patient's ability to tolerate pre-adjustment stresses.
Cervical Sprain/ Strain	• Should be reserved for acute traumatic sprain/ strain.	*Trauma*—Overstretch or overcontraction Hx as acute event *Radiation of pain*—Possible (referred) *Pain radiation with Valsalva-type activities*—No *Worse with Specific ROM*—Contraction of muscle or stretch of muscle or joint	*Ortho*—None *Neuro*—None *Active ROM*—Pain on active ROM that contracts involved muscles *Passive ROM*—Pain on endrange stretch of involved muscle or ligament	• Radiography not required for diagnosis. • With significant trauma or for med/legal purposes, radiographs may be required. • For specifics see radiographic guidelines.	• Myofascial therapy. • Limited orthotic support. • Ergonomic advice. • Preventive exercises and stretches (e.g., spinal stabilization exercises).
Neuritis or Radiculitis Due to Disc	• Requires hard neurological evidence of nerve root dysfunction. • Requires special imaging confirmation.	*Trauma*—Often Hx of similar events with resolution; major or minor trauma possible *Radiation of pain*—Often into arm/hand *Pain radiation with Valsalva-type activities*—Possible *Worse with Specific ROM*—Variable; may be related to disc protrusion	*Ortho*—Nerve compression or stretch tests positive (e.g., upper limb tension test) *Neuro*—Deficit in corresponding dermatome, myotome, and DTR *Active ROM*—Variable; weakness more in related upper limb muscle(s) *Passive ROM*—Variable	• Radiography may help initially in differentiating stenosis and disc. • MRI or electrodiagnostic studies may be needed after one month without resolution or if progressive.	• Emphasis may be placed more on "soft" techniques such as activator or traction. • Limited orthotic support. • When subacute, begin spinal stabilization.

(continues)

Neck Diagnosis Table (continued)

Diagnosis	Comments	History Findings	Positive Examination Findings	Radiography/Special Studies	Treatment Options
Non-Specific Cervical Spine Pain	• Used for patients with evidence of a myofascial cause. • Also used for patients without Hx of recent trauma. • May be used for unspecified neck pain.	*Trauma*—Not recent *Radiation of pain*—May radiate into shoulder or arm to hand *Pain radiation with Valsalva-type activities*—No *Worse with Specific ROM*—Variable	*Ortho*—None positive, however, may reproduce local symptoms *Neuro*—None (although patient may have neurological complaints such as numbness) *Active ROM*—Variable *Passive ROM*—Variable	• Radiography not necessary. • May be used to access biomechanical status or predisposition. • See PCCW Radiographic Guidelines.	• Myofascial therapy • Limited orthotic support • Ergonomic advice • Preventive exercises and stretches (e.g., spinal stabilization exercises)
Neuritis or Radiculitis Unspecified	• Used in cases where there are radicular signs/symptoms. However, not enough evidence to pinpoint disc vs other causes. • Used with radicular signs/symptoms where no specific nerve root is clearly involved.	*Trauma*—Variable presentation *Radiation of pain*—May radiate down shoulder and arm *Pain radiation with Valsalva-type activities*—Possible *Worse with specific ROM*—Variable	*Ortho*—Nerve compression or stretch tests positive (e.g., upper limb tension test) *Neuro*—Deficit in corresponding dermatome, myotome, and DTR *Active ROM*—Variable weakness *Passive ROM*—Variable	• Radiography may help in differentiating stenosis and disc. • MRI or electrodiagnostic studies may be needed after one month without resolution or if progressive.	• Limited orthotic support • Myofascial therapy • When subacute, begin deep flexor strengthening
Cervicobrachial Syndrome	• Used when neck pain with radiation is not radicular but referred.	*Trauma*—Variable presentation *Radiation of pain*—May radiate down shoulder and arm *Pain radiation with Valsalva-type activities*—No *Worse with specific ROM*—Variable	*Ortho*—Nerve compression or stretch tests negative *Neuro*—None *Active ROM*—Variable *Passive ROM*—Variable	• None needed initially.	• Limited orthotic support • Myofascial therapy • When subacute, begin deep flexor strengthening
Facet Syndrome	• Should be reserved for neck pain increased with hyperextension posture or movement (acute or chronic) with local pain.	*Trauma*—Variable *Radiation of pain*—Often into hand, or upper back *Pain radiation with Valsalva-type activities*—May be painful *Worse with Specific ROM*—hyperextension and rotation increases local or radiating pain	*Ortho*—Positions of rotation and/or hyperextension maneuvers may increase symptoms *Neuro*—None *Active ROM*—Variable *Passive ROM*—Variable *Motion palpation*—Endrange restriction to side of involved facet	• Radiography may be useful for determining biomechanical predispositions.	• Myofascial therapy • Limited orthotic support • Ergonomic advice • Preventive exercises and stretches • Avoid hyperextension/rotation
Thoracic Outlet Syndrome (TOS)	• Should be used only when TOS testing reproduces patient's complaint.	*Onset*—Traumatic onset in 40% of cases *Radiation of Pain/Neuro Symptoms*—Generally on medial aspect of arm (lower brachial plexus)	*Ortho*—Several provocative positions may reproduce symptoms: Adson's, Halstead's, Wright's, and Roos' tests	• Cervical spine films may reveal cervical ribs, however, this is not pathognomonic for TOS.	• Myofascial therapy • Preventive exercises and stretches • Postural training

Temporomandibular Complaints

# CHAPTER 3

Context

Although often viewed as the domain of the specialist, many temporomandibular joint (TMJ) disorders may be sufficiently screened and managed by the chiropractor. If the TMJ is conceptually approached like any other synovial joint, most common problems can be detected. These problems include synovitis, capsulitis, disc (meniscal) derangement, tendinitis, arthritis, and associated myofascial involvement. The complexity arises when multiple factors with regard to dentition occur. Comprehensive, yet cumbersome, approaches such as the craniomandibular index (74 separate items) generally are impractical and are not weighted toward items of most importance. Screening procedures are sufficient and can provide a baseline determination of the degree of involvement without sacrificing thoroughness.

Ambiguous terminology has always hampered discussions of TMJ disorders. In general, it is important to view (no matter what the terminology) TMJ conditions as intraarticular and extraarticular. Extraarticular involvement may range from cervical spine involvement (myofascial, postural, subluxation-related dysfunction) to dental abnormalities or pathologies. Some practitioners refer to the dysfunctional cervical spine–TMJ relationship as a TMJ syndrome. Intraarticular disorders center around familiar problems such as synovitis and capsulitis with a focus on the articular disc, which is often displaced or degenerated.

One study suggests that 85% to 90% of individuals will develop some TMJ-related symptom in their lifetime.[1] It appears that women are affected more commonly than men. Using a temporomandibular disorder (TMD) questionnaire, Nornura et al.[2] found that in a group of students, 53% showed some level of TMD, 36% had mild TMD, 12% had moderate, and 5.5% had severe TMD.

In evaluating the severe responders, women were about nine times more affected than men. Interestingly, many showing any level of TMD considered themselves tense people, clenched or ground their teeth, and reported clicking of the TMJ. Sixty-five percent reported frequent headaches and 61% had neck pain. Unfortunately, studies have shown a poor response to TMJ management, in the range of only 4% to 36%. An interesting subgroup of patients are professional violin and viola players who seem to have a higher than average predisposition toward TMJ problems.[3] Although osteoarthritis of the TMJ obviously is more prevalent in the elderly population, signs and symptoms of craniomandibular disorders tend to decrease in the elderly.[4] Although the TMJ may be the source of local pain, it has been accused of being a primary referral source for both neck and ear pain.[5]

Some additional complaints related to TMJ dysfunction include:

- Headache
- Ear pain
- Ipsilateral face pain
- TMJ pain on opening and closing the mouth
- Joint sounds
- Mandibular excursion restrictions
- Tinnitus/congestion/vertigo
- Neck stiffness
- Sinus congestion

Chronic headache unresponsive to treatment is a difficult scenario. First on the list of possibilities should be temporomandibular joint (TMJ) disorders.[6-8] Overlap with clinical indicators of tension-like headache is common. Some differentials include tenderness of the pterygoids, tenderness of the TMJ, clicking in the TMJ, and abnormal mandibular movement patterns on opening and closing.[6]

General Strategy

History

- Determine whether the patient's complaint is one of pain, clicking/popping, crepitus, inability to open fully, or fatigue with chewing.
- Determine whether there is any history of direct trauma, episodes of jaw locking, whiplash injuries, past diagnoses of an arthritis, or significant dental pathology.
- Determine whether there are other signs or symptoms suggestive of an underlying arthritis.
- Attempt to distinguish between an intraarticular and extraarticular problem.

Evaluation

- Determine dental status.
- Measure all aspects of mandibular gait.
- Perform provocative maneuvers of stretch (capsulitis), compression (synovitis), and contraction (myofascial).
- Palpate common tender areas indicating sites for specific, commonly involved structures.
- Radiographs are not helpful; magnetic resonance imaging (MRI) may be of benefit; however, it should be reserved for patients who have severe pain or are not responsive to several months of conservative care.

Management

- Management is multifactorial. Address myofascial issues with trigger-point massage, and muscle hyperactivity or hypertonicity with myofascial release techniques. Address compressive retrodiscal problems with a splint or stretching and breaking up adhesions with short-amplitude thrusts (except in those cases listed below).
- Refer patients to a dentist who specializes in TMJ problems if dental involvement is significant, an acute lock cannot be reduced, or treatment for chronic pain is unsuccessful. Refer to a medical doctor if fracture is suspected.

Relevant Anatomy and Biomechanics

The TMJ is best visualized by using both anterior-to-posterior and lateral-to-medial perspectives (**Figures 3–1** and **3–2**). These perspectives will assist when conceptualizing function and dysfunction. It is easiest to view the TMJ as a two-joint compartment. The

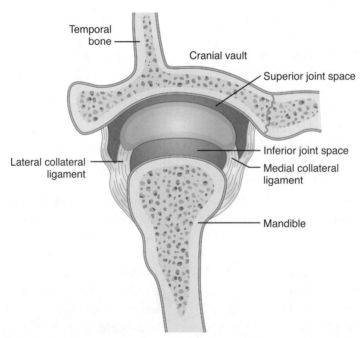

Figure 3–1 Frontal view of the TMJ showing the ligaments that tether the disc atop the condyle, dividing the TMJ space into two parts.

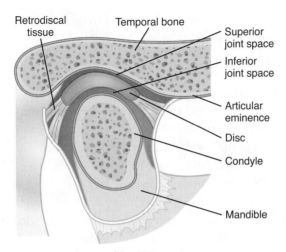

Figure 3–2 Lateral view of the TMJ.

superior compartment is bordered by the articular surface of the eminence of the temporal bone superiorly and the articular disc inferiorly. The superior compartment's function is to allow and govern linear movement or translation. The inferior compartment is bordered by the inferior surface of the articular disc and the superior surface of the condyle. The inferior compartment permits full rotary (open and closing) motion of the mandibular condyle if the condyle is seated under the articular disc. The articular disc, separating the TMJ into the superior and inferior compartments, is a necessary component for smooth jaw movement. If the disc is either degenerated or displaced (or both), limitation or popping/clicking of jaw movement will occur. The posterior attachment to the disc is the retrodiscal tissue. Although these two structures are connected, their composition and function are quite different. The disc is a biconcave structure consisting of dense fibrous connective tissue and, as such, is not vascularized or pain sensitive. The retrodiscal tissue, however, is mainly a large venous plexus covered with synovial membrane. It is well innervated and therefore a likely source of some TMJ pain. When irritated, the retrodiscal tissue is capable of producing synovial effusion.

The TMJ has a rich arterial supply arising from the branches of the anterior tympanic artery, the deep temporal artery, the auricular posterior artery, the transverse facial artery, the middle meningeal artery, and the maxillary artery. Of note is that the superficial temporal artery and the maxillary artery run along the lateral and medial sides of the condylar neck and may be at risk from soft tissue procedures or surgery for the TMJ.[9]

The disc is connected and stabilized by the collateral discal ligaments. Together with the capsular ligaments,

they are important in guaranteeing combined movement of the disc and condyle during jaw movement. Elongation or damage disengages this coupling and may allow anterior displacement of the disc.

A discussion of normal opening and closing of the jaw will illustrate the need for a balance among several structures to accomplish smooth and painless movement. As the mouth opens, there is relaxation of the closing muscles (mainly temporalis and masseters). After about 1 cm of opening, the inferior head of the external pterygoid muscle pulls on both the disc and the condyle. With the hyoid bone stabilized by the supra- and infrahyoid muscles, the digastric muscle helps pull the mandible downward and backward toward the end of opening. Rotation occurs primarily in the first third of opening. This movement occurs primarily between the inferior articular disc surface and the condylar head. Rotational movement is limited by tautness of the outer oblique band of the temporomandibular ligament. Further opening results in translation down the slope of the articular eminence to the point at which the condyle is slightly past the center of the eminence. During closing, the inferior head remains silent while the superior head of the pterygoid muscle stabilizes the disc and condyle as they translate posteriorly. The muscles that are primarily involved are the temporalis and masseter. Limitation of posterior movement of the condyle is provided, in part, by the inner horizontal band of the temporomandibular ligament.

Lateral movement of the mandible is caused by contraction of the ipsilateral temporalis and masseter muscles and contralateral contraction of the medial and lateral pterygoid muscles. Protrusion is the result of forward movement of the condyles through contraction of the lateral pterygoid muscle combined with forward mandible movement caused by contraction of the masseter and medial pterygoid muscles.

Abnormal movement may be asymptomatic or result in pain, popping/clicking, or crepitus. One of the most common functional problems with the TMJ is anterior displacement of the articular disc. When this occurs, the condylar head is positioned behind the posterior band of the disc. When viewed from the side, the articular disc looks like a stretched-out red blood cell. There is a thicker anterior band, a thin intermediate band, and a thickened posterior band. Normally, the condylar head rests in between the anterior and posterior bands in the depression formed by the intermediate area. This position is maintained from a closed-mouth to an open-mouth position. With anterior displacement, the condyle's starting position is behind the posterior band. With opening, if the condyle can override the posterior band to reach the intermediate area, a pop is often heard. When the pop is heard or felt close to full opening, marked anterior displacement and posterior ligament deterioration are suggested.[11] This characteristic pop is an indicator of anterior disc displacement with reduction. The condyle retains its normal position until full closing, when often it is again pulled back behind the posterior band of the disc. This may cause a pop or click, referred to as a reciprocal click. When the condylar head cannot reduce into the intermediate disc depression on opening, no pop is heard. This functional derangement is referred to as a closed lock. This unreduced displacement is referred to as a *lock* because condylar translation is limited by the disc–condyle relationship, preventing full opening. An open lock may occur when the condylar head extends far past the articular eminence and is not able to return posteriorly.

Although injury may be acute, many of the TMJ's problems are the result of chronic biomechanical dysrelationships. These may be complex, involving abnormalities of bone development or occlusal problems, yet many complaints are, at least in part, due to the indirect effects of soft tissue problems. As in any other joint, the capsule and ligaments are susceptible to acute or chronic stretching to the point that they no longer provide stability. In acute-stretch scenarios, further stretch often increases pain. One of the most common causes of overstretching of the capsule and ligaments is a distended joint. If this is a chronic process, the capsule and ligaments may be left in a poorly functioning overstretched position leading to hypermobility of the TMJ.

The pain-sensitive retrodiscal area is susceptible to compression. Both the compression itself and the resulting synovial fluid reaction that increases pressure in the joint may cause pain. Externally applied compression often increases the pain in this scenario. Compression of the retrodiscal tissue may be due to a number of reasons; however, there are some common culprits, as follows:

- Condylar compression due to anterior disc displacement, which forces the condyle posteriorly.
- A hypertonic temporalis muscle (posterior fibers) may pull the condyle back posteriorly.
- The vertical height of the teeth, when diminished (loss of teeth or attrition), causes the condyle to be displaced up and back into the retrodiscal material.
- A blow (or an overly aggressive adjustment) to the mandible in a superior/posterior direction may jam the condyle into the retrodiscal tissue.

Evaluation

History

It is important to determine any direct or indirect trauma to the TMJ (**Table 3–1**). Direct blows to the jaw can stretch or compress the same-side TMJ. A blow to the front of the jaw driving the jaw directly back will cause more of a compressive injury with a reactive synovitis. A blow to the lateral jaw may stretch the joint capsule, resulting in a capsulitis or disc derangement. Microtrauma may occur as a result of bruxism. Bruxism may be evident to the patient if he or she notices it during the day; however, if bruxism occurs at night, the patient may be unaware of grinding the teeth. A sleep partner may provide the answer.

If the patient has had a diagnosis of an inflammatory arthritis, such as rheumatoid arthritis, ankylosing spondylitis, psoriatic arthritis, Reiter's syndrome, or lupus erythematosus, it is likely that the TMJ pain is due to an inflammatory process. Patients with local infections such as measles, mumps, or infectious mononucleosis are similarly affected.

Asking about provocative maneuvers may help narrow the list:

- Clicking and popping—If the jaw clicks on opening, a disc displacement with reduction is often the cause; this occurs as the translating condyle slips into its normal position under the posterior edge of the disc; a closing click indicates that a weakened posterior ligament is failing to retract the disc.
- Locking—There are two general types of lock: (1) If the patient simply cannot open fully (closed lock), the disc is probably anterior to the condyle during jaw opening (recapture not possible). (2) If the patient is unable to close the mouth (open lock), the anterior condyle has dislocated; this may occur as the result of excessive joint laxity or blunt trauma.
- Pain with excessive opening—This is the hallmark of a capsulitis; additional accompanying complaints are pain with contralateral chewing and protrusion or lateral excursion of the mandible.
- Pain with chewing—The first possibility is a dental disorder; when the TMJ is involved, a synovitis is likely; this may be due to atypical chewing habits, chronic gum chewing, or any impact injury; the

Table 3–1 History Questions for Temporomandibular Joint Disorders

Primary Question	What Are You Thinking?	Secondary Questions	What Are You Thinking?
Was there a direct blow to the jaw?	Fracture, disc derangement, synovitis, capsulitis	Did you have a blow to the front of the jaw (directly back)? Did you have a blow to the outside of the jaw?	Fracture, synovitis, disc derangement Same-side capsulitis; opposite-side synovitis
Does your jaw lock?	Closed lock, acute open lock	Is the lock felt as a block to full opening? Does the jaw lock in full opening?	Closed lock (recapture of condyle to disc not possible) Anterior dislocation of condyle (often due to hypermobility of TMJ)
Is the complaint more one of popping or clicking?	Disc displacement, adhesions	Is there an opening and closing pop? Is there grinding or popping throughout opening or closing?	Disc displacement Adhesions
Is the pain worse when opening the mouth wide?	Capsulitis, hypermobility of TMJ	Did you have either a whiplash injury or a prolonged dental procedure? Do you often yawn widely?	Sudden or prolonged stretching of capsule leading to capsulitis Possible chronic stretching of capsule leading to hypermobility of TMJ
Is the pain worse with chewing?	Dental pathology, TMJ synovitis	Is the pain worse with cold, hot, or sweet foods? Is it worse when biting down on one side?	Dental pathology Same-side synovitis (ask about chronic gum chewing, grinding teeth at night, or habit of chewing on one side)
Are there other joints that hurt?	Referral from cervical spine, rheumatoid arthritis (RA), rheumatoid variants, connective tissue disease	Do you have cervical spine pain or headaches? Have you had a past diagnosis of another arthritis? Do your fingers or knees also hurt? Does your low back hurt (point to sacroiliac joint) or do your heels hurt?	Possible referral to TMJ (check for forward head position) More common with inflammatory arthritides Possible RA Reiter's syndrome, ankylosing spondylitis
Are there current signs of local or systemic infection?	Acute otitis media, measles, mumps, or mononucleosis	Do you have associated ear pain? Do you have sore throat and fatigue? Do you have swelling of the outer cheeks?	Ear infection Possible mononucleosis Mumps

patient may notice that he or she cannot close fully on the involved side so that the teeth touch.

Questioning the individual regarding associated neck pain, postural habits with regard to work and sleep, and any previous neck injuries may help establish a more myofascial or referred cause in those patients without specific complaints of clicking, popping, locking, or pain with chewing.

Examination

Examination of the TMJ focuses on two main bodies of information: (1) mandibular "gait" analysis with auscultation, and (2) palpation combined with provocative maneuvers including compressive, stretch, and contractile challenge. Secondary evaluation focuses on possible involvement of dental and cervical spine contributions.

The degree of opening is measured in two ways. One is measurement with a ruler (in millimeters). The other approach is to use the patient's own knuckles as a patient-specific (accounts for patient size) approach. The general rule of thumb is that if the patient can open two or two and a half knuckles' width, range of motion is considered normal. Less than two knuckles suggests hypomobility; an opening of three or more knuckles suggests hypermobility. It must be remembered that a hypermobile joint may be the result of posterior ligament stretching over a prolonged period of time.[12]

Mandibular gait analysis attempts to document visual range of motion on a cross-hair diagram. Measurement is made with a transparent straight-edge ruler in millimeters. With the horizontal line as an x-axis, laterotrusion (lateral movement to the left and right) from a starting position of neutral with the mouth closed may be documented. The vertical or y-axis line is used to document both maximum opening distance and deviation upon opening. An X placed next to the vertical line indicates a point at which clicking, crepitus, or pain occurs. Small notes indicating whether the clicking is on opening or variable should be added. The vertical line above the intersection point on the diagram represents the z-axis and is used to document the degree of protrusion of the jaw.

Muscle/tendon involvement is determined through the traditional approaches of palpation and contraction. There are distinct areas of tenderness that may correlate with involved structures. The masseter muscle may house several tender areas. The tendinous area is palpated under the zygomatic arch. Posterior to this are the deep vertical fibers of the masseter. The belly of the masseter is palpated just above the angle of the jaw. Cautious palpation should be used over the posterolateral aspect of the masseter because of the overlying parotid gland. Temporalis trigger points are not uncommon and often are found in a halo array above the ear in the belly of the muscle.

General testing of jaw opening and closing may give clues to muscle involvement due to an increased pain response. Resisting the patient's attempt at opening may cause pain when the inferior heads of the pterygoid muscles are involved. Resisted closing is accomplished by using a padded gauze contact over the incisors. Pain production implicates either the temporalis or masseter muscle.

Palpation of the TMJ should be performed both anterior and posterior to the tragus. Anterior to the tragus, a small depression is formed with jaw opening. Using a finger to palpate this depression, the examiner asks the patient to open and close the mouth. What may be appreciated is whether there is too much or too little condyle translation. Tenderness in the pretragus depression is an indicator of inflammation. Guided by the external auditory meatus to gain access to the posterior aspect of the TMJ, the examiner inserts a gloved fifth finger with the fingernail facing posteriorly. The patient is then asked to open and close slowly. The examiner may appreciate clicking or popping. If clicking or popping is felt, the examiner focuses on the involved joint and asks the patient to repeat opening until a pop or click is appreciated. Before closing, a tongue blade is placed between the teeth. The opening and closing sequence is repeated to determine whether the clicking or popping can be eliminated. If so, the disc has been recaptured, suggesting a mechanical cause of anterior disc displacement that may respond to a dental appliance. Tenderness on full closure suggests an inflamed posterior joint. Tongue blades placed posteriorly may reduce this tenderness.

One study by Kobs et al.[13] indicated that diagnosing anterior disc displacement clinically is not always possible. Special imaging is needed. This conflicts with an earlier study by Usumez et al.[14] In their study, MRI was used as the gold standard. The diagnostic accuracy overall was 83% for determining a normal disc–condyle relationship, 72% for diagnosing anterior disc displacement with reduction, and 81% for diagnosing anterior disc displacement without reduction. They conclude that not all patients with TMD symptoms require MRI.

Stretch testing is used to determine whether capsular irritation is present (**Figure 3–3**). An intraoral contact may be used to distract the mandible down and forward. An increase in pain is suggestive of capsular irritation. Compression testing is used to provoke pain

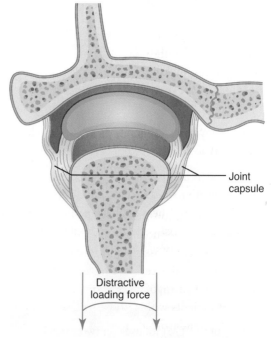

Figure 3–3 Stretch testing for capsular irritation.

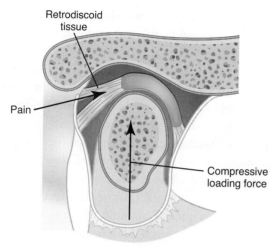

Figure 3–4 Compression testing for synovitis.

when synovitis is present (**Figure 3–4**). Pressure on the mandible in a superior posterior direction is likely to increase pain when the retrodiscal tissue is inflamed or a synovitis is present.

Postural evaluation is an important component of TMJ evaluation. The most common postural abnormality is a forward head position with a compensatory extension of the head to correct for visual requirements. Although the initial flexion component of the forward head position causes the mandible to translate down and forward, the compensatory extension forces the mandible posteriorly, potentially irritating the retrodiscal tissue.

Radiographic evaluation of TMJ disorders may be valuable when TMJ tomograms are employed. Standard radiography of the joint rarely provides any additional information. However, two studies indicate that the addition of tomogram findings had a significant effect on clinical decision making. The most common findings that influenced either diagnosis or treatment decisions were unanticipated osseous changes and unexpected condylar position.[15, 16]

Management

Several recent publications have demonstrated that some TMJ complaints can be successfully managed through a myofascial approach. One randomized study[17] evaluated in a private-practice setting the value of intraoral myofascial therapy or myofascial therapy plus exercise and advice for patients with TMJ pain. This research study utilized a standardized approach that included intraoral therapy to the pterygoids, temporalis, and a

technique called the sphenopalatine ganglion technique. Home exercises were also standardized and added to the management of half of the patients. The results indicate that intraoral myofascial therapy or intraoral myofascial therapy plus exercise and advice are superior to a control wait-and-see group. At a one-year follow-up, the groups with combined therapy of myofascial therapy plus exercise/advice had more success. Specific protocols are illustrated in the full-text article.

Osteopathic manual therapy was compared to standard conventional care of TMJ problems in a small randomized controlled trial.[18] Although patients in both groups improved, the group receiving osteopathic manual therapy required significantly less medication (nonsteroidal medication and muscle relaxants).

In a small randomized control trial,[19] researchers concluded that myofascial therapy to the muscles of mastication combined with the use of an occlusal splint led to an increase in mandibular ROM similar to a comparison asymptomatic group of patients.

One of the key distinctions in the determination of the appropriateness of TMJ adjustment (manipulation) is whether the joint is inflamed or whether there are adhesions. Compressive adjustments to an inflamed joint may provoke more pain. Adhesions are likely when the patient has opening clicks. The adjustment suggested by Curl and Saghafi[20] is to have the patient open to the point of the click. At this point the examiner loads the TMJ with a superior/anterior compression. A quick, small-amplitude thrust is then delivered parallel to the slope of the articular eminence. When the patient has an acute closed lock (not able to open fully, however, no joint clicking or popping) a distraction or gapping maneuver is used. The force is applied 90° to the slope of the articular eminence in an inferior posterior direction.

Splints are one form of conservative treatment with TMJ disorders. Splints should be considered as adjunctive therapy for TMJ disorders, given the observation that they are often no better than placebo.[21] There is a vast array of simple and complex splint products. In general, they are divided into hard and soft splints. The two types of hard splints are full occlusion or pivotal. Hard, full-occlusion splints are used for repositioning or stabilization. Repositioning splints attempt to alter the condylar position whereas stabilization splints do not alter dental alignment. Sato et al.[22] demonstrated in a small study group that 42% of patients with nonreducing TMJ disc displacement who opted for no treatment had resolution. Those treated with a stabilization splint had a 55% success rate. Those patients who did not have resolution naturally or respond to stabilization splinting after 19 months benefited most from surgery, with a success rate of 77%. Pivotal splints potentially are harmful and are rarely used.

In another study by Wassell et al.[23] a lower stabilizing splint was compared to a nonoccluding control. At six weeks, both splints provided similar relief. Those who preferred the nonoccluding (and switched over) were generally older and had more clicking in their TMJs. In total, 80% of the TMD patients were managed successfully using splinting.

Soft splints are used for protection and therefore are commonly used with a patient who grinds the teeth. The soft splints are similar to mouth guards made out of a latex type material. It appears that the use of a soft splint may be a helpful initial approach to patients with myofascial involvement of the temporalis or masseter muscle.[24, 25] The soft splint does not seem to cause occlusal changes. The most popular daytime soft splint is the Aqualizer. It is inexpensive and easy to use.

Surgery is often offered as an alternative for patients with chronic TMJ disc derangement. Although there are numerous approaches, three specific surgical treatments were compared to nonsurgical treatment with regard to pain reduction and long-term effects.[21] These surgical techniques included discoplasty, discectomy without replacement, and discectomy with replacement of the disc with a Teflon implant. The long-term success rate was between 52% and 71%; however, there was a very high incidence of osteoarthritis development (93% to 100% in the discectomy groups).

Algorithm

An algorithm for evaluation of TMJ complaints is presented in **Figure 3–5**.

Annotations

A. Always evaluate the cervical spine and head posture with regard to TMJ complaints. Forward head position or cervical dysfunction may affect TMJ function or cause referred pain.

B. Plain film radiographs are virtually useless, except perhaps for fracture. Tomograms have limited use. 3-D volume acquisition techniques with MRI are the most sensitive. Coronal images may be necessary if the integrity of the capsule or ligaments is believed compromised.

C. Open lock usually is the result of trauma or hypermobility of the TMJ. (See text for maneuver.)

D. Anterior disc displacement requires the condyle to snap past the posterior part of the disc to the intermediate area, causing a click. If a tongue blade eliminates clicking, the disc is recaptured. Consider use of dental appliance or specific adjustive maneuver (i.e., superior/anterior load and thrust).

E. Disc displacement with reduction causes a click also on closing as the condyle snaps back to the posterior aspect of the disc.

F. Acute closed lock indicates that the condyle cannot pass over the posterior aspect of the disc to reach the intermediate area. A distractive or gapping maneuver may be used.

G. Capsulitis due to trauma associated with marked swelling may indicate an underlying fracture.

H. Synovitis may be traumatic or the result of posterior displacement of the condyle due to anterior disc displacement, loss of vertical height of teeth, or a hypertonic temporalis muscle.

I. Tendinitis and trigger points may be found by increased tenderness in the belly and tendons of the masseter and temporalis.

J. Arthritides that should be considered are rheumatoid arthritis, psoriatic, Reiter's syndrome, ankylosing spondylitis, lupus, Lyme disease, and connective tissue disorders.

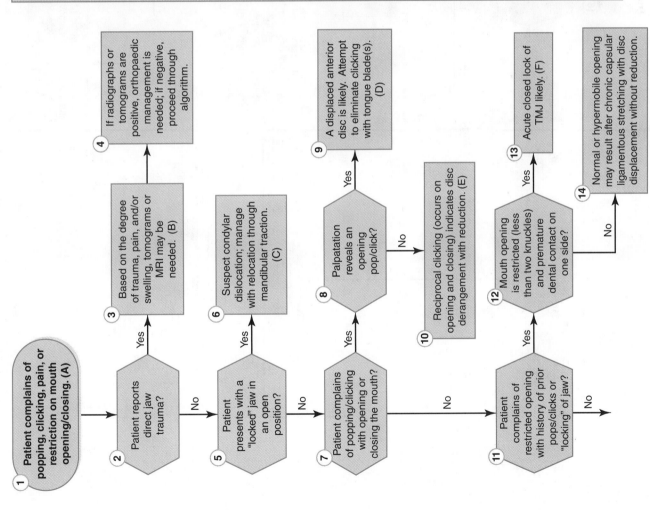

Figure 3–5 Evaluation of Temporomandibular Joint Complaints—Algorithm

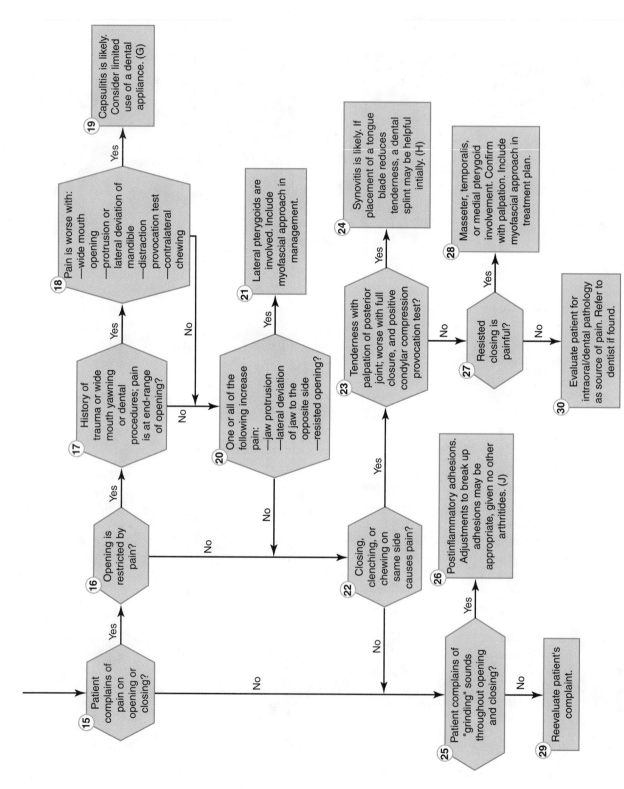

Figure 3–5 (Continued)

Selected TMJ Disorders

Capsulitis

Classic Presentation

The patient complains of pain or tenderness at the TMJ, especially with protrusion or lateral movement, chewing on the opposite side, or opening the mouth widely. There may be a history of trauma; however, most often there is not.

Cause

Overstretching of the capsule may be due to numerous causes, including wide yawning or dental procedures requiring prolonged wide opening. Microtrauma from poor chewing habits or occlusal problems may stretch and irritate the capsule.

Examination

Movements or positions that stretch the capsule often will increase pain. A condylar stretch test (pushing the mandible forward with the mouth open) may increase the pain (Figure 3–3), as will lateral deviation of the jaw to the opposite side, and wide mouth opening. Having the patient chew on the opposite side may also increase the discomfort.

Management

Avoidance of provoking maneuvers coupled with attention to proper dentition and re-education of jaw opening and chewing usually will resolve the problem. Ice and rest are used in the early stages.

Synovitis

Classic Presentation

The patient complains of TMJ pain that is worse with full closure on the ipsilateral side.

Cause

Either acute direct trauma or chronic malposition may cause synovitis of the posterior TMJ. Common causes of posterior displacement of the condyle are loss of vertical height of the teeth, anterior disc displacement, and a hypertonic temporalis muscle.

Examination

Condylar compression (Figure 3–4) by the examiner will often increase pain on the side of involvement. There may be lateral deviation to the opposite side with the mandible in the rest position. While palpating the posterior joint through the external auditory meatus, tenderness is increased on full closure. Using tongue blades, a distraction force is introduced. As the patient bites down, tenderness may decrease with one or two tongue blades placed between the teeth. Another approach is to have the patient open until a click or pop is heard, indicating an anteriorly displaced disc. A tongue blade is placed between the teeth and the patient is asked to open and close. Additional tongue blades may be added in an attempt to eliminate the click, indicating recapture of the disc.

Management

If the tongue blade addition eliminates or decreases the pain or clicking, a stabilization appliance may be useful.[26] During the acute stage of synovitis, the use of mild analgesics, ice, and a soft diet with relaxation of the masticatory muscles will be helpful. If adhesions have formed as a result of chronic synovitis, adjustive maneuvers along the slope of the articular eminence may free up movement and decrease pain.

Disc Derangement with Reduction

Classic Presentation

The patient complains of popping or clicking while opening and closing the mouth.

Cause

When the articular disc is displaced anteriorly or anteromedially, the condylar head rests posterior to the disc. An opening click occurs as the condyle translates into its normal central disc location. The closing click occurs because of weakness of the posterior ligament. The disc is not pulled backward, and the condyle slips into a posterior position behind the disc.

Evaluation

Palpation in front of or inside the ear will detect the opening and closing clicks. An attempt to reduce the click can be made through the use of tongue blades. After the opening click occurs, a tongue blade or blades can be placed between the posterior teeth on the same side. If the patient closes down on the blades and no click or pop is heard or felt, reduction has occurred, indicating an underlying disc derangement.

Management

A dental appliance may help prevent displacement of the condylar head posteriorly; however, this is a temporary solution. When adhesions are present, Saghafi and Curl[27] suggest using a quick, short-amplitude thrust maneuver. The patient opens until the click is felt. To stabilize the disc and condyle together, the doctor applies an axial compression through the angle of the jaw in a superior and anterior direction. Short-impulse thrusts can then be delivered along the slope of the articular eminence in a posterior superior direction.

Closed Lock

Classic Presentation

The patient complains of difficulty opening the mouth fully. There is pain and tenderness at the TMJ without current popping, although there may have been a history of prior popping on opening and/or closing. There may be an additional complaint of suboccipital pain, dysphagia, or tinnitus.

Cause

An anteriorly displaced (sometimes referred to as dislocated) articular disc is usually the cause. The condyle cannot translate to the intermediate portion of the disc. This may be due to hypermobility at the joint or trauma such as whiplash injury.[28] Often there is premature dental contact on the same side as disc displacement.

Examination

There often is tenderness at the TMJ and the patient is unable to open fully. He or she is unable to place two knuckles in between the front teeth. There is no popping on opening. The end-feel usually is soft. Overpressure is uncomfortable but usually not very painful.

Management

Manipulation is the treatment of choice. Several maneuvers are described in the literature. Curl[29] summarizes these gapping maneuvers into three main groups: (1) downward traction with a thrust 90° to the slope of the articular eminence, (2) forward traction of the condyle under the disc, and (3) gapping with active movement by the patient. Sedative or relaxation approaches often will assist these maneuvers. Contraindications include processes that would weaken the structure of the mandible or teeth, such as tumor, infection, periodontal disease, osteoporosis, fracture, or extreme muscle splinting.

Acute Open Lock

Classic Presentation

The patient presents with an acute locking of the jaw when it is fully open. The patient is extremely apprehensive. Pain is often due to the reactive spasm of the closing muscle. There may be history of trauma or previous occurrences when the mouth was opened too far.

Cause

Either trauma or hypermobility allows the condyle to be dislocated anterior to the articular eminence.

Examination

The patient presentation is pathognomonic: an apprehensive patient unable to close his or her mouth. If direct trauma has occurred, radiographs for fracture may be necessary.

Management

Bilateral manipulation with a downward traction is necessary to relocate the condyle.

APPENDIX 3–1

References

1. Solberg WK. Epidemiological findings of importance to management of temporomandibular disorders. In: Clark GT, Solberg WK, eds. *Perspectives in Temporomandibular Disorders.* Chicago: Quintessence; 1987:27–41.

2. Nomura K, Vitti M, Oliveira AS, et al. Use of the Fonseca's questionnaire to assess the prevalence and severity of temporomandibular disorders in Brazilian dental undergraduates. *Braz Dent J.* 2007;18(2):163–167.

3. Kovero O, Konomen M. Signs and symptoms of temporomandibular disorders and radiographically observed abnormalities in the condyles of the temporomandibular joints of professional violin and viola players. *Acta Odontol Scand.* 1995;53:81–84.

4. Ow RK, Loh T, Neo J, Khoo J. Symptoms of craniomandibular disorders among elderly people. *J Oral Rehabil.* 1995;22:413–419.

5. Blake P, Thorburn N, Stewart IL. Temporomandibular joint dysfunction in children presenting as otalgia. *Clin Otolaryngol.* 1982;7:237–244.

6. Graff-Radford SB. Temporomandibular disorders and headache. *Dent Clin North Am.* 2007;51(1): 129–144, vi–vii.

7. Svensson P. Muscle pain in the head: overlap between temporomandibular disorders and tension-type headaches. *Curr Opin Neurol.* 2007;20(3):320–325.

8. Lupoli TA, Lockey RF. Temporomandibular dysfunction: an often overlooked cause of chronic headaches. *Ann Allergy Asthma Immunol.* 2007;99(4):314–318.

9. Cuccia AM, Caradonna C, Caradonna D, et al. The arterial blood supply of the temporomandibular joint: an anatomical study and clinical implications. *Imaging Sci Dent.* 2013;43(1):37–44.

10. Berhardt O, Gesch D, Schwahn C, et al. Risk factors for headache, including TMD signs and symptoms, and their impact on quality of life. Results of the Study of Health in Pomerania (SHIP). *Quintessence Int.* 2005;36(1):55–64.

11. Farar WB. Characteristics of the condylar path in internal derangements of the TMJ. *Prosthet Dent.* 1978;39:319.

12. Freidman NH, Anstendig HS, Weisberg J. Case report: treatment of a disc dysfunction. *J Clin Orthodont.* 1982;16:408.

13. Kobs G, Bernhardt O, Kocher T, Meyer G. Critical assessment of temporomandibular joint clicking in diagnosing anterior disc displacement. *Stomatologija.* 2005;7(1):28–30.

14. Usumez S, Oz F, Guray E. Comparison of clinical and magnetic resonance imaging diagnoses in patients with TMD history. *J Oral Rehabil.* 2004;31(1):52–56.

15. Pullinger AG, White SC. Efficacy of TMJ radiographs in terms of expected versus actual findings. *Oral Surg Oral Med Oral Pathol.* 1995;79:367–374.

16. White SC, Pullinger AG. Impact of TMJ radiographs on clinician decision making. *Oral Surg Oral Med Oral Pathol.* 1995;79:375–381.

17. Kalamir A, Bonello R, Graham P, Vitiello AL, Pollard H. Intraoral myofascial therapy for chronic myogenous temporomandibular disorder: a randomized controlled trial. *J Manipulative Physiol Ther.* 2012;35(1):26–37.

18. Cuccia AM, Caradonna C, Annunziata V, Caradonna D. Osteopathic manual therapy versus conventional conservative therapy in the treatment of temporomandibular disorders: a randomized controlled trial. *J Bodyw Mov Ther.* 2010;14(2):179–184.

19. de Paula Gomes CAF, Politti F, Andrade DA, et al. Effects of massage therapy and occlusal splint therapy on mandibular range of motion in individuals with temporomandibular disorder: a randomized clinical trial *J Manipulative Physiol Ther.* 2013;xx:1–6.

20. Curl DD, Saghafi D. Manual reduction of adhesion in the temporomandibular joint. *Chiro Tech.* 1995;7:22–29.

21. Curl DD. The temporomandibular joint. In: Lawrence DJ, Cassidy JD, McGregor M, et al., eds. *Advances in Chiropractic.* St. Louis, MO: Mosby-Year Book; 1995; 2:143–181.

22. Sato S, Kawamura H, Motegi K. Management of nonreducing temporomandibular joint disk displacement: evaluation of three treatments. *Oral Surg Oral Med Oral Pathol.* 1995;80:384–388.

23. Wassell RW, Adams N, Kelly PJ. Treatment of temporomandibular disorders by stabilising splints in general dental practice: results after initial treatment. *Br Dent J.* 2004;197(1):35–41;discussion 31;quiz 50–31.

24. Wright E, Anderson G, Schulte J. A randomized clinical trial of intraoral soft splints and palliative treatment for masticatory pain. *J Orofac Pain.* 1995;9:192–199.

25. Visser A, Naieje M, Hansson TL. The temporal/masseter co-contraction: an electromyographic and

clinical evaluation of short-term stabilization splint therapy in myogenous CMD patients. *J Oral Rehabil.* 1995;22:387–389.

26. Friedman M H. Screening procedures for temporomandibular disorders. *J Neuromusculoskelet Sys.* 1994;2:163–169.

27. Saghafi D, Curl DD. Chiropractic manipulation of anteriorly displaced temporomandibular disc with adhesion. *J Manipulative Physiol Ther.* 1995;18:98–104.

28. Weinberg S, La Pointe H. Cervical extension-flexion injury (whiplash) and internal derangement of the temporomandibular joint. *J Oral Maxillofac Surg.* 1987;45:653–656.

29. Curl DD. Acute closed lock of the temporomandibular joint: manipulation paradigm and protocol. *Chiro Tech.* 1991;3:13–18.

Thoracic Spine Complaints

Context

Interest in the thoracic spine is often overshadowed by the more dramatic presentations of low back and cervical spine pain. Radicular pain into the arms and legs and its consequent functional limitations call more attention to the respective cervical and lumbar spine sources. Disc herniation is less common, as is nerve root compression in the thoracic spine, partly because of the restricted movement and stability provided by the direct attachment to the rib cage. Thoracic pain is probably as common as cervical or lumbar pain; however, it is less dramatic, due more often to the chronic consequences of postural imbalances. The pain is often of a low-grade nature and therefore less worrisome to the patient. When acute pain does occur, it is usually the result of acute muscle spasm or compression fracture. Compression fractures are usually the result of axial loading from a fall on the buttocks or, in osteoporotic individuals, minor or less memorable trauma.

Often there may be an age-related occurrence of thoracic pain or deformity. In children and adolescents scoliosis and hyperkyphosis are concerns (scoliosis is discussed in Chapter 5). The differential approach to hyperkyphosis should attempt to distinguish between simply poor posture habits and growth plate abnormalities as seen with Scheuermann's disease. In adults, the effects of chronic postural strain from seated work environments are predominant. Also, it appears that the long-term consequences of idiopathic scoliosis are more likely to result in pain in middle-aged adults. With senior patients, the primary concern is compression fracture, often the result of osteoporosis (osteoporosis is discussed in Chapter 30).

Although the cervical and lumbar regions require an evaluation of the limb plexuses, the thoracic spine is not involved directly (except for T1-T2). The thoracic spinal cord, however, is the home of the nerve cell bodies of the sympathetic nervous system. This relationship has not gone unnoticed by the chiropractic profession. Anecdotal stories regarding improvement of "visceral" conditions abound. The questions that still need research answers are: Do these outcomes represent the normal course of these disorders? Is the pain "referred" pain (somatovisceral) and to what degree can sympathetic innervation to organs be affected by vertebral subluxation? A review article by Nansel and Szlazak[1] discusses some of these issues. From this review it appears that there are many local regulating factors that can compensate for more proximal sympathetic dysfunction. It would appear that a more reflex or referred phenomenon may be the cause of those conditions that respond to manipulation. More research is needed to compare chiropractic management of commonly reported responsive conditions such as asthma, peptic ulcer, reflux esophagitis, gallbladder disease, and various gastrointestinal and gynecologic disorders.

General Strategy

History

- Determine whether the patient's complaint is one of pain, stiffness, midscapular fatigue, deformity, or a combination of complaints.
- Screen the patient for red flags such as a history of cancer, significant trauma, use of corticosteroids, or a history of infection suggestive of tuberculosis.
- Attempt to elicit a description of any inciting event or trauma, no matter how minor, if there is a history of sudden onset.

Examination

- Observe the patient for deformity: buffalo hump in the upper thoracic area (Cushing's syndrome), acute-angle kyphosis (compression fracture), kyphosis (Scheuermann's disease or postural), scoliosis (many causes; however, acute-angle painful scoliosis suggests osteoid osteoma or other local processes), and scapular winging (scoliosis or nerve damage causing weakness of the serratus anterior or trapezius muscle).

- Observe for skin lesions suggestive of herpes zoster (shingles) or skin cancer.
- Examine for active and passive range of motion and accessory motion.
- Perform a prone extension test on patients with a kyphosis to differentiate between a structural and a functional kyphosis.
- Perform an Adams' test (rib humping [angular rotation] suggests a structural curve) on patients with a scoliosis visible in the standing posture; also, observe the patient in the lying position in neutral and with maximum bending to the side of convexity (improvement indicates a functional component).
- Palpate and percuss the area in patients complaining of local pain.
- Remember that standard radiographs include anterior-to-posterior and lateral views; oblique films are used to evaluate the ribs for fracture and the vertebral bodies for trauma to the ring apophyses.
- Reserve special imaging, including bone scans and tomograms, for evaluation of metastatic lesions and osteoid osteoma or other tumors. Magnetic resonance imaging (MRI) is also helpful with spinal infection, tumor, and the rare disc herniation.

Management

- Patients with infection, primary tumor or metastasis, unstable fracture, severe or rapidly progressive scoliosis or kyphosis, and complications of corticosteroid use should be referred for medical evaluation and possible management.
- Patients with uncomplicated compression fractures, mild to moderate idiopathic scoliosis that is not rapidly progressing, uncomplicated Scheuermann's disease, facet syndrome, postural syndrome, T4 syndrome, and other mechanical causes should be managed conservatively. If unresponsive to care, further evaluation or referral for comanagement may be indicated.

Relevant Anatomy

The typical thoracic vertebrae are 2 through 8. They are heart-shaped bodies with shingle-like facets. The first thoracic vertebra is cervical-like, while the lower two thoracic vertebrae are more lumbar-like with a corresponding change in facet orientation. The typical vertebra has two attachment sites on the body for rib articulation. The costovertebral joint is at the intervertebral disc (IVD) of the typical vertebra, supported by a capsule and intrinsic radiate ligament. Another articulation occurs at the transverse process, with the tubercle of the rib supported by the costotransverse ligament. These ligaments are innervated by both the posterior primary rami and the anterior primary rami, indicating a neurologic priority for proprioceptive input. The superior costotransverse ligaments connect adjacent ribs. The thoracic kyphosis is a primary curve (as is the sacral angle). Thus, a structural kyphosis is created by the shape of the thoracic vertebrae, whereas in the cervical and lumbar regions the lordosis is acquired.

The facets are more shingle-like, overlapping at an angle of about 60° from the horizontal in the upper thoracics and up to 80° to 90° in the lower thoracics.[2] The medial branch of the dorsal rami supplies the joint capsules. The intervertebral discs are quite thin in the thoracic region. Innervation is from the sinuvertebral nerve. Nerve roots exit above the IVD, making nerve root compression from disc herniation less likely.

The muscles of the thoracic region may be divided generally into two types (**Figure 4–1**). The more superficial muscles such as the trapezius, rhomboids, levator scapulae, and latissimus dorsi are primarily extremity muscles assisting in direct movement of the arm or assisting through positioning of the scapulae. The deeper muscles act to extend the spine; they rotate segmentally and, to a lesser degree, flex laterally. Although the middle trapezius and rhomboids act directly on the scapulae, weakness allows forward displacement of the scapulae with a tendency toward an increased kyphosis.

There are some interesting neural connections between the thoracic spine and other regions:[3]

- Portions of the T1-T3(T4) nerve roots enter the brachial plexus, supplying the axillae and medial arm and forearm (may be clinically important with thoracic outlet syndrome [TOS]–like symptoms).
- The T12 nerve root enters the lumbar plexus as the iliohypogastric nerve, with lateral branches

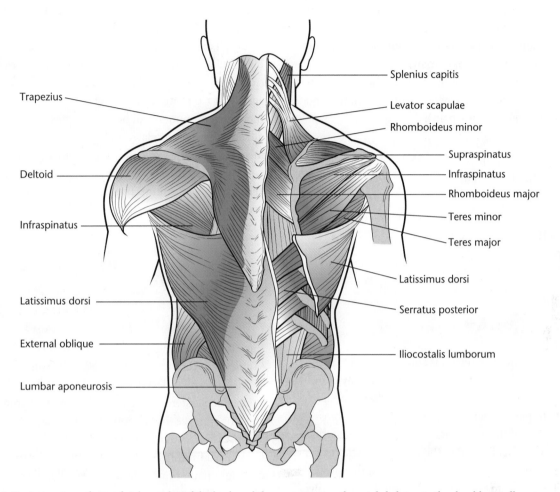

Figure 4–1 Posterior view of superficial muscles of the back and those connecting the axial skeleton to the shoulder girdle.

innervating the upper lateral thigh and an anterior branch innervating the pubic region.

- The lateral branch of the posterior primary rami of T2 descends paravertebrally to the level of T6 and then ascends to the acromion (considered with midthoracic or shoulder pain).
- The lateral branch of the posterior primary rami of T12 descends to the posterolateral iliac crest and lateral buttock (considered with "lumbar" or buttock pain).

The first branches of the posterior rami are descending branches. The medial branch of the posterior primary rami has recently been demonstrated to have an articular and nonarticular division with the articular supplying the facet joint and the nonarticular entering the connective tissue around the levator costalis with no direct connection to the facet joint.[4] The descending branches pass through a narrow space posterior to the superior costotransverse ligament. The lateral branch passes between

the superior costotransverse ligament and intertransverse ligament. It has been suggested that entrapment at these sites is a possible cause of thoracic spine pain.

The thoracic spinal cord houses the nerve cell bodies for the sympathetic nervous system. Access to other areas of the body is via the sympathetic chain. These ganglia are in close proximity to the heads of the ribs. The sinuvertebral nerve, which supplies the posterior longitudinal ligaments, epidural blood vessels, periosteum of the vertebra, and outer annulus, consists of a somatic branch and an autonomic branch. The autonomic branch comes from the gray rami communicantes or from the sympathetic ganglia near the nerve root and as the sinuvertebral nerve re-enters the intervertebral foramina. Branches of the sinuvertebral nerve may travel four or five segments in the neural canal before synapsing. Interestingly, the sympathetic neurons (for vascular supply) that follow somatic nerves into the arms may originate from as far down as T8.[5] This may account for a condition called the T4 syndrome reported in the literature on manipulation.[6] Although there is still a debate regarding the effect of manipulation on the sympathetic influence on visceral organ function, it is recognized that referred pain from organs is possible. Below are some specific organ innervations (approximate). The segmental levels specified may be painful when the organ is involved (viscerosomatic pain):

- heart—C8-T5(T8)
- lungs—T3-T5(T10)
- stomach—T5-T8(T9)
- pancreas—T7-T9
- gallbladder, liver, spleen, caecum, and duodenum—T6-T10
- appendix—T9-T11
- kidneys—T9-L2

Biomechanics

Mobility in the thoracic region is somewhat restricted by the rib cage attachments. The physiologic priority appears to be protection of visceral organs rather than mobility. Only 2° to 6° per segment of sagittal movement is possible, with 60% of this movement being flexion. Lateral flexion is somewhat limited in the upper thoracic region (5° to 6° per segment per side), increasing in the lower thoracic region (8° to 9° per side). Lateral flexion involves a coupled movement pattern with rotation.[7] In the upper thoracic region, lateral bending to one side causes the spinous processes to rotate into the convexity (opposite side; similar to the cervical region), while in the lower thoracic region the spinous processes rotate into the concavity (same side; similar to the lumbar region). Rotation occurs more in the upper thoracic spine (4° to 5° per side) than in the lower (2° per side), total of about 40° per side. Rotation also causes a coupled motion with lateral flexion to the opposite side and an accompanying extension (especially in the lower thoracics). In the upper thoracics, the coupled motion is lateral flexion and sagittal flexion.

During normal respiration, rib cage movement has been described as two patterns. In one description, the lower ribs (7 to 10) move in more of a buckethandle configuration due to costotransverse and costovertebral attachments and axis of motion. What this translates into is that the side-to-side dimension of the chest increases as the ribs become more horizontal (compared to the superior-to-inferior direction in the resting lung seen from a sagittal perspective). Others also describe a caliper movement of the lowest ribs, moving more posterior and lateral on inspiration and anterior and medial during expiration. For the upper ribs (2 to 6) a description of a pumphandle movement has been proposed. During inspiration the anterior aspect of the ribs moves superiorly and anteriorly. However, an in vivo study[8] suggests that rib motion at all levels is similar, meaning that there are components of both analogies of movement during inspiration related to lateral and anterior movement expansion. These movements are due in part to the type of articulation and angle of articulation with the vertebrae and sternum. Inspiration is more of an active process, whereas expiration is usually more passive due to the elastic recoil of the alveoli in the lungs.

Evaluation

History

Careful questioning during the history taking (**Table 4–1**) can point to the diagnosis. Some historical red flags include a history of drug or alcohol abuse, use of corticosteroids, diabetes, or direct trauma to the chest or rib cage. In patients older than age 70 years, a compression fracture or metastasis should be suspected. Combined findings of weight loss, a past history of cancer, night pain, or high fever (especially in a patient older than age 50 years) warrant a careful radiographic search for cancer or infection.

Trauma

Trauma to the thoracic area (e.g., a direct blow) should raise the suspicion of a rib fracture. The patient should be evaluated further with compression, percussion, vibration, and radiographs. A fall onto the buttocks with resulting thoracic pain is often due to a compression fracture. If the patient was involved in a car accident, a chance fracture may have occurred over the fulcrum of the seat belt.

Posture

Postural problems are common. There is a natural tendency for individuals who work at desks to accentuate the forward head—forward shoulder posture. Without frequent breaks or exercises to compensate, most individuals acquire a new "normal" posture. Asking the patient with an apparent kyphosis about his or her posture to determine the chronicity is important. It is possible that an adult had the predisposition to Scheuermann's disease as an adolescent. This will be evident radiographically.

Table 4–1 History Questions for Thoracic Spine Injury

Primary Question	What Are You Thinking?	Secondary Questions	What Are You Thinking?
Did you injure yourself (e.g., car accident, lifting, twisting, bending)?	Sprain/strain, fracture, subluxation	Did you have a sudden flexion	Compression or chance fracture
		(With older patient) Did you have pain after coughing, sneezing, stepping off a curb?	Compression fracture
		Did you suffer a blow to the chest?	Rib fracture
Does the pain radiate around to the chest?	Intercostal strain, intercostal neuritis, herpes zoster, diabetes, neurofibroma, degenerative joint disease	Do you have any associated skin lesions?	Herpes zoster
		Is the pain increased with stretching (e.g., yawning)?	Intercostal strain
		Do you have diabetes?	Diabetic neuropathy
Is the pain worse at night? Is it unrelieved with rest?	Osteoid osteoma, cancer, rib fracture	Is aspirin helpful?	Dramatic relief suggests osteoid osteoma; if no relief, consider cancer
		Is it more difficult to lie on your back?	Rib fracture
Is there associated chest or abdominal pain?	Referral or radiation from chest or abdominal disease	Is there associated epigastric pain?	Consider peptic ulcer, esophagitis, or pancreatitis
		Do you have upper right abdominal pain?	Cholecystitis or lithiasis
Do you have chronic pain?	Myofascial pain due to poor posture, ergonomic strain at work, fibromyalgia, or depression	Do you work in a seated, forward-head position? Do you have middle or upper scapular pain?	Postural syndrome
		Do you have pain all over your body? On both sides?	Fibromyalgia
		Do you have difficulty sleeping, loss of enjoyment in any activities?	Depression
		Is the pain associated with globally restricted thoracic spine movement?	Consider ankylosing spondylitis
Are you concerned about an observed deformity?	Postural kyphosis, Scheuermann's disease, compression fracture, scoliosis, scapular winging due to nerve damage	(In a senior) Did you have a sudden onset of a "hunched" appearance or gradual height loss?	Compression fracture (osteoporosis; traumatic, or pathologic)
		(In an adolescent) Are you constantly "hunched" forward?	Scheuermann's disease or postural syndrome
		Is there curving of back with a high shoulder or bulging ribs?	Scoliosis

For those who work at desks, it is important to determine the setup of the workstation. If the setup allows or encourages a forward head or slumped position, it is important to use this information in long-term planning for avoidance of postural pain. Adolescents often develop a slumped posture either because it is the posture of their friends or because of a lack of self-confidence.

Stiffness

Stiffness should be differentiated from a sensation or an objective loss of range of motion (ROM). Many patients who complain of stiffness have normal ROM, indicating that muscles are probably being posturally strained. When a young adult patient complains of difficulty in taking a deep breath or bending forward or to the sides, ankylosing spondylitis is suggested.

Deformity

On occasion an older patient or the parent of a child will notice a humping in the thoracic region. In the older patient, a compression fracture is likely and should be evaluated radiographically. In the child, deformity may represent simply a "bad" posture habit, Scheuermann's disease, scoliosis, or the rare Sprengel's deformity. The parent also may notice that the child with scoliosis has an unequal arm length evident by unequal sleeve length on shirts or blouses.

Examination

From a postural standpoint, there are several important clues for which to look. They include scapular winging, buffalo hump, acute-angle kyphosis, generalized hyperkyphosis, and scoliosis.

Scapular Winging

Scapular winging may be due to a scoliosis (convex side) or weakness of either the middle trapezius or serratus anterior (the muscle weakness is often secondary to nerve damage). Asking the patient to perform a push-up against the wall often will accentuate the winging. Winging that allows straight lateral drift of the scapula is due to weakness of the middle trapezius; flaring of the inferior border outward and of the upper border inward is indicative of serratus anterior weakness with probable damage to the long thoracic nerve. An unusually high scapula or small scapula may represent the uncommon Sprengel's deformity in which scapular muscles are underdeveloped or replaced by fibrous tissue.[9]

Buffalo Hump

A buffalo hump is the buildup of fat tissue in a patient with Cushing's disease or an individual on long-term corticosteroids; it should not be confused with a large lipoma or a Dowager's hump (compression fracture) or gibbous deformity (compression fracture or tuberculosis of the spine).

Acute-Angle Kyphosis

Acute-angle kyphosis is often seen in older women at the site of a compression fracture (called Dowager's hump or gibbous deformity); in younger athletes, an acute-angle kyphosis at the thoracolumbar region indicates atypical Scheuermann's disease.

Generalized Hyperkyphosis

A hyperkyphosis is common in adolescents for two major reasons: (1) poor posture, and (2) Scheuermann's disease. To differentiate between the functional (postural) type

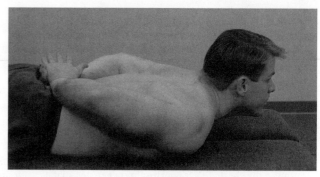

Figure 4–2 Prone extension is used to differentiate between a structural and a functional hyperkyphosis. If the kyphosis improves with extension, it is primarily functional; no improvement indicates a structural cause (e.g., Scheuermann's disease).

and the structural type, the patient is asked to lie prone and then to extend the trunk with the arms behind the back, lifting the chest off the table (**Figure 4–2**). If the kyphosis persists it is structural. A functional examination should include an evaluation of both the lumbar and cervical curves in an effort to determine their contribution or compensation for the thoracic kyphosis. The typical pattern is weak midscapular muscles, tight pectorals, weak deep neck flexors, tight deep neck extensors, weak abdominals, and tight lumbar paraspinals.

Scoliosis

The lateral curvature of a scoliosis is often visible in the standing patient; if present, ask the patient to flex forward at the waist at three levels (90° for the lumbar region, 60° for the midthoracic, and 30° to 45° for the upper thoracic), keeping the head down and the arms hanging loosely with no trunk rotation voluntarily acquired. Prominence of one side compared with the other is indicative of a structural curve (**Figure 4–3**). Measurement of the degree of trunk inclination may be performed with an inclinometer such as a scoliometer. A trunk angle greater than 7° is an indication of a structural curve of at least 20°.[10] Another test for scoliosis is to observe how much correction occurs when the patient lies prone. This can be evaluated further by asking the patient to bend maximally to the convex side of the curve. Some improvement will occur if there is a functional component to the curve.

The neurologic examination for the thoracic spine is brief, unless there is a suspicion of nerve root involvement. This rare occurrence will cause the patient to complain of pain that radiates to the front of the body, and there may be accompanying weakness of the abdominal

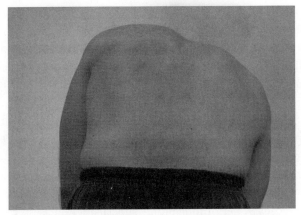

Figure 4–3 The Adams' test involves forward bending in an attempt to gain a skyline view of different areas of the back. This position of approximately 60° forward flexion demonstrates angular deformity (rib humping) in the midthoracic spine on the left.

muscles. It would be unusual for an upper motor neuron lesion to cause only isolated thoracic spine findings.

Because of the possibility of referral or radiation pain from a chest or abdominal source, it would be prudent to perform some chest and abdominal screening tests with patients complaining of both anterior and posterior pain. With costovertebral pain in the lower thoracic region, a kidney punch test might elicit a response with an inflammatory process such as pyelonephritis. If the pain is more in the middle thoracic or scapular areas, Murphy's sign for gallbladder disease may be elicited (see Chapter 31).

Palpation of the thoracic spine may be helpful in finding discrete areas of tenderness. Motion palpation is commonly used. Unfortunately, one small study indicated good intraexaminer reliability but poor interexaminer reliability.[9] It is important to challenge the midthoracic area in patients with diffuse arm complaints. Reproduction of arm complaints with pressure on the spinous or transverse processes suggests T4 syndrome.

Basic radiographic evaluation of the thoracic spine requires an anteroposterior (AP) and lateral view. Additional views are required in the following scenarios:

- If rib fracture is suspected, include AP and oblique views of the involved ribs.
- If associated chest pathology is suspected, include a posteroanterior and lateral view of the chest.
- If scoliosis is suspected, begin with a full spine (14 × 36) evaluation to determine involvement of the other spinal regions and, in younger patients, to determine the Risser sign. It has been recommended to take the film posterior-to-anterior to avoid increased radiation to the breasts

and genitals; however, it is suggested that the Risser sign is not as accurate on this view and, given the technology available with regard to collimation, filtering, film speed, and so on, the concern is not as strong as it once was. If a scoliosis is present, recumbent films with maximum bending into the curve convexity are important to determine the degree of functional versus structural curve (see Chapter 5). Measurements include the Cobb angle for degree of angulation, Nash-Mose measurement for degree of rotation, and the Risser sign for progression of the iliac crest apophysis (indicator of bone maturity). For the rare infantile idiopathic curve, the Mehta rib angle measurement may determine those likely to progress.

- If a compression fracture is evident, determination of stability is important. Collapse of the anterior margin to less than half the height of the posterior margin or more than 20° of wedging may indicate an unstable fracture. Loss of posterior vertebral height should raise the suspicion of a pathologic fracture often due to metastasis. Other clues may be a "missing pedicle" sign, indicating an osteolytic process such as breast cancer metastasis.

Special studies are required when tumor, unstable fracture, or osteoporosis is seen or suspected. Bone scans are helpful in determining metastatic sites in the spine and the location of osteoid osteomas. Dual x-ray absorptiometry is valuable for evaluating generalized bone mass status. MRI is valuable when nerve root compression, infection, or tumor is suspected and the degree of involvement or cause is uncertain.

Management

- Patients with infection, primary tumor or metastasis, unstable fracture, severe or rapidly progressive scoliosis or kyphosis, and complications due to corticosteroid use should be referred for medical evaluation and possible management or comanagement.
- Patients with uncomplicated compression fractures, mild to moderate idiopathic scoliosis that is not rapidly progressing, uncomplicated Scheuermann's disease, facet syndrome, postural syndrome, T4 syndrome, and other mechanical causes should be managed conservatively. If

unresponsive to care, further evaluation or referral for comanagement may be indicated.

- Patients with uncomplicated compression fractures will probably have pain for one to two months during the healing phase. Bracing or restraint in the thoracic region is not recommended because of its effect on normal breathing. The same is true for patients with cracked ribs or uncomplicated rib fractures (see Chapter 38, Chest Pain).

The recommendation of the Mercy Center Guidelines[12] is that a two-week trial of manipulative therapy at a frequency of three to five times per week (depending on severity) is appropriate for most uncomplicated mechanical problems. If unresponsive, a second two-week trial is suggested. If the patient is responsive to either treatment trial, a reduction in frequency of care over the following several weeks is appropriate. Maintenance care may be necessary in patients with chronic problems. If the patient is still not responding after a second two-week trial, laboratory testing, special imaging, or referral for medical evaluation should be given.

For most patients with chronic posturally induced pain, stretches, exercises, and modification of work or recreational activity patterns comprise the long-term approach to prevention. Stretching of tight pectoral muscles may be performed by leaning into a corner or doorway with the arm or arms elevated to shoulder level or above. Adding a slight contraction for a few seconds followed by relaxation may allow access to more ROM. Strengthening of the midscapular muscles can be performed prone or with the back against a corner. The emphasis is to keep the arms at shoulder level and elbows bent 90° and to maintain this position while the scapulae are squeezed together (no arm movement; only scapular movement). Patients with a kyphosis should also focus on strengthening of the lower trapezius by performing prone "superman" exercises. With the arms stretched out overhead and the hips stabilized, the patient attempts to lift the chest off the ground or table, holds for a few seconds, and slowly lowers. For generalized posture, stretching of the deep neck extensors, lumbar erector spinae, iliopsoas, and hamstrings should be coupled with strengthening of the deep neck flexors, midscapular muscles, abdominals, and gluteals.

Algorithm

An algorithm for the management of thoracic spine pain is presented in **Figure 4–4**.

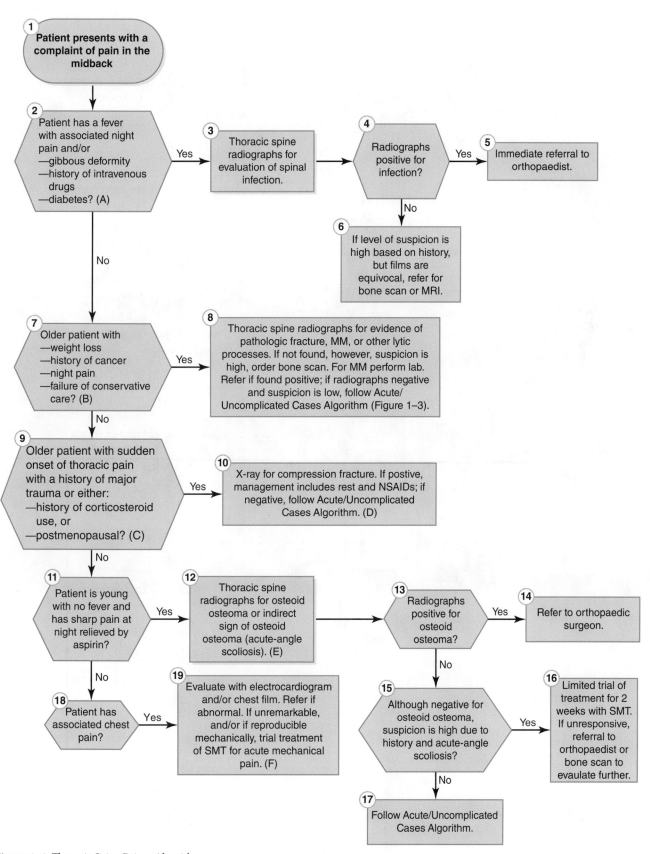

Figure 4–4 Thoracic Spine Pain—Algorithm

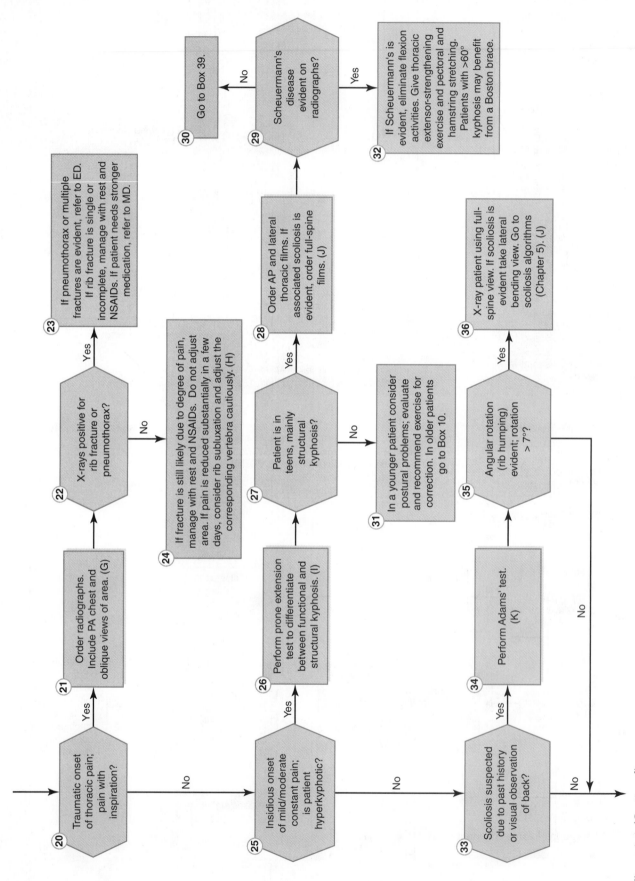

Figure 4–4 (Continued)

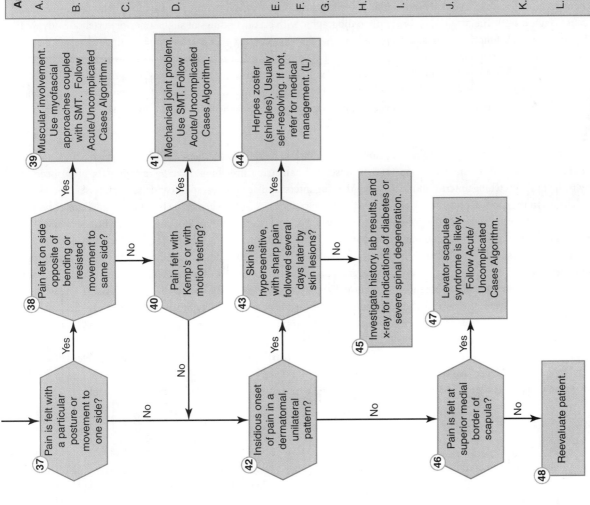

Annotations

A. Osteomyelitis is most common in diabetics and intravenous drug abusers. Fever may be present and tenderness to spinous percussion or deep pain.

B. Cancer or metastasis is suspected when there is a history of cancer, especially in patients over 50 who have experienced undesired weight loss or who have not responded to conservative care.

C. Osteoporosis-related compression fractures are most common in postmenopausal women or those on long-term steroid use without a history of significant trauma.

D. Fractures decreasing the anterior vertebral body height to <50% of posterior body height or causing more than a 20° angulation should be considered unstable and referred to an orthopaedist. Compression fractures are managed conservatively with rest and NSAIDs. Bracing/supports are not recommended for the thoracic area because of inhibition of normal breathing.

E. Osteoid osteoma may cause a small acute-angle scoliosis due to local muscle spasm.

F. Chest pain that is noncardiac is often sharp, localized, and reproduced by stretch, contraction or palpation.

G. Rib fracture management is generally rest and NSAIDs. Rib belts are not used because of inhibition of normal breathing.

H. Differentiating between rib fractures (cracked ribs) and subluxations of ribs is difficult; however, rib fractures do not feel substantially better in a few days.

I. A test to differentiate between structural and functional kyphosis is performed by having the patient extend the trunk from a prone position. If the kyphosis improves, the main component is functional.

J. Scoliosis x-rays are used to determine bone age using the Risser sign and the degree of curve using Cobb's angle. A lateral bending view with the patient bending as far into the convexity is used to compare Cobb's angles determining the functional amount of the curve.

K. The Adams' test coupled with scoliometer measurement is able to detect curves >20 when the angular rotation is >7°.

L. Herpes zoster usually follows a single nerve root in a dermatomal pattern; however, the appearance is patchy, not linear. Lysine and stress management may be helpful. Medical treatment may involve acyclovir.

Figure 4–4 (Continued)

Selected Disorders of the Thoracic Spine*

Scheuermann's Disease

Classic Presentation

The patient is a young male or female (age 13 to 17 years) who presents with a complaint of midback pain and fatigue. The patient has an increased kyphosis.

Cause

The cause of Scheuermann's disease has been debated for years. Scheuermann's disease is not an osteochondrosis. Currently, Scheuermann's is believed to be the result of vertebral growth plate trauma during the adolescent period with interruption or cessation of further growth.[13] It is generally agreed that wedging of greater than 5° in three consecutive vertebrae is the radiographic indicator of Scheuermann's. In addition, end-plate fractures (Schmorl's nodes) and anterior disruption (limbus bones) are evidence of discal extrusions. The midthoracic region is affected 75% of the time. The thoracolumbar region is affected 25% of the time. The incidence is as high as 8%.[14] There is a small male predominance and an increased incidence among family members. A unique type found in female gymnasts and adolescents performing heavy weight lifting is called atypical Scheuermann's (type II) disease or "apprentice kyphosis." There is an acute kyphotic angulation at one or two vertebral bodies in the area of T10-L4.[15] This represents trauma to the vertebral ring apophysis.

Evaluation

An examination for posture often will reveal an exaggeration of the cervical and lumbar lordosis with a hyperkyphotic thoracic region. If the patient is asked to lie prone and extend the chest off the table, persistence of the kyphosis will indicate a structural cause, most often Scheuermann's disease in a younger individual. If the kyphosis improves, a functional cause (poor habitual posture) is probably the cause (Figure 4–2). The diagnosis is primarily radiographic with classic findings of slight anterior vertebral body wedging (at least 5° per segment), Schmorl's nodes, and decreased disc height, all occurring over at least three contiguous vertebrae.[16] An alternate diagnostic criterion is a thoracic kyphosis greater than 45°. Additional findings include mild scoliosis and limbus bones (anterior marginal Schmorl's node representing ossification in the avulsed growth plate). The lordosis is measured using a modified Cobb angle taken off a lateral radiograph. The classic finding with atypical Scheuermann's is an anterior Schmorl's node occurring at only one or two levels at the thoracolumbar region. The anterior wedging with atypical Scheuermann's can be as much as 40% to 50%.

Management

Complications such as disc herniation or nerve root compression are rare. General management for uncomplicated Scheuermann's and kyphotic curves less than 60° should include postural exercises and hamstring stretching. Bracing or taping for proprioceptive awareness may be helpful. Stretching anterior muscles, strengthening interscapular muscles, spinal extension exercises, and attention to compensations in the cervical and lumbar curves are the primary focus. A Milwaukee brace is recommended for curves over 60°.[17] The most important period is during the growth spurt in males. For curves greater than 80°, surgery may be necessary. Atypical Scheuermann's requires restriction from all gymnastics participation and extension bracing for several months. With atypical Scheuermann's, radiographs should be retaken in three to four months to determine healing. The indication for surgery is a progressive kyphosis greater than 70° or for those who have had progression with bracing and finally intractable back pain. One common result from surgical correction is the development of a junctional kyphosis (a kyphosis adjacent to the arthrodesis). There is little literature evaluating the effectiveness of new surgical implants and the degree of junctional kyphosis. A recent study[18] indicates that:

- Correction of kyphosis is possible through either a combined anteroposterior or posterior approach. However, there is a higher rate of complication with the combined procedure.
- Proximal junctional kyphosis occurred in 32.1% of patients related to arthrodesis caudal to the proximal end vertebra. This is influenced by pelvic incidence (see spondylolisthesis).
- Distal junctional kyphosis occurs in 5.1% of patients associated with arthrodesis cephalad to the sagittal stable vertebra.

Compression Fracture

Classic Presentation

In older patients, the onset of sudden thoracic (or lumbar) pain occurs after a minor event such as sneezing or stepping off a curb. In younger patients, the history will usually involve a fall on the buttocks and/or a hyperflexion injury.

Cause

Compression fractures may be due to weakness in the bone, usually secondary to osteoporosis or cancer. Sufficient trauma may cause a fracture in normal bone. Approximately 35% of compression fractures in women over age 40 years are due to early menopause, 30% are due to long-term corticosteroid use, 8% are due to hyperthyroidism, and less than 2% are due to malignancy.[19]

Evaluation

A history of long-term corticosteroid use or age greater than 70 years is suggestive of compression fracture in patients with thoracic or lumbar complaints.[20] Pathologic fracture should be considered in patients older than 50 years with a past history of cancer or unexplained weight loss. There is often a sharp kyphotic angle at the area of fracture. The patient will have pain on percussion and deep pressure over the involved segment. The diagnosis is essentially radiographic. The lateral view is particularly helpful in determining important differentiating factors. An anterior step defect is most common, due to the increased stress imposed by the natural kyphosis, flexion, and gravity. Collapse of the anterior margin to less than half the height of the posterior margin or more than 20° of wedging may indicate an unstable fracture. Other indicators are based on the Denis criteria.[21] Using a three-column concept, if two or more columns are disrupted, the fracture is unstable. The three columns are the anterior column (anterior longitudinal ligament [ALL] to midvertebral body), middle column (midvertebral body to posterior longitudinal ligament [PLL]), and posterior column (PLL to suspraspinous ligament). Loss of posterior vertebral body height without a history of trauma should raise the suspicion of pathologic fracture, warranting a search for metastatic cancer or multiple myeloma. Healing of noncomplicated fractures should be evident within about three months.

Management

Fractures due to metastatic cancer or multiple myeloma require medical referral. Stable osteoporotic fractures can be managed conservatively with rest and over-the-counter pain medication. The acute pain is often severe for two weeks, with persistent pain for up to three months. At three months, if pain is persistent, reradiograph the area to determine the degree of healing. If the compression fracture is in the lumbar or thoracolumbar area, a restrictive corset may be helpful to remind the patient not to bend forward or make sudden movements. All patients with osteoporosis must avoid flexion exercises. There is a dramatic increase in compression fractures among those performing flexion versus extension exercises for low back pain (see also Chapter 30, Osteoporosis).

Minimally invasive procedures designed to fill the gap of the fracture and/or increase the height of the collapsed vertebrae have been utilized for a number of years, yet there still remains quite a degree of controversy. These procedures are performed by an orthopaedic surgeon or interventional radiologist and are generally outpatient procedures using a local anesthetic and minimal general anesthetic. The earliest procedure, called vertebroplasty, involves the injection of cement, usually polymethylmethacrylate (PMMA), into the vertebrae. There are two intentions. One is to fill in the gap and potentially relieve pain in those that fail conservative management. With the introduction of the next advance, balloon kyphoplasty, the second intention is to restore the height of the vertebrae and diminish the degree of kyphosis segmentally and across segments to improve cosmetic appearance. This is accomplished by inflating a balloon in the vertebrae to create a space into which the cement is injected. Several problems emerged. One is the potential leakage of the PMMA that may result in neurologic compromise. This may occur asymptomatically in as many as 65% of cases and symptomatically around 2% of the time. Pulmonary embolism from injection into the venous system is also possible, occurring in 2% to 26% of procedures.[22] Long-term effects are not known at this time. Additionally, randomized studies using control groups have not yet demonstrated a clinically significant difference between placebo and surgery other than some immediate improvement differences in pain with the surgical procedures.[23] Also, even though there have been improvements in the vertebral body height, at a segmental level, the differences are only a few millimeters at best. Reported as percentages of around 30% or so, these seem impressive but cosmetically not necessarily significant. No studies have demonstrated that there is prevention of future fracture and in fact it has been demonstrated that there may be an increase in fracture at adjacent levels. Specialty focused groups are inconsistent in their recommendations. The American Academy of Orthopaedic Surgeons in 2010[24] recommended against the use of vertebroplasty. Other groups such as the Australian Medical Services Advisory Committee recommend its use for those that have failed conservative management.[25] Others recommend its use for vertebral fractures other than compression fractures such as those due to cancer or other disease processes. Newer augmenting devices such as Kiva are being tested.[26] These devices are usually implants, often columns formed by coils, to form an intravertebral housing for the cement that is injected.

Osteoid Osteoma
Classic Presentation

The patient is usually a young male who presents with a complaint of well-localized midback pain. The pain is worse at night but relieved by aspirin (in 65% of patients).[27]

Cause

Osteoid osteomas are benign tumors affecting mainly the posterior elements of the vertebrae. They are not exclusive to the spine. In fact, 50% occur in the femur and tibia, and approximately 10% in the spine. Occurrence is most frequent in the lamina, followed by the pedicle, facet, and spinous processes.

Evaluation

The patient often has an acute-angle scoliosis at the site of the tumor (lesion on the concave side). The diagnosis is sometimes made from standard thoracic radiographs. The lesion is a small bony density that surrounds a smaller round, radiolucent nidus. Bone scans or tomograms often will be needed to confirm or identify the lesion.

Management

Refer the patient for surgical excision.

Postural Syndrome

Classic Presentation

The patient will present with a constant aching pain in the middle and upper thoracic regions. The pain is usually relieved by activity and made worse by working at a desk.

Cause

The natural imbalance between the anterior muscles and posterior muscles is often accentuated by various work postures that emphasize a "hunched," forward-head position. The large, tight muscles such as the pectorals become chronically shortened in adapting to the position, with associated weakness and constant strain of the midscapular muscles, which contract eccentrically.

Evaluation

Posturally the patient may present with a hyperkyphosis. There are often trigger points in the upper and middle trapezius, rhomboids, levator scapulae, and pectorals. Lower trapezius strength is minimal when the patient is asked to perform upper thoracic extension from a prone position with the arms held above the head (out in front of the body).

Management

The combination of manipulation of the thoracic and related regions with deep massage can be used initially to decrease discomfort. To prevent recurrence, exercises focusing on stretching the pectorals first, followed by strengthening of the midscapular muscles and lower trapezius should follow. Postural awareness may be increased with bracing or taping. The patient's work environment must be evaluated for ergonomic strengths. Redesign of the work environment and frequent breaks for stretching and mild isometrics often help.

T4 Syndrome

Classic Presentation

The patient complains of upper back stiffness and achiness with associated signs of upper extremity numbness and/or paresthesias (often in a stocking and glove distribution). There may be associated headaches.

Cause

The cause is unknown; however, it is postulated that sympathetic dysfunction somehow related to vertebral dysfunction in the upper thoracic region (T2-T7) causes a referred or reflex phenomenon in the arms or hands. Patients may report occurrence during the night or upon rising. This syndrome is more common in women (4:1 ratio) in the age range of 30 to 50 years. Prolonged sitting, sustained reaching and pulling activities, shoveling, and overhead cleaning have all been reported by patients.[28]

Evaluation

The patient will often have tenderness and restriction at the involved segment(s), most often T2-T7. Pressure or movement challenge at these areas may reproduce the patient's complaints. For all patients with arm complaints, a thorough neurologic examination should be performed in an attempt to differentiate nerve root, peripheral nerve, brachial plexus, or central nervous system disorders. The neurologic examination is normal in patients with T4 syndrome. Radiographs are not diagnostic for this syndrome.

Management

Manipulation or mobilization of the involved area, coupled with postural advice and exercise, will usually resolve the patient's complaints.

Herpes Zoster (Shingles)

Classic Presentation

A patient presents with isolated burning and pain that developed into skin lesions in a small patch on the chest and back. These vesicles crusted over a few days and cleared over the last few days. (Note: The presentation varies with the degree of involvement.) Small local lesions are most common although full body expression can occur in some individuals. Older patients more often have involvement of the forehead than younger individuals.

Cause

The cause is a latent varicella virus that resides in the dorsal root ganglion. Mechanical, emotional, or chemical stress causes activation along the corresponding dermatome. The formation of clusters of vesicles is preceded by pain, burning, and sensitivity. The average length of time for the whole process is one week.

Examination

The first visible appearance is a reddening in the area of involvement, followed by the formation of vesicles. The classic appearance of the lesions usually makes this a simple recognition without the need for testing. It is extremely important to recognize that if a dermatome is affected, it is often patchy involvement not extending along the full course of the dermatome (i.e., outlining the involved dermatome). This creates patches that may appear unconnected due to angulation of the ribs and corresponding dermatome.

Management

Localized involvement is self-limited and may be circumvented by avoiding recognizable triggers. Some practitioners recommend lysine; however, there is no evidence as yet to support that recommendation. For others with more involvement, acyclovir or implanted drug delivery systems are used. Seniors are at particular risk for the development of shingles. Recently, a new vaccine has been developed. Studies indicate that the new vaccine reduces the incidence by about 50%.[29, 30]

APPENDIX 4–1

References

1. Nansel D, Szlazak M. Somatic dysfunction and the phenomenon of visceral disease simulation: a probable explanation for the apparent effectiveness of somatic therapy in patients presumed to be suffering from true visceral disease. *J Manipulative Physiol Ther.* 1995;18:379–397.

2. Valencia F. Biomechanics of the thoracic spine. In: Grant R, ed. *Physical Therapy of the Cervical and Thoracic Spine.* New York: Churchill Livingstone; 1988:4.

3. Grieve GP. *Common Vertebral Joint Problems.* Edinburgh: Churchill Livingstone; 1981:15–17.

4. Ishizuka K, Sakai H, Tsuzuki N, Nagashima M. Topographic anatomy of the posterior ramus of thoracic spinal nerve and surrounding structures. *Spine (Phila Pa 1976).* 2012;37(14):E817–822.

5. Keele CA, Neil E, eds. *Samson Wright's Applied Physiology.* 12th ed. London: Oxford University Press; 1971.

6. DeFranca GG, Levine LJ. The T4 syndrome. *J Manipulative Physiol Ther.* 1995;18:34–37.

7. White AA, Panjabi MM. Kinematics of the spine. In: White AA, Panjabi MM, eds. *Clinical Biomechanics of the Spine.* Philadelphia: JB Lippincott; 1978:61–90.

8. De Groote A, Wantier M, Cheron G, Estenne M, Paiva M. Chest wall motion during tidal breathing. *J Appl Physiol.* 1997;83(5):1531–1537.

9. Carson WC, Lovell WW, Whitesides TE. Congenital elevation of the scapula. *J Bone Joint Surg Am.* 1981;63:1190.

10. Bunnell WP. An objective criterion for scoliosis screening. *J Bone Joint Surg Am.* 1984;66:1381–1387.

11. Love RM, Brodeur RR. Inter- and intra-examiner reliability of motion palpation for the thoracolumbar spine. *J Manipulative Physiol Ther.* 1987;10:1–4.

12. Haldeman S, Chapman-Smith D, Petersen DM, Jr. *Guidelines for Chiropractic Quality Assurance and Practice Parameters: Proceedings of the Mercy Center Consensus Conference.* Gaithersburg, MD: Aspen Publishers, Inc; 1993.

13. Yochum TR, Rowe LJ. Scheuermann's disease. In: Yochum TR, Rowe LJ, eds. *Essentials of Skeletal Radiology.* 2nd ed. Baltimore: Williams & Wilkins; 1996:1292–1295.

14. Lowe TG. Current concepts review: Scheuermann's disease. *J Bone Joint Surg Am.* 1990;72:940.

15. Blumenthal SL, Roach J, Herring JA. Lumbar Scheuermann's: a clinical series and classification. *Spine.* 1987;12:930.

16. Sorenson KH. *Scheuermann's Juvenile Kyphosis.* Copenhagen: Munksgaard; 1964.

17. Wenger DR, Frick SL. Scheuermann kyphosis. *Spine.* 1999; 24(4):2630–2639.

18. Lonner BS, Newton P, Betz R, et al. Operative management of Scheuermann's kyphosis in 78 patients: radiographic outcomes, complications, and technique. *Spine.* 2007;32(24):2644–2652.

19. Caplan GA, Scane AC, Frances RM. Pathogenesis of vertebral crush fractures. *J R Soc Med.* 1994;87:200.

20. Deyo RA, Rainville J, Kent DL. What can the history and physical examination tell us about low back pain? *JAMA.* 1992;268:760–765.

21. Denis F. Spinal stability as defined by the three-column concept in acute spinal trauma. *Clin Orthop.* 1984;189:65.

22. Bastian L, Schils F, Tillman JB, Fueredi G. A randomized trial comparing 2 techniques of balloon kyphoplasty and curette use for obtaining vertebral body height restoration and angular-deformity correction in vertebral compression fractures due to osteoporosis. *AJNR Am J Neuroradiol.* 2013;34(3):666–675.

23. Buchbinder R, Osborne RH, Ebeling PR, et al. A randomized trial of vertebroplasty for painful osteoporotic vertebral fractures. *N Engl J Med.* 2009;361(6):557–568.

24. Esses, Stephen I. et al. (September 2010), *The Treatment of Symptomatic Osteoporotic Spinal Compression Fractures: Guideline and Evidence Report,* American Academy of Orthopaedic Surgeons.

25. *Review of interim funded service: Vertebroplasty and New review of Kyphoplasty.* Medical Services Advisory Committee. 2011. ISBN 9781742414560.

26. Korovessis P, Vardakastanis K, Repantis T, Vitsas V. Balloon kyphoplasty versus KIVA vertebral augmentation—comparison of 2 techniques for osteoporotic vertebral body fractures: a prospective randomized study. *Spine (Phila Pa 1976).* 2013;38(4):292–299.

27. Helms CA, Hattner RS, Vogler JB III. Osteoid osteoma: radionuclide diagnosis. *Radiology.* 1984;151:779.

28. McGuckin N. The T4 syndrome. In: Grieve GP, ed. *Modern Manual Therapy of the Vertebral Column.* New York: Churchill Livingstone; 1986:370–376.

29. Oxman MN. Vaccination to prevent herpes zoster and postherpetic neuralgia. *Hum Vaccin.* 2007;3(2):64–68.

30. Oxman MN, Levin MJ, Johnson GR, et al. A vaccine to prevent herpes zoster and postherpetic neuralgia in older adults. *N Engl J Med.* 2005;352(22):2271–2284.

# CHAPTER 5

Scoliosis

Context

Scoliosis may be the result of detectable, cause-and-effect conditions. If scoliosis is found as part of a composite picture of a disorder (e.g., neurofibromatosis or polio-myelitis), it is categorized by cause. The list is long and includes neurologic, muscular, congenital bone anoma-lies, developmental (e.g., due to abnormal collagen), and several other recognizable disorders. The majority of scolioses, however, are idiopathic. The majority of scolioses do not progress; yet for those that do, cos-metic appearance, and occasionally cardiopulmonary compromise are concerns.

Idiopathic scoliosis is truly an enigma. Etiologically disguised by apparent causes that ultimately are revealed as effects, this seemingly simple spinal deviation has remained "idiopathic" for centuries despite astounding technologic advances. Sifting through the plethora of theories, it becomes apparent that no single causative factor is or probably ever will be identifiable.

The deformity seen with hyperkyphosis is an example of a sagittal plane disorder that progresses in one plane only. Scoliosis, on the other hand, causes spinal buckling resulting in a distortion into all planes. Idiopathic scoliosis radiographically masquerades as a lateral bending of the spine. In reality, the major components of the deformity in three dimensions include: (1) lordosis, (2) rotation and torsion, and (3) lateral deformity.[1] Rotation and lordosis are not as conspicuous on the standard anterior-to-posterior (or posterior-to-anterior) radiograph. The lateral deformity is not necessarily the major determinant of progression, yet the Cobb angle used to measure this component of the scoliosis has always been weighted as one of the, if not the major, factors upon which manage-ment decisions are based. Most important, concerns regarding cardiopulmonary dysfunction have been grossly misinterpreted, leaving the cosmetic deformity as the predominant concern for the patient.

There have been many shortcomings and misinterpre-tations with regard to the percentage of the population at risk for adolescent idiopathic scoliosis (AIS) and those at risk for progression. Generally, if the criterion of a 10° curve measured by the Cobb angle is used, the preva-lence of AIS (ages 10–16 years) is approximately 2–3%.[2] However, combining data from available epidemiologic and natural history studies, less than 1% of screened individuals and less than 10% of individuals positive for AIS on screening evaluation require treatment.[2]

For years chiropractors have claimed success in the management of scoliosis. Yet it is unclear whether all chiropractors were dealing with idiopathic scoliosis, or the type of scoliosis that is the painful consequence of muscle spasm, or the nonpainful scoliosis due to muscular imbalance that compensates for biomechani-cal asymmetry. Many chiropractors feel that by cor-recting asymmetry and keeping the spine segmentally and globally mobile, idiopathic scoliosis can be halted or reversed. Unfortunately, most studies indicate that although these biomechanical factors are potential fac-tors in curve progression, especially in larger curves, they are likely not the cause. Reflex mechanisms are proposed regarding proprioceptive input from the upper cervi-cal region.[3] These factors may play a role in setting the muscular response to a perceived "normal" that is false. Yet, again, more research must be done.

A study conducted with surgeons and chiropractors tested the feasibility of conducting a larger multicenter project to evaluate the effectiveness of chiropractor care for AIS compared to standard medical care including bracing.[4] The results of the study indicated that patient and doctor recruitment are indeed feasible. Hopefully, a more extensive study will be conducted in the near future.

General Strategy

History

- Determine whether the scoliosis onset was acute or slowly progressive.
- Determine whether there is associated acute pain at the apex (reflex muscle spasm due to a local process such as a tumor, a fracture, disc disease, etc.) or chronic pain (common in patients aged 40 years and above with idiopathic curves).
- Determine whether there was a previous diagnosis of scoliosis and whether radiographs were taken or treatment was rendered; if a brace or electrical stimulation was prescribed, determine whether the patient was compliant.
- Determine in children and young adults whether there is a family history, whether a female has reached menarche, whether a child has gone through a growth spurt, and whether indications of progression have been noticed by the parent or child.

Evaluation

- Determine whether there are any associated findings (congenital scoliosis), including clubfoot or other foot deformities, café au lait spots or patches (neurofibromatosis), or patches of hair along the spine (spina bifida).
- Observe the patient from behind for evidence of a scoliosis; perform an Adams' test; observe the patient with lateral bending into the convexity and lying prone (improvement indicates a functional component).
- Observe or measure any obvious asymmetries with regard to shoulder or hip height, winging of scapulae, or head tilt; measure with a plumb line to determine whether the scoliosis is compensated or uncompensated.
- Evaluate the patient for asymmetries of the lower extremities, including pronation, tibial torsion, femoral anteversion/retroversion, and leg length discrepancy; also test for asymmetric weakness or tightness of lower extremity musculature.
- Use a full-spine film to initially radiograph patients with scoliosis. The films should be evaluated for signs of congenital scoliosis (i.e., hemivertebrae, bar vertebrae), location of the curve, and pelvic unleveling. Measure the severity with a Cobb angle, rotation with the Nash-Moe method, and bone age with the Risser sign (iliac crest apophysis).
- Take films with the patient recumbent and laterally bending into the convexity (or with a push-prone technique) and the Cobb angle measured to determine the degree of flexibility of the curve. Subtraction of the recumbent Cobb angle from the standing Cobb angle will give an approximation of the functional component of the curve.

Management

- Most cases of congenital scoliosis should be sent for an orthopaedic consultation.
- Correlate history and examination findings to gauge the tendency to progression. The primary indicators are gender (females progress more often), severity of the curve, and the Risser sign; important secondary indicators are age at menarche, type of curve, flexibility of curve, and familial predisposition.
- Idiopathic scoliosis may be managed within given ranges (dependent on age, tendency to progress, patient/parent choice) if there is no progression. Progression should be monitored radiographically every three to four months unless there are signs of rapid progression. Nonradiographic monitoring is optional using Moire topography (not commonly in use anymore). Curves that show signs of progression prior to age of menarche in girls should be referred for bracing; in girls past the age of menarche, large curves may require surgical correction. With boys, the relationship to a growth spurt may be helpful in determining a tendency to progress (more progression during the growth spurt).
- Idiopathic curves may become painful in patients 40 years of age or older; management is for pain and correction of any obvious biomechanical or spinal dysfunction. Progression to instability or severe pain warrants an orthopaedic consultation.

Idiopathic Scoliosis Etiology

Although genetic factors have been proposed, it has not yet been determined what they are. Recurrence among relatives has been reported to be between 25% and 35%.[5]

With immediate relatives such as parents and grand-parents, the incidence appears to be three or four times higher. When both parents are affected, the number of children with significant curves was 40%, much higher than those without affected parents.[6]

The common thread running through many theories regarding the development and progression of idiopathic scoliosis is that sensory information is either aberrant or information processed at the spinal cord level, or more likely at higher levels such as the cortices, is misinterpreted, leading to inappropriate output information regarding body orientation in space.[7]

Several recent research studies shed some light on possible problems. In one study,[8] visuo-oculomotor and vestibulo-ocular functions were studied with video-oculography. Altered visuo-oculomotor functions were detected, especially for the saccadic latency for patients with a Cobb angle of 15° or more. The researchers propose that this may represent a dysfunction of oculomotor pathways at the cerebellar and/or brainstem level although it is unclear whether this is a cause or result of the scoliosis.

In another recent study,[9] measuring bioelectric activity of the brain in AIS patients matched to controls (i.e., those without AIS), patients with AIS appeared to demonstrate a premature shift of bioelectric focus to structures of the left hemisphere (including the left thalamus), which was increased with the severity of the curve. Although this shift is natural for older adolescents (aged 15–17 years) and healthy adults, it does not usually occur in healthy children (aged 7–14 years). This may represent a premature shift in postural control more representative and normal for older adolescents, but when occurring during pubescence may represent an altered output of muscle tone or even growth.

Regarding the potential effect of brainstem function in the progression of scoliosis, researchers have provided some preliminary evidence that vestibular dysfunction may have an asymmetrical effect on bone growth.[10] It is known that integration and interaction among the central nervous system, brainstem, and sympathetic nervous system help regulate bone remodeling. The type or severity of vestibular dysfunction is not known; further research is necessary to determine whether a specific type of dysfunction is identifiable and amenable to management.

Balance is often a problem in children with idiopathic scoliosis compared with those without.[11] Obviously, integration of proprioceptive, visual, and vestibular information is a factor.

It is known that curves greater than 30° are more likely to progress, having reached a point at which gravity has the advantage.[12] However, other concerns about progression center around the length of the spine, the length of the curve, and the size of the vertebrae.

One mechanical model that attempts to explain why females are prone to development of a progressive scoliosis has to do with the slenderness of their vertebrae. The model holds that the size of the vertebrae determines the load that can be accommodated. It is known that females, on average, have more slender spines than males. While their vertebral height increases by 50% during adolescent growth, the vertebral width increases by only 15%.[13] In addition, their growth spurt occurs during a time when their kyphosis is at a minimum, thereby decreasing the absorptive effect of the sagittal curves. In contrast, males have thicker vertebrae and achieve their growth spurt during a time when their kyphosis is at a maximum, which may explain why they are more prone to the development of Scheuermann's disease.[14]

Another important concept is that the spine has a critical load capacity past which it will begin to deform. When children grow, especially when they grow rapidly, the increase in height coupled with the increased slenderness of the spine causes a decrease in the critical load needed to cause deformation. This results in a 20% decrease in the critical load level for only a 10% increase in height. Add to that any weight gain and the critical load is more likely to be exceeded while the spine is most subject to deformity.

There are several biologic models regarding the cause and progression of idiopathic scoliosis. One model states that differential pressure on end-plates leads to asymmetric growth, which results in scoliosis development. Although the Hueter-Volkmann law states that increased pressure across a growing epiphysis (end-plate) will lead to decreased growth, it has been found that the disc is more fluid in growing individuals and is able to dissipate the forces more equally across the end-plates than in the adult spine. Therefore, the effects of increased pressure due to wedging are thought to be negligible, at least in smaller curves. Dickson et al.[15] feel that the posterior elements, in particular the facets, not having the advantage of disc cushioning, are more likely to change as a result and may then be more the cause for asymmetric growth. Two studies[16,17] have demonstrated pressure changes in the histologic structure of the intervertebral disc with effects in collagen and glycosaminoglycan content. This occurs after the scoliosis develops, indicating that it is a response rather than a cause.

One of the newest theories is that a defect in melatonin synthesis or metabolism is a cause of idiopathic scoliosis or is associated with its progression. The theory is based primarily on studies performed on pinealectomized chickens.[18] Later studies indicated that the effect of scoliosis development with removal of the pineal gland occurred only in bipedal animals.[19] Evidence for the role of melatonin in humans is less consistent. Machida et al.[20] demonstrated that with progressive cases of scoliosis, melatonin levels were lower compared with normals; however, progressive cases of congenital scoliosis had normal melatonin levels. Studies by Hillbrand et al.,[21] Fagan et al.,[22] and Bagnall et al.[23] were unable to demonstrate differences in melatonin levels between scoliosis patients and controls.

Another association may be between calmodulin and melatonin metabolism. It is proposed that the calmodulin-melatonin interaction represents a means by which regulation and synchronization of cell physiology occur. Calmodulin is a calcium-binding receptor protein and is a major mediator of cellular calcium function, including interaction with actin and myosin, regulation of a number of enzymatic processes, and cellular calcium transport across the cell membrane. Using the logic that the contractile protein synthesis systems of platelets and skeletal muscle (actin and myosin) are similar, an underlying systemic disorder might affect both. Increased calmodulin levels have been associated with adolescent idiopathic scoliosis. This role of calmodulin has recently been evaluated measuring platelet calmodulin levels in individuals with adolescent idiopathic scoliosis.[24] The findings indicate that levels correlate closely with curve progression and treatment results using bracing and surgical stabilization. However, correlation with curves that were nonprogressive was not consistent. It is known that there are transient changes in melatonin production based on age and that melatonin secretion is also governed by circadian rhythm.[25] At this time, it is likely that melatonin is related more to progression of AIS versus the cause or initiator of AIS.[26] Related theories are based on the role of serotonin and growth-producing hormones as associated with, but not causes of, idiopathic scoliosis.[27,28]

Finally, a recent study[29] calls into question the role of leptin. The researchers determined that there was abnormal leptin bioavailability in AIS girls. What this means diagnostically or therapeutically is still in need of investigation.

Although it may appear that an imbalance of muscular activity or strength may cause a scoliosis, the evidence suggests that any changes are reactions to the curve, not the causes. Asymmetric activity is found only in curves greater than 25°.[30] If asymmetric activity were the cause, these imbalances would be evident with lesser degrees of curvature. Comparison of bilateral muscle strength does not indicate any differences between scoliotic children and those without scoliosis.

Evaluation

The prime directive with scoliosis management is to prevent progression and reverse the deformity if possible. Making decisions regarding treatment may seem easy given the limited options available. The ingredients in this decision equation are not discrete, however, and they are based on risk-to-benefit ratios and outcome desires, which vary among doctors and patients. The primary concern for the patient is cosmetic. With severe scoliosis the physician may have additional concerns regarding cardiopulmonary function, although this is actually a rare complication.[31]

Recognition of the scoliosis at the earliest point is imperative. The first distinction that is requisite for management of a scoliosis is whether there is a known cause or whether it fits the larger group of idiopathic curves. Known causes often have associated nonspinal clues that should be screened for in all patients, not only those with an apparent curve. Bunch and Patwardhan[30] demonstrated how adequate compensation may camouflage the degree of distortion present. They use an analogy of a Christmas tree that appears to be symmetric; however, when stripped to the trunk it reveals a gross rotational distortion.

The next distinction is to determine whether a curve is primarily structural or functional. Structural curves are the end result of bone remodeling with a subsequent rotary distortion that then becomes evident superficially as a lateral curvature. This rotation is always into the concavity when using the spinous process as the reference point. In addition, structural curves do not correct with postural changes such as bending forward (Adams' test, **Figure 5–1**), lying down, or maximally bending into the convexity in a supine position (**Figure 5–2**).

Functional (nonstructural) curves have no permanent rotary component and correct or overcorrect with the positional changes noted above. Functional curves are usually compensatory to biomechanical problems or are the result of muscle spasm. The key difference is that scoliosis due to muscle spasm has a pain component that is often aggravated by bending forward. Idiopathic scoliosis is rarely the cause of spinal pain until later in life.

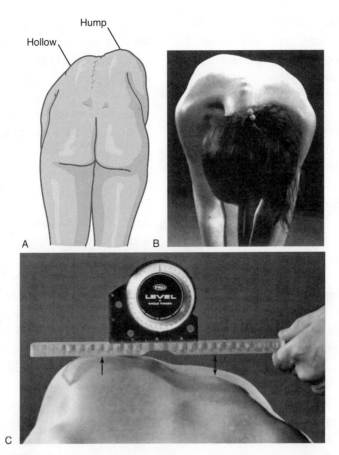

Figure 5–1 Rib hump in forward bending test. (A) Posterior view. (B) Anterior view. The two sides are compared. Note the presence of a right thoracic prominence. (C) Measurement of the prominence. The spirit level is positioned with the zero mark over the palpable spinous process in the area of maximal prominence. The level is made horizontal and the distance to the apex of the deformity (5 to 6 cm) noted. The perpendicular distance from the level to the hollow is measured at the same distance from the midline. A 2.4-cm right thoracic prominence is shown.

Reproduced from *Scoliosis and Other Spinal Deformities*, J.H. Moe, et al., p. 17, © 1978, with permission from Elsevier.

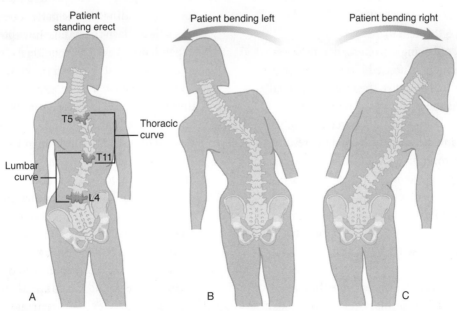

Figure 5–2 The value of the side bending to determine whether a curve is structural or nonstructural. (A) The patient is standing erect and both curves seem to be in balance. The question is: Are both curves structural, and therefore do both require treatment, or is one of the curves secondary and functional? (B) The patient bends to the left side and the lumbar curve straightens out and actually overcorrects. This curve is therefore a functional and nonstructural curve, and if surgery were required for the upper curve, this curve would not need to be fused. (C) The patient is bent to the right side and the upper curve does not correct completely. This indicates that the thoracic curve is structural and does require treatment.

Curves are named by the regional location of their apices. Single curves are relatively easy to identify; however, when two or three curves are present it is necessary to determine the major curve and compensatory (minor) curves. In general, the major curve is larger and more structural (greatest degree of rotation). Minor curves are generally smaller and more flexible.

Idiopathic scoliosis is also classified according to age: infantile—birth to 3 years (males predominate); juvenile—4 to 10 years of age (female ratio higher); and adolescent—more than 10 years of age (strong female to male ratio, 7:1 or higher).

Parents or guardians, a child's doctor, or school screening can detect scoliosis. Referral to one pediatric orthopaedic practice indicated that 42% of cases were discovered on school screenings, while 39% were discovered by the patient's primary care physician.[32] Detection by a parent is usually based on either noticing shoulder or scapula elevation or noticing that clothes hang unevenly. Unfortunately, this is not always readily apparent, and signs may be minimal where compensation has camouflaged the deformity. When scoliosis screening was introduced in the 1940s in the United States, the goal was to identify scoliosis due to poliomyelitis. As the program expanded, the goal changed to identification of children at a stage of scoliosis development early enough to allow a period of bracing in the hope of avoiding surgery. At present, school screenings are mandatory in approximately one third of the schools in the United States, with screening occurring between the ages of 10 and 16 years (grades 5 through 9).[33,34]

The statistical risk of having a scoliosis that progresses to the point that treatment is needed is only 0.2%. The referral rate averages 5%; however, the rate is suspected to be at least twice that because referral documentation forms are not available for a large percentage of patients.[35] Williams and Herbert[36] reviewed the results of several screening programs and found a false-positive rate of at least 60% and a false-negative rate of 23%. Viewed from a different perspective, Dickson[37] found that as few as 10% of children who screened positive for trunk asymmetry had a scoliosis that was progressive. These observations have raised serious concerns about the value of school screening. Given the low prevalence of progressive curves, given that at least one third of patients are detected by their primary care physician, and given that mainly girls with large curves premenarche are likely to progress, either modifications to screening or elimination of screening has been proposed.

Modifications would include: (1) use school screening only for those who do not have access to a primary care physician, (2) screen only premenarcheal girls, and (3) do not conduct school screening for boys. The U.S. Preventive Services Task Force (USPSTF) concluded that on the basis of available evidence, a recommendation for or against routine screening of asymptomatic adolescents for idiopathic scoliosis could not be made at this time.[38]

A consensus paper by Grivas et al.[39] lists some recommendations based on questions posed to experts. For school screenings, it was advised to screen with the patient seated to eliminate adding problems associated with lower extremity asymmetries.

The basis of screening is to check the standing patient for signs of asymmetry and scoliosis. The patient then bends forward to enable the examiner to check for humping (Adams' test) indicating the side of convexity of a structural curve. It is felt that this is a simple process, yet many screening personnel are not adequately trained. When faced with an equivocal case, the tendency is to refer. This purely observational (subjective) approach has no support from a quantifiable measurement. In addressing these concerns, several recommendations have been made to potentially reduce the false-positive referral rate:

- Train personnel. Have them screen in the presence of a trained supervisor before being allowed to screen alone.
- View the spine in at least three positions of forward bending. As the patient bends forward he or she is to clasp the hands and allow them to hang dependently. The examiner views from in front or behind first at about 45° to view the thoracic "skyline," then at a few degrees more of flexion for the thoracolumbar region, and finally at a right angle for the lumbar region.
- Use a scoliometer to measure the degree of rib "humping," or more preferably called the angle of inclination or trunk rotation. This device is basically an inclinometer that measures in degrees the amount of rotation of the trunk. The instrument is reliable and seems to allow discrimination between curves that are greater than 20°.[40] It has been determined that if 5° of inclination is found, it is likely that 20° of structural curve exists, requiring further evaluation. Bunnell[40] feels that using the scoliometer criterion of 5° of rotation would decrease the false-positive referral rate by half.

Some feel that this criterion should be extended to 7° to avoid false-positive results.

- Rescreen the child in six months when uncertain, instead of immediately referring.
- Establish several referral centers where an experienced examiner with access to radiographic facilities can examine the children at no cost. This suggestion is based on the observation that there is a very low rate (less than one third in one study) of compliance for follow-up evaluation.[32]

A presentation by Braun in 2007[41] indicates that a recent study identified 12 DNA markers that were used to accurately predict progression of curve severity in patients with adolescent idiopathic scoliosis by categorizing patients into high-risk and low-risk groups. If supported by future studies, this approach may revolutionize decision making with regard to conservative versus surgical correction.

Congenital Scoliosis

Congenital scoliosis, although not as common as idiopathic scoliosis, should always be screened for in a young patient. All children under the age of 10 years have an increased incidence of neuron axis deformities.[42] The most common causes generally may be divided into two categories: (1) failure of formation such as occurs with hemivertebrae, and (2) failure of segmentation such as occurs with unilateral bar vertebrae. It is more common for these to occur in various forms of combination as opposed to discrete entities. It is extremely important to remember that these congenital abnormalities occur in all three planes and may be underestimated with regard to progression when viewed on a single radiograph. In addition, cartilaginous tissue, not visible on the radiograph, may play a role in asymmetric growth.

Prognosis regarding progression is difficult; however, some generalizations may help guide the clinician with a warning that there are always exceptions to these generalities.[30]

- Single hemivertebrae in areas other than the thoracic spine are generally not rapidly progressive.
- Hemivertebrae on opposite sides with only a few normal vertebrae separating them are not likely to progress.
- Hemivertebrae may be further divided into fully segmented, partially segmented, or nonsegmented. The distinction is based on whether a disc space

exists on both sides (fully), one side (partially), or not at all (non). In general, the disc space represents the degree of growth potential and therefore the progression potential for the scoliosis. Nonsegmented hemivertebrae are the least likely to progress.

- Predictions of progression with unilateral bar vertebrae are less difficult. The presence of a unilateral bar is strongly suggestive of progression and warrants surgical referral.
- An example of a combination of congenital deformities likely to progress would be a unilateral bar vertebra with paired hemivertebrae on the opposite side.

Unlike idiopathic scoliosis, additional diagnostic clues exist outside the spinal column and musculoskeletal system. Interference with the development of the mesoderm in utero is usually associated with multiple affected areas.

- Twenty percent of patients with congenital scoliosis were found to have genitourinary abnormalities. Six percent had serious obstructive problems.[43]
- Heart defects were found in 15% of patients with a congenital scoliosis.[44]
- Ten percent of patients with congenital scoliosis will have spinal dysraphism, with half of these being diastematomyelia.[45] The rest will have anomalous bands, lipomas, or a tight filum terminale. Patients fall into three groups. The first group has the scoliosis as the prominent external sign. The other two groups may show excess hair growth, dimpling, or pigmentation problems (café au lait spots) over or around the spine. All patients should be observed for these subtle indicators. Other associated findings include a clubfoot, a congenitally dislocated hip, or an anatomically short leg.

Decision Making with Congenital Curves

The clinician must be aware of the different progression rates of congenital scoliosis. Given the significant numbers of extraspinal abnormalities that may coexist with congenital scoliosis, a thorough physical examination must be performed. It would then be appropriate to refer the patient to an internist if heart or genitourinary abnormalities are present or to a neurologist if there is a suspicion of neurofibromatosis or spinal dysraphism.

If the patient has a unilateral, nonsegmented hemivertebra or bilateral hemivertebrae separated by a few normal vertebrae, the patient should be monitored radiographically every three to six months. The least likely to progress are nonsegmented hemivertebrae. However, if there is a single segmented hemiverte-bra in the thoracic spine or a unilateral bar vertebra, refer for orthopaedic consultation because they are likely to progress.

If there are combined defects and the curve is less than 20° or less than 40° with a balanced trunk, the patient should be monitored radiographically every six months for progression. Refer if progressive. If there are combined defects and the curve is between 20° and 40° with an unbalanced trunk and flexible spine, bracing is appropriate. Curves with combined defects that are pro-gressive, and those greater than 40° should be referred for orthopaedic surgical consultation.

Idiopathic Scoliosis

Prognostications regarding the natural history of an indi-vidual's idiopathic scoliosis are primarily hinged on three primary and several secondary factors. The primary gauges of progression are the severity of the curve, the apex location, and the skeletal maturity of the individual. Secondary indicators include genetic tendencies, gender, and curve flexibility.

Although the severity of the curve is relatively easy to determine radiographically, skeletal maturity is a more complex variable. Two methods are used to determine skeletal maturity: (1) the Greulich-Pyle atlas, and (2) the Risser sign. The Greulich-Pyle atlas is a comparative refer-ence to match with a patient's left wrist radiographs. The Risser sign is a grading of iliac crest apophysis develop-ment (**Figure 5–3**). The upper pelvic rim is divided into four equal units. Radiographically the line of apophyseal growth progresses laterally to medially. It is believed that little growth (less chance for progression) occurs after a +4 Risser sign. Compared with a 36% progression with a Risser sign of 0, only 11% progressed with a Risser sign of 2.[46]

Various investigators have classified idiopathic curves into commonly occurring patterns. A widely accepted classification system by King[47] has not been shown to have a sufficient intraobserver or interobserver reliability to help guide decision making using spinal fixation surgery.[48,49] These curves are primarily structural and may lead to development of compensatory curves. The only way to distinguish among curves that appear to be of equal sever-ity is to note the degree of rotation and with side-bending films to determine which curves are flexible. A list of these patterns is given with some clues to recognition.

- Double major—This includes two curves of equal or close to equal size, both of which fail to correct

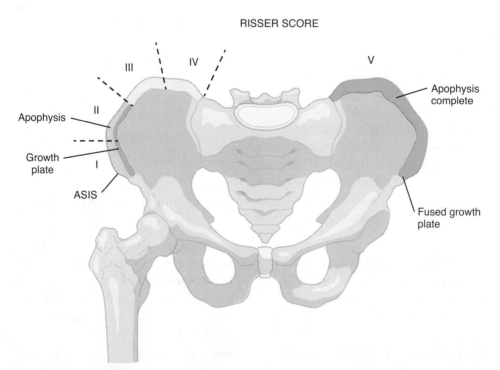

Figure 5–3 Grading the development of iliac crest apophysis according to the Risser sign. The iliac crest is divided into four quarters, and the excursion or stage of maturity is the amount of progression. In this example, the excursion is 50%; the Risser sign is 2.

much on lateral-bending films. The thoracic apices are at T7; the lumbar at L2. The upper end vertebra for the thoracic component is T5 or T6, with the lumbar being T11. The pattern is consistently right thoracic/left lumbar convexity. This is such a common pattern (90% of the time) that when the opposite is found it is suggested that consideration for further evaluation with magnetic resonance imaging (MRI) is necessary. A relatively common cause is syringomyelia or the type I Arnold-Chiari syndrome.[50] Arai et al.[51] found that although the incidence was only 4% for syringomyelia and Arnold-Chiari type I malformation each (total 8%), scoliosis was the only presenting complaint in 40% of these cases. Nineteen percent of these cases had a left convex thoracic curve. A recent study[52] attempted to determine the clinical indications for MRI of intraspinal abnormalities. The investigators found that if neck pain and headache (especially exertional headache) and neurologic findings such as ataxia, weakness, and a cavus foot were used as criteria for ordering MRI, all intraspinal abnormalities would be found.

- Right thoracic—This initially single curve extends from about T5 to T11 with the apex at about T8. Often confused with a double major curve, the right thoracic usually has a compensatory curve in the lumbar region that may at times be of equal size; however, it is flexible. The right thoracic curve is an excellent example that the thoracic curve is not commonly a mechanical compensation for a lumbar curve, but in fact it is the reverse. This demonstrates that an unlevel pelvis or sacrum is not often the stimulus for scoliosis formation with many curves.
- Lumbar—Usually extending from about T11-T12 to L3-L4; apices L1-L2. This curve is usually left convex (70% of time). Thoracic compensation is not uncommon; however, it occurs to a much smaller degree.
- Thoracolumbar—Extending from about T8 to L3; apices T11-T12. This single curve is less likely to have clearly compensatory curves associated with it. It is primarily right convex (80% of time).
- Double thoracic major—With an upper left curve extending from T2 to T7 and a lower right curve extending from T7 to L1, these two primary curves are usually compensated for in the cervical spine.

The standard King classification for scoliosis has been recently challenged by newer systems: the Conrad system[53] and the Lenke system.[54] The King system was developed in relation to decision making using Harrington rod surgery and is a uniplanar (coronal plane only), potentially outdated approach. One of the newer systems is the Conrad system, a coronal pattern classification system. There are 21 pattern categories further separated into 11 curve types (these include the King curve patterns). Another newer system is the Lenke system used primarily for surgical planning,[55] and although this system appears to be more reliable than the older King system, proper classification of high thoracic and lumbar curves may remain difficult. Lenke has made some recommendations for reducing these areas of disagreement on classification.[56] Generally, the Lenke system is based on three components:[57]

1. Curve types—Type 1 (main thoracic: MT), Type 2 (double thoracic: DT), Type 3 (double major: DM), Type 4 (triple major: TM), Type 5 (thoracolumbar/lumbar: TL/L), and Type 6 (thoracolumbar/lumbar main thoracic: TL/L-MT)
2. A lumbar spine modifier—based on severity of lumbar deformity (based on central sacral vertical line and the apical lumbar vertebrae; A = line between the pedicles, B = line between the medial aspect of the concave pedicle and the concave margin of the apical vertebral body, and C = line entirely medial to the concave aspect of the apical vertebral body)
3. A sagittal thoracic modifier—defined as the Cobb angle from T5-T12 (hypokyphotic [−], < 10°; normal [n], 10°–40°; and hyperkyphotic [+], > 40°)

The five most common curve patterns based on this system appear to be 1AN, 1BN, 2AN, 5CN, and 1CN, accounting for 58% of all operative curves.[56] Determining structural characteristics includes the use of bending and sagittal views. Proximal thoracic curves are determined to be structural, with a maximum residual Cobb measurement of ≥ 25° or T2-T5 kyphosis ≥ 20°. A main thoracic or thoracolumbar/lumbar curve is determined to be structural if there is a residual Cobb angle ≥ 25° or thoracolumbar T10-L2 kyphosis ≥ 20°.

Double curve patterns tend to progress more than single curve patterns. However, single curves with little compensation are more deforming, as are high thoracic curves. Lumbar curves are generally far less progressive compared with the other major curve patterns.[14]

The most important indicator of a good prognosis (slim chance of progression) is the closure of vertebral growth plates, generally indicating skeletal maturity. Because this event cannot currently be viewed directly, we are left, as often is the case, with indirect and therefore inaccurate clues.

Age is only an indirect measure of an individual's skeletal maturity. This is so primarily because hormonal factors are variable: one individual may achieve menarche and a growth spurt at a relatively early age while another may undergo these events two to three years later. This broad difference in growth spurt is an obvious normal distinction between boys and girls and in some ways may be one reason why scoliosis is less likely to progress in boys.

Growth potential is the critical factor. If the growth potential is known, the degree of concern for progression can be approximated. In other words, when the patient has attained most of his or her adult height, there is significantly less chance of progression. The end of the adolescent growth spurt, therefore, is a good indicator of relative stability in curve size.

The growth spurt is considered to be about a 3½-year period.[58] The peak height velocity when the rate of growth is greatest occurs during the first 1½ years. The rate decreases during the last two years. Several studies have pointed to an apparent difference in the timing of the growth spurt. Goldberg et al.[59] noted that girls with adolescent idiopathic scoliosis appear to have an early pubertal growth spurt, but no abnormality of total growth or development. Therefore, they simply reach the adult height at an earlier age than matched controls. Numerous studies[60–63] have demonstrated that girls with idiopathic scoliosis were significantly taller than matched controls. This was most apparent in the younger groups and much less apparent in the older groups. Final adult height comparisons showed no significant differences. Several studies[64–66] indicate that there may be increased growth hormone in girls with idiopathic scoliosis, particularly in the early stages of puberty.

A good indicator of the first rapid phase of height growth is the development of secondary sex characteristics. A staging for both girls and boys has been developed by Tanner.[67] Five stages for breast development and the development of pubic hair are used for girls; for boys, genitalia development and pubic hair growth (see Chapter 53). For modesty requirements, it may be necessary to use a modification of the Tanner criteria. This modification allows the patient to choose from a written description or pictorial rendition of each Tanner stage of pubic hair development.

In matching the Tanner staging to age, menarche, and peak height growth, a pattern appears. In the United States the average age for menarche is 12½ years (with a standard deviation of 1 year).[12] Menarche appears to occur earlier in girls with idiopathic scoliosis. It is significant that most authors[68] support Scoles et al.[69] in finding that height increased less than 3% after menarche. Therefore, it appears to signal the slowing of the growth spurt. Menarche corresponds to stage 4 breast and pubic hair growth using the Tanner criteria. This correlates with at least a year into the peak height growth phase. Boys, however, will usually reach peak height velocity in stage 4, later than girls.

It is often stated that idiopathic scoliosis is more common in females. When the data are examined more closely, however, it is clear that there is male predominance with infantile curves and that the ratio of males to females is generally equal with curves less than 20°.[70] Females dominate significantly with curves greater than 30°. Curves in need of surgical treatment show a dramatic female predominance of 7:1.

Flexibility is an important determination for distinguishing among the different curve patterns and may be a factor in the tendency to progress. Duval-Beaupere et al.[71] have determined two types of flexibility that must be considered: (1) collapse, the degree of increase in curvature when gravity acts as an axial force on the scoliosis (standing position), or the opposite is true, the degree to which the curve improves with recumbency; and (2) reducibility, the degree of correction that occurs with corrective forces such as bracing, laterally bending into the convexity, muscle stimulation, and so forth.

It was suggested that reducibility is not a constant that helps with prediction of which curves are likely to progress; however, it was suggested that those curves with the largest collapse tendencies (corrected most when lying) had the slowest evolution rates.

Although the flexibility of the curve is screened with an Adams' test, quantification is important to determine the degree of flexibility. Radiographically this is measured by comparing the Cobb angle from the standing anterior-to-posterior (AP) or posterior-to-anterior (PA) radiograph and a recumbent radiograph with the patient bending maximally into the convexity of the curve being evaluated. Another suggested approach, especially for surgeons estimating the degree of correction, is the "push-prone" technique.[72] It combines the above-described collapsibility and reducibility concepts by having assistants push on apical areas (using lead gloves) while the prone radiograph is taken. This approach was valuable for thoracolumbar and lumbar curve surgeries predicting the effects that correction of the primary curve has on curves above and below fusion.

Right and left lateral bending films are traditionally used to measure the flexibility of a scoliotic curve. A curve is classified as structural if it does not "bend out" or reduce to less than 20°. A study[73] determined that a single supine, non-effort-related radiograph is predictive of curve flexibility. Curves were classified using the Lenke classification system taken from measurements in the coronal plane for the proximal thoracic, main thoracic, and thoracolumbar Cobb angles. Sagittally, measurements were at T2–T5, T5–T12, and TL/L. Use of a formula allowed accurate determination of flexibility and reduced the large variation inherent in the older effort-based lateral bending films. Details are found in the article by Cheh et al.[73]

Summary of Scoliosis Evaluation

In an effort to synthesize the foregoing information, a summary approach to the young scoliotic patient is presented. Physical examination of all infants, children, and adolescents should include a screen for signs of both congenital defects in vertebral development and scoliosis. Congenital problems should be suspected when bony abnormalities are evident through deformity, hip dislocation, clubfeet, and the like, and dermatologic signs such as pigmentation changes and hair growth over affected areas.

Next, a standard standing observation for asymmetry should be performed followed by an Adams' test performed in three positions. Any humping should be quantified with a scoliometer. Radiographs should be obtained for patients whose angular rotation deformity (humping) is greater than 5°. If prior radiographs are available they should be ordered for comparison purposes. If radiographs are not recent and there is a suspicion of progression, new films should be ordered. If no films are available a baseline series must be ordered.

Radiographs should include a full-spine (14 × 36) posterior-to-anterior (PA) or anterior-to-posterior (AP) if the AP incorporates rare-earth screens and appropriate shielding. The suggestion of a PA view is based on the significant reduction in radiation exposure to developing breasts. A lateral full spine should complement the AP or PA in an effort to determine the degree of sagittal effect from the scoliosis (lordosis and kyphosis) and to glean a better idea of the degree of vertebral body involvement if a congenital defect is found. Cruickshank et al.[74] demonstrated that a lordosis or flattening is usually found at the apical region of structural curves rather than the visually perceived kyphosis. They demonstrated that this visual impression is incorrectly confirmed on the lateral radiograph. When a mean kyphosis of 41° was measured on the lateral view, it was found to represent an area of lordosis when the lateral view was corrected for rotation.

Finally, recumbent, laterally bending films should be included for each curve to determine the degree of curve flexibility. This involves the patient's maximally bending into the convexity of the curve. The Cobb angle is then compared between the standing and recumbent, laterally bending views. Subtraction of these two values indicates the functional aspect of the curve. This helps determine which curves are major curves and which are compensatory curves.

The Cobb angle is the standard measurement of the degree of curvature. Although there are some problems with this approach, its universal acceptance allows comparison with follow-up views taken in consultation and referral. The angle is based on determining the end vertebrae. These are the upper- and lowermost vertebrae that tilt last into the concavity of the curve and demonstrate no rotation based on pedicle location. By drawing lines along the end-plates of the vertebrae toward the concavity of the curve, it will be found that the first vertebra outside the curve will have lines that diverge from the other lines (**Figure 5–4A**). After choosing the end vertebra, a line across the top of the upper-end vertebra and across the bottom-end vertebra is drawn toward the concave side. Perpendicular lines are then drawn from each of these lines. The intersection of these lines equals the Cobb angle. It has been shown that there is some diurnal variation in the Cobb angle, as much as 5°.[75] This variation suggests repeating follow-up views at the same time of day if possible.

Determination of bone age (skeletal maturity) is made with the Risser sign.[76] With the iliac crest divided into four equal divisions, a determination is made regarding the extent of apophyseal fusion. Although the apophyseal advancement is from anterior-to-posterior and then medially, on a two-dimensional image such as a radiograph it appears as a lateral-to-medial growth. One study[77] demonstrated that the Risser sign may not be accurately viewed on a PA radiograph. When the line of

Cobb method

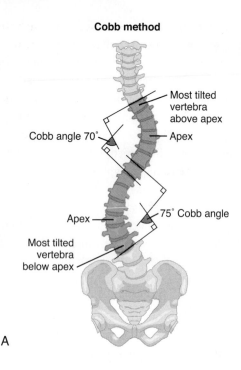

A

Nash-Moe method

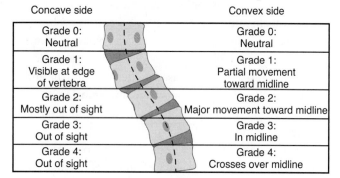

Concave side		Convex side	
Grade 0: Neutral		Grade 0: Neutral	
Grade 1: Visible at edge of vertebra		Grade 1: Partial movement toward midline	
Grade 2: Mostly out of sight		Grade 2: Major movement toward midline	
Grade 3: Out of sight		Grade 3: In midline	
Grade 4: Out of sight		Grade 4: Crosses over midline	

B

Figure 5–4 Measurement on a radiograph of degree of curvature in scoliosis according to the (A) Cobb angle and (B) Nash-Moe method.

growth has extended through the last quadrant, a Risser sign of 4 has been reached. At this stage there is still a radiolucent separation between the apophyseal line and the crest. Closure of this space is considered a Risser sign 5, indicating full skeletal maturity. There are some flaws with this measurement; however, it still is a major indirect indicator of vertebral end-plate closure, thereby indicating the end of scoliosis progression during adolescence. The time of appearance is relatively standard; however, the time of fusion is variable. It appears that vertebral end-plate closure has probably occurred by the time a Risser sign 4 is seen in some but not all individuals.[78] So, although a Risser sign 5 is a confirmation of closure, it appears that the Risser sign may be a

late indicator of end-plate closure. Still, the Risser sign is considered one of only three significant predictive factors with regard to scoliosis development.[79]

Rotation is another important observation made radiographically. The standard measurement is the Nash-Moe method. Using the pedicle shadows as reference points to a line drawn through the center of the vertebrae, the degree of deviation from the center line is determined (**Figure 5–4B**). A large rotational component to the curve suggests a structural type. The degree of rotation can be so great as to give the appearance of an oblique radiograph of the region.

Rotation that does not fit the pattern of a typical structural, idiopathic curve (body toward convexity, posterior elements toward the concavity) should suggest a functional, possibly muscle spasm, cause. Also if no rotation occurs, it is likely that the curve is more flexible. Both no rotation and body rotation into the concavity indicate a functional curve, and when coupled with a patient presenting with back pain, muscle spasm is likely the cause.

Nonradiographic evaluation for progression is usually topographically based. Moire topography and integrated shape investigation system (ISIS) screening are the two most commonly used instrumentations; however, they are not widely used in the United States. Moire topography is utilized primarily in Japan for school screening of idiopathic scoliosis.[80] It uses light sources that superimpose a grid on the patient's back.[81] A Polaroid photograph is taken of this surface distortion pattern. As on a geographic map, lines that diverge indicate higher elevations (posteriority) and lines that converge indicate less height (anteriority). Although designed as a tool to replace the positional examination at school screenings, Moire topography has not been found to be significantly valuable. Moire topography is most valuable as a nonradiographic monitoring tool for detecting scoliosis progression. Although there are some problems with false-positive results, it is helpful in indicating in most patients when a radiographic evaluation should be performed to determine the degree of progression. ISIS screening is more high-tech; therefore, it is more expensive and less available.[82] The principles are the same as those of Moire topography; however, a computer is used to generate an approximation of the coronal and sagittal curves. Again, it is not a good screening tool but may help with monitoring progression.

Recent advances have led to a genetic test called ScoliScore, which is a saliva-based test that incorporates 28 progression and 25 protection-associated markers.

Along with the patient's Cobb angle at the time of testing, the ScoliScore attempts to predict progression. In a recent study,[83] the ScoliScore risk distribution in the study population was 36% low risk, 55% intermediate risk, and 9% high risk. Using the clinical approach (i.e., the Lonstein/Carlson categorization) on the same patients, the risk distribution was 2% low risk, 51% intermediate risk, and 47% high risk, demonstrating that the clinical approach under-identified the low-risk and over-identified the high-risk group assuming the ScoliScore is a better predictor of progression. Only 25% of patients were in the same risk category for both systems. Only the Cobb angle showed significant correlation with ScoliScore. ScoliScore predicted nearly 16 times more low-risk patients and more than five times fewer high-risk patients. Practically, this means that the ScoliScore approach may rank patients more often in the low-risk category and remove some of the concern for patients categorized as high-risk using the older system. The problem is that ScoliScore testing is expensive and not very accessible.

Another recent study[84] indicated that the severity of the curve was the best predictor of progression. It was valuable only for low- and high-risk individuals, but not for intermediate-risk patients. The low-risk group had curves less than 18° on the day of presentation to the provider's office. The high-risk group were those with curves more than 26° on the day of presentation. This still leaves the grey zone of curves between 18°–26° where it is difficult to determine risk of progression either using the clinical approach or the ScoliScore approach.

Management

The literature regarding scoliosis development and progression, screening, and treatment is voluminous. The difficulty is that when criteria used for inclusion or exclusion are not held constant, meta-analysis and extrapolation based on this analysis are extremely difficult.

It would seem that decision making in scoliosis management would be a simple process. A curve exists where a straight line should be. Push on the apices of the curve (or curves), distract the curve to assist straightening, and finally level out the base on which the spine sits, avoiding any "compensatory" curve development. This "mechanical" approach fails for two major reasons: (1) the development of a curve or curves has a mechanical component that becomes a significant factor only after the curve

reaches 30°, and (2) the curve is not two-dimensional. A large rotational component is found with structural scoliosis also affecting the sagittal curves (kyphosis, lordosis). Individuals grow at different rates. In addition, one individual with a 30° curve may have progression while another may not for no known reason. Therefore, clinical decisions should err on the side of caution.

Prognosis is based on the following primary and secondary factors:[2]

- *Primary*
  - Double curve patterns progress more often than single curves (single curves cause more deformity).
  - The greater the curve at detection the greater the risk of progression.
  - There is a greater chance of progression if the onset is before menarche in females.
  - The lower the Risser sign at the time of diagnosis, the greater the chance of progression.
  - Males with similar sized curves have much less risk of progression than the corresponding female.
- *Secondary*
  - Curve progression may be higher for those with an associated thoracic kyphosis.
  - Risk of progression decreases significantly at skeletal maturity; however, it may progress based on the severity and location of the curve.

The risk of progression in skeletally mature individuals is fairly low; however, the following statistical predictors have been identified:[2]

- Thoracic curves—those greater than 50° Cobb angle, with apical vertical rotation greater than 30°, or a Mehta angle greater than 30° are more likely to progress.
- Lumbar curves—those greater than 30° Cobb angle, with apical vertical rotation greater than 30°, right convex curves, and those with translatory shifts (seen with a high intercrest line [an interiliac crest line falling at or above the fourth or fifth lumbar disc space allowing third lumbar shift on the fourth]) have a greater chance of progression.
- Thoracolumbar curves—those greater than 30° Cobb angle, those with apical vertical rotation greater than 30°, or those with translatory shifts are more likely to progress.
- Pregnant females have a chance of progression during pregnancy, only if curves are greater than 50° at time of pregnancy.

The key questions a clinician needs to ask in making a decision regarding management of idiopathic scoliosis are as follows:

- What is the risk of progression?
- What is the effectiveness of various conservative options versus operative options?
- What is the risk of using chiropractic methods versus bracing or surgery regarding progression?
- If bracing or surgery is needed, what are the criteria for referral (at what level of severity or age are they most effective)?
- What are the risks of surgery?
- What outcome is desired (reduction of curve, prevention of progression, improvement of cardiopulmonary function, etc.)?

The incidence of infantile scoliosis has decreased so markedly that the condition is rarely seen.[85] This fact, coupled with the finding of a left convex thoracic curve, suggests that infantile scoliosis may represent a form separate from idiopathic scoliosis. Environmental factors are believed to be the explanation. If a clinician does encounter an infantile scoliosis, congenital and paralytic causes should be ruled out. If the infantile form is still a consideration, an orthopaedist can predict progression using the Mehta rib-vertebra angle measurement.[86] The rib-vertebra angle measurement is formed by drawing a vertical line through the center of the vertebra. Lines drawn through the long axis of the right and left ribs intersect this line. If the difference between the right and left angles is greater than 20°, progression is likely. Conservative treatment using a serial elongation derotation flexion (EDF) cast approach has been demonstrated to be very effective in preventing progression with infantile scoliosis.[87]

Although it might be easy to set a cutoff point for conservative versus surgical care based on the severity of the curve, real life contains too many variables to allow such a clean black-and-white decision. Measurements of skeletal maturity must be included in an effort to determine likelihood of progression. Outcome desires are ultimately what guide the clinician in equivocal scenarios. Outcome predictability for orthotic treatment, adapted from Bunch and Patwardhan,[31] might include: (1) ability to halt progression, (2) chance of progression while braced, and (3) cost and complications associated with bracing (medical and psychologic). Outcome predictability for surgical management may include: (1) correction potential without complications, (2) infection and pseudarthrosis development, and (3) late complications.

In general, the predictability is fairly well known for each factor when matched with age (skeletal maturity) and curve severity. Still, there are scenarios where a "successful" outcome is fairly equal for both options. Then it is often the decision of the clinician based on the value he or she places on each of the outcome factors. For example, a 12-year-old girl with a 35° curve and a Risser sign of 3 might have an equal chance of a successful outcome with either treatment approach. However, the risk of infection, pseudarthrosis, and late complications is fairly low with surgery. A surgeon might consider this an acceptable tradeoff compared with one or two years of bracing, which carries with it about a 10% chance of progression, compliance issues, and psychologic complications. In the mind of the chiropractor or conservative orthopaedist, however, the lower cost of bracing and the avoidance of some of the rare but serious complications of surgery might be more appropriate. Neither is an incorrect choice. However, the desires of the parents and the child must be factored in before a decision is made. This requires a full discussion with the parents and the child of the options and their associated advantages and disadvantages.

Always keeping in mind the complexity that may exist in individual cases, the following is a suggested baseline approach to decision making based on severity of the curve and maturity. It is important to note that these are idiopathic curves, meaning that congenital and transient curves due to muscle spasm are not included.

- Curves less than 20° may be treated chiropractically.
  1. If the patient has not reached skeletal maturity, observation using nonradiographic means should be used to determine progression. Radiographs should be taken if there are signs of progression. Radiographs may be needed during periods of rapid growth to better gauge progression.
  2. If the patient has reached skeletal maturity, treatment for progression is not needed. If biomechanical faults are present, such as unilateral pronation or a significant leg length deficiency, correct them and obtain a radiograph to determine effectiveness. There is little chance of progression in this range of scoliosis, however.
- Curves between 20° and 40° are still within the conservative management range.
  1. If the patient has not reached skeletal maturity and the curve is less than 30°, initial chiropractic care may be applied; however, the clinician must be vigilant in monitoring for progression. Any signs of progression should result in

referral for bracing. This is the range at which bracing has been shown to be most effective.[68]

2. If the patient has reached skeletal maturity, progression is not likely. Correct biomechanical faults and observe periodically.

- Curves greater than 40° may require surgery.
 1. If the patient has a Tanner score of less than 2 and/or a Risser sign of less than 3, bracing should be tried for six months. If ineffective, refer for surgical consideration (see discussion below).
 2. If the patient has a Tanner 3 or a Risser 4, surgery is recommended.

A dilemma often exists for the chiropractor faced with a patient with a progressive or large curve who is seeking alternatives to bracing and surgery. The chiropractor is considered the last hope for the patient. It is important to explain fully to the patient and the parents the consequences of allowing the curve to progress and weigh against this the advantages of bracing or surgery. The consequences of progression are mainly cosmetic. The larger the curve at skeletal maturity, the more likely it will progress in adulthood. If cardiopulmonary function is normal as an adolescent, it is unlikely to become worse as an adult as a result of the scoliosis. In fact, forced vital capacity in nonsmokers does not decrease significantly until curves progress to 100° to 120° (a rare occurrence even in adulthood).[88] It is also likely that as an adult, chronic back pain is more likely. Therefore, with cosmesis as the central issue, it is a decision that is difficult to make not knowing an individual's future adult perspective on appearance. What might help put the decision in perspective is that it has been found that scoliotic patients have a high percentage of psychosocial adjustment problems, unemployment, delayed marriage, or no marriage.[31]

Comanagement with an orthopaedist is recommended when curves enter an equivocal range wherein decisions become difficult. Finding a knowledgeable and reasonable orthopaedist for comanagement guarantees that all alternatives are explained to the patient and the doctors understand each other's rationale and concerns. The patient is then able to make more educated choices not based on fear tactics from either camp.

Conservative Treatment Options

Lateral Surface Stimulation

The principle of electrical surface stimulation is based on providing a constant load through contraction of the larger trunk muscle via the lever arm of the ribs. It was hoped that by using stimulation for eight hours during the night the effects of creep and relaxation could be used in a positive way to effect change. The spine and its surrounding soft tissue support represent viscoelastic material. Viscoelastic material will undergo permanent change in length only when a constant load is applied over long periods of time. Although the initial reports[89] on electrical stimulation for scoliosis correction were extremely encouraging, subsequent studies have demonstrated an unacceptably low rate of success.[90]

Bracing

Bracing recently has come under attack as a viable conservative treatment option for progressive curves. The first doubts were raised when it was determined from school screening programs that curves in the 15° to 20° range that appeared to be successfully treated by bracing probably would have done as well without bracing. The study by Moe and Kettleson[91] initially indicated excellent results with bracing; however, the follow-up review of these patients by Carr et al.[92] indicated loss of correction the longer patients were off the brace. Finally, Emans et al.[93] reported on the effectiveness of part-time bracing as opposed to the tried-and-true full-time approach. A misrepresentation of who the braced group is compared with the control group may be a serious flaw in the interpretation of many studies. One study indicated that patients prescribed a brace actually were compliant to only 10% of the prescribed time-in-brace.[94] Comparison studies between groups that were braced and those that were not often inadvertently compared typically highly progressive curves that were not braced with curves less likely to progress that were braced (e.g., thoracic curves for nontreatment versus thoracolumbar curves that were braced). This bias toward bracing curves less likely to progress gave an unfair success ratio to the braced groups. A small group study and review of the literature by Goldberg et al.[95] suggests no difference between braced and non-braced skeletally immature adolescent girls. The Iowa Group report of 1996 indicated that it is still impossible to clearly state that bracing alters the natural history of idiopathic scoliosis in immature patients at high risk for progression.[96]

Many orthopaedists and chiropractors will still make the choice to brace or refer for bracing. If bracing is used, the following two factors, based on the current literature, may be important in patient selection:

1. Girls who were braced before and at the time of menarche had the best results. Those who were

braced months or more postmenarche had the least success. It is suggested that for this latter group bracing is little more than a "holding" device. (This may be true for most braced patients.)

2. The degree of curvature is crucial in determining the appropriateness of bracing. Curves less than 20° (and not progressing) probably will do as well without bracing. Curves greater than 40° are likely to lose substantial degrees of correction postbracing.

Therefore, girls who are at premenarche or menarche with curves in the 20° to 40° range have the greatest chance of success with bracing. It should be noted that although bracing was required for 23 hours a day in the past, bracing time is more commonly 16 to 18 hours with current prescriptions. A recent study indicated that bracing for 23 hours is more effective than the more commonly used 16- to 18-hour regimen.[97]

Bracing must be performed by an experienced orthotist at facilities that have experience in scoliosis brace fabrication. They are given specific design specifications by the orthopaedist. The corrective principles with bracing are based on applying pressure at the apices. This cannot be done directly, so the corrective pad is applied to the rib attached to the apical vertebra in the thoracic region. This places the pad below the apex from a surface perspective. The lumbar pad is applied to the paraspinal muscles over the transverse processes. Corrective pads are attached to the shell of the brace. Braces such as the Milwaukee brace may also apply distractive forces with a large metal superstructure extending to the occiput.

There are basically four types of brace designs:

1. Thoraco-Lumbo-Sacral Orthosis (TLSO) (also known as the Boston brace or "underarm" brace)—Fitted and custom molded from plastic. Basic principle is to apply three-point pressure to the curve.

2. Cervico-Thoraco-Lumbo-Sacral Orthosis (also known as the Milwaukee brace)—Similar to the TLSO brace but also includes a neck ring held in place by vertical bars attached to the brace. Worn 23 hours a day, it can be removed for swimming, sports, or gym class. More often used for thoracic spine curves.

3. Charleston Bending Brace—Called the "nighttime" brace because it is designed for limited use during sleeping. The brace is molded with the patient bending to the side thereby applying more pressure against the curve.

4. Dynamic Bracing (e.g. SpineCor)—Unlike rigid braces, these flexible braces use a system of corrective bands to accomplish derotation and other corrective forces. The idea is to allow more spinal mobility while being braced. Early results suggest that it may be an option for patients with small curves around 20 degrees. In one study,[98] 48% of patients were corrected, 28% were stabilized, and 14% progressed. In another study[99] for patients in the same severity range, it appeared that exercise fared as well as the SpineCor group with regard to curve improvement if determined as a change of 5°. The question of natural history is still unanswered due to lack of a control group.

A formal review by Rowe et al.[100] is similar to conclusions held by the Scoliosis Research Society—that the Milwaukee brace worn 23 hours is effective at halting progression. Lateral electrical surface stimulation was less effective than observation only. Wearing the brace for 8 to 16 hours a day was more effective than observation but less effective than 23 hours of use. In the brace manual for the Scoliosis Research Society, Rowe concludes from the available reviewed literature that curves kept under 45° tend not to progress over a lifetime. The average lifetime progression for braced curves was 7.9° compared to 23° in the untreated population. There was a subgroup that progressed more than 10° but this group could not be distinguished based on demographic indicators. He concludes that curves under 35° require full-time bracing. For curves greater than 40°, bracing will likely not be effective. A study published in 2013[101] demonstrated that for patients between the ages of 10 and 15 years, with a Risser grade 0, 1, or 2, and a Cobb angle between 20° and 40°, bracing was more effective at preventing progression to 50° (considered treatment failure in this study) when compared to an observation group. The success rate for bracing was 72% versus 48% in the observation group. This was dependent on length of time for wearing the brace. Although the mean time for brace wear was around 12 hours, those who wore the brace less than 7 hours had a treatment success equal to the observation group versus a 90% to 95% success rate for those who wore the brace around 13 hours per day.

One study by Katz and Duranni[102] indicated that 36% of a group of braced patients needed surgery. It would seem that for those patients in whom bracing is helpful the outcome is quite optimistic; however, not all braced patients will have success.

Exercise

It is still debated as to whether specific exercises alter the natural course of idiopathic scoliosis. A number of small studies by Weiss[103,104] indicate a potential; however, no large trial has demonstrated a significant difference between exercise versus natural history. In fact, a recent Cochrane review[105] concluded that there was insufficient evidence and that only one low-quality study suggested that exercises may be more effective than electrostimulation, traction, and postural training to avoid scoliosis progression. It is agreed that exercise as a single-therapy approach is not successful in reversing or slowing the progression of scoliosis. It is agreed that exercises are a necessary adjunct to bracing therapy with a focus on abdominal strengthening, strengthening of the muscles on the convex side of the curve, and stretching of the muscles on the concave side. An interesting study published a number of years ago by Mehta[106] indicated that the use of an active side-shift exercise had a beneficial effect on small curves. The exercise, called the side-shift, involves shifting the trunk (without laterally bending or rotating) away from the curve convexity as far as the spine will allow, holding for 10 seconds, and then relaxing. This is prescribed as an "as often as possible" exercise.

Chiropractic Adjustments

Four general concepts are used in defense of chiropractic manipulative treatment of scoliosis, as follows:

1. By freeing up movement at each segmental level, the spine is kept more flexible and scoliosis is less likely to progress.
2. By a reflex reaction, adjusting (manipulation) of the cervical spine may influence righting reflexes in an effort to balance the spine.
3. Removal of segmental dysfunction may eliminate sources of aberrant sensory input and consequent output problems such as pain and accompanying muscle spasm. Proprioceptive input would then be normalized, providing an appropriate database for higher cortical decisions of body positioning.
4. By leveling the pelvis and sacrum, a scoliosis can be corrected. It has been demonstrated previously, however, that although contributory, an unlevel pelvis or sacrum is not the cause of an idiopathic curve. If this were so, the first curve to develop would be a lumbar compensation followed by a thoracic curve. Another archaic belief is that by adjusting the apical vertebra toward the concavity the curve may be lessened. Force applied at this level would have to be applied for long periods of time (such as a brace) for any correction to occur. Viscoelastic tissue such as the spine has a tendency to return to its original shape unless a constant load is applied over long periods of time.

Troyanovich[107] has piloted a new approach to a thoracolumbar curvature based upon a determination of improvement radiologically using a sequential approach to correction based on the Codman's paradox principle (see Chapter 7 on the shoulder; sequence of movement patterns influences achieved final position). The flexibility of the curve is evaluated with a focus on the order of corrective exercises and position for inverse posture spinal adjustments. After a standard anterior-to-posterior view is taken, two follow-up views are performed with the patient attaining "corrective" positions in a predetermined sequence. One begins with thoracic translation and then thoracic lateral flexion. The second, a reverse in sequence, begins with thoracic lateral flexion followed by thoracic translation. The sequence that obtains the most correction is used in performing inverse posture adjustments and exercises. For example, if the neutral thoracolumbar view demonstrated right translation displacement of the thorax in relation to the pelvis and left lateral flexion malposition of the thorax in relationship to the pelvis, and if correction is most apparent with the sequence of right thoracic lateral flexion followed by left thoracic translation, the patient would be instructed to perform exercises that emphasize this pattern. Adjustments would be delivered with the patient in this position of "correction," usually using a drop table.

At this time there is no large-study research evidence (only a few isolated case reports) that chiropractic manipulative therapy (adjusting) affects the natural history of an idiopathic scoliosis. Certainly more research must be done to determine chiropractic's role in scoliosis management.

Romano and Negrini[108] performed a systematic review for manual therapy as a conservative treatment for idiopathic scoliosis and had to concede that no conclusions could be drawn based on the current paucity and quality of the available literature. Goldberg,[109] in a review of the etiology, detection, and management for idiopathic scoliosis, believes that it is difficult to draw any conclusions based on the current evidence.

Surgery

The use of surgery for AIS has been criticized recently with concerns that the tradeoff of complication rates to prevention of progression is not always justified and that natural history effects are not as serious as assumed. A critical appraisal by Weiss and Moramarco[110] expressed concern that surgeons do not always fully explain the potential consequences and potential benefits with all patients. They concluded that the complication rates over a lifetime may reach as high as 50%. A rebuttal[111] to this article states that although informing patients of potential risks is important, the statistics used to arrive at a 50% complication rate were including patients who had received older forms of surgery. They conclude that the newer forms with pedicle screws are more stable and less inclined to require re-surgery. They cite recent evidence that the infection rate of acute infections for AIS range from 0.5–6.7% and late onset infection (>12 months) range from 2.77–4.7%.

It is beyond the scope of this discussion to give a detailed description or recommendation for specific surgical techniques. Some general principles are outlined. The two main goals of surgery are to: (1) straighten the spine in the coronal plane and correct for sagittal contour (kyphosis or lordosis), and (2) stabilize the spine through arthrodesis. Various surgeons have developed an array of instrumentation for these corrective procedures. The original Harrington rod implantation has been modified over the years. The rods are used for distraction to straighten the spine and for compression to correct for kyphosis if appropriate.[109] To add stability to the rods, sublaminar wiring (Luque) or spinous-process wiring (Drummond et al.[113]) was devised. The sublaminar wiring carries with it a risk of neurologic complication.[114] It also did not produce a significant advantage in correction or stability. The Cotrel-Dubousset instrumentation focuses on correction of the rotational component in an effort to decrease rib humping.[115] This is accomplished through a cross-linking that connects the two rods. The apparatus is relatively stable in all planes.[116] Correction of sagittal plane deformity is at least as important as coronal correction. One study indicated that the Cotrel-Dubousset approach is successful in the correction and maintenance of sagittal plane deformity.[116] A 10-year follow-up study[121] of patients who had undergone surgery for idiopathic scoliosis with the Cotrel–Dubousset instrumentation found a very high rate of satisfaction. An interesting finding was that 45% of respondents indicated they had consulted a physician or physiotherapist for back pain during the last year before the follow-up.

It is finally feasible to test the long-term results of how AIS is managed. Studies have surfaced that measure quality of life, pain, and function in patients who have been managed either conservatively or with surgery. Taken together it appears as though 10 to as many as 60 years later, there are no significant differences. However, pain did seem to be a commonality for those with curvature progression and this was directly related to curve size.[118–121]

Adult Scoliosis

Although the main focus of this chapter is idiopathic scoliosis in the growing patient, the adult patient may present with unique management problems that warrant discussion. Adult scoliosis may be a residual from earlier idiopathic development or may develop in later years.[122] If, in fact, idiopathic scoliosis is not part of the patient's history, a search for cause should include the following:

- Scoliosis may be due to reactive muscle spasm. When muscle spasm is the cause, any pain-provoking entity is possible. Common causes include reactions to vertebral disc and facet injuries, visceral disorders, and spinal cord or nerve root involvement due to bony stenosis or tumor.
- Scoliosis may be due to degenerative and osteopenic disorders of the spine. When this results in instability, a mechanical (compensatory or buckling) scoliosis may develop.

It is important to consider that there are generally three periods in which scoliosis may be progressive: (1) infancy, (2) adolescence, and (3) after age 50 years. Past age 50 the most common causes are bone-softening disorders and degenerative instability. Although it is more common for scoliosis to be a residual to an earlier idiopathic or congenital beginning, it is possible for a new, progressive scoliosis to develop as a result of the above-mentioned structural disintegrations.

Adults have a higher incidence of nonflexible lumbar curves. In addition, pain is more likely to be a presenting complaint with adult scoliotic patients.[123] Some studies, however, demonstrate the incidence to be no higher than that in the general population.[124] If pain is reported, it is described as more of a dull, aching sensation or a sensation of fatigue in the area. Only with severe scoliosis have there been reports of direct nerve root compression.

Physicians traditionally have been instructed to be cognizant of several concerns. A brief description of each follows:

- Many physicians are concerned with cardiopulmonary function with an adult case. If the patient did not have difficulty as a child or adolescent, new problems are not likely to develop as an adult unless he or she smokes.
- Some investigators[125] suggest that an increase in mortality occurs with adult scoliosis. However, other studies[126] do not support this observation.
- Pregnancy is a concern due to the suspicion that the increase in weight and the hormonal influences of soft tissue relaxation will lead to progression. However, there is no indication that pregnancy acts as an accelerator of scoliosis development in the adult patient unless initially 50°.[127]
- Although progression of an adult idiopathic scoliosis curve is not as aggressive over short periods of time as an adolescent curve, progression may amount to 1° per year averaged over time, with the most progression occurring after age 50. Curves greater than 50° are more likely to follow this pattern, whereas curves of 30° and less are relatively stable.[128]

Decision Making with Adult Scoliosis

Management decisions for the adult patient with scoliosis are directed by the same outcome desires as for the adolescent patient with scoliosis, but with different response factors. Adult scoliosis is not generally as progressive, the curves are generally less flexible, pain may be a consequence of the deformity and an equal or dominant concern of the patient, correction is less dramatic, and complications of surgery are much higher, running in the range of 30% to 60%.[129]

Balancing these positive and negative factors results in a consensus that the major concern is to reduce the pain component and prevent progression. Correcting the deformity is not a primary goal not only because it is more difficult but also because it is limited severely by the maturity of the spine, eliminating any adaptive structural changes and the accompanying secondary structural degenerative changes. The only component that is amenable to correction is the soft tissue component, the functional component of the curve.

Conservative management focuses on pain amelioration and strengthening of spinal and abdominal muscles with caution in the osteoporotic patient, who should avoid flexion exercises. The postmenopausal osteoporotic patient should be given exercise and diet recommendations; however, the possibility of estrogen replacement therapy also should be discussed. Chiropractic manipulative therapy should be incorporated, but radiographic evidence of instability or osteopenia should alert the clinician to modify treatment approaches and refer the patient if unresponsive.

A formal system review of conservative treatment of adult scoliosis was performed by Everett and Patel.[130] They concluded that there is only Level IV evidence for physical therapy, chiropractic care, and bracing, and Level III evidence for injections. They state that the available literature does support further clinical research for conservative management.

Algorithms

Algorithms for evaluation and management of congenital, idiopathic, and adult scolioses are presented in **Figures 5–5** through **5–7**.

Summary

Understanding that not all scolioses are idiopathic focuses the examination first on identifiable causes. One of these causes is transient muscle spasm, which will present differently. In addition to contributing to back pain, the patient's scoliosis will not fit a typical pattern found in idiopathic scoliosis. Often there is little rotation or the spinous processes rotate into the convexity. When these signs are present, it is likely that chiropractic care will be beneficial. If unresponsive, consider that muscle spasm may occur as a result of serious neurologic and other pathologic processes. When a double curve pattern is evident but the apical pattern is left thoracic/right lumbar, consider referral for evaluation of possible brainstem or spinal cord abnormalities.

With idiopathic scoliosis it is important for the chiropractor to realize that justification for treating a progressive scoliosis is indefensible. Using the factors of age, skeletal maturity, severity of the curve, and location, the clinician should be able to determine adequately when to treat and monitor and when to refer. In equivocal situations it is prudent to obtain an orthopaedic consultation.

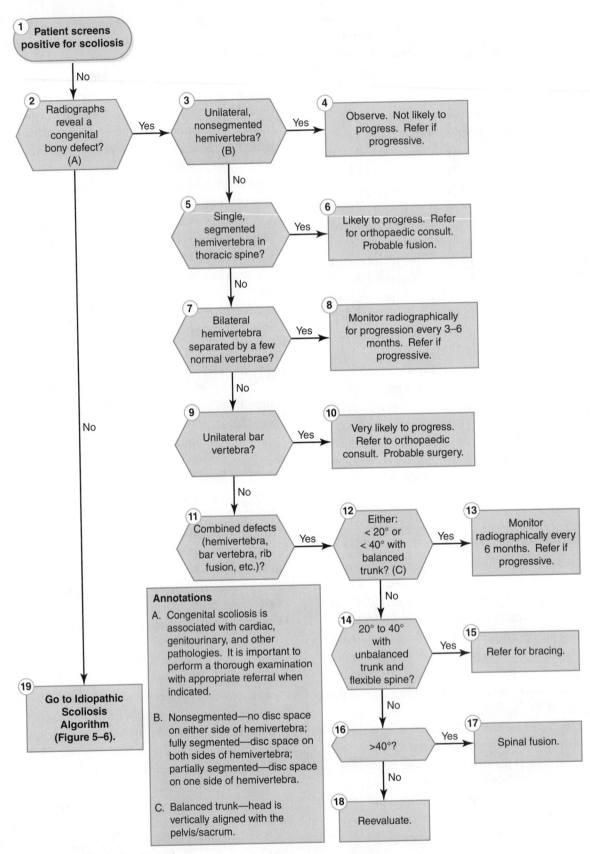

Figure 5–5 Congenital Scoliosis—Algorithm

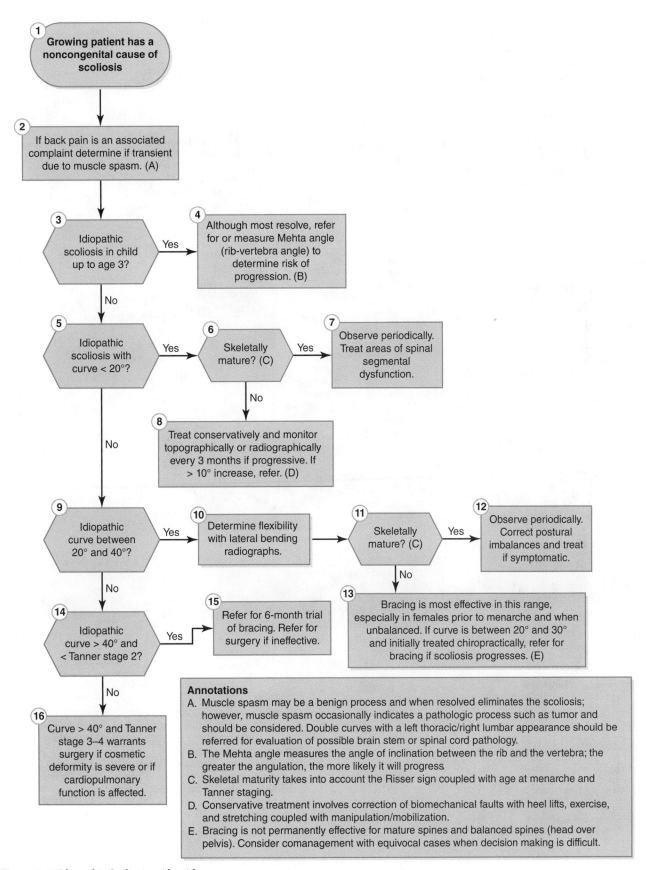

1 Growing patient has a noncongenital cause of scoliosis

2 If back pain is an associated complaint determine if transient due to muscle spasm. (A)

3 Idiopathic scoliosis in child up to age 3? — Yes → **4** Although most resolve, refer for or measure Mehta angle (rib-vertebra angle) to determine risk of progression. (B)

No

5 Idiopathic scoliosis with curve < 20°? — Yes → **6** Skeletally mature? (C) — Yes → **7** Observe periodically. Treat areas of spinal segmental dysfunction.

No (from 6) → **8** Treat conservatively and monitor topographically or radiographically every 3 months if progressive. If > 10° increase, refer. (D)

No (from 5)

9 Idiopathic curve between 20° and 40°? — Yes → **10** Determine flexibility with lateral bending radiographs. → **11** Skeletally mature? (C) — Yes → **12** Observe periodically. Correct postural imbalances and treat if symptomatic.

No (from 11) → **13** Bracing is most effective in this range, especially in females prior to menarche and when unbalanced. If curve is between 20° and 30° and initially treated chiropractically, refer for bracing if scoliosis progresses. (E)

No (from 9)

14 Idiopathic curve > 40° and < Tanner stage 2? — Yes → **15** Refer for 6-month trial of bracing. Refer for surgery if ineffective.

No

16 Curve > 40° and Tanner stage 3–4 warrants surgery if cosmetic deformity is severe or if cardiopulmonary function is affected.

Annotations
A. Muscle spasm may be a benign process and when resolved eliminates the scoliosis; however, muscle spasm occasionally indicates a pathologic process such as tumor and should be considered. Double curves with a left thoracic/right lumbar appearance should be referred for evaluation of possible brain stem or spinal cord pathology.
B. The Mehta angle measures the angle of inclination between the rib and the vertebra; the greater the angulation, the more likely it will progress.
C. Skeletal maturity takes into account the Risser sign coupled with age at menarche and Tanner staging.
D. Conservative treatment involves correction of biomechanical faults with heel lifts, exercise, and stretching coupled with manipulation/mobilization.
E. Bracing is not permanently effective for mature spines and balanced spines (head over pelvis). Consider comanagement with equivocal cases when decision making is difficult.

Figure 5–6 Idiopathic Scoliosis—Algorithm

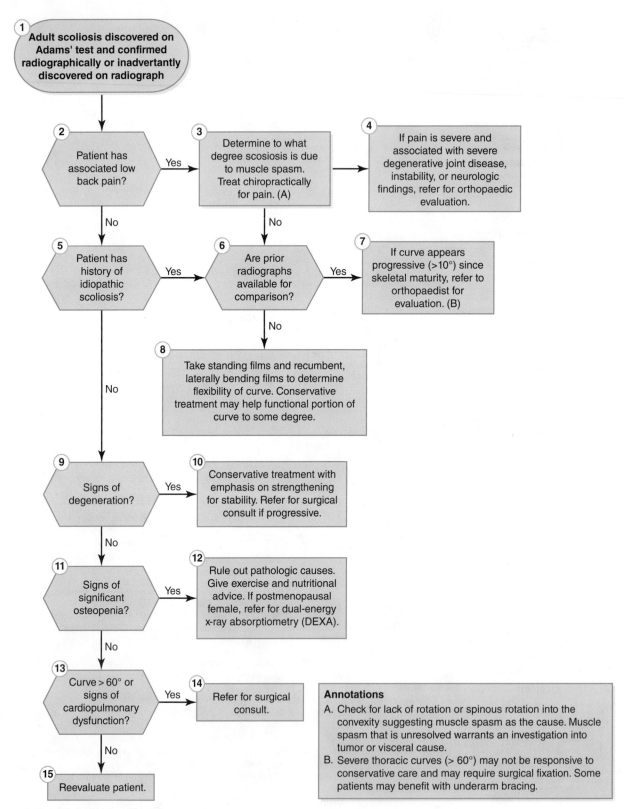

1 Adult scoliosis discovered on Adams' test and confirmed radiographically or inadvertantly discovered on radiograph

2 Patient has associated low back pain?

3 Determine to what degree scosiosis is due to muscle spasm. Treat chiropractically for pain. (A)

4 If pain is severe and associated with severe degenerative joint disease, instability, or neurologic findings, refer for orthopaedic evaluation.

5 Patient has history of idiopathic scoliosis?

6 Are prior radiographs available for comparison?

7 If curve appears progressive (>10°) since skeletal maturity, refer to orthopaedist for evaluation. (B)

8 Take standing films and recumbent, laterally bending films to determine flexibility of curve. Conservative treatment may help functional portion of curve to some degree.

9 Signs of degeneration?

10 Conservative treatment with emphasis on strengthening for stability. Refer for surgical consult if progressive.

11 Signs of significant osteopenia?

12 Rule out pathologic causes. Give exercise and nutritional advice. If postmenopausal female, refer for dual-energy x-ray absorptiometry (DEXA).

13 Curve > 60° or signs of cardiopulmonary dysfunction?

14 Refer for surgical consult.

15 Reevaluate patient.

Annotations
A. Check for lack of rotation or spinous rotation into the convexity suggesting muscle spasm as the cause. Muscle spasm that is unresolved warrants an investigation into tumor or visceral cause.
B. Severe thoracic curves (> 60°) may not be responsive to conservative care and may require surgical fixation. Some patients may benefit with underarm bracing.

Figure 5–7 Adult Scoliosis—Algorithm

APPENDIX 5–1

References

1. Dickson RA. Spinal deformity—adolescent idiopathic scoliosis: nonoperative treatment. *Spine*. 1999;24(24):2601–2606.

2. Weinstein SL. Natural history. *Spine*. 1999;24(24):2592–2600.

3. Nansel DD, Waldorf T, Cooperstein R. Effect of cervical spinal adjustments on lumbar paraspinal muscle tone: evidence for facilitation of intersegmental tonic neck reflexes. *J Manipulative Physiol Ther*. 1993;16:91–95.

4. Rowe DE, Feise RJ, Crowther ER, et al. Chiropractic manipulation in adolescent idiopathic scoliosis: a pilot study. *Chiropr Osteopat*. 2006;14:15.

5. Riseborough E, Wynne-Davies R. A genetic survey of idiopathic scoliosis in Boston. *J Bone Joint Surg Am*. 1973;55:974–982.

6. Czeizel A, Bellyei A, Barta O, et al. Genetics of adolescent idiopathic scoliosis. *J Med Genet*. 1978;15:424–427.

7. Herman RM, Mixon J, Fisher A, Maulucci R, Stuyck J. Idiopathic scoliosis and the central nervous system: a motor control problem. *Spine*. 1985;10:1–14.

8. Lion A, Haumont T, Gauchard GC, Wiener-Vacher SR, Lascombes P, Perrin PP. Visuo-oculomotor deficiency at early-stage idiopathic scoliosis in adolescent girls. *Spine (Phila Pa 1976)*. 2013;38(3):238–244.

9. Pinchuk D, Dudin M, Bekshayev S, Pinchuk O. Peculiarities of brain functioning in children with adolescence idiopathic scoliosis (AIS) according to EEG studies. *Stud Health Technol Inform*. 2012;176:87–90.

10. Vignaux G, Besnard S, Ndong J, Philoxene B, Denise P, Elefteriou F. Bone remodeling is regulated by inner ear vestibular signals. *J Bone Miner Res*. 2013;28(10):2136–2144.

11. Yamada K, Yamamoto H, Nakagawa Y, et al. Etiology of idiopathic scoliosis. *Clin Orthop*. 1984;184:50–57.

12. Bunnell WP. The natural history of idiopathic scoliosis. *Clin Orthop*. 1988;229:20–25.

13. Veldhuizen AG, Bass P, Webb J. Observation on the growth of the adolescent spine. *J Bone Joint Surg Br*. 1986;68:724–728.

14. Dickson R, Lawton I, Archer A, Butt W. The pathogenesis of idiopathic scoliosis. *J Bone Joint Surg Br*. 1984;66:8–15.

15. Dickson R, Lawton I, Archer A, Butt W. The pathogenesis of idiopathic scoliosis. In: Dickson RA, Bradford DS, eds. *Management of Spinal Deformities*. London: Butterworth; 1984.

16. Oegema TR, Bradford DS, Cooper KM, Hunter RE. Comparison of the biochemistry of proteoglycans isolated from normal, idiopathic scoliotic, and cerebral palsy spines. *Spine*. 1983;8:378–384.

17. Ghosh P, Bushnell GR, Taylor TK, et al. Distribution of glycosaminoglycans across normal and scoliotic spines. *Spine*. 1980;5:310–317.

18. Machida M, Dubousset J, Imamura Y, et al. Pathogenesis of idiopathic scoliosis: SEPs in chicken with experimentally induced scoliosis and in patient with idiopathic scoliosis. *J Pediatr Orthop*. 1994;14:329–335.

19. Machida M, Murai L, Miyashita Y, et al. Pathogenesis of idiopathic scoliosis: experimental study in rats. Presented at 32nd annual meeting of the Scoliosis Research Society; September 25, 1997; St. Louis, MO.

20. Machida M, Dubousset J, Imamura Y, et al. Melatonin: a possible role in pathogenesis of adolescent idiopathic scoliosis. *Spine*. 1996;22:1297–1301.

21. Hillbrand AS, Blackmore LC, Loder RT, et al. The role of melatonin in the pathogenesis of adolescent idiopathic scoliosis. *Spine*. 1996;21:1140–1146.

22. Fagan AB, Kennaway DJ, Sutherland AD. Total 24-hour melatonin secretion in adolescent idiopathic scoliosis. *Spine*. 1998;23:41–46.

23. Bagnall KM, Raso VJ, Hill DL, et al. Melatonin levels in idiopathic scoliosis: diurnal and nocturnal serum melatonin levels in girls with adolescent idiopathic scoliosis. *Spine*. 1996;21:1974–1978.

24. Lowe T, Lawellin D, Smith D, et al. Platelet calmodulin levels in adolescent idiopathic scoliosis: Do the levels correlate with curve progression and severity? *Spine* 2002;27(7):768–775.

25. Waldhauser F, Ehrhaut B, Forster E. Clinical aspects of the melatonin action: impact of development, aging and puberty, involvement of melatonin in psychiatric disease and importance of neuroimmunoendocrine interactions. *Experimentia*. 1993;49:671–681.

26. Machida M. Cause of idiopathic scoliosis. *Spine*. 1999;24(24):2576–2583.

27. Machida M, Miyashita Y, Murai L, et al. Role of serotonin for idiopathic deformity in pinealectomized chicken. *Spine*. 1997;22:1297–1301.

28. Wilmer S, Nilson KD, Kastrup K, et al. Growth hormone and somatomedin A in girls with

adolescent idiopathic scoliosis. *Acta Pediatr Scand.* 1976;65:547–552.

29. Liu Z, Tam EM, Sun GQ, et al. Abnormal leptin bioavail-ability in adolescent idiopathic scoliosis: an important new finding. *Spine (Phila Pa 1976).* 2012;37(7):599–604.

30. Bunch WH, Patwardhan AG. *Scoliosis: Making Clinical Decisions.* St. Louis, MO: CV Mosby; 1989.

31. Schultz A. Biomechanical studies of possible causes for the progression of idiopathic scoliosis—a reca-pitulation of research findings. In: Jacobs E, ed. *Pathogenesis of Idiopathic Scoliosis.* Chicago: Scoliosis Research Society; 1984.

32. Morrissy RT. School screening for scoliosis. *Spine.* 1999;24(24):2584–2591.

33. Bradford DS, Lonstein JE, Moe JH, et al. *Moe's Textbook of Scoliosis and Other Deformities.* 2nd ed. Philadelphia: WB Saunders; 1987.

34. Lonstein JE, Bjorkland H, Wamminger MH, et al. Voluntary school screening for scoliosis in Minnesota. *J Bone Joint Surg Am.* 1982;64:481–488.

35. Asher M, Beringer G, Orrick J, Halverbout N. The current status of scoliosis screening in North America. 1986. Results of a survey by mailed questionnaire. Presented to Scoliosis Research Society and British Scoliosis Society; September 1986; Hamilton, Bermuda.

36. Williams JI, Herbert MA. Is school screening reliable? *Orthop Trans.* 1985;9:110–111.

37. Dickson RA. Scoliosis in the community. *Br Med J.* 1983;286:615–618.

38. US Preventive Services Task Force. Screening for adolescent idiopathic scoliosis. In: *Guide to Clinical Preventive Services.* 2nd ed. Baltimore: Williams & Wilkins; 1996: 517–529.

39. Grivas TB, Wade MH, Negrini S, et al. SOSORT con-sensus paper: school screening for scoliosis. Where are we today? *Scoliosis.* 2007;2:17.

40. Bunnell WP. An objective criterion for scoliosis screening. *J Bone Joint Surg Am.* 1984;66:1381–1387.

41. Braun J. Twelve DNA markers accurately assess of progression in adolescent idiopathic scoliosis. Paper presented at 4th International Conference on Conservative Management of Spinal Deformities; May 2007; Boston, MA.

42. Goldberg CJ, Moore DP, Fogarty EE, Dowling FE. Left thoracic curve patterns and their association with disease. *Spine.* 1999;24(12):1228–1233.

43. MacEwen GD, Winter RB, Hardy JH. Evaluation of kidney anomalies in congenital scoliosis. *J Bone Joint Surg Am.* 1972;54:1341–1345.

44. Zorab P. Cardiac aspects of scoliosis. *J Bone Joint Surg Am.* 1974;56:442–447.

45. Dvonch BM, Bunch WH, Scarff TB. Spinal dysra-phism. In: Bradford D, ed. *The Pediatric Spine.* New York: Thieme-Stratton; 1985.

46. Lonstein JE, Carlson MJ. The prediction of curve progression in untreated idiopathic scoliosis during growth. *J Bone Joint Surg Am.* 1984;66:1061–1071.

47. King HA. Analysis and treatment of type II idiopathic scoliosis. *Orthop Clin North Am.* 1994;25(2):225–237.

48. Lenke LG, Betz RR, Bridwell KH, et al. Intraobserver and interobserver reliability of the classification of thoracic adolescent scoliosis. *J Bone Joint Surg Am.* 1998;80(8):1097–1106.

49. Cummings RJ, Loveless EA, Campbell J, et al. Interobserver reliability and intraobserver repro-ducibility of the system of King et al. for the classification of adolescent scoliosis. *J Bone Joint Surg Am.* 1998;80(8):1107–1111.

50. McGuire DJ, Keppler L, Kotagal S, Akbarnia BA. Scoliosis associated with type I Arnold-Chiari malfor-mations. *Orthop Trans.* 1987;11:122.

51. Arai S, Ohtsuka Y, Moriya H, Kitahara H, Minamia S. Scoliosis associated with syringomyelia. *Spine.* 1993;18:1591–1592.

52. Schwend RM, Henrikus W, Hall JE, Emans JB. Childhood scoliosis: clinical indications for mag-netic resonance imaging. *J Bone Joint Surg Am.* 1995;77(1):46–53.

53. Conrad RW, Murell GA, Morley G, et al. A logical coronal pattern classification of 2000 consecutive idiopathic scoliosis cases based on the Scoliosis Research Society—defined apical vertebra. *Spine.* 1998;23:1380–1391.

54. Ogon M, Geisinger K, Behensky H, et al. Interobserver and intraobserver reliability of Lenke's new scoliosis classification system. *Spine.* 2002;2(8):858–862.

55. Lenke LG, Betz RR, Harms J, et al. Adolescent idiopathic scoliosis: a new classification to grade extent of spinal arthrosis. *J Bone Joint Surg (Am).* 2001;83:1169–1181.

56. Lenke LG, Betz RR, Clements D, et al. Curve preva-lence of a new classification of operative adolescent idiopathic scoliosis: Does classification correlate with treatment? *Spine.* 2002;27:604–611.

57. Lenke LG, Betz RR, Bridwell KH, et al. Intraobserver and interobserver reliability of the classification of thoracic adolescent idiopathic scoliosis. *J Bone Joint Surg (Am).* 1998;80:1097–1106.

58. Marshall WA. *Human Growth and Its Disorders.* London: Academic Press; 1977.

59. Goldberg CJ, Dowling FE, Fogerty EE. Adolescent idiopathic scoliosis—early menarche, normal growth. *Spine.* 1993;18:529–535.

60. Wilmer S. A study of growth in girls with idiopathic structural scoliosis. *Clin Orthop.* 1974;101:129–133.

61. Wilmer S. A study of height, weight and menarche in girls with idiopathic structural scoliosis. *Acta Orthop Scand.* 1975;46:71–83.

62. Nicolopoulos KS, Burwell RG, Webb JK. Stature and its components in adolescent idiopathic scoliosis. *J Bone Joint Surg Br.* 1985;67:594–601.

63. Nordwall A, Wilmer S. Skeletal age in patients with idiopathic scoliosis. *J Bone Joint Surg Am.* 1974;56:1766–1769.

64. Wilmer S, Nilsson KO, Bergstrand CG. A study of growth hormone and somatomedin (sulfation factor) in girls with adolescent idiopathic scoliosis. *J Bone Joint Surg Am.* 1976;58:155.

65. Wilmer S, Nilsson KO, Kastrup K. Growth hormone and somatomedin A in girls with adolescent idiopathic scoliosis. *Acta Paediatr Scand.* 1975;65:547–552.

66. Ahl T, Albertsson-Wiklund K, Kalen R. Twenty-four hour growth hormone in pubertal girls with idiopathic scoliosis. *Spine.* 1988;13:139–142.

67. Tanner JM. *Growth at Adolescence.* 2nd ed. Oxford, England: Blackwell Scientific Publications; 1962.

68. Terver S, Kleinman R, Bleck EE. Growth landmarks and the evolution of scoliosis: a review of pertinent studies on their usefulness. *Dev Med Child Neurol.* 1980;22:675–684.

69. Scoles PV, Salvagno R, Vallalba K, Riew D. Relationship of iliac crest maturation to skeletal and chronological age. *J Paediatr Orthop.* 1988;8:639–644.

70. Rogala EH, Drummond DS, Curr J. Scoliosis incidence and natural history: a prospective epidemiological study. *J Bone Joint Surg Am.* 1978;60:173–176.

71. Duval-Beaupere G, Lespargot A, Grossiord A. Flexibility of scoliosis; what does it mean? Is the terminology appropriate? *Spine.* 1985;10:428–432.

72. Vedantam R, Lenke LG, Birdwell KH, Linville DL. Comparison of push-prone and lateral-bending radiographs for predicting postoperative coronal alignment in thoracolumbar and lumbar scoliotic curves. *Spine.* 2000; 25(1):76–81.

73. Cheh G, Lenke LG, Lehman RA, Jr., Kim YJ, Nunley R, Bridwell KH. The reliability of preoperative supine radiographs to predict the amount of curve flexibility in adolescent idiopathic scoliosis. *Spine.* 2007;32(24):2668–2672.

74. Cruickshank JL, Koike M, Dickson RA. Curve patterns in idiopathic scoliosis: a clinical radiographic study. *J Bone Joint Surg Br.* 1989;71:259–263.

75. Beauchamp M, Labelle H, Grimard G, et al. Diurnal variation of Cobb angle measurement in adolescent idiopathic scoliosis. *Spine.* 1993;18:1581–1583.

76. Risser JG. The iliac apophysis: an evaluation sign in the management of scoliosis. *Clin Orthop.* 1958;11:111–119.

77. Izumi Y. The accuracy of Risser staging. *Spine.* 1995; 20:1868–1871.

78. Bunch WH, Dvonch BM. Pitfalls in assessment of skeletal immaturity. *J Pediatr Orthop.* 1983;3:220–222.

79. Weinstein JN. Early results of scoliosis bracing study confirm efficacy of bracing, identify predictive factors. *Spine Lett.* 1994;1:2–8.

80. Porto F, Gurgel JL, Russomano T, Farinatti Pde T. Moire topography: characteristics and clinical application. *Gait Posture.* 2010;32(3):422–424.

81. Wilmer S. Moire topography for the diagnosis and documentation of scoliosis. *Acta Orthop Scand.* 1979;50:295–302.

82. Turner-Smith AR, Shannon TML, Hughston GR, Knopp DA. Assessing idiopathic scoliosis using a surface measurement technique. In: *Surgical Rounds for Orthopaedics.* Oxford, England: Orthopaedic Engineering Centre; 1988.

83. Roye BD, Wright ML, Williams BA, et al. Does ScoliScore provide more information than traditional clinical estimates of curve progression? *Spine (Phila Pa 1976).* 2012;37(25):2099–2103.

84. Lee CF, Fong DY, Cheung KM, et al. A new risk classification rule for curve progression in adolescent idiopathic scoliosis. *Spine J.* 2012;12(11):989–995.

85. Crossan JF, Wynne-Davies R. Research for genetic and environmental factors in orthopaedic disease. *Clin Orthop.* 1986;210:99–105.

86. Mehta MH. The rib-vertebra angle in the early diagnosis between resolving and progressing infantile scoliosis. *J Bone Joint Surg Br.* 1972;54:230–243.

87. Mehta MH, Morell G. The non-operative treatment of infantile idiopathic scoliosis. In: Zorab PA, Seigler D, eds. *Scoliosis: Proceedings of the Sixth Symposium.* London: Academic; 1979:71–84.

88. Weinstein SL, Zavala DC, Ponseti IV. Idiopathic scoliosis: long-term follow-up and prognosis in untreated patients. *J Bone Joint Surg Am.* 1981;63:702–712.

89. Axelgard J, Brown JC. Lateral surface stimulation for the treatment of progressive idiopathic scoliosis. *Spine*. 1983;8:242–260.

90. Sullivan JA, Davidson R, Renslaw TS, et al. Further evaluation of the Scolitron treatment of idiopathic adolescent scoliosis. *Spine*. 1986;11:903–906.

91. Moe JH, Kettleson DN. Idiopathic scoliosis: analysis of curve patterns and the preliminary results of Milwaukee brace treatment in one hundred sixty-nine patients. *J Bone Joint Surg Am*. 1970;52:1509.

92. Carr W, Moe J, Winter R, Lonstein J. Treatment of idiopathic scoliosis in the Milwaukee brace. *J Bone Joint Surg Am*. 1980;62:599–612.

93. Emans JB, Kaelin A, Bancel P, et al. The Boston bracing system for idiopathic scoliosis: follow-up results in 295 patients. *Spine*. 1986;11:792–801.

94. Houghton GR, McInerny A, Tew A. Brace compliance in adolescent idiopathic scoliosis. *J Bone Joint Surg Br*. 1987; 69:852.

95. Goldberg CJ, Dowling FE, Hall JE, Emans JB. A statistical comparison between natural history of idiopathic scoliosis and brace treatment in skeletally immature adolescent girls. *Spine*. 1993;18(7):902–908.

96. Noonan KL, Weinstein SL, Jacobson WC, Dolan LA. Use of the Milwaukee brace for progressive idiopathic scoliosis. *J Bone Joint Surg Am*. 1996;78:557–567.

97. Rowe DE, Bernstein SM, Riddick MF, et al. A meta-analysis of the efficacy of non-operative treatments for idiopathic scoliosis. *J Bone Joint Surg Am*. 1997;79:664–674.

98. Szwed A, Kolban M. Results of SpineCor dynamic bracing for idiopathic scoliosis. *Stud Health Technol Inform*. 2012;176:379–382.

99. Zaina F, Donzelli S, Negrini A, Romano M, Negrini S. SpineCor, exercise and SPoRT rigid brace: what is the best for Adolescent Idiopathic Scoliosis? Short term results from 2 retrospective studies. *Stud Health Technol Inform*. 2012;176:361–364.

100. Rowe DE, Bernstein SM, Riddick MF, Adler F, Emans JB, Gardner-Bonneau D. A meta-analysis of the efficacy of non-operative treatments for idiopathic scoliosis. *J Bone Joint Surg Am*. 1997;79(5):664–674.

101. Weinstein SL, Dolan LA, Wright JG, Dobbs MB. Effects of bracing in adolescents with idiopathic scoliosis. *N Engl J Med*. 2013. 369:1512–1521.

102. Katz DE, Durrani AA. Factors that influence outcome in bracing large curves in patients with adolescent idiopathic scoliosis. *Spine*. 2001;26(21):2354–2361.

103. Weiss HR, Weiss G. Curvature progression in patients treated with scoliosis in-patient rehabilitation—a sex and age matched controlled study. *Stud Health Technol Inform*. 2002;91:352–356.

104. Weiss HR, Weiss G, Petermann F. Incidence of curvature progression in idiopathic scoliosis patients treated with scoliosis in-patient rehabilitation (SIR): an age- and sex-matched controlled study. *Pediatr Rehabil*. 2003;6(1): 23–30.

105. Romano M, Minozzi S, Bettany-Saltikov J, et al. Exercises for adolescent idiopathic scoliosis. *Cochrane Database Syst Rev*. 2012;8:CD007837.

106. Mehta MH. Active correction by side-shift: an alternative treatment for early idiopathic scoliosis. In: Zorab PA, Seigler D, eds. *Scoliosis: Proceedings of the Sixth Symposium*. London: Academic; 1979:126–140.

107. Troyanovich SJ. Scoliosis: a special circumstance. In: Troyanovich SJ. *Structural rehabilitation of the spine and posture: a practical approach*. Huntington Beach CA, MPAmedia, 2001, p. 111–117.

108. Romano M, Negrini S. Manual therapy as a conservative treatment for adolescent idiopathic scoliosis: a systematic review. *Scoliosis*. 2008;3(1):2.

109. Goldberg CJ, Moore DP, Fogarty EE, Dowling FE. Scoliosis. a review. *Pediatr Surg Int*. 2008;24(2):129–144.

110. Weiss HR, Moramarco M. Indication for surgical treatment in patients with adolescent Idiopathic Scoliosis—a critical appraisal. *Patient Saf Surg*. 2013;7(1):17.

111. Bachmann KR, Goodwin RC, Moore TA. Indication for surgical treatment in patients with adolescent idiopathic scoliosis—a critical appraisal and counterpoint. *Patient Saf Surg*. 2013;7(1):21.

112. Harrington PR. Treatment of scoliosis, correction and internal fixation by spine instrumentation. *J Bone Joint Surg Am*. 1962;44:591–610.

113. Drummond D, Guadagni J, Keene JS, et al. Interspinous process segmental spinal instrumentation. *J Pediatr Orthop*. 1984;4:397–404.

114. Luque ER. Segmental spinal instrumentation for correction of scoliosis. *Clin Orthop*. 1982;163:192–198.

115. Cotrel Y, Dubousset J. New segmental posterior instrumentation of the spine. *Orthop Trans*. 1985;9:118.

116. De Jonge T, Dubousset JF, Illes T. Sagittal plane correction in idiopathic scoliosis. *Spine*. 2002;27(7):754–761.

117. Bjerkreim I, Steen H, Brox JI. Idiopathic scoliosis treated with Cotrel-Dubousset instrumentation: evaluation 10 years after surgery. *Spine.* 2007;32(19):2103–2110.

118. Haefeli M, Elfering A, Kilian R, Min K, Boos N. Nonoperative treatment for adolescent idiopathic scoliosis: a 10- to 60-year follow-up with special reference to health-related quality of life. *Spine.* 2006;31(3): 355–366; discussion 367.

119. Danielsson AJ. What impact does spinal deformity correction for adolescent idiopathic scoliosis make on quality of life? *Spine.* 2007;32(19 Suppl):S101–108.

120. Donaldson S, Stephens D, Howard A, Alman B, Narayanan U, Wright JG. Surgical decision making in adolescent idiopathic scoliosis. *Spine.* 2007;32(14):1526–1532.

121. Howard A, Donaldson S, Hedden D, Stephens D, Alman B, Wright J. Improvement in quality of life following surgery for adolescent idiopathic scoliosis. *Spine.* 2007;32(24):2715–2718.

122. Dawson EG, Moe JH, Caron A. Surgical management of scoliosis in the adult. *J Bone Joint Surg Am.* 1973;55:437.

123. Briard JL, Jegou D, Canchoix J. Adult lumbar scoliosis. *Spine.* 1979;4:526–532.

124. Nachemson A. Adult scoliosis and back pain. *Spine.* 1979;4:513–517.

125. Nilsonne U, Lundgren KD. Long term prognosis in idiopathic scoliosis. *Acta Orthop Scand.* 1968;39:456–465.

126. Collins DK, Ponseti IV. Long term follow-up of patients with idiopathic scoliosis not treated surgically. *J Bone Joint Surg Am.* 1969;51:425–445.

127. Bradford DS. Adult scoliosis: current concepts of treatment. *Clin Orthop.* 1988;229:70.

128. Weinstein SL, Ponseti IV. Curve progression in idiopathic scoliosis. *J Bone Joint Surg Am.* 1983;65:447–451.

129. Swank SM, Lonstein JE, Moe JH, Winter RB, Bradford DS. Surgical treatment of adult scoliosis: a review of 222 cases. *J Bone Joint Surg Am.* 1981;63:268–287.

130. Everett CR, Patel RK. A systematic literature review of nonsurgical treatment in adult scoliosis. *Spine.* 2007; 32(19 Suppl):S130–134.

Lumbopelvic Complaints

Context

Low back complaints account for a majority of presentations seen in chiropractic practice.[1] In the general population the estimated one-month prevalence for low back pain (LBP) is between 35% and 37%.[2] Approximately 80% of adults will have LBP at some time in their lives; however, only 14% will complain of pain lasting longer than two weeks.[3] It appears that adolescents with LBP are more likely to have problems as adults.[4] Although it is often quoted that 90% of patients with acute low back pain have resolution within four weeks (even without intervention), research indicates a more complicated natural history when viewed beyond the one-month window:

- Croft et al.[5] found that although 90% of patients had stopped consulting for LBP symptoms at three months, only 25% were symptom-free at one year.
- Von Korff[6] has shown that a significant amount of even acute LBP patients have persistent pain if followed for one to two years.
- Hestbaek and colleagues[7] systematically reviewed a number of papers and concluded that as many as 62% of patients will have one or more relapses during one-year follow-up of an index episode; 40% still with LBP at six months.[8] Initial relapses tend to occur at six- to seven-week intervals with a decreasing number of cases suffering renewed pain each time.
- Schiotzz–Christensen et al.[9] looked at the long-term prognosis for acute low back pain in general practice and found that in relation to sick leave, there was a 50% return to work within the first eight days and only 2% remained on sick leave after one year. It was noted though that 15% had been on sick leave during the following year and about half continued to complain of discomfort.

This indication of chronicity and recurrence varies partly on the measures used to indicate recurrence. A recent study by Marras et al.[10] evaluated this variance. Two hundred and six workers who reported low back pain were interviewed one year after return to full duty. Return to work was measured based on recurrent low back pain according to symptom reports, medical visits, self-reported lost days, and employer-reported lost days due to back pain. By measuring recurrent symptoms, the rate was 58% (P = 0.0001). Using medical visit as the recurrence criterion, the rate was 36% (P = 0.0001). The recurrence rate for self-reported lost time was 15%. Using employer-confirmed lost time as the indicator of recurrence, the rate was only 10% (P = 0.0077). Clearly, recurrence is dependent on the measure by which it is assessed. Of the 70% of individuals who have some back pain at some point in their lives, 25% will have symptoms of sciatica. The lifetime prevalence for lumbar disc herniation is between 1% to 5%.

In a study by Davis et al.[1] published in 2012, it was estimated that between the years 1997 and 2005, the total estimated expenditures for patients with spine problems in the United States increased 65%. Surgery for occupational back injury accounts for approximately 21% of these increased costs. Wasiak et al.[2] published in *Spine* in 2006 that 84% of total medical costs for LBP were related to recurrence. Approximately 13.6 million patient visits for spine care occurred in 2008. Despite population growth, only approximately 6% of adults sought medical care for a spine-related condition. The mean inflation-adjusted expenditure for medical care increased by 95% (from $487 in 1999 to $950 in 2008). For chiropractic care, the mean expenditure varied much less, fluctuating between a low of $473 in 1999 and a high of $662 in 2007. The annual combined direct and indirect costs for low back pain were estimated at $100 billion in 2000.[11] Clearly, given the current cost of health care, this amount has significantly increased.

Clinical determination of the specific tissue cause of LBP is often difficult, if not impossible. Literally any structure in the low back that is innervated could be a potential source of pain. Although clinically difficult, some diagnoses can be determined on the basis of a combination of radiographic or special studies. The traditional medical and chiropractic assumption of nerve root pressure as the primary source of low back and leg pain has not been supported in the literature. Clinically, only 1% of patients with LBP have neurologic deficits, and only one half of these patients elect for surgery.[12] Although the disc as a source of pain is still viable, the mechanism is rarely through compression of a nerve root. More often it is the result of an inflammatory process. Approximately 39% of patients will have LBP due to disc disruption.[13] Specifically, 5% of patients will have a disc herniation, 15% to 40% (dependent on study) will have facet involvement, 4% will have a compression fracture, 3% will have spondylolisthesis, and only 0.3% will have ankylosing spondylitis.[14] Malignant neoplasms account for only 1% of all causes of LBP.[15] Spinal infection accounts for only 0.01% of LBP cases.[16] Spinal stenosis represents what is considered a common cause in the older adult as a result of the above-mentioned disorders augmented by associated congenital causes or acquired degenerative processes. The role of the sacroiliac (SI) joints in causing low back and/or leg pain has only recently begun to be investigated. However, for most chiropractors SI joint subluxation (fixation) represents a common cause of LBP that appears to respond dramatically to manipulation.[17]

The chiropractor's initial role is to identify the patient with "ominous" signs. The evaluation may require special studies or referral to a specialist. If these signs are absent, it is imperative to distinguish the patient with LBP alone or LBP with radiation into the leg(s). For patients with low back and leg pain, it is important to determine those with frank neurologic signs indicating nerve root irritation versus those with referral of pain (no nerve root pathology). Focusing on the assessment of functional and neurologic status, decisions regarding management, comanagement, type of treatment, and prognosis can be broadly determined.

The effectiveness of chiropractic manipulation in the treatment of LBP has been recognized in several ways. Several past studies have demonstrated the cost effectiveness of chiropractic care.[18] Patient satisfaction has also been demonstrated.[19] The level of satisfaction for patients seeking care from a chiropractor versus a medical doctor was evaluated in the UCLA Low-Back Pain Study.[20] Satisfaction with chiropractic care was rated higher compared to medical care. The primary difference in satisfaction was the perception that chiropractors communicated more, giving advice and information about their low back pain. The appropriateness of chiropractic management of LBP was recognized by the Rand study.[21] More recently, recommendations made by the Agency for Healthcare Research and Quality (AHRQ) guidelines strongly favor manipulation as the primary delivered care to patients with acute LBP. The British randomized study by Meade et al.[22] has set the stage for the defense of long-term effectiveness of chiropractic manipulative therapy for LBP. In 2006, the European Guidelines for Low Back Pain were published in the *European Spine Journal*. A summary of recommendations for acute nonspecific low back pain included manipulation.[23] A series of articles appeared in a 2008 full issue of the *Spine Journal* devoted to evidence-informed management of chronic low back pain. Manipulation with exercise was judged as having moderate support in the literature.[24]

General Strategy

History

- Screen the patient for "red flags" that indicate need for immediate radiograph/special studies or referral to a specialist: severe trauma, fever or recent bacterial infection, saddle anesthesia, severe or progressive neurologic complaints, recent onset of bladder dysfunction in association with the LBP, unexplained weight loss, prior history of cancer, intravenous drug abuse or immunosuppression, or pain that is worse with recumbency or worse at night.
- Determine whether there was a history of trauma and determine the mechanism and severity.
- Determine whether the complaint is LBP alone or a combination of LBP and leg complaints such as pain, numbness or tingling, or weakness.
- If there are leg complaints, determine whether they are made worse with coughing, sneezing, or straining at stool.
- Determine the level of pain and functional capacity with a questionnaire (e.g., Oswestry, Roland-Morris).

Examination

- For patients with signs of cauda equina or rapidly progressing neurologic deficits, refer immediately for neurologic evaluation.
- For patients with suspected fracture (e.g., those in a motor vehicle accident, those who have fallen from a height, or those with osteoporosis), infection, or cancer, radiograph the area.
- For patients with LBP only, perform a thorough examination of the low back, including inspection, observation of patients' movements, palpation of soft and bony tissues, motion palpation of the spine, passive and active range of motion (using inclinometer or Schober method), functional assessment (e.g., Lewit/Janda and/or McKenzie approach), and orthopaedic examination.
- For patients with radiation of symptoms into the legs, add a thorough neurologic examination, including nerve stretch maneuvers, deep tendon reflexes, sensation testing (include pain, temperature, light touch, and vibration), and myotome testing.
- For patients with conflicting findings, inclusion of nonorganic testing may be helpful.
- Laboratory testing should be reserved for those patients suspected of having infection, cancer, or underlying diabetes.
- Patients with apparent multilevel neurological involvement should first undergo radiographic evaluation; consideration of computed tomography (CT) or magnetic resonance imaging (MRI) should be given if the patient is unresponsive to conservative care.
- If pain appears mechanical, the use of radiographs for three to four weeks can be delayed; however, if information gained from a radiographic evaluation is likely to change the treatment approach to the patient with regard to a specific technique or management approach, radiographs have value as an initial evaluation tool.
- For patients who are unresponsive to care after one month, consideration should be given to the use of MRI, CT, or electrodiagnostic studies.

Management

- Patients with clinical, radiographic, or laboratory evidence of tumor, infection, or fracture (other than a stable compression fracture) should be sent for medical evaluation and management.
- Patients who appear to have a mechanical cause of pain should be managed conservatively for one month; if unresponsive, further testing or referral for a second opinion is suggested.

Relevant Anatomy, Physiology, and Biomechanics

Many studies have attempted to localize tissues responsible for LBP and to determine where the pain is felt with regard to each of these structures. Approaches have included various relief and provocative injections, electrical stimulation, and pulling on surgically implanted strings, among others. It seems clear that when sciatica is present, it can occur only if the nerve root is already compromised by stretch, swelling, or compression.[25] This does not mean that sciatic pain cannot be mimicked by other tissues. Certainly, the intervertebral disc is a potential source of pain that in and of itself may lead to segmental referral of pain without frank neurologic findings (discussed below under "The Disk"). **Exhibit 6–1** illustrates the innervations of deep spinal structures including the disc, annulus, dura, posterior longitudinal ligament, and facet joints. The vascular structure for the dorsal root ganglia (DRG) includes primarily an internal arterialization with a superficial venous drainage. This anatomical arrangement may render the DRG vulnerable to ischemic consequences of external pressures and/or internal edematous swelling. A compartment-like syndrome may develop due to periforaminal degenerative changes or other space-occupying effects.[26]

The Three-Joint Complex

There are essentially three joints at each functional segment of the spine: the intervertebral joint and the two-facet or zygapophyseal joints. Kirkaldy-Willis[27] proposed a model of progressive dysfunction with regard to this three-joint complex whereby a shared functional relationship exists. The typical vertebra is composed of a body connected to a posterior arch via superiorly placed pedicles. The pedicles form the upper roof of the neural foramen. The vertebral canal is formed by the body, pedicles, and posterior arch. This canal can be

Exhibit 6–1 **Innervation of Deep Spinal Structures. The deepest structures are innervated by the sinuvertebral nerve (SVN) including the posterior annular fibers of the disc, the dura, the posterior longitudinal ligament, and the vertebral body. The posterior branch of the posterior primary rami (PPR) innervates the facet joints. The SVN has an anastamosis with the opposite side leading to the conscious perception of central pain when irritated. The facet joints are innerved by branches of the PPR that span several segments. Pain is more likely perceived as more localized and sided (i.e. right versus left). These deeper structures represent scleratogenous innervations which may lead to radiation of pain that is not radicular (e.g. non-dermatomal).**

Recurrent Meningeal Nerve (Sinuvertebral Nerve)	• Posterior vertebral body & internal and basivertebral veins • Posterior longitudinal ligament (PLL) and posterior intervertebral disc (IVD) • Anterior dura
Medial Branch of the Posterior Primary Rami (PPR)	• Facet joints & periosteum of posterior vertebral arch • Deep muscles • Interspinous, supraspinous, & intertransverse ligaments • Ligamentum flavum
Sympathetic Trunk & Gray Rami Communicantes	• Anterior & lateral vertebral body • Anterior & lateral aspects of intervertebral disc (IVD) • Anterior longitudinal ligament (ALL)

congenitally narrowed or narrowed through acquired projection of osteophytes or disc material or by thickening of the ligamentum flavum. The flaval ligaments serve as the attachments between adjacent laminae.

Neurology of the Disc and Deep Structures

The innervation of the lumbar area is primarily from the posterior ramus of the spinal nerve. The sinuvertebral nerve (also called recurrent meningeal nerve or nerve of Luschka) supplies the periosteum, posterior longitudinal ligament, the outer fibers of the annulus fibrosus, and the epidural vessels. There is a diffuse arrangement of anastomosis over several segments that may explain why localization to a specific level or side is difficult.

Discogenic pain is often sympathetic pain mediated by the sinuvertebral nerves. In numerous studies[28] in the rat model, lower lumbar discs and joint capsules have been demonstrated to be innervated by sensory neurons from the L1 and L2 dorsal root ganglia through the paravertebral sympathetic trunk. Also it has been demonstrated by Unimura et al.[29] that there is a "hole" in the segmental sensory innervation of L3 through L5 and that through the rami communicantes afferent information from these levels reaches the L2 spinal ganglion via the sympathetic chain; not from segmental dorsal root ganglia at each level of L3, L4, and L5. The afferent fibers are primarily nociceptive; the efferent fibers primarily vasomotor.

Also, Wakai et al.[30] have clearly demonstrated in the rat model that nerves that were thought to travel to a single structure can travel to other structures. Nerve cell bodies located in the DRG send two branches: one to the primary structure and the other to related structures. The sensory nerves that travel to the facet joints, SI joints, and IVD may also travel to the multifidi muscles. Although about 83% of fibers did not dichotomize, of the remaining 17% that do about 7% are from the facets, 7%

from the SI joints, but only 3% from the IVDs. Also, Sameda et al.[31] demonstrated that in rats, sensory nerves to the facet joints also travel to the sciatic nerve. This likely explains why referral pain mimics radicular pain.

The Disc

The lumbar intervertebral disc (IVD) is essentially divided into two parts: (1) an inner nucleus pulposus, and (2) an outer annulus fibrosus. The annulus fibrosus fibers cross each other at angles of 60° to 70° in successive layers, providing a strong resistance to rotational forces. Resistance to flexion and extension is strong with the nucleus pulposus bulging posteriorly on flexion while the annulus fibrosus bulges anteriorly.

The disc has been accused of being one of the major causes of LBP. It appears that it may play more of a primary role than that of direct compression of nerve roots. The outer third of the annulus fibrosus is supplied with nerve endings from branches of the sinuvertebral nerves, the gray rami communicantes, and the lumbar ventral rami.[32] Although it has been suggested that innervation is the result of ingrowth of granulation tissue only after disc injury, it has been demonstrated that the fetal and infant disc are innervated.[33] Correlated with the finding of outer annulus innervation, it has been demonstrated using discography that inner tearing of the annulus causes less pain than tearing that extends to the outer third of the annulus. Also, it has become clear that intervertebral discs do not fail by prolapsing (nucleus pulposus herniation). Even if an experimentally induced tear is created in the annulus, the nucleus does not herniate. Repeated flexion and extension also fail to induce herniation in partially herniated discs. Compression at the disc is more likely to result in vertebral end-plate fracture. It has been proposed that because the nucleus pulposus is without blood supply and therefore segregated from the body's immune system, end-plate fracture (exposure to the vertebral spongiosa) or prolapsed nuclear material that reaches the epidural space induces an immune response. Proteoglycans of the nucleus are, in essence, foreign material. The resulting immune inflammatory response causes further degradation of the nuclear matrix. It has been proposed that exposure of the nucleus pulposus to the vascular supply of the area activated the release of matrix metalloproteinases (MMPs). These include collagenases, gelatinase, stromelysin, and elastase. Now these are termed MMP-1, MMP-2, MMP-3, and MMP-12

respectively. This process is terminated by tissue inhibitors of metalloproteinases (TIMPs). MMP/TIMP balance is essential for restoring balance.

This degradation changes the biomechanical support provided by the nucleus. Also, erosion of the annulus fibrosus along radial fissures may occur. This inside-out process is referred to as "internal disc disruption." The combination of denaturing of the nucleus with loss of its normal cohesiveness and the erosion of the annulus may set the stage for the rare occurrence of herniating nuclear material with subsequent irritation or compression of nerve roots. Disc degeneration is associated with obliteration of the normal anastomosing arteries in the posterior longitudinal ligament with increased vascularity of the annulus (vertical orientation connecting to adjacent vertebrae).[34] Regression analysis demonstrated that these vascular changes occur prior to disc degeneration.

When the disc material is large enough to compress a nerve root, frank neurologic signs become evident. However, the most recent theory is that the herniated disc material causes more often an inflammatory reaction due to the release of irritating substances and/or as the result of an autoimmune inflammatory reaction.[35] A recent study[36] supported the growing opinion that disc herniations usually have a natural course of self-reduction through shrinkage. In this study, approximately 63% of patients had a natural reduction in the size of the disc herniation. The belief is that through resorption (caused by lack of nutrient supply), desiccation, and/or phagocytosis, the size of many disc herniations reduces over time. The old belief that herniations regress back into the annulus has not been supported. It is also true that in many cases where resolution of clinical symptoms occurs, there is no change in the size of the herniation.[37] When a disc "herniates" it can either be contained (annulus fibers are intact) or not contained (outer annulus failure allows prolapse into the vertebral canal). The terminology used to describe variations on this basic distinction is often confusing. Depending on whether the describer is a radiologist or a clinician, the same term may be used to describe different events, or a different classification system entirely may be developed.

The Facets

The facet joints of the lumbar spine allow a fair degree of flexion and some extension. Lateral bending and rotation are restricted by the mainly sagittal orientation of the facets. The orientation of segments L1-L4 has been compared to a J shape, where the anterior portion is oriented more medially. The L5-S1 facets are essentially coronal, allowing more freedom in flexion with rotation resisted by the iliolumbar ligaments. Facet tropism is a congenital anomaly in which there is a turning of the orientation of the facet articulation so that a facet that should be more sagittal, for example, is more coronal. Tropism is common, being found in 21% to 37% of the entire population, most occurring at the L4-L5 or L5-S1 facets.[38] Although this must alter biomechanics at that segmental level, it has not been demonstrated to cause a higher incidence of LBP in patients who have it. The facets take up approximately 16% to 18% of compressive loading on the lumbar spine; however, the facets accept approximately 33% of the shear force across a segment.[39]

The medial branch of the dorsal rami innervates the facets.[40] Thus, there is a unilateral distribution with some overlap between the inferior facets above and the superior facets below the segment. In other words, each facet theoretically has innervation from at least two levels. Therefore, it is theoretically possible for somewhat more localization to occur when the facet joint is the site of pain production as opposed to deeper pain-producing tissue that has an anastomosis innervation via the sinuvertebral nerve. The medial and lateral branches of the dorsal rami innervate the posterior muscles. Although the facet joints are possible sources of LBP, it is worth noting that facet joint blocks have been associated with a high placebo response rate (as much as 32%);[41] yet facet dysfunction seems to account for a significant number of low back complaints.

Degeneration of the facet proceeds from a nonspecific synovial reaction. Both distention of the joint capsule and degeneration of the hyaline cartilage that covers the facets follow, allowing for ligament laxity. The result is a joint that may potentially subluxate and cause narrowing of the lateral canal. If the process continues, older patients may have inferior facet enlargement that often occurs in a medial direction, causing central canal narrowing. Osteophytic superior facets usually project in an anterior direction to produce narrowing of the lateral recesses. Each process is a potential source of nerve root compression.

In addition to possible contribution to LBP through laxity of the joint capsule or bony hypertrophy with possible compressive effects, another possible facet pain source is the trapped meniscoid.[42] The meniscoid is an intra-articular joint inclusion that may become caught between the articular surfaces. It has been proposed that manipulation releases the meniscoid—relieving LBP.

Ligaments and Muscles

It is interesting that there are few ligaments in the lumbar region. The supraspinous ligament does not exist below L3 and above this level represents more or less the aponeurosis of the erector spinae or latissimus dorsi.[43] The interspinous ligament represents more of a tendinous extension of the erector spinae. Even the iliolumbar ligament is primarily muscle before age 30 years. The posterior longitudinal ligament is less broad than it is in the cervical region, posterolateral disc migration.

In simple terms, the muscles of the lumbar spine are divided into three layers: (1) those passing inside the ribs, (2) those passing outside the ribs, and (3) an intermediate layer. All three layers are supplied by the anterior primary rami with the exception of the erector spinae group, which is supplied by the posterior primary rami. The innermost layer is primarily composed of flexors such as the psoas. The intermediate layer is composed of the quadratus lumborum and the internal and external intercostal muscles. The erector spinae group is subdivided into three layers. Unlike the thoracic region, the lumbar region has no deep rotators. The multifidus in the middle layer of the erector spinae group attaches from the laminar and mammillary processes to the spinous processes of the vertebrae several levels above.

Biomechanics

As mentioned above, flexion is the most accessible movement pattern. Some extension and lateral bending are allowed; however, they are blocked by soft tissue and posterior joint orientation. Very little rotation occurs and is left primarily to the thoracic spine. When single-plane movements occur, there are often coupled motion patterns. With lateral flexion, there is a coupled movement of the segment so that the spinous process rotates toward the same side.[44] Also, a small amount of flexion occurs at the segment if the lumbar lordosis is in effect. Without a lordosis, there is slight extension at the segment. This coupling pattern may vary with posture.[45] In other words, laterally bending in flexion is not the same as it is in neutral. Most important, some investigators feel that abnormal coupled patterns may occur during flexion or extension and may be a predictor of low back problems.[46]

When an individual flexes forward at the waist, the paraspinal muscles support the trunk eccentrically through the first 30° to 60° while the gluteals and hamstrings keep the pelvis locked. Then the gluteals and hamstrings relax (eccentrically contract) to allow the pelvis to rotate at the hips to allow further flexion. This may be limited by tension in the hamstrings. At full flexion, the paraspinals are relaxed, with support provided mainly by ligaments. Lifting from this position can damage ligaments or strain muscles.

It appears that there are two general mechanisms for the cause of disc herniation: (1) sudden loading with the spine in flexion, and (2) degenerative failure of the annulus from repeated or prolonged mechanical stresses.[47, 48] The side-posture manipulation has often been accused as a possible cause of disc herniation. It is likely, though, that the limitation imposed by the restriction of the posterior facets is sufficient to prevent excessive rotation at the disc; however, Slosberg[49] cautions the doctor that this is true only if the facets are loaded in extension by maintaining a lordosis and the degree of rotation is controlled by the adjuster.

Sacroiliac Joint

The SI joint has, after much debate, regained the status of a true diarthrodial (synovial) joint capable of some movement.[50, 51] The joint is composed of an auricular-shaped surface with an upper vertical and a lower horizontal section. A synovial membrane covers the lower two thirds (ventral portion); the upper third (posterior) is mainly fibrous without synovial tissue. Stability is largely ligamentous. Movement has been described as nutation and counternutation. Nutation involves an anteroposterior movement around a transverse axis. Thus, when rising from a recumbent position, the sacral promontory moves forward a few millimeters.[52] This also occurs unilaterally, so that when standing on one foot, the SI joint on the side of weight-bearing reaches maximum nutation. SI joint innervation is from a broad area including both sacral and lumbar plexuses (L3-S2). This may explain the varied presentation of referred pain patterns with SI joint involvement.

Evaluation

History

Ominous Signs

Screening the patient for ominous signs can be performed quickly, yet relatively reliable information can be gained with regard to the need for further specialized evaluation or referral (**Table 6-1**). Cauda equina syndrome is a rare but serious condition. The most sensitive historical indicator is urinary retention (sensitivity = 0.90, specificity = 95%).[53] Therefore patients without urinary retention (or eventual overflow incontinence) are unlikely to have cauda equina syndrome. Although LBP is due to cancer only 1% of the time, it is obviously crucial to search for indicators of this possibility. Deyo[53] indicated in one study that the cancer patient will present with at least one of four historical findings: (1) older than age 50 (about 80% of patients with cancer-caused LBP), (2) previous history of cancer (specificity = 0.98), (3) unexplained weight loss, and (4) failure to respond to conservative therapy over a one-month period. It is important to remember, however, that only one third of patients eventually diagnosed with cancer as the cause of their LBP have a prior history of cancer (sensitivity = 0.31%). Another sensitive but nonspecific clue is that most patients with cancer report pain that is unrelieved by bed rest.

When screening for the extremely rare occurrence of a spinal infection, it is important to ask about urinary tract infections, an indwelling urinary catheter during a recent hospital stay, injection of illicit drugs, and any indications of skin infection.[53] A fever is highly specific for infection; however, 2% of patients with mechanical back pain may have a fever (possibly virus-related).[54]

Other Possibilities

In all older patients, a suspicion of compression fracture is warranted. The factor of age is most important for patients older than 70 years; the specificity is 0.96. Although it might seem logical that there would be a report of identifiable trauma, this finding has a low sensitivity (0.30); however, long-term corticosteroid use was highly specific (0.99). The sudden onset of pain with coughing, sneezing, or sudden flexion unassociated with radicular complaints should warrant a radiologic search for compression fracture.[14]

Combining four screening questions, a high level of suspicion may be gained for ankylosing spondylitis (AS): (1) Is there morning stiffness?, (2) Is there improvement in discomfort with exercise?, (3) Was the onset of back pain before age 40 years?, and (4) Has the pain persisted for at least three months? If at least three positive responses are given, AS should be suspected (sensitivity as high as 0.95 with specificity as high as 0.85).[55] However, it is always important to consider the

Table 6-1 History Questions for Low Back Pain

Primary Question	What Are You Thinking?	Secondary Questions	What Are You Thinking?
Did you injure yourself (car accident, fall, lifting, etc.)?	Disc lesion, muscle strain, facet injury, fracture	**Did you fall on your buttocks?**	Compression or coccygeal fracture
		Was this a sudden hyperflexion injury?	
		Did the pain appear while lifting or with sudden twisting?	Disc lesion or muscle strain
		Did you have a sudden extension injury?	Facet injury
Does the pain continue into the buttocks or leg?	Disc lesion, tumor, stenosis, referral from facet or trigger point (TrP)	**Does the pain extend below the knee?**	Nerve root pain due to disc, stenosis, or tumor; facet and TrP are less likely
		Does the pain extend into the buttocks or to the knee?	Lumbar facet, SI joint, and TrP
Do you have any difficulty with urination or defecation?	Cauda equina syndrome, prostate disease, disc lesion (Valsalva effect), constipation	**Do you have any numbness around the groin or genital area?**	Cauda equina syndrome
		Do you have leg pain when you defecate, cough, or sneeze?	Space-occupying lesion indicating tumor or disc lesion in most cases
		Do you have to urinate often and/or have difficulty stopping or starting?	Prostate cancer is possible.
Is there associated abdominal pain?	Genitourinary cause, abdominal aneurysm	**Is this associated with your menstrual period?**	Dysmenorrhea (if severe consider endometriosis), pelvic inflammatory disease
		Does the pain radiate around to the groin?	Kidney (infection or stone)
		Is there associated weakness in the legs?	Abdominal aneurysm
Is there marked weight loss?	Cancer, depression, diet	**Do you have a past history of cancer, night pain, pain unrelieved with rest?**	Cancer
Is there any weakness in the legs with activity?	Neurogenic or vascular claudication	**Is it relieved quickly with rest?**	Vascular claudication
		Is it better when flexed and/or relieved after 15–20 minutes of rest?	Neurogenic claudication (canal stenosis)

predictive value, which is dependent on the prevalence of the disorder. Because AS is relatively rare, the positive predictive value is quite low (0.04).

Low Back Pain with Radiation in the Leg(s)

One of the first historical discriminators between a disc and a referred (facet or muscular) source is whether or not the pain travels below the knee. Pain below the knee

is suggestive of a disc lesion with nerve root irritation. Paresthesia or numbness is more commonly found with disc lesions than with referred causes, especially in the foot or ankle area. Patients with disc lesions often will have a history of recurrent episodes of back pain without leg pain. It is likely that the patient will be between the ages of 30 and 50 years. This age range is due in part to the observation that the disc's nucleus pulposus dehydrates with aging, leaving little to herniate. The patient with a disc lesion may report a twisting injury accompanied by immediate leg pain. The leg pain is often more of a concern than the back pain. In the younger patient with a disc lesion, pain is often worse with sitting (due to increased disc pressure) and less with standing or walking. The older patient with leg pain is more likely to have compressive insult of a nerve root due to various forms of stenosis. The older patient has more difficulty with walking or standing because of the compressive effect created by the loading of the posterior elements (where most of the stenosis occurs).

In a study[56] published in 2013, a group of senior participants with low back pain and leg radiation were compared to determine if there were any findings that might help differentiate the cause. For patients identified as having a disc herniation as the cause, pain was experienced in the front of the thigh and shin more often. This reflects the finding that unlike a young population L3-L4 was one of the most common sites of herniation (40%). For patients with disc-related pain, unilateral leg pain was found in all, whereas for stenosis-related leg pain, bilateral leg complaints were found with 52% of patients. For patients with stenosis-related leg pain, they were more likely to experience pain in the posterior aspect of the knee.

Other Factors

It is always important to screen the patient with regard to medication use. Oral corticosteroid use would suggest the possibility of a compression fracture. Anticoagulant therapy may suggest epidural or spinal cord bleeding. Antidepressants may suggest an underlying psychologic component, especially in the patient with chronic pain. Increased body weight has been shown to be a possible weak risk indicator for LBP.[57] What may be surprising to the general public is that cardiovascular risk factors are significantly and independently associated with symptoms of lumbar disc herniation.[58] Smoking is the most significant, with a dose-dependent effect; the more cigarettes per day the higher the risk. A series of studies by Kauppila et al.[59–61] indicate that the blood supply to the lower lumbar vertebra is at risk compared to higher lumbar levels. Vascular anastomotic networks between vertebrae become obliterated with age and this process is likely accelerated with the occlusive effects of atherosclerosis.

If the patient is injured in a work-related accident or is involved in personal injury litigation, it is important to gain an appreciation of the patient's attitude toward employment and the desire to obtain compensation.

Patient questionnaires with regard to pain and functional capacity are important baseline data, especially with these patients.

Questionnaires

Although it may seem logical that improvement is better measured with apparent objective findings through clinical examination, outcome measures through the use of questionnaires may prove to be more reliable and reproducible. Deyo[62] reviewed the reliability and reproducibility of outcome measures used in back pain trials. Standard measures such as range of motion and ankle dorsiflexion strength were far less reliable (0.50/1.00) than a questionnaire measuring the ability to perform daily activities (sickness impact profile—0.90/1.00) or pain measurement (visual analog scale [VAS]— 0.94/1.00). Passive straight leg raising fared somewhere in between (0.78/1.00). The meta-analysis performed by Anderson and Meeker[63] also demonstrated better correlation between "functional" outcome assessment tools (questionnaires) than objective measures.

For patients with LBP, there are a number of questionnaires available. Two of the most popular that have been demonstrated to be valid and reliable are the Oswestry Disability Index for Low Back Pain and the Roland-Morris Low Back Pain Questionnaire.[64] The Oswestry Questionnaire (**Exhibit 6–2**) is a simple tool utilizing only 10 sections with six possible answers for each.[65] The answer choices are rated from 0 to 5, ranging from less to more disability. A percentage disability can be calculated by scoring and adding the answer choices and multiplying by 2 (**Exhibit 6–3**). For example, if a patient marked five answers that indicated moderate disability (e.g., $3 \times 5 = 15$) and five for more severe disability (e.g., $4 \times 5 = 20$) multiplying the total by 2 (2×35) results in a disability of 70%. This value could then be used as a comparison for future improvement. The Roland-Morris Questionnaire (**Exhibit 6–4**) is a behavioral measuring tool for patients with low back pain.[66] The 24-item survey is simple for the patient to complete by marking each description that fits his or her perceptions. For example, one statement is: I find it difficult to get out of a chair because of my back. When all the marked statements are added together, a score is generated. The higher the score, the greater is the disability. Many doctors add a visual analog scale (VAS) to the Roland-Morris.

A recent shift in thinking regarding the use of questionnaires has been based on the observation that

Exhibit 6-2 Oswestry Questionnaire

Please read

This questionnaire has been designed to give the doctor information as to how your back pain has affected your ability to manage in everyday life. Please answer every section, and mark in each section ONE BOX that applies to you. We realize you may consider that two of the statements in any one section relate to you, but please just mark the box that most closely describes your problem.

Section 1—Pain Intensity

- My pain is mild to moderate: I do not need painkillers.
- The pain is bad, but I manage without taking painkillers.
- Painkillers give complete relief from pain.
- Painkillers give moderate relief from pain.
- Painkillers give very little relief from pain.
- Painkillers have no effect on the pain.

Section 2—Personal Care (Washing, Dressing, Etc.)

- I can look after myself normally without causing extra pain.
- I can look after myself normally, but it causes extra pain.
- It is painful to look after myself, and I am slow and careful.
- I need some help but manage most of my personal care.
- I need help every day in most aspects of self-care.
- I do not get dressed; I wash with difficulty; and I stay in bed.

Section 3—Lifting

- I can lift heavy weights without extra pain.
- I can lift heavy weights, but it gives extra pain.
- Pain prevents me from lifting heavy weights off the floor, but I can manage if they are conveniently positioned (e.g., on a table).
- Pain prevents me from lifting heavy weights, but I can manage light weights if they are conveniently positioned.
- I can lift only very light weights.
- I cannot lift or carry anything at all.

Section 4—Walking

- I can walk as far as I wish.
- Pain prevents me from walking more than 1 mile.
- Pain prevents me from walking more than ½ mile.
- Pain prevents me from walking more than ¼ mile.
- I can walk only if I use a stick or crutches.
- I am in bed or in a chair for most of every day.

Section 5—Sitting

- I can sit in any chair as long as I like.
- I can sit in my favorite chair only, but for as long as I like.
- Pain prevents me from sitting more than 1 hour.

- Pain prevents me from sitting more than ½ hour.
- Pain prevents me from sitting more than 10 minutes.
- Pain prevents me from sitting at all.

Section 6—Standing

- I can stand as long as I want without extra pain.
- I can stand as long as I want, but it gives me extra pain.
- Pain prevents me from standing for more than 1 hour.
- Pain prevents me from standing for more than 30 minutes.
- Pain prevents me from standing for more than 10 minutes.
- Pain prevents me from standing at all.

Section 7—Sleeping

- Pain does not prevent me from sleeping well.
- I sleep well but only by using tablets.
- Even when I take tablets I have less than 6 hours sleep.
- Even when I take tablets I have less than 4 hours sleep.
- Even when I take tablets I have less than 2 hours sleep.
- Pain prevents me from sleeping at all.

Section 8—Sex Life

- My sex life is normal and causes no extra pain.
- My sex life is normal but causes some extra pain.
- My sex life is nearly normal but is very painful.
- My sex life is severely restricted by pain.
- My sex life is nearly absent because of pain.
- Pain prevents any sex life at all.

Section 9—Social Life

- My social life is normal and causes me no extra pain.
- My social life is normal but increases the degree of pain.
- Pain affects my social life by limiting only my more energetic interests (dancing, etc.).
- Pain has restricted my social life, and I do not go out as often.
- Pain has restricted my social life to my home.
- I have no social life because of pain.

Section 10—Traveling

- I can travel anywhere without extra pain.
- I can travel anywhere, but it gives me extra pain.
- Pain is bad, but I manage journeys over 2 hours.
- Pain restricts me to journeys of less than 1 hour.
- Pain restricts me to short necessary journeys under 30 minutes.
- Pain prevents my traveling except to the physician or hospital.

Reproduced with permission from J.C.T. Fairbank et al., The Oswestry Low Back Pain Questionnaire, *Physiotherapy,* Vol. 66, p. 271, © 1980, Chartered Society of Physiotherapy.

Exhibit 6–3 Scoring the Oswestry Questionnaire

The following are key points to scoring of the Oswestry:

- Generally, the patient fills out the questionnaire in approximately 5 minutes with scoring by the doctor taking approximately 1 minute.
- The patient attempts to mark the most relevant answer for each of the 10 sections.
- The scoring includes only those sections that have been marked by the patient.
- Scoring is on a scale of 0 to 5 with the first possible answer in the sequence being a "0" and the last in the sequence being a "5."
- For each section, the maximum possible score is 5. The total score is calculated by adding all the scores together and dividing by the total possible number of points.

For example, if all sections were marked (i.e., 10 × 5 = 50 points) and the total points were 20, then the following calculation would be performed:

$$\frac{20 \text{ (total score/points)}}{50 \text{ (total possible score/points)}} \times 100 = 40\% \text{ points}$$

If conversely only 8 out of the 10 sections were completed (i.e., 8 × 5 = 40 points) and the total points were 20, then the following calculation would be performed:

$$\frac{20 \text{ (total score/points)}}{40 \text{ (total possible score/points)}} \times 100 = 50\% \text{ points}$$

Although there is no real standard for the interpretation of these percentage points, the following is a commonly used reference for interpretation:

Percentage Points	Degree of Disability
0–20% points	Minimal disability
21–40% points	Moderate disability
41–60% points	Severe disability
Over 60% points	Patient is severely disabled due to pain in several aspects of life

A standard approach is to administer the questionnaire over time to determine changes in perceived function. An improvement in the index indicates an improvement in the patient's perception of function and may indicate changes not necessarily reflected in objective orthopaedic or neurological testing.

---

patients who develop chronic LBP impose an inordinate financial burden on society. It has also been observed that there are indicators and predictors of patients who develop chronic pain. The New Zealand guidelines for LBP contain a screening tool for what are termed "yellow flags" for psychosocial predictors of chronic pain (see **Figure 6–1**).[67] The guidelines attempt to screen for these psychosocial factors and suggest strategies for more appropriate management of acute LBP in an attempt to decrease risk for the development of chronic LBP and associated disability. The questionnaire and strategies for intervention are given in **Exhibits 6–5** and **6–6**.

Examination

General Evaluation

Examination "red flags" include the following:

- The patient has saddle paresthesia (cauda equina).
- Weight loss in an older patient with a prior history of cancer and associated neurologic findings on examination suggest cancer.
- Fever (specificity = 0.98) associated with spinal tenderness to percussion (percussion sensitivity = 0.86) suggests spinal infection in a patient who has

Exhibit 6–4 Roland-Morris Low Back Disability Questionnaire

Instructions

When your back hurts, you may find it difficult to do some of the things you normally do. This list contains some sentences that people have used to describe themselves when they have back pain. When you read them, you may find that some stand out because they describe you *today.* As you read the list, think of yourself *today.* When you read a sentence that describes how you feel *today,* check the box next to it. If the sentence does not describe you, then leave the box blank and go on to the next one. Remember, only check the sentence if you are sure that it describes you today.

☐   1.   I stay home most of the time because of my back.
☐   2.   I change position frequently to try to get my back comfortable.
☐   3.   I walk more slowly than usual because of my back.
☐   4.   Because of my back, I am not doing any of the jobs that I usually do around the house.
☐   5.   Because of my back, I use a handrail to get upstairs.
☐   6.   Because of my back, I lie down to rest more often.
☐   7.   Because of my back, I have to hold on to something to get out of an easy chair.
☐   8.   Because of my back, I try to get other people to do things for me.
☐   9.   I get dressed more slowly than usual because of my back.
☐ 10.   I only stand up for short periods of time because of my back.
☐ 11.   Because of my back, I try not to bend or kneel down.
☐ 12.   I find it difficult to get out of a chair because of my back.
☐ 13.   My back is painful almost all the time.
☐ 14.   I find it difficult to turn over in bed because of my back.
☐ 15.   My appetite is not very good because of my back.
☐ 16.   I have trouble putting on my socks (stockings) because of the pain in my back.
☐ 17.   I only walk short distances because of my back pain.
☐ 18.   I sleep less well because of my back pain.
☐ 19.   Because of my back pain, I get dressed with help from someone else.
☐ 20.   I sit down for most of the day because of my back.
☐ 21.   I avoid heavy jobs around the house because of my back.
☐ 22.   Because of my back pain, I am more irritable and bad tempered with people than usual.
☐ 23.   Because of my back, I go upstairs more slowly than usual.
☐ 24.   I stay in bed most of the time because of my back.

Rate the severity of your pain by checking one box on the following scale.

0	1	2	3	4	5	6	7	8	9	10

NO PAIN   UNBEARABLE PAIN

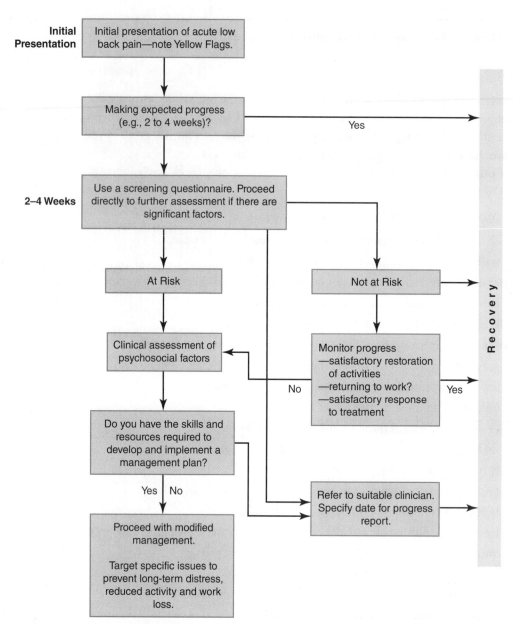

Figure 6–1 Assessing psychosocial yellow flags.
Courtesy of New Zealand Guidelines Group, Auckland, New Zealand.

a history of intravenous drug usage, has a urinary tract infection, or is immunocompromised.

The scope of the orthopaedic-neurologic examination often can be based on the distribution of a patient's complaint and a suspected underlying cause. The patient with LBP only (i.e., no leg pain) warrants an examination designed to determine whether the pain is reproducible and to what extent there is limitation in range of motion and/or function. If the pain is not reproducible mechanically, further tests to evaluate visceral possibilities such as genitourinary causes should be performed. Patients with radiation into the leg(s) must be categorized into those with nerve root lesions and those with referred signs or

symptoms. The primary distinction between these two broad categories is that patients with referred etiologies would rarely have hard neurologic evidence. For example, although the pain projection is in the distribution of the sciatic nerve, patients with referred causes often will have pain that does not extend below the knee. In addition, patients with referred pain would be highly unlikely to demonstrate myotome weakness, dermatome sensory abnormalities, or a decrease in reflexes (**Figure 6–2**).

It would seem logical that the clinical examination for radiculopathy (i.e., nerve root or spinal nerve compression) would be based on two principles: (1) reproduction of the radiation through mechanical maneuvers (i.e.

Exhibit 6–5 Guide to Assessing Psychosocial Yellow Flags in Acute Low Back Pain: Risk Factors for Long-Term Disability and Work Loss

PATIENT INFORMATION
SCREENING QUESTIONNAIRE (Linton & Halldén 1996)

Name: _____   ACC Claim Number: _____

Address: _____   Telephone (Home):(0) _____

_____   Telephone (Work):(0) _____

Job Title (Occupation): _____ Date stopped work for this episode: ____/____/____

These questions and statements apply if you have aches or pains, such as back, shoulder or neck pain. Please read and answer each question carefully. Do not take too long to answer the questions. However, it is important that you answer every question. There is always a response for your particular situation.

1. What year were you born? _____
2. Are you:
    ☐ male   ☐ female
3. Where do you have pain? Place a check (✓) for all the appropriate sites.
    ☐ neck   ☐ shoulders   ☐ upper back   ☐ lower back   ☐ leg
4. How many days of work have you missed because of pain during the past 18 months? Check (✓) one.
    ☐ 0 days [1]   ☐ 1–2 days [2]   ☐ 3–7 days [3]   ☐ 8–14 days [4]   ☐ 15–30 days [5]
    ☐ 1 month [6]   ☐ 2 months [7]   ☐ 3–6 months [8]   ☐ 6–12 months [9]   ☐ over 1 year [10]
5. How long have you had your current pain problem? Check (✓) one.
    ☐ 0–1 weeks [1]   ☐ 1–2 weeks [2]   ☐ 3–4 weeks [3]   ☐ 4–5 weeks [4]   ☐ 6–8 weeks [5]
    ☐ 9–11 weeks [6]   ☐ 3–6 months [7]   ☐ 6–9 months [8]   ☐ 9–12 months [9]   ☐ over 1 year [10]
6. Is your work heavy or monotonous? Circle the best alternative.
    Not at all   0 1 2 3 4 5 6 7 8 9 10   Extremely
7. How would you rate the pain that you have had during the past week? Circle one.
    No pain   0 1 2 3 4 5 6 7 8 9 10   Pain as bad as it could be
8. In the past three months, on average, how bad was your pain? Circle one.
    No pain   0 1 2 3 4 5 6 7 8 9 10   Pain as bad as it could be
9. How often would you say that you have experienced pain episodes, on average, during the past 3 months? Circle one.
    Never   0 1 2 3 4 5 6 7 8 9 10   Always
10. Based on all the things you do to cope, or deal with your pain, on an average day, how much are you able to decrease it? Circle one.
    Can't decrease it at all   0 1 2 3 4 5 6 7 8 9 10   Can decrease it completely
11. How tense or anxious have you felt in the past week? Circle one.
    Absolutely calm and relaxed   0 1 2 3 4 5 6 7 8 9 10   As tense and anxious as I've ever felt
12. How much have you been bothered by feeling depressed in the past week? Circle one.
    Not at all   0 1 2 3 4 5 6 7 8 9 10   Extremely
13. In your view, how large is the risk that your current pain may become persistent? Circle one.
    No risk   0 1 2 3 4 5 6 7 8 9 10   Very large risk
14. In your estimation, what are the chances that you will be working in 6 months? Circle one.
    No chance   0 1 2 3 4 5 6 7 8 9 10   Very large charge
15. If you take into consideration your work routines, management, salary, promotion possibilities and work mates, how satisfied are you with your job? Circle one.
    Not at all satisfied   0 1 2 3 4 5 6 7 8 9 10   Completely satisfied

(continues)

Here are some of the things which other people have told us about their back pain. For each statement please circle one number from 0 to 10 to say how much physical activities, such as bending, lifting, walking or driving, would affect your back.

16. Physical activity makes my pain worse
    Completely disagree   0   1   2   3   4   5   6   7   8   9   10   Completely agree
17. An increase in pain is an indication that I should stop what I am doing until the pain decreases.
    Completely disagree   0   1   2   3   4   5   6   7   8   9   10   Completely agree
18. I should not do my normal work with my present pain.
    Completely disagree   0   1   2   3   4   5   6   7   8   9   10   Completely agree
    Here is a list of 5 actvitities. Please circle the one number which best represents your current ability to participate in each of these activities.
19. I can do light work for an hour.
    Can't do it because of pain problem   0 1 2 3 4 5 6 7 8 9 10   Can do it without pain being a problem
20. I can walk for an hour.
    Can't do it because of pain problem   0 1 2 3 4 5 6 7 8 9 10   Can do it without pain being a problem
21. I can do ordinary household chores.
    Can't do it because of pain problem   0 1 2 3 4 5 6 7 8 9 10   Can do it without pain being a problem
22. I can go shopping.
    Can't do it because of pain problem   0 1 2 3 4 5 6 7 8 9 10   Can do it without pain being a problem
23. I can sleep at night.
    Can't do it because of pain problem   0 1 2 3 4 5 6 7 8 9 10   Can do it without pain being a problem

Courtesy of New Zealand Guidelines Group, Auckland, New Zealand.

Exhibit 6–6 Suggested Steps to Improve Early Behavioral Management of Low Back Pain Problems

1. Provide a *positive expectation* that the individual will return to work and normal activity. Organize for a regular expression of interest from the employer. If the problem persists beyond two to four weeks, provide a "reality-based" warning of what is going to be the likely outcome (e.g., loss of job, having to start from square one, the need to begin reactivation from a point of reduced fitness, etc.).

2. Be directive in scheduling *regular reviews of progress.* When conducting these reviews, shift the focus from the symptom (pain) to function (level of activity). Instead of asking "How much do you hurt?" ask "What have you been doing?" Maintain an interest in improvements, no matter how small. If another health professional is involved in treatment or management, specify a date for a progress report at the time of referral. Delays will be disabling.

3. *Keep the individual active and at work* if at all possible, even for a small part of the day. This will help to maintain work habits and work relationships. Consider reasonable requests for selected duties and modifications to the workplace. After four to six weeks, if there has been little improvement, review vocational options, job satisfaction, and any barriers to return to work, including psychosocial distress. Once barriers to return to work have been identified, these need to be targeted and managed appropriately. Job dissatisfaction and distress cannot be treated with a physical modality.

4. *Acknowledge difficulties* with activities of daily living, but avoid making the assumption that these indicate all activity or any work must be avoided.

5. Help to *maintain positive cooperation* between the individual, an employer, the compensation system, and health professionals. Encourage collaboration wherever possible. Inadvertent support for collusion between "them" and "us" can be damaging to progress.

6. *Make a concerted effort to communicate that having more time off work will reduce the likelihood of a successful return to work.* In fact, longer periods off work result in reduced probability of ever returning to work. At the

six-week point *consider suggesting vocational redirection, job changes,* the use of "knight's move" approaches to return to work (i.e., same employer, different job).

7. Be alert for the presence of individual beliefs that he or she should stay off work until treatment has provided a "total cure"; watch out for expectations of simple *"technofixes."*

8. Promote *self-management and self-responsibility.* Encourage the development of self-efficacy to return to work. Be aware that developing self-efficacy will depend on *incentives and feedback* from treatment providers and others. If recovery only requires development of a skill such as adopting a new posture, then it is not likely to be affected by incentives and feedback. However, if recovery requires the need to overcome an aversive stimulus such as fear of movement (kinesiophobia), then it will be readily affected by incentives and feedback.

9. Be prepared to ask for a second opinion, provided it does not result in a long and disabling delay. Use this option especially if it may help clarify that further diagnostic work-up is unnecessary. *Be prepared to say "I don't know"* rather than provide elaborate explanations based on speculation.

10. Avoid confusing the *report of symptoms* with the presence of emotional distress. Distressed people seek more help, and have been shown to be more likely to receive ongoing medical intervention. Exclusive focus on symptom control is not likely to be successful if emotional distress is not addressed.

11. *Avoid suggesting* (even inadvertently) that the person from a regular job may be able to *work at home,* or in their own business because it will be under their own control. This message, in effect, is to allow pain to become the reinforcer for activity—producing a deactivation syndrome with all the negative consequences. Self-employment nearly always involves more hard work.

12. Encourage people to recognize, from the earliest point, *that pain can be controlled and managed* so that a normal, active or working life can be maintained. *Provide encouragement for all "well" behaviors,* including alternative ways of performing tasks and focusing on transferable skills.

13. If barriers to return to work are identified and the problem is too complex to manage, referral to a multidisciplinary team as described in the *New Zealand Acute Low Back Pain Guide* is recommended.

Courtesy of New Zealand Guidelines Group, Auckland, New Zealand.

---

orthopaedic testing), and (2) objectively determining neurological deficit, the result of nerve damage (i.e., the neurological examination). However, recent reviews examining the value of the orthopaedic and neurological evaluation of patients with radiating complaints have revealed some consensus that may be different from what is taught and assumed by practitioners based on this logic.

The difficulty in reaching conclusions from the literature regarding the value of the clinical examination for patients with radiating complaints includes the following variables:

- Are the patients in a study evaluated in a primary, secondary, or tertiary care center? As patients progress through the staging of practitioner seen, a concentration effect results in a likelihood that there is a higher proportion of patients in the tertiary care setting with radiculopathy making the results of studies examining sensitivity/specificity more likely to demonstrate a higher detection ability.
- Do the patients seen in a study have confirmation from special imaging or surgery that they have a structural cause (i.e., disc herniation, tumor, stenosis) for their radiculopathy? Without this confirmation, patients assumed to have a radiculopathy may not.
- Are patients categorized by a specific level to determine the accuracy of the examination or are they categorized into general categories or radicular versus nonradicular? The value of the examination may be rated low if the outcome measure is accuracy of identifying a specific disc level or nerve root level versus whether the patient has a radiculopathy or not.
- Are orthopaedic tests, the neurological examination, or a combination of the two being tested for validity against a gold standard?
- Is there consistency of the orthopaedic tests being performed?
- Are the positives for a test the same in all studies?

Given that 98% of all disc lesions occur at the L4-L5 or L5-S1 discs, the likelihood of positive neurologic signs will be highest for the L5 or S1 nerve roots.[68] In earlier

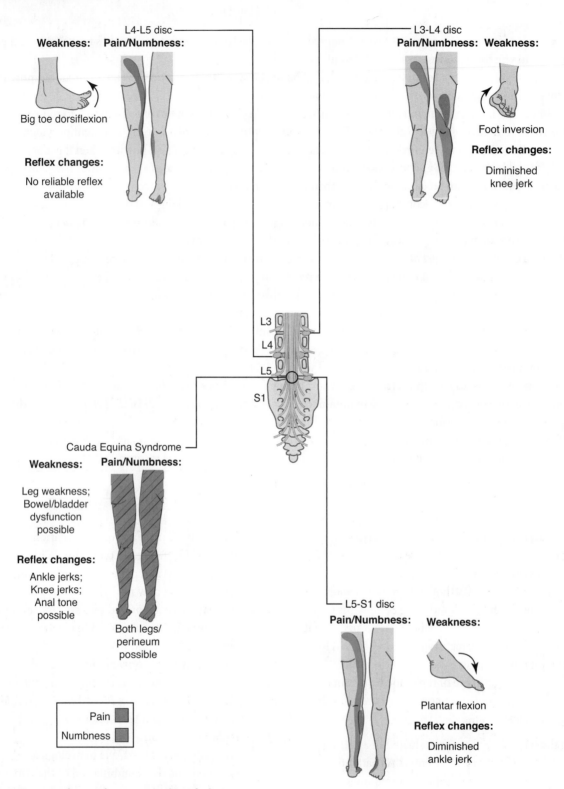

Figure 6–2 Common disc syndromes: neurologic findings.

studies, the ability to localize the nerve root and disc level was determined to be quite good. An L5-S1 disc rupture was 86% probable if all three S1 signs were found: (1) pain projection into the S1 area, (2) a pathologic Achilles reflex, and (3) a sensory defect in the S1 dermatome.[69] Localization to the L4-L5 disc was 87% probable with all three L5 signs: (1) extensor hallucis (EH) weakness, (2) pain projection into the L5 area, and (3) a sensory defect in the L5 dermatome. It is important to remember that pain projection into the S1 area can be found with any lumbar disc herniation; however, EH weakness and pain projection into the L5 area together are reliable indicators of an L5 nerve root lesion even when accompanied by S1 findings. With L5 nerve root involvement it is not uncommon also to find ankle dorsiflexion weakness with EH weakness. McCombe et al.[70] evaluated the reproducibility of several physical signs for LBP. Buttock wasting, toe standing, and heel standing were considered unreliable. The Achilles reflex was considered a reliable inter-examiner finding; however, the patellar reflex was not. The sensory examination was considered reliable. It is important to keep in mind that numbness is usually most evident distally. In other words, although the patient may complain of pain or numbness extending down the length of the leg to the foot, numbness may be demonstrated only distally at the foot.

More recently, the orthopaedic and neurological examination has come under attack for its poor diagnostic accuracy. In 2013, a study[71] published in *The Spine Journal* was a systematic review and meta-analysis of the value of the peripheral nervous system examination in patients with radiculopathy due to disc herniation. They utilized the three standard exam findings for detecting radiculopathy including motor testing, sensory testing, and deep tendon reflexes. The following summarizes their findings:

- For surgically and radiologically confirmed disc herniation, sensory testing demonstrated low diagnostic sensitivity at 0.40 and 0.32 respectively.
- Specificity was higher for all the three reference standards (0.59—sensory, 0.72—motor, and 0.64—deep tendon reflexes).
- Motor testing for weakness demonstrated diagnostic sensitivities of 0.22 for surgically confirmed and 0.40 for imaging confirmed disc herniation and moderate specificity values (0.79 and 0.62 respectively).
- The sensitivity for muscle atrophy was 0.31 and the specificity was 0.76 for surgically determined disc herniation.

- For reflex testing, specificity values were 0.78 and 0.75, respectively for surgically confirmed versus imaging confirmed herniation. Sensitivities for surgically and radiologically confirmed levels of disc herniation were 0.29 and 0.25; quite poor.
- The pooled positive likelihood ratios for all neurological examination components ranged between 1.02 and 1.26, indicating literally almost no value when looking across all testing.

Simply put, neurological examinations alone are not good for screening patients with suspected radiculopathy, but when positive, they have a moderate value of helping to rule in a radiculopathy. Said another way, you can more confidently know that someone has a radiculopathy when testing is positive but when negative, you cannot rule out a radiculopathy.

Although there are well over 50 orthopaedic tests listed in the literature for the low back and more than 15 for the SI joint, most are based on a common approach with some minor variations. Many tests can be classified as nerve tension tests, attempting to stretch a spinal nerve or nerve root. The second group of tests attempts to increase pressure or compression at various potential pain-producing sites (e.g., facet joints).

The most studied test is the straight leg raise (SLR).[72] This nerve tension test is considered quite valuable in distinguishing patients who have disc herniation from those who do not. A positive finding is reproduction of pain down the back of the leg to the foot with passive raising of the leg (**Figure 6–3**). Several observations are important to keep in mind while interpreting the response to an SLR:[73]

- A positive finding between 15° and 30° is a reliable indicator of disc herniation.

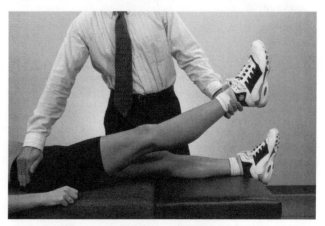

Figure 6–3 The straight leg raise test. Nerve root compression is likely when posterior leg pain is provoked below 45°.

- A positive finding above 60° provides little diagnostic information.
- A positive finding when adding either passive dorsiflexion of the ankle (Braggard's test), medial hip rotation, or flexion of the cervical spine.

It is important to question the patient about a positive response to better guarantee that the response is not due to hamstring stretching. Medial hip rotation may also call into question possible involvement of the piriformis muscle with referred leg pain consequences. Combining the SLR findings with neurologic findings will usually be sufficient. For example, an apparently positive SLR without hard neurologic findings would be more suspect of a referral source. The well-leg raise test is less sensitive; however, it is much more specific for a disc lesion. Therefore, a positive response is virtually diagnostic for a disc lesion. Additional testing may include a Valsalva maneuver in an attempt to increase intrathecal pressure. A space-occupying lesion such as a tumor or a disc may then increase the leg pain complaint of the patient. Disc lesions that are further lateral than the typical posterolateral herniation may be clinically confusing.[74-77] Far-lateral (sometimes called "far-out" lateral) lesions primarily cause leg complaints. Thecal signs are usually absent because the point of compression is beyond the dural sleeve. Higher lesions tend to cause anterior thigh pain and weakness with a decreased quadriceps reflex. S1 lesions are uncommon with far-lateral lesions unless there is an extra vertebra (L6). The degree of tropism may also be a factor and may be associated with far-lateral lesions.

In a cohort study using patients with signs and symptoms of radiculopathy confirmed with MRI results, researchers compared the sensitivity and specificity of a seated SLR compared to a supine SLR.[78] The results indicated that the supine SLR is more sensitive in reproducing leg pain than the seated SLR.

Poiraudeau et al.[79] performed an interesting study evaluating the ability of two lesser known clinical findings in differentiating patients who had "sciatica" into those with and without disc herniation. Unlike most studies, the gold standard was radiographic rather than surgical. Either MRI, CT, or myelography was used to determine disc involvement. The two clinical tests were the Bell test (BT) and the hyperextension test (HT). These were compared to the Lasegue's sign (LS: Straight Leg Raise) and the Crossed Lasegue's (CL) sign. There were several interesting observations. None of the tests demonstrated high degrees of interexaminer reliability using the interclass correlation coefficient (ICC). In fact, the range for the LS was 0.27–0.47. The most reliable among examiners was the CL with a range of 0.42–0.72. The BT ranged from 0.58–0.64 with the HT at 0.35–0.50. For sensitivity and specificity, the best performing tests were the LS with the best sensitivity, and the CL with the best specificity. The positive and negative predictive values for all four tests were similar. The combination of HT and the CL had the best PPV at 0.67–0.85. The BT was performed with the patient standing. The examiner exerted thumb pressure between the spinous processes of L4-L5 or L5-S1 or a nearby paraspinal area in an effort to reproduce the patient's leg pain. If only localized pain was produced, the test was regarded as negative. The HT was also performed with the patient standing. With the patient's knees kept straight, the examiner passively extended the patient slowly. If the patient's leg pain was reproduced, the test was positive; localized pain production was considered a negative test. It appears from this small study that adding the HT and correlating a positive finding with a CL sign may add some value in determining disc involvement with patients who have posterior radiation of pain down the leg.

There are many variations on neural tension testing, most of which have no literature support for or against their use. A sitting version is often called Bechterew's (**Figure 6–4**), but a newer test referred to as the flip test is similar. With passive extension of the knee with the

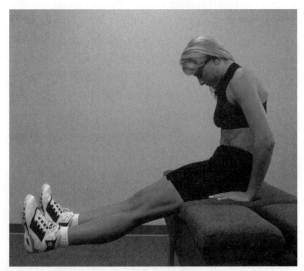

Figure 6–4 Bechterew's test. The seated patient is asked to extend the knees in an effort to determine whether leg pain is provoked. Having the patient flex the neck forward, hold his or her breath, and bear down (Valsalva maneuver) may increase the sensitivity of the test.

patient in the seated position, the flip test is supposed to cause a sudden falling of the leg or flipping back of the trunk due to pain. A study[80] evaluating the flip test concluded that due to the finding that only one third of patients demonstrated a "flip," the term "sitting SLR test," is a less misleading and more accurate name. In their study, 33% of patients felt no pain, 39% felt pain on full extension of the knee, and 28% resisted full extension of the knee due to pain.

Finally, a combination of provocation and relief testing is attempted with the slump test. The slump test (**Figure 6–5**) is performed with the patient seated with the arms behind the back. The patient is then asked to slump forward as much as possible while the examiner applies overpressure into flexion. The next step involves asking the patient to extend the involved knee (or in some descriptions the examiner extends the patient's knee). The examiner then applies passive dorsiflexion to the ankle. Neck flexion is then added to increase tension. If positive for radiation, neck flexion is released to

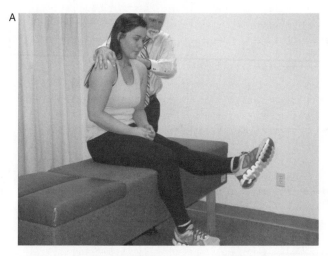

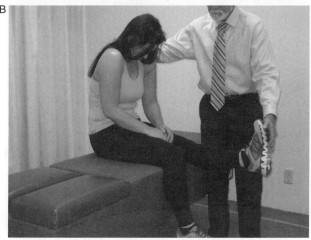

Figure 6–5 Slump test.

determine if there is a decrease or abatement of symptoms. Compared with the SLR, one study found that the slump test is more sensitive.[81]

A Cochrane review[81] published in 2010 summarized the literature to that date regarding the physical examination for lumbar radiculopathy. They found that:

- The SLR was highly sensitive (pooled estimate 0.92, 95% CI: 0.87 to 0.95) with a wide range for specificity (0.10 to 1.00, pooled estimate 0.28, 95% CI: 0.18 to 0.40) in *surgically confirmed* radiculopathy. Sensitivity was poorer for the SLR in *imaging confirmed* radiculopathy.
- The crossed SLR demonstrated high specificity (pooled estimate 0.90, 95% CI: 0.85 to 0.94) but consistently low sensitivity (pooled estimate 0.28, 95% CI: 0.22 to 0.35).
- Combining positive test results increased the specificity of physical tests, but few studies presented data on test combinations.

In a study[56] comparing leg-related complaints that were radicular versus stenosis-related in a senior group of participants, patients with herniation more often had positive nerve root tension signs with either or both straight-leg raising and femoral stretch signs positive in 58% of participants. Also, trunk flexion was more limited as compared to those with stenosis-related leg pain. Nerve root tension signs were found infrequently positive (8%). Patients with stenosis were more likely to have diminished Achilles reflexes. **Exhibit 6–7** demonstrates averaged likelihood ratios for some of the common orthopaedic and neurological examination findings to estimate the probability of lumbar radiculopathy.

Facets are often challenged through compression or stretch. In the supine patient, indirect pressure at the facets may occur with flexing the heel toward the buttocks, increasing the lordosis and consequently loading the facets. Another approach is the seated or standing Kemp's maneuver. While seated, the patient is taken passively into extension and rotation to each side in an attempt to determine whether local or radiating pain is reproduced (**Figure 6–6**). Local pain suggests a facet cause, whereas radiating pain into the leg is more suggestive of nerve root irritation, especially if the pain is below the knee. The standing Kemp's test is a less specific test because it involves an active attempt by the patient to bend back, running the contralateral hand down the opposite leg. Therefore, muscle activation may cause spasm that is unrelated to a neural compressive or stretch effect.

Exhibit 6-7 Likelihood Patient Has a Lumbar Radiculopathy

Approximating Probability: The likelihood ratios (LRs) in this graphical representation represent estimates of probability based on the aggregate of multiple reviews of each test finding. They are only approximations and only reliable indicators of a change in the context of a patient having an intermediate pre-test probability of between 20% to 80%. If the pre-test probability is very high or very low, the LR has little effect on changing the probability.

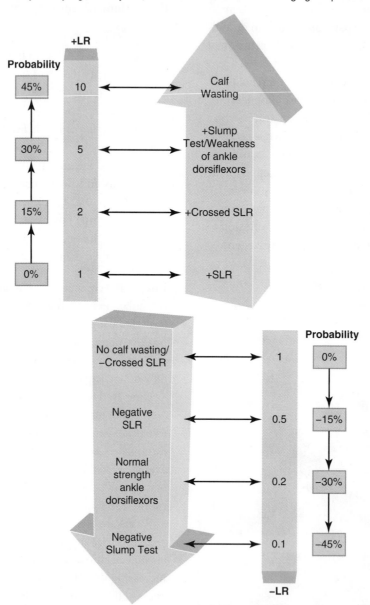

A recent study evaluated the intra- and interrater reliability of visual assessment of cervical and lumbar lordosis (without the use of a measurement instrument).[83] This study included chiropractors, physical therapists, physiatrists, rheumatologists, and orthopaedic surgeons. Subjects were divided into those with back pain and those without. Raters were asked to rate photographs placed in a PowerPoint presentation. Lateral views of relaxed individuals' cervical and lumbar curves were rated as normal, increased, or decreased. Interestingly, there was no difference in rating between those with or without back pain. The intrarater reliability was statistically fair ($\kappa = 0.50$) and the interrater reliability was poor ($\kappa = 0.16$).

Because leg length discrepancy has been often suspected as a biomechanical cause of LBP and other complaints, it is important to consider the reliability and validity of measurement of leg length in the physical

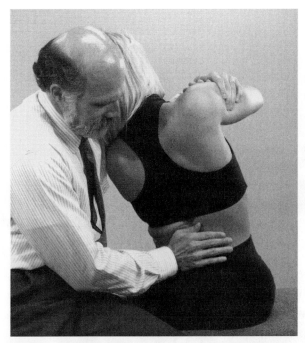

Figure 6–6 Kemp's test. Kemp's test may be performed with the patient seated or standing. While seated, the examiner applies pressure at the lumbar spine while extending and rotating the patient to one side and then the other.

examination. The reliability is good if the patient is measured supine and the difference in measurement allowed for agreement among examiners is extended to 12.5 mm, with the mean value of two measurements included.[84] Estimation through palpation of the iliac crests in the standing position is considered unreliable.[85] Leg length measurement is also used as an indicator and outcome measure for successful correction of biomechanical or neurologic dysfunction. Although some studies have indicated good reliability, others question the statistical analysis used in the studies, not to mention the design, which may include telling the examiners which is the short leg side.[86] More research is needed.

Motion palpation testing of the lumbar spine is commonly used in the evaluation of LBP. Studies have shown poor interexaminer reliability in some parts of the spine; however, Boline et al.[87] found interrater reliability at T12-L1 and L3-L4 and Mootz[88] found intrarater reliability at L4-L5.

Range of motion (ROM) may be evaluated through several procedures; however, there are problems with the reliability of all approaches.[89,90] Also, the correlation between ROM and functional impairment has been questioned.[91,92] Common methods are the modified (or modified-modified) Schober (**Figure 6–7**A) and

the inclinometer method (**Figure 6–7**, B and C).[93] The inclinometer approach uses either a single or double inclinometer; however, the principles are the same. Placing the inclinometers at the T12-L1 area and the sacrum, they are "zeroed out." The patient is then asked to flex, and the new readings are recorded. The same may be done with other movements. The bottom inclinometer readings are subtracted from the top inclinometer readings to obtain "true" lumbar participation (subtracting out the pelvic component). The modified Schober method uses a marking 5 cm and 10 cm above the lumbosacral junction (**Figure 6–7**A). With a tape measure held to the back, the patient is asked to flex. The difference is measured and recorded. The modified-modified Schober method involves connecting a line between the inferior margins of the posterior superior iliac spine and using a second skin marking 15 cm above the iliac line. The same procedure is then used to measure distance increases, using the closest millimeter. It is interesting to note that the old standard of measurement, the finger-to-floor method, is considered unreliable. A recent study[94] indicated that the change in the finger-to-floor results after the first month was a valid predictor of the change in self-reported disability using the Roland-Morris Disability Questionnaire over one year, outperforming the straight leg raise test as a measure of change in disability.

There are several commonly used approaches to functional testing of the low back. It is beyond the scope of this short discussion to cover all of these in any detail; however, the reader is encouraged to follow the references at the end of this chapter for more depth. The McKenzie approach to evaluation of LBP is to determine whether the patient has a postural problem, dysfunctional problem, or internal derangement.[95] This is accomplished by determining the position or movement that causes pain or relief. Patients who have no pain during, for example, flexion or extension (according to McKenzie) have a "postural" problem. This implies that the patient holds a particular posture during the day that needs to be interrupted to prevent the pain associated with holding any position for too long. The dysfunctional pattern is found when there is pain at end-range testing positions. McKenzie theorizes that this is due to shortened tissue. His solution is to stretch into the painful direction. The final category is the derangement syndrome. This patient has pain going through a movement pattern. More important, when the prone patient is asked to lift the trunk off the table by pushing up with

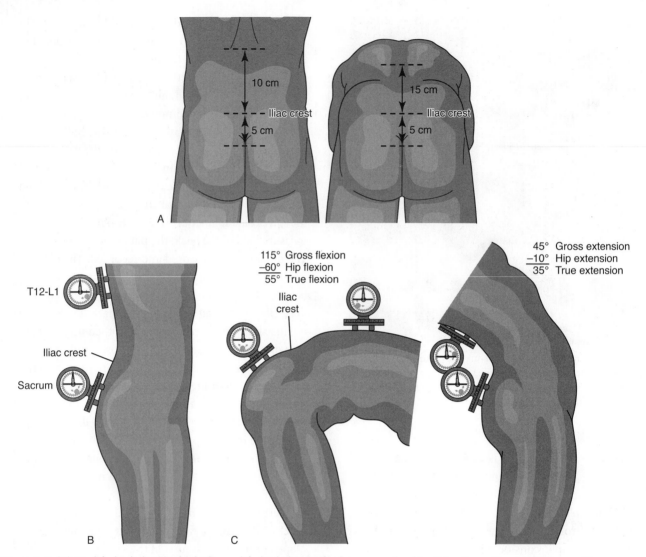

Figure 6–7 (A) Modified Schober Method. The modified Schober method measures the skin distraction with a tape measure. The modification of the Schober method test includes an additional third mark 5 cm below the lumbosacral junction. (B) and (C) Inclinometer Method. Lumbar spine range of motion is best measured with two inclinometers.

the hands and keeping the pelvis on the table, pain down the leg is increased (**Figure 6–8**). This is referred to as *peripheralization*. If the same maneuver is repeated after moving the pelvis to either side and the pain is felt more in the back (centralization), then a position of relief has been determined that is used as the main form of therapy for the patient. One study indicated poor intertester reliability for classification of these syndrome types in patients with LBP.[96] The interexaminer reliability of the McKenzie approach to evaluation of mechanical LBP has been questioned, yet a recent study[97] indicated that with a standardized protocol, the interexaminer reliability was high with the exception of identification of lateral shift.

Especially for patients with chronic LBP or for those interested in prevention, several functional approaches are helpful in determining exercise and stretching prescription. The Lewit/Janda approach is to search for "patterns" of muscle tightness and weakness and for dysfunctional patterns of movement.[98–100] These researchers focus on several patterns that seem to appear in layers. For the low back specifically, tight hip flexors and paraspinals associated with weak abdominals and gluteals are a common pattern. Function is also investigated by watching the timing of recruitment with specific movement patterns. For example, with active hip extension in the prone position, there is a sequential recruitment of hamstring, gluteals, and paraspinals. If the hamstrings and gluteals are dysfunctional requiring the paraspinals to contract early, facet impingement may occur as a result of the increase in lordosis.

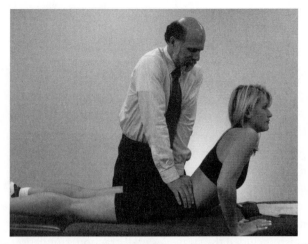

Figure 6–8 Prone extension is performed by asking the patient to lift the chest off the table by pushing up from the elbows first, if possible, then the hands. The examiner stabilizes the pelvis on the table.

Other approaches assess the patient's ability to perform predetermined exercises, rate the patient, and use the perceived weaknesses to prescribe an exercise program. Other testing involves expensive, sophisticated machines in an attempt to isolate certain muscle groups or to determine the patient's ability to lift.

Sacroiliac Tests

Palpatory tenderness over the posterior superior iliac spine (PSIS) has some degree of inter- and intraexaminer reliability.[101] Determination of iliac crest and PSIS heights as well as a sitting flexion test demonstrated only poor to fair intra- and interreliability concordance. Two tests that appear to be reliable for SI involvement are the iliac gapping test (**Figure 6–9**) and the compression test (**Figure 6–10**).[102] These tests require a patient response. Other tests that may be valuable are the distraction (SI

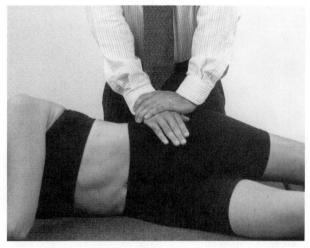

Figure 6–10 The sacroiliac compression (approximation) test.

stretch) test (not shown), Gaenslen's test (**Figure 6–11**), hip extension test (**Figure 6–12**), and Patrick-Fabere's test (not shown; see Chapter 11). The latter tests act as compression tests and require that the hip be considered as a possible contributor to a positive response. Localization of the patient's response coupled with ROM

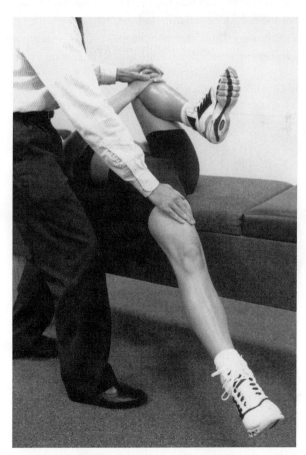

Figure 6–11 Gaenslen's test. The patient draws one leg up to the chest while the examiner distracts the opposite leg off the side of the examination, causing SI compression on the examiner's side.

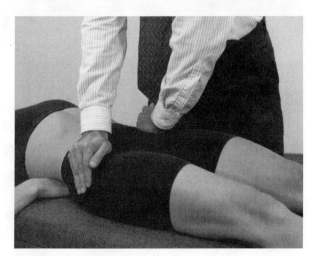

Figure 6–9 The Gapping test.

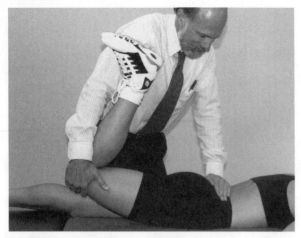

Figure 6–12 Passive hip extension may localize pain to the SI joint or lumbar facets.

of the hip may help localize the cause. In other words, if the pain is felt anteriorly and/or there is associated painful ROM in the hip, SI involvement is less likely. A common testing procedure used by manipulators is the Gillet or step test (**Figure 6–13**, A and B). Herzog et al.[103] reported that the test was reliable and a valuable indicator of the need for SI manipulation. A study by Mior et al.,[104] however, indicated poor kappa values. Furthermore, researchers in a study designed to test the interexaminer and intraexaminer reliability of the Gillet test for the SI joint found it to be unreliable.[105]

Nonorganic Signs

When a patient is a chronic LBP sufferer, has potential loss of job or family breakup, or is involved in litigation, it is important to consider the history with the clinical findings. In patients in whom there is a mismatch or an apparent overreaction is perceived, nonorganic testing should be included. Waddell et al.[106] originally designed these tests. They consist of five categories of inappropriate responses to various testing maneuvers, which included the strategies of distraction, simulation, and evaluation of tenderness, regional disturbances, and overreaction. Finding three or more of these positive findings would indicate that the patient is somatizing or malingering. McCombe et al.[70] and Fishbaine et al.[107] found that the regional disturbance category (abnormal regional sensory or motor disturbance such as the whole leg or overlapping dermatomal sensory complaints) and superficial tenderness (tenderness to light touch in a wide area) were unreliable. Part of the reason for less focus on regional disturbances is that it is possible for patients to have less discrete sensory or motor complaints with single nerve lesions, and it is always possible

A
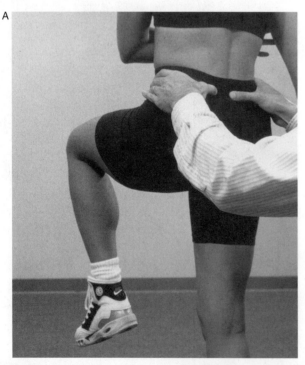

B
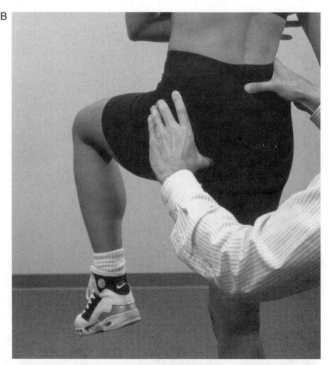

Figure 6–13 Testing for sacroiliac fixation. (A) The examiner palpates the sacral spine and the posterior superior iliac spine (PSIS). The patient then lifts the leg. If the joint is fixed, the PSIS will rise on that side. (B) The examiner palpates the sacral spine and the ischial tuberosity. With normal movement, the ischial tuberosity will move out laterally when the leg is lifted. If it moves upward, the joint is presumed fixed.

that they have a spinal stenosis, which often can present with unusual regional disturbances. Malingering or nonorganic testing maneuvers include axial loading in the standing patient, passive flexion of the hip with the knee flexed, rotational twisting of the trunk, and forward bending in the seated position, among others.

Screening for Risk Due to Strength/Endurance Weakness

A protocol based on studies·by Reger,[108] Rissanen,[109] Alaranta,[110] Schellenberg,[111] and others,[112,113] is in common use as a screening approach to evaluating strength and endurance. The observation from these studies is that simple in-office testing has some predictive value and, in place of more expensive isokinetic testing, provides a level of evidence for screening patients to determine specific weakness in either endurance or strength that can be used to prescribe rehabilitative exercises. Age- and gender-based normative data is then used to place the patient into one of five categories with five

being excellent, four: good, three: moderate, two: poor, and one: extremely poor.

The four screening exercises are:

- Repetitive arch-up test—performed supine off the edge of a high table with stability provided by examiner; maximum of 50.
- Repetitive sit-up test—performed on a high table with foot support provided by examiner; maximum of 50.
- Repetitive squatting test—patient performs with hand support next to table; maximum of 50.
- Static back endurance test—same position as arch-up test. However, patient holds as an isometric with the trunk parallel to the floor for as long as possible; maximum of 240 seconds.

A more recent modified version of this prescreening for risk based on endurance includes (see **Figure 6–14**):

- Side-bridge (right and left)—patient supports himself on one side with a flexed elbow and

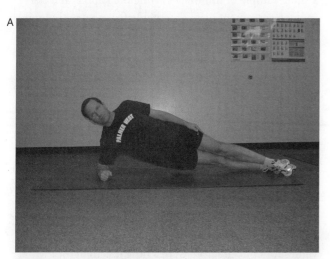
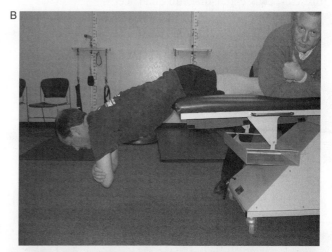
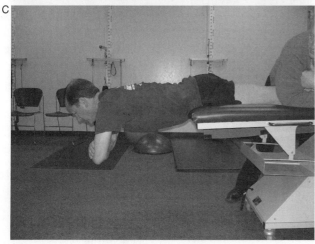
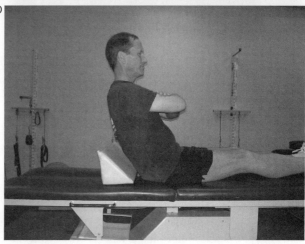

Figure 6–14 Strength/endurance screening for low back pain, (A) side-bridge, (B) arch-up, (C) back endurance (extension), (D) flexion (sit-up).

crossed feet (support at ankles). Generally should be held for about 1 to 1½ minutes in healthy young individuals.

- Flexion—patient is supine and supported by a jig or other device at 55° with hips and knees flexed to 90°. With the support removed, the patient is asked to hold the position for as long as possible. The average is about two minutes in healthy young individuals.

- Extension (same as static back endurance test above)—patient is supported at the ankles or lower legs in a prone position with the trunk suspended off of a high table. Patient is asked to hold a horizontal position to the ground with the arms crossed over the chest for as long as possible. The average length of time for healthy young individuals is about 2½ to 3 minutes.

One of the most commonly prescribed approaches to prevent low back pain is core stabilization. The principle is to provide "core" strengthening of the abdominal muscles, back extensors, and quadriceps.[112,113]

McGill,[114] in a series of experiments, has demonstrated that the typical "hollowing" approach used by some training methods is actually potentially dangerous because it causes some muscles to relax thereby decreasing stability. Stiffening is the recommended approach to abdominal support for spinal stability. McGill also cautions that the psoas muscle is used to create hip flexion torque and is minimally linked to the spine. However, he states that substantial spinal compression is caused by psoas contraction which may lead to injury. He recommends standard screening but includes provocative tests, stability, McKenzie, and endurance tests based on the type of patient and his or her specific life demands.

Radiography and Special Imaging
Plain Films

The use of plain film evaluation of the patient with LBP is dictated by several factors:

- Does the patient have either a history or physical examination findings of a "high risk"?
- To what degree does the information gained alter the treatment?
- What are the relative risk and cost for the patient?

If the intention is to search for contraindications to adjusting or need for referral, it is usually clear from the history or examination when radiographs are necessary.

If there are indications of cancer, infection, abdominal aneurysm, or fracture, radiographs are often the first screening test because of their high sensitivity.[115] Significant damage must occur, however, before these pathologic lesions are evident. When there are no high-risk indicators, the next need felt by many chiropractors is a biomechanical evaluation of the patient from both a gross and a segmental level. In other words, what are the relative imbalances with regard to symmetry? From a segmental perspective, static or active examination is used to search for restricted or excessive movement at a segmental level. The validity of this approach has been questioned; however, it may represent a potential source of information that may change the approach to the patient if used honestly. It is important to note that studies indicating poor reliability have had some methodological flaws. One study tested the reliability of chiropractors identifying common findings that may influence adjusting procedures such as disc degeneration, osteophytes, and spondylolisthesis, among others. Also included were a small sample of tumors.[116] While the kappas and percentage agreement were acceptable for most pathologies, they were not excellent. In particular, the identification of facet arthrosis was poor. Another study[117] emphasizes the need for radiologists' (chiropractic or medical) evaluation with questionable findings. Researchers recently conducted a comparative study evaluating examiners' ability to agree (interobserver agreement) and to detect abnormalities that would be possible contraindications to chiropractic treatment of the low back. These "contraindications" included infections, malignancies, inflammatory spondylitis, and spondylolysis-listhesis. The observers (examiners) were five chiropractors, three chiropractic radiologists, and five medical radiologists. The kappa values for chiropractors were a little less than for the specialists. Most importantly, the sensitivity and specificity for interpretation of pathologies were similar among all three groups, with the medical radiologists being more specific. The conclusion by the researchers is that for most radiographic indicators of contraindications to care, chiropractors might well be experienced enough to detect without the aid of a specialist.[118]

Numerous lines of mensuration are used to evaluate mainly facet loading, abnormal curve, or shear stresses to the spine. Gradings of spondylolisthesis and of central canal stenosis are also possible. Following is a limited description of some of these radiographic markings:

- Central canal stenosis. Two methods are used: (1) Beuler and (2) Eisenstein.[119] A magnification factor of 0.77 is used to compensate for the magnification effect of the radiograph. Both are relatively accurate. The Beuler method is more accurate at the L3 level. The normal sagittal diameter is approximately 15 mm or more. A diameter of 12 mm is considered relative stenosis; 10 mm or less is considered absolute. On the anteroposterior (AP) view, the interpendicular distance can be measured. An AP diameter of 11.5 mm and an interpendicular distance of less than 16 mm are considered diagnostic for spinal canal stenosis.[120]

- Facet syndrome. Several lines of mensuration are used to determine vertebral inclination on lateral films in an effort to uncover excessive weight distribution to the facets. The lumbar IVD disc angle varies at each level; however, any measurement greater than 15° is likely to indicate facet syndrome in those patients with correlated clinical symptoms. This is also true of the lumbosacral disc angle. The lumbosacral angle demonstrates wide variation of normal (26° to 57°) and is probably generally not helpful. The use of McNab's line is also not helpful because of the high incidence of abnormal findings in asymptomatic persons. Hadley's S curve is designed to indicate facet subluxation; however, displacements of 3 mm may not be visible. Although patients with LBP with a history of trauma have more severe facet degenerative signs on radiography than patients without a history of trauma, there appear to be no differences in pain and disability.[121]
- Spondylolisthesis: Meyerding's grading system is the standard for measuring the degree of spondylolisthesis. The superior surface of the base of the sacrum is divided into fourths (this can be performed with the segment below for higher spondylolisthesis). The degree of slippage is then measured and graded 1 through 4.

Some chiropractors feel that the identification of anomalies is an important reason for screening all patients with LBP. However, studies have not found a higher incidence of LBP in patients with facet tropism, transitional vertebrae, spina bifida, or Schmorl's nodes.[122,123] However, the identification of a transitional vertebra or facet tropism may alter the positioning of the adjustment (manipulation) or cause the doctor to choose a different manipulative approach. This has yet to be researched.

When pathology is suspected, it is important to begin with a limited series, including AP and lateral views. Lytic, blastic, and degenerative processes are usually well visualized on routine views. In addition, a calcified aortic aneurysm is visible on a lateral view. Special views should be reserved for specific concerns. For example, if the patient is seen to have a spondylolisthesis on the lateral film, oblique films may allow visualization of pars interarticularis discontinuity. If the SI joint is suspected of having a sclerotic focus (e.g., seronegative arthritides), angled spot-views may provide a clearer picture.

Computed Tomography

CT is usually reserved for suspected cases of fracture or stenosis. It may also be useful in imaging infection, tumor, the cause of pain in postoperative spines (recurrent disc herniation and fusion), and herniated discs in general. Because of the increased radiation exposure, MRI is often chosen as an alternative (also see Table 1–4).

Magnetic Resonance Imaging

MRI has the advantage of no ionizing radiation, yet it has a slightly higher cost. Soft tissue is well visualized. MRI is particularly valuable in evaluating disc pathology, the extent of tumor or infection invasion, and abnormalities involving the nerve root, thecal sac, or subarachnoid space. In differentiating between recurrent disc herniation or postsurgical fibrosis, MRI with gadolinium (injected) is often helpful (see also Table 1–4).

Bone Scan

Bone scan is quite sensitive to bone changes and is valuable in the detection of spinal metastasis and activity of a spondylolisthesis. However, it is not specific for the cause of the increased uptake pattern. In other words, any bony inflammatory condition may cause an increased uptake. The extent of damage is also not well visualized.

Discography and Pain Provocation/Relief Studies

For patients who have equivocal imaging studies or for patients with known pathology who are unresponsive to conservative care, various minimally invasive medical approaches have been suggested. These include discography, selective nerve root blocks, epidural blocks, sympathetic nerve blocks, and facet neurotomy (medial branch rhizotomy). **Table 6–2** summarizes each procedure, when it is most appropriate, and generally how it is performed.[32,124]

Table 6–2 Selected Nonsurgical Diagnostic and Therapeutic Procedures for the Discs, Nerve Roots, and Facet Joints

Procedure/Definition	Procedure	Expected Results
Discography: A diagnostic test used to view and assess the internal structure of a disc and determine if it is the source of a patient's complaint.	Under fluoroscopic guidance, a needle is advanced into the disc. Provocation discography attempts to identify a specific disc as the cause of a patient's complaint through injection of saline and radiopaque dye; analgesic discography attempts to relieve pain through injection of a local anesthetic into the suspected disc; computed tomography (CT) discography attempts to identify abnormal internal morphology and is used on the disc identified as the source of a patient's complaint.	The sedated patient is able to identify when his or her specific complaint is reproduced thereby identifying the disc causing the pain. Sometimes the procedure is quite painful. It should be used only when an anatomic diagnosis is needed.
Translaminar and Transforaminal Epidurals: A procedure in which epidural steroids are injected into the space outside the thecal sac (which contains the nerve roots) in an attempt to decrease any inflammatory process in that area. An anesthetic is used to block the pain muscle spasm cycle.	A local anesthetic is given. Then a spinal needle is introduced into the epidural space through either an interlaminar space (just lateral to the interspinous ligament) or a selected neuroforamen. An anesthetic and steroid are then injected.	The procedure takes about 30 minutes with 45 minutes recovery. The expected result is relief of pain. Complications are less for the transforaminal than the translaminar. There is more risk of needle-related trauma such as bleeding and intrathecal puncture with translaminar techniques.
Facet Block: A "block" is an anesthetic injection into the facet joint or capsule to determine if it is the source of a patient's complaint.	The patient is given a local anesthetic. A needle is guided to the facet joint or capsule under fluoroscopy. An anesthetic and steroid are injected into the area.	The procedure takes about 30 minutes. The patient should experience relief of pain. Patients who are either older than 65 years; have pain that is not worsened by either coughing, hyperextension, forward flexion, rising from flexion, extension with rotation; or relieved by recumbency have a high success rate with this procedure (92% initial pain relief).
Sympathetic Nerve Block: This test is primarily used to determine damage to the sympathetic nerve chain.	A local skin anesthetic is given, then a needle under fluoroscopic guidance is advanced next to the vertebral body. An anesthetic medication is then injected.	The procedure takes about 30 minutes with another 1 ½ hours for recovery. During the procedure the patient may experience redness and a feeling of warmth in the lower extremity.
Facet Neurotomy (Medial Branch Rhizotomy): This procedure involves denervation of the facet joint nerve supply by a radiofrequency probe. The two small medial branches are heated in an effort to interrupt nerve supply to the facet joint.	The prone patient is given a local anesthetic. Using fluoroscopy, the radiofrequency needle is directed to the base of the selected transverse process. The needle is heated to 80°C for 90 seconds. Two branches are treated.	If the facet is the source of pain, there is a 60% chance of pain relief until the nerves grow back (3 months to 1 ½ years). Risks are several days or weeks of increased pain and destabilization of the facet joint treated.

Some authors question the use of selective nerve blocks, citing little validation in randomized controlled trials.[125]

Thermography

There is much controversy with regard to the use of thermography. In general, thermography can be sensitive; however, it is nonspecific as to the cause of a patient's complaint. There are generally two types: (1) infrared, and (2) liquid crystal thermography. Electronic infrared thermography is more sensitive than liquid crystal; however, the cost and need for standardization of the testing environment make it relatively unavailable. In addition, thermography is between 78% and 94% sensitive for radiculopathy; however, it is nonspecific (20% to 44%).

Electrodiagnostic Studies

Electrodiagnostic studies (EDS) are used when there is a question as to the cause of a patient's low back and leg complaints. EDS consists of the following:

- Electromyography (EMG) is used to differentiate between nerve root causes, myelopathy, and myopathy. EMG does not become positive for three to four weeks following denervation. Positive findings include electrical hypersensitivity reactions such as fibrillation potentials and positive sharp waves.
- Nerve conduction velocity (NCV) is used to differentiate between entrapment neuropathies and radiculopathies; late responses such as the H-reflex are the electrodiagnostic equivalent of a decreased Achilles reflex and are found 90% of the time with S1 dysfunction.
- Sensory-evoked potentials (SEPs) are used to measure the sensory component of a patient's complaint in an attempt to localize the site of the pathologic lesion; dermatomal sensory-evoked potentials (DSEPs) may be useful in the assessment of patients with spinal stenosis.

The Council on Chiropractic Guidelines and Practice Parameters (CCGPP) has published a series of best-practices documents online. The low back chapter is available at www.ccgpp.com. It focuses primarily on management. Many of the conclusions and recommendations are similar to other published summaries.

Clinical guidelines[126] published by the American College of Physicians and the American Pain Society are consistent with current recommendations by similar groups including the National Council on Quality Assurance. The guidelines make seven recommendations, which are summarized as follows:

1. A focused history and examination should be performed to place patients in one of three broad categories: (a) nonspecific low back pain, (b) back pain associated with radiculopathy or spinal stenosis, or (c) back pain due to other specific causes. Also, the history should assess possible psychological risk factors.
2. Avoid routine imaging for patients with nonspecific LBP.
3. Perform diagnostic imaging for severe or progressive neurologic deficits, or when serious underlying conditions are suspected.

4. For patients with persistent LBP or signs of radiculopathy or stenosis, MRI or CT should be ordered only if they are potential candidates for surgery or epidural steroid injection.
5. Provide patients with evidence-based information on LBP with regard to natural history and activity, and provide information about self-care options.
6. Prescribing physicians should consider the use of medications with proven effect in conjunction with back- and self-care information.
7. For patients who do not improve with self-care options, consider the addition of non-pharmacological therapy including manipulation (for both acute and chronic LBP) and a host of other approaches including exercise, massage therapy, yoga, cognitive behavioral therapy, or progressive relaxation (less evidence than for manipulation).

It is interesting that no intervention had Grade A evidence (good quality evidence of substantial effect) for either acute or chronic LBP.

In 2006, the European Guidelines for Low Back Pain were published in the *European Spine Journal*. A summary of recommendations for acute nonspecific low back pain includes:[23]

- Give appropriate information and reassure the patient while being careful not to prescribe bed rest as a treatment.
- Advise patients to stay active and suggest working if possible.
- Pain medication may be necessary starting with NSAIDs, and then muscle relaxants for only short course prescription.
- Refer for spinal manipulation for patients failing to return to normal activities.
- Consider multidisciplinary treatment programs for those with subacute LBP and sick leave for more than four to eight weeks.

A series of articles appeared in a 2008 full issue of the *Spine Journal* devoted to evidence-informed management of chronic low back pain (CLBP). The intention was to bring together experts in various treatment strategy approaches who would summarize the existing literature and conclude with some statements about what is known and how well it is supported. Recommendations for further research were also included. A summary of those evidence-informed treatment conclusions is presented in **Table 6–3**.

Table 6–3 Evidence-Informed Summaries for Various Management Approaches to Chronic Low Back Pain (CLBP)

(Please note that these summaries are based on evidence-based criteria of the existing literature. Having no literature support for or against a given approach does not indicate that it is ineffective.)

Listed alphabetically

Tx Approach	Summary of Conclusions by Expert Panels for Chronic Low Back Pain
Acupuncture[127]	• Some evidence that acupuncture is effective immediately after a series of treatments for pain and functional improvement. • Evidence suggests that acupuncture is no more effective than other treatment methods. • The most consistent evidence suggests that the addition of acupuncture to other therapies improves outcomes. • Moderate evidence that acupuncture may be better than massage, especially if combined with exercise. • Inconclusive evidence for the effectiveness of acupuncture when compared to sham acupuncture.
Adjunctive analgesics[128]	• Evidence supporting the use of adjunctive analgesics is limited. • The panel suggests that it is reasonable to use tricyclic antidepressants (TCA) at low dosage for painful radicular syndromes when acetaminophen and NSAIDs have not helped.
Back school, brief education, fear avoidance[129]	Back School • Conflicting evidence about the effectiveness for back schools in reducing recurrences of LBP compared to usual care or no intervention. • Limited evidence that back schools are less effective than exercise. • Moderate evidence that back schools are not better than waiting, any intervention, placebo, or exercise for reduction of pain. However, there is conflicting evidence for the reduction of disability compared to the same interventions. • Limited evidence that back school is better than usual care or a cognitive behavioral-based back school. • Conflicting evidence that back schools are better than a waiting list, no intervention, or usual care for return to work. Brief Education • Limited evidence that brief education in the clinical setting (back book, pamphlet, etc.) is not more effective than usual care for reduction of pain but was more effective than usual care for return to work. • Conflicting evidence that brief education is more effective than usual care in reducing disability. • Limited evidence brief education is not as effective as yoga, massage, and exercise, but is more effective than a waiting list for pain reduction. • Limited evidence brief education is more effective than massage and no intervention, and less effective than yoga with massage for reduction of disability. • Panel recommended brief education in the clinical setting for return to work but not a back book or Internet discussion as an alternative to other treatments. Fear Avoidance Training • Moderate evidence that fear avoidance training emphasizing exposure to provocative maneuvers is more effective than graded activity for fear avoidance, pain, and disability. • Limited to moderate evidence that rehabilitation incorporating exposure to physical activities labeled "not recommended" is not different from spinal fusion with regard to pain, disability, and return to work. • The panel recommended fear avoidance training in a rehabilitative program as an alternative to spinal fusion and to include exposure as an important element of the training.
Cognitive behavioral training[130]	• Some evidence that cognitive behavioral therapy (CBT) is effective for chronic pain; generally helping with the pain experience, pain behavior and activity, cognitive coping and appraisal, and social functioning. • The recommendation is that the biopsychosocial approach to chronic pain is likely a multitherapy (interdisciplinary) approach that should include CBT.
Epidural steroid injection[131]	• For discogenic pain there are no well-designed studies that assess the efficacy of transforaminal epidural steroid injections (ESI). • Nonspecific ESIs have been demonstrated to have some short-term benefit. It appears that one to three appear effective.

Table 6–3 Evidence-Informed Summaries for Various Management Approaches to Chronic Low Back Pain (CLBP) (continued)

(Please note that these summaries are based on evidence-based criteria of the existing literature. Having no literature support for or against a given approach does not indicate that it is ineffective.)

Listed alphabetically

Tx Approach	Summary of Conclusions by Expert Panels for Chronic Low Back Pain
Extensor exercises[132]	• Lumbar extensor strengthening exercise (LESE), alone or with co-interventions, is more effective than passive modalities in improving pain and disability for CLBP. However, it has no clear benefit over other exercise programs. • The long-term benefits for LESE over other interventions is lost over time. • Hyperextension does not appear to offer additional benefit. • LESE alone or with co-intervention is more effective than stabilization exercise or home exercise in improving cross-sectional area of the paraspinal muscles. • LESE is more effective than no treatment and passive modalities in improving lumbar paraspinal muscle strength and endurance. However, there is no benefit compared to other exercise programs. • High-intensity lumbar strengthening appears to be more effective to low-intensity for improving strength and endurance. • Many methods of performing dynamic LSES. Panel did not recommend floor, stability ball, and free weight exercises. It felt that Roman chairs and benches are viable, although lumbar dynamometer machines appear to be the best option.
Facet injections and radiofrequency neurotomy[133]	• Some evidence that controlled lumbar medial branch blocks are the best diagnostic test for Z joint (facet) involvement. • Limited studies on medial branch neurotomy that indicate the majority of patients have pain relief lasting one year. • Controlled studies have shown that intra-articular injection of steroids is no more effective than placebo.
Functional restoration[134]	Functional restoration is a broad based approach drawing a team of multidisciplinary individuals together for formal quantification of physical deficits to guide an individualized approach. This includes psychosocial and socioeconomic components, multimodal disability management using cognitive behavioral training, and psychopharmacological use (for those in need) complemented by ongoing outcome assessment and communication among all involved. • Panel concludes that there is strong evidence that functional restoration reduces pain and improves function more than less intensive programs or usual care.
Herbs, vitamins, homeopathy[135]	• Strong evidence for 50 mg harpagoside per dose in aqueous extract of *H. procumbens* per day better than placebo. • Moderate evidence that 60 mg harpagoside is equal to 12.5 mg of rofecoxib. • Moderate evidence for 240 mg of salicin (extract of *S. alba*) per day is better than placebo. • Moderate evidence for intramuscular B12 when compared to placebo for pain reduction. • Moderate evidence that there is no difference in pain reduction among Spiroflor SRL, Cremor Capsici Compositus FNA, the capsici oleoresin gel. • Limited evidence for topical *C. frutescens* (Rado-Salil cream or Capsicum plaster), lavender, vitamin C, and manganese in addition to prolotherapy, and for homeopathy equivalent to physiotherapy.
IDET[136]	• Intradiscal electrothermal therapy (IDET) is a minimally invasive technique producing modest pain relief rather than functional improvement. • For patients with less functional impairment, well maintained disc height, and discogenic pain from annular tears or protrusions less than 3–4 mm IDET may be indicated as an alternative without the expectation of returning to demanding manual labor. • Success reported varies widely dependent on the type of study from only 14 (randomized) to 63% (nonrandomized studies).

(continues)

Table 6–3 Evidence-Informed Summaries for Various Management Approaches to Chronic Low Back Pain (CLBP) (continued)

(Please note that these summaries are based on evidence-based criteria of the existing literature. Having no literature support for or against a given approach does not indicate that it is ineffective.)

*Listed alphabetically

Tx Approach	Summary of Conclusions by Expert Panels for Chronic Low Back Pain
Lumbar stabilization exercises (LSE)[137]	• Moderate evidence that LSE are effective in improving pain and function in a heterogeneous group of patients with CLBP. • Strong evidence that LSE is no more effective than less specific, general exercise programs. • Strong evidence that LSEs are no more effective than manual therapy in the same population. • Caveat is that the few studies that qualified were comprised of heterogeneous patients. Suggestion for further research on homogeneous groups to determine any patient-specific effect.
Manipulation/ mobilization[24]	• Moderate evidence that spinal manipulative therapy (SMT) with strengthening exercise is similar in effect to prescription NSAIDs with exercise in both the short and long term. • Moderate evidence that flexion-distraction mobilization is superior to exercise in the short term and superior/similar in the long term. • Moderate evidence that a high-dose SMT regimen is superior to low-dose SMT in the very short term. • There is limited to moderate evidence that SMT is as good or better than chemonucleolysis for disc herniation in the short and long term. • There is limited evidence that mobilization is inferior to back exercise after disc herniation surgery.
Massage[138]	• Strong evidence that massage is effective for non-specific CLBP. • Moderate evidence that massage provides short- and long-term relief of symptoms. • Standard massage has the same effects as traditional Thai massage.
McKenzie method[139]	• The McKenzie method is primarily a system of assessment and classification. • Intervention studies have demonstrated that the McKenzie method produces better short-term outcomes than nonspecific, guideline-based care and equal or marginally better outcomes than stabilization or strengthening exercises for patients with CLBP.
Medicine-assisted manipulation[140]	• Generalizing medicine-assisted manipulation (MAM) is difficult because there are a variety of techniques which include manipulation under anesthesia (MUA), manipulation under joint anesthesia, and manipulation under epidural steroid injection. However, all studies to date have shown positive results regardless of specific technique used. • No recommendation can be made for a specific technique for MAM. • Generally the evidence for MAM is weak and consists mainly of observational studies.
NSAIDs, muscle relaxants, analgesics[141]	• No one drug or medication has been shown to be more effective than another. • No trials were available to compare the effectiveness of antispasmodic drugs to placebo or other treatments. • It is unpredictable which patient will respond to which medication and therefore it is recommended to apply a trial period of three to four days based on patient preference.
Nuclear decompression[142]	• Little evidence at this point in time; however, some indications that about 40% of patients obtain relief. • This procedure is suggested only for patients with disc protrusions less than 4–6 mm, minimal stenosis, and well-maintained disc height.
Opioid analgesics[143]	• Some evidence that opioid analgesics are effective in the short term compared to placebo. • Withdrawal rates are high due to side effects, however, among the remaining group, 1/3 respond well, 1/3 have a fair response, and 1/3 are nonresponders. • Improvement in pain is more substantiated than function. • No evidence of superiority among the opioids; addiction seems rare.
Physical activity, smoking cessation, weight loss[144]	• Moderate evidence that physical activity with general aerobic and strengthening exercise or aquafitness was more effective than nonactive controls for long-term reduction of disability and limited evidence for improvements in worst pain, medication use, work status, and mood. • Moderate evidence that different types of physical activity programs were equally effective. • No evidence yet for the efficacy of smoking cessation or nonoperative weight loss; however, there are few trials available.

Management

Prior to a discussion of the plethora of approaches to low back pain, a popular approach developed and tested by Murphy et al.[145] attempts to connect the examination to the management approach based on a diagnosis-based clinical decision rule (DBCDR). They are careful to point out that the DBCDR is not a clinical prediction rule but is an attempt to identify issues regarding the need for referral and when management is attempted, to consider factors related to the perpetuation of pain and the risk for disability so that all factors that affect patient recovery can be addressed. The sequence and focus of this approach is predicated on determining a cross-section of information including the answers to the following primary questions:

1. Are the symptoms with which the patient is presenting reflective of a visceral disorder or a serious or potentially life-threatening disease? Red-flag indicators would warrant referral.
2. From where is the patient's pain arising? The attempt is to use diagnostic clues to categorize patients into one of the following groups with different management approaches:
   - Centralization dominance—implying disc derangement possibly responsive to a McKenzie approach
   - Segmental pain—suggesting facet-related (subluxation) pain amenable to manipulation
   - Neurodynamic cause—implying a radiculopathy which may respond to manipulation or "neural" techniques
   - Myofascial/trigger point-related—potentially responsive to myofascial treatment approaches
3. What has gone wrong with this person as a whole that would cause the pain experience to develop and persist? The attempt is to determine factors that contribute to chronicity and recurrence including underlying dynamic instability (impaired motor control), central-mediated pain, fear avoidance of activity and catastrophizing behavior, and related, passive coping and depression.

Injections

Injection therapy for LBP takes many forms based on the underlying suspected cause. Trigger point injection, facet injection, and epidural injections are the most common. For radicular pain or for spinal stenosis, epidural injections are frequently recommended prior to surgery. Epidural injections involve anesthetics, steroids, or a combination of the two. Epidural steroid injections (ESI) are classified by type: (1) caudal, (2) interlaminar (also called translaminar), and (3) transforaminal (also known as a selective nerve root block). Caudal and interlaminar are referred to as nonspecific conducted without fluoroscopic guidance (i.e., a blind approach). Transforaminal ESIs are directed through fluoroscopic guidance. Recent studies indicate that the success of ESIs is based partly on the type and the location. A study[151] published in 2013 demonstrated a high response rate for lumbar ESI compared to caudal. Response rates for facet joints and the SI joint were substantially less. Also, a review[152] published in 2012 concluded that although limited for axial pain and pain secondary to surgery, transforaminal ESIs have good evidence for effectiveness for radiculitis secondary to disc herniation and fair evidence for effectiveness with spinal stenosis. Looked at another way, if ESIs are used not as a curative but to either allow other therapy such as manipulation or to prevent surgery, the statistics seem more favorable. A review[153] published in 2006 demonstrated that 71% of patients with a transforaminal ESI avoided surgery even at a five-year follow-up. What is not compared is the percentage of those who did not receive an ESI. Regarding safety, there was an unfortunate contamination event from a single compounding company (unregulated compared to normal pharmaceutical companies) in which 55 deaths occurred due to fungal infection. This isolated event is related to the production of the medication. A review by Epstein[154] in 2013 examined the risks related to adverse events in the literature. The most common were positional headache, adhesive arachnoiditis, allergic reactions, and spinal fluid leaks (which were less with transforaminal injections).

Surgery

Lumbar discectomy is performed over 480,000 times in the United States annually. Hospital costs for complex spine fusions can reach up to $80,000 per patient. The United States has the highest rate of low back surgery and these rates have increased by 55% from 1979 to 1990, with now 21 per 100,000 Medicare beneficiaries having a spine fusion annually.[155]

There are basically two types of spine surgery; decompression and fusion. Both may be utilized together in some procedures. Decompression may occur through discectomy or laminectomy/otomy or a combination of the two. The surgical techniques used are divided into two types: open and microscopic. By combining the two categorizations, different spine surgeries are named. Further differentiation is based on whether the surgery is instrumented or non-instrumented. Instrumented means the addition of screws, hooks, cable, cages, and so on. Noninstrumented implies that stabilization is primarily through bone, which is divided into autograph (also called autologous or autogenous), meaning from the patient or allograph, meaning from a donor.

One of the most common types of fusion surgeries is minimally invasive transforaminal lumbar interbody fusion (TLIF). Minimally invasive TLIF has been shown to be superior to the traditional open procedure in terms of postoperative back pain, total blood loss, need for transfusion, time to ambulation, soft-tissue injury, and functional recovery.

Under fluoroscopy in the anteroposterior and lateral views, a spinal needle is used to locate the level of lesion. Unilateral pedicle screws are placed percutaneously over a guide wire and then a laminectomy and TLIF are performed via a 21-mm nonexpandable tube. The advantage is the minimally invasive approach that preserves the midline muscular and ligamentous structures. Patients are usually released within 24 hours following the surgery, and are able to return to their daily routines and work within two to three weeks. Compared to the traditional four-hour procedure, this surgery takes only 45 to 60 minutes with minimal blood loss. There is also less pain because of the smaller incision

More recently, McMorland et al.[156] studied patients who were randomized to either microdiscectomy or manipulation. Microdiscectomy is a procedure where 1- to 2-cm incisions are made over midline at the level of the herniated disc. Laminotomies are performed as needed to allow visualization. Retraction of nerve roots is then used to allow access to the herniated disc. Both sequestrectomy and intra-annular discectomy are performed. Patients remained in the hospital for one to two days. Sixty percent of patients failing medical management for disc herniation-related sciatica demonstrated some benefit with side-posture manipulation equal to those who underwent microdiscectomy. Patients who failed to benefit from side-posture manipulation received benefit from subsequent surgical management. However, those patients failing to receive benefit from surgery did not benefit from subsequent management with manipulation. Based on this study, there is an implied care pathway that indicates that patients have no risk and possible benefit from manipulation and that those who fail to obtain relief have the option of microdiscectomy.

The older open surgeries require large incisions in the back or abdomen. For anterior approaches, vascular surgeons perform this portion of the surgery often requiring complicated dissection of muscles, nerves, and even organs so that the surgeon can gain access to the affected area. This preliminary process can take hours even before a spine surgeon begins. Patients are at a much higher risk for greater blood loss as well as nerve and muscle injury. Some surgeons still use this approach in select patients.

Obviously, one of the largest concerns about lumbar spine surgery other than cost is adverse events (AE) and complications. A past review[157] of complication rates for lumbar spine surgery included 11 studies with an overall mortality rate of <1%, but a complication rate of 3.7% to 12.8%. An adverse event is defined as any unexpected or undesirable event occurring as a result of spinal surgery, whereas a complication is defined as a disease or disorder that is a consequence of a surgical procedure. In one prospective observational study, this distinction was used and the researchers reported an overall AE rate of 14% and an overall complication rate of 3.2%. In the review by Street et al.[158] published in the *Spine Journal* in 2012, the first prospective approach to studying morbidity and mortality for spine surgery was conducted. There was an overall intraoperative AE rate of 12%. In the previous year, chart review retrospectively identified an intraoperative rate of 9.8% in 918 patients. The researchers also concluded that postoperative events appear to be grossly under-recorded by traditional methods.

The four most common intraoperative AEs were

- Dural tear (42 cases, 4.45%)
- Anesthetic related (32 cases, 3.4%)
- Blood loss, > 2 L (21 cases, 2.2%)
- Hardware malposition requiring revision (18 cases, 1.9%)

The total incidence of intraoperative AEs for the elective group was 14.65% compared with 9.3% for the emergency group (p. 01). The incidence of iatrogenic dural tear in the elective degenerative group was 12%, significantly higher to the incidence in all other groups. The incidence of infection for elective surgery was approximately 3%, similar to a recent previous publication by the Scoliosis Research Society, where they reported on 10,329 patients undergoing surgery for spinal stenosis with an overall complication rate of 7%, a mortality rate of 0.13%, a 3% dural tear rate, and a 2% infection rate.

In a recent publication about the incidence and mortality of thromboembolic events in lumbar spine surgery, we are reminded that when one thinks of spine surgery, it is easy to forget that in addition to local damage, other adverse events such as infection and vascular accidents occur. In this study[159] published in *Spine* in 2013, the researchers studied the incidence of deep vein thrombosis and pulmonary embolism as complications of lumbar spine surgery. They found an incidence for DVT of 2.4 per 1,000 cases for lumbar decompression surgery and an incidence of 4.3 per 1,000 cases for lumbar fusion. For pulmonary embolism the incidence for lumbar decompression was 1 out of 1,000 and 2.5 per 1,000 for lumbar fusion. These patients had higher preoperative pulmonary circulation disorders, coagulopathies, fluid-electrolyte disorders, anemia, and obesity. Also the rate was higher for large teaching hospitals.

A Cochrane review published in 2012 by Jacobs et al.[160] examined the effectiveness of total disc replacement for chronic discogenic low back pain. It was believed that artificial discs could act as low-friction devices allowing more spinal mobility. Articulating surfaces are either metal-on-polyethylene or metal-on-metal. Although such devices allow controlled motion, they do not replicate the elasticity of the normal human intervertebral disc. The researchers concluded that the reviewed studies indicated that compared to total disc replacement and traditional surgery, the effectiveness based on differences in the outcome measures used demonstrated very small advantages and that these differences did not exceed clinical relevance and/or the quality of evidence was low. For these reasons and the potential harm and complications that they suggest may occur years later, they warn the spine surgery community to be prudent about adapting this approach and to use it sparingly on select patients.

Although many studies examine the ability to predict chronicity following an acute episode of LBP, there are few that address prediction of lumbar spine surgery following occupational injury. In a study published in 2012 by Keeney et al.[161] among workers in Washington state with compensation for temporary total disability for occupational back injury, 9.2% underwent lumbar spine surgery within three years. Higher Roland-Morris Disability Questionnaire scores, greater injury severity, and first seeing a surgeon for the injury significantly increased the odds of having spine surgery. Forty-two percent of workers who first saw a surgeon had surgery. Participants younger than 35 years, females, Hispanics, and participants whose first visit for the injury was to a chiropractor had lower odds of surgery; only 1.5% of those who saw a chiropractor first had surgery. No other factors in the employment-related, health behavior, or psychological domains were significant. The odds of surgery were highest for workers with reflex, sensory, or motor abnormalities but odds were also high for workers with symptomatic radiculopathy without such abnormalities.

A quickly advancing field is the use of biologics in spine surgery. Biologics is based on the introduction of autologous or allogeneic stem cells or progenitor cells. Important characteristics of stem cells include the ability to (1) regenerate, and (2) differentiate into a variety of cell types. Generally, stem cells can be categorized several ways. Certainly, one obvious category is adult versus embryogenic. The advantage of embryologic stem cells (ESC) is their ability to differentiate into all three germ layer types of the mesoderm, endoderm, and ectoderm. However, ethical issues and the potential for the development of teratomas likely will restrict their usage in spinal surgery with perhaps the exception of treating spinal cord injury.

A specific type of adult, or somatic, stem cells called mesenchymal stem cells (MSCs) is more likely the group of cells of importance to standard spine surgery due to their limited potential to differentiate. The potentials include differentiation and development of bone, cartilage, muscle, and fat. The source of these cells is primarily from bone marrow and adipose tissue, and they are specifically referred to as mesenchymal progenitor cells (MPCs). Potential uses might include:[162]

- For fusion surgery and disc regenerative therapies based on MPCs' ability to differentiate into bone and disc.
- For stability postsurgically because MPCs secrete multiple bioactive factors such as multiple bone morphogenetic proteins (BMPs), which have a strong osteogenesis potential.
- For the treatment of both myelopathy and radiculopathy due to MPCs' production of immune modulatory factors, anti-inflammatory agents, and anti-fibrotic substances.

Direct culturing of existing spine tissue is already occurring. Cells from the nucleus pulposas (NP) and annulus fibrosis (AF) have been cultured from explanted tissue. A variety of stimulatory agents are used to cause growth; experiments have been conducted to test different bio-scaffolding for growth, including the use of three-dimensional printing devices. Interestingly, even cells from damaged discs retain the potential for activation. Cells cultured with total explanted discs retain more of the functional structure of the real disc. One study[163] in Europe specifically investigated regenerating the disc following microdiscectomy by extracting cells, expanding through culturing and stimulation, and replacing them through injection in a second procedure. The patients experienced a decrease in back pain in this study. The drawback is the need for two procedures. These techniques will likely require many years of testing and perfecting prior to use on humans on a regular basis.

Manipulation

Important screening questions or findings with regard to possible contraindication to manipulation of a specific area include the following:[164]

- use of anticoagulants
- recent back surgery (unstable spine)
- spinal infection
- spinal cancer
- severe osteoporosis
- signs of acute myelopathy or cauda equina syndrome
- acute inflammatory arthritis

In two separate reviews, Bronfort et al.,[165] found moderate evidence that for acute LBP, spinal manipulative therapy/mobilization is effective in the short term. For chronic LBP moderate evidence was shown again in the short term as compared to standard care, and in the long term as compared to physical therapy.

The evidence for manipulation is rather strong for acute LBP without radiation, but little research has been done to determine the effects on patients with "sciatica" or radiating pain into the leg below the knee. Two interesting studies have set the stage for further research based on their positive outcomes. One study by Santilli et al.[166] randomized patients with acute back pain and "sciatica" into either a true chiropractic manipulation group or a sham manipulation group. A total of 102 patients were treated with either true manipulation or sham manipulation for five days per week. Depending on pain relief, a "rapid thrust technique" similar to a diversified or Gonstead-like, side-posture treatment was applied for a maximum of 20 times. Standard outcome measures including visual analog scale, quality of life, use

of medication, and psychosocial findings were checked at 15, 30, 45, and 90 days. Manipulation was judged as more effective based on the percentage of pain-free cases. Interestingly, though, there were no significant differences in quality of life and psychosocial scores.

More recently, several studies indicate both safety and effectiveness for spinal manipulative therapy (SMT) in the management of lumbar radiculopathy. Regarding the conservative management of sciatica with clinical indicators of neurological dysfunction, a study[167] utilizing either the McKenzie approach or sham exercise demonstrated that although 65% of participants had three or four positive nerve root compression signs and would be considered by many medical physicians as surgical candidates, only 3% had symptoms so severe that they were referred to a neurosurgeon. At the end of the treatment period, 89% of patients reported being better or much better and at one-year follow-up, 91% of patients, surpassing the results indicated in the literature for surgical interventions.

In evaluating these studies, it is important that the patient population has an actual radiculopathy and not another cause of radiating leg pain.

As mentioned above in the discussion of surgery, in a study[156] published in 2010, patients who had failed usual medical care for LBP and sciatica were randomized to either microdiscectomy or SMT. At the end of the study, 60% of patients randomized to SMT demonstrated some benefit with side-posture manipulation equal to those who underwent microdiscectomy. Patients who failed to benefit from side-posture manipulation received benefit from subsequent surgical management. Those patients failing to receive benefit from surgery did not benefit from subsequent management with manipulation.

In 2011 a publication[168] in *Spine* compared the management of patients with sciatica through randomization to the McKenzie approach using directional exercise or manipulation. The McKenzie treatment method was "superior" to "manipulation" based on the number of patients who reported success following treatment (71%: McKenzie versus 59%: manipulation; odds ratio 0.58, 95% (CI) 0.36 to 0.91, P=0.018). The researchers concede though that the differences are statistically significant but unlikely to represent any clinically significant difference. There were some differences in response based on whether patients were categorized as centralizers, meaning their pain moved from the leg more toward the back versus peripheralizers who tended to have their pain radiate more into the leg with provoking maneuvers.

Seventy percent of the centralizers had success in the McKenzie group (105/151) whereas 59% of the centralizers had success in the manipulation group (92/156). And 67% of the peripheralizers had success in the McKenzie group (16/24) versus 37% of the peripheralizers who had success in the manipulation group (7/19). At one-year follow-up, of the original patients on sick leave, only 13% of patients in the manipulation group were still on sick leave compared to 21% of patients in the McKenzie group who were still on sick leave. We do not know whether or not the radiation in these patients was radicular.

For studies evaluating the effect of therapy for radiculopathy, it is important that the diagnosis of disc herniation and the level and type of herniation are documented for all participants using MRI. These MRI findings must match the clinical findings and correlate with the same nerve root and disc level. The following study was careful to exclude those that did not meet this inclusion factor.

A prospective study[169] performed in Switzerland, compared patients treated with nerve root injection (NRI) versus high-velocity, low-amplitude (HVLA) adjusting with a push move used for foraminal herniations and a pull move used for paramedian herniations. Improvement in the SMT group was 76.5% (39/51) compared with 62.7% (32/51) of the NRI group. Both treatment groups had significant decreases in their NRS scores at one month (P = 0.0001) with a 60% reduction for the SMT cohort and a 53% reduction for the NRI group. The cost effectiveness measured in both Swiss francs and U.S. dollars demonstrated an advantage for SMT over injection.

In 2014, for the first time in a major guideline recommendation, the North American Spine Society in their evidence-based guidelines for the management of LBP, stated that based on the literature evidence, spinal manipulation is an option for the relief of pain for patients with lumbar radiculopathy.[170]

For CLBP, Haas et al.[171] designed a study to evaluate the dose response of high-velocity, low-amplitude manipulation. Patients were randomized into several groups based on frequency. One group was manipulated one time per week, another group three times per week, and another group five times per week. At one month, the data suggest that there was a substantial linear effect of visits favoring a larger number of visits. More recently, Haas et al.[172] conducted a much larger study that included 400 patients with CLBP. One hundred patients were randomized into four groups

based on frequency, which included either 0, 6, 12, or 18 sessions of SMT delivered as HVLA manipulation. All participants were assigned 18 treatment visits, three per week for six weeks. So the range was from no real spinal manipulation in one group to as many as 18 treatments of SMT in another. The control was a light massage performed on the non-SMT visits. There was little real difference among groups but a modest effect for more treatments, with an optimal balance being 12 visits. It is common practice for chiropractors to recommend "maintenance" treatments for their patients with spinal pain including LBP. A survey by Rupert[173] indicated that approximately 95% of clinicians believe that maintenance treatments reduce the recurrence and exacerbation of symptoms. A preliminary study by Descarreaux et al.[174] evaluated the efficacy of preventive spinal manipulation for patients with CLBP. Both the treatment group and control group were given a high-intensity regimen of 12 visits over a one-month period. There was a one-month "washout period" for both groups. Following that period, the treatment group received maintenance spinal manipulation at three-week intervals for nine months while the other group did not. Although both groups had similar success with the initial high-intensity treatments and pain scores at the follow-up period, only the group with the maintenance spinal manipulations maintained their postintensive treatment disability scores. The control group reverted to their pretreatment levels.

For patients presenting with LBP, several studies suggest that some prediction can be made related to response to manipulation. Although many of these studies are small and are not randomized controlled studies, some common observations occur with most of them. One of these studies by Flynn et al.[175] suggests that if a patient presents with four out of five variables, the success rate approaches 95%. However, patients presenting with three or less of these same variables had a 50% or less chance of recovery. These variables are:

1. Segmental dysfunction/pain with springing palpation over the lumbar facets
2. Acute onset of pain < 16 days
3. No pain distal to the knee
4. Limited hip internal rotation
5. Low fear avoidance belief score

It is important to note that manipulation was performed by physical therapists in this study and therefore extrapolation to a chiropractic setting may not be similar.

Another report by Axen et al.[176] suggested that by the fourth visit the chance for recovery was only 30% if all of the following were present:

- No immediate improvement after first visit
- Pain was not decreased at second visit
- No decrease in disability reported at the second visit
- A reaction, such as local pain or fatigue, lasting more than 24 hours, new radiating pain, or other reactions to the first treatment

In a recent summary, Liebenson,[177] drawing on previous reports of predictability for LBP management, suggested the following approach to types of patients with chronic pain:

- Acute patients at risk of not responding to chiropractic care—Advise that gradually resuming activity, rather than prolonged rest, hastens recovery. Manipulate and mobilize other areas in addition to the low back, including hips or thoracic spine, and prescribe exercises, such as McKenzie or stabilization types, including instruction on how to perform them safely. Approximately 30% of patients may not respond to this approach.[178]
- Subacute patients at risk of not responding to chiropractic care—Assure patients that hurt does not mean harm and that pain is not the consequence of irreversible damage. In addition to the approach for acute patients, adding graded exposure to feared stimuli and following cognitive behavioral principles may be helpful. Linton[179] also suggests an emphasis on applied relaxation and promotion of a healthy lifestyle, including positive coping skills, controlling stress at home and work, good communication skills, assertiveness, and developing a plan for adherence.
- Chronic patients at risk of not responding to chiropractic care—Adding to the above approaches, advise the patient that pain is usually due to a central nervous system sensitization of pain due to lowered pain thresholds and tolerance. Also, consider involvement of a multidisciplinary team for comanagement, including a pain psychologist.

Cautions for the practitioner include:

- Passive treatment can be iatrogenic.
- Reinforcement of avoidance may occur if the focus is on pain relief prior to activation (return to activity).

- Psychosocial factors are an important and often ignored component.
- Job dissatisfaction is a significant predictor as to whether back injury and chronic disabling pain is reported.
- More success occurs with proactive policies that facilitate a return to work prior to total pain resolution.

Researchers in an interesting study comparing the psychological effects of spinal manipulation versus either physical treatment or verbal interventions used a meta-analysis of existing studies to compare psychological outcomes.[180] There appears to be some evidence that spinal manipulation improves psychological outcomes as compared with verbal interventions.

More studies must be performed to determine whether there is a global effect rather than effects that are segment-specific. The broader issues of passive and active care are applicable to any approach chosen by the chiropractor. Algorithms for these areas are given in Chapter 1. Algorithms for LBP screening and mechanical LBP are presented in **Figures 6–15** and **6–16**.

Mechanical Traction

There are a number of approaches to mechanical traction for LBP. The evidence for superiority of one type over another has not yet been demonstrated. A small study[181] published in 2009 identified some potential predictors of the likelihood of improvement using supine mechanical traction. The prediction rule includes the following four variables:

1. Fear Avoidance Belief Questionnaire – Work subscale < 21
2. No neurological deficits
3. > 30 years of age
4. Nonmanual work job status

If all four items were present, there was a LR of 9.4 that supine traction over three sessions would provide at least a 50% improvement in pain. The protocol included supine, intermittent traction applied with the patient's knees and hips flexed 90° and supported. The traction intensity was at 30% to 40% of the patient's body weight. Fifteen minutes of intermittent traction with a 30-second hold and a 10-second relaxation phase was utilized. Out of all study participants, only 20% met the four criteria that predicted success.

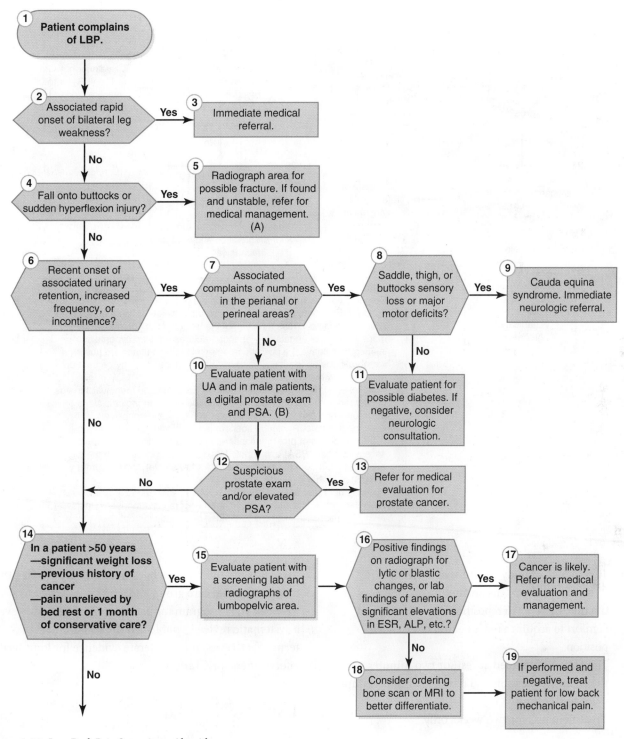

Figure 6–15 Low Back Pain Screening—Algorithm

A small study[182] published in 2007 compared the results of prone lumbar mechanical traction for patients with signs of nerve root compression. This preliminary study identified two predictors that, when both were present, discriminated between those who would and those who would not respond to traction. For those meeting the two variables of peripheralization with repeated lumbar extension and a positive crossed SLR there was a differentiation that identified 84% who responded to traction versus only 49% who recovered without traction. The protocol included the following:

- Static traction was applied in the prone position.
- The patient was positioned to maximize centralization of symptoms.

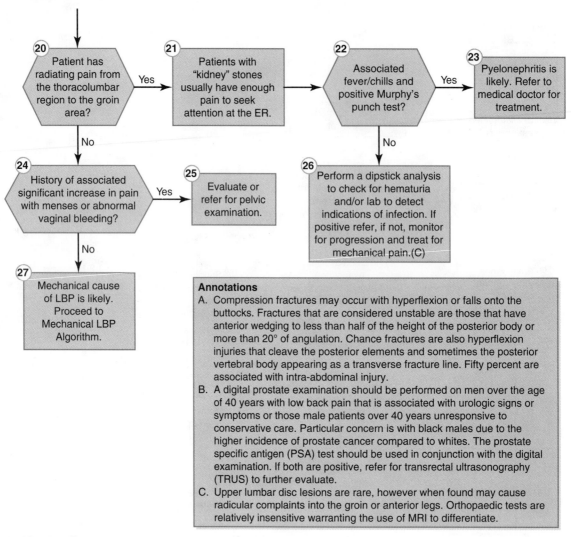

Annotations

A. Compression fractures may occur with hyperflexion or falls onto the buttocks. Fractures that are considered unstable are those that have anterior wedging to less than half of the height of the posterior body or more than 20° of angulation. Chance fractures are also hyperflexion injuries that cleave the posterior elements and sometimes the posterior vertebral body appearing as a transverse fracture line. Fifty percent are associated with intra-abdominal injury.

B. A digital prostate examination should be performed on men over the age of 40 years with low back pain that is associated with urologic signs or symptoms or those male patients over 40 years unresponsive to conservative care. Particular concern is with black males due to the higher incidence of prostate cancer compared to whites. The prostate specific antigen (PSA) test should be used in conjunction with the digital examination. If both are positive, refer for transrectal ultrasonography (TRUS) to further evaluate.

C. Upper lumbar disc lesions are rare, however when found may cause radicular complaints into the groin or anterior legs. Orthopaedic tests are relatively insensitive warranting the use of MRI to differentiate.

Figure 6–15 (Continued)

- 40% to 60% of body weight was utilized.
- If not initially in extension after three minutes of traction, there was a repositioning within patient comfort to acquire a more neutral or extended position.
- The patient remained at rest for two minutes after the treatment session and performed 10 press-ups prior to standing.
- Treatment was for two weeks only.

Even though there were no differences between groups at six weeks, it is notable that there were significant differences in favor of the tractioned group at two weeks, implying that these patients were able to function earlier than those without traction. More studies are needed.

Yoga

The evidence for yoga as an approach to LBP is still minimal. A study[183] published in 2011 demonstrated that there was no difference in back pain and general health between a usual care group and a group assigned to a 12-week yoga program for patients with CLBP. However, a systematic review[184] published in 2013 found short-term effectiveness and moderate evidence for long-term effectiveness for CLBP.

Exercise

Most exercise recommendations involve either prevention or rehabilitation after acute low back pain has subsided or for chronic low back pain patients. In a Cochrane review[185] evaluating the effect of exercise for the prevention of recurrences of LBP, it was found that at two to five years, the recurrence rate was 72% with an average of two recurrences over that time period. The researchers made an attempt to stratify exercises based on type but finding this difficult, divided exercise into a during-treatment type and a post-treatment intervention

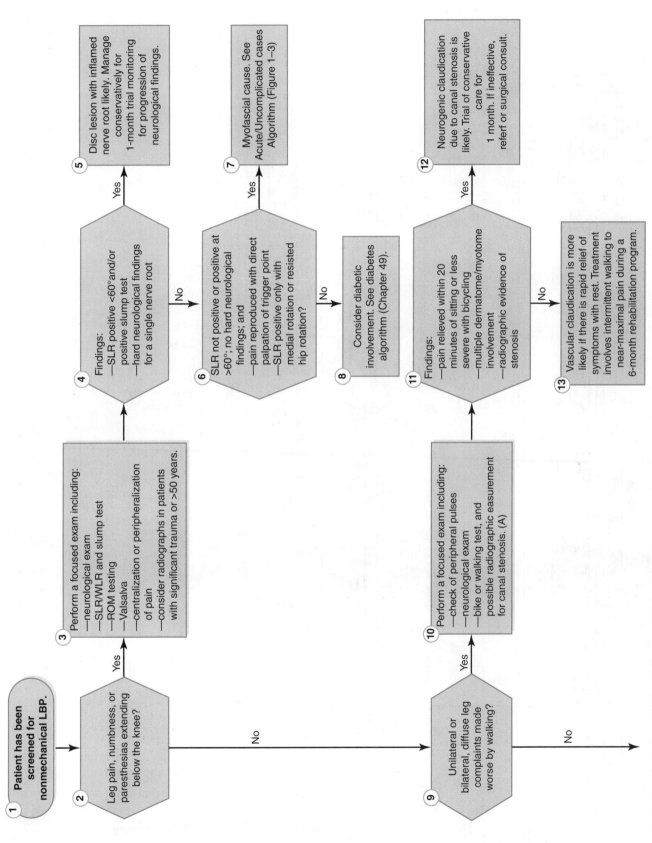

1 Patient has been screened for nonmechanical LBP.

2 Leg pain, numbness, or paresthesias extending below the knee? — Yes →

3 Perform a focused exam including:
—neurological exam
—SLR/WLR and slump test
—ROM testing
—Valsalva
—centralization or peripheralization of pain
—consider radiographs in patients with significant trauma or >50 years.

4 Findings:
—SLR positive <60° and/or positive slump test
—hard neurological findings for a single nerve root
— Yes →

5 Disc lesion with inflamed nerve root likely. Manage conservatively for 1-month trial monitoring for progression of neurological findings.

No ↓

6 SLR not positive or positive at >60°; no hard neurological findings; and
—pain reproduced with direct palpation of trigger point
—SLR positive only with medial rotation or resisted hip rotation?
— Yes →

7 Myofascial cause. See Acute/Uncomplicated cases Algorithm (Figure 1–3)

No ↓

8 Consider diabetic involvement. See diabetes algorithm (Chapter 49).

2 No →

9 Unilateral or bilateral, diffuse leg complaints made worse by walking? — Yes →

10 Perform a focused exam including:
—check of peripheral pulses
—neurological exam
—bike or walking test, and possible radiographic easurement for canal stenosis. (A)

11 Findings:
—pain relieved within 20 minutes of sitting or less severe with bicycling
—multiple dermatome/myotome involvement
—radiographic evidence of stenosis
— Yes →

12 Neurogenic claudication due to canal stenosis is likely. Trial of conservative care for 1 month. If ineffective, referr or surgical consult.

No ↓

13 Vascular claudication is more likely if there is rapid relief of symptoms with rest. Treatment involves intermittent walking to near-maximal pain during a 6-month rehabilitation program.

9 No →

Figure 6–16 Neruological and Mechanical Low Back Pain—Algorithm

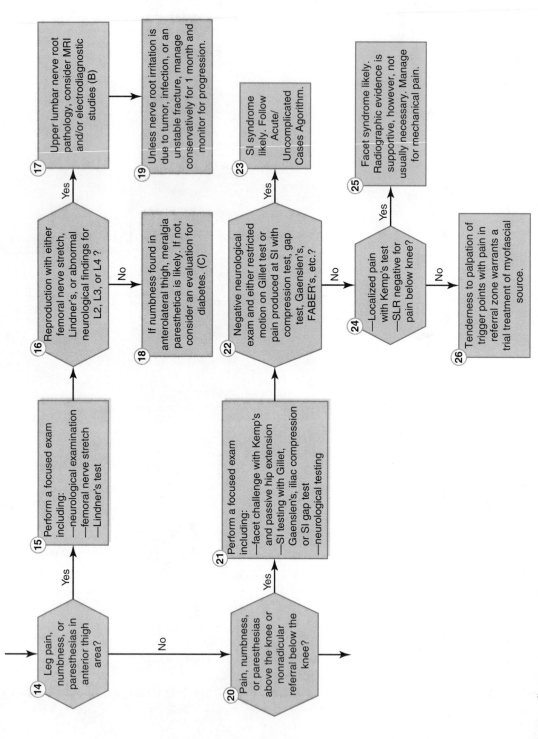

14 Leg pain, numbness, or paresthesias in anterior thigh area?

— Yes →

15 Perform a focused exam including:
— neurological examination
— femoral nerve stretch
— Lindner's test

16 Reproduction with either femoral nerve stretch, Lindner's, or abnormal neurological findings for L2, L3, or L4 ?

— Yes →

17 Upper lumbar nerve root pathology, consider MRI and/or electrodiagnostic studies (B)

→

19 Unless nerve root irritation is due to tumor, infection, or an unstable fracture, manage conservatively for 1 month and monitor for progression.

16 — No →

18 If numbness found in anterolateral thigh, meralgia paresthetica is likely. If not, consider an evaluation for diabetes. (C)

14 — No →

20 Pain, numbness, or paresthesias above the knee or nonradicular referral below the knee?

— Yes →

21 Perform a focused exam including:
— facet challenge with Kemp's and passive hip extension
— SI testing with Gillet, Gaenslen's, iliac compression or SI gap test
— neurological testing

22 Negative neurological exam and either restricted motion on Gillet test or pain produced at SI with compression test, gap test, Gaenslen's, FABER's, etc.?

— Yes →

23 SI syndrome likely. Follow Acute/ Uncomplicated Cases Agorithm.

22 — No →

24 — Localized pain with Kemp's test
— SLR negative for pain below knee?

— Yes →

25 Facet syndrome likely. Radiographic evidence is supportive, however, not usually necessary. Manage for mechanical pain.

24 — No →

26 Tenderness to palpation of trigger points with pain in referral zone warrants a trial treatment of myofascial source.

Figure 6–16 (Continued)

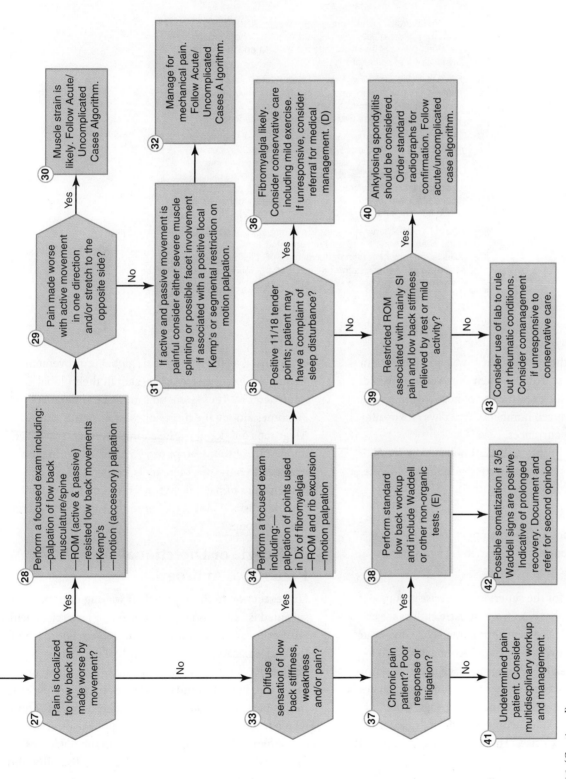

Figure 6–16 (Continued)

Annotations

A. Central canal stenosis may be estimated on a lateral lumbar radiograph using either Beuler's or Eisenstein's measurements. A normal canal is 15 mm; 12 mm is considered relative stenosis; 10 mm or less is considered absolute.

B. Upper lumbar disc lesions are rare, however, when they do occur, they often affect more than upper lumbar nerve roots. Therefore, the Achilles reflex may be affected and the patient may have some posterior leg pain.

C. Diabetes may cause distal sensory disturbances or cause unilateral peripheral nerve palsies such as in amyotrophy. With diabetic amyotrophy, involvement of the femoral nerve is most common with weakness and atrophy of the quadriceps.

D. Fibromyalgia is a more generalized, symmetric distribution of myofascitis. The American College of Rheumatology has set criteria for the diagnosis: pain in 11 of 18 tender sites in a patient with pain for at least 3 months. These bilateral points include suboccipital, lower cervical spine, trapezius, supraspinatus, second rib, lateral epicondyle, gluteals, greater trochanter, and medial fat pad of the knee.

E. Waddell's non-organic signs include generalized or non-anatomic tenderness, positive responses to simulated orthopaedic testing (axial loading, trunk rotation), distracted SLR (flip test), regional weakness and sensory abnormalities that are nonmyotomal and nondermatomal, and overreaction to testing.

Figure 6–16 (Continued)

type. Based on their review, there was no difference in the number of recurrences when exercise was given during treatment. However, the use of post-treatment exercises led to a reduced number of sick days and greater time between occurrences.

In a study by Bronfort et al.[186] published in *The Spine Journal*, patients with LBP were randomized into one of the following groups:

1. High-dose, supervised, low-tech trunk exercise
2. Spinal manipulative therapy
3. A short course of home exercise and self-care advice

The specifics for the supervised exercise group included an emphasis on trunk muscle endurance and trunk stability. There were approximately 20 one-hour sessions (about two per week) which included two to three sets of 15–20 repetitions for each exercise. Also included was a five-minute warm-up and six stretches including lumbar, gluteals, and hamstrings. Core strengthening included trunk extensions, leg extensions, and abdominal exercises. High-velocity, low-amplitude manipulation was performed on those patients in the spinal manipulative therapy group.

About 50% of patients in all groups experienced a 50% reduction in pain. About 60% of patients on average experienced a 50% gain in their global improvement. About 50% experienced a 75% gain in their global improvement. There were no significant differences in outcomes among the three approaches in this study. All groups did demonstrate an improvement; however, improvement to the point of a 75% reduction in pain was seen in only 30% of patients, on average, for all three groups of patients in the long term. Consistently, patient satisfaction was higher in the supervised exercise therapy group.

McKenzie or Directional Preference Approach

One exception to the approach of waiting until pain has subsided is "directional preference" (DP) exercises, which are a primary diagnostic and management approach of the McKenzie technique. A study by Long et al.[187] was designed as a randomized controlled study involving 312 acute, subacute, and chronic low back pain patients. In this particular study 74% of patients had a DP. Those who performed the DP versus the opposite direction of DP had immediate improvement in the outcomes measured, which included pain intensity, disability, and medication use, among others. DP is a particular position or repeated end-range movement that either centralizes a patient's radiating pain or eliminates or decreases lumbar spine pain. These motions include side-gliding/rotation or repeated end-range lumbar flexion or extension. The classic approach used by many practitioners is patient-performed prone-extension to determine if radiating pain centralizes to the low back or, if not, attempting side-shifting of the pelvis and repeating the position to determine effectiveness. The interrater reliability for identifying DP has been reported as high (kappa values between 0.79 and 1.00).

In a comparative study[188] published in 2012, patients with sciatica and some with clinical signs of radiculopathy were randomized to either a directional-exercise approach (i.e., McKenzie technique) or sham exercise. Participants in this study had, on average, severe pain with radicular findings. Over 50% had motor deficits or asymmetrical DTRs and 80% had sensory deficits. Sixty-five percent of them had three or four positive nerve root compression signs and 30% had two positive signs. Therefore, many medical physicians would classify most patients in this study as surgical candidates. A clinically significant change was set at a threshold of 30% change in the baseline Roland-Morris Disability Questionnaire and a 2-point decrease in a 10-point numerical pain score. At the end of the two-month treatment period, 89% of participants reported feeling better or much better and at a one-year follow-up, 91% of participants reported feeling better or much better. At the end of the treatment period, 74% of the symptom-guided group was back to work and 60% in the sham-exercise group had returned to work. There were no significant differences between groups for pain or RMDQ scores; however, with the exception of DTRs, there was a greater improvement in both motor deficits and sensory deficits after treatment and at one-year follow-up in the Symptom-Guided Exercise group that was statistically significant. In general, neurological findings improved significantly more in the symptom-guided exercise group versus the sham exercise group. The conclusion that is drawn for the participants in this study is that an active treatment approach results in significant improvement over eight weeks and these changes were sustained and improved over a one-year period for patients with acute, subacute, or chronic radicular pain.

A similar approach to determining a position of relief is proposed by Mulligan.[189] This dynamic approach to positionally based relief is based on assisting the vertebrae or sacrum into a position of accessory movement that may be blocked, and repeating a painful movement to determine if the pain is reduced or eliminated.

For example, if a patient has pain on forward flexion, the examiner contacts below the spinous process of a suspected segment and/or the articular pillar unilaterally. With pressure in an anterior superior direction, the patient is asked to flex forward to determine if decrease or relief of pain has occurred. Other positional stresses can be applied to the spinous processes pushing right or left. For the sacrum, pushing downward may relieve pain on flexion. The findings may help determine the spinal level to be adjusted.

Passive care involves procedures that are performed on the patient with the patient providing no more than cooperation. These include physical therapy modalities, passive ROM, massage/trigger point massage, mobilization, and manipulation. Criteria for passive care include a history of recent trauma, an acute or inflammatory condition, or dependency behavior. The primary goal is to control inflammation and pain. The frequency of manual therapy visits during the first 10 to 14 days may range from three to five visits per week dependent on the severity of the pain and disability. The patient should be reevaluated to determine whether therapy is effective. If not effective, a second two-week trial using a different treatment approach is warranted. If this is not successful, further evaluation with special imaging or comanagement with a medical doctor is recommended. Use of the New Zealand screening tool for psychosocial yellow flag indicators may help direct management for those at high risk for chronic pain and disability. Generally, if the patient has a preconsultation duration of symptoms greater than eight days or has severe pain, more than four previous episodes, or preexisting structural or pathologic conditions, the anticipated recovery time is often doubled.[190]

There is still and will continue to be some debate as to the appropriateness of side-posture manipulation in the treatment of disc herniations. The review of the literature by Cassidy et al.[191] supports the cautious application of this form of treatment. However, Slosberg's[49] review of the same literature points out some possible factors that may warrant a more cautious approach. Both reviews agree that low-grade mobilization attempts to determine the patient's response are a good screening procedure prior to the application of a thrust. In other words, if mild mobilization is applied at the involved segment, an increase in pain or reproduction of leg pain may be a caution against side-posture manipulation at that time.

Trigger point injection is advocated by some as a conservative alternative to surgery. Results indicate possible benefits for patients with chronic LBP.[192] A relatively new approach to chronic LBP is the use of connective tissue proliferants using injections of dextrose-glycerin-phenol and other substances (prolotherapy). Currently the literature is limited with regard to the effectiveness of this approach. The literature that does exist is mixed regarding prolotherapy's long-term efficacy.[193,194]

Medication

Through a systematic review of randomized, double-blind controlled trials, the Cochrane Collaboration Back Review Group evaluated the effectiveness of NSAIDs in the management of LBP.[195] The researchers also compared medications to determine whether one had demonstrable superior effectiveness. In a review of 51 studies, the group found that NSAIDs are effective for short-term symptomatic relief, but that no specific type of NSAID was clearly more effective. The group also stated that there was insufficient evidence to support the use of NSAIDs for chronic LBP.

Acupuncture

A systematic review[197] published in 2013 concluded that real acupuncture was slightly better than sham acupuncture for the treatment of acute LBP. The review of 11 randomized trials also indicated that acupuncture was as effective as medication for acute LBP. Another study[198] published in 2013 comparing acupuncture and sham acupuncture in the management of chronic LBP demonstrated that using the Oswestry Disability Index, the Beck Depression Inventory, and Short Form-36 scores, both groups improved without group difference. And yet another systematic review[199] published in 2013 evaluating the effectiveness of acupuncture in the management of nonspecific, chronic LBP concluded that acupuncture produced a clinically meaningful reduction in self-reported pain and improved function when compared to sham acupuncture or no treatment immediately post-intervention. It appeared that there was benefit to adding acupuncture to usual medical care but no significant differences between usual medical care and acupuncture alone.

Active Care and Prevention

Active care involves the patient in determining goals and objectives. Exercises and stretches, modification of diet or other lifestyle changes, and modification of work

or recreational environment or performance are among the targeted areas. Exercise takes into account the fitness level of the patient, pain-free ROM, strength, facilities, and motivation. In general, mild isometrics can be performed within pain-free ranges in an attempt to facilitate muscle activity and prevent atrophy. These are followed by various strategies involving isotonic exercises. The primary focus with the low back is strengthening abdominals and stretching the paraspinals. Information gained from a functional evaluation as discussed above can then lead to a more sophisticated approach at strengthening weak areas and stretching shortened areas. Although it is suggested that exercise is appropriate and helpful for subacute and chronic low back pain, the type of exercise that produces the best results has not surfaced in the literature.[187,200] Examples include core stabilization approaches,[112,113] Pilates,[201] and expensive equipment approaches such as MedEx. It would appear that results may be dependent on the patients and their individual needs for function. Following a strengthening phase, endurance and functional movement patterns are emphasized. Coupled with this approach is an attempt at proprioceptive stimulation through the use of balance exercises. For the low back, giant balance (Swiss) ball exercise protocols have been developed. A significant effect for exercise and acute low back pain compared to natural history has not been demonstrated.[202] The beneficial effects of exercise for chronic low back pain patients have been demonstrated.[203] A recent study[204] indicated that the success of three different active therapies for chronic low back pain did not differ; however, the cost of application did differ significantly. One of these active therapies was low-impact aerobics, which is associated with a very low cost when compared with muscle training devices or active physiotherapy.

Proper lifting is essential to avoid injury or reinjury. The primary focus is to maintain a slight lordosis when lifting. When possible, the patient should be instructed to lift lower objects by bending the knees first and lifting from the legs. To reduce the effect of increasing the extensor movement, the load should be kept as close to the body as possible. Twisting should be avoided while lifting. The spine is most vulnerable to lifting injury after holding a prolonged flexed position or after prolonged recumbency (in the morning). Finally, all lifting should be accompanied by co-contraction of the back and abdominal muscles. One controlled trial[205] failed to demonstrate any long-term benefit for an educational program designed to prevent work-associated low back injury.

Although it may seem counterintuitive, a systematic review by Martimo et al.[206] has concluded that there is no evidence to support the use of advice or training in working techniques with or without lifting equipment to prevent back pain and resulting disability. Additionally, in a recent study by Martimo et al.,[207] strong evidence was found that manual material handling advice or lifting assistant devices do not prevent low back injury.

The seated position causes significantly higher disc pressure than standing. When seated, the chair should be stable with a seat–backrest angle of 95° to 105°.[208] A lumbar support may help maintain a slight lordosis. A slightly forward-sloped seat may also be helpful. Too low a seat shifts more weight onto the ischial tuberosities. Proper desk height is considered about 27–30 cm higher than the seat, allowing the arms to rest with the elbows bent 90° with the hand relaxed on the desk surface.[209]

An active lifestyle provides many health benefits that are primarily regarded as cardiovascular and musculoskeletal, yet a study[210] published in 2007 indicates that seniors aged 70 years to 100 years who exercised vigorously were rewarded with a protective effect against LBP. Increasing levels of strenuous activity translated to an increasing magnitude of protection against LBP. Although no specific exercise or program could be determined from this study, intensity and frequency were the determinants of success.

A 2008 Cochrane review by Engers et al.[211] evaluated the literature for the effectiveness of individual patient education for LBP. This extensive review led the authors to conclude that there is strong evidence that an individual 2.5-hour oral educational session is more effective for short- and long-term return to work as compared to no intervention at all. Also, less educational time was not effective. This approach appears to be effective for acute and subacute LBP in improving long-term pain, as well as global improvement when compared to noneducational interventions. No specific type of individual education seemed to stand out as being more effective.

A Cochrane review[212] published in 2007 evaluated the effectiveness of herbal medicine for LBP. Three herbs were represented in the literature as having an effect greater than placebo, and in some cases equal to drug therapy. These were:

1. *H. procumbens* (Devil's Claw)—standardized daily dosage of 100 mg harpagoside.
2. *S. alba* (White Willow)—extract of *S. alba* at a standardized dosage of 120 mg of Salix per day.
3. Topical *C. frutescens* (Cayenne)—plaster application.

Selected Disorders of the Low Back

Disc Lesion with Radiculopathy

Classic Presentation

The patient complains of low back and leg pain below the knee, often of sudden onset from a bending and/or twisting maneuver. There is often a past history of several bouts of LBP that resolved.

Cause

Although in the past it was believed that all leg pain that was radicular was due to compression of a nerve root by a herniated nucleus pulposus, current thinking is that the nerve root is inflamed, but not always compressed.[213] Currently, it is theorized that herniated disc material causes the release of irritating substances or initiates an autoimmune inflammatory reaction. The disc, the corresponding inflamed nerve root, or compression of the nerve root by the disc may be the source of pain. When there is leg pain without objective neurologic evidence, the pain is often referred. When the nerve root is compressed, frank neurologic signs usually become evident. Only about 1% of LBP patients have frank neurologic findings.

Evaluation

Given that 98% of all disc lesions are at L4-L5 or L5-S1, the neurologic examination is focused to these areas. Although there are conflicting findings in systematic reviews regarding the value of the orthopaedic and neurologic evaluation for lumbar radiculopathy, the following might be considered a reasonable approach based on the literature. Use the SLR and the slump test as sensitive tests and the crossed-SLR as a more specific test. Combinations of orthopaedic findings with neurological testing may be helpful. An L5-S1 disc rupture is 86% probable if all three S1 signs are found: (1) pain projection into the S1 area, (2) a pathologic Achilles reflex, and (3) a sensory defect in the S1 dermatome.[69] Localization to the L4-L5 disc is 87% probable with all three L5 signs: (1) extensor hallucis (EH) weakness, (2) pain projection into the L5 area, and (3) a sensory defect in the L5 dermatome. It is important to note though that the patient's report of pain is *nondermatomal* in 64.1% of cases of lumbar radiculopathy according to the Murphy et al. study.[214] Also important to note is that in subjects with electrodiagnostic evidence of radiculopathy, 31% will have no weakness on examination and 33%–45% will have no sensory abnormalities.[215] And, although 64%–75% will have weakness on examination, only 15%–34% will complain of weakness.

Confirmation of nerve root involvement may be physiologic with electrodiagnostic studies or anatomic with MRI. These studies are rarely used during the first four weeks of a complaint unless severe, unremitting pain or progressive neurologic signs are present.

Management

Given the nucleus pulposus is avascular, when it is exposed to the body's normal defense mechanisms it is perceived as "foreign" and an immunological response is set in play to eliminate the disc material. As a result, it is likely in most cases of extrusion that many are "reabsorbed" over several months leading to a natural history of resolution.[216] This reabsorption process requires matrix metalloproteinases (MMPs). Previously these were called collagenases, gelatinase, stromelysin, and elastase. Now these are termed MMP-1, MMP-2, MMP-3, and MMP-12 respectively. This process is terminated by tissue inhibitors of metalloproteinases (TIMPs). MMP/TIMP balance is essential for resolution.

There is some debate as to whether side-posture adjusting should be used in the treatment of disc herniations.[49] The primary concern is the rotary component. If the patient is adjusted in a slightly extended side-lying position, the facets will more likely provide protection. If the rotary component is minimized and the patient is pretested with mild mobilization at the segment to determine aggravation of the leg complaint, cautious side-posture adjusting is a possible alternative.[190] In fact, in 2014, the North American Spine Society stated that manipulation was an option for patients with lumbar radiculopathy. Other studies listed above in the Management section of this chapter detail the evidence for which these conclusions were based. Manipulation under anesthesia is gaining support as an extension of the standard clinical approach in-office. Guidelines released in 2014 help advise the practitioner in patient selection. Practitioners also opt for "softer" approaches that involve no rotation, such as flexion-distraction, blocking, and activator adjusting.

In the event that nonsurgical management is ineffective, there are some middle-of-the-road medical approaches that involve either medication or injections. For example, many chiropractors refer their nonresponsive patients for a Medrol Dosepak prescription. A Medrol Dosepak is a medication card with twenty-one 4 mg pills. The medication is methylprednisolone (similar to prednisone). The patient starts with six pills (24 mg) and takes one less pill each day until finished. The pills are taken orally with a full glass of water before breakfast, after lunch, and after dinner.

Epidural injections are another approach. See the earlier discussion of epidural injections for the literature support and recommendations regarding this approach.

Surgery is rarely needed; however, when suggested, a number of procedures are used. **Table 6–4** summarizes the most common approaches. A new technique is currently being researched that attempts to heat and "shrink" the disc in patients who have discogenic pain.[217] This technique is called *intradiscal electrothermal annuloplasty* (IEA) and *intradiscal electrothermal therapy* (IDET). Using a radiofrequency probe, annular tissue is heated to 85°C for a mean duration of 14 minutes. The preliminary results are promising; however, further studies are needed. Data do not demonstrate a superior outcome for restored neurologic function for operative intervention compared to nonoperative over time. Yet, some authors still suggest that if there is a motor deficit after six months, operative intervention should be considered.[218] It is important to remember that with appropriate triage, the percentage of patients meeting the indications for surgical intervention is only between 2% and 4%.[219] A recent report from the Maine Lumbar Spine Study[220] presented data that suggested the five-year outcome for patients with sciatica secondary to lumbar disc herniation treated surgically was better for a larger percentage (70%) compared to those managed nonsurgically (56%). The researchers also reported that the patients treated surgically more commonly received disability compensation, and the relative benefit of surgery decreased over the five-year period. Macro and microdiscectomy have a reported success rate of 80% to 96%.[130] Comparisons between the outcomes of operative versus nonoperative medical management for lumbar disc herniation are difficult. Researchers[222,223] have attempted to determine long-term results but due to large numbers of crossover patients and the intention-to-treat analysis, conclusions were not possible. Generally speaking, both groups improve. However, there may be some slight benefit to surgical treatment. This was emphasized in a study by Mariconda et al.[224] who followed up on patients with an average of 27.8 post-surgery (discectomy) for their LBP and compared them to those who had not had surgery. There was a high satisfaction rate for those with surgery and a slight difference regarding pain, favoring those who had surgery over those who had not. The question is, if there is only a small difference, is the risk and cost of surgery worth it? The answer to this question will likely always depend to some extent on patient context and preference.

A new approach to the management of discogenic pain is being tested. This involves the use of an artificial lumbar disc. A two-year, follow-up, randomized trial[225] indicates good results for those that have failed other approaches. The concern, as was the case with early knee and hip replacements, is migration of the device. This approach may be an alternative for younger patients with less degeneration and is not a good option for those with considerable degeneration and poor bone quality. At this time, if surgery is considered, most surgeons would still recommend fusion for the majority of cases.

Table 6–4 Selected Surgical Procedures for Disc Lesions

Procedure	Comments
Intradiscal electrothermal therapy (IDET) or intradiscal electrothermal annuloplasty (IEA)	Using normal discographic technique, a catheter is inserted anteriorly into either the annulus or nucleus via a 17-gauge introducer. The active tip of this radiofrequency probe generates electrothermal heat starting at 65°C increasing in a stepwise process to 85°C for about 14 minutes. The intention is to shrink discal material and relieve discogenic pain.
Percutaneous/arthroscopic mechanical discectomy	A discoscope is used in either a biportal or single portal approach. Fluoroscopic monitoring is essential. On patients meeting selected criteria, the success rate is in the 90th percentile if those with increased mobility and reduced medication are included. However, only 66% had returned to work.
Percutaneous laser discectomy	Laser ablation for disc removal is a questionable technique due to the high cost of laser equipment and the potential for inadvertently injuring adjacent tissues such as the vertebral end-plate or spinal nerve, leading to chronic low back pain.
Percutaneous suction discectomy	Also called automated percutaneous lumbar discectomy, the nucleus pulposus is removed with a rotary cutting device attached to an aspiration probe. Studies have not shown consistent long-term results, and it is less cost-effective than microdiscectomy.
Open limited discectomy	A limited laminotomy with disc excision (also called microdiscectomy) is considered the treatment of choice by many surgeons.
Anterior discectomy and fusion	Anterior surgery is considered unnecessary given the less invasive limited laminotomy and fragment excision techniques available.

Fact Syndrome
Classic Presentation

The patient often will complain of well-localized LBP with some hip/buttock or leg pain above the knee. The onset is often sudden after a simple misjudged movement or arising from a flexed position.

Cause

The facet and its capsule may be the source of pain. Each facet receives innervation from two spinal levels, specifically from the medial branch of the posterior primary rami. Synovial folds (meniscoids) may become entrapped or pinched and cause pain. The synovium and capsule have specific substance P-sensitive nerves in addition to small-diameter nociceptors.[226] Another process that may predispose to facet-mediated pain is degeneration, seen more often in middle-aged and older adults.

Evaluation

Although there is often difficulty in distinguishing facet from disc/nerve root irritation, there is usually a cluster of findings that help support the differentiation. For facet syndrome, these include absence of neurologic deficits, absence of nerve root tension signs/tests, pain that is rather localized with Kemp's maneuver (extension and rotation; Figure 6–5), and when reproduced with an SLR does not extend below the knee. Radiographic evidence may include signs of facet imbrication using the lumbar or lumbosacral disc angle, or Hadley's S curve. The variability of normal findings in asymptomatic patients makes the use of these markings questionable. In general, any disc angle greater than 15° is strong evidence of facet imbrication.

Management

In a recent study[227] researchers measured the anterior to posterior position of the lumbar zygapophyseal joints using MRI scans taken before and after side-posture adjusting and before and after side-posture positioning. Spinal adjusting was demonstrated to produce increased gapping of the Z joints. Interestingly, side-posture positioning also produced some gapping, although less than the adjustment.

Facet syndrome appears to be particularly responsive to adjustment (manipulation). The mechanism is still not clear; however, two major proposals are that either the adjustment frees an entrapped meniscoid tab or large-fiber input causes reflex changes, reducing muscle spasm and reflex-mediated pain.

Medical approaches such as radiofrequency facet denervation and facet injections are often advocated. Facet denervation shows some promise for selected chronic low back pain sufferers.[228] Facet injection has mixed support in the literature.[229]

Canal Stenosis
Classic Presentation

Patients often are aged 50 years or older. They complain of back and leg pain. The pain can be unilateral and bilateral and often is diffuse. Patients may complain of the onset of leg complaints with walking (claudication) and relief after resting 15 to 20 minutes or by maintaining a flexed posture.

Cause

It is estimated that approximately 13% to 14% of patients with LBP seeking specialty physician consultation and 3% to 4% of those seeking general practitioner consultation have lumbar spinal stenosis.[230,231]

Stenosis may be central or lateral, caused by bony or soft tissue encroachment, and congenital or acquired. As a result, the signs and symptoms vary widely. For leg complaints to occur, it is usually true that there are multiple levels of stenosis. Congenitally, a trefoil shape of the spinal canal leads to central canal and lateral stenosis. Pedicogenic stenosis is due to anatomically short pedicles. Acquired stenosis is due to bony outgrowths from the facets, laminae, or pedicles, degenerative spondylolisthesis, or hypertrophied and/or calcified ligamentum flavum. Postoperative stenosis may also be a consequence of decompressive surgeries (e.g., laminectomies).

Evaluation

Neurologic deficits may be apparent, yet cross dermatomal and other nerve root boundaries. In an older patient with multilevel findings, stenosis should be considered. Often used is the bicycle or walking test to differentiate between neurogenic and vascular claudication. Patients with neurogenic claudication often find it possible to bicycle or walk farther when flexed. This theoretically opens up the canal and intervertebral foramina, taking pressure off the neural structures. One study[232] indicated that these tests may not be able to differentiate clearly between the two types of claudication. Although reasonably insensitive (0.60), improvement with flexion points strongly to canal stenosis. Central canal stenosis may be estimated on a lateral lumbar film using either the Eisenstein or Beuler method. A normal canal is 15 mm or greater; 12 mm is considered relative stenosis; 10 mm is considered absolute. CT scan is often used when bony canal stenosis is suspected. MRI is more valuable with soft tissue encroachment. Electrodiagnostic studies are often used when multiple nerve root levels appear to be affected. EMG is less valuable than dermatomal sensory-evoked potentials (DSEPs).[233]

Management

Treatment is based on the underlying type and cause of the stenosis. The natural history seems to suggest that many patients with stenosis may improve or remain stable (90%) without treatment.[234] If manipulative therapy is tried, caution should be used because of the possibility of increasing compression, causing an exacerbation or worsening of symptoms. The response to manipulative treatment is less predictable than for other causes of LBP. The positive response rate is approximately 36% according to a study by Cassidy et al.[17] If the patient has severe neurologic deficit or fails to respond to conservative management, surgical consultation is warranted for possible decompression of the area or areas. In one study,[235] a significant number of patients with spinal stenosis avoided surgery with aggressive therapies including exercise, analgesics, and epidural steroid injections. In a review comparing the four-year outcomes for surgical and nonsurgical management of lumbar spinal stenosis, it appears that both groups improve; however, 70% of the surgically treated group were free of their leg or back pain whereas only 52% of the nonsurgically managed group reported relief.[236] Those who went to surgery were at baseline reporting more severe symptoms and worse functional status. Therefore, it appears that those patients with the worst symptoms may be better candidates. It has been reported that patients who have surgery for lumbar stenosis have very good initial results but these are lost over one to two years so that they are comparable to conservative management. A study by Malmivaara et al.[237] indicates that although the effects decrease, disability, leg pain, and back pain are still more improved after two years compared with conservative management. A study by Weinstein et al.[238] published in 2008 concludes that there is significantly more improvement in all primary outcomes for those treated surgically compared to those treated non-surgically. For those who have radiographic evidence of stenosis yet do not have severe enough signs and symptoms to warrant surgical intervention, the evidence is unclear. One study[239] indicated that depression, cardiovascular comorbidity, dysfunction with walking (i.e., leg pain with walking), and scoliosis predicted poorer subjective outcome with surgery. It did appear that the more severe the stenosis, the more likely there would be a positive subjective outcome with surgery. There are some encouraging results from a randomized control study comparing two physical therapy approaches for lumbar spinal stenosis.[240] The data indicate that a six-week program including manual therapy, exercise, and bodyweight-supported treadmill walking resulted in recovery for 79% of patients.

Spondylolisthesis

Classic Presentation

There are several types of spondylolisthesis; however, the most common are isthmic, occurring in the young, and degenerative, occurring in the older patient. Patients may be asymptomatic or have LBP made worse with extension. In older patients, the degenerative spondylolisthesis may cause signs of stenosis.

Cause

Although congenital types and destructive (e.g., tuberculosis or cancer) types are possible, they are rare. The isthmic type is due to either a stress fracture of the pars interarticularis (spondylolysis) or an elongated pars; 90% of spondylotic spondylolisthesis occurs at L5.[241] The spondylolysis type is more likely to become symptomatic in children more than 5 years old. Although slippage is more common in girls, the isthmic type is one half as common as it is in boys. Sports such as gymnastics, which require repetitive hyperextension, are more likely to cause problems. There is a high incidence in Alaskan Eskimos. (Also see Chapter 53.) Degenerative spondylolisthesis was found to be associated with increased BMI, age, and angle of lordosis in women but not in men.[242]

Evaluation

Spondylolisthesis is primarily a radiographic diagnosis seen best on a lateral film. However, some patients may have increased back or leg pain with a one-legged balance test. The patient is asked to balance on one leg and hyperextend at the lumbar region. Palpation may reveal a prominent spinous process at the involved level with a steep sacral base angle. The radiographic grading of spondylolisthesis is based on dividing the sacrum (if L5) or the vertebrae below (if above L5) into fourths. Each slip of one fourth the length of the anterior to posterior body is considered a grade. Therefore, slippage of three fourths the AP length would be classified as a grade 3. The sacral table angle (STA) is one of several radiographic measures taken from a lateral radiograph to determine the biomechanical status of the sacrum and spine.[243] The STA is the angle in the sagittal plane subtended by a line on the anterior aspect of the superior end-plate of the sacrum to the posterior edge, and a line that starts from that point drawn down the posterior midline to the caudal end-plate of the sacrum. There is a strong association between a lower STA and the occurrence of pars defects that appears to be causative.

Developmental spondylolisthesis is in part due to the pelvic shape and support, which is radiographically measured by the pelvic incidence angle. A greater angle is found in those who develop a listhesis. Individuals also have a greater pelvic slope, sacral slope, and lumbar lordosis, while the thoracic kyphosis is reduced.[244] The pelvic incidence angle is measured on a lateral x-ray and is subdented by a line drawn through femoral head to the midline of sacral end-plate and a line drawn perpendicular to the sacral end-plate. Oblique radiographs may be used to assess the pars interarticularis integrity. Stability of the spondylolisthesis can be evaluated with a traction radiograph (the patient hangs from a bar) or a compression stress radiograph (20-kg rucksack on the shoulders). Another method involves using a measure referred to as the sagittal pelvic tilt index. This gives the examiner an objective measure quantifying the relationship between S2, the center of the hip, and L5. A decrease in the sagittal pelvic tilt index correlates with slip progression and risk of conservative treatment failure.[245] Single-photon emission tomography (SPECT) is often used to distinguish athletic patients who require an antilordotic brace and rest from those who do not have an "active" lesion.

Management

Most grade 1 spondylolistheses are asymptomatic and stable. Progressive slippage is rare, occurring in only 2% to 3% of patients.[246] The majority of slippage occurs in children under age 10 years. In adults with degenerative spondylolisthesis, progression is rarely greater than 18% anterior displacement. Grade 2 spondylolistheses may be symptomatic but are considered stable. Cassidy et al.[247] indicate a good response to manipulative management. Only when grade 3 or 4 spondylolistheses are discovered is there a need for surgical consultation. Patients with a hot SPECT bone scan are placed in a brace for several weeks. Follow-up scans should be performed in several weeks.

Sacroiliac Sprain and Subluxation

Classic Presentation

The patient presents with pain over one SI joint after straightening up from a stooped position, often lifting an object. The pain may radiate down the back of the leg. With a sprain the pain is often sharp and stabbing and is relieved somewhat by sitting or lying. The pain is less often affected by posture with an SI subluxation.

Cause

Although not often recognized in the medical literature as a source of LBP, two systematic reviews by McKenzie-Brown et al.[248] and by Hansen et al.[249] indicated that the prevalence of SI joint pain is between 10% to 19% of low back pain patients. The SI ligamentous support is strong; however, in younger patients, pregnant patients, or those with degenerative disease, prolonged or sudden lifting or bending may cause a sprain or subluxation. Movement at the SI joint is small but existent in younger patients. The movement is primarily an anteroposterior rotary movement around a transverse axis. This is an accessory movement (involuntary) occurring mainly when attaining a standing position. The sacral promontory moves forward approximately 3 to 6 mm.[250]

Evaluation

Either direct compression (Figure 6–9) or distraction (gapping; Figure 6–8) at the joint may increase the pain or in some cases decrease the pain. Other tests include Gaenslen's test (Figure 6–10) whereby the supine patient draws the uninvolved leg to the chest while the examiner extends the involved-side leg off the side of the table. An increase in posterior pain suggests SI involvement. The Gillet test (Figure 6–12) is essentially a motion test of the SI joints in an attempt to determine restricted movement. Although the sensitivity of these tests is questioned, the combination of patient presentation, history, and SI tests will usually help define the problem. Evaluation of the patient should include signs of seronegative arthritides (i.e., AS, Reiter's, or psoriatic). This would include a search for skin lesions, eye irritation, or heel/foot pain. A prior history of painful urination or eye pain suggests Reiter's syndrome. Marked decreases in forward flexion without significant pain suggest AS; extensor or scalp skin lesions suggest psoriatic arthritis. Radiographic discrimination is usually possible.

Management

Acute SI sprains are best managed with an SI support (brace). Adjusting of the SI joint should be performed cautiously, avoiding increased stretch to the ligaments. Patients with SI subluxation usually have dramatic pain relief with manipulation. One interesting study[251] found that isolated contraction of the transverse abdominals was effective at stabilization of the SI joint in those individuals found to have laxity and resulting pain. This contraction was through a "drawing-in" of the abdominal wall versus a "brace" pattern that incorporated all of the abdominal muscles. The McKenzie-Brown review concluded that evidence for the diagnostic value of SI joint injections was moderate, having a 20% false positive rate. Therapeutically, both reviews concluded that there is moderate evidence for short-term and limited evidence for long-term relief with intra-articular SI joint injections. They felt the evidence for the use of radiofrequency neurotomy was limited or inconclusive.

Piriformis Syndrome

Classic Presentation

The patient often complains of buttock and posterior leg pain with a nontraumatic onset.

Cause

The sciatic nerve may be compressed by the piriformis muscle. In most patients, the sciatic nerve runs under the muscle; however, in approximately 15% of the population, there are two muscle bellies with the sciatic nerve coursing between them.[252]

Evaluation

Either resisted external rotation of the hip or passive medial rotation of the hip may increase the pain. Some practitioners use an SLR test with internal rotation to distinguish between nerve root or piriformis involvement. This should be interpreted cautiously because nerve root irritation also may cause pain increase with this maneuver. Direct palpation of the piriformis may cause a referred pattern down the back of the leg. Predisposition to piriformis syndrome may be an anatomically short leg, pronation, or pelvic rotation.

Management

Postisometric relaxation techniques or myofascial release techniques are often helpful. In the acute stage, it may be necessary to use adjunctive physical therapy pain modalities. In rare cases, injection of the piriformis trigger point may be needed.

Ankylosing Spondylitis

Classic Presentation

The patient is usually a young man presenting with a complaint of chronic low back pain and stiffness with occasional radiation of pain into the buttocks, anterior, or posterior thighs. The patient feels the stiffness upon rising and has some relief of complaints with mild to moderate activity.

Cause

AS is an inflammatory arthritis that usually affects the SI joints with progressive spinal ankylosing. It is characterized by enthesopathy (inflammation at the site of ligamentous insertions). It affects about 1% of whites and 0.25% of blacks. Men are affected three times more often than women. Women are less likely to have disease as severe. In general, the earlier the onset, the more progressive the disease is. With progression there is gradual stiffening, loss of the lumbar lordosis, increase in the thoracic kyphosis, and decrease in chest expansion due to costotransverse joint involvement. Heart involvement may lead to atrioventricular conduction defects and aortic insufficiency in approximately 3% to 5% of patients with chronic, severe disease. Peripheral joint involvement occurs 50% of the time, with permanent changes occurring 25% of the time. The joints most affected are the hips, shoulders, and knees.

Evaluation

There are several formalized consensus criteria used to determine whether a patient has AS; some are specific to AS (i.e., Rome criteria and modified New York criteria) and some are more generalized as criteria used for the determination of spondyloarthropathies (Amor criteria and European Spondyloarthropathy Study Group [ESSG]).[253] Two validated outcome measures used in the evaluation and prognosis for AS patients are the Bath Ankylosing Spondylitis Radiology Index (BASRI) and the Bath Ankylosing Spondylitis Functional Index (BASFI).[254-257] In a recent study, researchers in search of long-term outcome predictors for patients with AS came to the following conclusions: 80% of the variations in radiological status and 50% of the variations in the functional capacities of AS patients are unknown.[258] These findings led the researchers to conclude that genetic factors are more important than environmental factors. Some of the standard predictors for a poor outcome—including age, early age of onset, lower socioeconomic status, positive family history, and associated inflammatory bowel disease—were not associated with a poorer outcome in this study. For patients who smoke, are male, have had iritis, hip involvement, and higher disease activity scores, the prognosis for a worse outcome is increased. Fatigue was a common complaint in patients with AS. In patients with advanced disease, osteopenia is a risk factor for compression fractures.

AS is suspected when a patient with chronic back pain and stiffness has a global decrease in ROM of the lumbopelvic area. This is best measured with an inclinometer (Figure 6–6, B and C) or with a tape measure using the Schober method (Figure 6–6A). Orthopaedic and neurologic tests are normal. Chest expansion may be decreased with chronic involvement. In approximately 15% to 20% of patients, an anterior uveitis is found. Although lab testing will reveal elevations in erythrocyte sedimentation rate (ESR) in 85% of cases and HLA-B27 in 90% of cases (compared with 6% to 8% of asymptomatic individuals) and a negative rheumatoid factor, these tests are nonspecific and not diagnostic. AS is primarily a radiographic diagnosis.[259] Early changes are seen at the SI joint with "pseudowidening," erosions, and sclerosis. In the spine, early changes include marginal sclerosis and erosion of the superior/inferior margins of the vertebral bodies, causing a "squaring" appearance on a lateral view. Calcification of spinal ligaments and the annulus fibrosus creates a "trolley track" sign and eventual fusion with a characteristic bamboo spine appearance. Peripheral joint involvement causes a periosteal reaction at ligament/tendon insertion points of the iliac crest, Achilles, and plantar fascia insertion points. Given that radiographic changes may not be visible for four to six years after the onset of symptoms, the use of HLA-B27 may be an early but nonspecific indicator. Elevated ESR has moderate sensitivity and specificity for AS; however, an elevated level is present in only 34% to 64% of patients with severe disease when radiographic changes are already evident.[260]

Management

AS, like other rheumatoid and rheumatoid-variant diseases, has an unpredictable course of remission and relapses.[261] Management includes manipulation to keep the spine flexible, stretching, and postural and breathing exercises. Manipulation should be as gentle as possible considering the inflammatory nature of this disease. In the early stages, the calcification present on the radiograph represents a "soft" ankylosing that allows for some intersegmental movement. With severe progression, monitoring for cardiac and pulmonary involvement should be performed. It is important that patients avoid long-term use of pain medication if possible because of the gastric and renal consequences. There are a few case study reports on the management of AS patients chiropractically.[262,263] These reports indicate varied responses and treatment approaches; therefore, no generalized statements can be made at this time regarding an agreed-upon approach. In a 2006 study,[264] a multimodal exercise program for AS patients was tested against a control group who did not perform any exercise. The program included aerobic exercise, stretching, and pulmonary exercises. Exercise was performed three times a week for three months. Physical work capacity and vital capacity values improved in the exercise group but decreased in the control group. This small study of 90 patients indicates that a multimodal approach may be of benefit to AS patients. The specifics of this program included:

- Prior to the step (aerobic) exercise, the target heart rates were calculated.
- A 10-minute warm-up of step exercises (using aerobic step device) was followed by 5 minutes of stretching, 20 minutes of step exercises, and 10 minutes of pulmonary exercise.
- The pulmonary exercises included twice the normal rate of respiration (inspiration through the nose; expiration through the mouth) and the use of deep breathing.

Reiter's Syndrome

Classic Presentation

A young male patient presents with a complaint of LBP that began after the onset of urethritis (burning on urination), conjunctivitis (eye pain), and skin lesions on the soles or palms.

Cause

Reiter's is a seronegative (negative for rheumatoid factor) arthropathy that follows an infection. *Chlamydia, Campylobacter, Salmonella,* and *Yersinia* have all been implicated. It appears that the HLA-B27 marker may indicate those individuals prone to a reactive arthritis following bacterial infection.

Evaluation

The diagnostic tetrad includes: (1) conjunctivitis that usually resolves in a day or two, (2) mucocutaneous lesions on the tongue, palate, and penis or plantar keratogenous lesions of the foot, (3) urethritis (often one of the first symptoms and often unresponsive to antibiotics), and (4) arthritis affecting the knees and ankles asymmetrically, but the SI joint is the most common symptomatic joint. Mechanical testing of the SI joint will usually increase pain. Laboratory testing may demonstrate increases in ESR and HLA-B271, but be negative for rheumatoid factor. Radiographic changes may be subtle at the SI joint in the early stages. Unilateral involvement with joint space narrowing, erosive changes, and eburnation of subchondral bone may be seen. "Sausage" fingers or toes due to marked swelling and ankylosis may also be seen.

Management

Antibiotics are ineffective. Management is primarily symptomatic. It must be remembered that this is an inflammatory disease, and manipulation of the SI joint may aggravate the patient's symptoms. Most of the nonarticular complaints resolve over days or weeks. Joint involvement may be progressive and permanent, however, especially in patients who have recurrent infection.

Multiple Myeloma

Classic Presentation

The patient is older (> 50 years) and complains of persistent back pain that is unrelieved by rest. The pain seems worse at night. There may be associated rib pain.

Cause

Multiple myeloma (MM) is a malignant disease characterized by proliferation of plasma cells with replacement of bone marrow, which results in osteoporosis, hypercalcemia, anemia, renal disease, and infection (often pneumonia) due to suppression of normal immunoglobulins.

Evaluation

In older patients with unexplained LBP, laboratory and radiographic evaluation may reveal signs of MM. Laboratory findings include anemia with normal erythrocyte morphology but increased rouleau formation, hypercalcemia, hyperuricemia, and increased globulins. A 24-hour urine test may reveal the presence of Bence-Jones protein (light chain). Electrophoresis will reveal a monoclonal spiking; immuno-electrophoresis usually demonstrates elevated immunoglobulin G (IgG). The definitive diagnosis is a bone marrow aspirate showing more than 20% plasma cells. Radiographic findings demonstrate osteopenia followed by widespread lytic lesions in the spine, ribs, and skull (punched out or rat-bite lesions). Unlike metastasis to the spine, MM does not usually affect the posterior elements such as the pedicles.

Management

Treatment is primarily palliative. Chemotherapy or radiation therapy is used primarily to relieve bone pain. Bone marrow transplant is curative, but the patient must be under age 55 years and therefore few patients with MM qualify. The survival rate is variable; however, some degree of prediction is based on the degree of IgG spiking on immunoelectrophoresis, anemia, and hypercalcemia. In general, patients with IgG less than 5 g/dL and no evidence of anemia, renal disease, or lytic lesions have a survival rate of 5 to 6 years.[265]

Metastatic Carcinoma

Classic Presentation

The patient is usually over age 50 years and complains of insidious onset of pain that is persistent, worse at night, and not mechanically affected. There is often a history of weight loss and fatigue. (*Note:* The patient may remain asymptomatic until late in the course of the disease or may become symptomatic after trauma because of the pathologic weakness of the vertebrae.)

Cause

Metastatic involvement of the spine accounts for only 1% of LBP. The most common metastases are from the breast, prostate, lung, and kidney. Prostate cancer spreads through Batson's plexus to the vertebrae. Metastasis from the above cancers may involve the vertebral bodies, pedicles, and, less commonly, the neural arches. The sequence of changes is usually replacement of fatty bone marrow with nonfatty tumor cells, followed by either destruction of the trabeculae with a periosteal response when a lytic metastasis is involved, or osteoblastic or sclerotic response such as with prostate cancer.

Evaluation

A history of prior cancer, unexplained weight loss, or unresponsiveness to conservative care for one month is highly suggestive of cancer, especially in patients older than 50 years of age. Radiographically, metastatic cancer may appear as an osteolytic process (such as the missing or one-eyed pedicle seen with breast cancer) or osteoblastic (such as the ivory vertebrae seen with prostate cancer). Compression fracture of the vertebrae with posterior collapse is highly suggestive of a cancer-induced pathologic fracture. Osteolytic processes may increase the serum calcium levels, whereas the osteoblastic process may increase the alkaline phosphatase levels. Determination of total and free prostate specific antigen (PSA) with a digital rectal examination should be performed in males suspected of prostate cancer. Bone scans may help determine the degree of spinal involvement with regard to location; MRI can determine the volume of involvement at any individual site. (For a list of spinal cord tumors, see **Table 6–5**.)

Management

Referral for an oncologic consult is necessary. Comanagement issues can then be discussed.

Infectious Spondylitis

Classic Presentation

Although there is no consistency regarding a typical patient and whether fever is present, the following is a presentation not to be missed: The patient presents with a complaint of deep back pain. There is a history of a recent respiratory or urinary tract infection (or intravenous drug use or diabetes). The patient is antalgic and complains of a fever and difficulty sleeping because of the pain.

Table 6–5 Malignancies of the Spine and CNS

Type	Summary Information
Astrocytomas	75% in cervical and thoracic areas
	20% in distal cord; 5% in the filum terminale
	Occur most frequently in ages thirties to forties
	50%–70% present with back, neck, or leg pain; 20%–30% have spasticity and stiffness of legs
	Survival period is from 1 to 8 years
Ependymoma	Slow-growing, benign tumors arising from ependymal cells in central canal (intramedullary), filum terminale, sacral area (extradural/extraspinal)
	Represent 60%–70% of spinal cord tumors
	60% occur in the conus, filum, or cauda equina
Hemangioblastoma	Benign tumor composed of dense network of capillary and sinus channels
	Usually intramedullary; may be intradural/extramedullary involving posterior roots of cauda equina
	Solitary or multiple; when multiple, associated with von Hippel-Lindau disease; patients develop renal cell carcinoma
Intradural lipomas	Benign neoplasms composed of fat cells
	Three types:
	1. filum terminale
	2. intradural
	3. lipomyelomeningocele
	Most common in thoracic spine; males more commonly affected
	The intradural type are not commonly a cause of radicular pain, unlike filum terminale lipoma
Intramedullary spinal cord metastasis	Found in only 1%–3% of tumor patients
	Lung and breast cancer most common
	Other non-CNS processes such as melanoma, leukemia, and lymphoma may metastasize to the cord
	CNS tumors that may involve cord are glioblastoma, ependymoma, and medulloblastoma
Extramedullary tumors: meningiomas	Meningiomas account for 25% of intraspinal tumors
	Occur from ages 20–60 years; peak in forties; female predominant (4:1)
	Predominance at exits of spinal nerves from dural sleeves
	Most common in T spine, they compress but do not invade spinal nerves or cord
Extramedullary tumors: neurinoma	Most common extramedullary (29%)
	Originate from sensory nerve roots; usually in C and T spine; however, 40% occur in L spine
	Peak incidence in fifties; male predominant
	Generally singular; when multiple, associated with von Recklinghausen's disease

Cause

Infection involving both the disc and the vertebral body is referred to as infectious spondylitis. This is more common in adults with a prior history of urinary tract infection, intravenous drug abuse, recent use of an indwelling catheter postsurgery, or skin infection. Children are more prone to discitis (usually benign) without vertebral body involvement. Infection is spread via the arterial system, Batson's venous plexus, and direct inoculation through surgery. There are generally two types: (1) pyogenic and (2) nonpyogenic. The pyogenic type is usually due to *Staphylococcus, Streptococcus,* and gram-negative organisms. The nonpyogenic type is usually due to tuberculosis; however, *Brucella* or fungi may be the cause.

Evaluation

Adults will usually have a deep pain made worse with pressure or percussion of the spinous process. Fever is often present. Although not particularly sensitive, it is relatively specific.[53] Radiographic indications often take three to four weeks to become evident. Pyogenic causes involve more than one vertebra, often leaving the disc unaffected. Bony lysis is followed by sclerosis in the vertebral bodies. Posterior elements are rarely affected. Nonpyogenic spondylitis centers around L1. On occasion, the posterior elements are involved. Laboratory findings include an increase in ESR, and occasionally changes are evident in leukocyte response.

Management

Refer for orthopaedic consultation and determination of course of care.

Abdominal Aneurysm

Classic Presentation

Most abdominal aneurysms are asymptomatic until rupture. The symptomatic patient may present with mild to severe middle abdominal or low back pain. There may be an associated complaint of leg pain with exertion (claudication).

Cause

Atherosclerotic aneurysms (weakening with dilation) occur primarily below the renal arteries (95% of the time). The incidence is between 2% and 4% with a 5:1 male predominance. It has become clear that smoking is an important risk factor for abdominal aneurysm.[265] In fact, the Agency for Healthcare Research and Quality has listed smoking as a screening question for men at risk for abdominal aneurysm.[266]

Evaluation

In asymptomatic patients the most common finding is a pulsatile mid- or upper abdominal mass. Palpation is most sensitive for abdominal aneurysms greater than 3.0 cm (50% for 3.0 to 3.9 cm and 76% for those > 5.0 cm) with an overall positive predictive value of 43%.[267] Auscultation may reveal a bruit. Peripheral pulses may be prominent (due to a reactive arteriomegaly). Lateral lumbar radiographs may reveal an enlarged calcific margin of the aorta, usually between L2 and L4. A diameter exceeding 3.8 cm is considered an aneurysm.[268] Other indirect findings may include erosion of the anterior vertebral bodies behind the aneurysm.

Management

Referral for abdominal ultrasonography is warranted to demonstrate the size and extent of involvement. Those patients with a documented diameter of 4–6 cm should have a surgical consultation. If not excised and grafted, most aneurysms will go on to rupture. However, one study[269] indicated that in patients 65 to 80 years old with aneurysms less than 6 cm, surgery was not necessary unless the aneurysm expanded more than 1 cm. Patients with acute rupture usually have a searing/tearing pain warranting immediate emergency management. Patients whose aneurysm proceeds to rupture have only a 10% to 20% survival rate.[270]

The Evidence—Lumbopelvic

Translation Into Practice Summary (TIPS)

The physical examination combined with the history is reasonably good at identifying disc disruption and/or lumbar radiculopathy, and stenosis. Neurologic testing in isolation is not as valuable as combined testing for numbness, weakness, and deep tendon reflex loss.

The literature on evaluation of the sacroiliac and pelvic regions is extensive but inconclusive. Pain provocation tests have been studied extensively and have been found individually to be poor, but as a group may rise to the level of value in ruling in sacroiliac involvement.

The Literature-Based Clinical Core

- The patient history is not good for identifying lumbar radiculopathy compared to other sources of radiating pain.

- The neurological examination consisting of sensation testing, muscle testing (myotome), and deep tendon reflex (DTR) testing is not good at identifying disc herniation and/or radiculopathy if used alone. The L5 reflex is unreliable and is not necessary to perform. The reliability of the DTR is best for L3/L4 spinal levels (i.e., patellar reflex), which is far less commonly involved than L4/L5 and L5/S1. The value of DTR findings is best for ruling in but not ruling out radiculopathy.

- Even with myotomal weakness, dermatomal numbness, a decreased or absent DTR, and a positive SLR, the positive LR is good but not great at identifying radiculopathy.

- The identification of a radiculopathy is increased when orthopaedic findings are combined with neurological findings. The combination of a positive slump test with findings of calf-wasting, a positive SLR and a crossed SLR when positive as a group is good at ruling in radiculopathy.

- Dermatomal radiation is inconsistent (i.e., radiation more often described as nondermatomal by patients) and is typical only for S1 involvement (although high-lumbar disc involvement does overlap sometimes with an S1 dermatomal patch).
- There are good indicators of spinal stenosis in the history including "no pain while seated." Decreases in sensation (vibration and pin-prick), decreased or absent DTRs, or weak muscle tests have only fair +LRs. Rombergs and/or a two-stage treadmill exam may be of value for detecting stenosis.
- The centralization phenomenon is good at identifying painful lumbar discs. The classification system for McKenzie has variable kappa values.
- Spinal instability may be detected with a combination of testing procedures, yet the value in determining management is still to be determined.
- The only valuable history indicator for sacroiliac (SI) involvement is pain relieved by standing, which has a good positive LR.
- Single pain-provocation tests are poor at either identifying or specifying SI involvement.
- Grouping a cluster of four or five tests including distraction, thigh thrust, sacral thrust, and compression after a repeated McKenzie approach is good at identifying SI involvement.
- Motion and static palpation tests demonstrate poor reliability.
- There are a number of orthopaedic tests designed to distinguish between SI versus lumbar involvement, but, there is no literature support for this function.

The Expert-Opinion-Based Clinical Core

- With radiculopathy, the area of numbness is patchy and does not extend throughout the radiation of pain pattern.
- Myotome weakness is painless weakness.
- There are no reliable tests for spondylolisthesis although the balance test is often used.
- Patients with insidious onset of SI pain should be evaluated radiographically for sero-negative arthritides given there are no orthopaedic tests that can discriminate these from other causes of SI pain.

- The reliability of leg-discrepancy testing is good and although there are no studies to indicate the validity for differentiating SI involvement, it may serve as an indicator of checking for SI involvement.

APPENDIX 6–1

References

1. Christensen M, Morgan D, eds. *Job Analysis of Chiropractic: A Project Report, Survey, Analysis, and Summary of the Practice of Chiropractic within the United States.* Greeley, CO: National Board of Chiropractic Examiners; 1993.
2. Papagerogiou AC, Croft PR, Ferry S, et al. Estimating the prevalence of low back pain in the general population: evidence from the South Manchester back pain survey. *Spine.* 1995;17:1889–1894.
3. Deyo RA, Tsui-Wu JY. Descriptive epidemiology of low back pain and its related medical care in the United States. *Spine.* 1987;12:264–268.
4. Hareby M, Neerguard K, Hesselsoe G, Kjer J. Are radiographic changes in the thoracic and lumbar spine of adolescents risk factors for low back pain in adults? *Spine.* 1995;20:2298–2302.
5. Croft PR, Macfarlane GJ, Papageorgiou AC, Thomas E, Silman AJ. Outcome of low back pain in general practice: a prospective study. *BMJ.* 1998;316(7141):1356–1359.
6. Von Korff M. Studying the natural history of back pain. *Spine.* 1994;19:2041S–2046S.
7. Hestbaek L, Leboeuf-Yde C, Manniche C. Low back pain: what is the long-term course? A review of studies of general patient populations. *Eur Spine J.* 2003;12(2):149–165.
8. Philips HC, Grant L. The evolution of chronic back pain problems: a longitudinal study. *Behav Res Ther.* 1991;29(5):435–441.
9. Schiottz-Christensen B, Nielsen GL, Hansen VK, Schodt T, Sorensen HT, Olesen F. Long-term prognosis of acute low back pain in patients seen in general practice: a 1-year prospective follow-up study. *Fam Pract.* 1999;16(3):223–232.
10. Marras WS, Ferguson SA, Burr D, Schabo P, Maronitis A. Low back pain recurrence in occupational environments. *Spine.* 2007;32(21):2387–2397.
11. Marras WS. Occupational low back disorder causation and control. *Ergonomics.* 2000;43(7):880–902.

12. Report of the Quebec Task Force on Spinal Disorders. *Spine*. 1987;12(suppl 1):51–59.

13. Schwarzer AC, April CN, Derby R, et al. The prevalence and clinical features of internal disc disruption in patients with chronic low back pain. *Spine*. 1995;17:1878–1883.

14. Deyo RA, Rainville J, Kent DL. What can the history and physical examination tell us about low back pain? *JAMA*. 1992;268:760–765.

15. Deyo RA, Diehl AK. Cancer as a cause of back pain: frequency, clinical presentation, and diagnostic strategies. *J Gen Intern Med*. 1988;3:230–238.

16. Sapico FL, Montgomere JZ. Pyogenic vertebral osteomyelitis: report of nine cases and review of the literature. *Rev Infect Dis*. 1979;1:754–776.

17. Cassidy JD, Kirkaldy-Willis WH, McGregor M. Spinal manipulation for the treatment of chronic low back and leg pain: an observational trial. In: Buerger AA, Greenman PE, eds. *Empirical Approaches to the Validation of Manipulative Therapy*. Springfield, IL: Charles C Thomas; 1985.

18. Manga P, Angus D, Papadopoulos C, Swan W. *A Study to Examine the Effectiveness and Cost-Effectiveness of Chiropractic Management of Low-Back Pain*. Richmond Hill, Ontario: Kenilworth Publishing; 1993.

19. Cherkin D, MacCormack F. Patient evaluations of low back pain care from family physicians and chiropractors. *West J Med*. 1989;150:151.

20. Hertzman-Miller RP, Morgenstern H, Hurwitz EL, et al. Comparing the satisfaction of low back pain patients randomized to receive medical or chiropractic care: result from the UCLA Low-Back Pain Study. *Am J Public Health*. 2002;92:1628–1633.

21. Shekelle PG, Adams AH, Chassin MR, et al. *The Appropriateness of Spinal Manipulation for Low-Back Pain: Project Overview and Literature Review*. Santa Monica, CA: Rand Publications; 1991.

22. Meade TW, Dyer S, Browne W, Townsend J, Frank AO. Low back pain of mechanical origin: randomised comparison of chiropractic and hospital outpatient treatment. *Br Med J*. 1990;300:1431–1437.

23. van Tulder M, Becker A, Bekkering T, et al. Chapter 3. European guidelines for the management of acute nonspecific low back pain in primary care. *Eur Spine J*. 2006;15 Suppl 2:S169–191.

24. Bronfort G, Haas M, Evans R, Kawchuk G, Dagenais S. Evidence-informed management of chronic low back pain with spinal manipulation and mobilization. *Spine J*. 2008;8(1):213–225.

25. Bozzao A, Gallucci M, et al. Lumbar disk herniation: MR imaging assessment of natural history in patients treated without surgery. *Neuroradiology*. 1992;185:135–141.

26. Parke WW, Whalen JL. The vascular pattern of the human dorsal root ganglion and its probable bearing on a compartment syndrome. *Spine*. 2002;27(4):347–352.

27. Kirkaldy-Willis WH. *Managing Low Back Pain*. New York: Churchill Livingstone; 1983.

28. Suseki K, Takahashi Y, Takahashi K, Chiba T, Yamagata M, Moriya H. Sensory nerve fibres from lumbar intervertebral discs pass through rami communicantes. A possible pathway for discogenic low back pain. *J Bone Joint Surg Br*. 1998;80(4):737–742.

29. Umimura T, Miyagi M, Ishikawa T, et al. Investigation of dichotomizing sensory nerve fibers projecting to the lumbar multifidus muscles and intervertebral disc or facet joint or sacroiliac joint in rats. *Spine (Phila Pa 1976)*. 2011;37(7):557–562.

30. Wakai K, Ohtori S, Yamashita M, et al. Primary sensory neurons with dichotomizing axons projecting to the facet joint and the low back muscle in rats. *J Orthop Sci*. 2010;15(3):402–406.

31. Sameda H, Takahashi Y, Takahashi K, Chiba T, Ohtori S, Moriya H. Primary sensory neurons with dichotomizing axons projecting to the facet joint and the sciatic nerve in rats. *Spine (Phila Pa 1976)*. 2001;26(10):1105–1109.

32. Palmgren T, Gronblad M, Virri J, et al. An immunohistochemical study of nerve structures in the annulus fibrosus of human normal lumbar intervertebral discs. *Spine*. 1999;24(20):2075–2079.

33. Bogduk N, April C, Derby R. Discography. In: *Spine Care*. St. Louis: CV Mosby; 1995.

34. Kauppila LI. Ingrowth of blood vessels in disc degeneration: angiographic and histological studies of cadaveric spines. *J Bone Joint Surg Am*. 1995;77(1):26–31.

35. McCarron RF, Wimpee MW, Hudkins PG, Laros GS. The inflammatory effect of nucleus pulposus: a possible element in the pathogenesis of low back pain. *Spine*. 1987;8:760–764.

36. Bozzao A, Gallucci M. Lumbar disk herniation: MR imaging assessment of natural history in patients treated without surgery. *Neuroradiology*. 1992;185:135–141.

37. d'Ornano J, Conrozier T, et al. Effects des manipulations vertebrales sur la hernie discale lombaire. *Rev Med Orthop*. 1990;19:21–25.

38. Giles LGF. *Anatomical Basis of Low Back Pain.* Baltimore: Williams & Wilkins; 1989:60–97.

39. Adams MA, Hutton WC. The mechanical function of the lumbar apophyseal joints. *Spine.* 1983;8:327.

40. Giles LGF, Taylor JR. Innervation of lumbar zygapophyseal joint synovial folds. *Acta Orthop Scand.* 1987;58:43–46.

41. Schwarzer AC, Wang S, Bogduk N, McNaught PJ, Laurant R. The prevalence and clinical features of lumbar zygapophyseal joint pain: a study in an Australian population with chronic low back pain. *Ann Rheum Dis.* 1995;211:356.

42. Bogduk N, Engel R. The menisci of the lumbar zygapophyseal joints: a review of their anatomy and clinical significance. *Spine.* 1984;9:454–450.

43. Bogduk N, Twomey LT. *Clinical Anatomy of the Lumbar Spine.* 2nd ed. Melbourne, Australia: Churchill Livingstone; 1991.

44. Pope MH, Wilder DG, Materri RE, Frymoyer JW. Experimental measurements of vertebral motion under load. *Orthop Clin North Am.* 1977;155:167.

45. Panjabi M, Yamamoto I, Oxland T, Crisco J. How does posture affect coupling in the lumbar spine? *Spine.* 1988;14:1001–1011.

46. Parmianpour M, Nordin M, Frankel V, Kahanovitz N. The triaxial coupling of torque generation of trunk muscles during isometric exertions and the effect of fatiguing isoinertial movements on the motor output and movement patterns. In: *Transaction of the Annual Meeting of the International Society for Study of the Lumbar Spine.* Miami, FL: International Society for Study of the Lumbar Spine; 1988:34.

47. Adams MA, Hutton WC. Prolapsed intervertebral disc: a hyperflexion injury. *Spine.* 1982;7:184–191.

48. Adams MA, Hutton WC. Gradual disc prolapse. *Spine.* 1985;10:524–531.

49. Slosberg M. Side posture manipulation for lumbar intervertebral disk herniation reconsidered. *J Manipulative Physiol Ther.* 1994;17:258–262.

50. Bellamy N, Park W, Rooney PJ. What do we know about the sacroiliac joint? *Semin Arthritis Rheum.* 1983;12:282–307.

51. Williams PL, Warwick R, eds. *Gray's Anatomy.* 36th ed. London: Churchill Livingstone; 1980:473.

52. Sturesson B, Selvik G, Uden A. Movements of the sacroiliac joints: a roentgen stereophotogrammetric analysis. *Spine.* 1989;14:162–165.

53. Deyo RA. Early detection of cancer, infection, and inflammatory disease of the spine. *J Back Musculoskel Rehabil.* 1991;1:69–81.

54. Waidvogel FA, Vasey H. Osteomyelitis: the past decade. *N Engl J Med.* 1980;303:360–370.

55. Calin A, Porta J, Fries JF, Schurman DJ. Clinical history as a screening test for ankylosing spondylitis. *Clin Rheumatol.* 1985;4:161–169.

56. Rainville J, Lopez E. Comparison of radicular symptoms caused by lumbar disc herniation and lumbar spinal stenosis in the elderly. *Spine (Phila Pa 1976).* 2013;38(15):1282–1287.

57. Leboeuf-Yde C. Body weight and low back pain: a systematic literature review of 56 journal articles reporting on 65 epidemiologic studies. *Spine.* 2000;25(2):226–237.

58. Jhawar BS, Fuchs CS, Colditz GA, Stampfer MJ. Cardiovascular risk factors for physician-diagnosed lumbar disc herniation. *Spine J.* 2006;6(6):684–691.

59. Kauppila LI. Ingrowth of blood vessels in disc degeneration. Angiographic and histological studies of cadaveric spines. *J Bone Joint Surg Am.* 1995;77(1):26–31.

60. Kauppila LI, Mikkonen R, Mankinen P, Pelto-Vasenius K, Maenpaa I. MR aortography and serum cholesterol levels in patients with long-term nonspecific lower back pain. *Spine.* 2004;29(19):2147–2152.

61. Kauppila LI, Penttila A. Postmortem angiographic study of degenerative vascular changes in arteries supplying the cervicobrachial region. *Ann Rheum Dis.* 1994;53(2):94–99.

62. Deyo RA. Measuring the functional status of patients with low back pain. *Arch Phys Med Rehabil.* 1988;69:1044–1053.

63. Anderson R, Meeker WC. A meta-analysis of clinical trials of spinal manipulation. *J Manipulative Physiol Ther.* 1992;15:181–194.

64. Hsieh CJ, Philips RB, et al. Functional outcomes of low back pain: comparison of four treatment groups in a randomized controlled trial. *J Manipulative Physiol Ther.* 1992;15:4–9.

65. Fairbanks J, Davies J. The Oswestry low back pain disability questionnaire. *Physiotherapy.* 1980;66:271.

66. Roland M, Morris R. Study of natural history of back pain, I: development of reliable and sensitive measure of disability in low back pain. *Spine.* 1983;8:141.

67. Kendall NAS, Linton SJ, Main CJ. *Guide to Assessing Psychosocial Yellow Flags in Acute Low Back Pain: Risk Factors for Long-Term Disability and Work Loss.* Wellington, New Zealand: Accident Rehabilitation & Compensation Insurance Corporation of New Zealand and the National Health Committee; 1997.

68. Kelsey JL, Golden AL, Mundt DJ. Low back pain/ prolapsed lumbar intervertebral disc. *Rheum Dis Clin North Am.* 1990;16:669–712.

69. Kortelainen P, Puranen J, Koivisto E, Larde S. Symptoms and signs of sciatica and their relation to the localization of the lumbar disc herniation. *Spine.* 1985;10:88–92.

70. McCombe PF, Fairbank JCT, Cockersole BC, Pynsent PB. Reproducibility of physical signs in low back pain. *Spine.* 1989;14:908–918.

71. Al Nezari NH, Schneiders AG, Hendrick PA. Neurological examination of the peripheral nervous system to diagnose lumbar spinal disc herniation with suspected radiculopathy: a systematic review and meta-analysis. *Spine J.* Jun 2013;13(6):657–674.

72. Urban LM. The straight-leg raising test: a review. *J Orthop Sports Phys Ther.* 1981;2:117–133.

73. Kosteljanetz M, Flemming B, Schmidt-Olsen S. The clinical significance of straight leg raising in the diagnosis of prolapsed lumbar disc. *Spine.* 1988;13:393–395.

74. Park JB, Chang H, Kim KW, Park SJ. Facet tropism: a comparison between far lateral and posterolateral lumbar disc herniations. *Spine.* 2001;26(6):677–679.

75. Erhard RE, Welch WC, Liu B, Vignovic M. Far-lateral disk herniation: case report, review of the literature, and a description of nonsurgical management. *J Manipulative Physiol Ther.* 2004;27(2):e3.

76. Tamir E, Anekshtein Y, Melamed E, Halperin N, Mirovsky Y. Clinical presentation and anatomic position of L3-L4 disc herniation: a prospective and comparative study. *J Spinal Disord Tech.* 2004;17(6):467–469.

77. Ozturk C, Tezer M, Sirvanci M, Sarier M, Aydogan M, Hamzaoglu A. Far lateral thoracic disc herniation presenting with flank pain. *Spine J.* 2006;6(2):201–203.

78. Rabin A, Gerszten PC, Karausky P, Bunker CH, Potter DM, Welch WC. The sensitivity of the seated straight-leg raise test compared with the supine straight-leg raise test in patients presenting with magnetic resonance imaging evidence of lumbar nerve root compression. *Arch Phys Med Rehabil.* 2007;88(7):840–843.

79. Poiraudeau S, Foltz V, Drape JL, et al. Value of the bell test and the hyperextension test for diagnosis in sciatica associated with disc herniation: comparison with Lasegue's sign and the crossed Lasegue's sign. *Rheumatology (Oxford).* 2001;40(4):460–466.

80. Summers B, Mishra V, Jones JM. The flip test: a reappraisal. *Spine (Phila Pa 1976).* 2009;34(15):1585–1589.

81. Majlesi J, Togay H, Unalan H, Toprak S. The sensitivity and specificity of the slump and the straight leg raising tests in patients with lumbar disc herniation. *J Clin Rheumatol.* 2008;14(2):87–91.

82. van der Windt DA, Simons E, Riphagen, II, et al. Physical examination for lumbar radiculopathy due to disc herniation in patients with low-back pain. *Cochrane Database Syst Rev.* 2010(2):CD007431.

83. Fedorak C, Ashworth N, Marshall J, Paul H. Reliability of the visual assessment of cervical and lumbar lordosis: how good are we? *Spine.* 2003;28(16): 1857–1859.

84. Beattie P. Validity of derived measurements of leg length differences obtained by the use of a tape measure. *Phys Ther.* 1990;70:150–157.

85. Mann M, Glasheen-Wray M, Nyberg R. Therapist agreement for palpation and observation of iliac crest heights. *Phys Ther.* 1984; 3:334–338.

86. Haas M. The reliability of reliability. *J Manipulative Physiol Ther.* 1991;14:199–208.

87. Boline PD, et al. Interexaminer reliability of palpatory evaluations of the lumbar spine. *Am J Chirop Med.* 1988;1:5–11.

88. Mootz RD. Intra- and interexaminer reliability of passive motion palpation of the lumbar spine. *J Manipulative Physiol Ther.* 1989;12:440–447.

89. Mayer TG, Kondraske G, Beals SB, Gatchel RJ. Spinal range of motion. Accuracy and sources of error with inclinometric measurement. *Spine.* 1997;22(17):1976–1984.

90. Chen SP, Samo DG, Chen EH, et al. Reliability of three lumbar sagittal motion measurement methods: surface inclinometers. *J Occup Environ Med.* 1997;39(3):217–223.

91. Nattrass CL, Nitschke JE, Disler PB, et al. Lumbar spine range of motion as a measure of physical and functional impairment: an investigation of validity. *Clin Rehabil.* 1999;13(3):211–218.

92. Nitschke JE, Nattrass CL, Disler PB, et al. Reliability of the American Medical Association guides' model for measuring spinal range of motion: its implication for whole-person impairment rating. *Spine.* 1999;24(3):262–268.

93. Souza TA. Which orthopaedic tests are really necessary? In: Lawrence DJ, Cassidy D, McGregor M, et al., eds. *Advances in Chiropractic.* St. Louis, MO: Mosby-Year Book; 1994;1:101–158.

94. Ekedahl H, Jonsson B, Frobell RB. Fingertip-to-floor test and straight leg raising test: validity, responsiveness, and predictive value in patients with acute/

subacute low back pain. *Arch Phys Med Rehabil.* 2012;93(12):2210–2215.

95. McKenzie R. *The Lumbar Spine: Mechanical Diagnosis and Therapy.* Waikanae, New Zealand: Spinal Publications; 1981.

96. Riddle DL, Rothstein JM. Intertester reliability of McKenzie's classifications of the syndrome types present in patients with low back pain. *Spine.* 1993;18(10):1333–1344.

97. Razmjou H, Kramer JF, Yamada R. Intertester reliability of the McKenzie evaluation assessing patients with mechanical low-back pain. *J Orthop Sports Phys Ther.* 2000; 30:368–389.

98. Lewit K. Manipulation and rehabilitation. In: Liebenson C, ed. *Rehabilitation of the Spine: A Practitioner's Manual.* Baltimore: Williams & Wilkins; 1995.

99. Janda V. Evaluation of muscular imbalance. In: Liebenson C, ed. *Rehabilitation of the Spine: A Practitioner's Manual.* Baltimore: Williams & Wilkins; 1995.

100. Lewit K. *Manipulative Therapy in Rehabilitation of the Locomotor System.* 2nd ed. Oxford, England: Butterworth-Heinemann; 1991.

101. Paydar D, Thiel H, Gemmell H. Intra- and interexaminer reliability of certain pelvic palpatory procedures and the sitting flexion test for sacroiliac joint mobility and dysfunction. *J NMS.* 1994; 2(2):65–69.

102. Potter NA, Rothstein JM. Intertester reliability for selected clinical tests for the sacroiliac joint. *Phys Ther.* 1985; 65:1671–1675.

103. Herzog W, Read LJ, Conway JW, et al. Reliability of motion palpation procedures to detect sacroiliac joint fixations. *J Manipulative Physiol Ther.* 1989;12:86–92.

104. Mior SA, McGregor M, Schut B. The role of experience in clinical accuracy. *J Manipulative Physiol Ther.* 1990;13(2):68–71.

105. Meijne W, von Neerbos K, Aufdemkampe G, von der Warff P. Intraexaminer and interexaminer reliability of the Gillet test. *J Manipulative Physiol Ther.* 1999;22:4–9.

106. Waddell G, McCulloch JA, Kummel E, Venner RM. Nonorganic physical signs in low-back pain. *Spine.* 1980; 5:117–125.

107. Fishbaine DA, Goldberg M, Rosomoff RS, Rosomoff H. Chronic pain patients and the nonorganic physical signs of nondermatomal sensory abnormalities (NDSA). *Psychosomatics.* 1991;32:294–302.

108. Reger SI, Shah A, Adams TC, et al. Classification of large array surface myoelectric potentials from subjects with and without low back pain. *J Electromyogr Kinesiol.* 2006;16(4):392–401.

109. Rissanen A, Alaranta H, Sainio P, Harkonen H. Isokinetic and non-dynamometric tests in low back pain patients related to pain and disability index. *Spine.* 1994;19(17):1963–1967.

110. Alaranta H, Luoto S, Heliovaara M, Hurri H. Static back endurance and the risk of low-back pain. *Clin Biomech (Bristol, Avon).* 1995;10(6):323–324.

111. Schellenberg KL, Lang JM, Chan KM, Burnham RS. A clinical tool for office assessment of lumbar spine stabilization endurance: prone and supine bridge maneuvers. *Am J Phys Med Rehabil.* 2007;86(5):380–386.

112. Barr KP, Griggs M, Cadby T. Lumbar stabilization: core concepts and current literature, Part 1. *Am J Phys Med Rehabil.* 2005;84(6):473–480.

113. Barr KP, Griggs M, Cadby T. Lumbar stabilization: a review of core concepts and current literature, Part 2. *Am J Phys Med Rehabil.* 2007;86(1):72–80.

114. McGill S. *Low Back Disorders: Evidence-Based Prevention and Rehabilitation: 3rd ed.* Champaign, IL: Human Kinetics; 2007.

115. Weinstein JN, McLain F. Primary tumors of the spine. *Spine.* 1987;12:843–851.

116. Assendelft WJJ, Bouter LM, Knipschild PG, Wilmink JT. Reliability of lumbar spine radiograph reading by chiropractors. *Spine.* 1997;22(11):1233–1241.

117. Taylor JAM, Clopton P, Bosch E, et al. Interpretation of abnormal lumbosacral spine radiographs: a test comparing students, clinicians, radiology residents, and radiologists in medicine and chiropractic. *Spine.* 1995;20(10):1147–1154.

118. De Zoete A, Assendelft WJ, Algra PR, et al. Reliability and validity of lumbosacral spine radiograph reading by chiropractors, chiropractic radiologists, and medical radiologists. *Spine.* 2002;27:1926–1933.

119. Dailey EJ, Beuler MT. Plain film assessment of spinal stenosis: method comparison with lumbar CT. *J Manipulative Physiol Ther.* 1989;12:192–199.

120. Ulrich CG, Binet EF, Sanecki MG, et al. Quantitative assessment of the lumbar spinal canal by computed tomography. *Radiology.* 1980;134:137–143.

121. Peterson CK, Bolton JE, Wood AR. A cross-sectional study correlating lumbar spine degeneration with disability and pain. *Spine.* 2000;25(2):218–223.

122. Nachemson AL. The lumbar spine: an orthopaedic challenge. *Spine.* 1976;1:59–71.

123. Hildebrandt RW. Chiropractic spinography and postural roentgenology, I. *J Manipulative Physiol Ther.* 1980;3:87–92.

124. Bogduk N, Aprill C, Derby R. Selective nerve root blocks. In: Wilson DJ, ed. *Interventional Radiography of the Musculoskeletal System*. London: Arnold Publishing; 1995.

125. Slosar PJ, White AH, Wetzel T. The use of selective nerve root blocks: diagnostic, therapeutic, or placebo? *Spine*. 1998;23(20):2253–2256.

126. Chou R, Qaseem A, Snow V, et al. Diagnosis and treatment of low back pain: a joint clinical practice guideline from the American College of Physicians and the American Pain Society. *Ann Intern Med*. 2007;147(7):478–491.

127. Ammendolia C, Furlan AD, Imamura M, Irvin E, van Tulder M. Evidence-informed management of chronic low back pain with needle acupuncture. *Spine J*. 2008;8(1):160–172.

128. Chang V, Gonzalez P, Akuthota V. Evidence-informed management of chronic low back pain with adjunctive analgesics. *Spine J*. 2008;8(1):21–27.

129. Brox JI, Storheim K, Grotle M, Tveito TH, Indahl A, Eriksen HR. Evidence-informed management of chronic low back pain with back schools, brief education, and fear avoidance training. *Spine J*. 2008;8(1):28–39.

130. Gatchel RJ, Rollings KH. Evidence-informed management of chronic low back pain with cognitive behavioral therapy. *Spine J*. 2008;8(1):40–44.

131. Depalma MJ, Slipman CW. Evidence-informed management of chronic low back pain with epidural steroid injections. *Spine J*. 2008;8(1):45–55.

132. Mayer J, Mooney V, Dagenais S. Evidence-informed management of chronic low back pain with lumbar extensor strengthening exercises. *Spine J*. 2008;8(1):96–113.

133. Bogduk N. Evidence-informed management of chronic low back pain with facet injections and radio-frequency neurotomy. *Spine J*. 2008;8(1):56–64.

134. Gatchel RJ, Mayer TG. Evidence-informed management of chronic low back pain with functional restoration. *Spine J*. 2008;8(1):65–69.

135. Gagnier JJ. Evidence-informed management of chronic low back pain with herbal, vitamin, mineral, and homeopathic supplements. *Spine J*. 2008;8(1):70–79.

136. Derby R, Baker RM, Lee CH, Anderson PA. Evidence informed management of chronic low back pain with intradiscal electrothermal therapy. *Spine J*. 2008;8(1):80–95.

137. Standaert CJ, Weinstein SM, Rumpeltes J. Evidence-informed management of chronic low back pain with lumbar stabilization exercises. *Spine J*. 2008;8(1):114–120.

138. Imamura M, Furlan AD, Dryden T, Irvin E. Evidence-informed management of chronic low back pain with massage. *Spine J*. 2008;8(1):121–133.

139. May S, Donelson R. Evidence-informed management of chronic low back pain with the McKenzie method. *Spine J*. 2008;8(1):134–141.

140. Dagenais S, Mayer J, Wooley JR, Haldeman S. Evidence informed management of chronic low back pain with medicine-assisted manipulation. *Spine J*. 2008;8(1):142–149.

141. Malanga G, Wolff E. Evidence-informed management of chronic low back pain with nonsteroidal anti-inflammatory drugs, muscle relaxants, and simple analgesics. *Spine J*. 2008;8(1):173–184.

142. Derby R, Baker RM, Lee CH. Evidence-informed management of chronic low back pain with minimally invasive nuclear decompression. *Spine J*. 2008;8(1):150–159.

143. Schofferman J, Mazanec D. Evidence-informed management of chronic low back pain with opioid analgesics. *Spine J*. 2008;8(1):185–194.

144. Wai EK, Rodriguez S, Dagenais S, Hall H. Evidence-informed management of chronic low back pain with physical activity, smoking cessation, and weight loss. *Spine J*. 2008;8(1):195–202.

145. Murphy DR, Hurwitz EL. Application of a diagnosis-based clinical decision guide in patients with low back pain. *Chiropr Man Therap*. 2011;19:26.

146. Poitras S, Brosseau L. Evidence-informed management of chronic low back pain with transcutaneous electrical nerve stimulation, interferential current, electrical muscle stimulation, ultrasound, and thermotherapy. *Spine J*. 2008;8(1):226–233.

147. Dagenais S, Mayer J, Haldeman S, Borg-Stein J. Evidence-informed management of chronic low back pain with prolotherapy. *Spine J*. 2008;8(1):203–212.

148. Don AS, Carragee E. A brief overview of evidence-informed management of chronic low back pain with surgery. *Spine J*. 2008;8(1):258–265.

149. Gay RE, Brault JS. Evidence-informed management of chronic low back pain with traction therapy. *Spine J*. 2008;8(1):234–242.

150. Malanga G, Wolff E. Evidence-informed management of chronic low back pain with trigger point injections. *Spine J*. 2008;8(1):243–252.

151. Galhom AE, al-Shatouri MA. Efficacy of therapeutic fluoroscopy-guided lumbar spine interventional procedures. *Clin Imaging*. 2013;37(4):649–656.

152. Manchikanti L, Buenaventura RM, Manchikanti KN, et al. Effectiveness of therapeutic lumbar

transforaminal epidural steroid injections in managing lumbar spinal pain. *Pain Physician*. 2012;15(3):E199–245.

153. Riew KD, Park JB, Cho YS, et al. Nerve root blocks in the treatment of lumbar radicular pain. A minimum five-year follow-up. *J Bone Joint Surg Am*. Aug 2006;88(8):1722–1725.

154. Epstein NE. The risks of epidural and transforaminal steroid injections in the Spine: commentary and a comprehensive review of the literature. *Surg Neurol Int*. 2013;4(Suppl 2):S74–93.

155. Mehra M, Hill K, Nicholl D, Schadrack J. The burden of chronic low back pain with and without a neuropathic component: a healthcare resource use and cost analysis. *J Med Econ*. 2012;15(2):245–252.

156. McMorland G, Suter E, Casha S, du Plessis SJ, Hurlbert RJ. Manipulation or microdiscectomy for sciatica? A prospective randomized clinical study. *J Manipulative Physiol Ther*. 2010;33(8):576–584.

157. Proietti L, Scaramuzzo L, Schiro GR, Sessa S, Logroscino CA. Complications in lumbar spine surgery: a retrospective analysis. *Indian J Orthop*. 2012;47(4):340–345.

158. Street JT, Lenehan BJ, DiPaola CP, et al. Morbidity and mortality of major adult spinal surgery. A prospective cohort analysis of 942 consecutive patients. *Spine J*. 2012;12(1):22–34.

159. Fineberg SJ, Oglesby M, Patel AA, Pelton MA, Singh K. The incidence and mortality of thromboembolic events in lumbar spine surgery. *Spine (Phila Pa 1976)*. 2013;38(13):1154–1159.

160. Jacobs WC, van der Gaag NA, Kruyt MC, et al. Total disc replacement for chronic discogenic low back pain: a Cochrane review. *Spine (Phila Pa 1976)*. 2013;38(1):24–36.

161. Keeney BJ, Fulton-Kehoe D, Turner JA, Wickizer TM, Chan KC, Franklin GM. Early predictors of lumbar spine surgery after occupational back injury: results from a prospective study of workers in Washington State. *Spine (Phila Pa 1976)*. 2012;38(11):953–64.

162. Goldschlager T, Oehme D, Ghosh P, Zannettino A, Rosenfeld JV, Jenkin G. Current and future applications for stem cell therapies in spine surgery. *Curr Stem Cell Res Ther*. Sep 2013;8(5):381–393.

163. Goldschlager T, Jenkin G, Ghosh P, Zannettino A, Rosenfeld JV. Potential applications for using stem cells in spine surgery. *Curr Stem Cell Res Ther*. 2010;5(4):345–355.

164. Haldeman S, Chapman-Smith D, Petersen DM, Jr. *Guidelines for Chiropractic Quality Assurance and Practice Parameters: Proceedings of the Mercy Center Consensus Conference*. Gaithersburg, MD: Aspen Publishers, Inc.; 1993.

165. Bronfort G, Haas M, Evans RL, Bouter LM. Efficacy of spinal manipulation and mobilization for low back pain and neck pain: a systematic review and best evidence synthesis. *Spine J*. 2004;4(3):335–356.

166. Santilli V, Beghi E, Finucci S. Chiropractic manipulation in the treatment of acute back pain and sciatica with disc protrusion: a randomized double-blind clinical trial of active and simulated spinal manipulations. *Spine J*. 2006;6(2):131–137.

167. Albert HB, Manniche C. The efficacy of systematic active conservative treatment for patients with severe sciatica: a single-blind, randomized, clinical, controlled trial. *Spine (Phila Pa 1976)*. 2012;37(7):531–542.

168. Petersen T, Larsen K, Nordsteen J, Olsen S, Fournier G, Jacobsen S. The McKenzie method compared with manipulation when used adjunctive to information and advice in low back pain patients presenting with centralization or peripheralization: a randomized controlled trial. *Spine (Phila Pa 1976)*. 2011;36(24):1999–2010.

169. Peterson CK, Leemann S, Lechmann M, Pfirrmann CW, Hodler J, Humphreys BK. Symptomatic magnetic resonance imaging-confirmed lumbar disk herniation patients: a comparative effectiveness prospective observational study of 2 age- and sex-matched cohorts treated with either high-velocity, low-amplitude spinal manipulative therapy or imaging-guided lumbar nerve root injections. *J Manipulative Physiol Ther*. May 2013;36(4):218–225.

170. Kreiner DS, Hwang SW, Easa JE, et al. An evidence-based clinical guideline for the diagnosis and treatment of lumbar disc herniation with radiculopathy. *Spine J*. 2014;14(1):180–191.

171. Haas M, Groupp E, Kraemer DF. Dose-response for chiropractic care of chronic low back pain. *Spine J*. 2004;4(5):574–583.

172. Haas M, Vavrek D, Peterson D, Polissar N, Neradilek MB. Dose-response and efficacy of spinal manipulation for care of chronic low back pain: a randomized controlled trial. *Spine J*. 2013:S1529–9430(13)01390–9.

173. Rupert RL. A survey of practice patterns and the health promotion and prevention attitudes

of US chiropractors. Maintenance care: Part I. *J Manipulative Physiol Ther.* 2000;23(1):1–9.

174. Descarreaux M, Blouin JS, Drolet M, Papadimitriou S, Teasdale N. Efficacy of preventive spinal manipulation for chronic low-back pain and related disabilities: a preliminary study. *J Manipulative Physiol Ther.* 2004;27(8):509–514.

175. Flynn T, Fritz J, Whitman J, et al. A clinical prediction rule for classifying patients with low back pain who demonstrate short-term improvement with spinal manipulation. *Spine.* 2002;27:2835–2843.

176. Axen I, Rosenbaum A, Robech R, et al. Can patient reactions to the first chiropractic treatment predict early favorable treatment outcome in persistent low back pain? *J Manipulative Physiol Ther.* 2002;25:450–454.

177. Liebenson C. Why some patients don't get better with traditional chiropractic care, and how rehabilitation can help. *Dynamic Chiropractic.* 2003;21:28–34.

178. Indahl A, Velund L, Eikeras O. Good prognosis for low back pain when left untampered: a randomized clinical trial. *Spine.* 1995;20:473–477.

179. Linton SJ, Anderson T. Can chronic disability be prevented? A randomized trial of a cognitive-behavior intervention and two forms of information for patients with spinal pain. *Spine.* 2000;25:2825–2831.

180. Williams NH, Hendry M, Lewis R, Russell I, Westmoreland A, Wilkinson C. Psychological response in spinal manipulation (PRISM): a systematic review of psychological outcomes in randomised controlled trials. *Complement Ther Med.* 2007;15(4):271–283.

181. Cai C, Pua YH, Lim KC. A clinical prediction rule for classifying patients with low back pain who demonstrate short-term improvement with mechanical lumbar traction. *Eur Spine J.* 2009;18(4):554–561.

182. Fritz JM, Lindsay W, Matheson JW, et al. Is there a subgroup of patients with low back pain likely to benefit from mechanical traction? Results of a randomized clinical trial and subgrouping analysis. *Spine (Phila Pa 1976).* 2007;32(26):E793–800.

183. Tilbrook HE, Cox H, Hewitt CE, et al. Yoga for chronic low back pain: a randomized trial. *Ann Intern Med.* 2011;155(9):569–578.

184. Cramer H, Lauche R, Haller H, Dobos G. A systematic review and meta-analysis of yoga for low back pain. *Clin J Pain.* 2013;29(5):450–460.

185. Choi BK, Verbeek JH, Tam WW, Jiang JY. Exercises for prevention of recurrences of low-back pain. *Occup Environ Med.* 2011;67(11):795–796.

186. Bronfort G, Maiers MJ, Evans RL, et al. Supervised exercise, spinal manipulation, and home exercise for chronic low back pain: a randomized clinical trial. *Spine J.* 2011;11(7):585–598.

187. Long A, Donelson R, Fung T. Does it matter which exercise? A randomized control trial of exercise for low back pain. *Spine.* 2004;29(23):2593–2602.

188. Albert HB, Manniche C. The efficacy of systematic active conservative treatment for patients with severe sciatica: a single-blind, randomized, clinical, controlled trial. *Spine (Phila Pa 1976).* 2012;37(7):531–542.

189. Mulligan B. *Manual Therapy: NAGS, SNAGS, MWMS, etc.* 5th ed. Wellington, New Zealand: Plain View Services Ltd.; 2005.

190. Hansen D. Determining how much care to give and reporting patient progress. *Top Clin Chiro.* 1994;1(4):1–8.

191. Cassidy JD, Thiel HW, Kirkaldy-Willis WH. Side posture manipulation for lumbar disc herniation. *J Manipulative Physiol Ther.* 1993;16:96–103.

192. Kovacs FM, Abraira V, Pozo F, et al. Local and remote sustained trigger point therapy for exacerbations of chronic low back pain. A randomized, double-blind, controlled, multicenter trial. *Spine.* 1997;22(7):786–797.

193. Klein RG, Eek BC, DeLong WB, Mooney V. A randomized double-blind trial of dextrose-glycerin-phenol injections for chronic, low back pain. *J Spinal Disord.* 1993;6(1):23–33.

194. Dechow E, Davies RK, Carr AJ, Thompson PW. A randomized, double-blind, placebo-controlled trial of sclerosing injections in patients with chronic low back pain. *Rheumatology.* 1999;38(12):1255–1259.

195. van Tulder MN, Scholten RJ, Koes BW, Deyo RA. Nonsteroidal anti-inflammatory drugs for low back pain: a systematic review within the framework of the Cochrane Collaboration Back Review Group. *Spine.* 2000;25: 2501–2513.

196. Cherkin DC, Eisenberg D, Sherman KJ, et al. Randomized trial comparing traditional Chinese medical acupuncture, therapeutic massage, and self-care education for chronic low back pain. *Arch Intern Med.* 2001;161:1081–1088.

197. Lee JH, Choi TY, Lee MS, Lee H, Shin BC, Lee H. Acupuncture for acute low back pain: a systematic review. *Clin J Pain.* 2013;29(2):172–185.

198. Cho YJ, Song YK, Cha YY, et al. Acupuncture for chronic low back pain: a multicenter, randomized,

patient-assessor blind, sham-controlled clinical trial. *Spine (Phila Pa 1976).* 2013;38(7):549–557.

199. Lam M, Curry P. Effectiveness of acupuncture for nonspecific chronic low back pain: a systematic review and meta-analysis. *Spine (Phila Pa 1976).* 2013;38(24):2124–2138.

200. Hayden JA, van Tulder MW, Malmivaara AV, Koes BW. Meta-analysis: exercise therapy for nonspecific low back pain. *Ann Intern Med.* 2005;142(9):765–775.

201. Rydeard R, Leger A, Smith D. Pilates-based therapeutic exercise: effect on subjects with nonspecific chronic low back pain and functional disability: a randomized controlled trial. *J Orthop Sports Phys Ther.* 2006;36(7):472–484.

202. Faas A, Chavannes AW, van Eijk, Gubbels JW. A randomized, placebo-controlled trial of exercise therapy in patients with acute low back pain. *Spine.* 1993;18(11):1388–1395.

203. Nelson BW, O'Reilly E, Miller M, et al. The clinical effects of intensive, specific exercise on chronic low-back pain: a controlled study of 895 consecutive patients with one year follow-up. *Orthopaedics.* 1995;10(10):971–981.

204. Mannion AF, Mentener M, Taimela S, Dvorak J. A randomized clinical trial of three active therapies for chronic low back pain. *Spine.* 1999;24(23):2433–2448.

205. Daltroy LH, Iversen MD, Martin SD, et al. A controlled trial of an educational program to prevent low back injuries. *N Engl J Med.* 1997;337:322–330.

206. Martimo KP, Verbeek J, Karppinen J, et al. Effect of training and lifting equipment for preventing back pain in lifting and handling: systematic review. *BMJ.* 2008.

207. Martimo KP, Verbeek J, Karppinen J, et al. Manual material handling advice and assistive devices for preventing and treating back pain in workers. *Cochrane Database Syst Rev.* 2007(3):CD005958.

208. Schmidt K, Ekholm J, Harris-Ringadahl K, et al. Effects of changes in sitting work posture on static neck and shoulder muscle activity. *Ergonomics.* 1986;29:1525.

209. Grandjean E. *Fitting the Task to the Man.* 4th ed. London: Taylor and Frances; 1988.

210. Hartvigsen J, Christensen K. Active lifestyle protects against incident low back pain in seniors: a population-based 2-year prospective study of 1387 Danish twins aged 70–100 years. *Spine.* 2007;32(1):76–81.

211. Engers A, Jellema P, Wnesing M, van der Windt D, Grol R, van Tudder M. Individual patient education for low back pain. *Cochrane Database of Systematic Review.* 2008(1):CD4004057.

212. Gagnier JJ, van Tulder MW, Berman B, Bombardier C. Herbal medicine for low back pain: a Cochrane review. *Spine.* 2007;32(1):82–92.

213. Kuslich SD, Ulstrom CL, Michael CJ. The tissue origin of low back pain and sciatica: a report of pain response to tissue stimulation during operation on the lumbar spine using local anesthesia. *Orthop Clin North Am.* 1991; 22:181–187.

214. Murphy DR, Hurwitz EL, Gerrard JK, Clary R. Pain patterns and descriptions in patients with radicular pain: does the pain necessarily follow a specific dermatome? *Chiropr Osteopat.* 2009;17:9.

215. Lauder TM. Physical examination signs, clinical symptoms, and their relationship to electrodiagnostic findings and the presence of radiculopathy. *Phys Med Rehabil Clin N Am.* 2002:451–467.

216. Jensen TS, Albert HB, Soerensen JS, Manniche C, Leboeuf-Yde C. Natural course of disc morphology in patients with sciatica: an MRI study using a standardized qualitative classification system. *Spine (Phila Pa 1976).* 2006;31(14):1605–1612; discussion 1613.

217. Derby R, Eek B, Ryan DP. Intradiscal electrothermal annuloplasty. *Scientific Newsletter of the International Spinal Injection Society.* 1998;3:1.

218. Saal JA. Natural history and nonoperative treatment of lumbar disc herniation. *Spine.* 1996;21:2S–9S.

219. Davis H. Increasing rates of cervical and lumbar spine surgery in the United States 1979–1990. *Spine.* 1994;19:117–124.

220. Atlas SJ, Keller RB, Chang Y, Deyo RA, Singer DE. Surgical and nonsurgical management of sciatica secondary to a lumbar disc herniation: five-year outcomes from the Maine Lumbar Spine Study. *Spine.* 2001;26:1179–1187.

221. McCulloch JA. Focus issue on lumbar disc herniation: macro- and microdiscectomy. *Spine.* 1996;21:45S–55S.

222. Weinstein JN, Lurie JD, Tosteson TD, et al. Surgical vs nonoperative treatment for lumbar disk herniation: the Spine Patient Outcomes Research Trial (SPORT) observational cohort. *JAMA.* 2006;296(20):2451–2459.

223. Weinstein JN, Tosteson TD, Lurie JD, et al. Surgical vs nonoperative treatment for lumbar

disk herniation: the Spine Patient Outcomes Research Trial (SPORT): a randomized trial. *JAMA.* 2006;296(20):2441–2450.

224. Mariconda M, Galasso O, Secondulfo V, Rotonda GD, Milano C. Minimum 25-year outcome and functional assessment of lumbar discectomy. *Spine.* 2006;31(22):2593–2599; discussion 2600–2601.

225. Sasso RC, Foulk DM, Hahn M. Prospective, randomized trial of metal-on-metal artificial lumbar disc replacement: initial results for treatment of discogenic pain. *Spine.* 2008;33(2):123–131.

226. Giles LGF. Pathoanatomical studies and clinical significance of lumbar zygapophyseal (facet) joints. *J Manipulative Physiol Ther.* 1992;15:36–40.

227. Cramer GD, Gregerson DM, Knudsen JT, et al. The effects of side-posture positioning and spinal adjusting on the lumbar Z joints: a randomized controlled trial with sixty-four subjects. *Spine.* 2002;27:2459–2466.

228. Van Kleef M, Barendse GA, Kessels A, et al. Randomized trial of radiofrequency lumbar facet denervation for chronic low back pain. *Spine.* 1999;24(18):1937–1942.

229. Goupille P, Fitoussi V, Cotty P, et al. Injection into the lumbar vertebrae in chronic low back pain. Results in 206 patients. *Rev Rheum Ed Fr.* 1993;60(11):797–801.

230. Fanuele JC, Birkmeyer NJ, Abdu WA, Tosteson TD, Weinstein JN. The impact of spinal problems on the health status of patients: have we underestimated the effect? *Spine.* 2000;25(12):1509–1514.

231. Hart LG, Deyo RA, Cherkin DC. Physician office visits for low back pain. Frequency, clinical evaluation, and treatment patterns from a U.S. national survey. *Spine.* 1995;20(1):11–19.

232. Turner JA, Ersek M, Herron L, Deyo R. Surgery for lumbar spinal stenosis: attempted meta-analysis of the literature. *Spine.* 1992;17:1–8.

233. Stolov WC, Slimp JC. Dermatomal somatosensory evoked potentials in lumbar spinal stenosis. In: *American Association of Electromyography and Electrodiagnosis and American Electroencephalography Society Joint Symposium.* San Diego, CA: American Association of Electromyography and Electrodiagnosis and American Electroencephalography Society; 1988:17–22.

234. Johnsson KE, Uden A, Rosen I. The effect of compression on the natural course of spinal stenosis: a comparison of surgically treated and untreated patients. *Spine.* 1991;16:615–619.

235. Simotas AC, Dorey FJ, Hansraj KK, Cammisa F, Jr. Nonoperative treatment for lumbar spinal stenosis: clinical and outcome results and a 3-year survivorship analysis. *Spine.* 2000;25(2):197–204.

236. Atlas SJ, Keller RB, Robson D, Deyo RA, Singer DE. Surgical and nonsurgical management of lumbar spinal stenosis: four-year outcomes from the main lumbar spine study. *Spine.* 2000;25:556–562.

237. Malmivaara A, Slatis P, Heliovaara M, et al. Surgical or nonoperative treatment for lumbar spinal stenosis? A randomized controlled trial. *Spine.* 2007;32(1):1–8.

238. Weinstein JN, Tosteson TD, Lurie JD, et al. Surgical versus nonsurgical therapy for lumbar spinal stenosis. *N Engl J Med.* 2008;358(8):794–810.

239. Aalto TJ, Malmivaara A, Kovacs F, et al. Preoperative predictors for postoperative clinical outcome in lumbar spinal stenosis: systematic review. *Spine.* 2006;31(18):E648–663.

240. Whitman JM, Flynn TW, Childs JD, et al. A comparison between two physical therapy treatment programs for patients with lumbar spinal stenosis: a randomized clinical trial. *Spine.* 2006;31(22):2541–2549.

241. McKee BM, Alexander WJ, Dunbar JS. Spondylolysis and spondylolisthesis in children: a review. *J Can Assoc Radiol.* 1971;22:100.

242. Jacobsen S, Sonne-Holm S, Rovsing H, Monrad H, Gebuhr P. Degenerative lumbar spondylolisthesis: an epidemiological perspective: the Copenhagen Osteoarthritis Study. *Spine.* 2007;32(1):120–125.

243. Whitesides TE, Jr., Horton WC, Hutton WC, Hodges L. Spondylolytic spondylolisthesis: a study of pelvic and lumbosacral parameters of possible etiologic effect in two genetically and geographically distinct groups with high occurrence. *Spine.* 2005;30(6 Suppl):S12–21.

244. Labelle H, Roussouly P, Berthonnaud E, Dimnet J, O'Brien M. The importance of spino-pelvic balance in L5-S1 developmental spondylolisthesis: a review of pertinent radiologic measurements. *Spine.* 2005;30(6 Suppl):S27–34.

245. Schwab FJ, Farcy JP, Roye DP, Jr. The sagittal pelvic tilt index as a criterion in the evaluation of spondylolisthesis. Preliminary observations. *Spine.* 1997;22:1661–1667.

246. Fredrickson BE, Baker D, McKollick WJ, et al. The natural history of spondylolysis and spondylolisthesis. *J Bone Joint Surg Am.* 1984;66:699.

247. Cassidy JD, Porter GE, Kirkaldy-Willis WH. Manipulative management of back pain patients with spondylolisthesis. *J Can Chiro Assoc.* 1978;22:15.

248. McKenzie-Brown AM, Shah RV, Sehgal N, Everett CR. A systematic review of sacroiliac joint interventions. *Pain Physician.* 2005;8(1):115–125.

249. Hansen HC, McKenzie-Brown AM, Cohen SP, Swicegood JR, Colson JD, Manchikanti L. Sacroiliac joint interventions: a systematic review. *Pain Physician.* 2007; 10(1):165–184.

250. Hendler N, Kozikowski JG, Morrison C, Sethuraman G. Diagnosis and management of sacroiliac joint disease. *J Neuromusc Syst.* 1995;3:169–174.

251. Richardson CA, Snijdera CJ, Hides JA, et al. The relation between the transversus abdominis muscles, sacroiliac joint mechanics and low back pain. *Spine.* 2002;27:399–405.

252. Pace JB, Nagel D. Piriformis syndrome. *West J Med.* 1976;124:435–439.

253. Amor B, Dougados M, Mijuyawa M. Critere diagnostique der spondyloarthopathies. *Rev Rheum Mal Osteoartic.* 1990;57:85–89.

254. van der Linden S, Valkenburg HA, Cats A. Evaluation of diagnostic criteria for ankylosing spondylitis. *Arthritis Rheum.* 1984;27:361–368.

255. Dougados M. Diagnostic features of ankylosing spondylitis. *Br. J Rheumatol.* 1985;34:301–303.

256. Calin A, MacKay K, Santos H, Brophy S. A new dimension to outcome application of the Bath Ankylosing Spondylitis Radiology Index. *J Rheumatol.* 1999;26:988–992.

257. Garrett S, Jenkinson T, Kennedy LG, et al. A new approach to defining disease status in ankylosing spondylitis: the Bath Ankylosing Spondylitis Disease Activity Index. *J Rheumatol.* 1994;21:2286–2291.

258. Doran MF, Brophy S, MacKay K, et al. Predictors of long-term outcome in ankylosing spondylitis. *J Rheumatol.* 2003;30:316–320.

259. Yochum TR, Rowe LJ. *Essentials of Skeletal Radiology.* 3rd ed. Baltimore: Williams & Wilkins; 1996;2:877–892.

260. ZN, Bilgie A, Kennedy LG, Calin A. Interleukin-6, acute phase reactants and clinical status in ankylosing spondylitis: a preliminary study. *Br J Rheumatol.* 1993;32:498–506.

261. Kennedy LG, Edmonds L, Calin A. The natural history of ankylosing spondylitis: does it burn out? *J Rheumatol.* 1993;20:688.

262. McDermaid C, Mior S. Ankylosing spondylitis presenting to a chiropractic office: a report of two cases. *JOCA.* 2000;44(2):87–97.

263. Henderson S. Rehabilitation techniques in ankylosing spondylitis management: a case report. *J Can Chiro Assoc.* 2003;47(3):161–167.

264. Ince G, Sarpel T, Durgun B, Erdogan S. Effects of a multimodal exercise program for people with ankylosing spondylitis. *Phys Ther.* 2006;86(7):924–935.

265. Mandelli F, Avvisati G, Tribalto M. Biology and treatment of multiple myeloma. *Curr Opin Oncol.* 1992;4:73.

266. Kakafika AI, Mikhailidis DP. Smoking and aortic diseases. *Circ J.* 2007;71(8):1173–1180.

267. USPSTF. *The Guide to Clinical Preventive Services.* McLean, Virginia: International Medical Publishing, Inc.; 2007.

268. LaRoy LL, Cormier PJ, Matalon TAS, et al. Imaging of abdominal aortic aneurysms. *Am J Roentgenol.* 1989;152:785.

269. Scott RA. Is surgery necessary for abdominal aortic aneurysm less than 6 cm diameter? *Lancet.* 1993;342:1395.

270. Ernst CB. Abdominal aortic aneurysms. *N Engl J Med.* 1993;328:1167.

APPENDIX 6-2

Low Back Diagnosis Table

Diagnosis	Comments	History Findings	Positive Examination Findings	Radiography/Special Studies	Treatment Options
Segmental dysfunction of: Thoracolumbar Joints Lumbar or Lumbosacral Joints SI Joint Pelvis	• Should be used when chiropractic manipulation is used as Tx for any low back problem/Dx. • Can be primary Dx if patient is asymptomatic or mildly symptomatic. • Must indicate chiropractic exam findings to support Dx.	Nonspecific	*Palpation*—local tenderness or other signs of subluxation *Ortho*—None *Neuro*—None *Active ROM*—Variable restriction *Passive ROM*—Endrange restriction *Motion palpation*—specific vertebral segmental restriction or symptoms produced on endrange	• Radiography not required for the diagnosis of subluxation. • Radiographic biomechanical analysis may assist in treatment decisions. • For specifics see radiographic guidelines.	• Chiropractic manipulative therapy (CMT). • Decisions regarding specifically which technique(s) is/are applied and modifications to the given approach will be directed by the primary Dx and patient's ability to tolerate preadjustment stresses.
Lumbosacral Sprain/Strain Sacroiliac Sprain/Strain Lumbar Sprain/Strain Note: sprain/strain is not synonymous with spasm or hypertonicity	• Should be reserved for acute traumatic	*Trauma*—Overstretch or overcontraction Hx as acute event *Radiation of pain*—Possible (referred) *Pain radiation with Valsalva-type activities*—No *Worse with specific ROM*—Contraction of muscle or stretch of muscle or joint	*Ortho*—None *Neuro*—None *Active ROM*—Pain on active ROM that contracts involved muscles *Passive ROM*—Pain on endrange stretch of involved muscle or ligament	• Radiography not required for diagnosis. • With significant trauma or for med/legal purposes, radiographs may be required. • For specifics, see radiographic guidelines.	• Myofascial therapy. • Limited orthotic support. • Ergonomic advice. • Preventive exercises and stretches (e.g., spinal stabilization exercises).
Ankylosing Spondylitis	• Dx is radiographic, directed by P.E. findings of restriction of LB ROM of gradual onset with progression.	*Onset*—Stiffness is progressive; pain is not major feature *Pain radiation*—Uncommon *ROM comments*—All ROM affected; stiffness alleviated by mild exercise/stretching	*Ortho*—None *Neuro*—None *Active & passive ROM*—Global restriction with mild endrange discomfort *Motion palpation*—Possible restriction globally and at SI joint	• Radiography required for Dx. • HLA-B27 not recommended due to non-specificity.	• Myofascial therapy. • Physiotherapy. • Daily exercises and stretches.

(continues)

Low Back Diagnosis Table (continued)

Diagnosis	Comments	History Findings	Positive Examination Findings	Radiography/Special Studies	Treatment Options
Neuritis or Radiculitis Due to Disc	• Requires hard neurological evidence of nerve root dysfunction. • Special imaging is required for diagnosis.	*Trauma*—Often Hx of similar events with resolution; major or minor trauma possible *Radiation of pain*—Often into leg down to foot *Pain radiation with Valsalva-type activities*—Possible *Worse with specific ROM*—Variable; may be related to position of disc protrusion	*Ortho*—Nerve stretch tests positive (e.g., SLR, WLR) *Neuro*—deficit in corresponding dermatome, myotome, and DTR *Active ROM*—Variable; weakness more in related lower limb muscle(s) *Passive ROM*—Variable	• Radiography may be used; however, not usually required initially. • MRI or electrodiagnostic studies may be needed after one month without resolution or if progressive.	• Limited orthotic support. • When subacute begin spinal stabilization.
General Code for Low Back Pain (Mechanical Low Back Pain)	• Used for patients with evidence of a myofascial cause. • Also used for patients without Hx of recent trauma. • May be used for unspecified low back pain.	*Trauma*—Not recent *Radiation of pain*—May radiate into buttocks or leg; not below knee *Pain radiation with Valsalva-type activities*—No *Worse with specific ROM*—variable	*Ortho*—None positive, however, may reproduce symptoms *Neuro*—None (although patient may have neurological complaints such as numbness) *Active ROM*—Variable *Passive ROM*—Variable	• Radiography not necessary. • May be used to access biomechanical status or predisposition. • See PCCW Radiographic Guidelines.	• Myofascial therapy. • Limited orthotic support. • Ergonomic advice. • Preventive exercises and stretches (e.g., spinal stabilization exercises).
Neuritis or Radiculitis Unspecified	• Used in cases where there are radicular signs/symptoms; however, not enough evidence to pinpoint disc vs. other causes. • Used with radicular signs/symptoms where no specific nerve root is clearly involved.	*Trauma*—Variable presentation *Radiation of pain*—May radiate down leg to foot *Pain radiation with Valsalva-type activities*—possible *Worse with specific ROM*—variable	*Ortho*—Nerve stretch tests positive (e.g., SLR, WLR) *Neuro*—Deficit in corresponding dermatome, myotome, and DTR *Active ROM*—Variable weakness *Passive ROM*—Variable	• Radiography suggested if spinal origin is suspected. • MRI or electrodiagnostic studies may be needed after one month without resolution or if progressive.	• Limited orthotic support. • When subacute begin spinal stabilization.

Condition	Indications/Notes	History	Examination	Imaging	Management
Facet Syndrome	• Should be reserved for LBP increased with hyperextension posture or movement (acute or chronic) with local pain or referred pain into the leg.	*Trauma*—Variable *Radiation of pain*—Often into leg down to knee (occasionally to the foot) *Pain radiation with Valsalva-type activities*—May be painful *Worse with specific ROM*—hyperextension increases local or radiating pain	*Ortho*—Kemps or hyperextension maneuvers *Neuro*—None *Active ROM*—Variable *Passive ROM*—Variable *Motion palpation*—Endrange restriction to side of involved facet	• Radiography may be useful in identifying various lines of mensuration indicating posterior weightbearing, facet arthrosis, or facet imbrication.	• Myofascial therapy. • Limited orthotic support. • Ergonomic advice. • Preventive exercises and stretches (e.g., spinal stabilization exercises). • Avoid hyperextension initially.
Neuralgia or Neuritis of Sciatic Nerve	• May be used for piriformis syndrome. • Not to be used for a discogenic cause of sciatica.	*Trauma*—Variable *Radiation of pain*—May radiate into buttocks or leg *Pain radiation with Valsalva-type activities*—No *Worse with specific ROM*—May be worse with internal or external rotation of hip	*Ortho*—Possible increase with SLR or other nerve root tension tests and internal rotation of hip *Neuro*—May be sensory abnormality, often hyperesthesia *Active ROM*—Internal or external rotation of hip may provoke *Passive ROM*—Internal rotation of hip	• Radiography not recommended.	• Myofascial therapy to piriformis muscle. • Strengthen and/or stretch of piriformis. • PT for acute pain; deep heat or interferrential.
Ankylosis or Instability of SI or Lumbosacral Joint	• Chronic instability or chronic sprain or strain of low back or SI. • Used with repetitive postural (occupational) mechanical stresses.	*Trauma*—Variable; report of repeated occurrences of pain *Radiation of pain*—Usually none *Pain radiation with Valsalva-type activities*—No	*Ortho*—Supported Adam's or belt test *Neuro*—None *Active ROM*—Variable *Passive ROM*—Variable *Motion palpation*—Hypermobility of SI joint when instability is present	• Radiography may be necessary in differential if there are repeated occurrences.	• Temporary SI support. • Exercises to strengthen lower back and pelvis.

Shoulder Girdle Complaints

Context

Shoulder pain in the general population has been reported to be as high as 50% in some countries.[1] The range is between 20%–50%. Chronic shoulder pain appears to be common. At six months following initial evaluation 34% to 79% of patients report still having shoulder symptoms[2-6] with 24% to 61% reporting pain 6 to 18 months beyond the initial six-month follow-up. Most disturbing is that only about half of the elderly who reported having shoulder symptoms sought treatment. Poor recovery from shoulder pain was associated with increasing age, severe or recurrent symptoms, restricted range of passive abduction, or with concomitant neck pain.[7] The presentation of mild trauma or overuse occurring before the onset of shoulder pain, acute onset, and early presentation to a caregiver indicated a favorable outcome.

The shoulder provides a unique diagnostic challenge. The shoulder's dependency on an integrated, position-dependent system of ligaments, muscles, and tendons for stability, coupled with the need for coordinated interaction of a number of joints, makes it a complex region to assess. When a single-event trauma occurs, soft tissue or bony damage is usually discovered by challenge on physical examination and/or radiographs. When trauma is not evident, however, it often becomes difficult to isolate a specific structure or cause. Many shoulder problems are, in fact, multidimensional. In other words, a patient with instability may develop an impingement phenomenon, or a patient with tendinitis or restricted mobility may overload the compensatory capacity of other structures, leading to further soft tissue involvement.

The unique design of the shoulder provides a great degree of mobility; however, as a result it cannot always provide substantial stability, especially at higher levels of elevation and/or extreme abduction. Therefore, local shoulder pain that occurs with these extremes of position is due to excessive demands on the stabilizing function of the muscles, ligaments, and capsule of the shoulder. In addition, mechanical or structural predisposition may narrow the variable space through which some tendons travel, resulting in an impingement phenomenon. These structures are rarely challenged in individuals whose work or play requires only minimal elevation.

Shoulder complaints are common in sports such as weight lifting, swimming, and throwing, or in an occupational setting requiring overhead work. In that context, injury, when not due to a single trauma, is often due to repetitive activity or overuse. These problems can often be linked to specific positional demands. Finally, the shoulder may be the site of injury when a fall onto an extended arm transforms the shoulder into a weight-bearing joint. Fracture, dislocation, tendon, or labrum damage must be considered.

The shoulder may be the site of pain originating or caused by a variety of sources, including the following:

- Referred pain from a variety of musculoskeletal sites such as cervical or thoracic spine facet joints or trigger points
- Referred pain from visceral sources such as the diaphragm, gallbladder, lungs, or heart
- Radicular pain from cervical nerve root compression
- Peripheral nerve and brachial plexus entrapments
- Local causes of pain
  - trauma (e.g., fracture, dislocation, tendon rupture)
  - overuse (e.g., tendinitis, capsular sprain, bursitis)
  - arthritide (e.g., osteoarthritis, rheumatoid arthritis, rheumatoid variants)
  - other (e.g., tumor or infection)

Although this list may seem overwhelming, the primary causes of shoulder complaints generally fall into several categories with some overlap, including the following:

- instability (traumatic or nontraumatic)
- impingement syndrome (anteromedial [subcoracoid]—subscapularis; anterolateral [subacromial]—biceps tendon, supraspinatus tendon, and subacromial bursa; posterolateral—posterior labrum and infraspinatus/teres minor tendons)
- tendinitis/bursitis
- osteoarthritis
- adhesive capsulitis
- acromioclavicular (AC) separations
- referred pain from the cervical spine

In the context of the chiropractic office setting, a common complaint is neck and shoulder/arm pain. With this presentation it is important to differentiate between neural referral versus radiculopathy. This differentiation requires a search for objective neurologic deficits. When not present, a mechanical or referral association is more likely. When the shoulder is part of a neck and arm complaint it is also important to consider brachial plexus involvement through overstretch (stinger) or compression (thoracic outlet syndrome) and a double-crush phenomenon.

Like all joints, the shoulder is susceptible to traumatic sequelae such as fracture, dislocation, and ligament or tendon rupture. When these are suspected, thorough radiographic and orthopaedic evaluations are necessary. If fracture or ligament/tendon rupture is found, an orthopaedic consultation is necessary. For most other conditions many practitioners[8] now recommend a conservative approach for at least six months.

In the elderly population, the accumulation of years of wear and tear leads to an end-stage of chronic irritation that results in osteoarthritis that may cycle into an impingement phenomenon. Degenerative labrum tears and rotator cuff tears are not uncommon in the senior, often becoming symptomatic with little or no trauma. The other common problem in the senior population is stiffening of the shoulder, sometimes due to adhesive capsulitis. Differentiating between the effects of osteoarthritis and adhesive capsulitis is an important element in approaching the stiffened senior shoulder.

Trauma, including surgery, may predispose the shoulder to early degenerative changes. Osteoarthritis may be more common than previously recognized.[9] Even when not evident radiographically, osteoarthritis has been demonstrated histologically. Therefore, osteoarthritis should be considered in the senior or posttraumatic patient. Arthritides that commonly affect the shoulder are ankylosing spondylitis and rheumatoid arthritis. Advanced rheumatoid arthritis often leads to rupture of the supraspinatus tendon. The shoulder may be a site of infection, although infrequently.

General Strategy

History

- Determine whether the patient's complaint is one of pain, stiffness, instability, weakness, numbness, or tingling.
- Localize the complaint to anterior, posterior, lateral, inferior, or superior.
- Determine whether there was a traumatic onset; if so, determine the mechanism and the need for immediate radiographic assessment before proceeding (possible fracture or dislocation).
- Determine any relationship to activity, with focus on position, degree of restriction, and amount of repetition (overhead position suggests possible impingement).
- Consider an acute calcific bursitis or the early phase of adhesive capsulitis if pain is the primary complaint with no history of trauma and all ranges of motion are painful. Also, Parsonage-Turner syndrome (i.e., brachial neuritis) may present with sudden, non-traumatic shoulder pain often following a respiratory infection.
- Determine whether there is a past injury if stiffness is the complaint; for specific ranges of restriction determine whether there was an antecedent period of moderate to severe pain that has gradually been replaced by stiffness (suggests adhesive capsulitis).
- If weakness is the complaint, determine whether the weakness is painless (suggests instability) or painful (inhibitory effect).
- Determine whether the patient has a history suggestive of damaged structures (i.e., anterior dislocation) or if the patient has a bilateral, multidirectional looseness indicative of generalized capsular laxity (nontraumatic) if instability is suspected.

- Determine the degree of functional impairment within the context of patient usage. Is the patient a high-end user, such as an athlete, or a low-end user such as a sedentary office worker?

Evaluation

- Perform a focus-based examination; however, begin with an evaluation of stability, given instability may be the cause of or contributor to other problems.
- Check for labrum damage, in particular, when instability or looseness is found or there is a history of trauma.
- Evaluate for impingement.
- Evaluate for specific muscle/tension involvement with palpation, muscle tests, and lag signs.
- Use findings to determine the need for further evaluation with regard to radiographic or special imaging, referral to a specialist, or initial management.

Management

- Dislocations should be relocated, preferably by an experienced individual; postreduction radiographs should be taken to determine whether an associated fracture is evident; rehabilitation of the shoulder is important to avoid recurrence.
- Infections, fractures, and tumors should be referred for orthopaedic consultation. Also, if the patient is in so much pain that it is interfering with the ability to sleep and is unaffected by over-the-counter medications, referral for prescribed pain medication should be made. This is most common with an acute subacromial bursitis and an early phase of adhesive capsulitis.
- All other shoulder disorders should be managed for six months with conservative approaches; if unresolved, consideration for special imaging should be given.

Relevant Anatomy and Biomechanics

The shoulder is capable of extreme mobility for the purpose of placing the upper limb in an almost infinite number of positions. For this mobility, a price is paid. From a bony support perspective, the shoulder is essentially unstable. As a result, the demand for constant integrated function is high for soft tissue structures delegated the job of providing that stability. This inherent instability becomes even more evident at higher degrees of shoulder elevation, making unusually high demands on coordinated muscular function. Damage to any of these soft tissue stabilizers results in increasing demands on the residual support structures. Add to this a repetitive demand from a sport or occupational perspective and the shoulder's ability to cope may be compromised (or overextended).

Depending on arm position and underlying pathologic processes, different aspects of the general capsular system are called into play. With the arm at the side, much of the support is ligamentous (superior glenohumeral ligament), with some contributions from a precarious glenoid ledge. Any relative abduction will cause an increased capsular and muscular contribution. A reciprocal contribution is most evident in the capsular structures, where stress is sequentially shared by the various capsular ligaments. With the arm at rest, the superior capsule contributes most. As the arm is elevated, the support management is shifted to the inferior capsular complex. This reciprocity also occurs with rotation. With the arm elevated, a hammock-like inferior capsule protects against inferior stress as well as anterior or posterior stress. With external rotation added to 90° abduction, the broad aspect of the capsule rotates in front of the humeral head while the posterior band of the complex supports posteriorly. The opposite occurs with internal rotation as posterior support is provided by the broad aspect of the inferior capsular complex and anterior support is provided by the cord-like anterior aspect of the complex. Another component of capsular control of movement is through a tension-dependent role in accessory movement of the humeral head. It has been found that capsular tightness contributes to an obligatory translation in the opposite direction of tension.[10] For example, in a normally functioning shoulder, the position of abduction with external rotation causes tension on the anterior capsule. In turn, this causes a posterior translation of the humeral head by approximately 4 mm.[11] This is also true with abduction, where tension in the inferior capsule and pull from the deltoid/supraspinatus couple cause a superior migration of the humeral head of approximately 3 to 6 mm. More is discussed under relevant clinical scenarios.

Additional support is provided passively by the fit of the humeral head into the glenoid. It is affected by the contact area, angle of the glenoid, and degree of adhesion or lack thereof. Active support is provided directly through the capsular integration of rotator cuff attachment. The biceps tendon also plays a crucial role in stability due to its position anteriorly as a mechanical block and its attachment to the superior labrum. The labrum is a fibrocartilaginous structure, analogous to the meniscus in the knee, which serves a primary function in stabilizing the shoulder, deepening the concavity within which the humeral head resides. Tears of the inferior labrum are common with dislocation. Tears of the superior labrum are classified based on type and cause. A specific type of superior labrum tear is referred to as superior labrum anterior to posterior (SLAP). There are four types of labrum tears: Type I lesions have primarily degeneration and fraying without instability. Type II SLAP lesions are by far the most common and demonstrate detachment of the superior labrum off the glenoid. Type III SLAP lesions are bucket-handle tears of the superior labrum; however, the remainder of the labrum is firmly attached to the glenoid. Type IV SLAP lesions have a bucket-handle tear that extends to the biceps tendon. Indirectly, movement of the scapula provides a stable platform upon which the humeral head can function at higher elevations. This is accomplished by an exquisite cooperation between the rotator cuff and the scapular muscles. A major player in this interaction is the serratus anterior muscle. The properly functioning scapula serves several roles, including:

1. Stabilization: Maintains the proper position to allow the instant center of rotation to be maintained within an optimum physiological range.
2. Retraction and protraction against the thoracic wall: Allows a greater range of shoulder/arm movement while maintaining a stabilized platform for the humeral head.
3. Elevation of the acromion: Allows for a greater range of abduction.
4. Serves as a base for muscle attachment: Connects the rib cage, upper extremity, and spine.

The shoulder is part of a complex of joints that function together to provide smooth movement of the upper extremity. This complex is composed of the sternoclavicular joint, the AC joint, the glenohumeral joint, and also the pseudojoint of the scapulothoracic articulation. The SC joint has a long axis superior to inferior and a short axis anterior to posterior. The joint faces slightly

posterior, outward and upward. It is not totally congruent, requiring an intra-articular disk (meniscus) similar to the AC joint. Although the joint axis indicates anterior to posterior and superior to inferior translation, 30° of axial rotation also occurs. Ankylosis at the SC severely limits elevation to only 90° of shoulder elevation. Through a series of levers and supports, the shoulder is allowed to function in many planes. The contribution of muscles may be categorized on the basis of several roles. First are the protectors. These are the inherently smaller rotator cuff muscles that act to compress the humeral head into the glenoid. Second are the pivoters. These are the scapular muscles that serve to pivot the scapula under the humeral head during elevation of the arm for proper muscle/tendon alignment and tension. The primary pivoters are the various fiber orientations of the trapezius and serratus anterior muscles. Next are the positioners. These act to position the shoulder in varying degrees of elevation. The deltoid complex and supraspinatus muscle play the major role. For purposes of strength or propulsion, there are the propellers. These are the much larger adductor/internal rotator muscles consisting mainly of the pectoralis and latissimus dorsi muscles.[12] There is a natural imbalance between the stronger internal rotators/adductors and weaker external rotators/abductors. This imbalance is often made worse by occupational posture and overdevelopment of the larger muscles.

The subscapularis, pectoralis, teres major, and latissimus dorsi are internal rotators (**Figure 7–1**). The external rotators include the infraspinatus, teres minor, and posterior deltoid. The abductors include the supraspinatus and deltoid group (**Figure 7–2**). Adduction is a large muscle movement accomplished by the pectoralis and latissimus dorsi. As stated previously, the rotator cuff musculature, in addition to a dynamic movement role, also serves to stabilize the shoulder through insertion into the capsule providing a tightening effect upon contraction. The need for stabilization increases with arm elevation. In an effort to determine which muscles contribute to stability, researchers conducted a cadaveric study with simulation.[13] In the midrange of motion, the supraspinatus and subscapularis provided the highest degree of stabilization. With the arm in external rotation and abduction, the cadaver shoulders were taken to end-range. In this end-range position (considered the most stressful for the anterior capsule of the shoulder), the subscapularis, infraspinatus, and teres minor provided more stability than the supraspinatus. The deltoid muscle takes on an

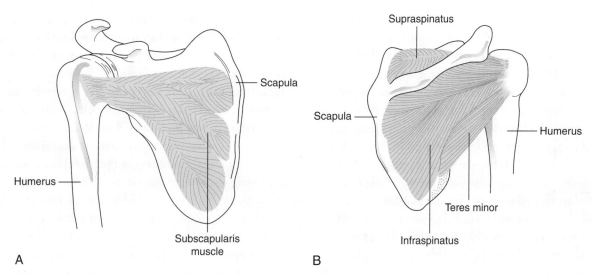

Figure 7–1 (A) The rotator cuff (anterior view); (B) the muscles of the rotator cuff (posterior view).

increasingly important role, especially the middle deltoid, as the shoulder becomes increasingly unstable.[14]

One of the more important anatomic or structural concepts with regard to efficient shoulder function has to do with the plane of the scapula. It is evident that the glenoid of the scapula does not face directly lateral. It faces between 30° and 45° forward because of the curved fit of the scapula on the bony thorax. The result is that more efficient muscle tension relationships exist in this plane.[15]

This is often apparent in the patient with a painful shoulder who unconsciously selects this scapular plane as his or her elevation plane of choice.

Several significant observations must be made with regard to shoulder elevation. The first is that with abduction of the arm with internal rotation, the arm can be abducted to only about 75° (if you eliminate scapular rotation or "shrugging" effects). With external rotation, the 45° angle between the axis of the humeral head and

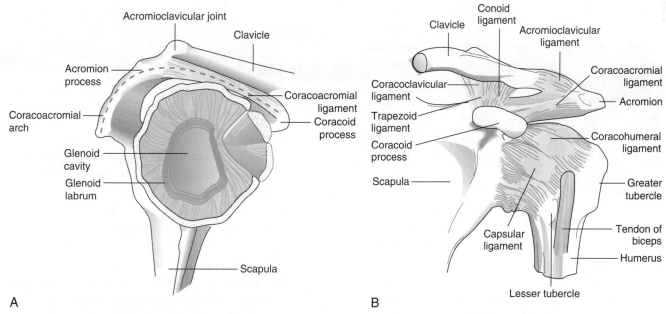

Figure 7–2 (A) The coracoacromial arch and glenohumeral joint (lateral view); (B) ligaments of the acromioclavicular and glenohumeral joints.

that of the axis of the shaft is moved out of the coronal plane automatically straightening the angle and adding the 45° angulation to the existing 75°, accomplishing a sleight of hand. In other words, it appears that the arm has been elevated to 120° of abduction when in fact it is due to the elimination of the angle between the humeral head and shaft. Jobe[16] also points out that to avoid impingement, the greater tuberosity must clear the glenoid rather than the acromion as more commonly believed. He feels that "impingement" may occur more as superior glenoid and labrum contact with the internal fibers of the rotator cuff and greater tuberosity. This occurs in shoulders with and without indicators of instability. Jobe describes four structures at risk of injury: (1) the internal fibers of the rotator cuff, (2) the superior labrum and biceps origin, (3) the greater tuberosity and posterosuperior glenoid, and (4) the inferior glenohumeral ligament and labrum complex (due to tension). It is also interesting to note that a similar theory is used to explain why patients experience relief with the relocation test (pain felt initially on a supine apprehension test). In other words, the anterior-to-posterior pressure used in the relocation test removes posterior impingement by repositioning the humeral head in relation to the glenoid.

Evaluation

History

A prognostic study by Thomas et al.[17] indicated that baseline characteristics, rather than treatment rendered, were a better predictor of outcome. Criteria that reduced the likelihood of recovery were: being female, reporting a gradual onset, or higher baseline disability scores. A study by Largacha et al.[18] attempted to determine, among other things, age at time of presentation for specific disorders. Those with instability seemed to present to a specialist around age 20–35 years. Patients with full-thickness tears present 15 years later than those with partial cuff tears. Those individuals with cuff tear arthropathy presented 13 years later than full-thickness tears. The conditions with greatest female prevalence were RA and adhesive capsulitis. All other conditions were male predominant, especially capsulorrhaphy arthropathy, degenerative joint disease (DJD), and traumatic instability. A study by Miranda et al.[19] indicated there was also an association found between mental stress, obesity, and older age; as well as physically

strenuous work and working with the trunk forward-flexed or with the hand above the shoulder level, and increased risk of shoulder pain. The more recent study by Leclerc et al.,[20] after adjustment for other risk factors, found that the presence of depressive symptoms was able to predict occurrence of shoulder pain. There was also an association between a low level of job control and shoulder pain. Men with repetitive tool use and women using vibrating tools and working with arms above shoulder level were also strong predictors of shoulder pain. All of these factors should be included, less for the diagnostic value, but for the predictive value of response to care or natural history.

In a systematic review of shoulder disability questionnaires, Bot et al. (2004)[21] evaluated 16 questionnaires focusing on those with the most evidence, which included the Disability of the Arm, Shoulder, and Hand Scale (DASH), the Shoulder Pain and Disability Index (SPADI), and the American Shoulder and Elbow Surgeons Standardized Shoulder Assessment Form (ASES). Properties scored included validity, reproducibility, responsiveness, interprobability, and practical burden. The results indicated that none of the questionnaires demonstrated satisfactory results for all properties. Only seven questionnaires showed adequate test/retest reliability (ICC > 0.70 with five questionnaires testing as inadequate). Most studies had small sample sizes ($n < 43$) and none had information on the interpretation of test results. The DASH received the best ratings for clinimetric properties.

Careful questioning may point to the diagnosis (**Table 7–1**).

Pain Localization

The following are possible causes of pain based on localization (see **Table 7–2** and **Figure 7–3**, A to C):

- Anterior
  1. traumatic—fracture, dislocation, subacromial bursitis, capsular sprain, rupture of long head of biceps, labrum tear
  2. nontraumatic or overuse—general impingement syndrome, subcoracoid impingement, biceps tendinitis, subacromial bursitis, subscapularis tendinitis, subluxation
- Lateral
  1. traumatic—contusion, supraspinatus rupture, referral from cervical spine or brachial plexus injury

Table 7–1 History Questions for Shoulder Complaints

Primary Question	What Are You Thinking?	Secondary Questions	What Are You Thinking?
Was there trauma? (Did you hurt your shoulder in an accident?)	Rule out fracture, subluxation, dislocation, separation, capsular or muscle tearing	Fall on an outstretched arm? Land on the top of your shoulder? Did you have your arm up and pulled back? Does your arm get stuck in certain positions that you can click back in place?	Clavicular fracture, posterior dislocation, supraspinatus, biceps, or labrum tear AC separation, distal clavicular fracture, shoulder pointer Anterior dislocation Glenoid labrum tear
Do you perform repetitive activities with your shoulder?	Impingement syndrome, capsular sprain, muscle strain, tendinitis	Do you work in overhead positions? Is it worse with lifting weights?	Impingement syndrome Osteolysis of distal clavicle with AC pain; labrum tear if mechanically locks or gives out, and muscle strain
Is there any associated neck pain?	Cervical spondylosis, disc lesion, referred facet pain	Trauma to the neck? Are the pains connected?	Whiplash, and the "lateral whiplash" of a cervical burner C5-C6 areas most commonly affected
Are there other problems that seemed to occur at the same time as your shoulder pain?	Arthritides, connective tissue disease, visceral referred pain	Any gastrointestinal symptoms (abdominal pain, etc.)? Any associated chest pain?	Gallbladder Cardiac referral
Is the complaint more of stiffness?	Adhesive capsulitis, subluxation, unrecognized posterior dislocation, arthritides	Past history of trauma? Did the stiffness get worse after a few weeks of pain?	Posterior directed force may have caused an unreduced posterior dislocation Adhesive capsulitis
Is there a sense of weakness or instability?	Capsular instability, glenoid labrum tear, neurologic weakness	Past history of trauma? Does it feel weak with your arm elevated?	Capsular, rotator cuff, or labrum damage Capsular looseness or damage
Have you ever been diagnosed with any kind of arthritis in the past?	Osteoarthritis uncommon unless previous surgery/trauma; RA, AS, pseudogout and others should be considered	Do you have other joint pains?	Finger joint pain might suggest RA, spine/S1 pain may suggest AS; knee/wrist pain may suggest pseudogout

2. nontraumatic or overuse—impingement syndrome, deltoid strain, supraspinatus tear or rupture, referral from cervical spine problem
- Superior
  1. traumatic—AC separation, distal clavicular fracture, shoulder pointer
  2. nontraumatic or overuse—osteoarthritis of the AC joint, osteolysis of the distal clavicle
- Posterior
  1. traumatic—scapular fracture, posterior dislocation
  2. nontraumatic or overuse—posterior impingement, infraspinatus or teres minor strain or tendinitis, posterior deltoid strain, triceps strain, suprascapular nerve entrapment

Traumatic and Overuse Injuries

With trauma, there are usually clear indicators of dislocation or separation. Fracture, too, may be implicated by the mechanism, magnitude of forces, and degree of pain. Common injury patterns for the shoulder include the following:

- Blow to the anterior shoulder—dislocation, subluxation, or contusion
- Fall onto top of shoulder—AC separation, distal clavicular fracture, shoulder pointer
- Fall on an outstretched arm (landing on hand with elbow extended)—AC separation, clavicular fracture, posterior dislocation, glenoid labrum or rotator cuff tear

Table 7–2 Shoulder Pain Localization

#	Structures	Overt Trauma	Insidious or Overuse
1	Acromioclavicular (AC) joint	AC separation, shoulder pointer, distal clavicular fracture	Osteoarthritis of AC joint, osteolysis of the distal clavicle
2	Deltopectoral triangle	Subscapularis rupture	Subscapularis tendinitis, capsulitis
3	Clavicle	Clavicular fracture	Pectoralis clavicular strain
4	Coracoid process	Coracoid fracture or bursitis	Pectoralis minor tendinitis
5	Biceps tendon	Biceps tendinitis	Biceps tendinitis
6	Pectoralis major	Pectoralis major rupture	Pectoralis major strain
7	Deltoid insertion (deltoid tubercle)	Bruise at or slightly below, possibility of hematoma and myositis ossificans	Common referral area for many shoulder conditions and C5 nerve root or facet irritation, deltoid strain
8	Supraspinatus insertion, subacromial bursa	Supraspinatus rupture	Impingement syndrome, bursitis, supraspinatus tendinitis
9	Infraspinatus/teres minor tendons and insertion	Contusion	Infraspinatus or teres minor tendinitis
10	Teres minor tendon, long head of triceps tendon, posterior circumflex artery, axillary nerve	Contusion	Teres minor or triceps tendinitis, quadrilateral space syndrome
11	Infraspinatus muscle, scapula	Scapular fracture	Atrophy due to suprascapular nerve entrapment
12	Levator scapulae, superior-medial border of scapula	Radiation zone for cervical disc lesions	Levator scapulae syndrome

Note: See Figure 7–3, A, B, and C, for localization of numbered areas.

- arm forced into external rotation and horizontal abduction with shoulder flexed to 90° or above—anterior dislocation, glenoid labrum tear
- sudden traction to the arm—medical subluxation or brachial plexus traction injury

- sudden pain with weight lifting (no apparent dislocation)—consider muscle/tendon rupture, labrum tear

With frank trauma excluded, the most fruitful approach is first to distinguish the patient's complaint.

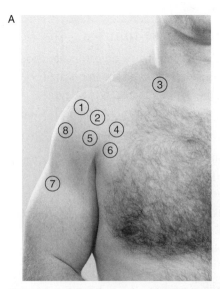
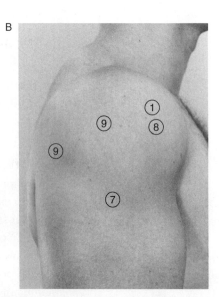
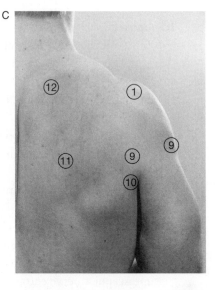

Figure 7–3 (A) Anterior shoulder; (B) lateral shoulder; (C) posterior shoulder.

Have the patient categorize his or her complaint into mainly pain, stiffness, instability, weakness, or numbness and/or tingling. Ascertain whether there are associated cervical or thoracic spine complaints. Although they are rare, determine whether there are any visceral complaints, in particular, right upper quadrant pain suggestive of biliary disease.

Pain

When pain is the chief complaint, it is important to determine whether it is chronic or acute. An attempt to define a positional relationship is important. For example, patients who feel most of their pain while working in overhead positions may have an impingement problem. Patients who find it difficult to throw a ball or otherwise attain the cocking position of abduction/external rotation often will have instability. With acute pain that is severe with no trauma, the inability to move the arm in all ranges of motion without pain is highly suggestive of an acute bursitis. With chronic and insidious cases, it is important to determine the extent to which overuse or misuse is a culprit.

Weakness

A sense of weakness or instability may be an isolated or associated complaint. It is important to discover past traumas, in particular dislocations or medical subluxations. If not rehabilitated, a progressive looseness of the capsule frequently develops. This may lead to concomitant damage to the labrum, resulting in a downward spiral. Another possibility is peripheral nerve damage such as suprascapular nerve involvement. Evidence is usually visually apparent with atrophy of the infraspinatus. When there is associated neck pain and painless weakness of the shoulder, consider and test for nerve root involvement. If there is no past trauma or surgery, consider the possibility of an inherent looseness of the shoulder capsule, which is likely a bilateral phenomenon. This is best determined with orthopaedic testing for instability.

Restricted Movement

With a complaint of stiffness, it is important to determine the sequence of events leading to the sense of restriction. For example, a patient complaining of an acute, unprovoked episode of incapacitating shoulder pain that lasted for weeks before resolving into stiffness is likely to have adhesive capsulitis. A patient with a past

traumatic history (especially a posteriorly directed force to the humerus) must be suspected of having a posterior dislocation. Those with a history of trauma or surgery might be expected to develop an early onset of osteoarthritic changes. In those with coexisting arthritides the shoulder may be a secondary area of involvement. In addition to osteoarthritis, the most common arthritides that involve the shoulder are rheumatoid arthritis and ankylosing spondylitis. All of the above causes are likely to result in stiffness in many planes. A single movement plane of stiffness must be qualified. Restriction due to pain and weakness is likely caused by a mechanical block resulting from bone or labrum pathology. If there is overuse or trauma to muscle, subsequent scarring may lead to an obvious restriction in the direction of stretch.

Other Complaints

Atrophy or deformity is sometimes the primary concern of patients. Atrophy of the infraspinatus is evident by a depression over the scapula. This is most often due to suprascapular nerve damage, not uncommon in overhead sports—in particular volleyball. If the patient complains of a mass in the distal arm, rupture of the long head of the biceps should be considered. The patient often will report an injury during which a pop was heard. Another cause of a mass in the arm is myositis ossificans. The patient will report having been struck on the arm, with subsequent swelling that never resolved. Radiographs will reveal the calcified muscle mass. Deformity at the top of the shoulder is often due to the instability of an AC separation or a distal clavicular fracture when trauma is reported. Without trauma and in an older individual, osteoarthritis of the AC joint is likely.

Examination

There is strong evidence that clinical tests for the rotator cuff:

- Are able to rule out full tears.
- Have questionable value for partial tears.
- Have moderate sensitivity and specificity for instability and labrum tears, but the quality of studies is still questionable.
- Indicate moderate reliability for ROM.
- Suggest that use of Cyriax testing of the shoulder has not been shown to be reliable.

An examination of the shoulder can be problem (diagnosis) focused or generic. If the intent of the examination is to reproduce a diagnostic impression leading to further evaluation such as radiographs or special imaging, then a diagnosis-focused examination may be appropriate. This is more likely in the acute setting. With a chronic problem, two aspects of the examination become important: (1) the diagnostic impression and (2) the comprehensive evaluation of the patient's biomechanical status. In other words, what are the limitations in active, active-resistive, and passive ranges of motion? How is the scapula participating in this motion? If the patient has signs of impingement, is there any underlying instability or looseness? The generic approach is best when multiple factors are suggested.

With an acute injury, mechanism of injury coupled with observation of patient positioning and shoulder contour often suggest an underlying cause:

- If the patient either was injured by a direct blow to the shoulder or was suddenly overstretched into a position of external rotation/abduction or extension, anterior dislocation is likely; significant pain causes the patient to hold the arm in slight abduction and external rotation; associated observational findings are a visibly flat deltoid, prominent humeral head anteriorly, and a prominent acromion with a posterior depression underneath.
- If the patient fell on an outstretched arm or any mechanism of posterior force was applied to a flexed arm, a posterior dislocation is likely; the patient holds the arm slightly adducted and internally rotated (sling position); a prominent coracoid with anterior shoulder flattening is an associated observational sign best seen from a bird's-eye view (looking down at the shoulder of a seated patient).

Palpation of the shoulder may be revealing for many common shoulder complaints. Tenderness and deformity at the AC joint are often secondary to trauma and may represent a second- or third-degree separation or distal clavicular fracture. If there is no deformity, consider a shoulder pointer (contusion of the local muscles) or a first-degree separation of the AC joint. If there is no trauma but there is deformity, consider an old AC separation or, in an older individual, osteoarthritis; tenderness may or may not be elicited. Discrete tenderness at the AC joint in a serious weight lifter suggests osteolysis of the distal clavicle.[22]

Tender areas often correlate well to specific tissue involvement. This is often position-dependent:[23]

- The supraspinatus tendon insertion is most palpable with the patient seated and the arm held behind the back with the elbow flexed; the arm is internally rotated as much as possible and the elbow is lifted away from the back as far as possible (maximum extension of the shoulder); the supraspinatus tendon is then palpable directly anterior-inferior to the AC joint.
- The infraspinatus and teres minor tendons are most palpable with the patient seated or prone with the shoulder flexed to 90°, adducted 10°, and externally rotated 20°; the elbow is bent to about 90° during positioning; the tendons are then palpable directly inferior to the posterior acromion.
- The subscapularis tendon is palpated with the shoulder held in neutral at the patient's side; the tendon is palpable deep under the area of the clavicle just medial to the medial border of the deltoid in the deltopectoral triangle.
- The tendon of the long head of the biceps is palpated with the patient's arm internally rotated 20°; the tendon is palpable in the same deltopectoral triangle as the subscapularis; however, the internal rotation has placed the biceps tendon in an overlying position.

Range of Motion

A small study by Hayes et al.[24] evaluated five methods including visual estimation, goniometry, still photography, "stand and reach," and hand-behind-back reach for six shoulder movements. For flexion, abduction, and external rotation, fair to good reliability was demonstrated for the interclass correlation coefficient (ICC) using visual, goniometry, and photography. The standard errors of measurement were between 14° and 25° (interrater) and 11° and 23° (intrarater). The hand-behind-back reach was the least reliable. While fair to good reliability was found for some approaches, the range of standard measurement errors indicates a large variation in precision.

Although active internal rotation of the shoulder is often tested with the patient being asked to reach behind the back and then to touch the highest point possible on the spine, this approach is fraught with misinterpretation. Both Wakabayashi et al.[25] and Ginn et al.[26] have determined that this is an inaccurate approach to measure, among other things, flexion of the elbow more than internal rotation of the shoulder. The contribution of internal rotation of the shoulder above the T12 vertebral level is very small.

Information from range of motion testing is often interpreted through a system developed by Cyriax sometimes referred to as a selective tension approach. Hayes et al.[27] performed a study on the reliability of resistive testing as proposed by Cyriax. The study included both the upper and lower extremities with the knee, shoulder, and elbow included. Examiners used maximum contraction testing and were unaware of previous testing results. The intrarater kappa values ranged from 0.44–0.82; the interrater kappa coefficients ranged from 0.00–0.46. A small number of patients who were classified as weak affected the kappa coefficients. In the intrarater evaluation percentages for the knee, evaluators averaged 91% of maximum kappa, while for the shoulder the average was 66.5%. For the interrater evaluation, the average was 60.4% of the maximum kappa for both the knee and the shoulder. The intrarater and interrater reliability were not acceptable for the shoulder.

Some characteristic movement pattern restrictions in range of motion (ROM) are as follows:

- Patients unable to perform most movements due to pain (and no history of trauma) are likely to have either an acute bursitis or the initial stage of adhesive capsulitis.
- If there is a history of trauma and the patient avoids any attempt at movement, consider dislocation and/or fracture.
- If there is a history of trauma and the patient is unable to lift the arm into flexion with a supinated arm, posterior dislocation should be considered.
- Pain in the midrange of abduction is referred to as a "painful arc." The painful arc is between 70° and 110° (**Figure 7–4**). To qualify as a painful arc, the

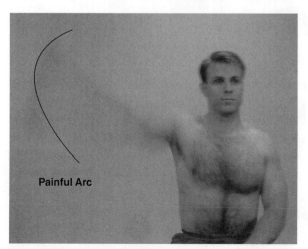

Painful Arc

Figure 7–4 The painful arc is between 70° and 110°. The patient will feel more pain in this range and less on either side of this arc.

pain must be less above this range. When patients cannot actively move beyond this range, the examiner should assist the patient to 120° and then ask the patient to continue if possible. In general, an active painful arc combined with a negative passive painful arc is suggestive of a contractile lesion (i.e., muscle/tendon). If a painful arc is felt on active and passive movement, the involved structures are less clear.

- Restriction in *both* active and passive ROM preferentially affecting external rotation, abduction, and then eventually extension and flexion suggests adhesive capsulitis.
- Pain felt at a discrete point with active ROM as a sharp pain is suggestive of a labrum tear, especially if it can be relieved by avoiding the specific position.
- Inability to lower from an abducted position (drop-arm test) is suggestive of a rotator cuff (specifically supraspinatus) tear.
- The use of body leaning or shoulder hunching is often visible when patients with adhesive capsulitis, rotator cuff tear, or osteoarthritis are compensating for weakness or loss of active movement.

When the patient performs abduction maneuvers, it is important to palpate the scapula for a normal glenohumeral to scapula ratio of movement. The ratio between humeral and scapular motion is often quoted as 2:1; however, this figure is an average. The ratio in the first 30° is closer to somewhere between 4:1 and 7:1; from 90° to 150° it is closer to 1:1.[28, 29] Thus, little movement occurs in the first 30°. Because the ratio changes with movement, it is often referred to as a rhythm. This rhythm changes with resistance.[30] With no resistance, the ratio starts at 7.9:1 and changes to 2:1 as the arm is raised. Light loads applied to the shoulder through the arm result in a rhythm ratio from 3:1 initially to 4.3:1 as the arm is raised. With heavy loading, the rhythm ratio starts at 1.9:1, going to 4.5:1 as the arm is raised. When excessive movement occurs at the scapula in the initial phase of abduction, weakness of the serratus anterior or other stabilizers is likely.

Scapular translation across the thoracic wall varies between 15 to 18 cm. A complex of abnormal positions or patterns has been referred to by various names, including scapulothoracic dyskinesis, floating scapula, and lateral scapular slide. A functional test for interscapular muscle weakness is to have the patient isometrically squeeze the scapulae together for 15 to 20 seconds, noting whether there is burning pain within 15 seconds. If so, this may indicate the need for strengthening. Another similar test is to have the patient hold a pencil between the shoulder blades for 30 to 60 seconds without dropping the pencil. In addition to static evaluation for scapular winging, a functional test called the lateral slide test is commonly performed.[31] The lateral slide test involves marking the inferomedial angle for each scapula with the reference point on the spine as the nearest spinous process (**Figure 7–5**). The distance is measured for each. In the second and third positions of the test, this measurement process is repeated. The three positions

are: (1) arm at side, (2) hands on hips with fingers facing forward, thumbs posterior, with about 10° of shoulder extension, and (3) arm at or below 90° of elevation with maximal internal rotation of the glenohumeral joint. Measurements are taken in each position. The interexaminer and intraexaminer reliability are generally good (about 0.84 to 0.88) for these measurements, with the least accurate position being the third (about 0.77 to 0.85).[32] Researchers have established a difference of 1.5 cm asymmetry as the threshold for abnormal.

Although the lateral scapular slide test has become a standard in detecting possible scapular dysfunction,

A
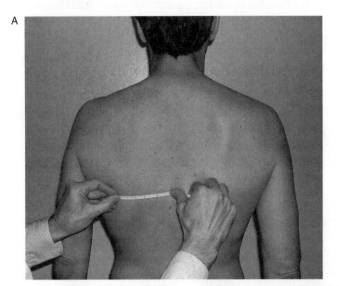

B
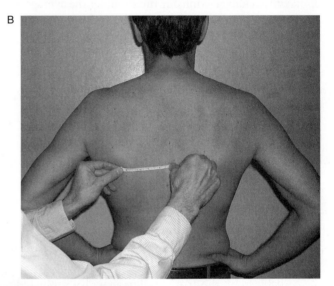

C
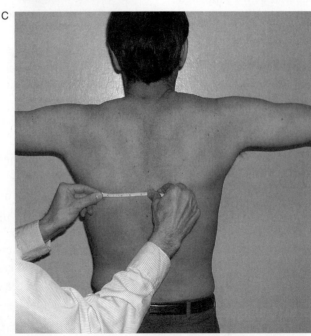

Figure 7–5 Lateral scapular slide measurement. (A) The first position, with arms at side; (B) the second position, with hands on hips; (C) the third position, with arms at or below 90° abduction, with glenohumeral internal rotation.

researchers in one study compared the findings in asymptomatic competitive athletes.[33] They found that scapular position was commonly asymmetrical in asymptomatic individuals, calling into question the value of this finding as a distinct indicator of a cause of shoulder problems in symptomatic patients.

If scapular muscle weakness or dyskinesia is suspected as a potential cause or aggravator of impingement, the examiner can perform a functional assist test by pushing laterally and upward on the inferior medial border of the scapula (simulating serratus anterior/lower trapezius function) while the patient raises the arm through various positions of elevation. If impingement symptoms are diminished, a relationship to scapular dysfunction is implied.

Instability

Testing for instability or looseness of the shoulder is not performed in the acute dislocation scenario. This testing is reserved for those patients with a past history of dislocation or medical subluxation and those individuals who are suspected of having generalized joint laxity. There are a number of tests; however, most examiners focus on three: (1) the load and shift (L&S) test, (2) the apprehension test, and (3) the relocation test.

The L&S test (**Figure 7–6**) is usually performed with the patient seated with the arm abducted slightly (20°) and the hand resting on the lap.[34] The examiner then loads the joint by compressing the humeral head into the glenoid. While stabilizing the scapula with one hand held over the spine of the scapula and clavicle, the other hand pushes the humeral head first forward to test for anterior instability, then backward for posterior stability (**Figure 7–6**A) and finally inferiorly (**Figure 7–6**B). It is also possible to test the patient supine with the arm in 20° horizontal adduction, 90° abduction, and neutral rotation. In general, when inferior laxity is present, a sulcus sign or depression will appear below the AC joint. It indicates not only inferior laxity but also multidirectional instability. It will usually be found on the opposite shoulder, indicating an inherent looseness of the individual's shoulder capsules. It is important to understand the amount of laxity that occurs in normal shoulders.

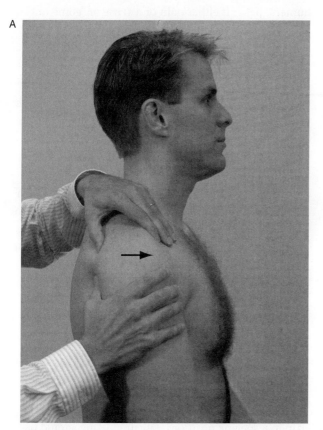
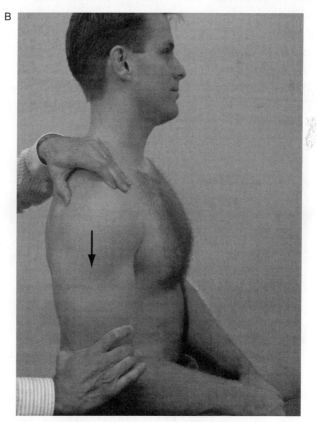

Figure 7–6 The L&S test involves stabilizing the scapula with one hand and grasping the humeral head with the other. Load the shoulder by pushing in toward the glenoid. (A) Then push forward to test anterior stability, and pull back to test posterior stability. (B) Pull downward on the arm to test inferior stability. A visible sulcus may appear under the acromion with a multidirectional loose shoulder.

Using an objective measurement device (e.g., KT-1000, Medmetric Corporation, San Diego, California) with asymptomatic individuals, for women the nondominant shoulder range of translation was 23.8 mm ± 4.2 mm; the dominant arm showed a translation of 22.6 mm ± 4.6 mm.[35] For men, significantly less translation occurred. The nondominant shoulder demonstrated translation of 18.3 mm ± 3.7 mm; the dominant shoulder demonstrated 17.1 mm ± 3.7 mm.

Instead of measuring in millimeters, grading is generally based on the relationship of the humeral head to the glenoid. The grading system developed by Altcheck et al.[36] uses a grading system of 0 to 3. A grade 0 indicates no instability, while a grade 1 involves movement to the rim of the glenoid. A grade 2 occurs when the examiner can feel the humeral head translate over the glenoid rim but it does not lock. A grade 3 indicates the humeral head locks over the rim. Another commonly used system by Cofield and Mansat[37] uses the same descriptors; however, the numbers 1 through 4 are used to indicate the same respective findings as the Altcheck et al. grades 0 to 3.

The apprehension test (**Figure 7–7**) may be performed with the patient seated or supine.[38] The advantage of performing the test supine is the ability to move directly into the relocation test, which can be used as part of a sequential approach. The patient's arm is abducted and externally rotated. A first attempt is simply to continue the arm into more horizontal abduction (extension) at about 90°. If there is no pain or sense of apprehension,

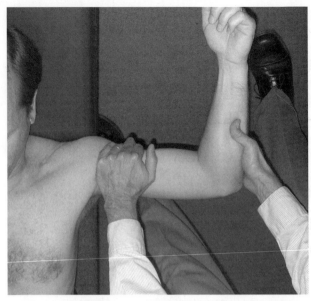

Figure 7–8 The relocation test is a repetition of the apprehension test; however, the examiner stabilizes the shoulder by applying an anterior to posterior force in an effort to relieve pain or a sense of apprehension.

continue testing at a higher elevation and add a cautious pressure in an anterior direction on the posterior humeral head. If either pain or a sense of "going out" is felt by the patient, the test is positive for anterior instability. The test is re-performed; however, by applying an anterior-to-posterior force (**Figure 7–8**), the sense of either pain or apprehension will usually be reduced (relocation test).[39] When apprehension is reduced with this relocation maneuver, instability is confirmed. If pain is reduced with this test, posterior glenoid impingement probably is present due to an underlying anterior instability. The presence of pain with the apprehension test that is relieved by the relocation test has been demonstrated by arthroscopic examination to correlate with articular surface pathology. When the shoulder is abducted to 110°, patients demonstrate rotator cuff contact with the posterosuperior labrum.[40]

Labrum Tears

One of the most difficult pathologies to determine on the clinical examination is a labrum tear. When instability is present or when an individual has complaints that sound like mechanical joint pain (e.g., shoulder gets "stuck" in certain positions or patient has a sharp pain in a specific position), labrum testing should be employed. There are two basic approaches with several variations. The original testing maneuver described in

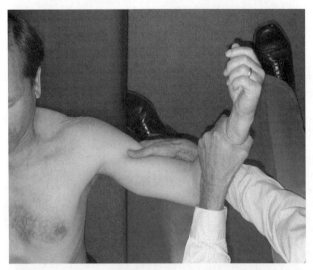

Figure 7–7 The apprehension test may be performed lying or standing. With the patient supine, the examiner extends the patient's shoulder while at 90° abduction and externally rotated while pushing the humeral head from posterior to anterior.

the literature is the clunk test. The patient is placed in the apprehension position with the examiner pressing the humeral head from posterior to anterior. The arm is then internally and externally rotated and circumducted in an attempt to elicit a deep "clunk" feeling or sound. Some examiners employ an axially compressive load (similar to Apley's compression test for the knee). One such test is called the Crank test (**Figure 7–9**), and it involves placing the patient's arm in maximum flexion, internally rotating and externally rotating the arm with an axial force applied. A positive response includes clicking with pain. The practitioners who developed the test found that when the Crank test, apprehension test, and L&S test findings were combined, the sensitivity of the clinical examination for labrum tears was better than with magnetic resonance imaging (MRI).[42]

More recent attempts at detecting labrum tears secondary to dislocation include the Kim test and the Jerk test. These may also indicate some underlying instability. The Kim test (**Figure 7–10**) is performed with the patient seated. Passively elevating the shoulder to 90°, the examiner applies an axial load while simultaneously lifting the distal humerus to impose a posterior inferior load to the shoulder. A positive would be a sudden onset of shoulder pain. The next test, the Jerk test (**Figure 7–11**) involves passive elevation of the shoulder to 90°; however, in this test, the scapula is stabilized. The examiner then imparts an axial compression while simultaneously horizontally adducting the shoulder across the chest. A positive result is an increase in shoulder pain that may or may not be associated with a click or clunk.

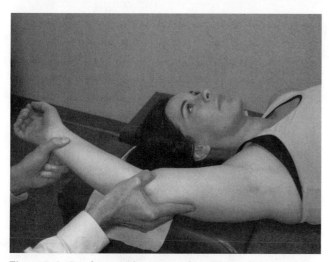

Figure 7–9 Crank test—This test involves placing the patient's arm in maximum flexion while internally rotating and externally rotating the arm with an axial force applied. A positive response includes clicking with pain.

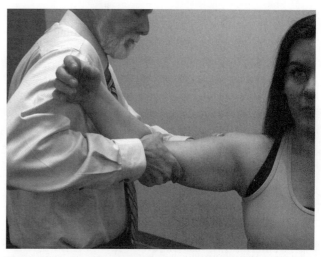

Figure 7–10 Kim test—Passively elevating the shoulder to 90°, the examiner applies an axial load while simultaneously lifting the distal humerus to impose a posterior-inferior load to the shoulder. A positive would be a sudden onset of shoulder pain.

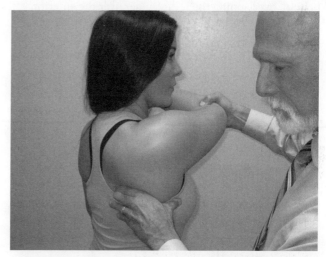

Figure 7–11 Jerk test—Involves passive elevation of the shoulder to 90°, however, in this test, the scapula is stabilized. The examiner then imparts an axial compression while simultaneously horizontally adducting the shoulder across the chest. A positive result is an increase in shoulder pain that may or may not be associated with a click or clunk.

Although it is often assumed that with an anterior dislocation an inferior labrum tear has occurred, another type of tear related to excessive contraction of the long head of the biceps referred to as a superior labrum anterior to posterior (SLAP) lesion is difficult to detect. The long head of the biceps originates off the superior glenoid with a conjoined insertion with the superior labrum. The logic of testing is to begin with sensitive tests related to instability and labrum tears in general, and if positive, to focus on biceps-specific tests to confirm. Sensitive tests for instability would include the apprehension test, relocation test, and the load-and-shift test. Sensitive tests generally for labrum tears without distinguishing which type of tear include some compressive tests such as the Crank test (utilizing axial compression through the humerus and rotation), and clunk test.

Specific biceps contraction tests to further test for SLAP lesions include:

- Anterior slide test
- Active compression test (O'Brien's sign)
- Biceps load test II
- Speed's test
- Yergason's test

The anterior slide test (**Figure 7–12**)[41] begins with the patient seated or standing with the hand of the involved arm placed on the posterolateral iliac crest (the thumb pointing posteriorly). The examiner, standing behind the patient, places one hand on the top of the shoulder from behind, overlapping the index finger over the anterior acromion. The examiner's other hand takes the patient's elbow and directs an axial force anterosuperior into the shoulder. The patient is asked to press back against this attempt. A pop/click or pain localized to the front of the shoulder is considered positive for a superior labrum tear. Labrum tears also are suggested when popping and clicking are found on L&S testing or any distractive maneuvers coupled with internal rotation.

Another testing strategy known as the active compression test (also known as the O'Brien sign) is performed with the patient standing (**Figure 7–13**).[42] The patient brings the arm to 90° of forward flexion with the elbow fully extended. The patient then adducts the arm 10°

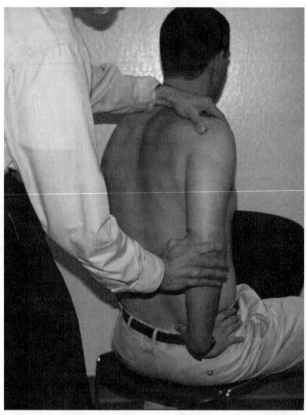

Figure 7–12 The anterior slide test involves the examiner stabilizing the shoulder joint while pressing through the long axis of the humerus in a superioranterior direction while the patient resists. A painful click, clunk, or pop is positive for a superior labrum tear.

to 15° across the chest. With the arm fully internally rotated (thumb down), the examiner (standing behind the patient) directs a downward force at the patient's forearm (patient's elbow remains extended). The test is

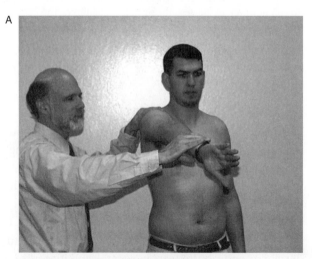
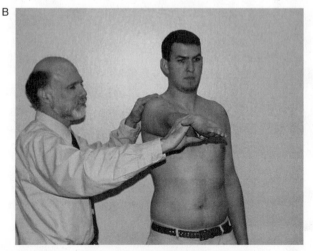

Figure 7–13 (A) First position of O'Brien sign. Patient's arm is in full internal rotation and 10° to 15° horizontally adducted. Examiner exerts a downward force while patient resists. (B) Test repeated with arm supinated. Pain felt in the first position and relieved or not produced during the second position is positive for a labrum tear if pain is felt deeply, or an acromioclavicular problem if felt superficially.

then repeated by directing a downward force with the forearm supinated (palm-up). For this study, a positive test occurred when the first test position caused pain that was reduced or eliminated with the second test position. The distinction between AC versus glenoid labrum injury was based on where the pain was felt. Pain felt "at the top" of the shoulder indicated AC injury, whereas pain felt "deep" in the shoulder indicated labrum injury. The authors point out that if pain is not reduced or eliminated by the second test, the test is not "positive." They also indicate that the patient should be resisting the examiner's downward force, not the opposite (examiner resisting patient's upward force). Surprisingly, this test sequence produced a very reliable detection of labrum tears and AC injury. For detecting labrum abnormalities, the sensitivity was 100%, the specificity was 98.5%, the positive predictive value was 94.6%, and the negative predictive value was 100%. For AC abnormalities, the sensitivity was also 100%, the specificity was 96.6%, the positive predictive value was 88.7%, and the negative predictive value was again 100%. These statistics were derived by comparing active compression test results with findings at surgery.

Kim et al.[49] developed a test referred to as the biceps load test for labrum tears. A redesign of this test was evaluated with better performance called the biceps load II test (**Figure 7–14**).[43] The test is performed by passively elevating the supine patients to 120° abduction and maximal, external rotated. The elbow is bent to 90°

of flexion and the forearm is supinated. The examiner then asks the patient to flex the elbow while the examiner resists this attempt. The test is positive for a SLAP lesion if the patient has pain during the resisted attempt. Some examiners introduce resistance to supination to further stress the biceps. The biceps II test yielded the following results: sensitivity of 89.7%, specificity of 96.9%, a positive-predictive value of 92.1%, a negative-predictive value of 95.5%, and a kappa coefficient of 0.815.

Two other tests utilized are not specific to labrum tears per se but do challenge the biceps. One is the standard muscle test for forearm flexion and supination called Yergason's test (**Figure 7–15**). The second test more often used for impingement testing is Speed's test (**Figure 7–16**). The original test was described as starting with the patient standing and the entire arm passively extended (elbow extended). The examiner then resists the patient's attempt at forward flexion and allows a full isotonic contraction into full flexion. The positive with either of these tests is shoulder pain that localized to the superior shoulder.

To evaluate the sensitivity, specificity, and positive and negative predictive value of tests used for SLAP lesions, three tests were studied:[45]

1. Anterior Slide (AS)
2. Active Compression (AC)
3. Compression Rotation (CR)

The sensitivity, specificity, and positive and negative predictive values were determined using arthroscopic comparison. The most sensitive test was the AC test at 47%; the most specific was the AS test at 84%. The

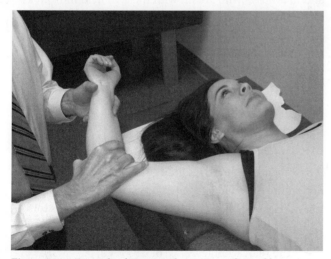

Figure 7–14 Biceps load II test—The test is performed by passively elevating the supine patients arm to 120° abduction and maximal, external rotation. The elbow is bent to 90° of flexion and the forearm is supinated. The examiner then asks the patient to flex the elbow while the examiner resists this attempt. The test is positive for a SLAP lesion if the patient has pain during the resisted attempt

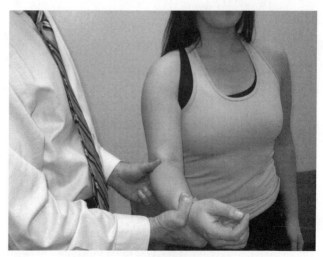

Figure 7–15 Yergason's test—The standard muscle test for the biceps with resisted forearm flexion and supination

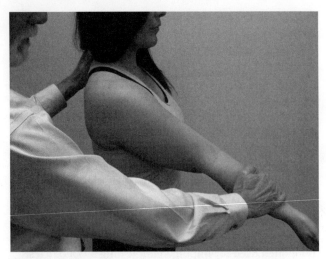

Figure 7-16 Speed's test—The examiner resists the patient's attempt at forward flexion and allows a full isotonic contraction into full flexion. A positive result is shoulder pain; localized to the superior shoulder.

highest positive predictive value was the AC test at 10%; and the highest overall accuracy was the AS test at 77%. The lowest accuracy was the AC at 54%. The AC test was not good at localizing or producing a click. There was an overlap of positives for impingement decreasing specificity.

Another study by Stetson et al.[46] compared the diagnostic value of the Crank test, O'Brien test, and MRI in detecting labrum tears. The results were:

- The Crank test positive predictive value (PPV) was 41% and the negative predictive value (NPV) was 61%. The Crank test was found to be 56% specific and 46% sensitive.
- The O'Brien test had a PPV of 34% and an NPV of 50%. The O'Brien test was found to be 31% specific and 54% sensitive.
- MRI had a PPV of 63% and an NPV of 83%. MRI was found to be 92% specific and 42% sensitive.

Combination findings were:

- MRI ± O'Brien had a PPV of 71% with 82% specific and 50% sensitive.
- MRI ± Crank had a PPV of 60% with 67% specific and 43% sensitive.

Some similar findings were reported in studies by Parentis et al.[47] and Guanche and Jones.[48] The findings of these studies, similar to the Stetson et al. study, conflict with initial reports by the developers of these tests. The primary difference is that Parentis et al. and Stetson et al. used a random population and used arthroscopy

to confirm findings. It seems that type I SLAP lesions are not as evident as type II SLAP lesions. Conclusions from the Parentis et al. study were that the two most sensitive tests for type II SLAP lesions were the active compression (65.2%) and the Hawkins' test (65.2%). The only other slightly valuable tests for sensitivity were Speed's test (40%), Neer's test (50%), and the relocation test (50%). The Yergason's, Crank test, pain provocation, and anterior slide were not sensitive. These same tests, though, had high specificity (Yergason's 93.5%, pain provocation test 90.2%, Crank test 82.6%, and anterior slide test 81.5%). Findings from the Guanche and Jones study are similar. The O'Brien test was 63% sensitive, 73% specific; and the Jobe relocation test was 44% sensitive, 87% specific. In their study, the Crank test, a test for tenderness of the bicipital groove, and the Speed test were not found to be useful in detecting labral tears.

Because many patients with anterior superior labral tears also have anterior supraspinatus tears, some authors coined the term SLAC lesion (superior labrum, anterior cuff). In one study, although impingement tests appeared to be generally negative with these patients, the Whipple test was positive in all 40 patients tested.[51] The Whipple test is a variation of the empty can test for the supraspinatus. The patient, holding the palm down and in front of the opposite shoulder, is asked to resist a downward force applied by the examiner.

Posterior labrum damage is common in weight lifters and in athletes who are hit with the arm held in front as a protection. Unfortunately, there are no tests for posterior labrum tears. About half of these patients experience clicking on load and shift testing.[52] Many patients possess full range of motion and demonstrate no indicators of instability.

Summary of Instability and Labrum Testing

A systematic review by Luime et al.[53] attempted to determine the value of six tests commonly used to evaluate instability and/or labrum tears. Results for each test were:

- The relocation test (LR, 6.5; 95% CI, 3.0–14.0).
- Anterior release (LR, 8.3; 95% CI, 3.6–19).
- Biceps load I and II (LR, 29; 95% CI, 7.3–115.0 and LR, 26; 95% CI, 8.6–80.0), respectively.
- Pain provocation of Mimori (LR, 7.2; 95% CI, 1.6–32.0).

- Internal rotation resistance strength (LR, 25; 95% CI, 8.1–76.0).
- The apprehension, clunk, release, load and shift, and sulcus sign tests proved less useful.

A prospective, cohort-study by Parentis et al.[54] evaluated provocative maneuvers for the diagnosis of SLAP tears of the shoulder. The study included 132 consecutive patients scheduled for diagnostic shoulder arthroscopy. The results indicated:

- The sensitivity for type II SLAP lesions was highest for the active compression test and Hawkins', followed by Speed's, Neer's, and Jobe's. They were statistically different from the other four tests ($P < 0.5$), but not from each other.
- The Hawkins' and active compression tests were the least specific. The most specific for type II lesions were the Yergason's and pain provocation tests ($P < 0.5$).
- Positive predictive values were low for all tests.
- Negative predictive values were in the 80% range for each test.

The authors concluded that finding negative test results might be valuable in ruling out a SLAP lesion.

A more recent review evaluated the reliability and diagnostic accuracy of the history and physical examination for diagnosing glenoid labral tears.[55] Although the diagnostic accuracy of individual tests is quite variable, it was found that by combining the history and exam, the reliability increased. The combination of popping or catching with either a positive Crank test or anterior slide test was suggestive of a labral tear and the absence of this combination suggests the absence of a tear (sensitive and specific). Additionally, the combination of a positive anterior slide with a positive active compression, or Crank test, suggests the presence of a labral tear.

Exhibit 7–1 is a graphical representation of determining the likelihood of instability and/or labrum tears based on aggregate likelihood ratios for each test and combination of test.

General Impingement

Impingement may occur under the subacromial arch, affecting mainly the supraspinatus, biceps, and subacromial bursa. Posterior impingement involves the posterior labrum, infraspinatus, and teres minor tendons. Subcoracoid impingement selectively impinges the subscapularis. Most tests designed for impingement focus on the subacromial arch. These are general tests and do not usually reveal a specific structure. One test is the painful arc discussed above in the ROM section. Other tests include the Neer test and the Hawkins-Kennedy test. The Neer test (**Figure 7–17**) is a passive test involving full forward flexion while holding down the shoulder (stabilizing with the other hand).[56] A positive result involves pain production at the end-range of full forward flexion, not in the midrange of motion. With the Hawkins-Kennedy test (**Figure 7–18**) the examiner places the patient's arm in an impingement position.[57] While standing behind the patient, it is important to prevent scapular elevation by hooking the hand over the top of the shoulder. The examiner's other hand lifts the arm into a position of 90° forward flexion, slight adduction, and internal rotation. The more internal rotation imposed in this position, the stronger the pain response. The positive pain response for impingement is anterior pain. Posterior stretch or pain implies involvement of posterior structures such as the infraspinatus and teres minor or posterior capsule. An interesting study by Pappas et al.[58] using three-dimensional open MRI evaluated the actual internal effects of the Hawkins' and Neer's tests to determine if their theoretical basis was, in fact, true. They found that subacromial contact occurred for the supraspinatus and infraspinatus with the Hawkins position but not with the Neer position. Intra-articular contact of the supraspinatus with the posterosuperior glenoid occurred with both positions. Subscapularis contact also occurred with the anterior glenoid with both positions.

A radiographic evaluation of testing positions using open MRI by Gold et al.[59] evaluated the glenoid contact by the supraspinatus and infraspinatus with the shoulder in external rotation and abduction loaded (resisted), and unloaded. This is the standard apprehension test performed supine. A positive test result of pain has been suggested to indicate posterosuperior rotator cuff pinching due to instability. This study indicated that both the supraspinatus and infraspinatus do, in fact, contact the glenoid in this position; loaded or unloaded.

Posterior capsular tightness can be determined by having the patient lie on his/her side with the shoulder to be measured on top (**Figure 7–19**). The examiner stands in front of the patient and, while stabilizing the scapula, lowers the shoulder (elbow bent) as far as it will move passively down toward the examining table. A measurement may then be taken from the medial epicondyle of the elbow to the tabletop. When the general impingement tests are positive it is important to attempt to localize which structures are involved by more specific testing.

Summary of Impingement Syndrome Testing

For impingement syndrome, diagnostic testing was evaluated in a cross-sectional study by Ardic et al.[60] and in a prospective study by Park et al.[61] In the Ardic study, comparison between clinical findings to diagnostic

ultrasonography and MRI was performed. The most painful shoulders had a more frequent finding of glenoid labral tear and this correlated with more restricted extension on physical examination. Subacromial bursal effusion/hypertrophy was correlated with shoulder disability and impingement test maneuvers. Clinical tests as a whole had modest accuracy for rotator cuff tears and biceps pathology. In the Park study,[61] 913 patients underwent physical examination and diagnostic arthroscopy. The physical examination included eight clinical tests:

Exhibit 7–1 Likelihood Patient Has Instability and/or a Labrum Tear

Approximating Probability: The likelihood ratios (LRs) in this graphical representation represent estimates of probability based on the aggregate of multiple reviews of each test finding. They are only approximations and only reliable indicators of a change in the context of a patient having an intermediate pre-test probability of between 20% and 80%. If the pre-test probability is very high or very low, the LR has little effect on changing the probability.

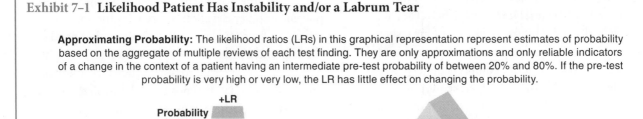
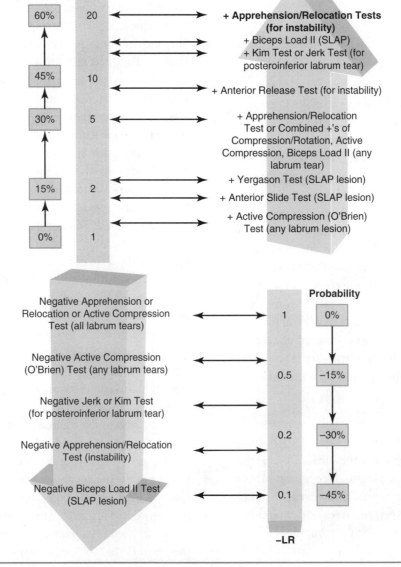

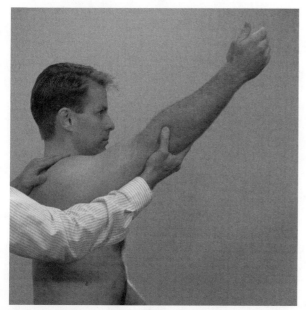

Figure 7–17 The Neer test is performed by passively elevating the arm into forward flexion to end-range. End-range pain is a positive sign of impingement.

Hawkins-Kennedy, Neer's, empty-can, Speed's, cross body adduction, infraspinatus strength test, drop-arm sign, and painful arc. Results indicated that the combination of the Hawkins-Kennedy, painful arc, and infraspinatus muscle tests yielded the best post-test probability (95%) for any degree of impingement.

Given the likelihood ratio for these patients (knowing that they were surgical candidates), test performance may appear inflated as far as sensitivity is concerned. If impingement has a functional rather than a structural

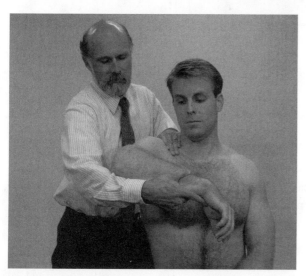

Figure 7–18 The Hawkins-Kennedy test for impingement involves passive internal rotation with the shoulder flexed forward 90°while the scapula is stabilized.

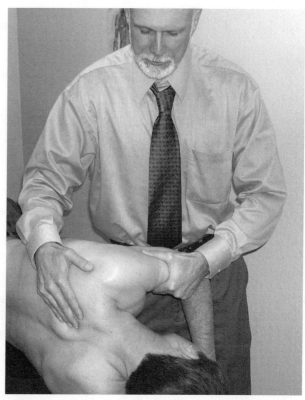

Figure 7–19 The maximum passive range of motion of the posterior capsule is determined by having the patient lie on his/her side and stabilize the scapula with the torso perpendicular to the table. The arm is brought toward the table in cross-body adduction (across the chest) until resistance is met. This may be visualized as an estimate or may be measured as the distance from the tip of the elbow to the examining table.

component, which is then not visible on arthroscopy, it is possible that arthroscopy may not be the gold standard for these functional cases.

Exhibit 7–2 is a graphical representation of determining the likelihood of subacromial impingement based on aggregate likelihood ratios for each test and combination of tests.

Rotator Cuff Tears (RCT)

One general approach is to test for external rotation or by using the Rent test as a screen for a rotator cuff tear.[62] Resisted external rotation is often weak regardless of which tendon is involved. The Rent test (**Figure 7–20**) involves the examiner passively extending the shoulder with the elbow flexed. The examiner then palpates in front of the AC joint while internally and externally rotating the humerus through the elbow. Palpation of a prominence (the greater tuberosity) and an adjacent rent (depression) indicates a full thickness tear.

Exhibit 7–2 Likelihood Patient Has Subacromial Impingement

Approximating Probability: The likelihood ratios (LRs) in this graphical representation represent estimates of probability based on the aggregate of multiple reviews of each test finding. They are only approximations and only reliable indicators of a change in the context of a patient having an intermediate pre-test probability of between 20% and 80%. If the pre-test probability is very high or very low, the LR has little effect on changing the probability.

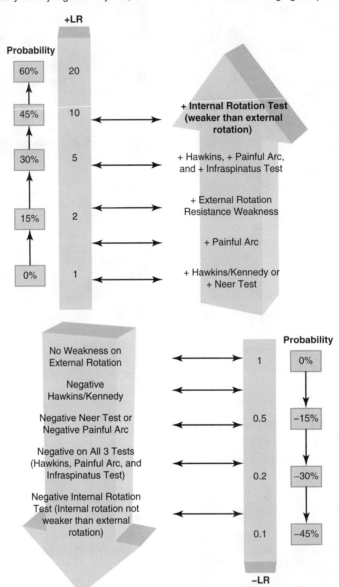

In a retrospective study by Ito et al.[63] common sites of pain were evaluated using clinical charts of 149 patients diagnosed with either rotator cuff tears or adhesive capsulitis confirmed by arthroscopic findings.

The results were that:

- The lateral and anterior shoulder were the most common sites of pain regardless of whether there was a tear or where the tear existed.
- Motion pain was more common than pain at rest for patients with rotator cuff tendinitis or tears.

The authors concluded that pain location was not useful in locating the site of a tear. However, the physical exam based on positive results to muscle tests with appropriate thresholds for muscle weakness was clinically useful. Specifically:

- Supraspinatus—the full can test and empty can test (**Figure 7–21**) showed higher accuracy when assessed with muscle weakness (78% and 79% respectively) than when assessed with pain (74% and 71% respectively).

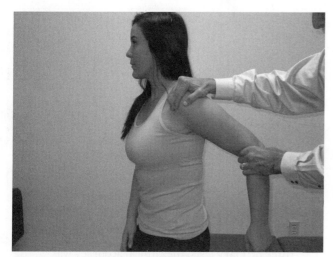

Figure 7–20 Rent test—The examiner passively extends the shoulder with the elbow flexed and internally rotated. The examiner then palpates in front of the AC joint while internally and externally rotating the humerus through the elbow. Palpation of a prominence (the greater tuberosity) and an adjacent rent (depression) indicate a full thickness tear.

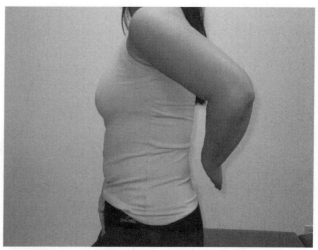

Figure 7–22 Lift-off test—The patient must have no pain on positioning the hand for the test to be specific for the subscapularis. If she or he is unable to lift the hand away from the back, the test is positive for a subscapularis tear.

- Infraspinatus—external rotation strength showed 50% accuracy using pain, and between 58% and 74% using weakness as a positive.
- Subscapularis—lift-off test (**Figure 7–22**) accuracy was 65% with pain and 62%–85% when using strength.

The researchers evaluated both pain reported by patients and pain provoked by muscle testing including the muscle grade at which a positive test occurred. Supraspinatus testing was the most accurate, with muscle strength at less than Grade V; infraspinatus testing was most accurate with the threshold of a positive at less than

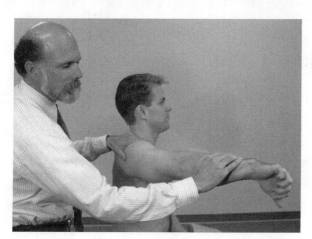

Figure 7–21 The empty can test for the supraspinatus is performed with the patient's shoulder abducted 90° in the plane line of the scapula (30° to 45° forward). With the shoulder in maximum internal rotation, the patient is asked to abduct further against resistance.

Grade IV; and for subscapularis, muscle strength at less than Grade III.

Kim et al.[64] evaluated how often partial subscapularis tears were found at surgery. It was discovered that about 19% of shoulders had partial subscapularis tears. These were not apparent clinically. They were associated with supraspinatus tendon tears, rotator cuff disease, and posterosuperior labral tearing. Independent risk factors were increasing age, dominant arm involvement, and infraspinatus tears.

Specific testing of contractile structures includes the following:

- Supraspinatus: Muscle testing of the supraspinatus is best performed as the empty can test (Figure 7–21). The patient attempts to lift the arm in the plane line of the scapula (scaption), which is 30° to 45° forward of straight abduction. The arm is maximally internally rotated. If this is not painful, the examiner adds resistance to the attempt at approximately 90° of scaption. Pain and weakness indicate a supraspinatus tear. It is important to remember that the intention of this test is to contract the supraspinatus in an impingement position; however, other muscles do participate, as with all resisted testing.[65] It has also been found that testing with the arm in a thumb's-up position recruits as much electromyographic activity; however, it is less painful than full internal rotation.[66]

- Biceps: Although there are a number of tests for the biceps, the one considered most sensitive by investigators is the Speed test.[67] Most biceps tests cause contraction of the biceps without movement of the tendon in the intertubercular groove. The Speed test involves an isotonic contraction into forward shoulder flexion with the elbow extended. The examiner resists this attempt through a full ROM. In so doing, the intertubercular groove travels under the tendon and therefore is more likely to cause irritation if there is an underlying inflammatory process or tendinitis.

- Infraspinatus/teres minor: Contraction into external rotation may cause pain if performed with the arm in the Hawkins-Kennedy position (90° forward flexion, forearm parallel to the floor).[68] This position places a stretch on the tendons prior to contraction. Kelly et al.[66] state that there is minimal pain produced, and therefore better test–retest reliability, when the infraspinatus is tested with the arm at the side (no elevation), 90° of elbow flexion, and the shoulder internally rotated 45° from the sagittal plane.

- Subscapularis: Although the subscapularis is an internal rotator, so are many other larger muscles; therefore, resisted internal rotation is a nonselective attempt at localization. If the subscapularis is involved, the lift-off test (Figure 7–22) may be positive. The patient places the hand behind the back and then attempts to lift the hand off the back.

The patient must have no pain on positioning the hand for the test to be specific for the subscapularis. If she or he is unable to lift the hand away from the back or the attempt is significantly painful, the test is positive.[69] Jemp et al.[68] found the best position for isolating the subscapularis from the pectoralis major was arm elevation to 90° in the scapular plane (scaption) position of 30° to 45° anterior to the coronal plane with the arm in neutral. The examiner supports the arm to allow a better attempt at internal rotation without any associated abduction or adduction attempts by the patient. A 2014 publication[70] indicated that by utilizing three primary tests, the clinical accuracy was quite good for detecting a full subscapularis tear. These included the lift-off test, the bear hug test (**Figure 7–23**), and the belly press test (**Figure 7–24**).

One would assume that muscle testing about the shoulder will indicate the presence of a partial tear or full rupture of the rotator cuff muscles. Logically, if there is a partial tear or full rupture, active resisted testing of the muscle should cause painful weakness with a partial tear and perhaps painless or minimally painful weakness with a full rupture. Given that rotator cuff musculature and tendon insertion is largely hidden by more superficial musculature, the observation of a displaced tendon or bulge of a retracted muscle tendon is not obvious.

A common testing procedure is the drop-arm sign where a patient's arm is elevated to above 90° and the

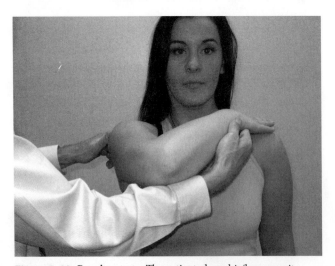

Figure 7–23 Bear hug test—The patient places his/her opposite hand on the top of the uninvolved shoulder. He/she then presses down on the shoulder imparting internal rotation while the examiner augments the resistance by pushing up on the wrist and hand. Extreme weakness or the inability to maintain without incorporating movement at the elbow indicates a subscapularis full-thickness tear.

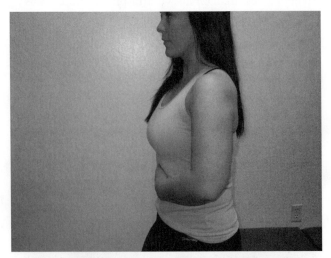

Figure 7–24 Belly-press (Napoleon test)— the patient places his/her palm against his/her abdomen at about the height of the xiphoid process. The elbow is aligned to the trunk. The patient presses maximally against the abdomen using internal rotation. Inability to maintain the position of the elbow due to weakness indicates a subscapularis tear.

patient is asked to hold the position. Inability to hold the position or lower through to the side without dropping indicates involvement of either the deltoid or supraspinatus, and given that the supraspinatus is more often torn, the assumption is that a tear of the supraspinatus has occurred. An extension of this concept is to add resistance to the position. This is often referred to as the Jobe sign. With the arm at 90° abduction, the examiner exerts a downward force while the patient attempts resistance. The obvious confounding factor is that this test is likely to cause pain with mainly shoulder conditions and the

pain is likely to cause a reflex inhibition of the muscles. The weakness, then, is more a neurologic response rather than a biomechanical inability to hold the position.

Park et al.[61] determined that there was a combination of three tests that taken together gave a high degree of diagnostic accuracy although taken individually, the tests were not very good. The combination of the painful arc, drop-arm sign, and infraspinatus muscle test produced the best post-test probability (95%) for a full-thickness rotator cuff tear when all are positive. **Exhibit 7–3** is a graphical representation of determining the likelihood

Exhibit 7–3   Likelihood Patient Has a Rotator Cuff Tear (General)

Approximating Probability: The likelihood ratios (LRs) in this graphical representation represent estimates of probability based on the aggregate of multiple reviews of each test finding. They are only approximations and only reliable indicators of a change in the context of a patient having an intermediate pre-test probability of between 20% to 80%. If the pre-test probability is very high or very low, the LR has little effect on changing the probability.

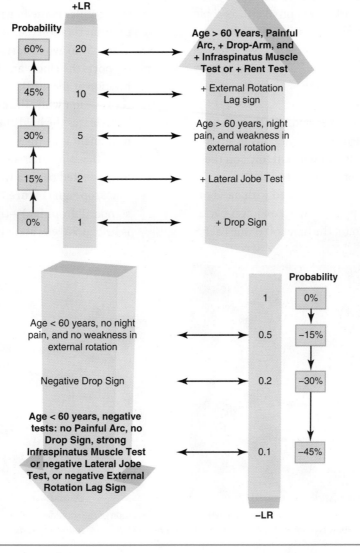

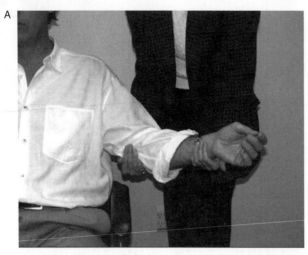 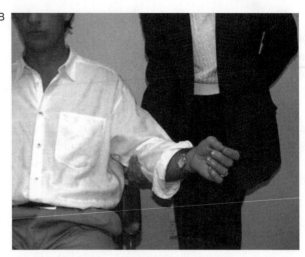

Figure 7–25 (A) First position of external rotation lag sign involves supporting the patient's elbow and externally rotating the shoulder, then backing off the end position by 5°. (B) Releasing the arm contact while continuing to support at the elbow may allow a "drift" of the arm into internal rotation if the test is positive.

of a full thickness RCT based on aggregate likelihood ratios for each test and combination of tests. Hertel et al.[71] performed an evaluation of 100 consecutive patients. The results of those patients who went on to arthroscopic or open repair of any rotator cuff muscle/tendon were examined to determine the effectiveness of several tests in detecting a partial or full rupture. The tests incorporated into the study evaluation were:

- The Jobe sign—shoulder elevated to 90° abduction with internal rotation; patient maintains position with examiner exerting a downward force on the arm (similar to the empty can test).
- The lift-off test—the patient is seated with hand of involved arm placed palm outward on lower back; the patient is asked to lift the hand off of the back.

- The external rotation lag sign (**Figure 7–25**)—the patient is seated, the elbow is passively flexed to 90° and the shoulder is held at 20° elevation in the scapular plane in a position of near maximum external rotation (i.e., maximum external rotation minus 5° to avoid elastic recoil); the examiner supports the elbow and holds the arm in external rotation at the wrist; the patient is asked to hold the position while the examiner supports the elbow but releases the hold at the wrist; the degree of movement is estimated and is referred to as the "lag" (i.e., the difference between supported and unsupported passive ROM).
- The drop sign (**Figure 7–26**; different from the standard drop sign)—the patient is seated, the arm is held at 90° elevation (in the scapular plane) and

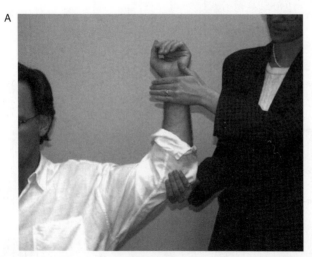 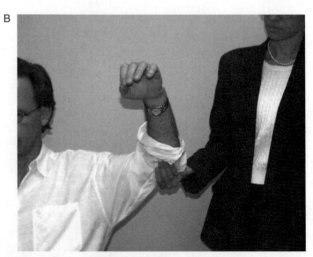

Figure 7–26 (A) First position of the drop sign involves abduction and external rotation of the shoulder while supporting the patient's elbow. Back off of the end position by 5°. (B) Elbow is supported while forearm contact is released. A "drift" into internal rotation indicates a positive lag response.

almost full external rotation with the examiner supporting the elbow and holding the arm in external rotation at the wrist; the patient is asked to hold the position while the examiner supports the elbow but releases the wrist hold; the degree to which the arm falls into internal rotation is the degree of lag.

- The internal rotation lag sign (**Figure 7–27**)—the patient is seated; the patient is asked to bring the arm behind the back with the palm facing outward; the arm is held in near maximum internal rotation and with the hand away from the back by approximately 20° of extension; the patient is asked to hold the position while the examiner supports the elbow but releases the wrist hold; if the patient is unable to hold the position, the lag sign is positive.

The biomechanical principle used in the design of the lag sign was to place the muscle/tendon in the most disadvantaged position possible, thereby requiring full function of the muscle. Also, the position was designed to eliminate, as much as possible, contribution from other synergists. False negatives may occur if there is a restricted passive movement pattern. False positives may occur if the arm is held in maximum rotation or if the patient has an excessive passive range of motion.

The results of the study indicate the following:

- For rupture of the supraspinatus and infraspinatus tendons, the external rotation lag sign was less sensitive but more specific than the Jobe sign; this is probably because the Jobe sign is often painful.

- The drop sign was the least sensitive but was as specific as the external rotation lag sign.
- Partial ruptures of the supraspinatus were not revealed with the external rotation lag sign.
- For the subscapularis, the internal rotation lag sign was as specific as but more sensitive than the lift-off sign.
- Partial ruptures of the subscapularis tendon could be missed with the lift-off sign but detected with the internal rotation lag sign.

Acromioclavicular Joint

AC joint problems are usually evident from the history, observation, and direct palpation. A maneuver that may assist is compression, which is performed by cupping the shoulder from anterior and posterior with both palms and pressing together. Distraction using the spine of the scapula and clavicle may also cause some pain. The O'Brien sign, as described above, is also an important test for AC involvement. The sulcus sign, used to indicate instability of the shoulder, is also present with second- and third-degree AC separations.

Radiography and Special Imaging

Radiographic examination of the shoulder is based on the suspected underlying pathology. General screening involves an anterior-to-posterior (AP) radiograph performed with the patient's arm internally and externally rotated. Some suggested views based on the structures or conditions suspected follow. Discussion of these views

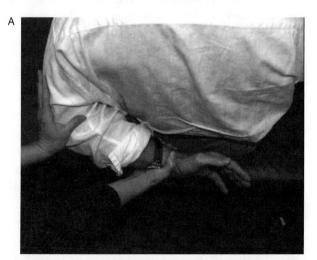
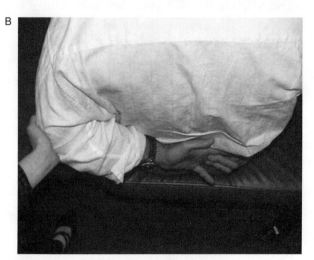

Figure 7–27 (A) First position of internal rotation lag sign involves supporting the patient's elbow and internally rotating the shoulder with the arm behind the back, then backing off the end position by 5°. (B) Releasing the arm contact while continuing to support at the elbow may allow a "drift" of the arm toward the back if the test is positive.

with illustrations of how to perform them may be found in the author's text *Sports Injuries of the Shoulder*.[72]

- Impingement: Evaluation of the subacromial outlet may be seen with the anterior oblique or outlet view (Y view); other helpful views for acromial morphology include the AP view with 30° caudal tube tilt and the AP acromial view (15° cephalad tube tilt) (Zanca view).

- Anterior dislocation: An anterior dislocation is usually visible on an AP neutral; however, the AP internal rotation or anterior oblique (Y) view is best.

- Posterior dislocation: The best view is the Y view; supplementary views are the transthoracic and Velpeau or other axial projections.

- AC joint separation: Weighted and nonweighted anterior projections are often used to determine the degree of separation; these are bilateral shots; a coracoclavicular distance greater than 1.3 cm indicates third-degree separation.

- Instability: If traumatic instability is suspected, several modified axillary projections are of potential benefit in demonstrating residual Hill-Sachs and Bankart (glenoid lip avulsions associated with labrum tears) lesions; these include the West Point view and Didiée view for Bankart lesions, and the AP with internal rotation and the Stryker notch view for Hill-Sachs lesions.

- Osteolysis or fractures of the distal clavicle: The Zanca projection taken with 10° to 15° cephalad tube tilt (about half the technique of an AP shoulder projection) is used.

- Sternoclavicular (SC) joint: Two views are used to evaluate the SC joint—the Hobbs' view and the serendipity view.

- Humeral head fractures: Most fractures are visible on an AP radiograph with internal and external rotation.

Newly released radiographic guidelines for the chiropractic profession provide a very useful approach to determining both the need and type of imaging appropriate for a given patient scenario. In general, special imaging of the shoulder should be reserved for cases where conservative care has failed to resolve the problem. Available tools include MRI, computed tomography (CT), arthrography, and ultrasonography. The strengths of each are outlined below.

- MRI: MRI is a valuable tool when patients are unresponsive to conservative care. However, asymptomatic individuals may have partial or full-thickness tears. As many as 54% of asymptomatic individuals older than age 65 years were found to have partial thickness tears and 26% had full thickness tears.[73] Therefore, caution should be used when using MRI as the only indicator for need of operative repair. Full-thickness tears of the rotator cuff are readily apparent (sensitivity and specificity at 90% or above), whereas partial-thickness tears (sensitivity, 74%; specificity, 87%) may require fat saturation or other techniques to help differentiate them.[74] Glenoid labrum tears are less recognizable, and the sensitivity and specificity vary depending on the investigator. It is generally accepted, however, that the sensitivity is in the range of 75% or less.[75] This varies depending on the site. Superior tears are the most discernible, followed by a poor ability to visualize inferior tears (around 40% sensitivity), and even less ability to visualize posterior tears (about 7%).[76] New approaches being investigated and used in some facilities include the use of kinematic MRI and also performing standard MRI with the addition of gadolinium.[77]

- CT arthrogram: CT arthrograms are used mainly for glenoid labrum and rotator cuff tears; many consider them the imaging tool of choice. The difficulty is finding facilities that will perform them. The accuracy of CT arthrography with rotator cuff tears has been reported to be as high as 95% to 100%.[78] However, other studies have not demonstrated an advantage over MRI.[79]

- Ultrasonography: Ultrasonography (diagnostic ultrasound) can be an excellent tool for detecting full-thickness cuff tears. Partial tears are sometimes detectable.[80] Interpretation may be the weak point because of the major variations in findings due to operator skill.

In an extensive systematic review by Dinnes et al,[81] studies involving clinical examination, ultrasonography, MRI, and MR arthrography (MRA) were evaluated. The review was specific to impingement syndrome and rotator cuff tear (full or partial). Cohort studies for clinical examination indicated that physical examination used by specialists can rule out the presence of a rotator cuff tear.

The interobserver agreement in the classification of rotator cuff tears using MRI was examined in a recent study.[82] Although there was good agreement in predicting full-thickness rotator cuff tears and the number of tendons involved, there was moderate agreement in predicting the involved side of partial-thickness tears, and poor agreement in predicting the grade of a partial tear compared at surgery.

One recent study[83] evaluated the classification systems used by surgeons in determining rotator cuff tears. Agreement was high for full-thickness tears and whether partial tears were articular or bursal. However, the study showed disagreement on the depth of the tear. For full-thickness tears, the highest agreement was found when they were classified by topography (degree of retraction) in the frontal plane.

Management

In the event of an acute dislocation, relocation is accomplished with several maneuvers; the easiest to perform is the Milch maneuver.[84] This procedure involves slowly elevating the arm while maintaining external rotation and superior pressure on the humeral head. Another approach is to use two relocators. One provides traction or stabilization while the other uses long-arm traction of the involved arm. This distraction will significantly relieve pain. An attempt at relocation through adduction and internal rotation may be attempted. If unsuccessful, maintaining traction will reduce pain until emergency help arrives. Relocation may be difficult, and when not possible requires emergency department referral. A postreduction radiograph should be obtained to determine if there are any associated fractures. The chiropractor can play a valuable role in rehabilitation, which has been shown to substantially reduce the risk of recurrence.[85]

If radiographs reveal signs of infection, fracture, or tumor, the patient should be referred for orthopaedic consultation. All other problems can be addressed conservatively unless the patient's pain threshold does not allow a nonmedicated course. Acute pain may be managed by various physical therapy approaches, including high-voltage galvanic or interferential. Over-the-counter medications may be necessary.

Support and stabilization are needed in several scenarios: AC separations, postrelocation, atraumatic instability, and acute bursitis. These may be provided by supportive strapping using various types of elastic tape or a sling. The advantage of taping is that it allows function, whereas a sling prevents use of the arm. The pain level and degree of injury dictate the better approach.

Rehabilitation of the shoulder generally proceeds through a sequential approach, beginning with a focus on the stabilizers (rotator cuff), followed by the scapular stabilizers (serratus anterior and trapezius). The large movers such as the pectoralis major and latissimus dorsi muscles can then be addressed. Without proper stabilization, the larger muscles may cause more damage due to abnormal glenohumeral motion; without proper scapular stabilization, impingement is more likely. Muscle inhibition and altered patterns of muscle activation may be the cause or the result of shoulder disorders. Two muscles that are commonly inhibited are the serratus anterior and lower trapezius muscles.[86] The functional consequences are more likely to be evident in athletes than in an average sedentary individual.

Some recent important findings that may assist in choosing the appropriate exercise include the following:

- The work of Clisby et al.[87] and Britter et al.[88] suggests that to maximize infraspinatus activation it is important with isometric exercises to keep the load to 40% of a maximum contraction. When using concomitant adduction, keep the adduction component to a very mild contraction (10%) to avoid incorporation of the middle deltoid over the infraspinatus. With the arm at the side, the posterior deltoid may act as an adductor.
- It appears from Werner et al.[86] that the highest subacromial pressures occur with a combination of internal rotation, flexion, and abduction. Interestingly, paralysis of the supraspinatus or infraspinatus had no effect on subacromial pressure at rest, or with active shoulder movement. In a separate study by Gerber et al.[89] paralysis of the supraspinatus and infraspinatus resulted in a loss of external rotation strength by 80% and abductor strength by 75%.
- Regarding exercise performed with the shoulder in an immobilizer, Smith et al.[90] found the following. Scapular depression produced large serratus anterior activity with small rotator cuff, biceps, and anterior deltoid activity. Upper subscapularis activity was quite high with all exercises. The authors suggest that exercise is appropriate for patients postsurgically with the exception of those with initial subscapularis repair.
- Smith et al.[91] also evaluated the effect of protraction on shoulder strength. They found that internal rotation strength was reduced by 13% to 24%. External rotation increased mildly in the internally rotated position while decreasing in the neutral, or externally rotated position. It is not clear whether this is clinically detectable.

A facilitation phase using mild isometrics in various movement patterns such as internal and external rotation is helpful. Another effective tool for facilitation and stabilization is use of rapid elastic tube exercises limited to about a 20° to 30° arc (back and forth) for 60 seconds or until fatigue or pain occurs. The general program begins with light weights (5 to 10 lb) and high repetition (15 to 20), using perhaps three sets performed every day. A core group of exercises has been recommended, including the following:[92, 93]

- scaption (abduction in the scapular plane of 30° to 45° forward) or flexion
- horizontal abduction with external rotation performed prone
- seated press-up
- bent-over row
- push-up with a plus (extending the arms at the top of the push-up)

Newer recommendations still include the exercises above with some recommended modifications and the addition of only a few new exercises based on recorded EMG activity. Following is a summary of more recent conclusions:

- The infraspinatus and teres major generated moderate to high activity with both the prone horizontal and prone external rotation exercises.[94]
- Using the proprioceptive neuromuscular facilitation (PNF) approach, a D1 and D2 diagonal pattern are good overall exercises with a focus on the serratus anterior. These combination maneuvers use the entire upper extremity in a pattern of adduction, extension, and internal rotation for the D2 and abduction, flexion, and external rotation for the D1 exercise (lawnmower exercise).[95]
- Performing the push-up with a plus with the hands externally rotated and on an unstable surface provided the most stimulation for the serratus anterior.[96, 97]
- Only the press-up and push-up with a plus activate both the lower trapezius and the serratus anterior.[98]
- The side-lying wiper is a new exercise. The participant lies on his or her side, flexes the elbow 90°, abducts the shoulder 90° and supports the elbow with the opposite hand. The participant then proceeds to internally and externally rotate from this support position. Researchers found that this isolated infraspinatus activity without

significantly incorporating the upper trapezius or posterior deltoid.[99]

The importance of the posterior cuff has been overshadowed by the interest in rehabilitating the supraspinatus. Yet due to the possibility of superior humeral head translation with the supraspinatus, it is considered more important to first focus on posterior rotator cuff strengthening.

The prime concern with impingement, though, is to avoid abduction or scaption above about 70° due to the force couple of the supraspinatus and deltoid that causes an increase superior translation of the humeral head on the glenoid, increasing subacromial impingement. This superior translation may be position-dependent. Blackburn et al.[100] evaluated exercises for the supraspinatus and posterior rotator cuff. Prone horizontal abduction with the shoulder abducted 100° and externally rotated (elbow extended) caused the most activity in the supraspinatus (**Figure 7–28**). With the patient prone and the glenohumeral joint at 90° and the elbow bent to 90°, external rotation caused maximum electromyographic activity of the infraspinatus and teres minor.

A recent study by Horrigan et al.[101] used MRI to evaluate activity of muscles while individuals performed three exercises: (1) scaption with internal rotation (SIR), (2) side-lying abduction (SLA; moving from neutral or adduction to 45° abduction with 8% of body weight for males and 5% of body weight used for females), and (3) the military press. The SLA exercise (**Figure 7–29**) demonstrated the most activity (determined by signal intensity increase on MRI) for the supraspinatus, deltoid, infraspinatus, subscapularis, and trapezius. The SIR exercise showed the second highest activity for these muscles.

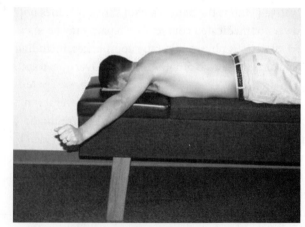

Figure 7–28 Prone arm elevation toward the ceiling with the shoulder abducted 90 to 120° is an excellent all-around rotator cuff exercise.

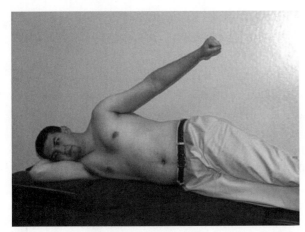

Figure 7–29 Side-lying abduction of the arm to 45° is an excellent exercise for the rotator cuff without risk of impingement. Muscles activated include the supraspinatus, deltoid, infraspinatus, subscapularis, and trapezius.

None of the exercises caused significant increased activity in the teres minor. In addition to the Horrigan study[92] that used MR relaxation time, researchers in a recent study evaluated the most effective exercise for the supraspinatus using the same measurement approach.[102] Using MRI T2 relaxation time to determine which exercise stimulated the supraspinatus most, the empty can, full can, and horizontal abduction (prone) were compared. The empty can and full can exercises had similar stimulation profiles, both demonstrating high levels of activity for the supraspinatus. Horizontal abduction was far less stimulating.

Electromyographic evaluation of a series of shoulder exercises using elastic tubing yielded the following results:[103]

- Shoulder shrug—this was considered the most effective exercise with regard to how many muscles were active; high activity was noted for the subscapularis (especially during the retraction phase), trapezius, and latissimus dorsi; other muscles that were stimulated included the supraspinatus, infraspinatus, and serratus anterior.
- Internal rotation—low levels of activity for a number of muscles including the subscapularis (which had higher activity with the shoulder shrug and narrow- and middle-grip seated rows) and pectoralis major as the two main muscles with lesser activity of the biceps, latissimus dorsi, and serratus anterior.
- External rotation—infraspinatus was the primary muscle activated; moderate activity of supraspinatus, subscapularis, pectoralis major, and serratus anterior.

- Forward punch—also considered a very effective exercise with the greatest activity from the supraspinatus, serratus anterior, and anterior deltoid; pectoralis major and infraspinatus were also stimulated.
- Seated row (middle-grip)—main activity in the supraspinatus and subscapularis.
- Seated row (wide-grip) (**Figure 7–30**)—same activity as middle-grip with addition of trapezius and infraspinatus.
- Seated row (narrow-grip)—primarily the subscapularis.

The authors suggest that for the subscapularis it might be appropriate to begin with internal rotation due to the low activity of the subscapularis and then progress to more demanding exercises such as the wide-grip seated row than progressing to the narrow- and medium-grip seated row. In contrast, for all other muscles, the wide-grip seated row is considered a more advanced exercise. In a recent study using needle EMG, nine men and six women were evaluated while performing a series of exercises, including the standard push-ups with a plus, internal rotation at the side, and diagonal exercises.[104] The findings indicated that upper subscapularis activity was greater than lower subscapularis activity for all exercises except internal rotation at the side. The push-up plus and diagonal exercises stressed both upper and lower portions of the muscle to the greatest extent. The researchers concluded that the two sections of the subscapularis may have different functional responses with exercise.

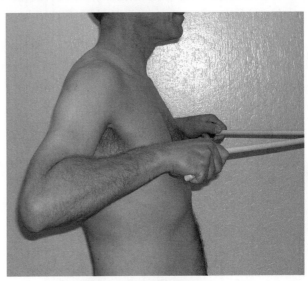

Figure 7–30 Seated rowing with a wide grip is an excellent exercise for the subscapularis, supraspinatus, and trapezius.

One recent study[105] determined surface electromyographic (EMG) activity of the serratus anterior in 20 healthy subjects performing the following exercises:

- Shoulder extension—elastic tubing is used; subject is standing with elbow flexed 90° and starting at waist height (tubing in front of body); subject extends shoulder while flexing the elbow and then returns to start position.
- Forward punch—elastic tubing is used; subject stands with tubing behind, then with starting position at side, elbow flexed 90°, subject then punches forward, flexing shoulder to shoulder height and extending elbow.
- Serratus anterior punch—elastic tubing, which is attached behind subject, is used; with the shoulder at shoulder height and elbow extended, the subject starts with the humerus internally rotated 45° and scapula retracted, then the subject protracts the scapula moving the fist forward and then retracts to the starting position.
- Dynamic hug (**Figure 7–31**)—elastic tubing, which is attached behind subject, is used; subject is standing with elbows flexed 45°, arms abducted to 60°, and the shoulders internally rotated to 45°; the subject then horizontally flexes following an imaginary arc until hands touch, then returns to the starting position.
- Scaption with external rotation—a small dumbbell is used; subject is standing and lifts the shoulder in the scapular plane to shoulder height with shoulder externally rotated (thumbs up).
- Press-up—subject is seated with hands on chair at level of buttocks, then extends elbows to lift the body off the chair; position is held for 3 seconds.

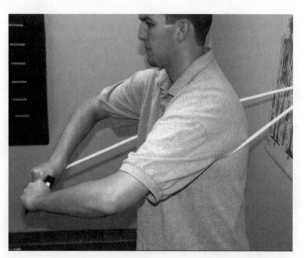

Figure 7–31 The dynamic hug exercise has been shown to be an excellent exercise for the serratus anterior (along with push-up with a plus and forward punching).

- Push-up plus—prone subject performs a standard push-up with hands shoulder-width apart, then protracts the scapula to rise higher vertically.
- Knee push-up plus—same as push-up; however, patient is supported by knees.

The serratus anterior punch, scaption with external rotation dynamic hug, knee push-up plus, and push-up plus exercises demonstrated muscle activity greater than 20% of a maximal voluntary contraction. The greatest activity was demonstrated for the push-up plus and the dynamic hug. Both accentuated scapular protraction while maintaining an upwardly rotated scapula. The advantage of these exercises is they are all performed at or below 90° of abduction avoiding potentially painful or damaging higher elevations. These exercises were ranked primarily by average amplitude, and they represent low resistance, high reps emphasizing an endurance training approach. The serratus anterior is also maximally stimulated at all higher ranges of elevation including abduction, scaption, and flexion; however, these higher positions may be unattainable or dangerous with an injured or painful shoulder.

Low Energy Laser and Shockwave Therapy

Given the current interest in low-energy laser (cold laser) treatment of soft tissue disorders, a brief description of the current evidence is warranted. Low energy laser is purported to activate the electron transport chain and thereby enhance the synthesis of ATP, which would then activate membrane ion carriers altering the flow of calcium between mitochondria and the cytoplasm. Taken as a whole, these changes theoretically speed healing through cellular mechanisms. This is accomplished without the thermal effects of higher energy lasers. There have been some small studies[106, 107] with patients suffering from myofascial chronic neck pain that suggest that low-level laser at 830 nm or 904 nm may be effective alone or in combination with other treatments compared to a sham laser treatment. Short-term effects of real shockwave therapy (SWT) include analgesic and anti-inflammatory results likely due to removal of inflammatory mediators coupled with nociceptive inhibition through a gate-control mechanism. Longer term healing effects may be related to acute vessel rupture and subsequent angiogenesis in soft tissues. EFD between 0.04 and 0.22 mJ/mm^2 have very few side effects as reported in the literature, including pain, erythema, local soft tissue swelling, and local subcutaneous hematomas among others. High-energy SWT is quite uncomfortable without local anesthetic.

At the current time, based on literature evidence, treatment parameters appear empirical. The clinician weighs the advantage of high-energy treatment with the comfort level of low-energy treatment. It does appear that both high- and low-energy protocol procedures are equally effective if the total energy applied is approximately the same. The compensation, then, is to utilize a low-energy protocol but use more impulses over more treatment sessions to achieve a similar result to high-energy treatment protocols, especially when administered by chiropractors who are not able to use local anesthetic in-office.

A Cochrane review[108] which examined the value of low-level laser on rheumatoid arthritis suggests that there may be some benefit for short-term relief. They did conclude that success was influenced by several variables, such as wavelength, treatment duration, dosage, and site. More recent evidence seems to support the use of SWT for calcific tendinitis, adhesive capsulitis, and rotator cuff tendinosis.[109, 110]

Manipulation

The literature on manipulation for the shoulder is both sparse and complex. Most studies that use the term manipulation are utilizing what chiropractors would consider mobilization (e.g., Maitland: Grade I–IV). Studies on manipulation include the cervical spine as much, or more than, the shoulder joint itself.

The largest randomized controlled study (RCT) on manipulation and the shoulder was conducted by Winters et al.[111] Their group performed a follow-up study two years later.[112] In the original study, patients from general practices in the Netherlands were included. There were 198 patients with shoulder complaints divided into diagnostic groups: a shoulder girdle group ($n = 58$) and a synovial group ($n = 114$). These diagnostic groups were based on testing that indicated for the synovial group that pain or limited movement was due to the synovial structures about the shoulder including subacromial structures, the acromioclavicular joint, the glenohumeral joint, or any combination of these. Patients in the shoulder girdle group had pain and sometimes slightly limited range of active movement of the glenohumeral joint. The assumption was, for patients with shoulder problems without specific shoulder findings, that the source was unrelated to the synovial structures but could be due to functional

disorders of the cervical spine, upper thoracic spine, or the upper ribs. Manipulation was performed by physical therapists and could include manipulation of the cervical spine, upper thoracic spine, the upper ribs, the acromioclavicular joint, or the glenohumeral joint. The method of manipulation was not clearly described. The shoulder girdle group was randomized to either manipulation or physiotherapy. Patients in the synovial group were randomized to corticosteroid injection, manipulation, or physiotherapy. In the shoulder girdle group, at five weeks, 70% of the manipulation group considered themselves cured compared to only 10% of the physiotherapy group. In the synovial group, at five weeks, 75% of patients in the injection group, 20% of the physiotherapy group, and 40% of the manipulation group reported a "cure." There was a shift of patients from the synovial group to the shoulder girdle group as a result of treatment success with nonsteroid anti-inflammatory drugs (NSAIDs). Drop-out rates due to treatment failure in the synovial group were high in the manipulation group (59%) and in the physiotherapy group (51%). In the shoulder girdle group drop-out was 20% in the manipulation group, and 45% in the physiotherapy group. The large drop-out rates are of concern, particularly with regard to the "manipulation" approach in this study. The first concern is that there is no description of the method used. Secondly, the treatment was not standardized, in that any given patient might have had manipulation of the cervical spine only, the glenohumeral joint only, or multiple joints. There is no indication of who received which method. The advantage to this approach is that it may be more representative of clinical practice where the approach varies from patient to patient based on their specific needs. However, drawing conclusions about specific manipulation approaches is not possible with this method. The follow-up study two years later[112] indicated that the advantage of manipulation or corticosteroid injection was lost over time. Part of the reason may have been the high attrition rate and a failure of "success" cases to respond.

A more recent RCT by Bergman et al.[113] studied the effectiveness of manipulative therapy for the shoulder girdle in addition to usual medical care for relief of shoulder pain and dysfunction. The premise that cervicothoracic spine dysfunction is a cause or risk factor for shoulder pain was based upon one systematic review by Sobel et al.[114] and two studies by Norlander et al.[115, 116] All patients received usual medical care from general practitioners. Only the intervention group received additional manipulative therapy to the cervicothoracic area or adjacent ribs (but not to the shoulder). Treatment consisted of up to six sessions in a 12-week period. Follow-up was over a one-year period. At six weeks, no differences between groups were demonstrated. At 12 weeks, 43% of the intervention group (manipulation plus usual medical care), and 21% of the control group reported full recovery. At 52 weeks, the same difference in recovery rate was reported. Of these groups, 16% had manipulation of a vertebral segment or joint outside the shoulder region.

In a small RCT by Conroy et al.,[117] patients were assigned to either a joint mobilization/comprehensive treatment group or a comprehensive treatment group that consisted of only the administration of hot packs, active ROM, physiologic stretching, muscle strengthening, soft tissue mobilization, and patient education. The joint mobilization utilized in the first group was of the Maitland type. Maitland mobilization involved applying oscillatory pressure of two to three oscillations per second. There was no indication of a Grade V Maitland (manipulation) being used. The experimental group (the one with joint mobilization) improved on all variables, while the control group improved only with mobility and function. The mobilization group had less 24-hour pain, and pain with a subacromial compression test when compared to the comprehensive treatment group. No differences in ROM and function were reported.

A very specific manipulation approach was evaluated in a study by Kebl et al.[118] The study involved 29 elderly patients with preexisting shoulder problems including tendinitis, bursitis, osteoarthritis, healed fracture, or neurologic impairment, and chronic pain in one or both shoulders. They were randomized to either an osteopathic manipulation therapy (OMT) group or a control group for 14 weeks. The OMT was a technique utilizing end-range isometric contractions against doctor resistance. The control group received a placebo treatment, which involved positioning only, with no contractions. Both groups had significantly increased ROM and decreased perceived pain. Those receiving the OMT demonstrated continued improvement in their ROM, while ROM in the placebo group decreased over several months. The manipulative technique was a specific approach called the Spencer technique. It is not "true" manipulation but in fact a mobilization technique involving seven end-range positions held as an isometric contraction against resistance.

A case report by Vermeulen et al.[119] involving several patients diagnosed with adhesive capsulitis tested the effects of three months of end-range mobilization on increases in range of motion and increases in joint capsule volume. Out of the seven participants, four patients rated their improvement as excellent, two rated it as good, and one rated it as moderate as related to shoulder function. At the nine-month follow-up, all patients appeared to maintain some gain in joint mobility.

A small randomized, single-blinded, placebo-controlled trial of 30 participants was conducted to determine the effect of shoulder adjusting (high-velocity, low-amplitude) on patients with a diagnosis of shoulder impingement syndrome.[120] Patients were randomized to either a de-tuned ultrasound group or a shoulder adjustment group. At the one-month follow-up, there were significant positive treatment effects with regard to a visual analog scale and Short-Form McGill Pain Questionnaire. All other studies were case studies that tended to either be general,[121-123] specific to spinal adjusting for shoulder problems,[124-126] or specific to disorder.[127-135]

The Council on Chiropractic Guidelines and Practice Parameters (CCGPP) Upper Extremity team concluded that there is moderate evidence that manipulation (i.e., mobilization including Grade V Maitland [cavitation]) may be of short-term benefit and limited evidence for long-term benefit for patients with shoulder pain.[136]

The CCGPP expert panel made recommendations for use of high-velocity, short-amplitude (HVSA) manipulation that include avoidance of any anticipated risk. Further evaluation and management may be required for patients with a failure to respond to treatment within a reasonable period of time.

- For all patients who have fracture, suspected fracture, dislocation, severe generalized or local osteoporosis, infection, tumor, or infection, HVSA manipulation is contraindicated.
- For patients who have had surgery of the shoulder, consider date of surgery, extent of surgery, type of procedure, and other related factors in making decisions about use of HVSA manipulation.
- For all patients, an evaluation for joint stability must be performed. Based on the findings, it is recommended that no HVSA manipulation be used for patients with medical subluxation, hypermobility syndromes (e.g., Marfan's, Ehlers–Danlos syndrome), or gross looseness indicating multidirectional instability. Mobilization such as applying a load-and-shift or Maitland Grade I–IV type of translational movement may be appropriate in these case settings.
- For patients with adhesive capsulitis or any acute inflammatory condition such as rheumatoid

arthritis, active hemarthrosis or extensive swelling, rheumatoid variant disease, crystalline disease (e.g., gout), or acute bursitis, it is recommended not to use HVSA. There is some literature evidence that aggressive mobilization may worsen or prolong the natural history of adhesive capsulitis.[146] Based on this evidence and the experience of our panel, it is felt that an HVSA approach is highly risky, certainly in the early stages of adhesive capsulitis. For the middle and later stages of adhesive capsulitis, chiropractors should consider a progressive application of increasing the grade of amplitude of manipulation. It is recommended that by using patient feedback and response as a guide, increasing grades of amplitude may be applied.

- For patients with impingement syndrome with a known structural cause (e.g., type 3 acromion, arthritis), it is strongly recommended that any HVSA manipulation not be applied in a superior direction.

Disorder-Specific Recommendations

Prior to prescribing a rehabilitation program for any patient it is important to understand the restrictions imposed by any underlying pathology. Some general recommendations for patients with specific shoulder problems follow:

- Instability—Although instability may either result from trauma or can be due to developmental or acquired "looseness" of the shoulder joint, the imposed restrictions in movement patterns are often similar. For anterior instability it is important to avoid the extremes of abduction, external rotation coupled with horizontal abduction (horizontal extension). This fits the general rule of thumb with any ligament/capsular injury: avoid the position of injury. Common weight-lifting maneuvers that may violate this rule are those that allow the elbow to drift behind the body, often as the starting or ending position of a given exercise. Common examples include the beginning stretch position of a "butterfly" maneuver for the pectorals. This may be imposed either by machinery (e.g., Cybex machine) or with free weights. Overhead presses with dumbbells or bars may also be dangerous if in the higher levels

of elevation the elbows drift behind the body. The lat pulldown, which uses an overhead bar attached to a pulley, begins with the shoulders in a fully stretched position of elevation. Unfortunately, the shoulders are often relaxed prior to a sudden effort to adduct the arms. This does not allow proper stabilization of the shoulder.

- Impingement—Impingement may be secondary to instability or due to other functional or mechanical causes. When secondary to instability, it is important to use the above guidelines prior to focusing on impingement restrictions. Subacromial impingement is likely to be aggravated by the position of abduction (specifically 90°–110°) and internal rotation. The most common offensive lifting maneuver is the lateral raise when the arm is in neutral or internal rotation. All overhead presses and Nautilus-type deltoid machines should be initially avoided.

- Biceps tendinitis—Given that with standard biceps exercises the tendon of the biceps is relatively stationary in relation to the intertubercular groove, these exercises are not usually the offenders. What does aggravate a biceps tendinitis is either excessive weight with traditional biceps curls, or more commonly, exercises that cause the tendon to travel up and down through the groove during the exercise. These exercises include forward flexion maneuvers such as forward raises and bench presses.

- Osteolysis of the distal clavicle—Repetitive grinding or compressive/shear forces may cause erosion of the distal end of the clavicle. Most often, the weight lifter is using a very heavy weight. It is important to avoid several exercises with this condition: bench presses using a wide grip, dips, and dead lifts. Some weight lifters also complain of pain with overhead presses. Substitution with narrow-grip bench presses, cable cross-overs, or incline or decline benching with lighter weights is suggested as an initial approach.

Algorithms

Algorithms for evaluation and management of traumatic shoulder pain, nontraumatic shoulder pain, and shoulder complaint other than pain are presented in **Figures 7–32** to **7–34**.

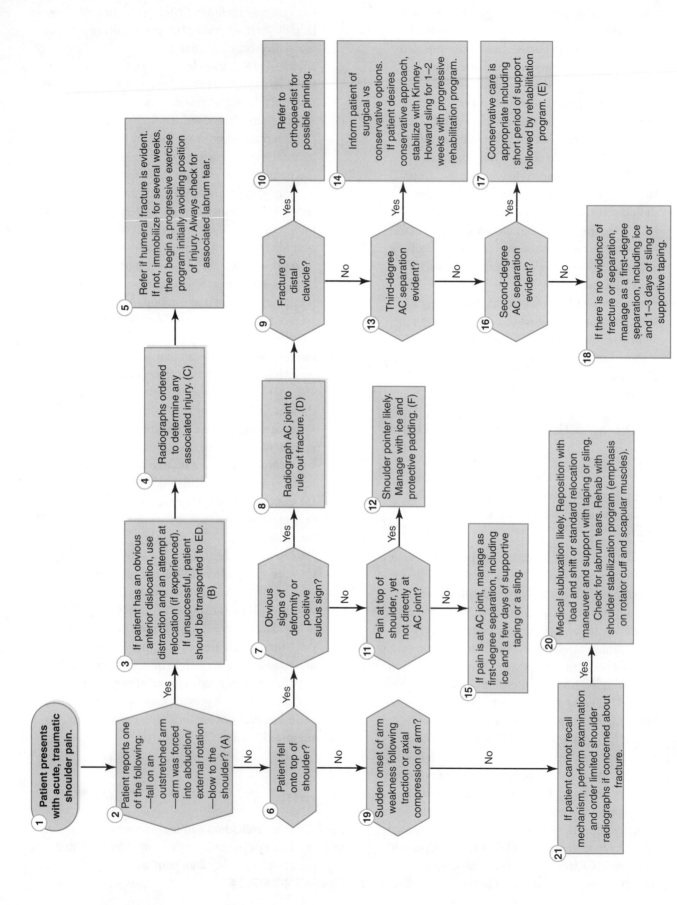

Figure 7-32 Traumatic Shoulder Pain—Algorithm

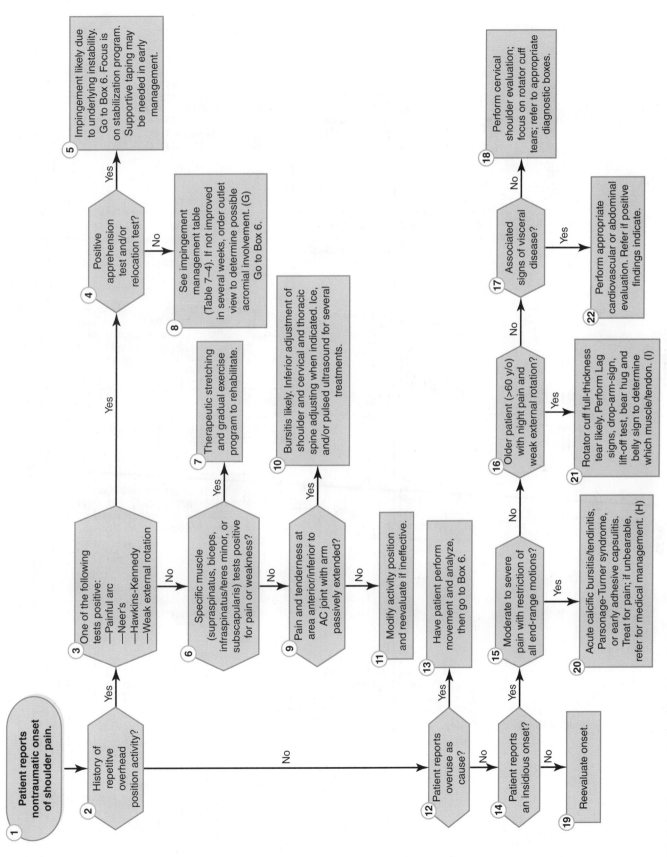

Figure 7–33 Nontraumatic Shoulder Pain—Algorithm

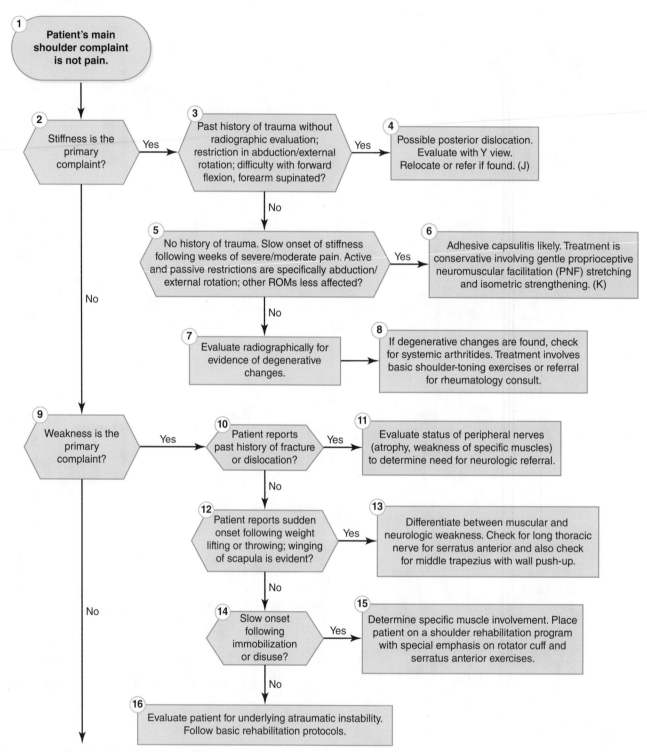

1 Patient's main shoulder complaint is not pain.

2 Stiffness is the primary complaint?
— Yes →
3 Past history of trauma without radiographic evaluation; restriction in abduction/external rotation; difficulty with forward flexion, forearm supinated?
— Yes →
4 Possible posterior dislocation. Evaluate with Y view. Relocate or refer if found. (J)

(3 → No ↓)

5 No history of trauma. Slow onset of stiffness following weeks of severe/moderate pain. Active and passive restrictions are specifically abduction/external rotation; other ROMs less affected?
— Yes →
6 Adhesive capsulitis likely. Treatment is conservative involving gentle proprioceptive neuromuscular facilitation (PNF) stretching and isometric strengthening. (K)

(5 → No ↓)

7 Evaluate radiographically for evidence of degenerative changes.
→
8 If degenerative changes are found, check for systemic arthritides. Treatment involves basic shoulder-toning exercises or referral for rheumatology consult.

(2 → No ↓)

9 Weakness is the primary complaint?
— Yes →
10 Patient reports past history of fracture or dislocation?
— Yes →
11 Evaluate status of peripheral nerves (atrophy, weakness of specific muscles) to determine need for neurologic referral.

(10 → No ↓)

12 Patient reports sudden onset following weight lifting or throwing; winging of scapula is evident?
— Yes →
13 Differentiate between muscular and neurologic weakness. Check for long thoracic nerve for serratus anterior and also check for middle trapezius with wall push-up.

(12 → No ↓)

14 Slow onset following immobilization or disuse?
— Yes →
15 Determine specific muscle involvement. Place patient on a shoulder rehabilitation program with special emphasis on rotator cuff and serratus anterior exercises.

(14 → No ↓)

16 Evaluate patient for underlying atraumatic instability. Follow basic rehabilitation protocols.

Figure 7–34 Shoulder Complaint (Other Than Pain)—Algorithm

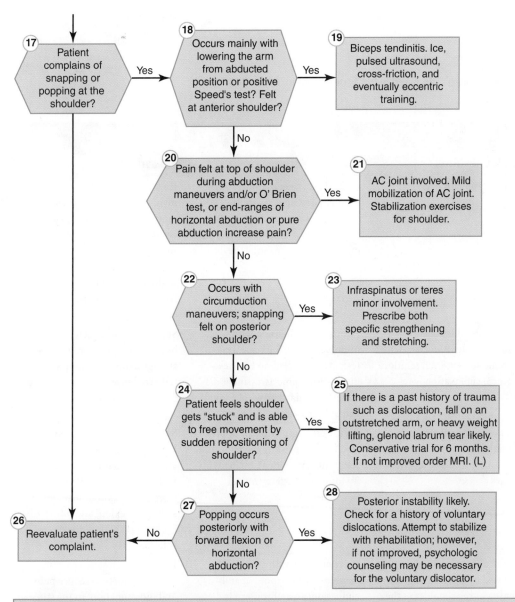

Annotations

A. Anterior dislocations are usually due to a fall or a blow to the arm when it is in a position of abduction and external rotation.

B. The Milch maneuver is an attempt to lift the arm through abduction with the arm externally rotated and at the same time maintaining superior pressure on the humeral head. Other approaches use distraction coupled with adduction and internal rotation.

C. Dislocation is usually readily apparent without films; however, complications including Hill-Sachs lesion and Bankart lesions are visible on apical oblique films or Stryker notch films. Posterior dislocation and Hill-Sachs are visible on the Y view.

D. If a deformity is present, take a Zanca (unilateral AC) radiograph (10°–15° degs. cephalad). Bilateral weighted views are rarely necessary because the distinction between second- and third-degree injuries does not alter management.

E. Second- and third-degree separations are immobilized for 1–2 weeks with a Kinney-Howard sling. Progressive exercises focus on forward flexion and shrugs.

F. A shoulder pointer is a contusion to the top of the shoulder usually involving the upper trapezius or deltoid muscle. Ice initially. Protect with doughnut padding if patient is involved in sports.

G. The outlet view is a Y view with a 10° to 20° caudal tube tilt.

H. Parsonage-Turner syndrome is a neurological inflammation probably due to a virus which often results in atrophy of involved muscles.

I. The combination of an older patient with night pain and weakness in external rotation is sensitive for full-thickness rotator cuff tears. The lift-off test, bear hug, and belly press are sensitive for subscapularis tears. The drop-arm sign is more sensitive for supraspinatus or infraspinatus tears.

J. The Y view is essentially a lateral scapular view positioning the scapula perpendicular to the bucky; central beam through the glenoid.

K. A combination of mild PNF stretching called rhythmic stabilization and ultrasound is the primary treatment. Home stretches and pendulum exercises are also helpful.

L. Labrum tests include the Crank, O'Brien, Anterior Slide, Jerk, Kim, and Biceps Load II tests (see text).

Figure 7–34 (Continued)

Selected Disorders of the Shoulder

A summary of most of the shoulder disorders discussed below is presented in **Table 7–3**.

Table 7–3 Summary of Shoulder Disorders

Condition	Signs/Symptoms	Exam Findings	Treatment
Impingement syndrome	Shoulder pain with overhead activities	Painful arc, Neer's, and Hawkins-Kennedy tests positive with secondary impingement, positive relocation test; radiographic assessment may include outlet view or Zanca view	Ice, rest from inciting activity, myofascial release to involved muscles; crossfriction to tendons; stretch posterior capsule; possible superior-to-inferior adjustment; exercise begins with arm slightly abducted, progressing from isometrics to isotonics with emphasis on rotator cuff
Traumatic anterior instability	History of shoulder dislocation (usually shoulder is overstretched into abduction/external rotation) or medical subluxation	Positive apprehension with improvement using relocation test; laxity evident on L&S testing; radiographic assessment may include standard views plus modified axillary views	Support in initial stage with bracing or taping; progressive strengthening program with initial avoidance of coupled abduction and external rotation
Nontraumatic instability	May have history of medical subluxation or simply overuse pain with overhead or repetitive activities	Positive for pain with the apprehension test; relieved by the relocation test; multidirectional, bilateral laxity found on L&S testing	Support in initial stage with bracing or taping; progressive strengthening program with emphasis on rotator cuff strengthening first; include scaption, flexion, and prone horizontal abduction/external rotation
Adhesive capsulitis	A period of pain lasting for weeks is followed by a period of gradual stiffening of the shoulder as the pain resolves	Restriction in both active and passive external rotation and abduction; an arthrogram is diagnostic in some cases but usually not necessary	Dependent on stage: pain stage requires efforts to reduce pain and inflammation; in the stiffening phase, rhythmic stabilization-based stretching and ultrasound are helpful
Rotator cuff tear	Sudden shoulder pain with overhead or lifting activity	Usually supraspinatus is involved—positive empty can test; tear visible with MRI, diagnostic ultrasound, or arthrography	Rest, ice, and support followed by a gradual strengthening program; with total rupture in an athletic patient, surgery is necessary.
AC separation	Patient fell on the shoulder or outstretched arm	Visible bump at AC joint; weighted and nonweighted views may indicate the degree of laxity and damage	Shoulder support for one to two weeks with gradual strengthening program for shoulder; focus on rotator cuff and trapezius
Labrum tear	Usually mechanical signs/symptoms with painful locking and "clunking" with a specific movement pattern	Various tests are available including the clunk test, Crank test, O'Brien sign, anterior slide test, and biceps load test (see text for description)	Some small tears may heal and respond to conservative management. Most require surgical debridement and repair.

Impingement Syndrome

Classic Presentation

The patient reports shoulder pain that is worse with overhead activities. The patient often will have a positive history for a sports or occupational requirement to work in an overhead position.

Cause

Impingement of several structures may occur. The biceps tendon, superior labrum supraspinatus tendon, and the subacromial bursa are all vulnerable to this anterolateral type of impingement. Structural causes include variant acromial types that are hooked or lengthened, degenerative changes on the undersurface of the acromion, and an inflammatory process in the subacromial space.[137] More recently, an MRI study revealed a significant number of patients with lateral, downward angulation of the acromion. In addition, medial osteophyte formation at the AC joint was found. Most of the lateral sloping acromia and medial AC joint osteophytes cannot be seen on standard radiography.[138] Functional considerations are primarily due to decreases in available subacromial space that occur with elevation and internal rotation, especially at 90°. Instability is often a coexisting problem, allowing excessive superior movement of the humeral head. There may also be a component of posterior capsular tightness that causes superior-anterior migration with arm abduction. Subcoracoid impingement may cause irritation of the subscapularis. Posterior impingement may be caused by a repetitive "cocking" position of the arm, irritating the infraspinatus or teres minor.

Evaluation

The site of tenderness varies depending on the site of impingement. Subacromial impingement causes tenderness and pain at the anterior joint at the biceps tendon, supraspinatus insertion at the greater tuberosity, or under the AC joint. More posterior tenderness suggests impingement of the infraspinatus/teres minor tendons. Tenderness or pain at the coracoid process that is made worse by passive horizontal adduction may indicate subcoracoid impingement of the subscapularis. The traditional tests include demonstration of a painful arc, the Hawkins-Kennedy test, and Neer's test.[139] The painful arc (Figure 7–4) is evident when a patient has an increase of pain in the mid-range of 70° to 110° of abduction with less or no pain above or below this range. The Hawkins-Kennedy test (Figure 7–12) passively places the patient's arm in forward flexion 90° with the elbow flexed to 90° and passively rotated internally. Neer's test (Figure 7–11) is a passive forward flexion test that is positive for pain at full end-range flexion. Another confirmatory test in patients with underlying instability is relief of pain with anterior-to-posterior support in the apprehension position, the relocation test (Figure 7–8).

Management

The management approach is based on the severity of symptoms; however, the long-range goal is to stabilize the shoulder with a progressive rehabilitation program, stretching of the posterior capsule, and modification of sport or occupational activities (**Table 7–4**). If the patient is not responsive in several months, an MRI may be helpful in differential diagnosis or planning any surgical management. One study was based on the premise that there may be a delay in muscle activation with sudden movement of the shoulder that may lead to impingement.[140] The researchers used surface EMG and found muscle recruitment to sudden movement. The sequence was an initial activation of the middle deltoid followed by simultaneous contraction of all three heads of the trapezius. This pattern was not altered but was delayed in fatigued muscles. These findings may be used as part of a strategic prevention plan for impingement.

Researchers in another study focused on an approach to prevent impingement by affecting the position of the scapula through stretching and strengthening.[141] Researchers evaluated scapular position using a three-dimensional electromechanical digitizer that determined both thoracic inclination and scapular orientation and position. Twenty asymptomatic volunteers with a forward shoulder posture were given pectoral muscle stretching and also strengthening exercises for the scapular retractors and elevators and the glenohumeral abductors and external rotators. Exercises and stretching were performed three times per week for six weeks. Strength of horizontal abduction and internal and external rotation increased while anterior inclination of the thoracic spine decreased. The glenohumeral contribution to elevation increased. At 90° abduction, the scapula showed less upward rotation and less superior translation after the exercise test period.

A study evaluating the relationship between patients with impingement and posterior capsular tightness and any related effects on range of motion found that patients with impingement of the nondominant arm had posterior capsular tightness and restrictions in both internal and external rotation as compared to the control group (patients without impingement).[142] Patients with impingement of the dominant arm had posterior capsular tightness and limitation in internal rotation only as compared to the control group.

Borstad et al.[143] have demonstrated a possible relationship between a shortened pectoralis minor muscle and impingement. Shortening appears to alter scapular kinematics causing more anterior tipping and internal rotation. In a second study, Borstad et al.[144] evaluated three approaches to stretching the pectoralis minor. One approach was the self-stretch in the doorway with the arm

Table 7–4 Management of Impingement Syndrome and Tendinitis

Parameter	Acute Stage	Subacute Stage	Symptom-Free Stage
Criteria	Painful arc, +Hawkins-Kennedy and Neer's tests, pain with overhead activity; for isolated tendinitis, pain with specific muscle action	Tests are less positive for pain	Tests are no longer positive
Goals	Decrease inflammation and pain	Increase rotator cuff strength while avoiding impingement position	Train through impingement range; functionally train for occupational or sport activity
Concerns	May be caused by a mechanical irritation from os acromiale or type III acromion	Overzealous athlete or worker unable or unwilling to rehabilitate the rotator cuff	Overzealous with progressing through exercise routine or not maintaining improvement with a routine shoulder exercise program
Requirements for progression to next stage; approximate time needed	Able to perform isometrics throughout ROM without pain, pain-free passive ROM; 1 week	Able to perform three sets of 15 repetitions of primary exercises pain-free for several days in a row; 3–6 weeks	Able to perform functional exercises without pain
Manipulation/ mobilization	Superior-to-inferior manipulation or mobilization may be helpful; check cervical spine and scapula for fixation	Superior-to-inferior manipulation or mobilization may be helpful; check cervical spine and scapula for fixation	Superior-to-inferior manipulation or mobilization may be helpful; check cervical spine and scapula for fixation
Modalities	Inferential at 80–150 pps/20 minutes daily with ice	Ultrasound at 1.4 wt/cm2 for 5 minutes; ice after exercise	Ice after exercise
External brace, support, etc.	Usually not necessary; however, shoulder support taping may be of benefit	None	None
ROM/flexibility	Codman/pendulum exercises; begin stretching of posterior shoulder capsule	Continue posterior capsular stretching	Continue posterior capsular stretching
Open-chain exercise	Isometrics performed every 20° to 30°	Begin with midrange, short arc, fast reciprocating motions into internal and external rotation. Perform daily exercise with light weight (1–5 lb), working up to 3 sets of 15 repetitions; exercises include scaption or flexion, prone horizontal abduction, bent-over rowing, internal rotation	Perform plyometric exercises if patient is an athlete and uses upper body; plyoball tosses against a wall or mini trampoline
Closed-chain exercise	None	Wall push-ups, press-ups, push-ups with a plus	Balance ball and wobble board push-ups; stair-step machine using hands
Proprioceptive training	Passive PNF diagonal patterns into flexion and extension	Begin PNF diagonal patterns with accommodated resistance	Incorporate PNF functional patterns specific to sport or occupation
Associated biomechanical items	Scapular immobility, cervical or thoracic spine dysfunction	Scapular immobility, cervical or thoracic spine dysfunction	Incorporate lower body training to reduce stress on shoulder; include balance exercises on balance boards
Lifestyle/activity modifications	Avoid overhead activities; maintain aerobic capacity with bicycling or running	Gradually introduce minimal overhead activities; maintain aerobic capacity with bicycling or running	Perform every-other-day shoulder exercise routine

Key: PNF, proprioceptive neuromuscular facilitation.

at 90° abduction and the patient rotating the trunk outward to stretch. The other doctor-assisted stretches included a supine stretch with the arm in the apprehension position and the other seated with scapular stabilization with the back hand while the front hand pushed posteriorly at the AC joint. The most effective approach was the self-stretch in the doorway.

In a prospective, randomized trial by Walther et al.,[145] it appears that patients with impingement syndrome managed with either conventional physiotherapy, a self-training program, or functional brace had the same significant improvement in function and pain at 12 weeks. A new approach being used for chronic tendinosis throughout the body is a sclerosing of neovessels that develop in the involved area of the tendon. For the supraspinatus, one study's results indicate a potential use for recalcitrant patients.[146]

Traumatic Instability

Classic Presentation

The patient has a past history of shoulder dislocation. The patient currently complains of pain or weakness when the arm is placed in either an overhead position or the apprehension position of 90° flexion coupled with external rotation and horizontal abduction (horizontal extension).

Cause

Dislocation of the glenohumeral joint causes significant damage to the capsule, some ligaments, often the glenoid labrum, and the humerus itself. The result is a diminished static support system that must rely on dynamic support from the surrounding muscula-ture. A common acronym used for this type of instability is TUBS, which stands for Traumatic, Unilateral, Bankart (a Bankart lesion represents anterior-inferior labrum damage), and Surgery. This implies that this traumatically induced type of instability causes a labrum tear often requiring surgery. This is also referred to as Torn Loose instability. Anterior instability due to an anterior disloca-tion is the most common, accounting for 90% to 95% of cases.[147] Posterior instability is found in patients who chronically self-dislo-cate or patients who have seizures.

Evaluation

Stability should be evaluated with an L&S test and the apprehension tests and its variants.[34] The L&S test (Figure 7–6) is a push–pull maneuver applied to the neutral shoulder in an attempt to determine in which direction instability is present. Inferior instability is suggestive of multidirectional instability. In other words, for there to be significant inferior displacement, much of the capsule must be damaged. The apprehension position (Figure 7–7) tests the patient for the reproduction of apprehension (a sense that the shoulder may go out of place) and pain. If either sensation is found, an anterior-to-posterior force is applied to the patient in the supine posi-tion as the apprehension position is acquired (the relocation test) (Figure 7–8). If the apprehension is ameliorated, instability is likely. If pain is reduced, a coexisting impingement syndrome may be causing discomfort. Glenoid labrum testing should also be included. Several tests exist, including the Crank test, the O'Brien sign (Figure 7–10), and various shear tests in search of painful snapping or clunking felt deep in the shoulder.[43] Other tests include the jerk test and the Kim test, both described in the examination section of this chapter. Superior labrum anterior to posterior (SLAP) tears are further tested with specific tests challenging the origin of the long head of the biceps off of the superior labrum including Yergason's, biceps load test II, and Speed's test.

Management

Results from a recent study suggest that patients who have a first-time dislocation are at risk for dislocation within the first six weeks.[148] Patients with substantial pain, a visible shoulder deformity, or restriction in movement at one-week post reduction should be reevaluated with radiographs to exclude redislocation.

A study by Itoi et al.[149] demonstrated a significant decrease in redislocation for first-time dislocators (anterior) if the arm is immo-bilized in an externally rotated (26% versus 42%) instead of the traditional internally rotated position. It was recommended for those 30 years of age or younger.

Unfortunately, shoulders with traumatic instability are less amenable to conservative management (**Table 7–5**). These shoulders often have underlying mechanical interference with normal movement. Until the mechanical factor is surgically removed or repaired, the patient may continue to experience symptoms. The need for surgery is based entirely on activity level and degree of incapacita-tion. Prior to surgical consultation, most patients should be taken through a six-month trial of conservative care with a focus on shoulder stabilization. In patients with instability, the middle and posterior deltoid, in addition to the scapular muscles, should be the focus.[150] The anterior head may provide significant shear force and should initially be de-emphasized.

Shoulder bracing for instability has been classified into three types.[151] The first uses a checkrein to keep the shoulder in a "safe-zone." The other two apply direct or indirect posterior forces to the shoulder, usually through neoprene or similar materi-als. However, it appears that the stabilizing effect is probably not related to restriction of shoulder external rotation and is likely

Table 7–5 Management of Chronic Anterior or Multidirectional Shoulder Instability

Parameter	Initial Stage	Intermediate Stage	Advanced Stage
Criteria	Instability evident on L&S or other stability tests; pain or apprehension with apprehension test; relieved by relocation test	Instability testing remains unaffected; however, pain or apprehension is reduced when performing apprehension test	Full pain-free ROM present; all muscles test strong in all ROMs
Goals	Initiate shoulder stabilization program while avoiding positions of risk	Focus on rotator cuff and scapular stabilization exercises, protected return to sporting activity if support is worn	Functionally train the shoulder to meet the demands of a given sport or occupational activity
Concerns	May be an associated glenoid labrum tear that will interfere or prevent successful rehabilitation	Possible glenoid labrum tear or too early a return to activity, noncompliance of patient with exercise program requirements and restrictions	Patient compliance with continuing exercises in a preventive program
Requirements for progression to next stage; approximate time needed	Strength present within lower ranges of shoulder movement; scapula demonstrates stability with resisted abduction or protraction; no "mechanical" pain block in active movement patterns; 1–2 weeks	Pain-free shoulder ROM; muscles test strong without pain; able to perform three sets of 10 reps for 2–3 weeks without pain; 3–6 weeks	Pain-free performance of sport or occupational activity; 3–6 months
Manipulation/mobilization	Mild mobilization into restricted accessory motion; however, manipulation is contraindicated; cervical spine adjusting may be helpful	Mild mobilization into restricted accessory motion; however, manipulation is contraindicated; cervical spine adjusting may be helpful	Mild mobilization into restricted accessory motion; however, manipulation should be employed with caution; cervical spine adjusting may be helpful
Modalities	Ice after exercise	Ice after exercise	Ice after exercise
External brace, support, etc.	Shoulder support taping or bracing may be needed in the earlier stages while performing exercises	Shoulder support taping or bracing may be needed in the earlier stages while performing exercises	Exercises performed without bracing or taping; for high-level competition, it may be necessary to continue wearing a restriction brace for an extended period of time
ROM/flexibility/massage	Passive PNF diagonal patterns to facilitate functional movement patterns	Myofascial release technique for scapular and anterior chest muscles	As needed
Open-chain exercise	Isometrics in multiple arcs throughout a range of motion; then rhythmic stabilization in multiple arcs (reciprocal motion in a short arc performed as quickly as possible until pain or fatigue limits)	Core exercises include scaption or flexion, prone abduction, prone rowing, pressup, and prone flies (for midscapular muscles) performed with light weights or elastic tubing, performing 3–5 sets of 12–15 reps	Plyometric exercises using plyoballs against wall and mini trampoline (size of ball based on functional activity requirements)
Closed-chain exercise	None	Wall push-ups progressing to ground push-ups to push-ups with a plus	Balance on palms using balance ball stabilization approach; use balance devices to perform push-ups on; use stair-stepping machine using hands

Table 7–5 Management of Chronic Anterior or Multidirectional Shoulder Instability (continued)

Parameter	Initial Stage	Intermediate Stage	Advanced Stage
Proprioceptive training	Taping or support is primary proprioceptive stimulus plus PNF passive diagonals	Resisted PNF diagonal patterns (incorporates patterns that combine either flexion/extension with external rotation/internal rotation, with abduction/adduction)	Accomplish to some degree by plyometrics; PNF sport-specific patterns can be emphasized; PNF exercises can be performed in various body positions that simulate the sport or occupational requirements
Associated biomechanical items	Address spinal posture as contributing factor, including hyperlordotic cervical and lumbar curves, and a hyperkyphotic thoracic curve creating a slumped position of the shoulder	Continue to address spinal posture with focus on reduction of thoracic kyphosis; begin strengthening lower extremity and trunk for need in reducing stress on shoulder muscles with throwing and other activities	Continue to address spinal posture with focus on reduction of thoracic kyphosis; begin strengthening lower extremity and trunk for need in reducing stress on shoulder muscles with throwing and other activities
Lifestyle/activity modifications	Avoid carrying objects that drag down on the arm; avoid overhead and abduction/external rotation positions	Avoid abduction and external rotation against resistance such as ball throwing or racquet hitting	Make shoulder exercises a part of every-other-day exercise routine

proprioceptive in nature (similar to the effect of taping on stability).[152] The decision as to which is appropriate is dictated by cost, comfort, and if a sport is played, which one.

The standard for symptomatic TUBS patients is an open Bankart procedure (patients have torn the anterior-inferior labrum [Bankart lesion]). The procedure involves suturing of the capsulolabral complex to the anterior glenoid rim. Failure rates were originally reported at about 2% (redislocations). This study indicated that the failure rate was 11% with patient follow-up after four to nine years. (Subluxation [medical] was included in the criteria for failure.)[153]

In recent studies, researchers have attempted to determine the long-term effects of various surgical procedures for instability. One study[154] compared open to arthroscopically performed surgery and the outcome of redislocation rates, and researchers found that open surgery using suture anchors compared with arthroscopically placed bioabsorbable tacks (Suretac fixators) demonstrated a redislocation rate of 10% for the open and 15% for the arthroscopically performed procedures using a follow-up of two to five years. There appeared to be more limitation in external rotation with the open procedure than with the arthroscopic procedure.

One of the concerns with surgery is the loss of proprioception due to nerve damage. In one study[155] researchers evaluated the role of surgery in actually restoring proprioceptive reflex activity for patients with shoulder instability. Surgical interventions, whether arthroscopic, open, or thermal, seem to restore proprioceptive defects that existed after joint injury.

Thermal capsulorrhaphy, or thermal-assisted capsular shrinkage (TACS), is the delivery of thermal energy in the form of a laser or radiofrequency device used to shrink the capsule in individuals with capsular laxity without tearing (AMBRI patients). The primary change that occurs is conversion of collagen to a homogenous sheet of protein (hyalinization). A normal histologic appearance has been reported to take approximately 12 weeks to occur; however, in one study, patients who had failed procedures and were treated operatively had reported attenuation (thinning) of the capsule, making surgery more difficult. Also, researchers found that histologic abnormalities can exist for up to 16 months post-capsulorrhaphy.[156]

Although many TACS procedures were performed without long-term information about outcome, in a recent study researchers reported the results of a 15- to 47-month follow-up.[157] Over time, 231 consecutive overhead athletes were followed. Of these, 87% returned to competition and 88% reported good to excellent long-term outcomes using the athletic shoulder outcome rating scale. With the recent advent of thermal-assisted approaches to tightening loose shoulder capsules, several concerns have developed. Due to reported failures, one study attempted to determine whether there were indicators of failure based on a follow-up study of 106 patients receiving TACS procedure.[158] Concomitant surgical procedures at the time of TACS were not associated with failure. The researchers found that TACS may have limited value for the following patients:

- Those who have had prior operations
- Those with multiple dislocations

- Those with multidirectional instability
- Those involved in contact sports

A more recent two-year, follow-up study by Hawkins et al.[159] evaluated the long-term effects of TACS. They concluded that the failure rates are still quite high for multidirectional and posterior instability. They recommend capsular placation and/or rotator interval closure if used in the treatment of these cases. They also recommend lengthening the initial immobilization period. Articles by Wilk et al.[160] and Tyler et al.[161] review a theoretical approach to rehabilitation following TACS based on type of patient and procedure. For overhead athletes, they recommend not allowing excessive external rotation or elevation and no shoulder extension post-op. For those with congenital laxity, they recommend no passive ROM until after 14 days of immobilization. And for those with labrum procedures, they recommend avoidance of isolated biceps training for six to eight weeks post-op.

Nontraumatic Instability or Looseness

Classic Presentation

The patient is usually asymptomatic. When symptoms occur, they often are the result of a sudden traction on the arm that results in pain and weakness felt in the entire arm (subluxation); supporting the arm relieves symptoms. Another common presentation is difficulty working in overhead positions due to a sense of fatigue rather than pain.

Cause

Most patients have an inherent looseness to their shoulder capsules (born loose).[162] This may be accentuated by sporting activities that constantly stretch the capsule, such as with throwing sports and swimming. The acronym for this type of instability is AMBRI: Atraumatic, Multidirectional, Bilateral, often responds to Rehabilitation, and does not require an Inferior capsular shift surgical stabilization procedure. Patients are asymptomatic unless the shoulder is subluxated with a distraction force or they develop impingement secondary to a loose capsule.

Evaluation

The L&S tests (Figure 7–6) are the most practical ones. Pulling the humeral head forward or backward usually indicates a large degree of movement, sometimes enough to almost subluxate the joint. Most important, inferior traction often causes the development of a sulcus sign or depression under the AC joint. These findings are bilateral. Researchers in one study were interested in determining whether there were differences in translation between patients who had the traumatic type of instability (TUBS) versus the acquired (AMBRI).[163] Also, they wanted to determine any differences between symptomatic and asymptomatic shoulders. Open MRI was used with the shoulder in various positions with and without muscle activity. Results showed that those with TUBs had increased translation at 90/90 position; however, muscle activity helped to recenter the humeral head. Interestingly, those with AMBRI had increased translation of both shoulders that was not recentered with muscle activity.

Researchers evaluating swimmers versus other athletes who do not use shoulder elevation as a prominent feature of the sport (i.e., soccer) indicated that significantly more translation occurred in swimmers as compared to soccer players. However, there was no "instability" related to these findings in asymptomatic patients.[164] If the patient has developed secondary impingement, another finding (in addition to positive impingement tests) is pain that is produced by the apprehension test (Figure 7–7). The pain is reduced by the relocation test (Figure 7–8), in which an anterior-to-posterior force is applied to the proximal humerus as the arm is abducted and externally rotated (supine patient).

Management

A standard strengthening program involving initial focus on the rotator cuff and serratus anterior is necessary to substitute for the laxity of the joint capsule (Table 7–4). This may be assisted by functionally taping the shoulder. Avoidance of positions that further stretch the capsule is important. Surgical stabilization is rarely necessary.

Adhesive Capsulitis

Classic Presentation

The presentation varies depending on the stage at which the patient presents. The patient is usually over age 40 years. In the acute phase, the patient complains of moderate to severe pain that limits all shoulder movement. In most instances, the patient cannot recall any specific event that triggered the pain. The pain interferes with sleep and in many instances causes the patient to seek prescribed pain medication. In the middle phase, the patient may present with a past history of the acute phase one to three months previously; now the pain is much less, but she or he notices that lifting the arm or turning it out is severely restricted. In the final phase, the patient may report a very slow increase in ROM, but he or she still has significant reduction.

Cause

The prevalence of adhesive capsulitis is 0.5% of the general patients while 4.3% of the diabetic patients meet the criteria for adhesive capsulitis.[165] The cause is unknown. The most accepted theory is that adhesion development occurs between or within the capsule of the shoulder; however, this is not always visible at surgery. Also, the patient often responds to stretching techniques that place little stretch on the capsule. Some individuals may be predisposed, such as those with diabetes, hyperthyroidism, or chronic obstructive or other lung disease, and those who have had a myocardial infarction.[166] It has been shown that, contrary to logic, this process is not due to immobilization. The process begins as an inflammatory process that resolves with fibrosis. The three stages are: (1) an acute inflammatory stage that causes a presentation that overlaps with other conditions, leading to (2) a stiffening stage, and months to years later (3) a thawing phase wherein some of the ROM is recovered.

Evaluation

Most patients present in the stiffening phase. The classic restriction pattern is a significant and equal loss of active and passive ROM. The movements most affected are abduction and external rotation. Flexion is usually the least restricted. Muscle testing is usually strong within the available range. Loss of abduction is often substituted by shoulder shrugging or trunk leaning. Improvement of motion restriction following mild reciprocal isometric contractions (rhythmic stabilization) is confirmatory for adhesive capsulitis. Lack of improvement suggests a bony blockage possibly due to osteoarthritis or an undiagnosed posterior dislocation (if there is a history of trauma).

Management

As noted in previous studies, Levine et al.[167] reiterate that conservative management of adhesive capsulitis has similar clinical outcomes to surgical management (manipulation under anesthesia). Patients treated conservatively generally showed significant improvement over a period of three to six months. Those who went on to surgery were generally younger patients and had usually attempted conservative management for about one year. Conservative management in this study included physical therapy with a large percentage of patients (37%) who received a corticosteroid injection at some time in their treatment. Supporting this observation was the study by Kivimaki et al.[168] Patients were randomized into a manipulation under anesthesia (MUA) group or a control group of home exercise only. After a one-year follow-up, there were no significant differences in pain or function.

Another approach to adhesive capsulitis is arthrographic distension therapy where fluid is introduced into the shoulder joint to distend the capsule and break up adhesions. Either steroids or a saline solution is typically used. In a 2008 Cochrane review,[169] there was fairly strong evidence that saline and steroid distension provided short-term benefits for pain, range of motion, and function; however, there was no indication that this was better than alternative treatments.

Yet another study[170] compared manipulation under anesthesia to distension therapy with steroid injection. The results, using standardized outcome measures such as a Constant Score, visual analog scale, and Short Form-36 (SF36), found no difference in the two groups after two years, with the researchers concluding that the higher risk of manipulation under anesthesia was a reason to preferentially use distension therapy. This was a small study and limited in strength for that reason. In a study[171] comparing not only pain relief but increases in external rotation, researchers found that in addition to a higher percentage of patients being pain-free following distension (88%) compared to MUA (67%), a higher percentage of patients with distension therapy had an increase in external rotation compared to those with MUA. Again, the conclusions are limited by the small sample size of patients.

Exhibit 7–4 **Treatment of Adhesive Capsulitis**

Stage I (acute)

In-office
- Treatment in the acute stage focuses on pain relief through the use of aspirin or nonsteroid anti-inflammatory drugs and transcutaneous electrical nerve stimulation.
- Avoid aggressive mobilization or adjustive techniques.

Home
- Use passive Codman's exercises and mild isometrics (25% contraction for 5 to 8 seconds).
- Sleep on unaffected side with affected side supported by a pillow to avoid excessive internal rotation.

(continues)

Exhibit 7–4 **Treatment of Adhesive Capsulitis (continued)**

Stages II and III (subacute and chronic)

In-office
- Continue treatment for pain.
- Use ultrasound for palliative pain relief and use prior to stretching.
- Use rhythmic stabilization and hold–relax techniques to increase ROM.
- Use passive stretching with moist heat pack and gravity assistance.

Home
- Do further stretching with self-mobilization with an emphasis on inferior glide.
- Do "giant ball" exercises, pulley exercises, and wand exercises for later stages of stretching.

Most patients in the acute phase do not respond to physical therapy attempts at pain control. During this phase, the pain is often disabling, requiring prescribed pain medication. The chiropractor is most effective in the later stages. In the stiffening phase, use of rhythmic stabilization, coupled with ultrasound, is usually effective in increasing ROM (Exhibit 7–1). This is supported by home exercises, including continuation of rhythmic stabilization, pendulum, and proper wall-walking exercises. Rhythmic stabilization involves taking the patient's arm to the available end-range of abduction/external rotation. The patient is then instructed to apply a minimal (15% to 25%) contraction into further abduction/external rotation for five or six seconds, followed by an immediate switch to the opposite pattern. This reciprocates back and forth several times. The patient relaxes, and the new range is passively acquired by the doctor. Mild mobilization at the joint may be helpful; however, forceful adjusting is likely to cause an inflammatory flare-up. Significant improvement should occur over a one- to three-month period. Failure to improve warrants referral for MUA.

Rotator Cuff Tear

Classic Presentation

There are two possibilities, dependent on age. For the younger patient, the patient is likely to give a history of an acute traumatic event such as lifting a heavy weight or a fall on an outstretched arm. Older patients may not recall the inciting event, complaining of insidious onset of pain felt at night. Patients usually complain of pain with overhead activities or weakness in lifting the arm.

Cause

The most common tears are in the supraspinatus. There are generally two areas where tears occur—articular sided and bursal sided. Most partial tears are articular sided and may be related to poor vascularity.[172] Tears may be due to a sudden trauma (especially a pincer action) or more likely occur secondary to chronic degenerative changes in the tendon.

Evaluation

The patient often has signs similar to those of the patient with impingement. The patient usually has difficulty raising or lowering the arm actively. The combination of a painful arc, drop-arm sign, and weak external rotation is diagnostic of rotator cuff tear if all are positive. For the supraspinatus, weakness is found with the empty can test (Figure 7–14) or the drop-arm sign. External rotation is weak for both supraspinatus and infraspinatus tears. For the subscapularis, weakness is found with the lift-off test, the internal rotation lag sign, the belly press, and the bear hug tests. More recently, a number of "lag" signs have been evaluated (see description in the main text). Radiographically, there may be apparent superior head migration on an AP view. Further imaging can be accomplished with ultrasonography, MRI, or an arthrogram. Ultrasonography is accurate but operator-dependent, MRI is sensitive but may require fat suppression to distinguish rotator cuff tear from other changes, and an arthrogram cannot evaluate bursal-sided partial tears.[173]

Management

Partial tears can be rehabilitated gradually, beginning with isometrics and gradually progressing through a strengthening program (Exhibit 7–2). A rest period from sports or occupational activities is required. Full-thickness tears are usually surgically repaired in younger individuals.

Acute Calcific Bursitis and Tendinitis
Classic Presentation

The patient presents with severe shoulder pain that increases with any shoulder movement, either with an insidious onset or subsequent to a fall or other major trauma.

Cause

The prevalence of calcific tendinitis ranges from 7% to 36% of the population with a reported incidence of between 2.5% and 20%.[174] The calcified tendon is visible on radiographs and was thought to represent a degenerative process. Rowe,[175] however, found that calcific tendinitis did not occur in patients under age 30 years or over age 60 years and that many patients with radiographic evidence of calcification were asymptomatic. For calcific tendinitis, there are intratendinous deposits of carbonated apatite. It appears that pain occurs on resorption of the calcium deposition. This is an inflammatory phase and causes pain that lasts about two weeks in the acute phase and up to three months in the chronic form of the disorder. Direct trauma and trauma subsequent to cuff rupture are other more obvious causes.

Evaluation

The patient exhibits a supportive posture, holding the arm against the side to avoid movement. All movement, active and passive, is painful. If possible, the bursa may be palpated by passively extending the shoulder and palpating in front of the AC joint for tenderness and swelling. There are two classifications utilized to rank calcifications based on size and clinical presentation. The Bosworth system[176] classifies calcium deposition as tiny (0.5 cm), medium (0.5–1.5 cm) and large (1.5 cm). The Gartner and Simons[177] classifications include: Type 1, pasting and not clear on radiographs; Type 2, pasting and clear on radiographs; and Type 3, without clear limits and a tendency toward spontaneous resolution. These classification systems are utilized in studies of effectiveness when utilizing ultrasound, shockwave therapy, or corticosteroid injection.

Management

An attempt at sling support and palliative physical therapy application may be made. Evidence suggests that ultrasound helps in resorption of the calcific deposits.[178] In a recent study,[179] researchers randomized symptomatic patients with verified calcific tendinitis into one group treated with ultrasound (15-minute session with frequency of 0.89 MHz and intensity of 2.5 watts square centimeter on pulsed mode 1:4) while the other group received a sham insonation. Treatment was for six weeks, with daily treatments for the first three weeks and then three times/week for three weeks. After a nine-month follow-up period, 42% of patients had calcific deposition resolution and 23% had partial resolution if they had been treated with the pulsed ultrasound regimen. There was only 2% to 3% resolution in the sham group. There were greater decreases in pain at the end of treatment phase for the pulsed ultrasound-treated group versus the sham. However, at nine months the difference between the groups was no longer significant, suggesting that there may be a role in short-term management only.

Another approach to calcific tendinitis is the use of extracorporeal shockwave therapy. This approach is also used for lateral epicondylitis and plantar fasciitis, among other similar conditions. Researchers in one study evaluated the difference between two protocols, one using a low-energy density (1,500 impulses of 0.06 mJ/mm² compared to 1,500 impulses of 0.28 mJ/mm²), requiring the use of local anesthesia.[179] In the high-intensity group, 68% of patients rated the results of treatment good or excellent compared to only 52% in the low-energy group at a six-month follow-up. In a more recent publication,[180] in a small randomized trial, groups were also assigned to different energy levels. One group received extracorporeal shock wave therapy (ESWT) at an energy level of 0.20 mJ/mm², and the other group received ESWT at an energy level of 0.10 mJ/mm². Both groups received 2,400 pulses once a week for four weeks. Although calcific deposits resolved in the same percentage of patients in both groups, an energy level of 0.20 mJ/mm² appeared to be more effective than an energy level of 0.10 mJ/mm² if matched to the outcomes of pain relief and functional improvement again supported by the previous study's findings.

Exhibit 7–5 Treatment of Acromioclavicular Joint Injury

AC Separations

Type I—Sprain (first-degree separation)

- Use ice and analgesics for pain control.
- Rehabilitative exercises may begin quickly because the AC joint is stable.
- Protective doughnut pad should be worn during contact sport participation.

(continues)

Exhibit 7–5 Treatment of Acromioclavicular Joint Injury (continued)

Type II—Partial subluxation (second-degree separation—torn AC ligament)

- Use ice and analgesics.
- Immobilize with a Kinney-Howard sling with following recommendations:
  1. Two slings are used so that the athlete may shower with support.
  2. Changing slings should be done only with the elbow supported.
  3. Tightening of the sling also should be done with elbow support.
  4. The sling is worn for about two weeks, depending on extent of injury.
- Isometrics may be performed while in the sling, using the opposite hand (elevation of the arm or shoulder is avoided).
- After the sling, rehabilitate the shoulder muscles with emphasis on:
  1. deltoid with shrugs and raises (limited to below 90° initially)
  2. trapezius with shrugs and front rows
  3. biceps
  4. pectorals with light weights and avoiding extremes of horizontal adduction initially
- Return to sport requires protective pad sewn or taped into place.

Type III—Total separation (third-degree separation—torn AC and coracoclavicular ligaments)

- Use ice and analgesics for pain.
- Options suggested by various practitioners:
  1. Immobilization for two to four weeks in a Kinney-Howard sling with above rehabilitation (author's choice).
  2. No immobilization with use of progressive exercises and sports participation with protection in two to four weeks.
  3. Surgical repair including the following options:
     —stabilization of clavicle to coracoid with a screw
     —resection of lateral clavicle
     —transarticular AC fixation with pins
     —use of coracoacromial ligament as substitute AC ligament

Osteolysis of the distal clavicle

- Athlete retires from competitive weight lifting.
- Modify weight-lifting activities, including the following:
  1. Substitute bench press with incline or decline press, or cross-cable exercises.
  2. Modify bench press using close grip instead of wide grip; reduce weight used.
  3. Eliminate dips and substitute with above pectoral exercises and triceps extensions.
- Athlete undergoes surgery, usually resection of lateral/distal clavicle.

Shoulder pointer and acromial apophysitis

- Use ice and analgesics for pain.
- Avoid overhead activities for several weeks, in particular with weights.
- Protect the lesion with an acromial (doughnut) pad.

Many patients with acute bursitis, however, are in severe pain requiring prescription medication in the early stages.

Acromioclavicular Separation

Classic Presentation

The patient presents with a traumatic onset of shoulder pain following either a fall on an outstretched arm or a fall onto the top of the shoulder.

Cause

AC separations are classified into three grades (however, six types have been described by Rockwood et al.[181]). Grade I (first degree) indicates some tearing of the AC ligament, but no instability. Grade II (second degree) indicates rupture of the AC ligament. Grade III (third degree) involves tearing of the AC ligament and the coracoclavicular (conoid and trapezoid) ligaments. Both grades II and III are unstable.

Evaluation

The mechanism of injury and the pain/tenderness and swelling or deformity at the AC joint are classic findings. Radiographs should be obtained to rule out a distal clavicular fracture or to determine degree of injury. Weighted and nonweighted bilateral views are used to demonstrate an increased coracoclavicular space. A space greater than 1.3 cm is usually consistent with a third-degree (grade III) separation. The displacement is due less to superior migration of the distal clavicle than to inferior displacement of the glenohumeral joint.[182] In other words, this represents a different form of shoulder instability and as a result requires stabilization and support more than replacement of the clavicle into its normal position.

Management

All AC separations can be managed conservatively (see Exhibit 7–2).[183] As in previous studies, Calvo et al.[184] found that conservative management of third-degree separations result in the same successful, long-term clinical outcomes as surgical management. Those treated surgically had a higher incidence of osteoarthritis and coracoclavicular ligament ossification. Grade III separations will leave a permanent bump at the shoulder, and for some patients may be a persistent site of minor discomfort. For those patients who require cosmetic perfection, or for those in whom conservative management has not sufficiently returned to normal function, surgery is an option. The standard treatment of AC separations includes a short period of support with a Kinney-Howard sling (shoulder support on same side as arm sling). Mild isometrics followed by isotonics with emphasis on deltoid and upper trapezius exercises followed by biceps and pectoral exercises are usually sufficient to return to near full function. Padded protection should be worn in sports activities.

Osteolysis of the Distal Clavicle

Classic Presentation

Osteolysis may be secondary to AC trauma or excessive weight lifting. The weight lifter is usually a young man complaining of diffuse pain felt with the bench press, clean and jerk, or dip. The patient is a serious weight lifter who benches 300 pounds or more.

Cause

The cause is unknown. However, direct trauma to the AC joint, as occurs with AC separations or repetitive compression from specific weight-lifting maneuvers, causes a resorption of the distal end of the clavicle.[22]

Evaluation

Although the patient may complain of pain when abducting beyond 90°, the orthopaedic shoulder examination findings are usually unremarkable. This fact, combined with finding a discrete area of tenderness at the AC joint or distal clavicle, should raise the suspicion. Instead of a shoulder series, the radiographic view of choice is the AC spot (Zanca) view. This involves a 10° to 15° cephalad tube tilt shot, with about half of the technique used for a general shoulder radiograph. Resorption is usually evident with an increased widening of the joint space or subchondral defects.

Management

Osteolysis requires a period of modification in weight-lifting activities. Modification includes switching to narrow-grip bench presses (instead of wide grip), cable cross-overs, and incline or decline presses. The dip should be avoided. If the pain persists, however, the only conservative solution is to stop lifting heavy weights for at least six months. If not effective or the patient is noncompliant, resection or acromioplasty may be somewhat effective.

Little Leaguer's Shoulder

Classic Presentation

A 14-year-old male baseball pitcher complains of shoulder pain that occurs mainly when throwing hard. The pain has come on gradually. He points to a tender area that is located at the proximal humerus.

Cause

Rotational stresses on the growth plate of the proximal humerus result in a Salter-Harris Type 1 injury in pitchers who over-pitch or who pitch too frequently. More rarely, this may cause a Salter-Harris Type 2 fracture with a triangular metaphyseal avulsion.

Evaluation

Researchers in a recent article attempted to determine whether those individuals with Little Leaguer's shoulder had similar characteristics given that there is no specific clinical test for this condition.[185] The problem is that, according to this study, the average child with Little Leaguer's shoulder had symptoms for over seven months before being diagnosed! The profile that developed follows:

- Male pitcher around 14 years of age (basemen were second most common, with outfielders and catchers least affected)
- Involved in youth or adolescent baseball
- Either playing continuously for 12 months on a single team or playing for six months on more than one team
- Pain of gradual onset (small percentage had sudden onset)
- Pain at the proximal humerus felt only when throwing hard
- Pain unrelated to a specific phase of throwing (in most cases)
- Pain for an average of seven months (wide range, from one week to two years in the current study)

Examination findings included:

- Swelling and loss of range of motion are uncommon findings.
- Tenderness over the proximal humerus is the most consistent finding. (Specific tenderness over the lateral aspect of the proximal humerus was found in 70% of patients in this study.)
- In this study, the only weakness detected was in external rotation.
- Various muscle testing positions increased the pain; however, the two most common were external rotation testing and the empty can test (thumbs-down abduction).

Radiographic findings included:

- The most consistent finding is widening of the proximal humeral physis.
- Additional findings include demineralization, sclerosis of the proximal humeral metaphysis, and fragmentation of the lateral aspect of the proximal humeral metaphysis.
- Bilateral views are recommended due to the variation in the "look" of epiphyses.
- AP internal and external views are recommended. (*Souza note: Always consult with a chiropractic or medical radiologist if there is any doubt.*)
- It may take several months for the widening of the proximal humeral physis to "heal" radiographically.

Management

Although there is no agreed-upon management recommendation, it is clear that rest is essential, although how long is debatable. In the current study, an average of three months was used, with three caveats:

1. The radiographic "healing" may take longer than three months; however, this should not prevent the initial rehabilitation phase of return to easy throwing.
2. A gradual return to throwing is needed, with pain as the limiting factor.
3. Recovery time varies, and in some cases it may take as long as 12 months (until the next season) before the pitcher can return to throwing full force.

In the current study, resistance exercises often caused pain and therefore were not used as a primary approach to the return-to-play rehabilitation prescription. An interval training approach has been developed by Axe et al.[186] These recommendations are based on age and pitch speed. Although there are Little League rules regarding how often a pitcher can pitch, what often is not taken into consideration are practice sessions and that a player may play for more than one team. Also, adherence to the rules is variable. A good resource for coaches and parents is an article (written for parents) by Andrews and Feisig[187] about how many pitches should be allowed. Complications of Little Leaguer's shoulder include the rare avascular necrosis, loose bodies, and early closure of the epiphysis.

The Evidence - Shoulder

Translation Into Practice Summary (TIPS)

The literature on evaluation of the shoulder is extensive. It provides some strong direction as to what is and is not helpful in the diagnosis of specific conditions; however, overlap of terms and conditions makes a specific diagnosis sometimes difficult. Distinction between neck and shoulder pain versus shoulder pain alone is an important discriminator prior to testing the patient. Many of the diagnostic tests in the literature have been designed and tested in orthopaedic or sports centers and may not reflect the patient population of a practice environment that is not specialized. There is agreement in the literature that the diagnostic evaluation is very good at ruling-out serious conditions.

The Literature-Based Clinical Core

- Age gives a helpful starting point in determining the risk of specific disorders.
- For labrum tears the history is neither sensitive nor specific except for a minimally helpful support when a patient reports popping, clicking, or catching.
- Range of motion is highly reliable but of unknown diagnostic value; however, it may provide some indications of functional capacity.
- Manual muscle testing is reliable with certain weakness thresholds indicative of specific pathologies:
  a. Weak abduction and/or external rotation—subacromial impingement and/or full thickness rotator cuff tears
  b. Weak internal rotation—subscapularis tears
- Evaluation of muscle or posterior capsular tightness is moderately reliable but is not helpful in distinguishing between symptomatic and asymptomatic patients, and is therefore of unknown value.
- For instability:
  a. The apprehension test is most valuable for identifying instability when "apprehension" is the positive finding.
  b. Labrum tear tests are highly variable; however, there is some evidence that the Kim and the jerk test may be helpful in ruling-in a labrum tear,

with the biceps load test II useful in identifying SLAP lesions. None of the tests are good at ruling out a labrum tear.

  c. The combination of the Anterior Apprehension Test and Jobe Relocation Test may be of value in identifying but not ruling-out labrum tears.
  d. For ruling-in and ruling-out labrum tears, the combination of the crank, apprehension, relocation, load-and-shift, and inferior sulcus sign may be of value.
  e. For ruling-in or ruling-out SLAP lesions, combining two highly sensitive tests (compression rotation, anterior apprehension, and O'Brien tests) with one specific test (Yergason's, biceps I & II, and Speed's tests) may be helpful, whereas individually the tests are of little value.
- For subacromial impingement:
  a. The Hawkins-Kennedy and Neer tests together may be helpful in ruling-in or ruling-out impingement.
  b. The painful arc may add useful support for a diagnosis of impingement but is not specific.
  c. The combination of a painful arc, Hawkins-Kennedy, and weak external rotation has a good post-test probability of detecting impingement.
- For rotator cuff tendinitis:
  a. The Hawkins' and Neer's tests alone may provide some value in ruling-in a rotator cuff tendinitis but they are specific to a particular tendon and may overlap with subacromial impingement test findings.
  b. The combination of a positive response for both the Hawkins' and Neer's tests is more valuable than each test alone for identifying rotator cuff tendinitis.
- For rotator cuff tears:
  a. The combination of the history of a patient age 65 years or older suffering from night pain with weak external rotation is helpful in ruling-in rotator cuff tear if all are positive; if none are positive, good at ruling-out rotator cuff tear.
  b. The combination of a painful arc, weakness in external rotation, and a positive drop-arm sign together are good at ruling-in a rotator cuff tear though not any specific tendon. Ruling-out is strongest with the absence of positives on all the tests.
  c. Nonspecific tests for ruling-in but not ruling-out rotator cuff tears are the belly press, bear

hug, and Napoleon tests. The hornblower sign may be a good ruling-in and ruling-out test.

d. Specific tests may identify some specific muscles if there is a full-thickness tear:

  i. Subscapularis—the lift-off test, internal rotation lag-sign are good for ruling-in a full-thickness tear.

  ii. Infraspinatus—resisted external rotation weakness is reasonably good at ruling in a full-thickness tear. The drop-arm test is a good rule-in and rule-out test for full-thickness tears.

  iii. Supraspinatus – the drop-arm test is a good rule-in and rule-out test for full thickness tears.

- For the AC joint:

  a. Findings of AC tenderness or positives for AC compression, the O'Brien sign, Paxinos sign, or palpation of the AC joint are not helpful in ruling-in or ruling-out AC disorders.

  b. There may be some value for the AC resisted extension test in ruling-in or ruling-out AC disorders.

The Expert-Opinion-Based Clinical Core

- The observation of deformity with a history of trauma is useful in determining the need for radiographs.
- The limitation of forward flexion of the shoulder with the arm supinated is a good indicator of posterior dislocation.
- The limitation of abduction/external rotation and/or internal rotation that is the same with both active and passive ROM testing is a strong indicator for middle-phase adhesive capsulitis.

APPENDIX 7–1

References

1. Van der Heijden GJ. Shoulder disorders: a state-of-the-art review. *Ballieres Clin Rheumatol.* 1999;2:287–309.

2. Croft P, Pope D, Silman A. The clinical course of shoulder pain: prospective cohort study in primary care. Primary Care Rheumatology Society Shoulder Study Group. *BMJ.* 1996;313:601–602.

3. Bartolozzi A, Andreychik D, Ahmad S. Determinants of outcome in the treatment of rotator cuff disease. *Clin Orthop Relat Res.* 1994;308:90–97.

4. van der Windt DA, Koes BW, de Jong BA, Bouter LM. Shoulder disorders in general practice: incidence, patient characteristics, and management. *Ann Rheum Dis.* 1995;54:959–964.

5. Chard MD, Sattelle LM, Hazleman BL. The long-term outcome of rotator cuff tendinitis—a review study. *Br J Rheumatol.* 1988;27(5):385–389.

6. van der Windt DA, Koes BW, Boeke AJ, Deville W, De Jong BA, Bouter LM. Shoulder disorders in general practice: prognostic indicators of outcome. *Br J Gen Pract.* 1996;46:519–523.

7. Croft P, Pope D, Silman A. The clinical course of shoulder pain: prospective cohort study in primary care. Primary Care Rheumatology Society Shoulder Study Group. *BMJ.* 1996;313(7057):601–602.

8. Souza TA, ed. *Sports Injuries of the Shoulder: Conservative Management.* New York: Churchill Livingstone; 1994.

9. Ratcliffe A, Flatow EL, Roth N, et al. Biochemical markers in synovial fluid identify early osteoarthritis of the glenohumeral joint. *Clin Orthop.* 1996;330:45–53.

10. Harryman DT, Sidles JA, Clark JM, et al. Translation of the humeral head on the glenoid with passive glenohumeral motion. *J Bone Joint Surg Am.* 1990;72:1334–1343.

11. Howell SM, Galinat BJ, Benzi AJ, et al. Normal and abnormal mechanics of the glenohumeral joint in the horizontal plane. *J Bone Joint Surg Am.* 1988;70:227–232.

12. Perry J. Muscle control of the shoulder. In: Rowe CR, ed. *The Shoulder.* New York: Churchill Livingstone; 1988;17.

13. Lee SB, Kim KJ, O'Driscoll SW, Morrey BF, An KN. Dynamic glenohumeral stability provided by the rotator cuff muscles in the mid-range and end-range of motion: a study in cadavera. *J Bone Joint Surg Am.* 2000;82-A(6):849–857.

14. Kido T, Itoi E, Lee SB, et al. Dynamic stabilizing function of the deltoid muscle in shoulders with anterior instability. *Am J Sports Med.* 2004;31(3):399–403.

15. Nuber CW, Bowman JD, Perry JP, et al. EMG analysis of classical shoulder motion. *Trans Orthop Res Soc.* 1986;11:186–189.

16. Jobe CM. Superior glenoid impingement. *Orthop Clin North Am.* 1997;28(2):137–143.

17. Thomas E, van der Windt DA, Hay EM, et al. Two pragmatic trials of treatment for shoulder disorders in primary care: generalisability, course, and prognostic indicators. *Ann Rheum Dis.* 2005;64(7):1056–1061.

18. Largacha M, Parsons IM, Campbell B, Titelman RM, Smith KL, Matsen F, 3rd. Deficits in shoulder function and general health associated with sixteen common shoulder diagnoses: a study of 2674 patients. *J Shoulder Elbow Surg.* 2006;15(1):30–39.

19. Miranda H, Viikari-Juntura E, Martikainen R, Takala EP, Riihimaki H. A prospective study of work related factors and physical exercise as predictors of shoulder pain. *Occup Environ Med.* 2001;58(8):528–534.

20. Leclerc A, Chastang JF, Niedhammer I, Landre MF, Roquelaure Y. Incidence of shoulder pain in repetitive work. *Occup Environ Med.* 2004;61(1):39–44.

21. Bot SD, Terwee CB, van der Windt DA, Bouter LM, Dekker J, de Vet HC. Clinimetric evaluation of shoulder disability questionnaires: a systematic review of the literature. *Ann Rheum Dis.* 2004;63(4):335–341.

22. Scavenius M, Iversen BF. Nontraumatic clavicular osteolysis in weight lifters. *Am J Sports Med.* 1992;20:463.

23. Mattingly GE, Mackarey PJ. Optimal methods for shoulder tendon palpation: a cadaver study. *Phys Ther.* 1996;76:166–174.

24. Hayes K, Walton JR, Szomor ZR, Murrell GA. Reliability of five methods for assessing shoulder range of motion. *Aust J Physiother.* 2001;47:289–294.

25. Wakabayashi I, Itoi E, Minagawa H, et al. Does reaching the back reflect the actual internal rotation of the shoulder? *J Shoulder Elbow Surg.* 2006;15(3):306–310.

26. Ginn KA, Cohen ML, Herbert RD. Does hand-behind-back range of motion accurately reflect shoulder internal rotation? *J Shoulder Elbow Surg.* 2006;15(3):311–314.

27. Hayes KW, Petersen CM. Reliability of classifications derived from Cyriax's resisted testing in subjects with painful shoulders and knees. *J Orthop Sports Phys Ther.* 2003;33(5):235–246.

28. Doddy SG, Waterland JC, Freedman L. Scapulohumeral goniometer. *Arch Phys Med Rehabil.* 1970;51:711.

29. Jobe FW, Moynes DR, Brewster CE. Rehabilitation of shoulder instabilities. *Orthop Clin North Am.* 1987;18:473.

30. McQuade KJ, Smidt GL. Dynamic scapulohumeral rhythm: the effects of external resistance during elevation of the arm in the scapular plane. *J Orthop Sports Phys Ther.* 1998;27(2):125–133.

31. Kibler WB. The role of the scapula in athletic shoulder function. *Am J Sports Med.* 1998;26:325–337.

32. Odom CJ, Hurd CE, Denegar CR, et al. Intratester and intertester reliability of the lateral scapular slide test: Master's thesis. Slippery Rock University, Slippery Rock, PA, 1994.

33. Koslow PA, Prosser LA, Strony GA, et al. Specificity of the lateral scapular slide test in asymptomatic competitive athletes. *J Orthop Sports Phys Ther.* 2003;33:331–336.

34. Hawkins RJ, Schutte JP, Huckell GH, et al. The assessment of glenohumeral translation using manual and fluoroscopic techniques. *Orthop Trans.* 1988;12:727.

35. Pizzari T, Kolt GS, Remedios L. Measurement of anterior-to-posterior translation of the glenohumeral joint using the KT-1000. *J Orthop Sports Phys Ther.* 1999;29:602–608.

36. Altcheck DA, Warren RF, Oritz G, et al. T-Plasty: a technique for testing multidirectional instability in the athlete. *J Bone Joint Surg.* 1991;73A:105–112.

37. Cofield RH, Mansat P. Examination under anesthesia. In: Warren RF, Craig EV, Altcheck DA, eds. *The Unstable Shoulder.* Philadelphia: Lippincott-Raven; 1999:133–139.

38. Rockwood CA. Subluxations and dislocations about the shoulder. In: Rockwood CA, Green DP, eds. *Fractures in Adults.* 2nd ed. Philadelphia: WB Saunders Company; 1984:722.

39. Jobe FW, Kvine RS. Shoulder pain in the overhand and throwing athletes: the relationship of anterior instability and rotator cuff impingement. *Orthop Rev.* 1989;18:963.

40. Hammer DL, Pink MM, Jobe FW. A modification of the relocation test: arthroscopic findings associated with a positive test. *J Shoulder Elbow Surg.* 2000;9(4):263–267.

41. Kibler WB. Specificity and sensitivity of the anterior slide test in throwing athletes with superior glenoid labral tears. *Arthroscopy.* 1995;11:296–300.

42. O'Brien SJ, Pagnani MJ, Fealy S, et al. The active compression test: a new and effective test for diagnosing labral tears and acromioclavicular joint abnormality. *Am J Sports Med.* 1998;26:610–613.

43. Kim SH, Ha KI, Han KY. Biceps load test: a clinical test for superior labrum anterior and posterior lesions (SLAP) in shoulders with recurrent anterior dislocations. *Am J Sports Med.* 1999;27(3):300–303.

44. Liu SH, Henry MH, Nuccion S, et al. Diagnosis of glenoid labral tears: a comparison between magnetic resonance imaging and clinical examinations. *Am J Sports Med.* 1996;24:149–154.

45. McFarland EG, Kyum Kim T, Savino RM. Clinical assessment of three common tests for superior labral anterior-posterior lesions. *Am J Sports Med.* 2002;30(6):810–815.

46. Stetson WB, Templin K. The Crank test, the O'Brien test, and routine magnetic resonance imaging scans in the diagnosis of labral tears. *Am J Sports Med.* 2002;30(6):806–809.

47. Parentis MA, Mohr KJ, ElAttrache NS. Disorders of the superior labrum: review and treatment guidelines. *Clin Orthop Rel Res.* 2002;400:77–87.

48. Guanche CA, Jones DC. Clinical testing for tears of the glenoid labrum. *Arthroscopy.* 2003;19(5):517–523.

49. Kim SH, Ha KI, Ahn JH, et al. Biceps load test II: a clinical test for SLAP lesions of the shoulder. *Arthroscopy.* 2001;17(2):160–164.

50. Kim YS, Kim JM, Ha KY, Choy S, Joo MW, Chung YG. The passive compression test: a new clinical test for superior labral tears of the shoulder. *Am J Sports Med.* 2007;35(9):1489–1494.

51. Savoie FH, Field LD, Atchinson S. Anterior superior instability with rotator cuff tearing: SLAC lesion. *Ortho Clin Am.* 2001;32(3):457–461.

52. Mair S, Zarzour R, Speer K. Posterior labral injury in contact athletes. *Am J Sports Med.* 1998;26:753–759.

53. Luime JJ, Verhagen AP, Miedema HS, et al. Does this patient have an instability of the shoulder or a labrum lesion? *JAMA.* 2004;292:1989–1999.

54. Parentis MA, Glousman RE, Mohr KS, Yocum LA. An evaluation of the provocative tests for superior labral anterior posterior lesions. *Am J Sports Med.* 2006;34(2):265–268.

55. Walsworth MK, Doukas WC, Murphy KP, Mielcarek BJ, Michener LA. Reliability and diagnostic accuracy of history and physical examination for diagnosing glenoid labral tears. *Am J Sports Med.* 2008;36(1):162–168.

56. Neer CS. Anterior acromioplasty for chronic impingement syndrome in the shoulder: a preliminary report. *J Bone Joint Surg Am.* 1972;54:41.

57. Hawkins RJ, Kennedy JC. Impingement syndrome in athletes. *Am J Sports Med.* 1980;8:151.

58. Pappas GP, Blemker SS, Beaulieu CF, McAdams TR, Whalen ST, Gold GE. In vivo anatomy of the Neer and Hawkins sign positions for shoulder impingement. *J Shoulder Elbow Surg.* 2006;15(1):40–49.

59. Gold GE, Pappas GP, Blemker SS, et al. Abduction and external rotation in shoulder impingement: an open MR study on healthy volunteers initial experience. *Radiology.* 2007;244(3):815–822.

60. Ardic F, Kahraman Y, Kacar M, Kahraman MC, Findikoglu G, Yorgancioglu ZR. Shoulder impingement syndrome: relationships between clinical, functional, and radiologic findings. *Am J Phys Med Rehabil.* 2006;85(1):53–60.

61. Park HB, Yokota A, Gill HS, El Rassi G, McFarland EG. Diagnostic accuracy of clinical tests for the different degrees of subacromial impingement syndrome. *J Bone Joint Surg Am.* 2005;87(7):1446–1455.

62. Wolf EM, Agrawal V. Transdeltoid palpation (the rent test) in the diagnosis of rotator cuff tears. *J Shoulder Elbow Surg.* 2001;10(5):470–473.

63. Itoi E, Minagawa H, Yamamoto N, Seki N, Abe H. Are pain location and physical examinations useful in locating a tear site of the rotator cuff? *Am J Sports Med.* 2006;34(2):256–264.

64. Kim TK, Rauh PB, McFarland EG. Partial tears of the subscapularis tendon found during arthroscopic procedures on the shoulder: a statistical analysis of sixty cases. *Am J Sports Med.* 2003;31(5):744–750.

65. Rowlands LK, Wertsh JJ, Prinack SJ. Kinesiology of the empty can test. *Am J Phys Med Rehabil.* 1995;74:302–304.

66. Kelly BT, Kadmas WR, Speer KP. The manual muscle examination for rotator cuff strength: an electromyographic investigation. *Am J Sports Med.* 1996;24:581–593.

67. Grenshaw AH, Kilgore WE. Surgical treatment of biceps tenosynovitis. *J Bone Joint Surg Am.* 1966;48:1496.

68. Jemp YN, Malanga G, Growney ES. Activation of the rotator cuff in generating isometric shoulder rotation torque. *Am J Sports Med.* 1996;24:477–485.

69. Greis PE, Kuhn JE, Schultheis JM, et al. Validation of the lift-off test and analysis of subscapularis activity during maximal internal rotation. *Am J Sports Med.* 1996;24:589–593.

70. Faruqui S, Wijdicks Foad A. Sensitivity of physical examination versus arthroscopy in diagnosing subscapularis tendon injury. *Orthopedics.* 2014;37:E29–E33.

71. Hertel R, Ballmer FT, Lambert SM, Gerber CH. Lag signs in the diagnosis of rotator cuff rupture. *J Shoulder Elbow Surg.* 1996;5:307–313.

72. Davis J. Radiography. In: Souza TA, ed. *Sports Injuries of the Shoulder: Conservative Management.* New York: Churchill Livingstone; 1994:257.

73. Sher JS, Uribe JW, Posada A, et al. Abnormal findings on magnetic resonance images of asymptomatic shoulders. *J Bone Joint Surg Am*. 1995;77(1):10–15.

74. Tuite MJ, Yandov DR, DeSmet AA, et al. Diagnosis of partial and complete rotator cuff tears using combined gradient echo and sine echo imaging. *Skeletal Radiol*. 1994;23:541–545.

75. Green MR, Christensen KP. Magnetic resonance imaging of the glenoid labrum. *Am J Sports Med*. 1990;18:229–234.

76. Legan JM, Burkhard TK, Golf WB, et al. Tears of the glenoid labrum: MR imaging of 88 arthroscopically confirmed cases. *Radiology*. 1991;179:241–246.

77. Bonutti PM, Norfray JF, Friedman RJ, Genez BM. Kinematic MRI of the shoulder. *J Comput Assist Tomogr*. 1993;17:666–669.

78. Hunter JC, Blatz DJ, Escobedo EM. SLAP lesions of the glenoid labrum: CT arthrographic and arthroscopic correlation. *Radiology*. 1992;184:513–518.

79. Neumann CH, Petersen SA, Jahnke AH, et al. MRI in the evaluation of patients with suspected instability of the shoulder joint including comparison with CT arthrography. *Rofo*. 1991;154:593.

80. Introcaso JH. Sonography. In: Souza TA, ed. *Sports Injuries of the Shoulder: Conservative Management*. New York: Churchill Livingstone; 1994:291.

81. Dinnes J, Loveman E, McIntyre L, Waugh N. The effectiveness of diagnostic tests for the assessment of shoulder pain due to soft tissue disorders: a systematic review. *Health Technol Assess*. Vol 7; 2003:iii,1–166.

82. Spencer EE, Jr., Dunn WR, Wright RW, et al. Interobserver agreement in the classification of rotator cuff tears using magnetic resonance imaging. *Am J Sports Med*. 2008;36(1):99–103.

83. Kuhn JE, Dunn WR, Ma B, et al. Interobserver agreement in the classification of rotator cuff tears. *Am J Sports Med*. 2007;35(3):437–441.

84. Milch H. Treatment of dislocation of the shoulder. *Surgery*. 1938;3:732.

85. Aronen JG, Rehan K. Decreasing the incidence of recurrence of first-time anterior shoulder dislocations with rehabilitation. *Am J Sports Med*. 1984;12:283.

86. Glousman R, Jobe FW, Tibone JE, et al. Dynamic electromyography analysis of the throwing shoulder with glenohumeral instability. *J Bone Joint Surg*. 1988;70-A:220–226.

87. Clisby EF, Bitter NL, Sandow MJ, Jones MA, Magarey ME, Jaberzadeh S. Relative contributions of infraspinatus and deltoid during external rotation in patients with symptomatic subacromial impingement. *J Shoulder Elbow Surg*. 2007;17(1S):S87–S92.

88. Bitter NL, Clisby EF, Jones MA, Magarey ME, Jaberzadeh S, Sandow MJ. Relative contributions of infraspinatus and deltoid during external rotation in healthy shoulders. *J Shoulder Elbow Surg*. 2007;16(5):563–568.

89. Gerber C, Blumenthal S, Curt A, Werner CM. Effect of selective experimental suprascapular nerve block on abduction and external rotation strength of the shoulder. *J Shoulder Elbow Surg*. 2007;16(6):815–820.

90. Smith J, Dahm DL, Kaufman KR, et al. Electromyographic activity in the immobilized shoulder girdle musculature during scapulothoracic exercises. *Arch Phys Med Rehabil*. 2006;87(7):923–927.

91. Smith J, Dietrich CT, Kotajarvi BR, Kaufman KR. The effect of scapular protraction on isometric shoulder rotation strength in normal subjects. *J Shoulder Elbow Surg*. 2006;15(3):339–343.

92. Townsend H, Jobe FW, Pink M, Perry J. Electromyographic analysis of the glenohumeral muscles during a baseball rehabilitation program. *Am F Sports Med*. 1991;19:264.

93. Moseley JB, Jr, Jobe FW, Pink M, et al. EMG analysis of the scapular muscles during a shoulder rehabilitation program. *Am J Sports Med*. 1992;20:128.

94. Sciascia A, Kuschinsky N, Nitz AJ, Mair SD, Uhl TL. Electromyographical comparison of four common shoulder exercises in unstable and stable shoulders. *Rehabil Res Pract*. 2012;783–824.

95. Escamilla RF, Yamashiro K, Paulos L, Andrews JR. Shoulder muscle activity and function in common shoulder rehabilitation exercises. *Sports Med*. 2009;39(8):663–685.

96. Lee S, Lee D, Park J. The effect of hand position changes on electromyographic activity of shoulder stabilizers during push-up plus exercise on stable and unstable surfaces. *J Phys Ther Sci*. 2013;25(8):981–984.

97. Seo SH, Jeon IH, Cho YH, Lee HG, Hwang YT, Jang JH. Surface EMG during the push-up plus exercise on a stable support or Swiss ball: scapular stabilizer muscle exercise. *J Phys Ther Sci*. 2013;25(7):833–837.

98. Andersen CH, Zebis MK, Saervoll C, et al. Scapular muscle activity from selected strengthening exercises performed at low and high intensities. *J Strength Cond Res*. 2012;26(9):2408–2416.

99. Ha SM, Kwon OY, Cynn HS, Lee WH, Kim SJ, Park KN. Selective activation of the infraspinatus muscle. *J Athl Train*. 2013;48(3):346–352.

100. Blackburn TA, McLeod WD, Whilte B, Wolford L. EMG analysis of posterior rotator cuff exercises. *Athletic Training*. 1990;25(1):40–45.

101. Horrigan JM, Shellock FG, Mink JH, Deutsch AL. Magnetic resonance imaging evaluation of muscle usage associated with three exercises for rotator cuff rehabilitation. *Med Sci Sports Exerc*. 1999;31(10):1361–1366.

102. Takeda Y, Kashiwaguchi S, Endo K, et al. The most effective exercise for strengthening the supraspinatus muscle: evaluation by magnetic resonance imaging. *Am J Sports Med* 2002;30(3):374–381.

103. Hintermeister RA, Lange GW, Schultheis JM, Bey MJ, Hawkins RJ. Electromyographic activity and applied load during shoulder rehabilitation exercises using elastic resistance. *Am J Sports Med*. 1998;26(2):210–220.

104. Decker MJ, Tokish JM, Ellis HB, Torry MR, Hawkins RJ. Subscapularis activity during selected rehabilitation exercises. *Am J Sports Med*. 2003;31(1):126–134.

105. Decker MJ, Hintermeister RA, Faber KJ, Hawkins RJ. Serratus anterior muscle activity during selected rehabilitation exercises. *Am J Sports Med*. 1999;27:784–791.

106. Gur A, Sarac AJ, Cevik R, Altindag O, Sarac S. Efficacy of 904 nm gallium arsenide low level laser therapy in the management of chronic myofascial pain in the neck: a double-blind and randomize-controlled trial. *Lasers Surg Med*. 2004;35(3):229–235.

107. Chow RT, Heller GZ, Barnsley L. The effect of 300 mW, 830 nm laser on chronic neck pain: a double-blind, randomized, placebo-controlled study. *Pain*. 2006;124(1–2):201–210.

108. Brosseau L, Robinson V, Wells G, et al. Low level laser therapy (Classes I, II and III) for treating rheumatoid arthritis. *Cochrane Database Syst Rev*. 2005(4):CD002049.

109. Galasso O, Amelio E, Riccelli DA, Gasparini G. Short-term outcomes of extracorporeal shock wave therapy for the treatment of chronic non-calcific tendinopathy of the supraspinatus: a double-blind, randomized, placebo-controlled trial. *BMC Musculoskelet Disord*. 2012;13:86.

110. Speed C. A systematic review of shockwave therapies in soft tissue conditions: focusing on the evidence. *Br J Sports Med*. 2013. doi: 10.1136/bjsports-2012-091961

111. Winters, JC, Sobel, et al. Comparison of physiotherapy, manipulation, and corticosteroid injection for treating shoulder complaints in general practice: randomised, single-blind study. *BMJ*. 1997 3;314:1320-5.

112. Winters JC, Jorritsma W, Groenier KH, Sobel JS, Meyboom-de Jong B, Arendzen HJ. Treatment of shoulder complaints in general practice: long-term results of a randomised, single-blind study comparing physiotherapy, manipulation, and corticosteroid injection. *BMJ*. 1999; 318(7195):1395.

113. Bergman GJD, Winters JC, Groenier KH, et al. Manipulative therapy in addition to usual medical care for patients with shoulder dysfunction and pain: a randomized, controlled trial. *Ann Intern Med*. 2004;141(6):432.

114. Sobel J, Kremer I, Winters J, Arendzen J, de Jong B. Reviews of the literature. The influence of the mobility in the cervicothoracic spine and the upper ribs (shoulder girdle) on the mobility of the scapulohumeral joint. *J Manipulative Physiol Ther*. 1996;19:469–474.

115. Norlander S, Gustavsson BA, Lindell J, Nordgren B. Reduced mobility in the cervico-thoracic motion segment—a risk factor for musculoskeletal neck-shoulder pain: a two-year prospective follow-up study. *Scand J Rehabil Med*. 1997;29(3):167–174.

116. Norlander S, Aste-Norlander U, Nordgren B, Sahlstedt B. Mobility in the cervico-thoracic motion segment: an indicative factor of musculoskeletal neck-shoulder pain. *Scand J Rehabil Med*. 1996;28(4):183–192.

117. Conroy DE, Hayes KW. The effect of joint mobilization as a component of comprehensive treatment for primary shoulder impingement syndrome. *J Orthop Sports Phys Ther*. 1998;28(1):3–14.

118. Knebl JA, Shores JH, Gamber RG, Gray WT, Herron KM. Improving functional ability in the elderly via the Spencer technique, an osteopathic manipulative treatment: a randomized, controlled trial. *J Am Osteopath Assoc*. 2002;102(7):387–396.

119. Vermeulen HM, Obermann WR, Burger BJ, Kok GJ, Rozing PM, van Den Ende CH. End-range mobilization techniques in adhesive capsulitis of the shoulder joint: A multiple-subject case report. *Phys Ther*. 2000;80(12):1204–1213.

120. Munday S, Jones A, Brantingham J, Globe G, Jensen M, Price J. A randomized, single-blinded, placebo-controlled trial to evaluate the efficacy of chiropractic shoulder girdle adjustment in the treatment of shoulder impingement syndrome. *J Am Chiro Assoc*. 2007; 44(8):6–15.

121. Donahue T, Bergmann T, Donahue S, Dody M. Manipulative assessment and treatment of the shoulder complex: case reports. *J Chiro Med.* 2003;2:145–152.

122. Kaye M. Evaluation and treatment of a patient with upper quarter myofascial pain syndrome. *J Sports Chiro Rehabil.* 2001;15:26.

123. Pribicevic M, Pollard H. A multi-modal treatment approach for the shoulder: a 4 patient case series. *Chiropr Osteopat.* 2005;13:20.

124. Sharp J. Treatment of shoulder and cervical dysfunction in an infant. *Chiropr Technique.* 1999;11:53–56.

125. Smith T. Cervical manipulation for shoulder injury. *JNMS.* 2000;8:24–26.

126. Sobel JS, Winters JC, Groenier K, Arendzen JH, Meyboom de Jong B. Physical examination of the cervical spine and shoulder girdle in patients with shoulder complaints. *J Manipulative Physiol Ther.* 1997;20(4):257–262.

127. Feeley K. Conservative chiropractic care of frozen shoulder syndrome: a case study. *CRJ.* 1992;2:31–37.

128. Polkinghorn BS. Chiropractic treatment of frozen shoulder syndrome (adhesive capsulitis) utilizing mechanical force, manually assisted short lever adjusting procedures. *J Manipulative Physiol Ther.* 1995;18:105–115.

129. Moreau CE, Moreau SR. Chiropractic management of a professional hockey player with recurrent shoulder instability. *J Manipulative Physiol Ther.* 2001;24:425–430.

130. Gimblett PA, Saville J, Ebrall P. A conservative management protocol for calcific tendinitis of the shoulder. *J Manipulative Physiol Ther.* 1999;22:622–627.

131. Kiner A. Diagnosis and management of grade II acromioclavicular joint separation. *Clin Chiropr.* 2004;7:24–30.

132. Stoddard J, Johnson C. Conservative treatment of a patient with a mild acromioclavicular joint separation. *J Sports Chiropr Rehabil.* 2000;14:118.

133. Shrode LW. Treating shoulder impingement using the supraspinatus synchronization exercise. *J Manipulative Physiol Ther.* 1994;17:43–53.

134. Pribicevic M, Pollard H. Rotator cuff impingement. *J Manipulative and Physiol Ther.* 2004;27(9):580.

135. Kazemi M. Adhesive capsulitis: a case report. *J Canadian Chiropr Assoc.* 2000;44:169–176.

136. Brantingham JW, Cassa TK, Bonnefin D, et al. Manipulative therapy for shoulder pain and disorders: expansion of a systematic review. *J Manipulative Physiol Ther.* Jun 2011;34(5):314–346.

137. Penny JN, Welsh RP. Shoulder impingement syndromes in athletes and their surgical management. *Am J Sports Med.* 1981;9:11.

138. McGillivray J, Fealy S, Potter HG, O'Brien SJ. Multiplanar analysis of acromion morphology. *Am J Sports Med.* 1998;26:836–840.

139. Souza TA. History and examination of the shoulder. In: Souza TA, ed. *Sports Injuries of the Shoulder: Conservative Management.* New York: Churchill Livingstone; 1994:167–219.

140. Cools AN, Witvrounv EE, DeClercq GA, et al. Scapular muscle recruitment pattern: electromyographic response of the trapezius muscle to sudden shoulder movement before and after a fatiguing exercise. *J Orthop Sports Phys Ther.* 2002;32:221–229.

141. Wang CH. McClure P, Pratt NE, Nobilin R. Stretching and strengthening exercises: their effect on three-dimensional scapular kinematics. *Arch Phys Med Rehabil.* 1999;80:923–929.

142. Tyler TF, Nicholas SJ, Roy T, Clenn GW. Quantification of posterior capsule tightness and motion loss in patients with shoulder impingement. *Am J Sports Med.* 2000; 28(5):668–673.

143. Borstad JD, Ludewig PM. The effect of long versus short pectoralis minor resting length on scapular kinematics in healthy individuals. *J Orthop Sports Phys Ther.* 2005;35(4):227–238.

144. Borstad JD, Ludewig PM. Comparison of three stretches for the pectoralis minor muscle. *J Shoulder Elbow Surg.* 2006;15(3):324–330.

145. Walther M, Werner A, Stahlschmidt T, Woelfel R, Gohlke F. The subacromial impingement syndrome of the shoulder treated by conventional physiotherapy, self-training, and a shoulder brace: results of a prospective, randomized study. *J Shoulder Elbow Surg.* 2004;13(4):417–423.

146. Alfredson H, Harstad H, Haugen S, Ohberg L. Sclerosing polidocanol injections to treat chronic painful shoulder impingement syndrome-results of a two-centre collaborative pilot study. *Knee Surg Sports Traumatol Arthrosc.* 2006;14(12):1321–1326.

147. Post M. *The Shoulder—Surgical and Non-Surgical Management.* Philadelphia: Lea & Febiger; 1978.

148. Robinson CM, Kelly OM, Wakefield AE. Redislocation of the shoulder during the first six weeks after a primary anterior dislocation: risk factors and results of treatment. *J Bone Joint Surg.* 2002;84–A(9):1552–1559.

149. Itoi E, Hatakeyama Y, Sato T, et al. Immobilization in external rotation after shoulder dislocation reduces the risk of recurrence. A randomized controlled trial. *J Bone Joint Surg Am.* 2007;89(10):2124–2131.

150. Lee SB, An KN. Dynamic glenohumeral stability provided by three heads of the deltoid muscle. *Clin Orthop Rel Res.* 2002;400:40–47.

151. Harding III WG, Nowicki KD, Perdue PS, et al. Managing anterior shoulder instability with bracing. *J Musculoskel Med.* 1997;14(6):50–58.

152. Chu JC, Kane EJ, Arnold BL, Gansneder BM. The effect of a neoprene shoulder stabilizer on active joint reposition sense in subjects with stable and unstable shoulders. *J Athl Train.* 2002;37(2):141–145.

153. Magnusson L, et al. Kartus J, Ejerhed E, et al. Revisiting the open Bankart experience: a four- to nine-year followup. *Am J Sports Med.* 2002;30(6):778–782.

154. Karlsson J, Magnusson L, Ejerhed E, et al. Comparison of open and arthroscopic stabilization for recurrent shoulder dislocation in patients with a Bankart lesion. *Am J Sports Med.* 2001;29(5):538–542.

155. Myers JB, Lephart SM. Sensorimotor deficits contributing to glenohumeral instability. *Clin Orthop Relat Res.* 2002;400:98–104.

156. McFarland EG, Kim TK, Banchaseuk P, McCarthy EF. Histologic evaluation of the shoulder capsule in normal shoulders, unstable shoulders, and after failed thermal capsulorrhaphy. *Am J Sports Med.* 2002;30(5):636–642.

157. Reinold MM, Wilk KE, Hooks TR, et al. Thermal-assisted capsular shrinkage of the glenohumeral joint in overhead athletes: a 15- to 47-month follow-up. *J Orthop Sports Phys Ther.* 2003;33(8):455–467.

158. Anderson K, Warren RF, Altchek DW, et al. Risk factors for early failure after thermal capsulorrhaphy. *Am J Sports Med.* 2002;30(1):103–107.

159. Hawkins RJ, Krishnan SG, Karas SG, Noonan TJ, Horan MP. Electrothermal arthroscopic shoulder capsulorrhaphy: a minimum 2-year follow-up. *Am J Sports Med.* 2007;35(9):1484–1488.

160. Wilk KE, Reinold MM, Dugas JR, Andrews JR. Rehabilitation following thermal-assisted capsular shrinkage of the glenohumeral joint: current concepts. *J Orthop Sports Phys Ther.* 2002;32(6):268–292.

161. Tyler TF, Calabrese GJ, Parker RD, Nicholas SJ. Electrothermally-assisted capsulorrhaphy (ETAC): a new surgical method for glenohumeral instability and its rehabilitation considerations. *J Orthop Sports Phys Ther.* 2000;30:390–400.

162. Matsen FA, Thomas SG. Glenohumeral instability. In: Evans CM, ed. *Surgery of the Musculoskeletal System.* 2nd ed. New York: Churchill Livingstone; 1989.

163. Von Eisenhart-Rothe RM, Joger A, Englmeier KH, et al. Relevance of arm position and muscle activity on three-dimensional glenohumeral translation in patients with traumatic and atraumatic shoulder instability. *Am J Sports Med.* 2002;30(4):514–522.

164. Tiborne JE, Lee TQ, Csintalan RP, et al. Quantitative assessment of glenohumeral translation. *Clin Orthop Rel Res.* 2002;400:93–97.

165. Thomas SJ, McDougall C, Brown ID, et al. Prevalence of symptoms and signs of shoulder problems in people with diabetes mellitus. *J Shoulder Elbow Surg.* 2007;16(6):748–751.

166. Souza TA. Frozen shoulder. In: Souza TA, ed. *Sports Injuries of the Shoulder: Conservative Management.* New York: Churchill Livingstone; 1994:441–455.

167. Levine WN, Kashyap CP, Bak SF, Ahmad CS, Blaine TA, Bigliani LU. Nonoperative management of idiopathic adhesive capsulitis. *J Shoulder Elbow Surg.* 2007;16(5):569–573.

168. Kivimaki J, Pohjolainen T, Malmivaara A, et al. Manipulation under anesthesia with home exercises versus home exercises alone in the treatment of frozen shoulder: a randomized, controlled trial with 125 patients. *J Shoulder Elbow Surg.* 2007;16(6):722–726.

169. Buchbinder R, Green S, Youd J, Johnston R, Cumpston M. Arthrographic distension for adhesive capsulitis (frozen shoulder). *Cochrane Database Syst Rev.* 2008(1):CD007005.

170. Jacobs LG, Smith MG, Khan SA, Smith K, Joshi M. Manipulation or intra-articular steroids in the management of adhesive capsulitis of the shoulder? A prospective randomized trial. *J Shoulder Elbow Surg.* 2009;18(3):348–353.

171. Ibrahim T, Rahbi H, Beiri A, Jeyapalan K, Taylor GJ. Adhesive capsulitis of the shoulder: the rate of manipulation following distension arthrogram. *Rheumatol Int.* 2006;27(1):7–9.

172. Ozaki J, Fujimoto S, Nakagawa Y, et al. Tears of the rotator cuff of the shoulder associated with pathological changes in the acromion: a study of cadavers. *J Bone Joint Surg Am.* 1988;70:1224.

173. Unger HR, Neumann CH, Petersen SA. Magnetic resonance imaging. In: Souza TA, ed. *Sports Injuries*

of the Shoulder: Conservative Management. New York: Churchill Livingstone; 1994:299–321.

174. Hurt G, Baker CL, Jr. Calcific tendinitis of the shoulder. *Orthop Clin North Am.* 2003;34(4):567–575.

175. Rowe CR. Tendinitis, bursitis, impingement, "snapping" scapula, and calcific tendinitis. *The Shoulder.* New York: Churchill Livingstone; 1988:105.

176. Bosworth BM. Calcium deposits in the shoulder and subacromial bursitis: a survey of 12,122 cases. *JAMA.* 1941;116:2477–2482.

177. Gartner J, Simons B. Analysis of calcific deposits in calcifying tendinitis. *Clin Orthop Relat Res.* 1990(254):111–120.

178. Ebenbichler GR, Erdogmus CB, Resch KL, et al. Ultrasound therapy for calcific tendinitis of the shoulder. *N Engl J Med.* 1999;340:1533–1538.

179. Rompe JD, Burger R, Hopf C, Eysel P. Shoulder function after extracorporeal shock wave therapy for calcific tendonitis. *J Shoulder Elbow Surg.* 1998;7:505–509.

180. Ioppolo F, Tattoli M, Di Sante L, et al. Extracorporeal shock-wave therapy for supraspinatus calcifying tendinitis: a randomized clinical trial comparing two different energy levels. *Phys Ther.* 2012;92(11):1376–1385.

181. Rockwood CA, Williams GR, Young DC. Injuries to the acromioclavicular joint. In: Rockwood CA, Green DP, Bucholz RW, eds. *Fractures in Adults.* 3rd ed. Philadelphia: WB Saunders; 1991:1192.

182. Souza TA. Sternoclavicular, acromioclavicular, and scapular disorders. In: Souza TA, ed. *Sports Injuries of the Shoulder: Conservative Management.* New York: Churchill Livingstone; 1994:409–439.

183. Calvo E, Lopez-Franco M, Arribas IM. Clinical and radiologic outcomes of surgical and conservative treatment of type III acromioclavicular joint injury. *J Shoulder Elbow Surg.* 2006;15(3):300–305.

184. Bjerneld H, Hovelius L, Thorling J. Acromioclavicular separations treated conservatively: a 5-year followup study. *Acta Orthop Scand.* 1983;54:743.

185. Carson WG, Gasser SI. Little Leaguer's Shoulder: A report of 23 cases. *Am J Sports Med.* 1998;26(4):575–580.

186. Axe MJ, Snyder-Mackler L, Konin JG, et al. Development of a distance-based interval throwing program for Little League-Aged athletes. *Am J Sports Med.* 1996;245:94–602.

187. Andrews JR, Feisig G. How many pitches should I allow my child to throw? *USA Baseball News,* April 1996, p. 5.

APPENDIX 7–2

Shoulder Diagnosis Table

Diagnosis	Comments	History Findings	Positive Examination Findings	Radiography/Special Studies	Treatment Options
Subluxation or Fixation of: Glenohumeral Joint Acromioclavicular Joint Sternoclavicular Joint Scapulothoracic Joint (functional)	• Should be used when chiropractic manipulation is used as Tx for any shoulder problem/Dx • Can be primary Dx if patient is asymptomatic or mildly symptomatic (e.g., mild stiffness or pain level >2/10) • Must indicate chiropractic exam findings to support Dx	*Nonspecific*	*Palpation*—Local tenderness or other signs of subluxation *Ortho*—None *Neuro*—None *Active ROM*—Variable restriction *Passive ROM*—End-range restriction *Motion palpation*—Specific articular restriction or symptoms produced on end-range	• Radiography not required for the diagnosis of subluxation • Radiographic biomechanical analysis may assist in treatment decisions	• Chiropractic adjustive technique • Decisions regarding specifically which technique(s) is/are applied and modifications to the given approach will be directed by the primary Dx and patient's ability to tolerate pre-adjustment stresses
Infraspinatus or Teres Minor sprain/strain Subscapularis sprain/strain Supraspinatus sprain/strain Biceps Sprain/Strain Note: Sprain/strain is not synonymous with spasm or hypertonicity	• Requires an inciting event of trauma or overuse.	*Mechanism*—Overstretch or overcontraction Hx as acute event *Worse with specific ROM*—Contraction of muscle or stretch of muscle or joint	*Ortho*—Specific tests for each muscle, including tenderness at muscle/tendon: • Supraspinatus—empty can or lag sign • Subscapularis—lift-off test or lag sign • Infraspinatus/teres minor—lag sign *Biceps*—Speed's *Neuro*—None *Active ROM*—Pain on active ROM that contracts involved muscles *Passive ROM*—Pain on end-range stretch of involved muscle or ligament	• Radiography not required for diagnosis • With significant trauma or for med/legal purposes, radiographs may be required • If calcific tendinitis (726.11) is suspected, radiographs may be indicated • If associated with impingement, an outlet view is suggested	• Myofascial therapy • Limited orthotic support (taping or brace) • Ergonomic advice • Strengthening and preventive exercises

Condition	History/Mechanism	Examination	Imaging	Treatment
Adhesive Capsulitis	In early stages, adhesive capsulitis appears as an acute process indistinguishable from other processes such as acute bursitis or tendinitis	*Onset*—Acute onset of pain that may or may not be traumatic. Stiffness is progressive; pain is not major feature in later stages. *ROM comments*—Abduction and external rotation decreased first followed by internal rotation	*Ortho*—No specific tests. *Neuro*—None. *Active & Passive ROM*—Equal restriction in both passive and active ROM, specifically in abduction and external rotation. *Motion palpation*—Possible restriction globally	Radiography not used for Dx; however, may be used in ruling out other conditions such as calcific tendinitis in acute stages and OA in later stages. Arthrogram most sensitive test for adhesive capsulitis	• Myofascial therapy • Physiotherapy such as ultrasound • Daily exercises and stretches based on rhythmic stabilization; also wall-walking and pendulum exercises • Adjusting contraindicated in acute stage; mobilization possible
Subdeltoid Bursitis	• Subdeltoid (same as subacromial) bursitis is often found associated with impingement syndrome or may be found as an isolated condition • Calcific bursitis is particularly acute and painful, limiting all ROM and difficult to control pain	*Mechanism*—Hx of trauma, except with chronic bursitis where chronic repetitive microtrauma may occur. *Worse with specific ROM*—All ROM are often affected with acute bursitis, especially end-range forward flexion	*Palpation*—Tenderness found anterior to AC joint on passive extension of shoulder. *Ortho*—None; most movement is painful, precluding most ortho testing; there may be some positives on impingement testing in subacute cases. *Active ROM*—Most movements are painful, in particular forward flexion. *Passive ROM*—End-range forward flexion and abduction are painful	• Radiography not usually necessary initially except to rule out fracture/dislocation with acute trauma or when calcific bursitis is suspected	• Limited orthotic support • Physiotherapy for pain and swelling control • Herbal recommendations for pain and swelling • If pain is intolerable, referral for medical prescription for pain meds • Mobilization possible
Impingement Syndrome	• Impingement may be primarily mechanical (i.e., subacromial spurs) or primarily functional (e.g., related to instability)	*Mechanism*—Variable; however, most commonly overhead activities over time produce impingement. *Limited activities*—Overhead activities most restricted	*Ortho*—Neer's, Hawkins-Kennedy, and painful arc; more specific tests may then be used for specific structures. *Neuro*—None	• Radiography may be used, including an outlet view (for subacromial spurs or anomalies) and a Zanca view for the AC joint	• Myofascial therapy • Limited orthotic support • Ergonomic advice for sport or occupation • Preventive and strengthening exercises and stretches

(continues)

Shoulder Diagnosis Table (continued)

Diagnosis	Comments	History Findings	Positive Examination Findings	Radiography/Special Studies	Treatment Options
AC Separation (indicate degree)	• AC separations are another form of instability (especially with 2nd and 3rd degrees) • Always consider associated distal clavicular fracture in acute cases and osteolysis in chronic cases (when pain is still present)	Mechanism—Direct fall onto AC or fall on outstretched arm/hand are most common causes	Observation/palpation—With 2nd and 3rd degree there is an obvious step-deformity; palpation reveals localized tenderness and swelling Ortho—Compression or distraction at AC are painful (used for 1st-degree tears only)	• Radiography must include weighted and nonweighted bilateral views of the AC joints; degree based on coracoacromial distance • In chronic pain cases, consider a Zanca view for possible osteolysis	• Limited orthotic support using principle of Kenney-Howard sling; time frame based on degree of injury • Use isometrics while patient is in sling; progress to isotonics when pain permits • Consider referral for surgical stabilization when patient concerned about cosmetic appearance
Anterior Dislocation Posterior Dislocation	• Anterior, by far, is the most common • Posterior dislocations are often undiagnosed for at least one month following occurrence	Mechanism—Arm pulled back into abduction/external rotation (anterior dislocation) or direct anterior blow to shoulder or fall on outstretched arm (posterior dislocation)	Observation—Arm locked in external rotation (anterior); prominent coracoid, flat anterior shoulder (posterior) Neuro—Check motor/sensory function distally Active ROM—Patient unable to fully supinate and raise the arm with posterior dislocation	• Radiography required to determine any associated fractures; views vary based on presentation, although specialized views such as the Stryker view are valuable • Scapular or Y view for posterior dislocation	• Limited orthotic support in a sling for approximately 2–3 weeks followed by tape/support for several weeks • Avoid abduction/external rotation • Preventive and strengthening exercises
Glenoid Labrum Tear	• Labrum tears may be obviously traumatic (usually anterior/inferior) or less obvious (SLAP lesions; anterior/superior) • Types of tears are classified similarly to meniscus tears	Mechanism—May be associated with anterior dislocation (anterior/inferior) or sudden contraction of biceps or fall on forward flexed arm (SLAP lesion)	Ortho—Instability testing may be positive in addition to specific testing incuding: Crank test, O'Brien sign, slide test, or pronation provocative test Active ROM—May have a painful "sticking" in movement relieved by repositioning and a "clunk"	• Radiography may assist if there is bony involvement of the glenoid; these are best seen on modified axillary views • MRI is less sensitive than CT arthrograms	• Conservative trial of strengthening and modified work or sports activities • Patients unresponsive to conservative trial should be referred for surgical debridement and stabilization if necessary

Myofascitis	• Also may be used if a strain is not evident from the history; however there are indicators of muscle tenderness, stiffness, or pain	*Onset*—Nonspecific regarding onset *Symptoms*—Patient usually complains of pain, aching, and/or tenderness in specific muscle or tendon areas that may radiate pain in nondermatomal pattern	Trigger points are evident as localized tenderness in a muscle that corresponds to traditional (Travell/Simons) trigger point charts; these points may be local or refer pain when compressed	• Not required or recommended	• Mysofascial approaches, such as myofascial stripping, trigger point massage, or spray and stretch approaches, are the standard • Home stretching and modification of activity suggestions
Laxity Hypermobility	• Requires physical examination confirmation.	History of a single event, traumatic injury to the joint is not found; however, either overuse (micro-trauma) or generalized inherent looseness is/are evident	Capsular or ligament testing reveals "looseness" that falls within the physiologic range of normal	• Not usually recommended unless when differentiating pathological laxity from congenital or overuse acquisition	• Strengthening program • Bracing or functional taping during rehabilitation or during strenuous activities

Elbow Complaints

Context

Although anatomically analogous to the knee, the elbow is injured far less often. In large part, this is due to the non-weight-bearing function of the elbow. As the link between the shoulder and the wrist/hand, the elbow is functionally challenged with repetitive activities. These overuse mechanisms account for the majority of complaints. Overstrain is common at the origin of the wrist extensors (lateral elbow) and the wrist flexors (medial elbow). With athletes, valgus stress predominates, in particular in throwing sports and in activities requiring the use of an arm extension such as a bat, racquet, or club. These devices increase the medial stress across the elbow by increasing the length of the lever arm. As with the rest of the upper extremity, the elbow becomes weight-bearing when an axial force is applied acutely during a fall, or chronically with gymnastic maneuvers and with some chiropractors due to adjusting maneuvers.

General Strategy

History

- Clarify the type of complaint.
  1. Is the complaint one of pain, stiffness, looseness, crepitus, locking, or a combination of complaints?
  2. Localize the complaint to anterior, posterior, medial, or lateral.
- Clarify the mechanism if traumatic.
  1. Did the patient fall on an outstretched hand? Consider fracture or dislocation (in children, consider a supracondylar fracture).

  2. Did the patient fall on the tip of the elbow (olecranon)? Consider olecranon fracture.
  3. Did the patient have hyperextension of elbow? Consider dislocation and supracondylar fracture.
  4. Did the patient have sudden stretch to the inside of the elbow? Consider medial collateral ligament sprain or lateral compressive injury to the radial head or capitellum.
  5. Did the patient have sudden traction to the elbow? Radial head subluxation is likely.
- Determine whether the mechanism is one of overuse.
  1. In what position does the patient work?
  2. Does the patient perform a repetitive movement at work or with sports involving pronation and supination? Consider muscle strain, trigger points, or peripheral nerve entrapment.
  3. Does the patient perform a repetitive movement at work or with sports involving cocking or medial stretch to the elbow? Consider medial collateral ligament sprain, flexor muscle strain, or ulnar nerve stretch irritation.
- Determine whether the patient has a current or past history/diagnosis of his or her elbow complaint or other related disorders.
  1. Are there associated neck or shoulder complaints or diagnoses?
  2. Does the patient have gout, rheumatoid arthritis, chronic renal pathology, or psoriasis?

Evaluation

- With trauma, palpate for points of tenderness and obtain a radiograph for the possibility of fracture/dislocation.

- Challenge the ligaments of the elbow with varus and valgus stress.
- When nontraumatic, challenge the musculotendinous attachments with stretch, contraction, and a combination of contraction in a stretched position.
- When trauma or overuse is not present, evaluate the patient's elbow for swelling and deformity (olecranon bursitis, gouty tophi, osteoarthritis).

Management

- Refer fracture/dislocation for orthopaedic management.
- Refer cases of infection, unresolving bursitis, and gout.
- Manage soft tissue disorders and articular disorders with conservative care.

Relevant Anatomy and Biomechanics

The elbow joint performs two movement patterns: (1) extension/flexion, and (2) pronation/supination of the forearm. The "hinge" function of extension/flexion occurs primarily at the ulnotrochlear joint, the articulation between the distal humerus and proximal ulna and the olecranon process of the ulna and the distal fossa of the humerus. Most daily activities require elbow participation in a range of motion (ROM) between 30° and 130°.[1] Functionally, flexion is accomplished by the biceps, brachialis, and brachioradialis. Extension is primarily due to triceps contraction. As one might guess, the larger muscular contribution to flexion makes it the stronger movement. Extension is approximately 70% as strong as flexion.[1] Supination and pronation occur at the proximal radioulnar joint and the radiocapitellar joint, the articulation between the radial head and the capitellum of the distal humerus. Functionally, supination is accomplished through contraction of the biceps brachii and the supinator muscles. Supination is more effective with the elbow flexed because of the prestretch of the supinator muscle and mechanical advantage of the biceps. Pronation is accomplished by the pronator teres and less effectively by the pronator quadratus. Pronation is more effective with the elbow extended, placing a prestretch on the pronator teres. Supination is slightly stronger (15%) than pronation due to the contribution of the biceps. The

biceps and triceps cross both the shoulder and elbow joints. Flexion of the shoulder decreases effectiveness of the biceps with elbow flexion and supination; extension decreases effectiveness of the triceps with extension.

As with all joints, stability is provided by a contribution of position-dependent ligamentous and capsular tension, bony congruity, and static/dynamic muscle/tendon support. Similar to the knee, a bony lock occurs in full extension, providing some protection from varus and valgus forces. In the elbow, the fit of the olecranon process of the ulna into the olecranon fossa of the distal humerus provides some stability with extension. This tongue-and-groove lock is aided by tension in the anterior capsule and collateral ligaments. The main restraint to valgus strain in extension is from the anterior oblique portion of the medial collateral ligament (**Figure 8–1**).

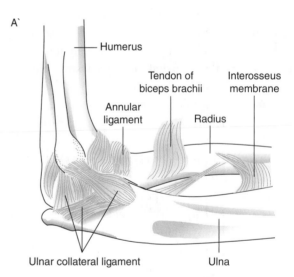

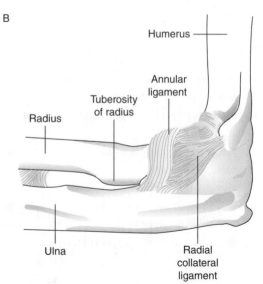

Figure 8–1 The elbow joint: (A) medial view; (B) lateral view.

With the elbow flexed to between 10° and 60°, the medial collateral ligament becomes lax. It is in this midrange position that most medial-sided injuries occur. When the elbow is flexed to 90° and beyond, the posterior aspect of the medial (ulnar) collateral ligament becomes tight. Medial stability is statically and dynamically provided by the flexor/pronator muscle group, which takes its origin off of the medial epicondyle of the humerus. Lin et al.[2] evaluated the role that muscles and tendons play in stabilizing the elbow. They found that the flexor carpi ulnaris (FCU), flexor carpi radialis (FCR), and flexor digitorum superficialis (FDS) act as dynamic stabilizers for valgus stress with the static protection provided by the FCU. The extensor carpi ulnaris and extensor digitorum communis increased medial ulnar collateral ligament strain and valgus at both 45° and 90°. Lateral stability is provided by a very weak lateral collateral ligament, and more significantly from the anconeus muscle.[3] Lateral stability is assisted statically and dynamically by the extensor wad of muscles that take their origin off the lateral epicondyle.

Restriction to overextension is provided by stretch of the anterior capsule and biceps tendon in addition to the bony block of the olecranon in the olecranon fossa. Flexion is restricted by muscle contact, tension in the posterior capsule and the triceps tendon, and radial head and humerus contact. Pronation is restricted by the crossing of the radius and the ulna. Supination is limited by tension in the pronator muscle group.

Evaluation

History

First, determine the type of complaint or complaints the patient has: pain, stiffness, locking, etc. Determine if there is a history of trauma (recent or distant), whether there is an overuse component, or whether the complaint had an insidious onset. Attempt to localize the complaint to the anterior, posterior, lateral, or medial aspect of the elbow. The answers to these questions should sufficiently narrow the possibilities to allow for a more focused examination (**Table 8–1**).

Table 8–1 History Questions for Elbow and Forearm Complaints

Primary Question	What Are You Thinking?	Secondary Questions	What Are You Thinking?
Was there an injury?	Fracture, dislocation, sprain (capsular/ligamentous)	**Hyperextended (overextended)?**	Anterior capsule sprain
			Elbow dislocation
			Supracondylar fracture in children
		Fell on hand with elbow extended?	Radial head fracture
		Fell on tip of elbow?	Olecranon fracture or bursitis
		Overstretched inside of elbow?	Medial collateral ligament sprain or rupture
			Damage to ulnar nerve
			Medial epicondyle avulsion
			Capitellum fracture
		Sudden traction on arm?	Radial head subluxation
Was there any repetitive activity?	Overuse leading to tendinitis, trigger points (TrPs), osseous reactive changes	**Throwing?**	Compression injuries on lateral side; stretch on medial
		Racquet sport?	Lateral pain—lateral epicondylitis or supinator TrP
			Medial pain—medial epicondylitis or pronator TrP
		Pain on outside of elbow with typing, hammering, using a screwdriver?	Lateral epicondylitis or supinator TrP

(continues)

Table 8–1 History Questions for Elbow and Forearm Complaints (continued)

Primary Question	What Are You Thinking?	Secondary Questions	What Are You Thinking?
Do you have weakness at the elbow?	Biceps rupture or strain, cervical disc, neural compression/entrapment	Associated with pain? Any associated neck pain and/or radiation?	Possibly due to pain inhibition Cervical disc or subluxation
Do you have stiffness or restricted movement?	Osteoarthritis (OA) or other arthritide, flexor contracture, osteophytes, effusion	History of excessive throwing? Early-morning stiffness? Swelling with blocked extension?	Flexor contracture, osteophytes, loose bodies OA Effusion or bursitis
Do you have superficial swelling?	Bursitis or tophi (gout)	Back of elbow? Also big toe swelling?	Olecranon bursitis Gout

Pain Localization

The following are possible causes of pain based on location (**Figure 8–2**, A and B, and **Table 8–2**):

- anterior
  1. traumatic—anterior capsular sprain, distal biceps tendon strain, fracture, or dislocation
  2. nontraumatic—capsular sprain, biceps tendinitis, and pronator teres strain
- posterior
  1. traumatic—olecranon fracture, bursitis, triceps strain
  2. nontraumatic—olecranon bursitis, triceps tendinitis, degenerative joint disease
- medial
  1. traumatic—ulnar collateral ligament sprain, ulnar nerve traction, epicondyle avulsion, flexor/pronator strain

  2. nontraumatic—minor ulnar collateral ligament sprain, chronic ulnar nerve irritation, flexor/pronator strain (medial epicondylitis)
- lateral
  1. traumatic—radial head fracture, radial head subluxation, osteochondritis dissecans of the capitellum
  2. nontraumatic—lateral epicondylitis, osteocartilaginous fragments from the radial head or capitellum

Traumatic and Overuse Elbow Pain

As with all traumatic onsets, a search for dislocation or fracture and the possible complications associated with each is the first order of business. Dislocation and fracture are often the consequence of hyperextension of the elbow. In particular in children, the possibility of a supracondylar fracture should always be considered with

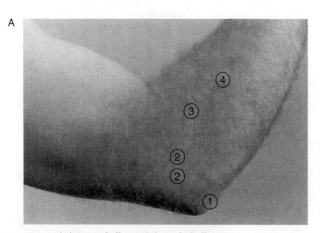
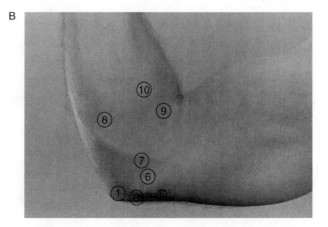

Figure 8–2 (A) Lateral elbow; (B) medial elbow.

Table 8–2 Elbow Pain Localization

#	Structures	Overt Trauma	Insidious or Overuse
1	Olecranon, triceps insertion	Olecranon fracture, olecranon bursitis	Triceps tendinitis, valgus-extension overload
2	Lateral epicondyle of humerus, origin of extensor wad	Supracondylar fracture (or slightly above)	Lateral epicondylitis
3	Radial head, capitellum	Radial head fracture, radial head subluxation	Radial head subluxation, osteochondritis dissecans of the capitellum
4	Supinator, proximal radius	Proximal radius fracture	Supinator syndrome, posterior interosseous nerve syndrome (palpation point)
5	Ulnar nerve	Damage from associated fracture	Ulnar neuritis, subluxating ulnar nerve
6	Medial epicondyle of humerus, origin of flexor quad	Supracondylar fracture, ulnar collateral ligament sprain	Medial epicondylitis, Little League/pitcher's elbow (apophyseal injury)
7	Ulnar collateral ligament	Collateral ligament sprain	Collateral ligament sprain
8	Wrist flexors	Contusion	Flexor tendinitis
9	Biceps tendon insertion/tuberosity of radius	Biceps avulsion	Distal biceps strain
10	Pronator teres	Contusion	Pronator teres syndrome (palpation point)

Note: See Figure 8–2 for localization of numbered areas.

a history of a hyperextension injury due to a fall on an outstretched hand or a direct blow just above the antecubital fossa.[4] These fractures account for two thirds of children's elbow fractures; one third of adult elbow fractures are distal humeral.[5] Unfortunately, these types of fractures resemble dislocations, but they are often more serious. Dislocations at the elbow are usually posterior. They also occur with hyperextension and are the result of a leverage effect. As the olecranon is blocked by the olecranon fossa, the trochlea is levered over the coronoid process. The medial collateral ligament is ruptured, and there may be associated radial head or capitellar fractures. These types of injuries are usually seen in an acute, on-the-field or playground scenario. Attempts at relocation should be tempered by the possibility that a dislocation is in fact a fracture. Attempts at relocation may cause neurovascular injury.

Valgus stress to the elbow is less often an acute injury; more often it is a chronic overuse phenomenon. If a sudden valgus force is applied to the elbow, avulsion of the medial epicondyle, medial collateral ligament sprain, and capitellum fracture should be considered. A direct fall onto the tip of the elbow with the elbow flexed may result in either an olecranon fracture or olecranon bursitis. Sudden traction on the forearm of a young child may result in a radial head entrapment phenomenon often called nursemaid's elbow.

Overuse injuries account for many of the problems presenting as medial or lateral elbow pain. Disorders associated with repetitive flexion maneuvers and medial elbow pain are suggestive of medial epicondylitis. Repetitive extension maneuvers associated with lateral elbow pain are suggestive of lateral epicondylitis. Repetitive pronation maneuvers associated with medial anterior elbow and forearm pain suggest pronator involvement, especially if associated with distal neurologic signs and symptoms. These are discussed in more detail in Chapter 9.

Repetitive sports activities are probably the most common cause of persistent elbow pain. Throwing sports or sports that require leverage at the elbow through an arm extension such as a bat, racquet, or club are the main instigators. The cocking portion of the throwing act places enormous medial stretch and lateral compression stress into the elbow joint. The forearm contributions to various pitches in baseball may selectively strain the pronator or wrist flexor group of muscles. At the end of acceleration, there may be a posterior compressive force component that should be considered in athletes complaining of pain on passive and active end-range extension.

Weakness

Weakness at the elbow without associated pain should suggest the possibility of a biceps tendon rupture. There should be a history of a sudden flexion contraction with an associated proximal migration of the biceps muscle belly. Most other causes of localized elbow weakness are due to pain. Some patients with elbow flexion contracture may perceive elbow movement as weak.

Instability

Instability will be the consequence of a past fracture, dislocation, or sudden valgus force. Following elbow dislocations, only about 1% to 2% of patients have significant instability.[6] More frequently, instability is the result of constant valgus loading of the immature athletic elbow. It is important to ask about other joints. A generalized looseness of all joints first may be noticed in the elbow. Most of these are "normal" variants based on age and female gender; however, some connective tissue disorders such as Ehlers-Danlos syndrome and Marfan syndrome must be considered.

Restricted Motion

Restriction to passive flexion or extension coupled with a traumatic history suggests joint effusion or fracture. A nontraumatic restriction to passive extension suggests a tight biceps or anterior capsule. A history of overuse is usually found. A nontraumatic restriction to passive flexion suggests a tight triceps or posterior capsular adhesions.

Locking or Crepitus

Locking or crepitus in a young patient is suggestive of osteochondritis dissecans, whereas in an older patient it is suggestive of degenerative changes. If the patient complains of crepitus or locking with pronation and supination, a search for radiocapitellar involvement is warranted. If the patient complains of crepitus on extension of the elbow, osteophytic involvement of the medial epicondyle or olecranon is possible. If there appears to be a pop with extension, the radial head is likely the source at the lateral elbow and a subluxating ulnar nerve at the medial elbow.

Superficial Complaints

The most common superficial complaints at the elbow are the skin lesions associated with psoriasis. Swellings are usually due to either gouty tophi (also seen with chronic renal failure) or an olecranon bursitis. A history of resting on the elbow or an occupation requiring constant support onto the elbow is often found.

Numbness and tingling complaints are almost always associated with a pattern including the forearm and wrist or neck and shoulder. A search for specific peripheral nerve localization findings or nerve root findings is presented in Chapter 9 and Chapter 2, respectively.

Examination

In an acute scenario, a quick check of distal neural and vascular integrity should be made with simple wrist and finger movements coupled with palpation of distal pulses while the history is being elicited.

Observation of the carrying angle of the elbow may indicate past or current bony derangement. The carrying angle for males is between 5° and 10°; for females, 10° and 15°. Cubitus valgus (greater than 20°) suggests laxity of the medial joint or possible compression injury to the lateral joint at the radial head or capitellum. Cubitus varus (less than 5°) is sometimes referred to as a gunstock deformity and may indicate fracture or epiphyseal damage. When the patient assumes a pain-relief position of about 70° of flexion and 10° of supination, joint effusion is often the cause. Note proper alignment of the posterior elbow with the elbow flexed. The three bony landmarks, the medial epicondyle, lateral epicondyle, and olecranon, should form a triangle of points; with extension they are horizontally aligned.

Swelling about the elbow is unusual unless there is an underlying fracture, bursitis, or gouty tophi deposit. Olecranon bursitis is the most common and is unmistakable due to its posterior location and size. Superficial skin lesions that are isolated to the elbow (and perhaps knees and scalp) are most often psoriatic. These lesions are silver, scaly patches found mainly on the extensor aspect of the forearm or elbow.

Palpation is useful in locating common bony or soft tissue damage sites. The olecranon process posteriorly may be tender due to a traumatic fracture (history of a fall on the elbow) or a stress fracture (excessive elbow extension). The medial epicondyle may be tender to palpation with ligament tears or flexor muscle strain. The lateral epicondyle may be tender to palpation with lateral epicondylitis or, more rarely, lateral collateral ligament sprain. Tenderness at the radial head is found with both fracture and subluxation.

Orthopaedic testing focuses on stability, internal derangement, nerve entrapment, and muscle/tendon problems. Additional testing may incorporate cervical spine testing for nerve root or referral pain sources, and biomechanical factors due to shoulder or wrist dysfunction. Following are the standard orthopaedic tests for the elbow:

- Valgus testing:[7] By flexing the elbow to 15° or 20°, the stability provided by the olecranon is eliminated and the anterior joint capsule is relaxed (**Figure 8–3**). The shoulder is then externally rotated to prevent any shoulder rotation during the stability testing. A valgus force is applied to the medial elbow while palpating for instability or restrictions. Opening at the joint indicates damage to the primary stabilizer, the anterior bundle of the medial collateral ligament. Pain with no instability may occur as a result of minor and/or chronic medial collateral ligament sprains or flexor/pronator muscle strains.
- Valgus/extension overload: With the elbow slightly flexed, a valgus force is applied. The elbow is then extended while maintaining the valgus force. Pain indicates an impingement phenomenon that occurs between the olecranon and posteromedial aspect of the humerus or olecranon fossa.[8]
- Varus testing: By flexing the elbow to 20° or 30°, a varus force will be focused more on the lateral collateral complex (**Figure 8–4**). The shoulder should be internally rotated to eliminate any shoulder contribution that could be misinterpreted as coming from the elbow.

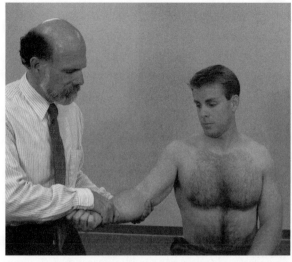

Figure 8–4 Varus testing for stability is performed with the elbow bent to 20° to 30° flexion and the arm internally rotated. A medial to lateral force is applied.

- Mill's test: Lateral epicondylitis will usually be more painful with passive stretching of the extensors. This is accomplished through passive wrist flexion with the elbow extended (**Figure 8–5**).

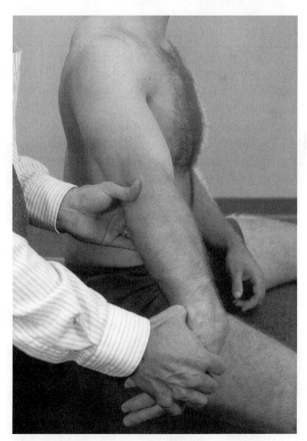

Figure 8–5 Mills' maneuver for lateral epicondylitis involves passive stretching of the extensors through passive flexion of the wrist with the elbow extended.

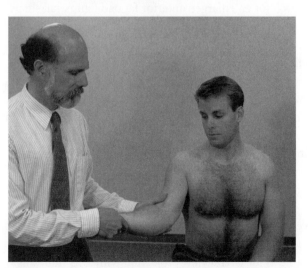

Figure 8–3 Valgus testing for stability is performed with the elbow held at 15° to 20° flexion and the forearm supinated. A force is applied from lateral to medial.

- Reverse Mill's test: Medial epicondylitis will usually be more painful with passive stretching of the flexors. This is accomplished through passive wrist extension with the elbow extended.
- Cozen's test: Resisted wrist extension (with the elbow both flexed and extended) will usually increase the pain of lateral epicondylitis (**Figure 8–6**). Weakness on wrist extension is more indicative of radial nerve or C7 nerve root involvement.
- Tinel's test: With ulnar nerve irritation due to compression or hypermobility (subluxating or dislocating ulnar nerve), tapping over the nerve at the posterior elbow may cause pain or paresthesias down the medial forearm. This should be compared with the opposite elbow to determine the patient's sensitivity to this maneuver.
- Ulnar compression test: Full elbow flexion held for 3 to 5 minutes may cause pain, paresthesias, or a numbness down the medial arm when the ulnar nerve is irritated. A complementary test is to palpate for ulnar nerve subluxation/dislocation when the elbow is taken from extension to full flexion.

Functional patterns that are suggestive of specific disorders include the following:

- **Triceps tendinitis**—Posterior pain on resisted extension with full shoulder flexion and/or pain

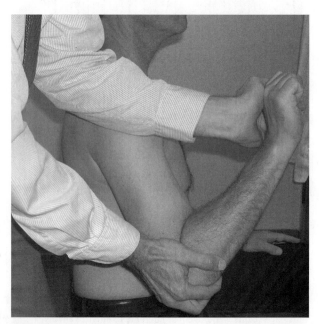

Figure 8–6 Cozen's maneuver for lateral epicondylitis is performed with the elbow flexed or extended. The patient is asked to extend the wrist against resistance.

with passive flexion of the elbow with the shoulder fully flexed.
- **Distal biceps tendinitis or avulsion**—Anterior pain on resisted flexion/supination with the shoulder fully extended and/or pain with passive wrist and elbow extension with the shoulder fully extended.
- **Pronator teres strain**—Anterior pain on resisted pronation with the elbow in neutral and extended and/or pain with passive supination with the elbow extended.
- **Supinator strain**—Anterolateral pain on resisted supination and/or passive pronation (sometimes with a Yergason test).
- **Lateral epicondylitis**—Lateral pain on resisted wrist extension and/or passive flexion of the wrist with the elbow extended/forearm pronated and/or resisted finger extension.
- **Medial epicondylitis**—Medial pain on resisted wrist flexion with the elbow extended and/or passive wrist extension with the elbow extended/forearm supinated and/or resisted finger flexion.

Radiographic evaluation of the elbow begins with two standard views: the anterior-to-posterior (AP) and lateral. In addition to obvious signs of fracture, indirect indicators of intra-articular fracture are positive fat pad signs. On a normal lateral view a small anterior fat pad may be visible as a small radiolucent triangle at the distal humerus. The posterior fat pad is not usually visible because of the overlap of the humeral condyles. When a patient presents with acute elbow trauma, a diligent search for an enlarged anterior fat pad (ship's sail shape) and a posterior fat pad should be made. A positive fat pad sign is indicative of intracapsular bleeding, usually due to intracapsular fracture.[9] When a positive fat pad sign is evident yet a fracture is not obvious on the two standard views, additional views should be utilized until the fracture is located. If still not visible, the patient should be supported for five to seven days and reexamined radiographically to be sure.[10] A false-positive fat pad sign may occur if the lateral view is not positioned properly caused by even slight rotation.[11]

When the radial head and neck are the areas of concern, a lateral oblique view is helpful.[12] Another excellent view is the radial head-capitellum view (patient position same as for lateral view projection with a 45° tube angle toward the patient).[13] This view is also valuable in finding osteochondritis dissecans of the capitellum (Panner's), and radial head, capitellum, and coronoid process fractures. Coronoid process fracture or pathologic lesion is best visualized with the medial (internal) oblique projection. When restriction to extension is found on examination, an axial view is helpful in demonstrating osteophytes of the olecranon-trochlear joint.[14] Patients who demonstrate ulnar nerve signs should be evaluated with a cubital tunnel view in an effort to visualize medial trochlear osteophytes. This is similar to the axial view; however, the elbow is positioned in 15° of external rotation (maximally flexed).[15]

Approximately 25% of patients who appear clinically to have either lateral or medial epicondylitis may demonstrate soft tissue calcification at the attachment sites of the respective muscle groups on standard elbow views.[16] However, this is not necessary for establishing a diagnosis. It is essentially an incidental finding.

Management

- Fractures and dislocations require referral to prevent neurovascular or long-term biomechanical complications.
- Tendinitis disorders are treated with protected rest, icing, and physical therapy (PT) modalities for pain. Nonsteroid anti-inflammatory drugs (NSAIDs) or alternatives might be helpful in the acute stage. Cross-friction massage with the tendon under stretch, and myofascial release techniques to the involved muscles every other day for two to three weeks should resolve most problems. Modification or elimination of an inciting activity is required for prevention of future recurrence.
- Little League elbow without radiographic evidence of damage may be managed conservatively with rest and ice. Slow return to pitching with strict adherence to Little League rules and avoidance of curve balls and side-arm pitching will usually control the problem.
- Little League elbow with radiographic evidence of medial stress or lateral compression injury should be referred or comanaged.
- Valgus-extension overload may be managed initially with taping or bracing to prevent extension. Avoidance of any forceful extension activities is required. If the patient wants to pursue the activity (usually sports), referral for decompression of the posterior elbow is suggested.

Lateral Epicondylitis (LE)

Lateral epicondylitis (LE) is a relatively common disorder. Although prevalence studies are limited, the most commonly reported study is from 1974.[17] The range reported is between 1% to 10% with a range of 1% to 3% quoted most often. The incidence of LE in general practice is estimated between 4–7 per 1,000 patients.[18] For chiropractic practice, the incidence is less clear.

Lateral epicondylitis is a condition characterized by the development of lateral elbow pain worsened by resisted wrist extension and gripping. It is a degenerative process, not an inflammatory condition as once thought. Even though LE is also referred to as tennis elbow and accounts for between 75% to 80% of the 50% of recreational tennis players who complain of lateral elbow pain, tennis players account for only 5% of all LE patients.[19-22] By far, the most commonly reported causes are work-related.[23-26] Between 35% and 61% are related to work, and 27% with leisure activities. Unknown precipitating cause accounts for 30%.[27] Among workers, LE results in an average time off from work of 12 weeks in as many as 30% of those affected.[28]

A U.S. National Institute for Occupational Safety and Health (NIOSH)[29] review found no evidence for an association between repetitive work and LE, or postural factors with LE. The study did find strong evidence for a relationship between a combination of risk factors (i.e., force, repetition, and posture) and LE. Lateral epicondylitis is seen more often in individuals between the ages of 40 to 60 years, with an equal distribution between men and women.[28, 30] Lateral epicondylitis appears to be self-limiting with a reported duration per episode of between six months and two years.[31]

In a prospective study of patients with LE, Waugh et al.[32] indicated that women were more likely than men to have work-related onset, repetitive keyboarding jobs, and cervical joint signs. Among women, these factors were associated with higher final disabilities of the arm, shoulder, and hand (DASH) and visual analog scale (VAS) scores. Women and patients who report nerve symptoms are more likely to experience a poorer short-term outcome after physiotherapy management of LE.[33] There were two recent systematic reviews for LE: one by Bisset et al.[34] and one by Smidt et al.[35] It is clear from these reviews that although there are a large number of studies, many have insufficient power and some have conflicting results. Also, there are a low number of quality studies per intervention. There were no clinical studies found on the diagnostic accuracy or reliability for the clinical examination of LE.

In an RCT evaluating cost effectiveness for interventions for LE, Korthals-de Bos et al.[36] determined that the success rate for a physiotherapy group was 91%, 69% for a corticosteroid injection group, and 83% for a wait-and-see group; 83% at one year. They concluded that from a cost perspective a wait-and-see approach should be the first approach. Similar to the Korthals-de Bos study, Smidt et al.[37] randomized patients to corticosteroid injection, physiotherapy, or a wait-and-see group. Follow-up was at 3, 6, 12, 26, and 52 weeks. There was a clear advantage at six weeks for corticosteroid injection. However, there was a high recurrence rate in the injection group. At 52 weeks, there was no advantage, with 69% of the injection group reporting success, compared to 91% of patients reporting success with physiotherapy, and 83% of patients in the wait-and-see group reporting success. As a long-term approach, it was suggested that either physiotherapy or wait-and-see are more effective; however, dependent on pain levels, injection may be needed.

Although the Bisset[34] review indicated lack of evidence for long-term benefit using physical interventions for lateral epicondylitis, there was limited evidence that exercise may have an effect on pain reduction but not on maximum grip strength. Also, some limited evidence was found for an effect using a combination treatment that included ultrasonography, exercise, and transverse friction massage when compared to a corticosteroid injection. The one study included in the Bisset review was a follow-up, prospective study by Pienimake et al.[33] of an RCT conducted in 1996.[38] The program utilized in this study consisted of a four-step exercise for eight weeks with a 36-month follow-up (*n* = 30 patients). The exercise group improved more when compared to a pulsed-ultrasound group with lower pain scores on a visual analog scale. At the three-year follow-up, the exercise group had pain scores and pain drawings that had improved significantly more than the ultrasonography group. Five patients in the ultrasonography group had resorted to surgery, whereas only one patient in the exercise group had surgery. In the Smidt[35] review, only ultrasonography demonstrated a clinically and statistically relevant positive effect, although the evidence was rated as weak. They did conclude, though, that one study determined that exercise was significantly better than ultrasonography combined with friction massage.

Braces or splints are commonly used for LE. These range from small "counter-force" braces to larger braces, and even wrist braces. There is some disagreement as to whether the imposed rest by bracing/splinting is beneficial or detrimental to either the initial or overall outcome. This concern arises from conflicting results in the literature. In a retrospective study by Derebery et al.[39] of 4,614 workers,

those who were splinted had higher rates of limited duty, more medical visits and charges, higher total charges, and longer treatment durations compared to patients who were not splinted. One criticism of the study is that, as a retrospective study, the pretreatment differences between patients would not have been randomly allocated, although the study attempted to neutralize some of the effect using propensity score methodology. Another criticism is that the types of braces were not standardized. In an RCT by Struijs et al.,[40] a brace-only group was compared to a combination group that received both a brace and physiotherapy. At six weeks, physiotherapy was superior to brace only for pain, disability, and satisfaction. The brace-only group was superior on ability of daily activities. At six months and one-year follow-ups, there were no significant differences between treatment approaches. A more recent RCT by Faes et al.[41] used a specialized dynamic extensor brace custom-made for each patient. They compared a brace group to a no-brace group. Brace treatment resulted in significant pain reduction, improved functionality of the arm, and improvement in pain-free grip strength. After the treatment period, the brace group maintained beneficial effects at a one-year follow-up. Unfortunately, this specific brace is not necessarily available, and the cost of the brace was not stated or considered.

Takasaki et al.[42] evaluated numerous positions to determine the best stretch for the extensor carpi radialis longus and brevis. They found the combination of elbow extension, forearm pronation, and wrist flexion/ulnar deviation to be most effective.

As with other chronic tendinopathies, lateral epicondylitis may be approached using an eccentric training program. There are few studies specific to this area. However, one study[43] incorporating an isokinetic eccentric approach has been published. The control group in this study was treated with cross-friction, stretching, ice, TENS, or ultrasonography, but was not given any exercise program. The exercise group performed their program on a Cybex isokinetic machine. Focus was placed on the wrist extensors and forearm supinators. The elbow flexion angle was maintained at 60°. Progression through the program involved an initial submaximal contraction of about 38% and a speed of 30° per second. Subjects were treated three times per week for an average duration of about nine weeks. There were marked improvements in pain and function in the exercise group as compared to the control group.

The literature includes studies on both local manipulation/mobilization of the elbow and nonlocal manipulation for lateral epicondylitis. The nonlocal manipulative approaches included cervical and/or cervicothoracic spine manipulation and manipulation of the wrist. The systematic reviews by Smidt[35] in 2003, which included all physiotherapy approaches, concluded that there was insufficient evidence for mobilization techniques, specifically for the wrist for LE. The systematic review by Bisset[34] in 2004 indicated that there was some evidence that local manipulation may have an immediate effect; however, the study was a single-treatment approach without follow-up. The study referred to by Bisset was by Vicenzino.[44] He demonstrated a substantial increase in pain-free grip during treatment using a lateral-glide mobilization (Mulligan-type). Patients were randomized to a lateral-glide treatment group or a position-only (no gliding) group. As mentioned above, the study indicates only the immediate effect but had no follow-up to determine how long effects lasted.

The Bisset review also concluded that wrist manipulation did not demonstrate a significant difference when compared to a treatment group that included cross-friction massage, exercise, and pulsed-ultrasound. The study referred to was an RCT by Struijs et al.,[45] that utilized a Lewit-type mobilization of the wrist. This study demonstrated a similar positive outcome for both groups in visual analog scale, grip strength, and pain threshold at the end of six weeks. This study was rated low by our group.

Specific studies related to chiropractic management of lateral epicondylitis include only one randomized, prospective study[46] and an occasional case report.[47] In the randomized, prospective report by Langen-Peters et al.,[46] patients were treated with either adjusting (manipulation) of the elbow with associated stretching or ultrasonography. Both groups demonstrated improvement; however, there was no control group for comparison. This small study indicated that either manipulation of the elbow with stretching/strengthening or ultrasonography is effective in the short term.

An RCT by Vicenzino et al.[48] utilized a lateral-glide mobilization at the C5-C6 vertebral segments. This small study of 15 patients demonstrated significant improvements in pain threshold, pain-free grip strength, and pain scores, relative to placebo or control. There was no measure of duration of effect in any short- or long-term follow-up. The second study was a retrospective evaluation by Cleland et al.[49] This study compared ultrasonography, soft tissue mobilization, and elbow joint mobilization versus a group treated with cervical spine manual therapy, which included passive accessory mobilization and movement techniques. Data were derived from a telephone interview over an undesignated time period that appears to be at least one to three years. Seventy-five percent of the local treatment group, and 80% of the local-plus-manual therapy group had a successful outcome. The local-plus-manual therapy to the cervical spine group achieved a successful long-term outcome in fewer visits (mean of 9.6 visits for local versus a mean of 5.6 visits for the local plus C-spine manipulation group).

There is moderate evidence to suggest that mobilization of either the elbow, cervical spine, or wrist may produce some immediate benefit but no evidence for or against long-term benefit. There is no evidence for or against high-velocity, short-amplitude (HVSA) adjusting of the elbow in the management of LE. The CCGPP Upper Extremity Team expert opinion supports the use of HVSA manipulation (adjustment) of the elbow with some recommendations for use that include avoidance of risk. Further evaluation and/or management are required for patients who fail to respond to treatment within a reasonable period of time.

- For all patients who have fracture, suspected fracture, dislocation, active hemarthrosis or extensive swelling, severe generalized or local osteoporosis, infection, or tumor, HVSA manipulation is contraindicated.
- For patients who have had surgery of the elbow, consider date of surgery, extent of surgery, type of procedure, and other related factors in making decisions about the use of HVSA manipulation.
- Cautious or modified application of manipulation should be considered for the following: known joint mice, traction spurs, or olecranon arthrosis.
- For all patients, an evaluation for joint stability must be performed. Based on the findings, it is recommended that no HVSA manipulation be used for patients with hypermobility syndromes (e.g., Marfan, Ehler–Danlos), or gross looseness indicating multidirectional instability. Mobilization such as applying a Maitland Grade I–IV type of translational movement may be appropriate in these case settings.
- For patients with any acute inflammatory condition such as rheumatoid arthritis, crystalline disease (e.g., gout), or acute bursitis it is recommended not to use HVSA. For some patients with olecranon bursitis, HVSA manipulation may be safely applied if the bursitis is chronic, or the application is not specific to the olecranon.

Algorithm

An algorithm for evaluation and management of elbow/forearm pain is presented in **Figure 8–7**.

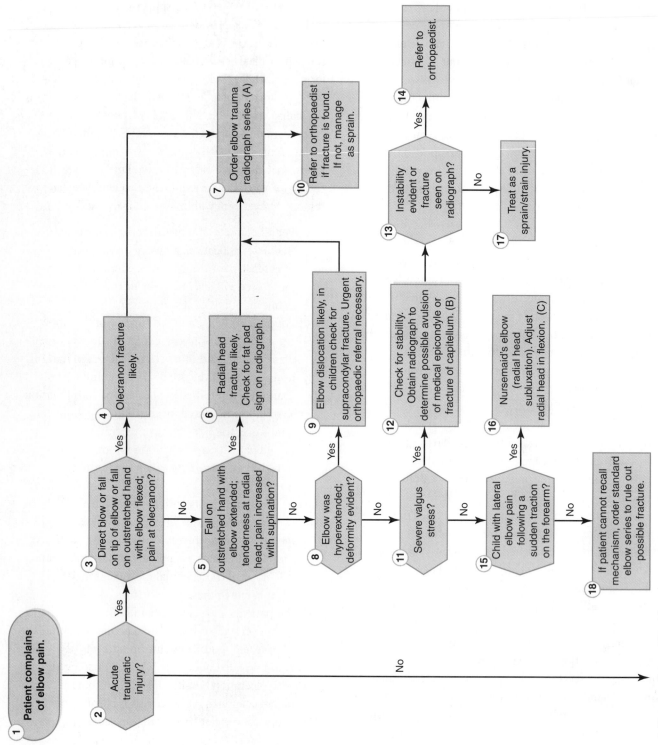

Figure 8–7 Elbow/Forearm Pain—Algorithm

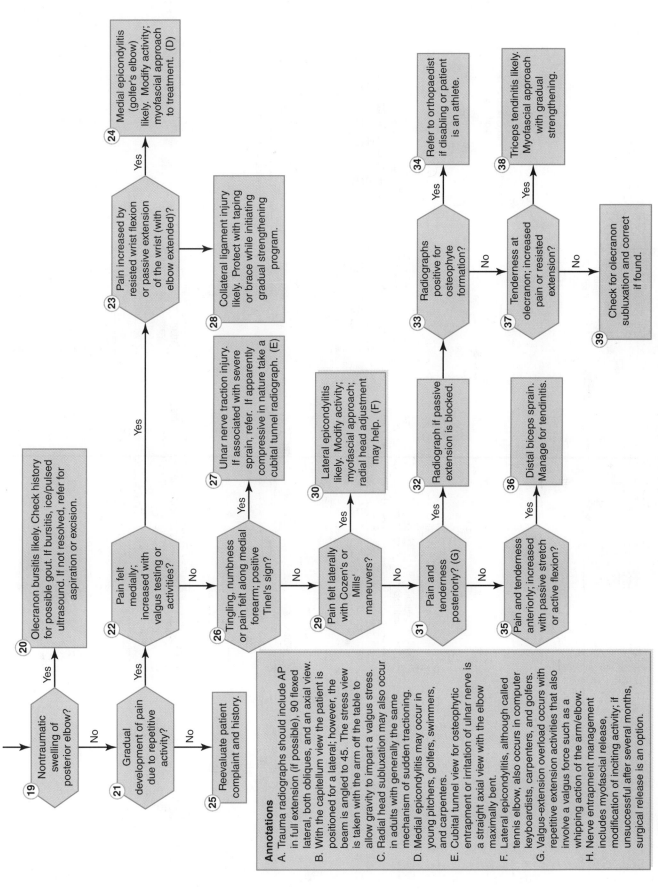

Annotations

A. Trauma radiographs should include AP in full extension (if possible), 90 flexed lateral, both obliques, and an axial view. With the capitellum view the patient is positioned for a lateral; however, the beam is angled to 45. The stress view is taken with the arm off the table to allow gravity to impart a valgus stress.

B. Radial head subluxation may also occur in adults with generally the same mechanism of sudden tractioning.

C. Medial epicondylitis may occur in young pitchers, golfers, swimmers, and carpenters.

D. Cubital tunnel view for osteophytic entrapment or irritation of ulnar nerve is a straight axial view with the elbow maximally bent.

E. Lateral epicondylitis, although called tennis elbow, also occurs in computer keyboardists, carpenters, and golfers.

F. Valgus-extension overload occurs with repetitive extension activities that also involve a valgus force such as a whipping action of the arm/elbow.

G. Nerve entrapment management includes myofascial release, modification of inciting activity; if unsuccessful after several months, surgical release is an option.

Figure 8–7 (Continued)

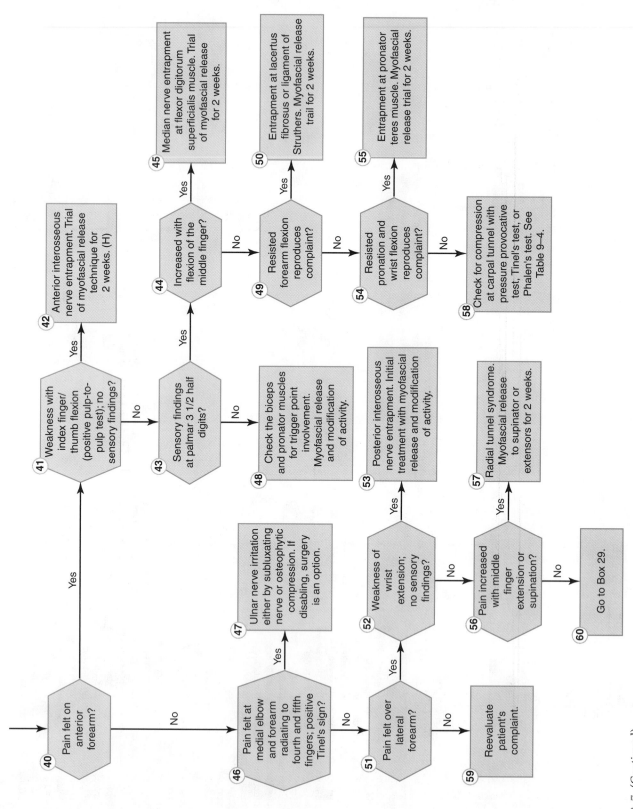

Figure 8–7 (Continued)

Selected Disorders of the Elbow

Lateral Epicondylitis (Tennis Elbow)

Classic Presentation

The patient presents with lateral elbow pain associated with a repetitive sport or occupational activity.

Cause

Many theories have been proposed and many structures have been implicated; however, the currently accepted theory is that initially there is tearing of the extensor carpi radialis brevis (ECRB) origin.[50] This process may extend to the extensor digitorum communis (EDC) or the extensor carpi radialis longus (ECRL). The histologic description of the change in tissue is called angiofibroblastic hyperplasia.[51] Repetitive movements requiring forceful wrist extension, radial deviation, and supination are the most common causes. Although it is associated with tennis, other sports and occupational activities are also possible causes. Meat cutters, plumbers, and weavers are examples of those who may be affected. With tennis, novice players with poor backhand technique account for most cases. With professional players, the forehand or the serve may be the cause. The more frequently an individual plays, the higher the risk of developing tennis elbow.

Evaluation

Tenderness is elicited at the lateral epicondyle, specifically at the origin of the ECRB. Tenderness 5 mm anterior and distal to the lateral epicondyle is most common. Provocative maneuvers include contraction of the wrist extensors with the elbow flexed or extended (Cozen's maneuver [Figure 8–6]) and stretching of the wrist extensors with passive wrist flexion with the elbow extended (Mill's maneuver [Figure 8–5]). Painful resisted middle or ring finger extension implicates the EDC. Wrist extension with radial deviation implicates the ECRB or ECRL. Another suggested test is the chair lift test. The patient is asked to pick up a light chair by the chair back. The patient's elbow is extended with the forearm pronated. This is usually impossible for the patient with lateral epicondylitis because of the pain. Radiographs may demonstrate calcification in as many as 25% of patients with lateral epicondylitis, although they are rarely indicated.[16] Synovial plicae of the elbow may mimic lateral epicondylitis. Some distinctions are that the point of maximum tenderness is posterior to the lateral epicondyle and centered more at the posterior radiocapitellar joint. There may be a small loss of extension range of motion. Diagnostically, MRI may be helpful. To date, the literature is only on arthroscopic treatment revealing good short-term results.[52]

Management

In the acute phase, ice and rest from the inciting activity are essential. Imposed rest through the use of a splint with the wrist in 30° to 45° of extension may relieve tension on the ECRB.[53] Through a graded program of slow stretching and isometric exercise progressing to isotonic exercise of the wrist extensors with an eccentric focus, resolution and prevention may be initiated. Myofascial release techniques are effective. Cross-friction massage, manipulation, and mobilization are helpful in the subacute phase.[54] During the subacute phase, the use of a tennis elbow brace may help redistribute forces distal to the ECRB. Recommendations are to use a pneumatic or Velcro type that is 3.0- to 3.5-in. wide.[55] If tennis is the culprit, recommend a midsize ceramic or graphite racquet with natural gut strings. The string tension should be 3 to 5 lb below what the athlete is used to (usually 52 to 55 lb).[56] Use the Nirschl approach to proper grip size.[57]

A common approach to tendon problems is eccentric rehabilitation exercises. A standard protocol involves usually three sets of ten with the last set being uncomfortable. A systematic review in 2014 indicates that eccentric exercise is an effective approach for LE.[58]

In a review of treatment approaches to lateral epicondylitis, researchers compared corticosteroid injections, physiotherapy, and a wait-and-see approach.[59] Although short-term benefits for corticosteroid injection were far superior (92% success rate) compared to physiotherapy (47%) and the wait-and-see policy (32%), the differences between injections and physiotherapy were lost in long-term follow-up, indicating physiotherapy at one year was far superior (91%). In fact, the wait-and-see policy patients were significantly better at one year (83%) compared to injection (69%). Contrasting this study is a systematic review by the same researcher[59] that indicated there was insufficient evidence for the use of most physiotherapy interventions for lateral epicondylitis due to contradicting results, insufficient power, and a small number of studies.[60] Only ultrasound had weak evidence for efficacy.

Injectables have become more recently popular; in particular, platelet-rich plasma (PRP) injections. The theory is that by creating a concentrate of platelets from the patient's own blood, growth factors will help stimulate healing. A comparison study for various injectables including corticosteroid, PRP, sclerosing agents, and sodium hyaluronate concluded that sodium hyaluronate compared with placebo showed consistently better results.[61] The study also found that corticosteroids were effective for short-term relief but may be worse than other treatments over the long run. Another similar study found value for prolotherapy and sodium hyaluronate.[62] Yet another study in 2013 using a double-blinded randomized approach found no difference between patients' pain relief at three months when treated with saline as compared with glucocorticoids or PRP.[63] Another study not only confirmed this but said that none provided an acceptable level of pain relief for those with LE.[64] There has been an increased use of shockwave therapy for lateral epicondylitis over the last few years. In one recent review study, researchers found a mixed report based on two studies using similar protocols.[65] The researchers recommended further study prior to drawing conclusions or making recommendations. The older studies include the following and their conclusions:

- A double-blinded, randomized controlled trial using shockwave therapy compared to a sham therapy: Results indicated a significant placebo effect with no evidence of benefit using shock therapy.[66]
- A small one- and two-year follow-up study with a control group (sham treatment): Results indicated that 61% of patients treated with shockwave therapy were free of complaints while the control group patients were unchanged.[67]
- A randomized, double-blind study with 74 patients: Results indicated that all patients improved significantly over time and that there was no evidence that shockwave therapy was better than placebo.[68]

Yet the preponderance of newer studies find value in the use of shockwave therapy for both acute and chronic LE.

- A 2013 study found value for patients with recalcitrant LE.[69]
- A 2012 study found that using an initial treatment with shockwave for acute LE was also effective.[70]
- A publication in 2012 indicated that shockwave therapy was effective for short-term relief.

Although used for years, only recently has there been support for the use of low-level laser treatment (LLLT) for tendinopathies.[71]

A small, recently published study compared manipulation of the wrist with a second protocol of ultrasound, friction massage, and muscle stretching and strengthening for the management of lateral epicondyitis.[72] Short-term success was better for manipulation of the wrist compared to the traditional ultrasound, friction massage, and muscle stretching/strengthening approach. Long-term studies are needed to determine whether these benefits are maintained.

An investigative approach is topical nitric oxide application. Researchers in a randomized, double-blinded, placebo-controlled clinical trial compared a combination of a routine rehabilitation program with either a transdermal patch of glyceryl trinitrate or a placebo patch in the management of chronic extensor tendinosis.[73] This topical application of nitric oxide is believed to stimulate collagen synthesis in fibroblasts. It appears that the treated group had a good response with regard to reduction in elbow pain with activity at two weeks and decreased tenderness at six and 12 weeks. Follow-up at six months demonstrated that 81% of the treated patients were asymptomatic during activities of daily living compared to 60% who had performed the rehabilitation program but received the placebo patch. It appears that both are effective, with some advantage to using the patch.

Medial Epicondylitis

Classic Presentation

The patient complains of medial elbow pain following a repetitive activity such as hammering or use of a screwdriver. In athletes, the inciting activity usually involves wrist flexion and pronation such as in serving and overhead and forehand strokes. Golfing ("golfer's elbow"), climbing ("climber's elbow"), or throwing may also cause symptoms. Patients may also complain of pain or weakness on gripping.

Cause

Medial epicondylitis is believed to be a tendinopathy of the origin of the wrist flexors and pronator teres.

Evaluation

Tenderness is found at the medial epicondyle. Pain is reproduced with resisted wrist flexion and pronation. Passive stretching of the wrist flexors with wrist extension, keeping the elbow straight, may also elicit pain (reverse Mill's test).[7] In chronic cases, an elbow flexion contracture may occur, leading to restriction of extension and/or supination. An ulnar neuropathy may coexist with medial epicondylitis.[74] Tinel's sign may be positive over the ulnar nerve. Routine radiographs may reveal calcifications in close proximity to the medial epicondyle in 20% to 30% of patients with epicondylitis.

Management

In the acute phase, ice and rest from the inciting activity are essential. Imposed rest through the use of a splint with the wrist in 10° of flexion may relieve tension on the flexor muscle group. If the flexor carpi radialis is involved, 10° of radial deviation should be added. For pronator involvement, a splint that blocks forearm rotation may be needed. In most cases, however, myofascial release of the flexor muscle mass and pronator teres is sufficient to alleviate the patient's problem. Through a graded program of slow stretching and isometric exercise progressing to isotonic exercise of the wrist extensors with an eccentric focus, resolution and prevention may be initiated. Cross-friction massage, manipulation, and mobilization may be helpful in the subacute phase. During the subacute phase, the use of a tennis elbow brace may help redistribute forces. Other treatment approaches are similar to lateral epicondylitis. There is evidence for the use of shockwave therapy for both.

Triceps Tendinitis (Posterior Tennis Elbow)

Classic Presentation

The patient complains of pain at the tip of the elbow after a repetitive extension activity or a single event involving forceful elbow extension.

Cause

Strain of the triceps insertion on the olecranon is usually due to common athletic endeavors performed by boxers, weight lifters, pitchers, shot-putters, and occasionally tennis players.[75]

Evaluation

Tenderness is found at the olecranon process. Pain is increased with resisted elbow extension, especially with a starting position of elbow flexion.

Management

Myofascial release techniques are used for the triceps. Cross-friction may be applied to the insertion point at the olecranon. Ice and rest from the inciting activity are essential. Decrease the amount of weight used in elbow extensions if the patient is working out.

Posterior Impingement Syndrome

Classic Presentation

The patient is usually an athlete complaining of a sharp posterior elbow pain, especially on quick extension of the elbow. There may be associated complaints of popping or clicking with extension or an occasional complaint of locking.

Cause

Repetitive extension leads to posterior compression between the olecranon trochlea and olecranon fossa, which may simply cause a reactive synovitis or progress to degeneration and the production of osteophytes or loose bodies.

Evaluation

There is often a blockage to active and passive extension at end-range accompanied by pain. The valgus-extension overload test involves applying a valgus stress while extending the elbow.[8] Pain and often crepitus are produced with this maneuver. Radiographically, an axial view is required. A cubital tunnel view may also be revealing. If the radiographs are negative, computed tomography or arthrography may be necessary to reveal cartilaginous loose bodies.

Management

If loose bodies are evident, referral for surgical consultation should be made. If there appears to be primarily synovial hypertrophy or pinching, an acute pain program should be initiated with rest, ice, and use of an extension-block brace or taping.

Nursemaid's Elbow

Classic Presentation

A parent presents a child (usually between ages two and four years) with lateral elbow pain after either swinging the child by his or her arms or sudden jerking of the child's arm.

Cause

The radial head is not fully formed, allowing damage or entrapment of the annular ligament by a distraction/rotation force.

Evaluation

Exquisite lateral elbow pain and tenderness in a child without obvious trauma such as a fall or a blow to the elbow are indicative of nursemaid's elbow. Palpation may reveal the malpositioned radial head.

Management

Reduction is accomplished by elbow flexion and rotation. Radiographic confirmation of reduction should be performed.

Little League Elbow

Classic Presentation

The patient is usually an adolescent baseball pitcher who complains of either medial or lateral elbow pain.

Cause

Little League elbow is really a syndrome.[76] The repetitive valgus stress incurred with pitching causes stretch injury to the medial elbow and possible compression injury to the lateral elbow. Medial elbow pain is due to microtrauma to the medial anterior oblique ligament as well as accelerated growth and fragmentation of the medial epicondylar epiphysis. Laterally an osteochondritis dissecans of the capitellum and various degrees of radial head injury, including premature closure, may occur.[77]

Evaluation

Tenderness may be found at both the medial and the lateral elbow. Valgus testing (**Figure 8–3**) may reveal laxity and/or pain that must be distinguished radiographically to determine whether ligament damage or epiphyseal damage is the cause. Alternating supination and pronation performed actively or passively may cause palpable or audible crepitus at the head of the radius when osteochondritis dissecans or radial head damage is present.[78] A flexion contracture may be evident on passive ROM evaluation. Popping and clicking or locking may occur on full-range active movement. Radiographically it is important to include specialized views, including the radial head-capitellum view and the valgus stress view.[13]

Management

If radiographically confirmed, referral for an orthopaedic consultation is warranted. If clinically apparent, yet radiographically normal, modification or elimination of the inciting activity is needed. Modification of pitching should include decreased time pitching (following Little League rules), avoidance of throwing curve balls, and teaching proper mechanics. Proper mechanics would include use of trunk and legs with less dependence on the elbow and wrist, avoidance of whipping or snapping of the elbow, and slow practice to accentuate proper form. The typical acute pain modalities should be used initially, and proper warm-up and stretching should be used prior to any activity.

Osteochondrosis (Panner's Disease)

Classic Presentation

The patient is usually a young male complaining of unilateral (dominant arm) lateral elbow pain and stiffness. Associated complaints may include clicking and locking. The patient is often involved in a sport activity several times a week.

Cause

Osteochondrosis of the capitellum is caused by avascular necrosis. This may be due to trauma or other causes disturbing the circulation to the chondroepiphysis of the capitellum.[79] The vessels that supply this area pass through unossified epiphyseal cartilage and may be compressed. Also, there may be an anomalous distribution with no anastomosis decreasing the available blood supply. Other names for osteochondrosis of the capitellum include Panner's disease,[80] osteochondrosis deformans, osteochondritis, and aseptic/avascular necrosis.

Evaluation

A history of excessive throwing, as occurs in Little League pitching, or repeated weight bearing, as occurs in gymnastics, should always dictate the need for radiographs in any child with elbow pain. The diagnosis of Panner's disease is largely radiographic. The examination should include passive and active supination and pronation with the elbow extended in an effort to palpate or hear crepitus at the radial capitellar joint. Radiographs must include obliques and a radial head-capitellum view. Fragmentation or loose body formation is a clear indicator of this condition.

Management

The best prognosis is for children with an open epiphysis. Reducing or eliminating any identifiable causative activity is required. A period of rest and splinting for two to three weeks should be followed by gradual stretching and strengthening. Gradual return to the activity is allowed if symptoms do not persist. If there are loose fragments or a locked elbow, referral for orthopaedic consultation is necessary. Failure of a conservative trial of several months should also warrant an orthopaedic consultation.

A management approach used for osteochondral problems of the knee and ankle is also being used for the elbow. Autologous osteochondral mosaicplasty is an approach that uses osteochondral grafts from the patient's body (femoral condyles) to implant in the capitellum in an effort to repair the articular defect. Recent evidence[81] suggests that this is a viable approach for advanced lesions in Little League pitchers. Long-term effects are not known at this time.

Olecranon Bursitis

Classic Presentation

The patient presents with an obvious swelling just distal to the point of the elbow.

Cause

The olecranon bursa acts as a cushion when the elbow is in contact with any surface. Therefore, a single fall on the elbow, or more commonly, repeated weight bearing or dragging of the elbow on the ground as occurs in wrestling causes irritation and swelling.

Evaluation

The goose-egg sized swelling at the elbow is difficult to miss. It must be differentiated from other swellings such as tophi in patients with gout and kidney failure. It is also crucial to distinguish between an infected or simply an inflamed bursa. Infection is more likely when there is an obvious wound near the bursitis. Additionally, the infected bursa will be warm and more tender than a simple bursitis.

Management

Protection with a doughnut support taped to the elbow, avoidance of the inciting activity when chronic, and ice or pulsed ultrasound are usually sufficient. When unsuccessful, referral for aspiration and possible excision should be made. Bursas usually grow back in six to 24 months. Patients with an infected bursa should be referred immediately for aspiration and antibiotic treatment.

The Evidence—Elbow

Translation Into Practice Summary (TIPS)

There is little literature evidence on evaluation of the elbow. Although there is some evidence for tests that tend to rule-in or rule-out fracture, medical collateral ligament damage, and cubital tunnel disorders, there is no evidence for or against the use of diagnostic tests for lateral epicondylitis (LE), proximal median nerve entrapment or radial nerve entrapment syndromes.

The Literature-Based Clinical Core

- Supine elbow-extension may be helpful in making decisions about possible fracture at the elbow.
- The moving valgus-stress test is good at ruling-out MCL involvement and moderately good at ruling-in.
- Tinel's and elbow flexion are valuable for ruling-in or out cubital tunnel entrapment of the ulnar nerve.
- Range of motion testing is reliable for flexion, extension, and forearm pronation/supination but its clinical utility is not known.
- There are no studies evaluating the value of tests for lateral epicondylitis.

The Expert-Opinion-Based Clinical Core

- Deformity, crepitus at the radiocapitellar joint, and inability to extend post-trauma suggest the need for radiographs.
- Severe pain with pronation and supination following trauma suggests fracture (if compression injury) and nursemaid's elbow if in a child and distraction is the mechanism.
- Valgus extension testing may provoke pain and crepitus with olecranon joint pathology (especially in athletes).
- Mill's, Cozen's, resisted finger extension, and/or the chair lift test may be valuable for identifying lateral epicondylitis.
- For pronator syndrome, the following may be of value:
  - Resisted forearm pronation with elbow extended, wrist flexed (repeated)
  - Resisted elbow flexion and forearm supination with elbow fully flexed
  - Resisted finger flexion
- For supinator syndrome, the following may be of value:
  - Resisted middle finger extension with elbow extended
  - Extreme forearm pronation with wrist flexion
  - Elbow flexion
  - Resisted supination with elbow flexed (repeated)

APPENDIX 8–1

References

1. Morrey BF, Askew LJ, An KN, et al. A biomechanical study of normal elbow motion. *J Bone Joint Surg Am.* 1981;63:872.
2. Lin F, Kohli N, Perlmutter S, Lim D, Nuber GW, Makhsous M. Muscle contribution to elbow joint valgus stability. *J Shoulder Elbow Surg.* 2007;16(6):795–802.
3. Schwab GH, Bennett JB, Woods GW, et al. Biomechanics of elbow instability: the role of the medial collateral ligament. *Clin Orthop.* 1980;186:44.
4. Whiteside JA. Field evaluation of common athletic injuries. In: Grana WA, Kalenak A, eds. *Clinical Sports Medicine.* Philadelphia: WB Saunders; 1991:130–151.
5. Griggs SM, Weis APC. Bone injuries of the wrist, forearm and elbow. *Clin Sports Med.* 1996;15:373–400.
6. Linschied RL, Wheeler DK. Elbow dislocation. *JAMA.* 1965;194:1171.
7. Bennett JB, Tullos HS. Ligamentous and articular injuries in the athlete. In: Morrey BF, ed. *The Elbow and Its Disorders.* Philadelphia: WB Saunders; 1985:502–522.
8. Wilson FD, Andrews JR, Blackburn TA, McCluskey G. Valgus extension overload in the pitching elbow. *Am J Sports Med.* 1982;1:83–88.
9. Murphy WA, Seigel MJ. Elbow fat pads with new signs extended differential diagnosis. *Radiology.* 1977;124:659.
10. Smith DN, Lee JR. The radiological diagnosis of posttraumatic effusion of the elbow joint and its clinical significance: the displaced fat pad sign. *Injury.* 1978;10:115.
11. Griswold R. Elbow fat pads: a radiographic perspective. *Radiol Technol.* 1982;53:303.
12. Ballinger PW. *Merril's Atlas of Radiographic Positions and Procedures.* 6th ed. St. Louis, MO: CV Mosby; 1986:82–93.
13. Greenspan A, Norman A. The radial-head-capitellum view: useful technique in elbow trauma. *Amer J Radiol.* 1982;138:1186.

14. Bontrager KL, Anthony BT. *Textbook of Radiographic Positioning and Related Anatomy*. 2nd ed. St. Louis, MO: CV Mosby; 1987:112–115.

15. St. John JN, Palmaz JC. The cubital tunnel in ulnar nerve entrapment neuropathy. *Radiology*. 1986;158:119.

16. Nirschl RP, Petrone FA. Tennis elbow: the surgical treatment of lateral epicondylitis. *J Bone Joint Surg Am*. 1979;61:832–839.

17. Allander E. Prevalence, incidence, and remission rates of some common rheumatic diseases or syndromes. *Scand J Rheumatol*. 1974;3(3):145–153.

18. Hamilton PG. The prevalence of humeral epicondylitis: a survey in general practice. *J R Coll Gen Pract*. 1986;36(291):464–465.

19. Gruchow HW, Pelletier D. An epidemiologic study of tennis elbow. Incidence, recurrence, and effectiveness of prevention strategies. *Am J Sports Med*. 1979;7(4):234–238.

20. Maylack FH. Epidemiology of tennis, squash, and racquetball injuries. *Clin Sports Med*. 1988;7(2):233–243.

21. Wadsworth TG. Tennis elbow: conservative, surgical, and manipulative treatment. *Br Med J (Clin Res Ed)*. 1987;294(6572):621–624.

22. Coonrad RW, Hooper WR. Tennis elbow: its course, natural history, conservative and surgical management. *J Bone Joint Surg Am*. 1973;55(6):1177–1182.

23. Dimberg L. The prevalence and causation of tennis elbow (lateral humeral epicondylitis) in a population of workers in an engineering industry. *Ergonomics*. 1987;30(3):573–579.

24. Kivi P. The etiology and conservative treatment of humeral epicondylitis. *Scand J Rehabil Med*. 1983;15(1):37–41.

25. Kurppa K, Viikari-Juntura E, Kuosma E, Huuskonen M, Kivi P. Incidence of tenosynovitis or peritendinitis and epicondylitis in a meat-processing factory. *Scand J Work Environ Health*. 1991;17(1):32–37.

26. Roto P, Kivi P. Prevalence of epicondylitis and tenosynovitis among meatcutters. *Scand J Work Environ Health*. 1984;10(3):203–205.

27. Binder AI, Hazleman BL. Lateral humeral epicondylitis—a study of natural history and the effect of conservative therapy. *Br J Rheumatol*. 1983;22(2):73–76.

28. Verhaar JA. Tennis elbow. Anatomical, epidemiological and therapeutic aspects. *Int Orthop*. 1994;18(5):263–267.

29. Bernard B. *Musculoskeletal Disorders (MSD) and Workplace Factors: A Critical Review of Epidemiologic Evidence for Work-Related Musculoskeletal Disorders of the Neck, Upper Extremity, and Low Back*. Cincinnati, OH: NIOSH, Centers for Disease Control and Prevention National Institute for Occupational Safety and Health; 1997.

30. Nirschl RP. The etiology and treatment of tennis elbow. *J Sports Med*. 1974;2(6):308–323.

31. Hudak PL, Cole DC, Haines AT. Understanding prognosis to improve rehabilitation: the example of lateral elbow pain. *Arch Phys Med Rehabil*. 1996;77(6):586–593.

32. Waugh EJ, Jaglal SB, Davis AM. Computer use associated with poor long-term prognosis of conservatively managed lateral epicondylalgia. *J Orthop Sports Phys Ther*. 2004;34(12):770–780.

33. Pienimaki T, Karinen P, Kemila T, Koivukangas P, Vanharanta H. Long-term follow-up of conservatively treated chronic tennis elbow patients. A prospective and retrospective analysis. *Scand J Rehabil Med*. 1998;30(3):159–166.

34. Bisset L, Paungmali A, Vicenzino B, Beller E. A systematic review and meta-analysis of clinical trials on physical interventions for lateral epicondylalgia. *Br J Sports Med*. 2005;39(7):411–422; discussion 411–422.

35. Smidt N, Assendelft WJ, Arola H, et al. Effectiveness of physiotherapy for lateral epicondylitis: a systematic review. *Ann Med*. Vol. 35; 2003:51–62.

36. Korthals-de Bos IB, Smidt N, van Tulder MW, et al. Cost effectiveness of interventions for lateral epicondylitis: results from a randomised controlled trial in primary care. *Pharmacoeconomics*. 2004;22:185–195.

37. Smidt N, Van der Windt D, Assendelft WJJ, Deville W, Bouter LM. Corticosteroid injections, physiotherapy or a wait-and-see policy for lateral epicondylitis: a randomised controlled trial. *Nederlands Tijdschrift Voor Fysiotherapie*. 2004;114(1):14.

38. Pienimaki TT, Tarvainen TK, Siira PT, Vanharanta H. Progressive strengthening and stretching exercises and ultrasound for chronic lateral epicondylitis [corrected] [published erratum appears in PHYSIOTHERAPY 1997;83(1):48]. *Physiotherapy*. 1996;82(9):522.

39. Derebery VJ, Devenport JN, Giang GM, Fogarty WT. The effects of splinting on outcomes for epicondylitis. *Arch Phys Med Rehabil*. 2005;86(6):1081–1088.

40. Struijs PAA, Kerkhoffs GMMJ, Assendelft WJJ, van Dijk CN. Conservative treatment of lateral epicondylitis: brace versus physical therapy or a combination of both—a randomized clinical trial. *Am J Sports Med*. 2004;32:462–469.

41. Faes M, van den Akker B, de Lint JA, Kooloos JG, Hopman MT. Dynamic extensor brace for

lateral epicondylitis. *Clin Orthop Relat Res.* 2006;442:149–157.

42. Takasaki H, Aoki M, Muraki T, Uchiyama E, Murakami G, Yamashita T. Muscle strain on the radial wrist extensors during motion-simulating stretching exercises for lateral epicondylitis: a cadaveric study. *J Shoulder Elbow Surg.* 2007;16(6):854–858.

43. Croisier JL, Foidart-Dessalle M, Tinant F, Crielaard JM, Forthomme B. An isokinetic eccentric programme for the management of chronic lateral epicondylar tendinopathy. *Br J Sports Med.* 2007;41(4):269–275.

44. Vicenzino B, Paungmali A, Buratowski S, Wright A. Specific manipulative therapy treatment for chronic lateral epicondylalgia produces uniquely characteristic hypoalgesia. *Man Ther.* 2001;6(4):205–212.

45. Struijs PA, Damen PJ, Bakker EW, Blankevoort L, Assendelft WJ, van Dijk CN. Manipulation of the wrist for management of lateral epicondylitis: a randomized pilot study. *Phys Ther.* 2003;83:608–616.

46. Langen-Pieters P, Weston P, Brantingham JW. A randomized, prospective pilot study comparing chiropractic care and ultrasound for the treatment of lateral epicondylitis. *Eur J of Chirop.* 2003;50(3):211.

47. Kaufman RL. Conservative chiropractic care of lateral epicondylitis. *J Manipulative Physiol Ther.* 2000;23(9):619–622.

48. Vicenzino B, Collins D, Wright A. The initial effects of a cervical spine manipulative physiotherapy treatment on the pain and dysfunction of lateral epicondylalgia. *Pain.* 1996;68(1):69–74.

49. Cleland JA, Whitman JM, Fritz JM. Effectiveness of manual physical therapy to the cervical spine in the management of lateral epicondylalgia: a retrospective analysis including commentary by Vicenzino B. *J Ortho Sports Phys Ther.* 2004;34(11):713.

50. Plancher KD, Hallbrecht J, Lourie JM. Medial and lateral epicondylitis in the athlete. *Clin Sports Med.* 1996;15:283–305.

51. Regan W, Wold LE, Conrad R. Microscopic histopathology of chronic, refractory lateral epicondylitis. *Am J Sports Med.* 1992;20:746–749.

52. Ruch DS, Papadonikolakis A, Campolattaro RM. The posterolateral plica: a cause of refractory lateral elbow pain. *J Shoulder Elbow Surg.* 2006;15(3):367–370.

53. Sailer SM, Lewis SB. Rehabilitation and splinting of common upper extremity injuries in athletes. *Clin Sports Med.* 1995;14:411–446.

54. Kushner S, Reid DC. Manipulation in the treatment of tennis elbow. *J Orthop Sports Phys Ther.* 1986;7:264.

55. Froimson AI. Treatment of tennis elbow with forearm support band. *J Bone Joint Surg Am.* 1971;53:183.

56. Legwold G. Tennis elbow: joint resolution by conservative treatment and improved technique. *Physician Sportsmed.* 1984;12:168.

57. Nirschl RP. Elbow tendinosis/tennis elbow. *Clin Sports Med.* 1986;11:856–860.

58. Cullinane FL, Boocock MG, Trevelyan FC. Is eccentric exercise an effective treatment for lateral epicondylitis? A systematic review. *Clin Rehabil.* 2014;28(1):3–19.

59. Smidt N, van der Windt DA, Assendelft WJ, et al. Corticosteroid injections, physiotherapy, or a wait-and-see policy for lateral epicondylitis: a randomized controlled trial. *Lancet.* 2002;359:657–662.

60. Smidt N, Assendelft WJ, Arola H, et al. Effectiveness of physiotherapy for lateral epicondylitis: a systematic review. *Ann Med.* 2003;35:51–62.

61. Hart L. Corticosteroid and other injections in the management of tendinopathies: a review. *Clin J Sport Med.* 2011;21(6):540–541.

62. Krogh TP, Bartels EM, Ellingsen T, et al. Comparative effectiveness of injection therapies in lateral epicondylitis: a systematic review and network meta-analysis of randomized controlled trials. *Am J Sports Med.* 2013;41(6):1435–1446.

63. Krogh TP, Fredberg U, Stengaard-Pedersen K, Christensen R, Jensen P, Ellingsen T. Treatment of lateral epicondylitis with platelet-rich plasma, glucocorticoid, or saline: a randomized, double-blind, placebo-controlled trial. *Am J Sports Med.* 2013;41(3):625–635.

64. Shiple BJ. How effective are injection treatments for lateral epicondylitis? *Clin J Sport Med.* 2013;23(6):502–503.

65. Buchbinder R, Green S, White M, et al. Shock wave therapy for lateral elbow pain. *Cochrane Database System Rev.* 2002; (11):CD003524.

66. Speed CA, Nichols D, Richards C, et al. Extracorporeal shock wave therapy for lateral epicondylitis: a double blind randomized controlled trial. *J Orthop Res.* 2002;20:895–898.

67. Wang CJ, Chen JA. Shock wave therapy for patients with lateral epicondylitis of the elbow. *Am J Sports Med.* 2002;30:422–425.

68. Melikyan EY, Shahin E, Miles J, Baimbridge LC. Extracorporeal shock-wave treatment for tennis-elbow: a randomized double-blind study. *J Bone Joint Surg Br.* 2003;85:852–855.

69. Ilieva EM, Minchev RM, Petrova NS. Radial shock wave therapy in patients with lateral epicondylitis. *Folia Med (Plovdiv).* 2012;54(3):35–41.

70. Lee SS, Kang S, Park NK, et al. Effectiveness of initial extracorporeal shock wave therapy on the newly diagnosed lateral or medial epicondylitis. *Ann Rehabil Med.* 2012;36(5):681–687.

71. Tumilty S, Munn J, McDonough S, Hurley DA, Basford JR, Baxter GD. Low level laser treatment of tendinopathy: a systematic review with meta-analysis. *Photomed Laser Surg.* 2010;28(1):3–16.

72. Struins PA, Damen PJ, Bakker EW, et al. Manipulation of the wrist for management of lateral epicondylitis: a randomized pilot study. *Phys Ther.* 2003;83:608–616.

73. Paoloni JA, Appleyard RC, Nelson J, Murrell GAC. Topical nitric oxide application in the treatment of chronic extensor tendinosis at the elbow: a randomized, double-blinded, placebo-controlled clinical trial. *Am J Sports Med.* 2003; 31:915–920.

74. Nirschl RP. Treatment of medial tennis elbow tendinitis. Presented at the Annual Meeting of the American Academy of Orthopaedic Surgeons; New Orleans; February, 1986.

75. Nirschl RP. Soft tissue injury about the elbow. *Clin Sports Med.* 1986;5:638–644.

76. Grana WA, Girshkin A. Pitcher's elbow in adolescence. *Am J Sports Med.* 1980;82:333–336.

77. O'Neil DB, Micheli LJ. Overuse injuries in the young athlete. *Clin Sports Med.* 1988;7:602.

78. American Academy of Orthopaedic Surgeons. *Joint Motion: Method of Measuring and Recording.* Chicago: American Academy of Orthopaedic Surgeons; 1965.

79. Singer KM, Roy SP. Osteochondrosis of the humeral capitellum. *Am J Sports Med.* 1984;12:351.

80. Panner JH. A peculiar affection of the capitellum humeri resembling Calve-Perthes' disease of the hip. *Acta Radiol.* 1929;10:234.

81. Iwasaki N, Kato H, Ishikawa J, Saitoh S, Minami A. Autologous osteochondral mosaicplasty for capitellar osteochondritis dissecans in teenaged patients. *Am J Sports Med.* 2006;34(8):1233–1239.

APPENDIX 8-2

Elbow and Forearm Diagnosis Table

Diagnosis	Comments	History Findings	Positive Examination Findings	Radiography/Special Studies	Treatment Options
Subluxation or Fixation of: Radioulnar Joint Ulnohumeral Joint Radiohumeral Joint	• Should be used when chiropractic manipulation is used as Tx for any elbow/forearm problem/Dx. • Can be primary Dx if patient is asymptomatic or mildly symptomatic (e.g., mild stiffness or pain level < 2/10). • Must indicate chiropractic exam findings to support Dx.	*Nonspecific*	*Palpation*—Local tenderness or other signs of subluxation *Ortho*—None *Neuro*—None *Active ROM*—Variable restriction *Passive ROM*—End-range restriction *Motion palpation*—specific articular restriction or symptoms produced on end-range	• Radiography not required for the diagnosis of subluxation. • Radiographic biomechanical analysis may assist in treatment decision. • For specifics see radiographic guidelines.	• Chiropractic adjustive technique. • Decisions regarding specifically which technique(s) is/are applied and modifications to the given approach will be directed by the primary Dx and patient's ability to tolerate preadjustment stresses.
Radial Collateral Ligament (RCL) Sprain Ulnar Collateral Ligament (UCL) Sprain Radiohumeral Joint Sprain/ Strain Ulnohumeral Joint Sprain/ Strain Note: Sprain/strain is not synonymous with spasm or hypertonicity.	• Used for either strain of a muscle tendon or sprain of a ligament/capsule in an acute setting.	*Mechanism*—Overstretch or overcontraction Hx as acute event *Worse with Specific ROM*—Contraction of muscle or stretch of muscle or joint	*Ortho*—Varus testing for UCL; valgus testing for RCL may reveal tenderness or laxity dependent on degree of injury. Specific tests for each muscle including tenderness at muscle/tendon: *Active ROM*—Pain on active ROM that contracts involved muscles *Passive ROM*—Pain on end-range stretch of involved muscle or ligament	• Radiography and stress radiographs may be used to determine if bony avulsion has occurred or damage to epiphyseal plate in younger patients. • For specifics see radiographic guidelines.	• Limited orthotic support (taping or brace) for first- and second-degree injuries. • Strengthening and preventive exercises. • Third-degree injury and/or those with bony avulsion or epipheryseal injury should be referred for orthopaedic consult.

Medial Epicondylitis Lateral Epicondylitis	• These conditions must be differentiated from local peripheral nerve entrapments and trigger point disorders.	*Mechanism*—For lateral epicondylitis repetitive movements requiring forceful dorsiflexion, radial deviation, and supination are often cause for medial epicondylitis overuse of wrist flexors *Symptoms*—Pain and tenderness at respective epicondyle	*Palpation*—Tenderness at respective epicondyle *Ortho*—Positive Mill's and/or Cozen's for lateral epicondylitis and reverse Mill's and/or Cozen's for medial epicondylitis *Neuro*—None	• Radiography not recommended.	• Myofascial therapy. • Physiotherapy such as ultrasound. • Daily exercises and stretches. • Ergonomic advice for sports or occupational activities.
Olecranon Bursitis	• Although this is often due to trauma, idiopathic and secondary to gout or chronic kidney disease is also possible.	*Mechanism*—If no Hx of direct trauma, careful questioning may reveal a posture that involves prolonged pressure on bursa such as leaning on elbow	*Palpation*—Large swelling at tip of elbow with variable tenderness	• Radiography not usually necessary initially except to rule out fracture with acute trauma.	• Physiotherapy for pain and swelling control. • Usually not self-resolving and requires surgical excision (bursa grows back).
Peripheral Neuritis (Entrapment) Median Nerve Ulnar Nerve Radial Nerve	• Peripheral neuropathies may be secondary to overuse and therefore misdiagnosis as myofascial or sprain/strains is common. • Multiple sites of entrapment are possible for each nerve and must be specified. • Neurological positives may vary if entrapment or compression is transient.	*Mechanism*—If due to muscle/myofascial entrapment overuse or hypertrophy of related muscle may cause compression, in particular, if nerve runs through muscle or two heads of muscle *Symptoms*—Varied symptoms; however, numbness/tingling, pain, and if motor branch of nerve involved, weakness may be reported	*Palpation*—If nerve is superficial enough Tinel's (ulnar) or compression of nerve may reproduce complaint(s) *Ortho*—Tests for specific site of entrapment are utilized including: Median—Resisted pronation, or resisted finger flexion, passive elbow flexion Radial—Resisted supination or wrist extension *Ulnar*—Passive elbow flexion	• Radiography not usually needed unless for ulnar nerve osteophytes are suspected cause of entrapment. • Electrodiagnostic studies may be needed if clinical signs are equivocal or patient is unresponsive to care.	• Myofascial management of involved muscles. • Physiotherapy. • Referral for acupuncture or surgical care if conservative trial is ineffective.

(continues)

Elbow and Forearm Diagnosis Table (continued)

Diagnosis	Comments	History Findings	Positive Examination Findings	Radiography/Special Studies	Treatment Options
Myofascitis	• Used when specific trigger points are identified on physical examination. • Also may be used if a strain is not evident from the history; however, there are indicators of muscle tenderness, stiffness, or pain.	Onset—Nonspecific regarding onset Symptoms—Patient usually complains of pain, aching, and/or tenderness in specific muscle or tendon areas that may radiate pain in nondermatomal pattern	• Trigger points are evident as localized tenderness in a muscle that corresponds to traditional (Travell/Simons) trigger point charts. These points may be local or refer pain when compressed.	• Not required or recommended.	• Myofascial approaches such as myofascial stripping, trigger point massage, or spray and stretch approaches are the standard. • Home stretching and modification of activity suggestions.
Laxity Hypermobility	• Used to identify causation or the result of a patient's primary diagnosis such as a sprain or strain due to hypermobility.	A history of a single event, traumatic injury to the joint is not found; however, either overuse (microtrauma) or generalized inherent looseness is/are evident.	• Capsular or ligament testing reveals "looseness" that falls within the physiologic range of normal.	• Not usually recommended unless differentiating pathological laxity from congenital or overuse acquisition.	• Strengthening program. • Bracing or functional taping during rehabilitation or during strenuous activities.

Wrist and Forearm Complaints

Context

The wrist is a complex of multiple joints that are required to function as the flexible link between the hand and the forearm. In essence, there are no tendon attachments that function at the wrist. Tendons cross the wrist to insert into the hand, fingers, and thumb. Stability, therefore, is inherently ligamentous. Problems affecting muscles that originate off the elbow and forearm may be manifested clinically as pain at the wrist. Biomechanical friction or inflammatory processes may affect the tendons as they cross the wrist.

Wrist complaints are often the result of direct trauma, falls, overuse, and arthritides. With trauma, the most likely possibilities other than sprains are fractures and instability due to ruptured ligamentous support. Unfortunately, it is far too common for wrist pain to be dismissed as a simple sprain if no fracture is evident radiographically. Varying degrees of instability, however, may occur without associated fracture, and unless the examiner is testing for possible instability or is radiographically focused on the signs of instability, chronic pain and dysfunction may result from mismanagement.

In the athletic and computer operator population, overuse is common. Positions that strain muscles repetitively are likely to result in an insidious onset of wrist pain. Weight lifting, rowing, and racquetball are among the common activities that may overstrain the wrist. Cumulative trauma in the workplace has become an important Occupational Safety and Health Administration concern. Most injury is due to assembly-line movement patterns and computer use.[1] The ergonomics of these overuse problems have been studied extensively, and technologic advances in design have provided a proactive approach to these patients.

When the wrist becomes a weight-bearing joint, injury occurs. Two common scenarios of transformation from a non-weight-bearing joint to a weight-bearing joint are bracing the body for a fall and the chronic demands placed on the gymnast or chiropractor. The injury mechanism for gymnasts is obvious when handstands and other support or balance maneuvers add an element of forced, dorsiflexed weight-bearing, often with torque added.[2] The mechanism for the chiropractor is repeated extension/compression injury with side-posture or double-transverse adjusting. Some chiropractors also experience wrist pain with cervical chair adjusting if the wrist is not kept straight (in neutral).

Forearm pain and wrist pain are often concomitant complaints. With a history of trauma, fracture should be ruled out. Insidious onset of forearm and wrist complaints is often due to overuse. When a complaint of pain is associated with either weakness or numbness/tingling, peripheral nerve entrapment is likely.[3] A history of overuse or misuse is usually evident, often involving repeated pronation/supination or flexion/extension. Patients who are pregnant or have metabolic disorders or rheumatoid conditions are also prone to develop reactions at the wrist, including median nerve entrapment and tendinopathies.

Chiropractors are often confronted with the patient who has been diagnosed with or is suspicious he or she has carpal tunnel syndrome. Carpal tunnel syndrome is a common diagnosis in the United States with an increase in reported cases from the 1980s to the 1990s. More than 200,000 carpal tunnel release procedures are performed each year in the United States. The direct medical costs are estimated at $1 billion per year.[4] It is hoped that through proper evaluation, differentiation from other causes of hand pain and numbness, and initial conservative management, this financial impact may be lessened.

General Strategy

History

- Clarify the type of complaint.
  1. Is the complaint one of pain, stiffness, looseness, crepitus, or a combination of complaints?
- Clarify the mechanism if traumatic (see **Table 9–1**).
  1. For a fall on an outstretched hand, consider scaphoid fracture, carpal instability, and/or distal forearm fractures; for patients younger than age 12 years, consider epiphyseal damage or torus fracture.

- Determine whether the mechanism is one of overuse.
  1. In what position does the patient work?
  2. Does the patient perform a repetitive movement at work or during sports activity?

Evaluation

- With trauma, palpate for points of tenderness and obtain radiographs to evaluate possibility of fracture/dislocation or dissociation.
- If radiographs are negative for fracture, challenge the ligaments of the wrist, in particular the scapholunate (Watson's test) and the lunotriquetral (ballottement test) articulations; if unstable include stress views to the radiographic series.

Table 9–1 Fractures of the Upper Extremity

Fracture Site	Common Mechanisms	Radiographs	Management
Scaphoid	Fall on outstretched hand or blow to an object with the palm (60% to 70% of all carpal bone fractures)	Scaphoid series—PA, lateral, 45° pronation PA, ulnar deviation PA; optional Stecher view (PA, 20° angle from vertical, distal to proximal)	Nondisplaced fracture—cast immobilization including distal interphalangeal (DIP) joint of thumb; change every two weeks; switch to short-arm thumb spica (DIP of thumb not included) at six weeks; displaced—screw or wire fixation
Hamate	Hook of hamate due to striking a stationary object (e.g., golf swing hits the ground)	Carpal tunnel view and 45° supination oblique; computed tomography (CT) may be necessary	Excision of fragment in older patient; adolescents—initial trial of cast (short arm cast with fourth and fifth metacarpophalangeal joints in flexion include base of thumb); no union after six weeks, needs excision of fragment
Triquetral	Dorsiflexion or direct trauma; impingement of the ulnar styloid into the triquetrum (second most common carpal fracture)	Routine series including obliques	Nondisplaced fracture—short arm cast with mild extension for four weeks; displaced—open reduction and wired
Capitate	Forced dorsiflexion of the wrist	Routine radiographs; check for associated scaphoid fracture	Nondisplaced fracture—cast immobilization for six to eight weeks; displaced—open reduction and wired
Trapezium	5% of carpal fractures; due to direct blow or forced extension of the transverse arch	Routine wrist views plus carpal tunnel and a Bett's view of the carpometacarpal (CMC) joint; CT may be needed	When associated with a dislocation or subluxation of the CMC joint reduction, excision of any fragments and casting are required
Pisiform	Direct trauma to the thenar eminence	Pisiform view (lateral view with wrist in 30° of supination); check for injury to distal radius	Immobilization in short arm cast; 30° of flexion and mild ulnar deviation for four to six weeks
Kienbock's	Shear stress due to ulnar minus variance leads to avascular necrosis of the lunate from repetitive activity or direct trauma in a young patient	Visible on routine views; gradual progression to lunate sclerosis with collapse and intercarpal arthritis	Surgery is an option; cast immobilization considered useful in some cases. Ulnar lengthening or radial shortening is used. All surgical correction leads to restricted wrist motion.

Table 9–1 Fractures of the Upper Extremity (Continued)

Fracture Site	Common Mechanisms	Radiographs	Management
Distal radius: Galeazzi	Distal radial fracture with dislocation or subluxation of the distal radioulnar joint (6% of forearm injuries)	Radiographic clues are fracture at ulnar styloid base, dislocation/subluxation of ulna on true lateral view, and shortening of the radius 5 mm relative to the distal ulna	Compressive plate fixation with a minimum of five screws
Distal ulnar: Monteggia's	Fracture of the ulna with associated dislocation of the radial head; fall on an outreached hand with forearm forced into pronation or a direct blow	AP and true lateral elbow; radial head dislocation is missed 16% to 52% of the time	Closed reduction and long arm cast with forearm in supination with children. Adolescents and adults require internal fixation of ulna with a compression plate; radial head is a closed reduction.
Capitellum	Often associated with a medial collateral ligament injury	AP and true lateral view	Open reduction and internal fixation; if more severe, excision of fragments
Coronoid	Rare	Best seen on a true lateral	Surgical fixation
Radial head	Common fracture; fall on an outstretched hand with the forearm pronated	Radial-capitellum view is the most specific	Immobilization sometimes requires surgical fixation

- When the injury is nontraumatic, challenge the musculotendinous attachments with stretch, contraction, and a combination of contraction in a stretched position.
- When trauma or overuse is not present, evaluate the patient's wrist for swelling and deformity (discrete nodules are likely ganglions, deformities are likely arthritides: osteoarthritis [OA] or rheumatoid arthritis [RA]).

Management

- If radiographs are negative for fracture or dissociation but there is a high level of suspicion, place a soft cast on the patient for two to three weeks and reradiograph in two weeks to determine callus status.
- Refer fracture/dislocation and dissociation for orthopaedic management.
- All other soft tissue and articular disorders may be managed for a two- to three-month trial treatment period if necessary.

Relevant Anatomy and Biomechanics

The wrist, as the connection between the hand and the forearm, requires a demanding degree of sophisticated movement. As always, this tradeoff of increased movement is somewhat compromised by lack of strong muscular support. Although there are many interosseous ligaments that support and connect individual carpal bones, there is relatively little or no muscular support, save the support provided by tendons on their way to finger/hand attachment. As a result, when the ligamentous support is damaged, muscular support is less effective than it might be in other joints.

There is an inherent imbalance of the muscles controlling the hand and wrist. The flexors are stronger than the extensors. Few movements require the strength of the extensors; however, the flexors are required for gripping, and from an evolutionary protective standpoint, for survival. As a result, activities that do require extensor activity often result in strain.

The carpal bones have been functionally divided various ways by different investigators, yet the basic division is into a distal row (trapezium, trapezoid, capitate, and hamate) and a proximal row (scaphoid, lunate, triquetrum, and pisiform). Extrinsic (connection between the radius/ulna and carpals or metacarpals) and intrinsic (carpal to carpal) ligaments provide support.[5] The primary extrinsic support is from the volar intracapsular ligaments. Posterior intracapsular ligaments are thinner and less supportive. Intrinsic support is an intricate overlapping of different length ligaments. The short intrinsic scapholunate, lunotriquetral, and capitolunate are the most important. Disruption of any of these ligaments will result in a destabilizing effect, allowing independent movement of other carpals. Because these intrinsic ligaments are shorter than the extrinsic ligaments, the reserve ability for stretch is less, leaving them more likely to be damaged.[6] The radius absorbs approximately 80% of an axial load; the ulna, 20%.[7]

The proximal and distal rows of carpal bones function together to provide a variety of precision maneuvers of the hand and fingers. With ulnar deviation, the triquetrum moves under the lunate, which dorsiflexes, taking the lunate with it; the scaphoid follows. With radial deviation, the scaphoid, lunate, and triquetrum move into palmar (volar) flexion while the distal carpal row dorsiflexes. Coupling between the proximal and distal carpal rows is guided by the scaphoid. With ligamentous damage, carpal bones are uncoupled, allowing some bones to become intercalated (unconnected).

The triangular fibrocartilage complex (TFCC), which consists of the triangular fibrocartilage (articular disc), the meniscus, the ulnar collateral ligament, the dorsal and volar radioulnar ligaments, and the extensor carpi ulnaris tendon, stabilizes the ulnar side of the wrist.[8] Although anatomically on the ulnar side, this complex is extremely important for stability of the radiocarpal joint. The TFCC is usually an intact structure well into age 30 years or older; however, in gymnasts the rate of degeneration is quite high.[9, 10]

TFCC perforations (traumatic or degenerative) and avulsions may occur with repetitive weight-bearing or, more rarely, in a single traumatic event. A predisposition to TFCC injury appears to be related to ulnar length. *Ulnar variance* is the term used to describe the relationship between the distal ends of the radius and the ulna. When the ulna extends past what is in essence a parallel line drawn across the distal radius, positive variance is demonstrated. Palmer and Werner[11] found that 81% of subjects with a positive variance had perforations of the TFCC whereas only 17% of those with negative variance had perforations. Fatigue fractures and Kienbock's disease (avascular necrosis) of the lunate have been associated with a negative ulnar variance. Hypermobility and forceful repetitive wrist motions seem to be the other significant cofactors.

Muscular control of the wrist is dependent on a muscle mass that arises from the elbow and proximal forearm (**Figures 9–1** A, B, and C; **Figure 9–2**). Because

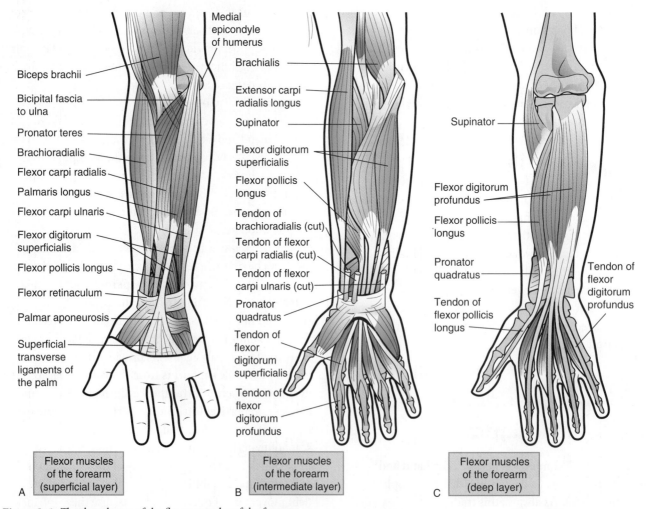

Figure 9–1 The three layers of the flexor muscles of the forearm.

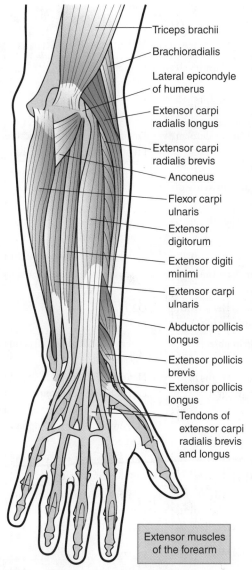

- Triceps brachii
- Brachioradialis
- Lateral epicondyle of humerus
- Extensor carpi radialis longus
- Extensor carpi radialis brevis
- Anconeus
- Flexor carpi ulnaris
- Extensor digitorum
- Extensor digiti minimi
- Extensor carpi ulnaris
- Abductor pollicis longus
- Extensor pollicis brevis
- Extensor pollicis longus
- Tendons of extensor carpi radialis brevis and longus

Extensor muscles of the forearm

Figure 9–2 Extensor muscles of the forearm.

of the need for carpal bone mobility, the insertion of the extensors is primarily on the metacarpals. The primary flexors of the wrist are the flexor carpi ulnaris and flexor carpi radialis. Each also will assist in deviating the wrist toward the named direction (i.e., radialis toward the radial direction). The rotatory movements of pronation and supination are primarily forearm movements, with the wrist along for the ride. The primary pronators are the pronator teres and pronator quadratus. Pronation is more effective with the elbow straight, due to prestretch, and therefore there is a mechanical advantage for the pronator teres. Supination is accomplished by the supinator muscle and the biceps brachii. Supination is more effective with the elbow flexed because of the mechanical advantage of the biceps with flexion and the prestretch of the supinator with flexion.

Neural control of wrist movement is via the radial, median, and ulnar nerves. Wrist extension and supination are due primarily to the radial nerve. Flexion of the wrist is divided between the ulnar and median nerves. Pronation is primarily dependent on median nerve innervation. Entrapment of each of these nerves or its branches will result in weakness of related muscles, numbness/tingling, or pain in the distribution of the respective nerve. The classic entrapment neuropathy of the wrist is carpal tunnel syndrome; however, entrapment may occur proximal to the carpal tunnel, mimicking carpal tunnel syndrome. Patients who complain of numbness/tingling, weakness, or forearm pain should be suspected of having peripheral nerve entrapment, or if bilateral, a systemic neuropathy (e.g., diabetic neuropathy).

Evaluation

History

Careful questioning of the patient during the history taking can point to the diagnosis (**Table 9–2**).

Pain Localization

The following are possible causes of pain based on location (**Figure 9–3** A, B, and C; **Table 9–3**):

- Anterior
  1. Traumatic—lunate dislocation, radial fracture, hook of hamate fracture, or distal forearm fracture
  2. Nontraumatic—median or ulnar nerve entrapment
- Posterior
  1. Traumatic—navicular fracture (anatomic snuffbox), carpal dissociation, or distal forearm fracture
  2. Nontraumatic—de Quervain's syndrome, intersection syndrome, extensor tendinitis, carpal subluxations, radial nerve entrapment

Traumatic and Overuse Injuries

With trauma, the main concern is ruling out fracture or dislocation. This requires various radiographic imaging approaches. Determining which standard radiographic views to include is based in large part on the specific area of pain, swelling, or deformity. In addition, the mechanism of injury may suggest a specific possibility.

Table 9–2 History Questions for Wrist and Forearm Complaints

Primary Question	What Are You Thinking?	Secondary Questions	What Are You Thinking?
Did you fall on an outstretched hand?	Fracture, dislocation, ligamentous instability	**Is there pain on the thumb side of your wrist?**	Scaphoid fracture likely
		Is there any painful popping or clicking?	Ligament instability
		Is there any swelling or deformity at the wrist?	Distal radial or ulnar fracture; lunate dislocation
Did the pain begin after repetitive activity?	Tendinitis, peripheral nerve entrapment, trigger points	**Do you have any associated numbness, tingling, or sense of weakness?**	Peripheral nerve entrapment
		Is the pain on the thumb side of the wrist?	de Quervain's or intersection syndrome is likely
Is the complaint mainly stiffness or restricted movement?	QA, other arthritides such as pseudogout	**Is there swelling in the joint?**	Synovitis, traumatic or arthritic
		Have you had any past injuries or surgeries to the wrist?	Posttraumatic or surgical adhesion or accelerated OA
		Is the pain worse in the morning and improved with activity?	OA likely
Is there a chief complaint of weakness?	Painful process, neurologic cause	**Does it hurt to grip objects?**	Often associated with fracture and TFC damage
		Are there associated signs of numbness or tingling?	Neural involvement may be local at carpal tunnel, entrapment of motor nerve such as anterior interosseous, or from nerve root compression at the neck
		Is the weakness worse with overhead activity?	Thoracic outlet syndrome or shoulder instability likely
Do you have any known disorders such as diabetes, hypothyroidism, or arthritis?	Diabetes or hypothyroidism may predispose the patient to carpal tunnel syndrome	**Do you have a diagnosis of any arthritis or pain in other joints?**	Bilateral or symmetric joint involvement suggests an RA or connective tissue problem

Following are some common injury patterns and potential sites of damage (also see Table 9–1):

- Fall on an outstretched hand. Axial loading usually occurs to the ulnar, palmar side of the wrist, creating compressive and shearing forces. Common injuries include scaphoid and distal radius fractures, scapholunate and lunotriquetral ligament damage leading to varying degrees of instability, and triangular fibrocartilage injury at the ulnar side of the wrist.
- Fall on a flexed hand. Compression injury occurs to the flexor (palmar) wrist with avulsion or stretch injury to the dorsal wrist. Structures involved are similar to those involved in dorsiflexion injuries, with slightly different fracture patterns; in addition, dorsal capsule avulsion may occur.

Accumulative trauma may occur when the wrist is used as a weight-bearing or partial weight-bearing joint. Commonly, the dorsal aspect of the wrist is irritated, leading to various degrees of dorsal impaction syndromes. Local synovitis, hypertrophied and/or pinched synovium, and osteocartilaginous fracture are possible with dorsal impaction.

Weakness

Weakness may be present for several reasons. Most commonly, a patient will report pain as the limiting factor with gripping. If the pain is well localized or a specific movement other than gripping is weak and painful, a specific anatomic structure may be detected through palpation and specific testing.

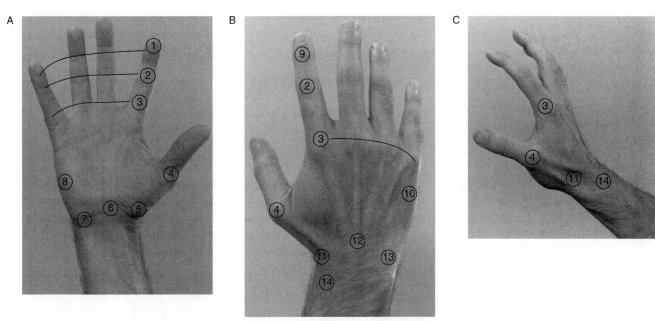

Figure 9–3 (A) Anterior wrist and hand; (B) posterior wrist and hand; (C) radial wrist and hand.

Table 9–3 Wrist and Hand Pain Localization

#	Structures	Overt Trauma	Insidious or Overuse
1	Flexor digitorum profundus (FDP) insertion	Avulsion of FDP, fracture of distal phalanx	Psoriatic arthritis
2	Proximal interphalangeal (PIP) joint	Capsular sprain or dislocation at PIP	RA, OA, psoriatic arthritis, Reiter's syndrome
3	Metacarpophalangeal (MCP) joint	Dislocation, collateral ligament sprain, capsular sprain	Mild capsular sprain, OA, trigger finger (on palmar surface)
4	First MCP joint	Dislocation, gamekeeper's thumb (ulnar collateral ligament sprain)	OA, bowler's thumb (digital neuritis), trigger thumb
5	First metacarpal base, abductor pollicis longus insertion	Bennett's fracture/dislocation	de Quervain's tenosynovitis
6	Carpal tunnel, lunate	Lunate dislocation, dissociation, subluxation	Carpal tunnel syndrome (palpation/pressure point)
7	Flexor carpi ulnaris, ulna	Distal ulna fracture or dislocation	Tendinitis
8	Pisiform/hamate, tunnel of Guyon	Hook of hamate fracture	Tunnel of Guyon compression of ulnar nerve
9	Distal interphalangeal (DIP) joint and distal phalanx	Fracture of distal phalanx, mallet finger (avulsion of extensor tendon)	Psoriatic arthritis
10	Metacarpals	Metacarpal fracture	Subluxation or extensor tendinitis
11	Anatomic snuff-box, abductor policis longus (APL), extensor policis brevis (EPB) of the thumb	Scaphoid fracture, radial styloid fracture	de Quervain's, Wartenberg's syndrome (entrapment of radial sensory nerve)
12	Lunotriquetral joint, extensor tendons	Lunotriquetral dissociation, dislocation, distal	Ganglion, lunate subluxation, extensor tendinitis
13	Ulnar styloid process, extensor carpi ulnaris (ECU) tendon	Ulnar styloid fracture	ECU tendinitis or tendon subluxation
14	Intersection of extensor tendons and APL, EPB	Distal radial fracture	Intersection syndrome, RA

Note: See Figure 9–3 for localization of numbered areas.

Most patients with a complaint of weakness will indicate some difficulty with gripping activities. Reid[12] categorized these activities. The two main grip maneuvers are power grip and precision grip. Each grip maneuver requires the strength and coordination of specific joints and muscles. By determining the specific grip that feels weak (often painless), the examiner may focus on potential neural involvement. A list of specific grip patterns and the main muscle/nerve control for that grip follows (also consider nerve root involvement when associated with neck and arm pain):

- Power grip includes grasping a ball, bat, bottle, or briefcase. The ulnar nerve is important for this grip as the primary innervation for the ulnar aspect of the wrist, for both flexion and sensation.
- Precision grip includes holding a pen, a key, or fingertip-to-thumbtip maneuvers. The median nerve is important for this grip as the primary innervation to the radial side of the wrist.

The thumb may be important for stability with both grip patterns and is supplied by both the median and ulnar nerves. Opening of the hand from the grip position or extension is largely dependent on the radial control of extensor action.

Instability

Instability may be associated with a sense of weakness. It may also be the misinterpretation of a sense of clumsiness that is more suggestive of a neural cause. Finally, the patient may assume instability exists because of constant popping and clicking about the wrist; however, clicking and popping are not necessarily pathologic unless accompanied by pain.

Restricted Motion

Restriction of both active and passive range of motion should raise the suspicion of joint effusion. With trauma, the suspicion is fracture or dislocation as the underlying cause. Without a history of trauma, it is more likely that an inflammatory arthritis is the cause. End-range passive restrictions are suggestive of subluxation.

Superficial Complaints

One of the most common superficial complaints is the presence of painful nodules on the dorsal or volar wrist. A history of chronic repetitive motion is often found, which suggests the mostly likely diagnosis—ganglions. It is also common to find a history of fluctuation in size

over time. A classic presentation with established RA is multiple nodules and swelling over the dorsum of the wrist associated with wrist pain and stiffness.

Skin lesions, when isolated to the wrist, are more likely an indication of a systemic process such as rheumatic fever (erythema marginatum) or RA. Associated signs or symptoms of each disease should be sought.

Examination

Wrist

Examination of the wrist is a standard procedure involving observing for deformities and swellings, palpating for areas of tenderness, stressing of ligamentous structures for instability, testing range of motion with overpressure, testing muscle, and palpating accessory motion. By combining these findings with the history, a preliminary working diagnosis can usually be determined.

Orthopaedic testing of the wrist focuses mainly on carpal instability due to stretching or disruption of interosseous ligaments. Positive test results include a combination of popping or clunking with pain. Painless pops and clicks are common and do not represent pathologic damage or a source of a patient's wrist pain. Tests include the following:

- Watson's test (**Figure 9–4**) for scapholunate stability. The examiner presses the scaphoid from anterior (volar) to posterior (dorsal) with the wrist first in ulnar deviation. By moving the wrist passively into the radial direction, a painful clunk or pop may be produced, indicating that the proximal pole of the scaphoid subluxated over the posterior rim of the radius.
- Lunotriquetral ballottement (**Figure 9–5**) test. The examiner stabilizes the lunate between the thumb and index finger and does the same with the triquetrum. A shearing between the bones is accomplished by moving the bones in opposite directions (i.e., the lunate is forced posteriorly while the triquetrum is forced anteriorly). A painful clunk or pop is indicative of lunotriquetral joint instability.
- Midcarpal instability. By having either the patient actively or the examiner passively pronate and ulnar deviate the wrist, a painful pop is felt on the ulnar aspect of the wrist. This indicates midcarpal instability.
- Axial load testing. The examiner applies an axial load through the first metacarpal of the thumb and the trapezium while adding a shear force. Fracture

or joint arthrosis often will result in painful crepitus with this maneuver.

- Dynamometer testing. Although the dynamometer is most often used when trying to measure the degree of strength loss with a nerve root or peripheral nerve entrapment or compression, when a past history of wrist trauma is elicited, dynamometer testing may reveal weakness due to instability.

Soft tissue assessment of the wrist is based on a combination of palpation at the sites of insertion of major tendons, coupled with contraction, stretch, and contraction in a stretched position. For example, for the extensors carpi radialis longus and brevis, one or a combination of the following will usually increase the patient's pain complaint:

- Stretching into flexion and ulnar deviation
- Contraction from the above position into radial deviation and wrist extension
- Palpation over the second and third metacarpals dorsally

By simply applying this approach to the remainder of tendons crossing the wrist, soft tissue involvement of a specific tendon is usually made apparent. A specific test involving the stretching concept is Finkelstein's test (**Figure 9–6**)

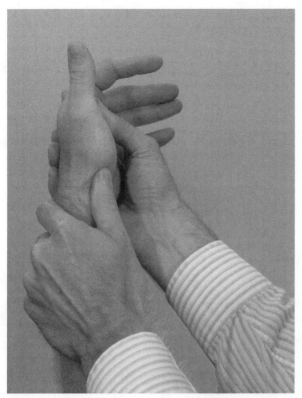

Figure 9–4 Watson's test for scapholunate dissociation. The radius is stabilized while the tubercle of the scaphoid is pushed from anterior to posterior. The wrist is then passively moved from ulnar deviation into radial deviation. A painful clunk or pop is a positive finding.

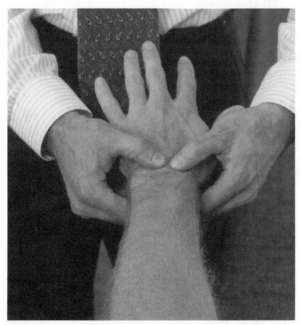

Figure 9–5 The ballottement test for lunotriquetral dissociation. The examiner stabilizes the lunate while shearing the triquetrum. A positive finding is the production of a painful clunk or pop.

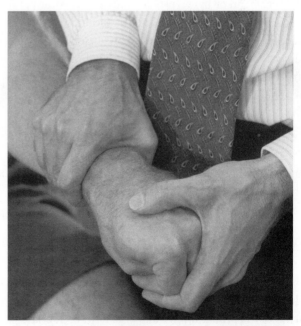

Figure 9–6 Finkelstein's test for de Quervain's tenosynovitis. The patient grasps the thumb while the examiner passively ulnar deviates the wrist. Pain at the radial wrist is a positive finding when it is notably more than the opposite wrist pain response.

for de Quervain's syndrome.[13] The patient is asked to clench the fingers over the thumb. The examiner then passively ulnar deviates the wrist, taking care not to press on the metacarpophalangeal joint of the thumb. Although this maneuver is uncomfortable, it is usually not painful. Compare results with those for the opposite (hopefully uninvolved) side. This maneuver illustrates some general orthopaedic testing principles. Although the intent is to stretch the abductor policis longus and the extensor policis brevis, the position also stretches the superficial branch of the radial nerve (Wartenberg's syndrome), the flexor carpi radialis (tendinitis), and the extensors carpi radialis longus and brevis (intersection syndrome) and compresses the scaphoid (scaphoid fracture) and the metacarpophalangeal joint of the thumb (arthritis). Localization of pain and tenderness coupled with mechanism of injury should differentiate among these possibilities.

Forearm/Wrist

Patients who present with either forearm pain or forearm pain with associated hand or wrist numbness/tingling or weakness should be evaluated for peripheral nerve entrapment. Each of three peripheral nerves (median, ulnar, and radial) may be compressed or entrapped at several sites. Depending on the site of entrapment, motor weakness or sensory abnormalities may be found specific to the nerve. In addition, if the site of entrapment is a fibrous band or hypertrophied muscle, provocative maneuvers focused on these contractile and noncontractile structures may reproduce or worsen the patient's subjective complaints. Following are some common tests, structural sites of entrapment, and findings specific to a peripheral nerve or its branches.

Median Nerve Pronator Syndrome

The median nerve may be compressed or entrapped at several locations proximal or local to the pronator teres. The most proximal site is the ligament of Struthers, an anomalous ligament that connects to the supracondylar process of the distal medial humerus. This is a rare anomaly occurring in only 1% of individuals.[14] Another site is entrapment at the lacertus fibrosus (bicipital aponeurosis) as it attaches to the pronator teres muscle. The most common entrapment sites are between the two heads of the pronator teres and also at the arch of the flexor digitorum superficialis. Hypertrophy or fibrous bands are the cause in most cases. Each site may be localized with specific positional testing.

- Lacertus fibrosus or ligament of Struthers: Symptoms of proximal forearm aching pain with possible hand pain may be provoked by resisted elbow flexion at 120° to 130° with supination.[15]
- Pronator teres: Resisted pronation with wrist flexion may increase symptoms of proximal forearm pain; passive stretching of the proximal forearm with the elbow and wrist extended or direct deep palpation of the pronator teres may provoke symptoms.[16]
- Flexor digitorum superficialis: Resisted flexion of the middle finger may increase forearm pain symptoms.

Anterior Interosseous Syndrome

Compression of the motor branch of the median nerve may cause proximal forearm pain and thumb and finger weakness.[17] Numbness and tingling complaints and objective sensory loss are not found. Weakness may occur in the flexor policis longus, pronator quadratus, and flexor digitorum profundus of the second and third fingers. The result is an inability to perform the "OK" sign of tip-to-tip apposition of the thumb and index finger.[18] With weakness the patient presses pulp to pulp and cannot flex enough to contact the thumb and fingertips. Motor nerve compression can cause an aching pain because these peripheral nerve branches carry sensory fibers to the joints and muscles, and occasionally to skin receptors. Entrapment may be due to anomalous vessels or muscle slips; however, the most common sites are at the pronator teres and flexor digitorum superficialis muscles after the median nerve has given off the anterior interosseous motor branch.

Carpal tunnel syndrome: The median nerve passes through the carpal tunnel formed by the transverse carpal ligament superiorly, the pisiform-hamate bones medially, and the navicular-trapezium bones laterally. The carpal tunnel contains the flexor tendons for the fingers and thumb and occasionally anomalous vessels or muscles such as the palmaris longus. Pressure in the tunnel is increased with swelling in the tunnel or the extremes of flexion or extension. Symptoms include numbness and paresthesias over the radial three and one half digits with sparing of the thenar eminence. Weakness or clumsiness in gripping may be reported. Eventually thenar atrophy may occur. Sensory symptoms are reproduced with several provocative tests:

- Tinel's sign: Tapping over the carpal tunnel at the wrist may elicit distal feelings of numbness or paresthesias (sensitivity, between 60% and 74%; specificity, 80%).[19]

- Phalen's test: Forced passive flexion at the wrist (pressing the backs of the hands together) or reverse Phalen's with forced passive extension (palm to palm) may elicit symptoms (sensitivity, between 49% and 64%; specificity, 55%).
- Pressure provocative test: Instead of tapping, direct pressure with a cuff or with thumb pressure at the carpal tunnel will elicit symptoms (sensitivity, close to 100%).[20]

Ulnar Nerve Cubital Tunnel Syndrome

The ulnar nerve is rarely trapped in the fascia covering the triceps and an aponeurosis called the arcade of Struthers or at the ulnar groove. Entrapment more frequently occurs in the tunnel just distal to where the ulnar nerve travels through the posterior condylar groove on the medial epicondyle of the humerus.[21] The floor consists of the medial trochlea and the ulnar collateral ligament; the roof consists of the triangular arcuate ligament that bridges the origins of the flexor carpi ulnaris (FCU). With flexion the arcuate ligament stretches, narrowing the tunnel, and the proximal edge of the FCU tightens; the ulnar collateral ligament can then bulge into the tunnel.[22] Excessive valgus angulation from throwing or acute trauma may stretch the nerve. Provocative tests[23] include the following:

- Holding the elbow flexed between three and five minutes
- Tinel's tapping sign at the posterior elbow (this is inconsistent; however, it is occasionally helpful if compared with the opposite side)
- Possible snapping or popping of the nerve with rapid extension or flexion (subluxating the ulnar nerve)

Ulnar Tunnel or Tunnel of Guyon Syndrome

At the wrist the ulnar nerve (and artery) pass through an osseofibrous tunnel formed by the groove between the pisiform and hook of the hamate. The floor is the pisohamate ligament; the roof is an extension of the FCU tendon. The ulnar nerve divides into a superficial nerve that is primarily sensory and a deep nerve that is exclusively motor. Sensory supply is to the fifth and ulnar half of the fourth digit. Motor supply is primarily to the hypothenar muscles, all the interossei, two medial lumbricals, the

deep head of the flexor policis brevis, and the abductor policis.[24] Anastomosis between the ulnar and median nerve may lead to mixed findings. Provocation testing is with Tinel's sign or pressure at the pisiform hamate area (just distal/medial to the pisiform). Sensory testing also should be performed.

Radial Nerve. Radial tunnel syndrome (RTS): At the elbow the radial nerve lies on the anterior capsule just lateral to the lateral epicondyle. It then passes between the two heads of the supinator muscle. Prior to entering the supinator muscle the radial nerve can be compressed by fibrous bands off the anterior radial head, the sharp medial edge of the extensor carpi radialis brevis (ECRB), a fan-shaped vascular arcade, and the arcade of Frohse (the thickened edge of the superficial head of the supinator).[25] Provocative maneuvers and related sites of entrapment include the following:

- ECRB—resisted middle-finger extension with the elbow extended (positives found also with lateral epicondylitis) or extreme forearm pronation with passive wrist flexion
- Radial head—resisted elbow flexion and forearm supination
- Arcade of Frohse—extreme forearm pronation with passive wrist flexion

Posterior Interosseous Nerve Syndrome (PINS)

The literature often overlaps the description of RTS and PINS. RTS is considered more a mixed-nerve syndrome, with wrist or forearm pain as the main patient complaint. PINS is considered a pure entrapment of the motor branch of the radial nerve.[26] Testing is specifically searching for weakness in wrist extension or thumb and index finger extension. Compression of the posterior interosseous nerve may also occur at the distal radius.[27] Pain is often reproduced with forceful wrist extension or palpating the forearm with the wrist flexed.

Cheiralgia paresthetica (Wartenberg's syndrome):[28] The superficial radial nerve is susceptible to trauma between the tendons of the extensor carpi radialis longus (ECRL) and the brachioradialis. Trauma or repetitive pronation and supination may cause irritation. The patient's complaints are mainly numbness and paresthesia over the dorsolateral wrist and hand. Finkelstein's test is usually negative; however, Tinel's test performed over the dorsolateral wrist may reproduce the symptoms.

Imaging

Radiographic decision making for the wrist is dictated by the degree of trauma or whether there is any suspicion of arthritis involvement based on the history and physical examination. Some common examples follow:

- A combination of anatomic snuff-box tenderness in a patient with a history of a fall on an outstretched hand suggests scaphoid injury. A scaphoid series includes a posteroanterior (PA) view, a true lateral view, a 45° pronation PA view, and an ulnar deviation PA view.[29] Another view that may be helpful is the Stecher view.[30] This is a PA shot with an angle of 20° to the vertical, angled from distal to proximal. When suspicion is high but no fracture is evident, additional angled views may help catch the fracture line. Initially, radiographs are often unrevealing even when a fracture is present. When the suspicion is high yet radiographs are negative, immobilization for two to three weeks in a thumb spica cast is recommended, followed by a second radiographic evaluation. Most fractures become apparent at this time. If immediate determination is necessary because of a particular patient's high level of use (e.g., professional athlete) a bone scan should be performed at three days postinjury. A negative bone scan rules out fracture.[31] Computed tomography (CT) scans may also be beneficial in equivocal presentations.
- If a patient has joint line tenderness coupled with a history of a fall on a dorsiflexed hand and a positive Watson's test (scapholunate dislocation or subluxation), ballottement test (lunotriquetral dissociation), or midcarpal stability test (midcarpal instability), respectively, is likely. The lateral view will show a disrelationship between the radius, lunate, capitate, and third metacarpal. Two patterns may be evident: the dorsal intercalated segmental instability (DISI) pattern or the volar intercalated segmental instability (VISI) pattern (sometimes called PISI). These instability patterns are based on the position of the lunate in relationship to the radius. Several angles can be measured; however, the most common is the scapholunate angle, which normally ranges between 30° and 60°; greater than 70° indicates scapholunate dissociation. If not evident statically, stability or stress views should be added. These include the clenched fist (AP) view or a traction

view, lateral views in flexion and extension, and anteroposterior (AP) views in radial and ulnar deviation.[32]

- A combination of trauma to the pisiform with local tenderness coupled with any sensory abnormalities into the fourth and fifth fingers is suggestive of a hook of hamate fracture. The PA view may demonstrate subtle signs such as absence of the hook or cortical ring or sclerosis in the area of the hook.[33] A carpal tunnel view and/or a 45° supinated oblique view is suggested.[34] When these views are unrevealing yet the suspicion is high, referral for a CT scan is warranted.[35]

Management

- Referral for orthopaedic consultation or management is necessary for fractures, dislocations, and carpal dissociations.
- Entrapment or compression syndromes may benefit from a conservative approach employing myofascial release and/or bracing and patient education regarding modification of the inciting activity.
- Tendinitis not associated with an inflammatory arthritis is best managed with conservative care emphasizing rest, ice, cross-friction massage to the tendon, or myofascial release to the respective muscle. On occasion, splinting may be necessary. An eccentric exercise program may also be useful.
- Caution should be exercised when using soft-tissue approaches to inflammatory arthritis problems. Referral to a rheumatologist may be necessary.

The CCGPP Upper Extremity Team expert opinion supports the use of high-velocity, short-amplitude (HVSA) manipulation (adjustment) of the wrist with some recommendations for use that include avoidance of risk. Further evaluation and/or management is required for patients who fail to respond to treatment within a reasonable period of time.

- For all patients who have fracture, suspected fracture, dislocation, active hemarthrosis or extensive swelling, severe generalized or localized osteoporosis, infection, or tumor HVSA manipulation is contraindicated.
- For patients who have had surgery of the wrist/hand, consider date of surgery, extent of surgery,

type of procedure, and other related factors in making decisions about the use of HVSA manipulation.

- For all patients, an evaluation of joint stability must be performed. Based on the findings, it is recommended that no HVSA manipulation be used for patients with dissociation (i.e., instability), hypermobility syndromes (e.g., Marfan's, Ehlers-Danlos syndrome), or gross looseness indicating multidirectional instability. Mobilization such as applying a Maitland Grade I–IV type of translational movement may be appropriate in these case settings.

Algorithm

An algorithm for the evaluation and management of wrist pain is presented in **Figure 9–7**.

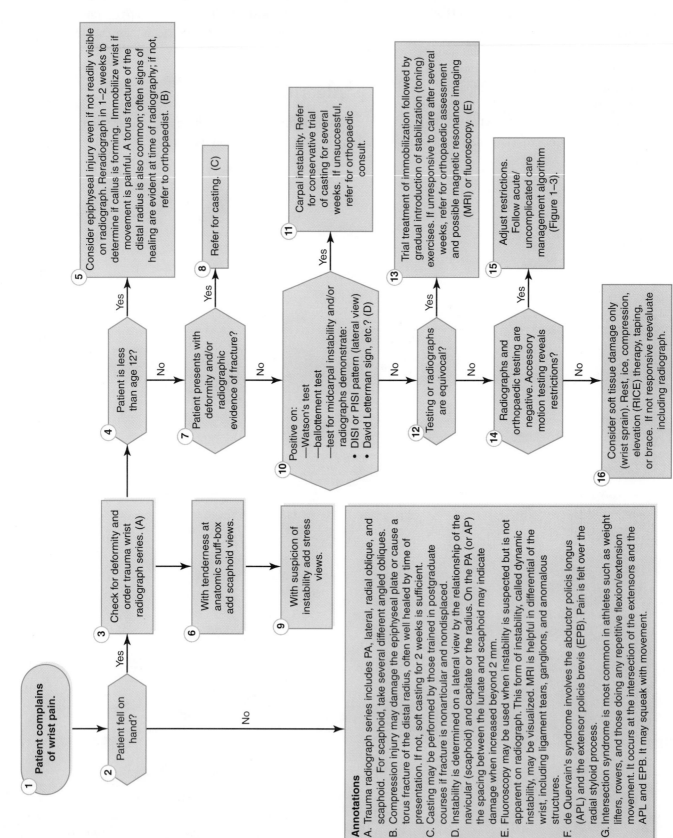

Annotations

A. Trauma radiograph series includes PA, lateral, radial oblique, and scaphoid. For scaphoid, take several different angled obliques.

B. Compression injury may damage the epiphyseal plate or cause a torus fracture of the distal radius, often well healed by time of presentation. If not, soft casting for 2 weeks is sufficient.

C. Casting may be performed by those trained in postgraduate courses if fracture is nonarticular and nondisplaced.

D. Instability is determined on a lateral view by the relationship of the navicular (scaphoid) and capitate or the radius. On the PA (or AP) the spacing between the lunate and scaphoid may indicate damage when increased beyond 2 mm.

E. Fluoroscopy may be used when instability is suspected but is not apparent on radiograph. This form of instability, called dynamic instability, may be visualized. MRI is helpful in differential of the wrist, including ligament tears, ganglions, and anomalous structures.

F. de Quervain's syndrome involves the abductor policis longus (APL) and the extensor policis brevis (EPB). Pain is felt over the radial styloid process.

G. Intersection syndrome is most common in athletes such as weight lifters, rowers, and those doing any repetitive flexion/extension movement. It occurs at the intersection of the extensors and the APL and EPB. It may squeak with movement.

Figure 9–7 Wrist Pain—Algorithm

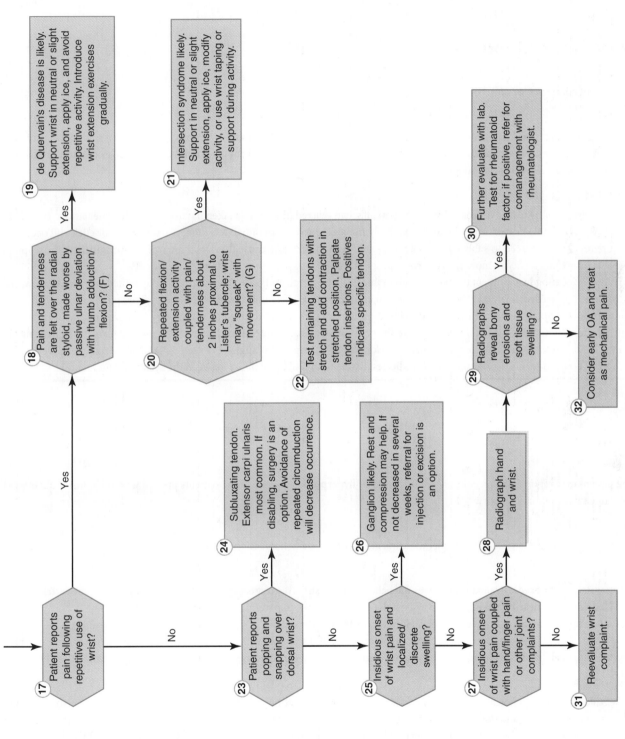

Figure 9–7 (Continued)

Selected Disorders of the Wrist and Forearm

INSTABILITY

Scapholunate Dissociation

Classic Presentation

The patient complains of radial or dorsal wrist pain following a fall on an outstretched hand.

Cause

By falling onto the thenar eminence, the wrist is forced into hyperextension, ulnar deviation, and intercarpal supination, which forces the capitate between the scaphoid and lunate.[36] The result is tearing or stretching of the scapholunate interosseous and radioscaphoid ligaments, which leads to various degrees of instability.

Evaluation

The standard stability test is Watson's.[37] With the patient's arm relaxed, the wrist is taken passively into ulnar deviation. The examiner presses the distal pole posteriorly as he or she passively moves the wrist into radial deviation. A painful pop or click will occur as the proximal pole is forced to subluxate dorsally. This subluxation occurs because the dorsal force of the examiner on the scaphoid prevents its normal ability to move into a vertical position.

When evaluating instability of the wrist radiographically, AP, lateral, and oblique views are supplemented with an AP clenched-fist view and, if needed, a lateral view taken in flexion and extension.[38] Scapholunate dissociation appears on the PA or AP as a 3-mm or greater space between the lunate and the scaphoid; it is sometimes referred to as the Terry Thomas[39] or David Letterman sign. In addition, there is a vertical orientation to the scaphoid that also creates a cortical overlap, referred to as the signet ring sign. On the lateral view, a DISI pattern may be visible.[40] Normally, the scaphoid is angled between 30° and 60°. Angulation greater than 65° to 70°, coupled with a dorsiflexed lunate, indicates dissociation (lack of stability between the scaphoid and lunate).

Management

Surgery is usually necessary.

Triquetrolunate Dissociation

Classic Presentation

The patient may report a fall on either a palmar-flexed or hyperpronated wrist. Some patients present with only dorsal ulnar wrist pain and a nontraumatic history.

Cause

Stretching or disruption of the lunotriquetral ligaments allows palmar subluxation of the lunate.

Evaluation

The standard orthopaedic evaluation involves the ballottement test.[41] This test is performed by stabilizing the lunate or triquetrum and "shucking" or shearing the other bone against the stabilized bone. A painful pop is considered a positive test.

Radiographic evaluation is usually normal. However, with a static instability a PISI (also known as VISI) deformity on the lateral wrist view is seen. The PISI pattern is palmar subluxation of the lunate and scaphoid with a dorsiflexed triquetrum. When the radiographs are negative for instability, either fluoroscopic evaluation or an arthrogram is necessary to reveal an underlying dynamic instability.

Management

If the ballottement test is positive, but radiographs are negative, initial treatment is immobilization in a long arm cast for six to eight weeks (wrist in ulnar deviation and dorsiflexion). If instability is radiographically evident (static instability), there is some disagreement as to management. Some practitioners suggest surgery; others suggest repositioning of the lunate and scaphoid followed by immobilization.

Triquetrohamate Instability (Midcarpal)

Classic Presentation

A patient may present with a history of a fall or blow to the medial (anatomic) side of the hand with hyperpronation. Some patients may have wrist pain without a specific traumatic event.

Cause

Ligamentous tearing disrupts the osseous coupling between the hamate and triquetrum.

Evaluation

Reproduction may occur on either passive or active pronation coupled with ulnar deviation. Unfortunately, a host of other ulnar-sided problems may also respond with a painful click,[42] including TFCC damage, lunotriquetral ligament tears, and distal radioulnar subluxation. Axial compression may also produce a click with midcarpal and other instabilities. Radiographic evaluation is usually normal. With a static instability, a DISI pattern may be visible. Videofluoroscopic evaluation is most sensitive, often revealing a sudden movement of the proximal carpal row from the normal PISI pattern in radial deviation to a DISI pattern near the end-range of ulnar deviation.

Management

Initially, immobilization may be effective for six weeks. If ineffective in reducing instability or pain, various forms of surgery are recommended.

Triangular Fibrocartilage Injury

Classic Presentation

A patient presents with pain on the ulnar side of the wrist made worse by pronation and supination. She or he may have a traumatic history such as a fall on an outstretched hand or no obvious trauma.

Cause

The TFCC is the fibrocartilaginous structure at the distal end of the ulna. It is part of the complex that supports the ulnar side of the wrist. The TFCC is injured through several mechanisms that result in either perforations (traumatic and degenerative) or avulsions. Degenerative changes occur by the third decade. Other factors include the poor blood supply limited to the peripheral 15% to 25% of the disc[43] and the association of ulnar positive variance (along ulna) that causes compression and thinning of the TFCC.

Evaluation

To differentiate between damage to the distal radioulnar joint (DRUJ) and the TFCC, the examiner may stabilize the radius and ulna by compressing them together proximal to the DRUJ. Passive movement of the forearm into pronation and supination should be uneventful if only the TFCC is involved. Second, ulnar deviation, axial loading, and shearing distal to the DRUJ often will produce pain and crepitus when the TFCC is damaged. Radiographic evaluation is largely an attempt to determine whether the patient has positive ulnar variance. For standardization it is recommended that the PA film be taken with 90° of elbow and shoulder flexion with the hand as flat as possible.[44] A line drawn perpendicularly across the distal end of the radius should be even with the distal ulna. Referral for an arthrogram or magnetic resonance imaging (MRI) may confirm the diagnosis of TFCC damage.

Management

Initial management is to immobilize the wrist in neutral for several weeks, obviously avoiding any ulnar deviation or compression maneuvers subsequent to splint removal. Failure to resolve requires arthroscopic evaluation and repair that includes resection of the distal ulna.

TENDINITIS/TENDINOSIS

de Quervain's Tenosynovitis

Classic Presentation

A patient presents with a complaint of radial wrist pain with a history of activities that require either forceful gripping with ulnar deviation or repetitive use of the thumb.[45]

Cause

Stenosing tenosynovitis of the abductor pollicis longus (APL) and extensor pollicis brevis (EPB) occurs as a result of chronic microtrauma to either the tenosynovium or sheath.[46]

Evaluation

Pain is reproduced with resisted thumb extension with the wrist in radial deviation or with the standard Finkelstein test.[47] The Finkelstein test begins by having the patient grasp his or her thumb with the same side fingers. The examiner passively deviates the wrist ulnarly. Tenderness is often found 1/2 inch proximal to the radial styloid.

Management

Initially, a conservative trial of activity modification, ultrasound, and nonsteroid anti-inflammatory drugs (NSAIDs) should be attempted. Failure to improve within two to three weeks requires immobilization with a thumb spica for another two to three weeks. If ineffective, referral for local steroid injection should be made. Rarely, surgery is needed.

Intersection Syndrome

Classic Presentation

A patient (often an athlete) presents with a complaint of pain and crepitus two inches or so above the wrist on the dorsoradial aspect. There is usually a history of repeated flexion/extension movement with either occupational or sports activity.[48]

Cause

An inflammatory response and possible adventitial bursitis occur at the crossing of two groups of tendons: the APL and EPB crossing over the wrist extensors. This condition is more common in canoeists, weight lifters, and recreational tennis players.

Evaluation

There is usually tenderness and swelling 4 to 6 cm proximal to Lister's tubercle.

Management

Rest, NSAIDs, and ice may help initially. Myofascial release techniques applied proximal to the tendon crossing may also be of benefit. If unsuccessful, splinting for two weeks may help enforce a rest period. Prevention includes modification or elimination of the inciting activity.

Other Tendinopathies

Following is a list of tendinopathies/tendinosis and the patient population most often associated with each:

- Extensor pollicis longus tendinitis/tendinosis—seen in drummers, athletes involved in racquet sports, and patients with rheumatoid arthritis.
- Extensor indices proprius syndrome and extensor digiti minimi tendinitis/tendinosis—due to trauma and overuse.
- Extensor carpi ulnaris tendinitis/tendinosis—relatively common tenosynovitis found in occupations or sports requiring repetitive wrist movement such as racquet sports, rowing, golf, and baseball. The tendon has its own sheath separate from the extensor retinaculum, which may rupture following forced supination, flexion, and ulnar deviation. This will lead to a painful snapping over the back of the wrist.

Evaluation

Palpation of the tendon or its insertion is usually painful, and there may be associated swelling. Full stretching of the tendon or contraction in a stretched position may reproduce the patient's complaint.

Management

Avoidance of the inciting activity coupled with myofascial release of the involved muscle may be helpful. If ineffective, a short period of soft cast immobilization may be necessary. For patients with RA, referral for medical management is prudent.

PERIPHERAL NERVE ENTRAPMENTS
MEDIAN NERVE

Carpal Tunnel Syndrome

Classic Presentation

The patient presents with a complaint of pain and numbness/tingling in the palmar surface of the thumb and radial two and one half fingers; the symptoms are worse at night that may be relieved by shaking the hand (Flick sign). The patient typically complains of clumsiness with precision gripping.

Cause

The median nerve runs through an osteofibrous tunnel created by the transverse carpal ligament and carpal bones. Although direct compression from ganglions, fractures, and dislocations is possible, it is more common to have a history of direct external pressure on the tunnel or a history of prolonged wrist use in full flexion or extension. Pressure inside the tunnel increases in these extreme positions. Additional factors may have to do with fluid retention, as in pregnancy, RA, diabetes, and connective tissue disorders. Patients deficient in B vitamins may be predisposed. The prevalence of CTS is not entirely clear. The most often quoted percentage is 3.7% from a population-based study by Atroshi et al.[49] One of the lowest reported prevalence is by Katz et al.[50] and Levine et al.[51] at 1%. The range, however, is between 0.7% to 9.2% for women and from 0.4% to 2.1% for men in the general population.[52-54] Certainly in some high-risk populations, this percentage is higher[55-57] with a prevalence as high as 61%. Tanka's[58] study on self-reported CTS indicated that approximately 0.5% of the population has been diagnosed with CTS. Atroshi[49] found that obesity is associated with an increased incidence of CTS. They found that women in their forties and fifties are four times more likely to suffer from CTS than men. Further confusing the identity, and therefore management, of CTS is the variable and unpredictable course. Some studies[59] indicate a cyclic, unpredictable occurrence of "silent" periods alternating with periods of exacerbation. Other studies[60] indicate spontaneous improvement without management. There is strong evidence for an association between exposure to a combination of risk factors and CTS. Carpal tunnel syndrome is an important contributor to work-related healthcare costs. There was some concern when the U.S. Department of Labor, Bureau of Labor Statistics reported a tenfold increase in the number of disorders "associated with repeated trauma" between 1981–1991.[61] CTS is reported as the most frequent of these disorders.[62] There was some speculation about the introduction of computer use including keyboard and mouse usage. Recent studies contradict the assumption of a causative relationship to keyboard use. The evidence points to a combination of highly repetitive work or, in combination with forceful work, and work involving hand and wrist vibration. Specifically, risk is high for work that demands intensive manual exertion[58, 63] such as automobile assembly, meatpacking, and poultry processing, but not necessarily frequent computer users (when compared to the general population).[53] There is no evidence in published literature at this time between posture and CTS.

Evaluation

There is no clear "gold standard" for the diagnosis of CTS. Although the clinical examination is used as a standard which is then often "confirmed" by electrodiagnostic (ED) studies, it is clear that there is overlap among other neurological conditions and that ED studies may produce false positives and false negatives for patients with CTS.[64] A recent study[65] emphasizes that the relationship between ED findings and patient symptoms and function are independent measures and may not be related. More confounding is that the sensitivity and specificity for ED has been based on the standard of a positive clinical evaluation, such as a positive Tinel's sign. This is worrisome considering the convincing evidence in the Kuschner et al.[66] review questioning the value of Tinel's sign and of Phalen's test that clearly demonstrated a wide range of sensitivity and specificity. Sensitivity for Phalen's ranged from 40% to 88% with an overall average sensitivity of 60% or 80% dependent on the inclusion of a study by Posch et al.[67] Specificity was 80% overall. Tinel's sign had an overall sensitivity of 49% with the Posch[19] data and 64% without. Overall specificity was 55%. On the other hand a more recent review by LaJoie et al.[68] applies a different statistical approach to determine the sensitivity and specificity of these commonly used tests. The authors claim that latent class analysis is necessary if there is no reference standard (gold standard). In other words, if there is an assumption that the reference test is 100% sensitive and specific, underestimation may occur when evaluating other tests in comparison. With that approach, these authors reevaluated Tinel's and Phalen's and found them to be highly sensitive (0.97 and 0.92, respectively) and specific (0.91 and 0.88, respectively). The sensitivity and specificity of nerve conduction velocity testing was 0.93 and 0.87, respectively. A systematic review and narrative review by MacDermid et al.[69, 70] are somewhat intermediate to the conclusions drawn in the LeJoie and Kuschner reviews. They agree with Kuschner[66] stating that the quality of many of the studies was poor. The overall estimate for Phalen's was 68% for sensitivity and 73% for specificity. Tinel's estimated sensitivity was 50% and specificity, 77%. The carpal compression test had estimates of 64% and 83% for sensitivity and specificity, respectively. Specific, but not sensitive, were two-point discrimination testing and atrophy or testing of strength of the abductor pollicis brevis.

A prospective study by Nora et al.[71] demonstrated a wide range of findings that seemed to vary based on overlapping disease and patient subjectivity. Out of a total of 1,528 hands that were diagnosed with CTS, the severity was considered mild in 42% of cases, moderate in 18%, and severe in 40%. Patients had a female-to-male predominance of 5.6:1. Symptoms were restricted to the hand and wrist in 51.8% of cases with paresthesia and in 18.5% of cases with pain. In 92.5% of the partially affected hands, paresthesia was present in at least one of the three first fingers, while pain affected the three first fingers in 78.8% of these hands. Matching to the Katz's hand diagram revealed a classic pattern in 12.6% of affected hands with a pattern rated as probable CTS in 66.3%. Tinel's and Phalen's sign were positive in 34.2% and 56.3% of these hands, respectively.

- A patient diagram called the Katz diagram is valuable in establishing the location and extent of the patient's hand complaint (**Exhibit 9–1**).[72] There are three diagrams that the patient can match including classic, probable, and unlikely. The classic is not what most would assume based on the classic description. It illustrates symptoms that are quite diffuse involving all fingers and thumb on both surfaces and forearm involvement also on posterior and anterior aspects. Classic is ≥2 out of digits 1, 2, 3; no palm involvement but radiation into forearms allowed as part of description. Probable is ≥2 out of digits 1, 2, 3; however, the palm is involved. Possible is ≥1 out of digits 1, 2, 3; palm is involved. Unlikely is 0 out of digits 1,2,3 with possible medial palm involvement. The "unlikely" pattern illustrates more ulnar nerve involvement.

Exhibit 9–1 **The Katz Diagram**

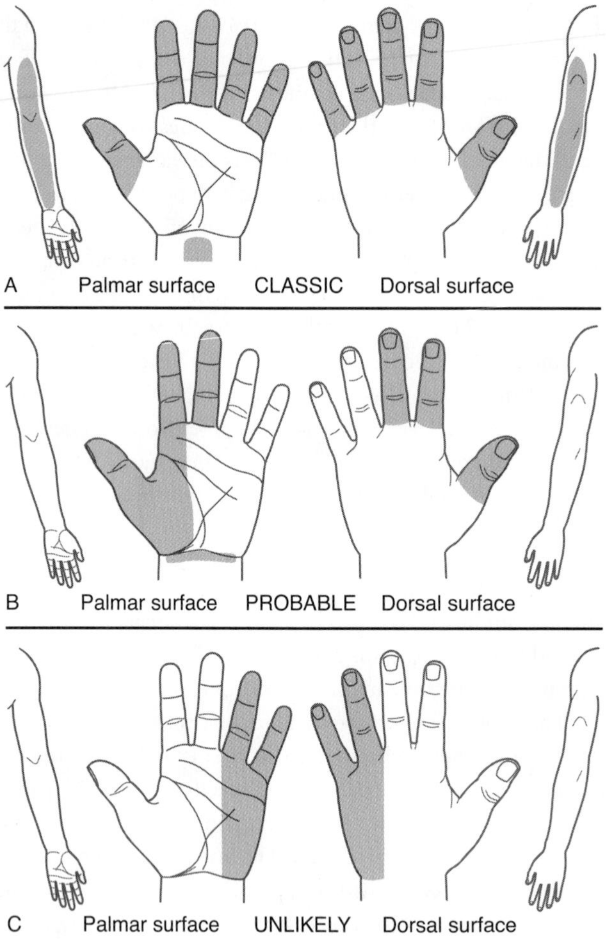

A   Palmar surface   CLASSIC   Dorsal surface

B   Palmar surface   PROBABLE   Dorsal surface

C   Palmar surface   UNLIKELY   Dorsal surface

Reproduced from Katz JN, Stirrat C, Larson MG, et al. A self-administered hand symptom diagram in the diagnosis and epidemiologic study of carpal tunnel syndrome. *J Rheumatol.* 1990;17:1495-1498.

D'Arcy et al.[73] performed a systematic review of history taking and physical examination for diagnosing CTS, and used ED testing as the comparative standard. In the studies that met the inclusion criteria, the following were indications of the value of history and physical examination findings confirmed by ED testing:

- Hypalgesia in the median nerve territory (LR, 3.1, 95% CI, 2.0–5.1)
- Classic or probable Katz hand diagram[74] results (LR, 2.4, 95% CI, 1.6–3.5)
- Weak thumb abduction strength (LR, 1.8, 95% CI, 1.4–2.3)

Findings arguing against CTS were:

- Unlikely Katz hand diagram results (LR, 0.2, 95% CI, 0.0–0.7)
- Normal thumb abduction strength (LR, 0.5, 95% CI, 0.4–0.7)
- Some standard tests such as Phalen's and Tinel's signs, thenar atrophy, and nocturnal paresthesia had little or no diagnostic value for positive ED test findings.

It is important to note that the degree or severity of CTS in these patients was likely beyond that seen by many primary care physicians or chiropractors. These were patients seen by orthopaedic surgeons, physical therapists, and ED laboratories, further questioning the value of these standard clinical examination approaches in less severe cases. With regard to nerve conduction studies, a sensitivity and specificity analysis was performed in a study by Lew et al.[75] in 2005. The results indicate that measurement of a single short-nerve segment tended to be superior to results obtained by either long-segment studies, or differential subtraction between two segments of the same nerve. Short-segment, onset-latency transcarpal mixed NCV yielded the highest sensitivity (75%).

Management

Both the surveys by Bernard[63] and Andersen[76] clearly demonstrated no association between keyboard use and CTS. However, there is still some question regarding mouse usage and CTS. On the other hand, the Verhagen et al.[77] Cochrane systematic review indicated some evidence for the effectiveness of some specific types of keyboards for patients with CTS.[78] Evidence for expensive ergonomic interventions was not clearly demonstrated in their review. In Cochrane reviews on nonsurgical management of CTS by Verdugo et al.[79] only two RCTs met the criteria for inclusion. One by Garland[80] was published in 1964 when surgical treatment would be different from current standards. The other study by Gerritsen[81] compared splinting to surgery for the management of CTS. Both studies produced evidence in favor of surgery. However, while the Gerritsen study showed a statistically significant advantage for surgery, it also demonstrated a CI that was quite low and close to nonsignificant with an RR of 1.38 (95% CI 1.08–1.75). The surgery rated in this study was an open carpal tunnel release, which would currently not be the standard.

Newer studies indicate that 90% of CTS patients fully recover within a few weeks after surgical release of the carpal tunnel, whereas only between 30% and 70% of CTS patients fully recover with conservative interventions within a few weeks to a few months.[82] The standard of conservative care is nocturnal neutral splinting or a cock-up splint worn for several weeks to determine effect. It is important to make an early referral for EDS and/or specialist consult if related to the workplace environment if: (1) symptomatic for over 6–12 months prior to claim acceptance, as conservative care is less likely to benefit; (2) time-loss exceeds two weeks; or (3) significant improvement, including ability to work, is not attained within the first several weeks of conservative care.[82]

It is clear that the term manipulation is not synonymous with an "adjustment" or Grade V mobilization. Only one randomized controlled trial by Davis[83] evaluated chiropractic management versus usual medical care. Even this study is not specific to manipulation/adjustment of the wrist including manipulation of the spine as part of the overall management. In both Cochrane reviews on conservative management of CTS by O'Connor[84] and Verdugo,[79] the Davis study was included, but the conclusions reached were inconsistent. This is partly due to the different outcome measures used, but also because the determination was to focus on whether chiropractic management was of benefit beyond usual medical care. The Davis study, in fact, indicated that in the short term, both approaches were essentially equal. The improvement reported was in perceived comfort and function, and nerve conduction and finger sensation overall, but showing no significant differences between groups. In the Davis study, medical treatment consisted of medication and nocturnal wrist supports. Chiropractic treatment included nocturnal wrist support, myofascial massage/loading, and ultrasonography in addition to "manual thrusts" to the wrist and spine. No other high-quality studies on chiropractic management were found other than case reports.[85]

In addition to manipulation/mobilization for carpal tunnel syndrome, chiropractors may utilize other management approaches including wrist supports/splints, ultrasonography, and/or B6 vitamins (pyridoxine). Other approaches that have been studied include laser therapy, nerve/tendon gliding/stretching, or yoga. In the O'Connor[84] Cochrane systematic review, all of the above approaches were evaluated for evidence. In the Verdugo[79] Cochrane review, only splinting was compared to surgery.

Table 9–4 Conservative Management of Carpal Tunnel Syndrome

Parameter	Acute Stage	Subacute Stage	Symptom-Free Stage
Criteria	Numbness/tingling in palmar thumb, index, and radial half of middle finger; positive Tinel's, Phalen's, or compression test.	Frequency of numbness/tingling event is decreasing.	No complaints with moderate daily use of wrists; limited work activity does not provoke symptoms.
Goals	Reduce any internal swelling, decrease pain or numbness/tingling frequency.	Gradually retrain patient to perform activities with less stress to carpal tunnel; wean patient off daytime use of support.	Maintain proper ergonomic work environment; wean patient off night support.
Concerns	If condition progresses, atrophy of thenar muscles is likely and the need for surgery increases; patient may have irritation of the median nerve at more proximal sites; patient with diagnosis from other doctor may not have carpal tunnel syndrome.	Patient is unable to avoid aggravating activities or shows signs of progression.	Patient returns to work activities without proper ergonomic support.

(continues)

Table 9–4 Conservative Management of Carpal Tunnel Syndrome (Continued)

Parameter	Acute Stage	Subacute Stage	Symptom-Free Stage
Requirements for progression to next stage; approximate time needed	Improvement of frequency and intensity of numbness/tingling complaint; no progressive atrophy of thenar muscles; 1–3 weeks.	Able to perform daily activities (without brace) with minor symptoms; 2–3 weeks.	No symptoms with work activity; 2–3 months.
Manipulation/mobilization	Adjustments of the lunate and radioulnar articulation may help; evaluate the cervical spine for possible fixation.	Adjustments of the lunate and radioulnar articulation may help; evaluate the cervical spine for possible fixation.	Adjustments of the lunate and radioulnar articulation may help; evaluate the cervical spine for possible fixation.
Modalities	Ice, rest, electromyographic stimulation (bipolar for 20 min/d with ice; 80–120 Hz first few days, 1–150 Hz next few days, 1–15 Hz next few days).	Underwater ultrasound at 1.5–2 wt/cm² for 5–7 minutes; ice after strengthening exercises for 10 minutes.	Ice after exercises.
External brace, support, etc.	Consider use of splint in neutral or slight extension.	Continue use of splint, gradually decreasing daytime use.	Continue night splinting if necessary; attempt gradual reduction of use.
ROM/flexibility massage	Mild stripping massage to flexor and extensor groups of muscles.	Grade 3 or 4 myofascial release to extensors or flexors based on findings.	Maintain flexibility with mild postisometric relaxation technique.
Open-chain exercise	Mild isometrics in pain-free ranges with focus on extension.	Isometrics progressing to isotonic exercises with a focus on wrist extensors, pronators, and supinators; flexor exercises should be performed but not emphasized.	Continue isotonic exercises on an every-other-day routine for maintaining wrist strength and preventing recurrence.
Associated biomechanical items	Evaluate the patient's work posture, especially with keyboard and mouse positions and padding; attempt to isolate provoking maneuvers or positions.	Follow-up of modification of workstation for patient; gradually introduce patient to activity beginning with short periods of work and frequent rest periods.	
Lifestyle/activity modifications	Avoid activities that compress the anterior wrist, such as wrist-supported typing, use of a mouse, or activities that require lifting; this may require a work restriction request to the patient's employer. Decrease salt intake; consider use of B6 with a B-complex vitamin; consider use of bromelain or NSAIDs.	Continue to avoid postures that compress the anterior wrist or force the wrist into hyperflexion or extension; avoid carrying heavy objects or repeated pronation supination.	

Splinting has been used as a treatment approach for CTS with the theoretical purposes of both preventing use and also decreasing pressure within the carpal tunnel. Additional variations include neutral/extension splinting and nocturnal versus full-time usage. Braces/splints can be custom-made or stock. The findings in the Verdugo[79] systematic review are similar to other reviews such as Gerritsen,[86] D'Arcy,[73] and Feurstein,[87] and RCTs such as Gerritsen[81] that indicate outcomes that favor surgery. Gerritsen's RCT indicated that at the end of an 18-month follow-up, 41% of patients in a splint group had eventually resorted to surgery. However, in this prospective evaluation for splinting, Gerritsen et al.[81] found a 31% success rate for splinting. Only two prognostic indicators were identified. For patients with both a short duration of CTS complaints (one year or less) and a score of 6 or less for severity of paresthesia baseline at night, the predicted probability of success was 62%. The percentage of patients correctly identified by this model was 78% (95% CI, 69–87%).

Ultrasonography was evaluated in two trials, one by Ebenbichler[88] and the other by Oztas,[89] which demonstrated that two weeks of treatment was not beneficial. However, these trials did demonstrate significant improvement following seven weeks of treatment. A newer study using dexamethasone demonstrated improvement with phonophoresis.[91] Interestingly, O'Connor pooled the data for these studies even though one trial used continuous ultrasound while the other used pulsed-ultrasound. In the Goodyear-Smith[90] systematic review of nonsurgical management for CTS, they conclude that the Ebenbichler and Oztas studies provide conflicting evidence with a high drop-out rate. They state that there is limited evidence for ultrasonography in the short- and medium-term (up to six months). A more recent study supports this finding.[93] Numerous approaches may be included in the conservative management of CTS. The evidence is limited for each.

- B6—Two RCTs on the effects of 10–12 weeks of vitamin B6 therapy have been evaluated.[94,95] There is limited evidence for improvement of finger swelling and movement discomfort with 12 weeks of treatment. However, there is also limited evidence that B6 does not improve any of the symptoms or signs of CTS.
- One study by Akalin et al.[95] on nerve/tendon gliding exercises compared these exercises to wrist splint only, or wrist splint combined with the exercises. Although there was some improvement with static two-point discrimination, there was no advantage over wrist-splint-only treatment for improving hand symptoms and signs.
- One study by Garfinkel et al.[96] evaluated yoga stretching as compared to wrist splinting for CTS. There was limited evidence that yoga improved pain and decreased Phalen's sign findings better than wrist splinting. There was limited evidence that yoga and wrist splinting were similar in providing short-term improvement with Tinel's sign, grip strength, and nocturnal awakening.
- There is limited evidence that low-level laser treatment has not been shown to have an advantage over a sham laser treatment.[98] More recent studies show mixed results in other joints.

Pronator Syndrome

Classic Presentation

The patient presents with a complaint of volar forearm pain. There is usually no history of trauma; however, there is often a history of repetitive pronation and wrist flexion such as incurred by carpenters, assembly line workers, and weight lifters.

Cause

Compression may occur at several sites, including the bicipital aponeurosis (lacertus fibrosus) that connects with the pronator teres, between the two heads of the pronator teres, and at the flexor digitorum superficialis by a thickened, fibrotic arch. Compression between the heads of the pronator is often due to hypertrophy. Other (rarer) sites are beneath the ligament of Struthers (supracondylar arch), the median artery, and a bicipital tuberosity bursa.[99]

Evaluation

- Reproduction of the patient's complaint is based on a direct or an indirect search for the compression site.
- Provocation with resisted elbow flexion and supination with maximum elbow flexion implies the lacertus fibrosus or less often the ligament of Struthers.
- Provocation with resisted pronation, keeping the elbow extended and the wrist flexed, suggests pronator teres compression (hypertrophy common).
- Provocation with resisted middle finger flexion suggests that the site of compression is the flexor digitorum superficialis.

When the lacertus fibrosus is involved, active pronation may reveal indentations in the pronator teres. Direct pressure over the pronator teres often will reproduce symptoms. Electrodiagnostic studies are of little value.

Management

Initial management involves a trial of myofascial release and/or rest. If unresponsive to myofascial release after two to three weeks, splinting for two to three weeks may be necessary. If symptoms persist beyond six months, surgical exploration may be necessary.

Anterior Interosseous Syndrome

Classic Presentation

The patient presents with a complaint of anterior proximal forearm pain that occurred either acutely after a single violent forearm muscle contraction or from repetitive activity. There is an associated complaint of weakness, usually isolated to pinch of the thumb and index finger and usually within 12 to 24 hours after the onset of pain.

Cause

Compression sites are similar to those for pronator teres syndrome; however, they are most commonly at the flexor digitorum superficialis or deep head of the pronator teres. At these sites, the anterior interosseous nerve, a motor branch of the median nerve, is compressed or entrapped. It may also be seen with stingers (acute stretch injuries to the brachial plexus) or after an interscalene block.

Evaluation

Inability to pinch the tips of the thumb and index finger together results in a pulp-to-pulp pinch. This is due to weakness of the flexor policis longus (FPL) and index finger flexor digitorum profundus (FDP). The pronator quadratus may be weak when tested with resisted forearm pronation with full elbow flexion. On occasion, there may be weakness of the hand intrinsics due to a Martin-Gruber anastomosis, which is found in 15% of the population (connection between median and ulnar nerves). Electrodiagnostic studies are considered the gold standard with denervation of the FPL and index finger FDP and pronator quadratus.

Management

Conservative treatment should be attempted for up to eight weeks, at which time surgery should be considered. Conservative care involves myofascial release, rest, and anti-inflammatory medication.

ULNAR NERVE

Cubital Tunnel Syndrome

Classic Presentation

The patient presents with a complaint of medial forearm pain and paresthesia into the ring and little finger. There is often a history of activities, such as throwing, that medially stretched the elbow.

Cause

Compression or stretch may cause irritation of the ulnar nerve. Stretch is usually due to valgus force to the elbow. Compression may be at the two heads of the flexor carpi ulnaris or may be due to osteophytes in the cubital tunnel. Less common causes include lipomas, ganglions, and anomalous soft tissue structures. Pressure in the tunnel is increased with elbow flexion and wrist extension (threefold), and the cocking position of throwing (sixfold).[100]

Evaluation

The symptoms are often reproduced by passive or resisted elbow flexion with the elbow in a maximally flexed position. The Tinel's sign is variable and somewhat unreliable. Electrodiagnostic studies are rarely necessary but may be helpful in differentiating among other medial forearm pain syndromes.

Management

Conservative management includes rest, ice, and anti-inflammatories. In addition, if entrapment is at the flexor carpi ulnaris, myofascial release may be of help. Night splinting with the elbow flexed to 45° in neutral rotation is recommended. Failure of conservative care should warrant a surgical consultation.

Tunnel of Guyon

Classic Presentation

The patient complains of numbness/tingling or pain in the fourth and fifth digits.

Cause

The ulnar nerve may be compressed in the tunnel of Guyon, which is an osseofibrous tunnel formed by the groove between the pisiform and the hook of the hamate. Activities that cause chronic compression at this site may result in ulnar nerve dysfunction. Constant compression on handlebars, as with cyclists, may cause this problem (handlebar or cyclist's palsy). Other causes include vascular abnormalities, fractures of the hook of the hamate, and ganglions.[101]

Evaluation

Provocation testing includes either Tinel's or pressure at the pisiform hamate area (just distal and medial to the pisiform). Compression may occur at several areas, causing either mixed motor and sensory findings or isolated motor or sensory findings. Sensory testing may reveal abnormalities in the fourth and fifth digits. Two-point discrimination may be affected in the same region. Motor involvement may be evident by testing grip strength. Weakness of the adductor policis may be evident with Froment's sign.

Grasping a piece of paper between the thumb and the index finger, the patient flexes the distal thumb to substitute for the weak adductor policis. Wartenberg's sign is positive when the patient cannot fully adduct all fingers.

Management

Protection with padding and modification of any inciting activity that adds pressure to the area, such as a change in handlebar or bicycle position with cyclists, are usually sufficient. If there is an obvious neural deficit, refer to an orthopaedist when the problem persists for longer than a few weeks.

RADIAL NERVE

Radial Tunnel Syndrome

Classic Presentation

The patient complains of a dull, aching pain over the lateral forearm.

Cause

There is a disagreement with regard to whether radial tunnel syndrome (RTS) should be considered an entity separate from posterior interosseous nerve syndrome (PINS).[102] The distinction is mainly clinical when entrapment occurs at a site where the PIN is selectively affected, leading to motor findings with no sensory deficits. As the radial nerve enters and traverses the forearm, it may be compressed or entrapped at several locations, including the radial head, the medial edge of the ECRB, a fan-shaped vascular arcade, the arcade of Frohse (thickened edge of the superficial head of the supinator), and the two heads of the supinator muscle.

Evaluation

Tenderness is distal to the lateral epicondyle (approximately four fingerbreadths below the lateral epicondyle). Provocative maneuvers are based on the site of entrapment: ECRB—resisted middle finger extension with the elbow extended; radial head—elbow flexion; supinator muscle—resisted, repeated supination with the forearm flexed; arcade of Frohse—extreme forearm pronation with wrist flexion. Weakness of the wrist extensors is often found when the PIN is involved.

Management

If the syndrome is due to repeated pronation/supination, rest from the activity and modification of the activity are required. Myofascial release technique is particularly helpful when the entrapment is at the supinator muscle. Adjusting the radial head may be of benefit in some cases.

Cheiralgia Paresthetica (Wartenberg's Syndrome)

Classic Presentation

The patient complains of numbness or tingling over the dorsolateral aspect of the wrist and hand.

Cause

The superficial branch of the radial nerve is susceptible to trauma between the tendons of the ECRL and the brachioradialis. Repetitive movements such as pronation and supination are often the cause. Wearing a wrist band or a brace or taping may cause compression. Direct blows to the dorsolateral forearm/wrist may also cause this disorder.

Evaluation

Tinel's sign is often positive over the point of compression at the dorsolateral wrist. Pain may be caused by passive ulnar deviation and flexion of the wrist.

Management

If there is a compressive culprit such as a wrist brace, support, or taping, modify use to avoid compression. If there is a repetitive movement cause, initially rest from the activity and modify the movement to avoid further irritation. Myofascial release above the area may be helpful; however, release at the area often reproduces the problem.

FRACTURES

Scaphoid

Classic Presentation

The patient presents with pain at the anatomic snuff-box after a fall on an outstretched hand. The patient often is seen three to six months after the trauma.

Cause

An impact injury with the wrist in maximum dorsiflexion (greater than 90°) will fracture the scaphoid. The radial styloid may impact the midportion of the scaphoid. The vascular supply to the scaphoid runs distal to proximal and therefore distal fractures generally heal without incident. Proximal pole fractures, however, usually result in avascular necrosis. Proximal pole fractures account for about 20% of all scaphoid fractures.

Evaluation

The clinical examination is often more revealing than radiographs. There are several tests, including axial compression of the index or middle finger, percussion on the extended thumb, forced dorsiflexion, and resisted pronation. One of the most sensitive tests is to stretch the patient's pronated hand carefully into maximum ulnar deviation. A positive test result is obtained when pain is produced at the anatomic snuff-box. The positive predictive value is 52%.

Although it may appear that radiographs are the definitive tool for detecting a scaphoid fracture, initial films are often negative. In addition, follow-up films (two to three weeks postinjury) are not always helpful. One study[103] indicated an interpretation error of 40%. However, it is prudent to use multiple views, including several oblique films at the time of injury and in two to three weeks. A scaphoid series includes the standard PA, lateral, right and left obliques, and a PA view with radial and ulnar deviation with the fingers flexed. When the suspicion is high but films are unrevealing, a bone scan or CT scan is usually diagnostic.

Management

Initial treatment of nondisplaced fractures is cast immobilization, which includes the forearm and the proximal interphalangeal joint of the thumb. If there is no visible fracture line on initial radiographs, the patient should be managed as if a scaphoid fracture is present when there is a positive scaphoid fracture test, especially if there is any associated swelling at the dorsal radial wrist. Follow-up films are taken in about two weeks with the cast removed. If a fracture is evident, cast immobilization is continued to 8 to 12 weeks. Out-of-cast films are taken in 6 and 12 weeks. If further healing is necessary, continue immobilization for two to four weeks. Referral is necessary if healing is not progressing or if there is a displaced fracture. Another referral scenario is an associated perilunar dislocation where the capitate dislocates off the lunate.

Hook of Hamate

Classic Presentation

The patient presents with pain just distal and radial to the pisiform following impact to the area from a fall, a bat, racquet, or golf club.

Cause

The hook of the hamate is susceptible to direct trauma. A fall on or blow to the hypothenar eminence may result in fracture. The fracture is unstable because of the pull from the flexor carpi ulnaris (through the pisohamate ligament), the opponens digiti and flexor digiti quinti, and the transverse ligament.

Evaluation

Pain is felt 1 to 2 cm distal and radial to the pisiform. Radiographs include the carpal tunnel view and 20° supinated view. When a fracture is not visible but suspected, a bone scan or CT scan may be valuable.

Management

Fragment excision is usually successful, followed by a short arm cast for three to four months.

Kienbock's Disease

Classic Presentation

The patient presents with a stiff and painful wrist. Often there is no history of trauma.

Cause

Kienbock's disease is avascular necrosis of the lunate due to a stress or compression fracture. Repetitive minor trauma is suspected as the common initiator.

Evaluation

Diagnosis is usually difficult until the lunate becomes more radiopaque than the surrounding carpal bones. CT or MRI is more sensitive, yet should be used only when the suspicion is high and radiographic confirmation is equivocal.

Management

If Kienbock's disease is detected, cast immobilization for about eight weeks is necessary to allow revascularization. When this fails, surgery is used to decompress the area before collapse of the lunate. This may also include osteotomy of the radius to equal out a relatively short ulna. Following collapse, replacement with a prosthetic or autogenous material is used. Intercarpal fusion is the least desirable procedure. One study indicated that conservative care may provide a similar long-term outcome compared to surgery.

FOREARM

Following is a list of forearm fractures. These fractures are usually due to a fall on an outstretched hand or a blow to the area.
- Monteggia—shaft fracture of the ulna with an associated dislocated radial head.
- Galeazzi—fractured distal radius and dislocated ulna.
- Greenstick—an incomplete fracture, often of both the radius and the ulna, in a skeletally immature patient; healing usually occurs in six to eight weeks.
- Colles'—distal radial fracture with dorsal and radial angulation.
- Smith's—distal radial fracture with volar (palmar) angulation.

MISCELLANEOUS CONDITIONS

Dorsal Impaction Syndrome

Classic Presentation

The patient presents with a complaint of dorsal wrist pain. There is a history of repeated forced dorsiflexion with some component of concomitant weight-bearing (the two groups most commonly affected are gymnasts and chiropractors).

Cause

Repeated dorsiflexion causes compression of the dorsal wrist structures, leading to a capsulitis and a number of reactive changes, including localized hypertrophic synovitis (meniscoid of the wrist) and osteocartilaginous changes in the dorsal rim of the scaphoid, lunate, capitate, or radius.

Evaluation

Tenderness is found at the middorsal aspect of the wrist, specifically at the lunocapitate area. Unfortunately, unless radiographic changes are evident, there are no indicators other than the history.

Management

Essentially an overuse (and misuse) condition, the dorsal impaction syndrome is managed by avoidance of the offending position, forced dorsiflexion. Blockage of forced passive dorsiflexion can be accomplished by the use of a wrist brace with a limiter such as taping the front of the wrist and forearm or placing padding on the back of the wrist (thick felt or multiple layers of moleskin). Flexion exercises also may be helpful. If ineffective, splinting in a soft cast for two to three weeks may allow healing. For the chiropractor, use of non-weight-bearing adjusting techniques or substitution with other soft techniques for a period of time may be the final answer.

Ganglions

Classic Presentation

The patient presents with a complaint of dorsal wrist pain. Passive dorsiflexion often makes it worse. The patient may have found a small tender nodule or knot. There is usually a history of a repetitive wrist activity occupationally or with sports. Most often, the patient is under age 35 years.

Cause

Ganglions are soft tissue tumors that arise from either the capsule or tendon sheaths. They are most common at the dorsal scapholunate ligament or at the metacarpal heads. Ganglions represent mucinous degeneration into multiple intraligamentous cysts or larger, sometimes palpable cysts.

Evaluation

Unfortunately, not all ganglions are palpable. It has been observed that often the more occult (smaller ganglion), the more symptomatic. Radiographs are useless except to rule out other causes. MRI may be useful.

Management

If the ganglion is visible, an initial attempt at compression to rupture the capsule is sometimes made. However, ganglions tend to reappear unless surgically excised. The need for surgery is based on the degree of discomfort and effect on daily activities, occupation, or sport. Ganglions often fluctuate in size.

APPENDIX 9–1

References

1. Bureau of National Affairs. OSHA advance notice of proposed rulemaking for ergonomic safety and health management. (57 FR34192, August, 1992) OSHA Rep. 1992; 310–318.

2. Weiker GG. Hand and wrist problems in the gymnast. *Clin Sports Med.* 1992;11:189–202.

3. Weinstein SM, Herring SA. Nerve problems and compartment syndromes in the hand, wrist, and forearm. *Clin Sports Med.* 1992;11:161–188.

4. Levine DW, Simmons BP, Koris MJ, et al. Self-administered questionnaire for the assessment of severity of symptoms and functional status in carpal tunnel syndrome. *J Bone J Surg Am* 1993;75:1585–1592.

5. Taleisnik J. *The Wrist.* New York: Churchill Livingstone; 1985.

6. Pin PG, Nowak M, Logan SE, Young VL, et al. Coincident rupture of the scapholunate and lunotriquetral ligaments without perilunate dislocation: pathomechanics and management. *J Hand Surg Am.* 1990;15:110–119.

7. Green DP. *Operative Hand Surgery.* New York: Churchill Livingstone; 1988.

8. Kauer JMH. The distal radioulnar joint. *Clin Orthop.* 1992;275:37–45.

9. Mikic ZD. Age changes in the triangular fibrocartilage of the wrist joint. *J Anat.* 1978;126:367–384.

10. Mandelbaum BR, Bartolozzi AR, Davis CA, et al. Wrist pain syndrome in the gymnast: pathogenetic, diagnostic, and therapeutic considerations. *Am J Sports Med.* 1989;17:305–317.

11. Palmer AK, Werner FW. The triangular fibrocartilage complex of the wrist: anatomy and function. *J Hand Surg.* 1981;6:153–162.

12. Reid DC. *Sports Injury Assessment and Rehabilitation.* New York: Churchill Livingstone; 1992:1061.

13. Thorson E, Szabo RM. Common tendinitis problems in the hand and forearm. *Orthop Clin North Am.* 1992; 23:65–74.

14. Tubiana R. *The Hand.* Philadelphia: WB Saunders; 1981.

15. Spinner M. *Injuries to the Major Branches of the Peripheral Nerves of the Forearm.* 2nd ed. Philadelphia: WB Saunders; 1978:194.

16. Spinner M, Linscheid RL. Nerve entrapment syndromes. In: Morrey BF, ed. *The Elbow and Its Disorders.* Philadelphia: WB Saunders; 1985:73–91.

17. Spinner M. The anterior interosseous nerve syndrome with special attention to its variations. *J Bone Joint Surg Am.* 1970;52:84–94.

18. McCue FC III, Miller GA. Soft-tissue injuries of the hand. In: Petrone FA, ed. *Symposium on Upper Extremity Injuries in the Athlete.* St. Louis, MO: CV Mosby; 1986:84.

19. Kuschner SH, et al. Tinel's sign and Phalen's test in carpal tunnel syndrome. *Orthopedics.* 1992;15:1297–1302.

20. Williams TM, et al. Verification of the pressure provocative test in carpal tunnel syndrome. *Ann Plast Surg.* 1992;29:8–11.

21. Long RR. Nerve anatomy and diagnostic principles. In: Pappas AM, ed. *Upper Extremity Injuries in the Athlete.* New York: Churchill Livingstone; 1995:47–48.

22. Vanderpool SW, Chalmers J, Lamb DW, et al. Peripheral compression lesions of the ulnar nerve. *J Bone Joint Surg Br.* 1968;50:792–803.

23. Eversmann WW. Compression and entrapment neuropathies of the upper extremity. *J Hand Surg.* 1983;8:759–766.

24. Shea JD, McClain EJ. Ulnar nerve compression syndromes at and below the wrist. *J Bone Joint Surg Am.* 1969;61:1095–1103.

25. Regan WD, Morrey BF. Entrapment neuropathies about the elbow. In: Delee JC, Drez D, Jr, eds. *Orthopedic Sports Medicine: Principles and Practice.* Philadelphia: WB Saunders; 1994:844–859.

26. Spinner M. The arcade of Frohse and its relationship to posterior interosseous nerve paralysis. *J Bone Joint Surg Br.* 1968;50:809–812.

27. Carr D, David P. Distal posterior interosseous syndrome. *J Hand Surg Am.* 1985;10:873.

28. Wartenberg R. Cheiralgia paresthetica (Isolierte neuritis des ram superficialis nerve radialis). *Z Gesamte Neurol Psychiatry.* 1932;141:145–155.

29. Leonard RN. Fractures and dislocations of the carpus. In: Brown BG, Jupiter JB, Levine AM, et al., eds. *Skeletal Trauma.* Philadelphia: WB Saunders; 1992.

30. Stechers WR. Roentgenography of the carpal navicular bone. *Amer J Radiol.* 1937;37:704–705.

31. Jorgenson TM, Anderson J, Thammesen P, et al. Scanning and radiology of the carpal scaphoid bone. *Acta Orthop Scand.* 1979;50:663–665.

32. Dobyns JH, Linscheid RL, Chao EYS, et al. *Traumatic Instability of the Wrist.* Chicago: American Academy of Orhopaedic Surgeons Instructional Course Lectures; 1975;24:182.

33. Norman A, Nelson J, Gren S. Fracture of the hook of the hamate: radiographic signs. *Radiology.* 1985;154:49–53.

34. Nisenfield FG, Neviasser RJ. Fracture of the hook of the hamate: a diagnosis easily missed. *J Trauma.* 1974;14:612–616.

35. Polivy KD, Millender LH, Newberg T, et al. Fractures of the hook of the hamate: a failure of clinical diagnosis. *J Hand Surg Am.* 1985;10:101–104.

36. Mayfield JK. Wrist ligamentous anatomy and pathogenesis of carpal instability. *Orthop Clin North Am.* 1984;15:209.

37. Watson HK, Dhillon HS. Intercarpal arthrodesis. In: Green DP, ed. *Operative Hand Surgery.* 3rd ed. New York: Churchill Livingstone; 1993;1:113.

38. Gilula LA, Weeks PN. Post-traumatic ligamentous instability of the wrist. *Radiology.* 1978;129:641.

39. Frankel VH. The Terry Thomas sign. *Clin Orthop.* 1977;129:121.

40. Linsheid RL, Dobyns JH, Beckenbaugh RD, et al. Instability patterns of the wrist. *J Hand Surg Am.* 1983;8:682.

41. Reagan DS, Linsheid RL, Dobyns JH. Lunotriquetral sprains. *J Hand Surg Am.* 1984;9:502.

42. Brown DE, Lichman DM. Midcarpal instability. *Hand Clin.* 1987;3:135.

43. Mikic Z. The blood supply of the human distal radio-ulnar joint and the microvasculature of its articular disk. *Clin Orthop.* 1992;275:19.

44. Bowers WH. The distal radioulnar joint. In: Green DP, ed. *Operative Hand Surgery.* 2nd ed. New York: Churchill Livingstone; 1988.

45. Wood MB, Dobyns JH. Sports related extra-articular wrist syndromes. *Clin Orthop.* 1986;202:93–102.

46. Keifhaber TR, Stern PJ. Upper extremity tendinitis and overuse syndromes in the athlete. *Clin Sports Med.* 1969;67:116–123.

47. Finkelstein H. Stenosing tenovaginitis at the radial styloid process. *J Bone Joint Surg Am.* 1930;12:509–540.

48. Grundberg AB, Reagan DS. Pathologic anatomy of the forearm: intersection syndrome. *J Hand Surg Am.* 1985;10:299–302.

49. Atroshi I, Gummesson C, Johnsson R, Ornstein E, Ranstam J, Rosen I. Prevalence of carpal tunnel syndrome in a general population. *JAMA.* 1999;282(2):153–158.

50. Katz JN, Lew RA, Bessette L, et al. Prevalence and predictors of long-term work disability due to carpal tunnel syndrome. *Am J Ind Med.* 1998;33(6):543–550.

51. Levine DW, Simmons BP, Koris MJ, et al. A self-administered questionnaire for the assessment of severity of symptoms and functional status in carpal tunnel syndrome. *J Bone Joint Surg Am.* 1993;75(11):1585–1592.

52. Stevens JC, Sun S, Beard CM, O'Fallon WM, Kurland LT. Carpal tunnel syndrome in Rochester, Minnesota, 1961–1980. *Neurology.* 1988;38(1):134–138.

53. Stevens JC, Witt JC, Smith BE, Weaver AL. The frequency of carpal tunnel syndrome in computer users at a medical facility. *Neurology.* 2001;56(11):1568–1570.

54. de Krom MC, Knipschild PG, Kester AD, Thijs CT, Boekkooi PF, Spaans F. Carpal tunnel syndrome: prevalence in the general population. *J Clin Epidemiol.* 1992;45(4):373–376.

55. Hagberg M, Morgenstern H, Kelsh M. Impact of occupations and job tasks on the prevalence of carpal tunnel syndrome. *Scand J Work Environ Health.* 1992;18(6):337–345.

56. Thomsen JF, Hansson GA, Mikkelsen S, Lauritzen M. Carpal tunnel syndrome in repetitive work: a follow-up study. *Am J Ind Med.* 2002;42(4):344–353.

57. Stevens E. Carpal tunnel syndrome: a dental hygienist's fate? Facts you should know and practice. *Nda J.* 1996;47(1):14–15.

58. Tanaka S, Wild DK, Seligman PJ, Behrens V, Cameron L, Putz-Anderson V. The US prevalence of self-reported carpal tunnel syndrome: 1988 National Health Interview Survey data. *Am J Public Health.* 1994;84(11):1846–1848.

59. Braun RM, Davidson K, Doehr S. Provocative testing in the diagnosis of dynamic carpal tunnel syndrome. *J Hand Surg [Am].* 1989;14(2 Pt 1):195–197.

60. Padua L, Padua R, Aprile I, D'Amico P, Tonali P. Carpal tunnel syndrome: relationship between clinical and patient-oriented assessment. *Clin Orthop Related Res.* 2002;395:128.

61. BLS reports on survey of occupational injuries and illnesses in 1989. *Am Ind Hyg Assoc J.* 1991;52(2):A92.

62. Abbas MA, Afifi AA, Zhang ZW, Kraus JF. Meta-analysis of published studies of work-related carpal tunnel syndrome. *Int J Occup Environ Health.* 1998;4(3):160–167.

63. Bernard B. *Musculoskeletal Disorders (MSD) and Workplace Factors: A Critical Review of Epidemiologic*

Evidence for Work-Related Musculoskeletal Disorders of the Neck, Upper Extremity, and Low Back. Cincinnati, OH: NIOSH, Centers for Disease Control and Prevention National Institute for Occupational Safety and Health; 1997.

64. Goodgold J. A statistical problem in diagnosis of carpal tunnel disease. *Muscle Nerve.* 1994;17(12):1490–1491.

65. Chan L, Turner JA, Comstock BA, et al. The relationship between electrodiagnostic findings and patient symptoms and function in carpal tunnel syndrome. *Arch Phys Med Rehabil.* 2007;88(1):19–24.

66. Kuschner SH, Ebramzadeh E, Johnson D, Brien WW, Sherman R. Tinel's sign and Phalen's test in carpal tunnel syndrome. *Orthopedics.* 1992;15(11):1297–1302.

67. Posch JL, Prpic I. Surgical treatment of the carpal tunnel syndrome. *Handchirurgie.* 1975;7(2):95–98.

68. LaJoie AS, McCabe SJ, Thomas B, Edgell SE. Determining the sensitivity and specificity of common diagnostic tests for carpal tunnel syndrome using latent class analysis. *PlastReconstr Surg.* 2005;116(2):502–507.

69. MacDermid JC, Wessel J. Clinical diagnosis of carpal tunnel syndrome: a systematic review. *J Hand Ther.* 2004;17(2):309–319.

70. MacDermid JC, Doherty T. Clinical and electrodiagnostic testing of carpal tunnel syndrome: a narrative review. *J Orthop Sports Phys Ther.* 2004;34(10):565–588.

71. Nora DB, Becker J, Ehlers JA, Gomes I. Clinical features of 1039 patients with neurophysiological diagnosis of carpal tunnel syndrome. *Clin Neurol Neurosurg.* 2004;107(1):64–69.

72. Golding DN, Rose DM, Selvarajah K. Clinical tests for carpal tunnel syndrome: an evaluation. *Br J Rheumatol.* 1986;25(4):388–390.

73. D'Arcy CA, McGee S. Does this patient have carpal tunnel syndrome? *JAMA.* 2000;283(23):3110–3117.

74. Katz JN, Stirrat CR. A self-administered hand diagram for the diagnosis of carpal tunnel syndrome. *J Hand Surg [Am].* 1990;15(2):360–363.

75. Lew HL, Date ES, Pan SS, Wu P, Ware PF, Kingery WS. Sensitivity, specificity, and variability of nerve conduction velocity measurements in carpal tunnel syndrome. *Arch Phys Med Rehabil.* 2005;86(1):12–16.

76. Andersen JH, Thomsen JF, Overgaard E, et al. Computer use and carpal tunnel syndrome: a 1-year follow-up study. *JAMA.* 2003;289(22):2963–2969.

77. Verhagen AP, Bierma-Zeinstra SM, Feleus A, et al. Ergonomic and physiotherapeutic interventions for treating upper extremity work related disorders in adults. *Cochrane Database Syst Rev;* 2004:CD003471.

78. Tittiranonda P, Rempel D, Armstrong T, Burastero S. Effect of four computer keyboards in computer users with upper extremity musculoskeletal disorders. *Am J Ind Med.* 1999;35(6):647–661.

79. Verdugo RJ, Salinas RS, Castillo J, Cea JG. Surgical versus non-surgical treatment for carpal tunnel syndrome. *Cochrane Database Syst Rev;* 2003:CD001552.

80. Garland H, Langworth EP, Taverner D, Clark JM. Surgical treatment for the carpal tunnel syndrome. *Lancet.* 1964;13:1129–1130.

81. Gerritsen AA, Korthals-de Bos IB, Laboyrie PM, de Vet HC, Scholten RJ, Bouter LM. Splinting for carpal tunnel syndrome: prognostic indicators of success. *J Neurol Neurosurg Psychiatry.* 2003:1342–1344.

82. The Department of Labor & Industries' Work-Related Carpal Tunnel Syndrome Diagnosis & Treatment Guideline. 2013. www.lni.wa.gov/ClaimsIns/Providers/Treatment/TreatGuide/default.asp

83. Davis PT, Hulbert JR, Kassak KM, Meyer JJ. Comparative efficacy of conservative medical and chiropractic treatments for carpal tunnel syndrome: a randomized clinical trial. *J Manipulative Physiol Ther.* 1998;21(5):317.

84. O'Connor D, Marshall S, Massy-Westropp N. Non-surgical treatment (other than steroid injection) for carpal tunnel syndrome. *Cochrane Database Syst Rev.* 2003(1): CD003219.

85. Valente R, Gibson H. Chiropractic manipulation in carpal tunnel syndrome. *J Manipulative PhysiolTher.* 1994:246–249.

86. Gerritsen AA, de Krom MC, Struijs MA, Scholten RJ, de Vet HC, Bouter LM. Conservative treatment options for carpal tunnel syndrome: a systematic review of randomized controlled trials. *J Neurol.* 2002;249:272–280.

87. Feuerstein M, Burrell LM, Miller VI, Lincoln A, Huang GD, Berger R. Clinical management of carpal tunnel syndrome: a 12-year review of outcomes. *Am J Ind Med.* 1999;35(3):232–245.

88. Ebenbichler GR, Resch KL, Nicolakis P, et al. Ultrasound treatment for treating the carpal tunnel syndrome: randomized "sham" controlled trial. *BMJ.* 1998;316(7133):731.

89. Oztas O, Turan B, Bora I, Karakaya MK. Ultrasound therapy effect in carpal tunnel syndrome. *Arch Phys Med Rehabil.* 1998;79(12):1540–1544.

90. Goodyear-Smith F, Arroll B. What can family physicians offer patients with carpal tunnel syndrome other than surgery? A systematic review of nonsurgical management. *Ann Fam Med.* 2004;2:267–273.

91. Bakhtiary AH, Fatemi E, Emami M, Malek M. Phonophoresis of dexamethasone sodium phosphate may manage pain and symptoms of patients with carpal tunnel syndrome. *Clin J Pain.* 2012;29(4):348–353.

92. Bakhtiary AH, Rashidy-Pour A. Ultrasound and laser therapy in the treatment of carpal tunnel syndrome. *Aust J Physiother.* 2004;50(3):147–151.

93. Spooner GR, Desai HB, Angel JF, Reeder BA, Donat JR. Using pyridoxine to treat carpal tunnel syndrome. randomized control trial. *Can Fam Physician.* 1993;39:2122–2127.

94. Stransky M, Rubin A, Lava NS, Lazaro RP. Treatment of carpal tunnel syndrome with vitamin B6: a double-blind study. *South Med J.* 1989;82(7):841–842.

95. Akalin E, El O, Peker O, et al. Treatment of carpal tunnel syndrome with nerve and tendon gliding exercises. *Am J Phys Med Rehabil.* 2002;81(2):108–113.

96. Garfinkel MS, Schumacher HR, Jr., Husain A, Levy M, Reshetar RA. Evaluation of a yoga based regimen for treatment of osteoarthritis of the hands. *J Rheumatol.* 1994;21(12):2341–2343.

97. Irvine J, Chong SL, Amirjani N, Chan KM. Double-blind randomized controlled trial of low-level laser therapy in carpal tunnel syndrome. *Muscle Nerve.* 2004;30(2):182–187.

98. Posner MA. Compressive neuropathies of the median and radial nerves at the elbow. *Clin Sports Med.* 1990;9:343.

99. Glousman RE. Ulnar nerve problems in the athlete's elbow. *Clin Sports Med.* 1990;9:365.

100. Rettig AC. Neurovascular injuries in the wrists and hands of athletes. *Clin Sports Med.* 1990;9:389.

101. Plancher KD, Peterson RK, Steichen JB. Compressive neuropathies and tendinopathies in the athletic elbow and wrist. *Clin Sports Med.* 1996;15:331.

102. Corley FH. Commonly missed fractures in the hand and wrist. *J Musculoskel Med.* 1993;10:55–68.

103. Almquist EA. Kienbock's disease. *Clin Orthop.* 1986;202:68.

Finger and Thumb Complaints

Context

Finger and thumb complaints reflect a wide spectrum of disorders ranging from local pathology to distal manifestations of systemic disease. Local pathology is usually due to trauma. Localization of pain or tenderness coupled with mechanism of injury substantially narrows down the possibilities. Radiographs are usually necessary to discover subtle bone damage not accessible through clinical examination. When a history of trauma is not evident, local finger/thumb pain is often associated with clues of systemwide involvement. Conditions such as arthritides, connective tissue disease, or vascular problems such as Raynaud's disease or reflex sympathetic dystrophy must be considered.

When a hand complaint is an extension of pain from another site, a peripheral nerve, nerve root, or spinal cord involvement must be differentiated. When numbness, tingling, or weakness is reported, peripheral nerve entrapment is likely, especially when the forearm or wrist is part of the pattern. When the neck and shoulder are part of the pathway of complaint, nerve root compression by a disc, nerve entrapment by osteophytes, or referral from the cervical facets should be considered. For a more detailed discussion of each of these possibilities see the specific section for each in this chapter.

The chiropractor's role with hand trauma is clearly to determine the degree of injury. The degree of injury often is not severe and all that is needed is appropriate splinting, taping, or a cast. Articular or displaced fractures; tendon detachments or severage; deep lacerations with risk of infection; and animal, spider, or human bites must be referred. Most nontraumatic complaints reflect chronic processes that may benefit from conservative management.

General Strategy

History

- Localize the complaint and determine whether it is one of pain, stiffness, numbness/tingling, weakness, popping/snapping, coldness, deformity, or a combination.
- If traumatic, determine whether the mechanism was compressive or rotational, or caused by excessive flexion, extension, abduction, or adduction.
- If traumatic, consider radiographs in most cases to determine whether there is any underlying fracture.
- If nontraumatic, determine whether there are associated complaints such as other joint complaints (arthritides), deformities (arthritides), or cervical spine or arm complaints (facet referral, nerve root, brachial plexus, or peripheral nerve).

Evaluation

- If traumatic, test for neurovascular status; examine for lacerations, swellings, or deformity; test ligamentous stability.
- If nontraumatic, examine for sites of local tenderness over joints and tendon insertions; test for accessory motion.

Management

- Displaced or articular fractures, severed or avulsed tendons, and infection should be referred for orthopaedic consultation and management.

- Many ligament injuries can be managed with taping or splints unless there is an associated articular fracture.
- Rheumatoid and connective tissue disorders may require comanagement.

Relevant Clinical Anatomy

The fingers and thumb participate in not only simple survival functions such as gripping but also complex actions that require amazing dexterity. The mechanical and neurologic integration necessary for this high functional demand is complex (**Figure 10–1**, A and B). An ingenious system of pulleys, redundant muscular and neural support, and varying joint design allows for an enormous degree of subtlety of motion. The general arrangement of the hand is similar to that of many joints, with a system of muscles that allows for flexion, extension, abduction, and adduction. Rotational movements are largely due to elbow/forearm and thumb movement.

Fingers

Flexion of the digits is accomplished mainly through extrinsic muscle control provided by the flexor digitorum superficialis (FDS) and flexor digitorum profundus (FDP) with assistance from the intrinsic lumbricals and interossei. The lumbricals, in fact, originate off the radial

side of the FDP tendons. The FDS tendon splits at the proximal end of the first phalanx, allowing the FDP to pass through and insert onto the distal phalanx.[1] The FDS then reunites and splits again to insert on either side of the middle phalanx. The volar interossei originate off the radial side of the fourth and fifth metacarpals and the ulnar side of the second and first metacarpal, allowing adduction of the fingers (in relation to the middle finger). The dorsal interossei originate off the metacarpals and abduct the fingers. The second and third dorsal interossei abduct toward the thumb. This is important for pinch-grip stability. A complex system of annular pulleys allows the flexor tendons to generate the greatest amount of force. There are five of these with one at each joint (MCP, PIP, and DIP) and two approximating the proximal and middle phalanx. The three at the joints are numbered proximal to distal A1, A3, and A5. The two fibro-osseous pulleys are numbered A2 and A4 proximal to distal. There are also three cruciform pulleys: two at the middle phalanx and one at the proximal phalanx. The cruciforms are not often injured or damaged; however, the A pulleys, in particular A2 and A4, are often partially or completely torn in rock climbing injuries.

Extension of the fingers is accomplished by the extensor digitorum (ED) muscle/tendons. The fifth finger is assisted by the digiti quinti and the index finger by the extensor indices. The primary insertion of the ED is onto the dorsum of the proximal phalanx. As the tendon continues distally it connects to lateral bands

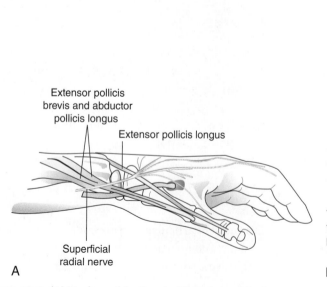

Extensor pollicis brevis and abductor pollicis longus

Extensor pollicis longus

Superficial radial nerve

A

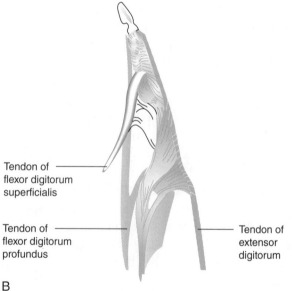

Tendon of flexor digitorum superficialis

Tendon of flexor digitorum profundus

Tendon of extensor digitorum

B

Figure 10–1 (A) Tendons of the thumb; (B) tendons of the finger.

that are the continuation of the interossei and lumbrical muscles. The lateral bands continue distally to unite into a combined insertion into the distal phalanx. The ED tendon also inserts into the middle phalanx. Although there is an insertion into each distal phalanx, the primary functional insertion is at the proximal phalanx. When the ED tendon pulls, most of the action is at the proximal phalangeal insertion. When the proximal phalanx is extended, the interossei and lumbrical connections to the lateral bands cause these intrinsic muscles to be the primary extensors of the middle and distal phalanges. When the ED relaxes, these same muscles act as flexors. With the metacarpophalangeal (MCP) joint flexed to 90°, tension on the ED pulls the distal interphalangeal (DIP) and proximal interphalangeal (PIP) joints passively into extension without the aid of the interossei.[2]

The index and middle fingers are stable, whereas the fourth and fifth fingers are mobile (the fifth being the most mobile). This is in large part due to the unique articulation at each joint. In particular, the articulation between the fifth metacarpal and the hamate is similar to the saddle configuration at the thumb and, like the thumb, allows for greater mobility.[3] This is visible while observing the metacarpal heads during flexion and extension. The heads are in alignment with extension, allowing the palm to rest flat. With full flexion (clenched fist), the fourth and fifth heads flex beyond that of the second and third, creating a curved arch. Clinically, this is important with fracture management where more rotational or varus/valgus angularity is allowed with fourth and especially fifth metacarpal fractures. Additionally, the overlap of support provided by the intrinsic ligaments and interossei muscles makes the metacarpals quite stable even with fracture or ligament injury.

Thumb

The thumb's mobility is due to its position and the articular configuration at the carpometacarpal and MCP joints. Nine muscles act on the thumb to allow not only flexion/extension and abduction/adduction, but also opposition (abduction, rotation, and flexion). Although flexion and extension may occur at all the thumb joints, abduction and adduction occur mainly at the carpometacarpal joint (some at the MCP joint).

Flexion, extension, and abduction of the thumb are accomplished through a muscle couple made up of a long

extrinsic muscle/tendon and a short intrinsic muscle. Flexion is due to the flexor pollicis longus (FPL) and the flexor policis brevis (FPB). Extension is accomplished with the ED and the extensor pollicis brevis (EPB) muscles. Abduction is governed by the abductor pollicis longus (APL) and abductor pollicis brevis (APB). The short muscles are part of the thenar group and are joined by the adductor pollicis and opponens pollicis muscles. Adduction is controlled by the first palmar interosseous muscle and adductor pollicis. The tendons of the EPB and the APL outline the anatomic snuff-box, a common location of tenderness with scaphoid fractures. These tendons may be involved in de Quervain's disease. Ligamentous support is provided by two collateral ligaments (similar to the other phalanges), one on each side, with assistance by paired accessory ligaments. The collateral ligament on the inside web is the ulnar collateral ligament. This is often injured with a hyperextension or abduction injury referred to as gamekeeper's thumb. Support at the MCP joint is provided by the volar ligaments and plate.

Evaluation

History

Careful questioning of the patient during the history taking can point to the diagnosis (**Table 10–1**).

Pain Localization (see Figure 9–3, A–C)
Finger

- Metacarpophalangeal (MCP) joint
  1. Traumatic—dislocation, collateral ligament sprain or rupture
  2. Nontraumatic—capsular sprain, osteoarthritis (OA)
- Proximal interphalangeal (PIP) joint
  1. Traumatic—dislocation (coach's finger), boutonnière deformity (hyperflexion injury)
  2. Nontraumatic—rheumatoid arthritis (RA), Reiter's syndrome, psoriatic arthritis, or OA
- Distal interphalangeal (DIP) joint
  1. Traumatic—mallet finger (hyperflexion), flexor digitorum avulsion (jersey finger)
  2. Nontraumatic—psoriatic arthritis

Table 10–1 History Questions for Finger and Thumb Complaints

Primary Question	What Are You Thinking?	Secondary Questions	What Are You Thinking?
Was there an injury?	Fracture, dislocation, ligament sprain, tendon avulsion, capsular sprain	Hit on end of finger?	Fracture
			PIP joint dislocation
		Finger bent back?	Capsular sprain
			Sprain
			Volar plate tear
			Avulsion of FDP (jersey finger)
			PIP or MCP joint dislocation
		Thumb pulled back?	Gamekeeper's thumb (injury to DIP)
		Finger forced into flexed position?	Mallet finger (injury to DIP)
			Boutonniere deformity (tearing of central slip)
		Hit an object with a clenched fist?	If thumb is involved rule out metacarpal fracture
			If hand is involved rule out metacarpal fracture
Does your finger feel stiff?	Arthritis (OA or RA), capsular effusion or adhesion, subluxation, trigger finger	Does your finger get stuck in a flexed position?	Trigger finger likely (check for nodule)
			Capsular effusion or adhesion
		Can't close finger(s)?	Retinacular tightness
		Worse in morning; better with mild activity?	OA
		Associated swelling or deformity?	RA
			OA
			Psoriatic arthritis
Is there a sense of weakness?	C8-T1 nerve roots, peripheral nerve entrapment	Associated neck pain and/or radiation into hand?	Cervical disc, tumor, or spondylosis
		Associated elbow or forearm pain?	Peripheral nerve entrapment (distinguish by which muscles)
Do you routinely perform repetitive activity with your fingers?	Tendinitis, peripheral nerve entrapment	Is the pain at your thumb or slightly above?	de Quervain's disease
			Intersection syndrome

Thumb

- Traumatic—gamekeeper's thumb (ulnar collateral ligament [UCL] sprain or rupture), Bennett's fracture (first MCP base)
- Nontraumatic—OA, bowler's thumb (digital neuritis)

Traumatic Finger Pain

As distal joints, the fingers are vulnerable to all order of outside forces. Hand and finger injuries are particularly common in sports.[4] General patterns of injury occur with "hyper" movements:

- Hyperextension may simply strain the palmar surface of the fingers or hand or result in tendon avulsion of the flexor digitorum profundus, volar plate damage, or dislocation or fracture.[5]
- Hyperflexion may cause dislocation, central extensor tendon slip damage at the PIP joint, or extensor tendon avulsion at the DIP joint.
- Rotational or valgus/varus forces will often result in collateral ligament damage. With more force a dislocation or fracture is possible.
- Direct axial forces to the extended fingers may cause a synovitis or fracture. An axial force to the knuckles often results in a metacarpal fracture or

simply a local contusion to the knuckle (boxer's knuckle). The examiner may need to be persistent in determining whether the patient, in a fit of anger, punched an inanimate (or animate) object.

- When the patient has a cut or laceration, a tendon or nerve may be severed. Wounds are open to infection, and questions about animal, insect, or object penetration, and recent tetanus shots should be asked.

Weakness

Weakness in the fingers may be a generalized or local problem. Clarify whether the patient feels pain with movement or gripping. Pain localization when associated with a weakness complaint may be helpful; however, a complaint of weakness with pain is itself nonspecific because of the reflex or voluntary inhibition that occurs with painful movement. The patient should be asked about weakness that relates to a specific movement. It is important to remember that a perception of weakness may be due to stiffness or inflexibility at a joint or joints. Passive range of motion testing will often reveal this component.

Weakness in a single digit following trauma should suggest tendon avulsion, especially if associated with deformity. Weakness with specific finger/thumb gripping or pinching suggests a peripheral nerve entrapment or damage. Gross weakness with hand gripping is possible with any number of problems; however, the problem usually is neural. Ulnar or median nerve involvement will affect grip strength, as will nerve root compression. Radiation of a complaint from the forearm suggests peripheral nerve entrapment, whereas pain or paresthesia radiating from the neck suggests nerve root or a referral phenomenon. Weakness in grip may also be the result of instability at the wrist. Remember that grip strength is usually decreased with the use of thick gloves. Grip strength is also position-dependent. Gripping is most efficient in neutral or slight wrist extension (less than 30°). Beyond these limits the mechanical advantage of the finger flexors is reduced.

Restriction in Movement

Movement restriction in the fingers should be divided into posttraumatic or insidious. Stiffness, especially with flexion, is not uncommon after an axial load injury to the finger with a resultant capsular sprain and reactive synovitis. Because of the inability to immobilize the fingers as easily as more proximal joints, the fingers are constantly stressed. As a result, capsulitis of the digits often takes two months or more to resolve.

An insidious onset suggests an arthritis. The two most common are OA and RA. Historically, there is often a distinction between the two. OA often causes the patient to complain of early-morning stiffness that improves after 20 to 30 minutes of activity. RA is often more restrictive and takes several hours to improve. Exacerbations with movement are more common with RA. A search for corroborative evidence includes the age of the patient, family history, and involvement of other joints. In an elderly patient with unilateral complaints of knee or hip pain, OA is more likely. In a middle-aged woman with a positive family history and bilateral, diffuse involvement of the PIP joints, RA is more likely.

Restriction to movement may be localized to the fourth and fifth fingers with an associated flexion contracture evident. This is likely to be Dupuytren's contracture.[6] Questioning regarding alcohol consumption or possible diabetes should be included. A unique restriction complaint is snapping of a finger or thumb upon extension. This is often due to a trigger finger or thumb. Initially, the patient may report the ability to overcome an extension restriction actively. As the condition progresses, she or he may have to extend the finger passively past the restriction, often with an audible snap.

Superficial Complaints

As the distal point of the upper extremity, the fingers and hands are often indicators of more proximal and often systemic conditions. Complaints range from numbness/tingling, coldness, skin and nail lesions, and burning sensations. If one or two fingers appear blanched and cause the patient pain when exposed to cold, Raynaud's disease or phenomenon is likely. Nail lesions are often indicators of various systemic processes. Longitudinal nail lines are seen with anemia, clubbing with chronic pulmonary disorders, and pitting with psoriasis. Many complaints of numbness or tingling are connected to a wrist, forearm, or neck complaint. See the related section in this text for a more thorough discussion. When there is localized numbness in the thumb, compression of the ulnar digital nerve of the thumb is often the cause; it is called bowler's thumb. A "sausage finger" (swelling of the PIP joint) suggests psoriatic arthritis or Reiter's syndrome.

Examination

Traumatic Injury

When evaluation is immediately posttraumatic, a quick check of neurovascular status is warranted.[7]

Vascular

- Allen's test for radial and ulnar arteries: The patient is instructed to open and close the hand several times. He or she is then instructed to keep the hand tightly closed in a fist. The examiner occludes both the radial and ulnar arteries at the wrist. The patient is then asked to open the hand. The examiner releases pressure on the artery and observes for filling; the distal hand reddens within a few seconds. Repeat with the opposite artery. This test may also be used for the digital arteries at the fingers: The examiner gently squeezes the radial and ulnar sides of the volar tip with finger and thumb, sliding them proximally while maintaining the squeeze. The finger should become pale. Release pressure with the finger to determine whether the finger fills. Repeat with release of thumb pressure to check the patency of the other artery.

Neural

- Two-point discrimination: This is the minimal distance at which a patient can discriminate between two points of stimulation. A paper clip bent to expose two points 4 mm apart may be used (testing is on the palmar surface). The two points must touch the skin simultaneously. Although the distance varies over the hand, an average of 4 to 5 mm is used for a quick check.
- Sensory testing (use a pin; check for pain perception)
  1. Ulnar nerve—volar tip of little finger
  2. Radial nerve—dorsum of thumb web
  3. Median nerve—volar tips of index and middle fingers
- Motor (gross check)
  1. Ulnar nerve—cross middle finger over the back of the index finger
  2. Radial nerve—extend thumb
  3. Median nerve—point thumb toward ceiling (palm up on table)

- Muscle/tendon check (inability to perform may indicate a severed or avulsed tendon)
  1. Flexor digitorum profundus—with MCP and PIP joints held in extension (or held down with the patient's palm up), ask the patient to flex the DIP (often the result of a hyperextension injury).
  2. Flexor digitorum superficialis—with patient's palm up, hold down all untested fingers into extension and ask the patient to flex the unrestrained finger.
  3. Flexor pollicis longus—with the thumb held in extension at the MCP joint, ask the patient to flex the IP joints.
  4. Extensor digitorum—with the wrist in extension, ask the patient to extend at the MCP and IP joints.

Observation should focus on a search for deformity and swelling. This search is occurring as the above neurovascular check is being performed. Note that if there is an apparent dislocation, depending on the joint involved, an attempt at relocation should be made. See specific joints in the selected disorders section. Next, check for a rotational deformity of a finger, best seen with flexion of the fingers to the palm. Rotational or angular deformity is an indication of fracture. Tapping on an extended finger often will increase the pain if a fracture is present.[8] Further evaluation with radiographs is necessary. Tapping at the knuckle with the fingers flexed to the palm may reveal a metacarpal fracture. Swelling localized to a joint may indicate ligamentous rupture or capsular sprain with an associated synovitis. Stability testing of the PIP and MCP joints is performed in two positions: 30° and 70° of flexion. In each of these positions, a varus and valgus stress is applied to the joint.

Radiographic evaluation is necessary with most finger injuries. Standard anteroposterior (AP) and lateral views will reveal most fractures or dislocations. It is important to search for an associated dislocation when a fracture is evident. This is often best seen on a lateral view. For fractures of the metacarpal, it is useful to add a lateral view with the hand pronated about 20°. Otherwise, metacarpal fracture lines may be obscured.[9] For the thumb, AP and lateral views are required. Stress views (pulling the thumbs into abduction) are often necessary to determine the degree of injury with a gamekeeper's thumb. Greater than 30° difference between the two sides indicates rupture of the ulnar collateral ligament, as does an avulsion fracture of the proximal base.[10]

Nontraumatic

Observation of the fingers may reveal deformities or swellings. Deformities at the distal and proximal joints are most commonly associated with two arthritides, OA and RA. DIP joint involvement is referred to as Heberden's nodes; PIP involvement is referred to as Bouchard's nodes when associated with OA or RA.[11] Involvement with either arthritis is often bilateral and involves more than one digit. MCP joint involvement is rare with OA but may occur with RA and psoriatic and gouty arthritis. Psoriatic arthritis affects mainly the DIP joint and is usually associated with skin lesions on the extensor surfaces of the extremities and pitting and ridging of the nails. Swelling and tenderness of the entire involved finger (sausage finger) is found with psoriatic arthritis and Reiter's syndrome (check for associated sacroiliac pain). Clubbing of the fingers may occur with a variety of pulmonary diseases, including tuberculosis and bronchogenic carcinoma.

Severe RA will present with fusiform swelling of the PIP joints, ulnar deviation of the fingers at the MCP joints, interosseous muscle atrophy, extensor tenosynovitis, and subcutaneous nodules over the extensor surfaces of the forearm and wrist. Laboratory testing is most useful for RA, checking for rheumatoid factor (immunoglobulin [Ig] M and anti-IgG) and increases in the erythrocyte sedimentation rate. However, rheumatoid factor is found in only 70% to 80% of patients with RA.

Observation and palpation of the fingers/hand may reveal vascular compromise.

- Reflex sympathetic dystrophy—A combination of shiny, swollen skin is present (the whole arm is often involved in shoulder-arm-hand syndrome).
- Raynaud's phenomenon or disease—Often one or two fingers are "white" compared with other fingers; the condition is worse upon exposure to cold. Raynaud's disease is idiopathic; Raynaud's phenomenon is associated with an identifiable connective tissue disorder such as scleroderma or systemic lupus erythematosus.

When stiffening is the main complaint, it is important to distinguish between intrinsic muscle and capsular/collateral ligament tightness. This is accomplished by joint positioning that either tightens or relaxes these structures. For the PIP joint, the Bunnel-Littler test (**Figure 10–2**) is used.[12] With the MCP joint held in slight extension, the PIP joint is passively flexed toward

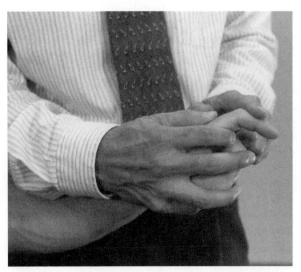

Figure 10–2 Bunnel-Littler test. With the MCP joint stabilized the examiner attempts to flex the PIP joint. If not flexible, the MCP joint is flexed and the test is repeated. Ability to flex indicates tight intrinsic muscles. Inability to flex in the second position indicates joint contracture or swelling.

the palm. Inability to flex fully is indicative of either joint capsule contracture or tight intrinsic muscles. If the PIP joint can be flexed after moving the MCP joint into slight flexion, the intrinsic muscles are tight. If the PIP joint cannot be flexed with MCP joint flexion, joint contracture is likely the cause. For the DIP joint, the retinacular test is used. Here the distinction is between the retinacular ligaments and the joint capsule. The retinacular test (**Figure 10–3**) is the distal extension of the Bunnel-Littler

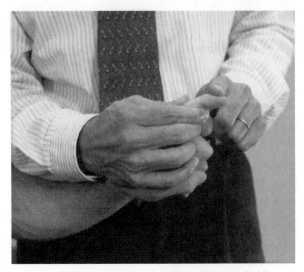

Figure 10–3 The Retinacular test. With the PIP joint held in neutral, the examiner attempts to passively flex the DIP joint. If unable to flex, the DIP is flexed slightly and the DIP is again flexed. If unable to flex in the second position, a joint contracture is present; able to flex indicates retinacular tightness.

concept. While the PIP joint is held in neutral, the examiner attempts to flex the DIP joint passively. If it cannot be flexed, either retinacular or capsular tightness is the cause. If after flexion of the PIP joint the DIP joint can be passively flexed, retinacular tightness is the cause. If the DIP joint still cannot be passively flexed, a joint capsule contracture is likely.

Radiographic evaluation of the hand is often a search for either fracture or typical clustered findings suggestive of each arthritis.[13]

- RA: Early signs are of soft tissue swelling; progression results in periarticular demineralization, loss of joint space, erosions of the joint margins (rat-bite lesions), and malalignment of the fingers (especially ulnar deviation at the MCP joints).
- OA: Joint space narrowing, sclerosis, subchondral cysts, and osteophytes are the hallmarks of OA. Bony enlargement of the DIP joints is typical (Heberden's nodes) and occasionally at the PIP joints (Bouchard's nodes). The CMC joint of the thumb is also often affected.
- Psoriatic: Bone resorption of the tufts of the distal phalanges may be seen; progression to the rest of the phalange may occur with the most severe form of psoriatic arthritis, arthritis mutilans.

There is some overlap between wrist, hand, and forearm complaints and testing. See the specific sections for each. Neurologic involvement from a proximal source is described in Chapters 2 and 9.

Management

Acute Traumatic Injury

Management of acute injury is as follows:

- Dislocations of the PIP and DIP joints should be relocated if possible; clinical testing for instability and radiographs for associated fracture should be performed.

- Fractures involving more than 20% to 30% of the articular surface should be referred for orthopaedic consultation.
- Nondisplaced fractures are casted (specific position-dependent on joints involved).
- Displaced fractures are referred for surgical stabilization.
- Flexor tendon avulsion (mallet finger) or a suspected severed tendon requires orthopaedic referral.
- Ligament damages to the volar plate, central extensor slip, or collateral ligaments are splinted (see Related Conditions section for specifics).

Nontraumatic Conditions

- Rheumatoid or connective tissue disorders warrant comanagement with a rheumatologist.
- Osteoarthritic involvement requires a mild finger/hand strengthening program; physical therapy heating modalities may be transiently beneficial; mobilization and manipulation of the involved joints when performed cautiously may also be of benefit.
- Peripheral nerve causes of numbness/tingling or pain should first be treated with a myofascial release approach for two to three weeks to determine treatment effectiveness, modification of any identifiable inciting activity, and, when necessary, splinting or soft casting for a short course of imposed rest.
- Soft tissue contracture of the intrinsic muscles may also benefit from postisometric relaxation and myofascial release.
- Joint contracture may benefit from mobilization and deep heat with passive stretching when subacute or chronic.

Algorithms

Algorithms for evaluation and management of thumb pain, traumatic hand pain, and nontraumatic hand pain are presented in **Figures 10–4** to **10–6**.

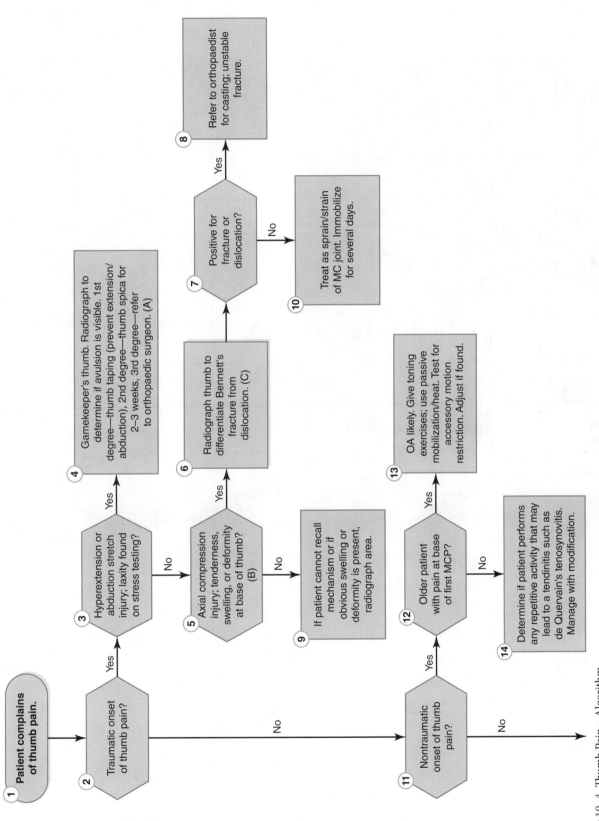

Figure 10-4 Thumb Pain—Algorithm

1. Patient complains of thumb pain.

2. Traumatic onset of thumb pain?

3. Hyperextension or abduction stretch injury; laxity found on stress testing?

4. Gamekeeper's thumb. Radiograph to determine if avulsion is visible. 1st degree—thumb taping (prevent extension/abduction), 2nd degree—thumb spica for 2–3 weeks, 3rd degree—refer to orthopaedic surgeon. (A)

5. Axial compression injury; tenderness, swelling, or deformity at base of thumb? (B)

6. Radiograph thumb to differentiate Bennett's fracture from dislocation. (C)

7. Positive for fracture or dislocation?

8. Refer to orthopaedist for casting; unstable fracture.

9. If patient cannot recall mechanism or if obvious swelling or deformity is present, radiograph area.

10. Treat as sprain/strain of MC joint. Immobilize for several days.

11. Nontraumatic onset of thumb pain?

12. Older patient with pain at base of first MCP?

13. OA likely. Give toning exercises; use passive mobilization/heat. Test for accessory motion restriction. Adjust if found.

14. Determine if patient performs any repetitive activity that may lead to a tendinitis such as de Quervain's tenosynovitis. Manage with modification.

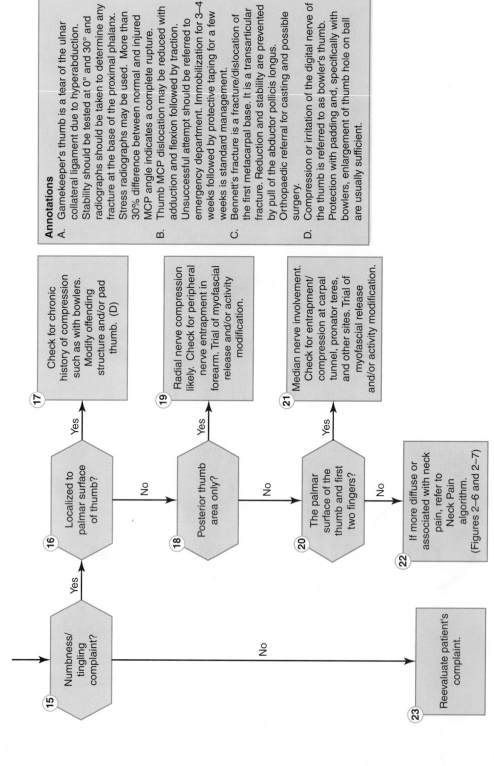

Annotations

A. Gamekeeper's thumb is a tear of the ulnar collateral ligament due to hyperabduction. Stability should be tested at 0° and 30° and radiographs should be taken to determine any fracture at the base of the proximal phalanx. Stress radiographs may be used. More than 30% difference between normal and injured MCP angle indicates a complete rupture.

B. Thumb MCP dislocation may be reduced with adduction and flexion followed by traction. Unsuccessful attempt should be referred to emergency department. Immobilization for 3–4 weeks followed by protective taping for a few weeks is standard management.

C. Bennett's fracture is a fracture/dislocation of the first metacarpal base. It is a transarticular fracture. Reduction and stability are prevented by pull of the abductor pollicis longus. Orthopaedic referral for casting and possible surgery.

D. Compression or irritation of the digital nerve of the thumb is referred to as bowler's thumb. Protection with padding and, specifically with bowlers, enlargement of thumb hole on ball are usually sufficient.

15 Numbness/ tingling complaint?

Yes →

16 Localized to palmar surface of thumb?

Yes → 17 Check for chronic history of compression such as with bowlers. Modify offending structure and/or pad thumb. (D)

No →

18 Posterior thumb area only?

Yes → 19 Radial nerve compression likely. Check for peripheral nerve entrapment in forearm. Trial of myofascial release and/or activity modification.

No →

20 The palmar surface of the thumb and first two fingers?

Yes → 21 Median nerve involvement. Check for entrapment/ compression at carpal tunnel, pronator teres, and other sites. Trial of myofascial release and/or activity modification.

No →

22 If more diffuse or associated with neck pain, refer to Neck Pain algorithm. (Figures 2–6 and 2–7)

No (from 15) →

23 Reevaluate patient's complaint.

Figure 10–4 (Continued)

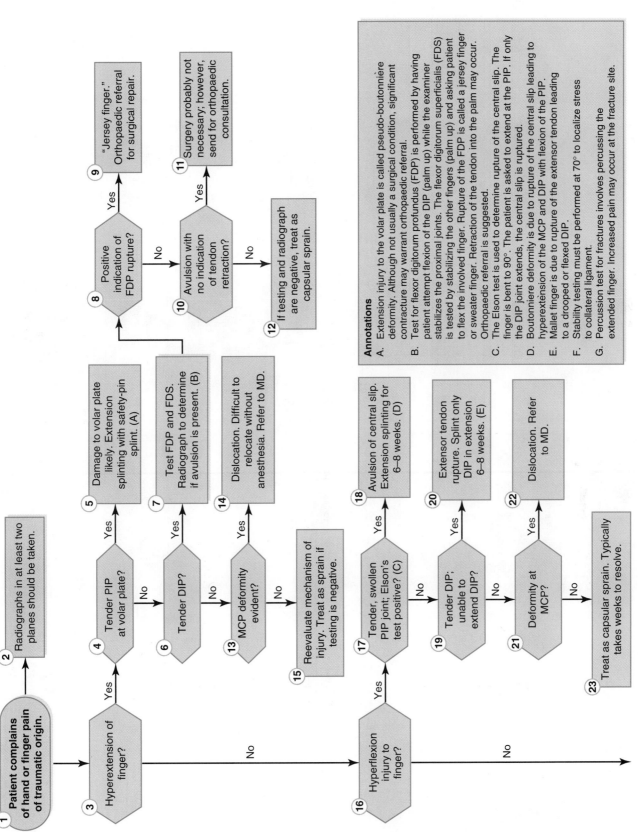

Figure 10–5 Traumatic Hand Pain—Algorithm

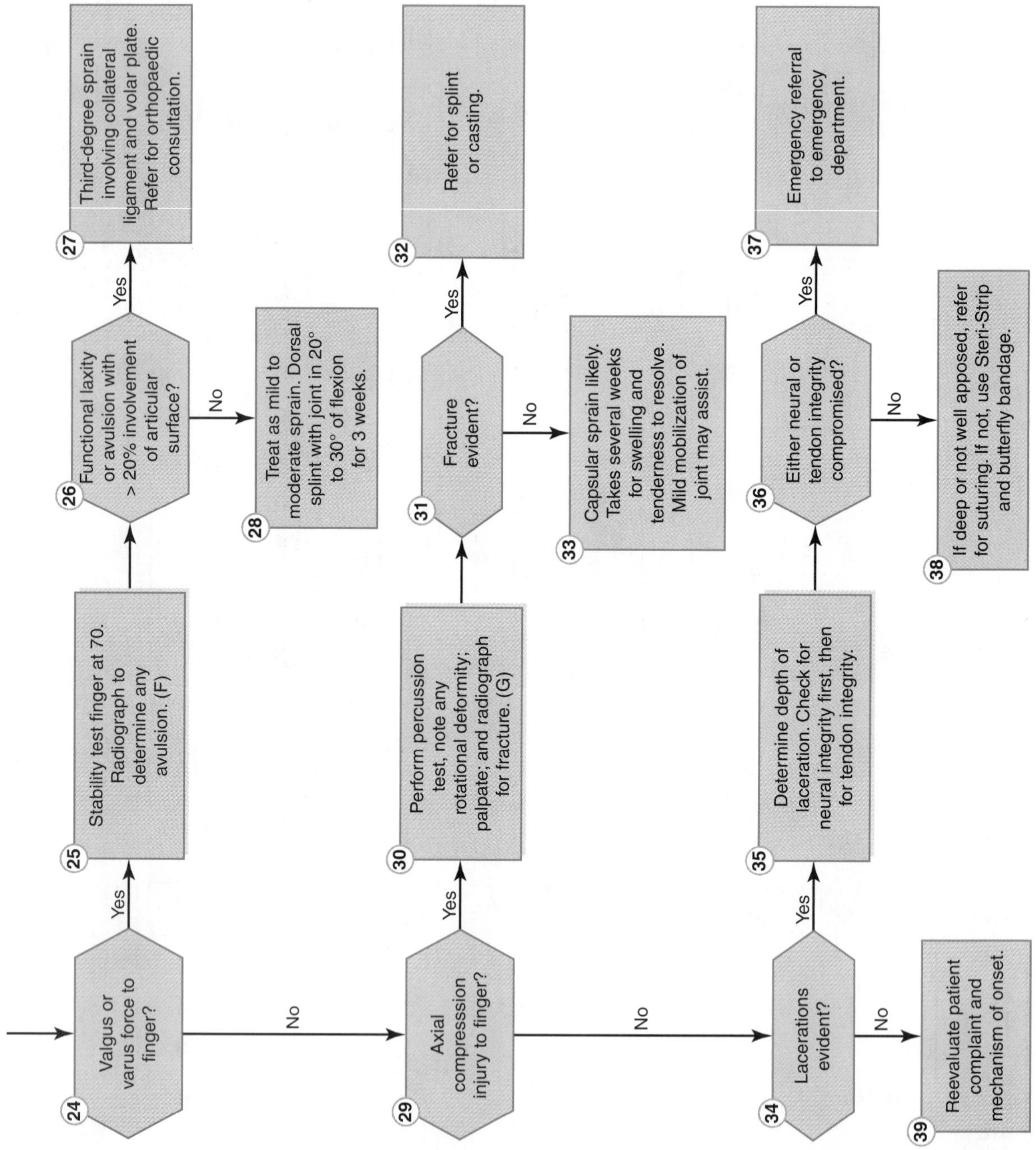

Figure 10–5 (Continued)

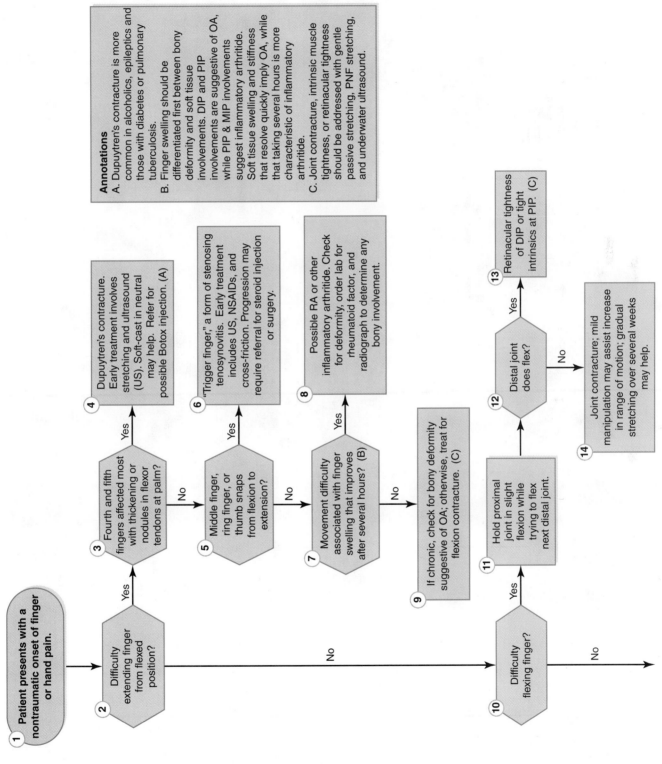

Figure 10–6 Nontraumatic Hand Pain—Algorithm

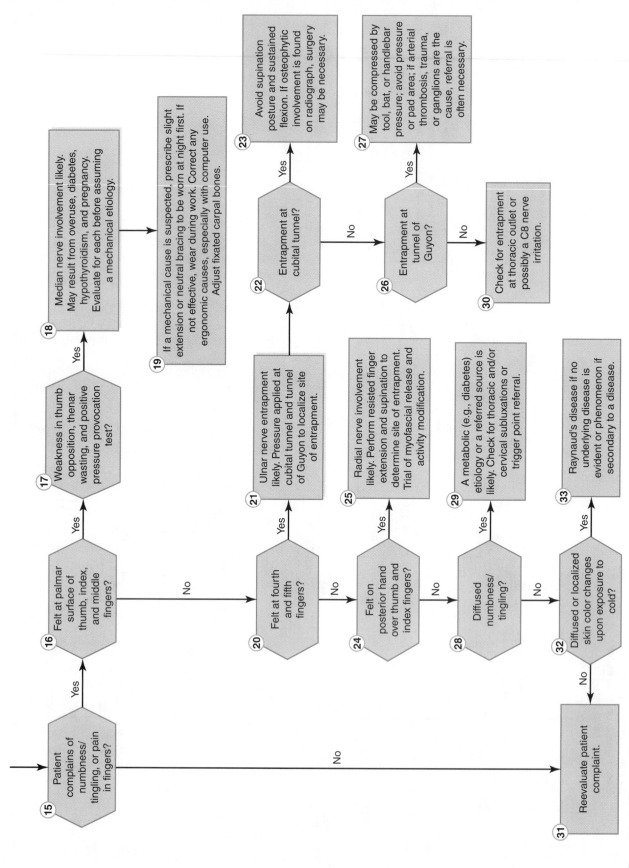

Figure 10–6 (Continued)

Selected Disorders of the Finger, Thumb, and Hand

A summary of the disorders discussed below is presented in **Table 10–2**.

FINGER

DISTAL INTERPHALANGEAL JOINT

Mallet Finger: Extensor Tendon Avulsion

Classic Presentation

A patient complains of distal finger pain after being hit on the end of the finger with a ball. The distal finger is dropped into a flexed position.

Cause

A compressive force on the tip of an extended finger, forcing it into flexion, causes avulsion of the extensor digitorum tendon. Commonly, this is due to a ball hitting the finger; often called "baseball finger."[14] Because of the drooping deformity, another pseudonym is drop finger.

Table 10–2 Summary of Hand Conditions

Name of Condition	Injury	Treatment
Boutonnière deformity	Flexion injury of PIP, tearing central slip; deformity is hyperextension of MCP and DIP with flexion of PIP.	PIP is splinted in extension for several weeks.
Pseudoboutonnière deformity	Extension injury of DIP with damage to volar plate.	Extension splinting; safety-pin splint.
Jersey finger	Avulsion of flexor digitorum profundus; hyperextension injury.	Usually surgery.
Mallet finger (baseball finger)	Hyperflexion injury to DIP.	Extension splinting of DIP for six to eight weeks.
Collateral ligament injury	Usually ulnar stress to a flexed MCP.	Remember to stress test at 70° and radiograph for possible fracture fragment. Splint PIP at 30° of flexion.
PIP joint dislocation (coach's finger)	Axial or extension force to middle phalanx.	Immobilize at 20°–30° of flexion for several weeks.
MCP dislocation	Dorsiflexion injury, usually tearing the volar plate.	Difficult to reduce; often requires anesthesia. Immobilize for three to four weeks.
Gamekeeper's thumb	MCP joint sprain of ulnar collateral ligament, usually due to hyperabduction or extension.	Tape with a cinch between thumb and first finger for several weeks.
Bennett's fracture	Fracture/dislocation of first metacarpal base.	Difficult to reduce due to pull of abductor pollicis longus. Usually need open reduction with fixation of fracture fragment.
Boxer's fracture (overlap definition with bar-room fracture dependent on source)	Hitting an object with an unprotected fist, usually fracture of the fifth or fourth metacarpal. Look for rotation or angular deformity. Percuss distal end of finger.	Gutter splint or hand cast for six weeks.

Evaluation

Active extension of the DIP joint is impossible; however, passive extension is usually accessible with some associated tenderness over the dorsum of the joint. Radiographic evaluation must include two planes of view to visualize clearly any degree of avulsion or epiphyseal fracture in immature athletes. The lateral view may also demonstrate subluxation (medial) at the joint. Two points of caution are, first, that the DIP joint may also be injured (central slip damage) and should always be included in the examination, and second, if a large piece of bone is avulsed, surgery may be necessary.

Management

Treatment involves splinting of the DIP joint in extension (not hyperextension) for up to six weeks.[15] Gradual active and passive range of motion exercises may then begin. This is followed by another six weeks of night and, if applicable, athletic splinting.[16] The PIP joint must not be included in the splinting to prevent contracture. It is imperative that the patient always keep the DIP joint in extension. He or she must remember this when changing finger splints.

Football or Jersey Finger: FDP Rupture

Classic Presentation

A patient complains of distal finger pain after getting his or her finger forcefully extended while grabbing a moving object.

Cause

Hyperextension of the DIP joint may result in rupture of the FDP tendon. Because of a common mechanism, this is often referred to as football or jersey finger, in which the finger (often the ring finger) is caught in an opponent's jersey.[17] While the athlete is grabbing the jersey, the opponent pulls away, exerting an extension force on the flexing finger. The degree of injury is based in part on how far the tendon has migrated, which may be as far as the palmar crease.

Evaluation

Acute evaluation requires testing of FDP function. This is accomplished by asking the patient to flex the DIP joint fully while the PIP joint is held in extension by the doctor. Inability to flex is diagnostic for rupture.

Management

Unlike many finger injuries, this injury requires immediate referral for surgical repair. Surgery has a better prognosis within the first three to four days postinjury.

Dislocation

Classic Presentation

A patient reports having the distal finger pulled out of place by a hyperextension injury. Pain and some deformity may be evident at the DIP joint. If the patient is an athlete, he or she may have had the dislocation reduced prior to presentation.

Cause

Disruption of the volar plate allows dorsal dislocation of the distal phalanx. Associated tendon or collateral ligament damage is possible.

Evaluation

Tenderness and dorsal deformity of the distal phalanx are seen in the acute presentation. Radiographs should always be taken to rule out any associated fractures. After reduction, it is imperative to check for damage to the collateral ligaments and for flexor/extensor tendon function.

Management

Reduction is accomplished with long-axis traction while gently increasing the deformity. After reduction, immobilization in a dorsal or volar splint (not including the PIP joint) for two to three weeks is sufficient. There is debate as to whether to splint in 30° of flexion or full extension. Following splinting, flexion exercises are begun while maintaining protective splinting during any sporting activities.[18]

PROXIMAL INTERPHALANGEAL JOINT

Central Slip Tear (Boutonnière Deformity)

Classic Presentation

The patient presents with pain at the PIP joint and an associated deformity after having an injury that involved forced flexion of the finger.

Cause

A hyperflexion injury of the PIP joint may result in tearing of the central slip of the extensor digitorum tendon. The lateral bands drop anteriorly and maintain the PIP in flexion while the DIP joint is extended.

Evaluation

There is pain and point tenderness at the PIP with associated swelling. Functionally, the PIP joint cannot be actively extended. Eventually, a boutonnière deformity occurs as hyperextension of the DIP and flexion of the PIP. At this point the DIP cannot be actively extended. Due to volar slippage of the lateral bands, active and passive flexion is not possible at the distal joint.[19]

Management

It is imperative that the PIP joint be immobilized with a finger splint in full extension for approximately six weeks. If not splinted properly, there will be no apposition of the torn ends of the central slip and deformity will result. This is often the case when loss of active extension is attributed to pain and the athlete is splinted in flexion for a collateral ligament sprain by an inexperienced coach/trainer/doctor. Due to the severity of the injury, an additional four to six weeks of splinting is necessary at night and during athletic activity (if applicable). When 45° of flexion and full extension are attained, the splinting may be discontinued.

Volar Plate Injury

Classic Presentation

The patient (often an athlete) complains of finger pain after his or her finger was pulled back or overextended by a ball or from a fall on an outstretched finger.

Cause

The volar plate on the anterior surface of the PIP is injured by a hyperextension injury to the finger.[20]

Evaluation

Pain and tenderness are found at the PIP joint. If chronic, a pseudoboutonnière deformity may result due to scar tissue formation and subsequent contracture with the PIP joint held in flexion. The distinction between a boutonnière and a pseudoboutonnière deformity is that normal mobility is present at the DIP with pseudoboutonnière deformity.[21]

Management

The PIP joint is splinted in 30° of flexion for four to five weeks. If unsuccessful, surgical referral should be made.

Dislocation

Classic Presentation

The patient complains of middle finger pain following a hyperextension injury (often in ball-handling sports). It is not unusual for a coach or trainer to reduce the joint with an assumption that the individual simply "jammed" the finger.

Cause

Hyperextension with some axial loading while the PIP joint is in extension causes volar plate rupture and often an avulsion fracture of the base of the middle phalanx.

Evaluation

Tenderness and deformity are found at the PIP joint if acute. After reduction, the MCP joint should be tested for active and passive range of motion. Static stability testing for collateral ligament and volar plate integrity must also be included. Radiographs are requisite to rule out associated fractures (especially when associated with an axial load or rotation injury).

Management

Reduction is accomplished by long-axis traction with gentle hyperextension of the PIP joint. If unsuccessful, refer for reduction with a local digital nerve block. Following reduction, ice and splint. A volar splint is applied with the finger held in 20° to 30° of flexion for two to three weeks. This is followed by buddy-taping for an additional two weeks, especially if participating in sports. Gentle active range of motion should be prescribed after the initial three weeks of splinting.

Collateral Ligament Sprain

Classic Presentation

A patient presents with a sports-related injury whereby the finger was pulled sideways (usually ulnar). The patient often reports that the finger "went out," but it either reduced spontaneously or was reduced by the patient.

Cause

A varus or valgus force stretches and tears the collateral ligament support at the PIP. The index finger is most often involved. The force is often sufficient to subluxate the joint medically; however, it often reduces spontaneously or is reduced by the patient, a coach, or a trainer.[22] Associated partial or complete rupture of the volar plate is possible depending on the magnitude of force.

Evaluation

Tenderness is found over the PIP collateral ligament and volar plate. Swelling is often rapid, leaving little time to test for stability. Stability testing should include varus and valgus attempts at two positions of flexion, 30° and 70°. Like all ligamentous injuries, there are varying degrees of damage. Radiographic demonstration of an avulsion fracture involving the volar plate is indicative of a rupture.

Management

With first- and second-degree sprains, the PIP is immobilized with a dorsal splint for two to four weeks in a 20° to 30° flexed position and may be buddy-taped to an adjacent finger for more stability. If a volar plate avulsion involves more than 20% of the articular surface, surgery may be indicated.[23]

Flexor Pulley Injuries (Rock Climber's Finger)
Classic Presentation

Patients present with a sudden onset of finger pain while rock climbing using a "crimp" position or shock-loading the fingers when they lost their footing.

Cause

A complex system of annular pulleys allows the flexor tendons to generate the greatest amount of force. There are five of these with one at each joint (MCP, PIP, and DIP) and two approximating the proximal and middle phalanx. These two fibro-osseous pulleys are designated A2 and A4 numbered from proximal to distal. These are loaded the most with climbing, and more eccentrically when the climber uses a crimp position of 90° to 100° of PIP flexion with hyperextension of the DIP. The A2 is the strongest able to withstand up to 400 N; however, strains can exceed 450 N when climbers fall and catch their weight by their fingers.

Evaluation

There is a report of sudden pain and swelling with occasionally a report of a pop at the time of injury. Tenderness is found over the involved areas. Like all soft tissue injuries, there are varying degrees of damage from partial tears to full rupture. Bowstringing, meaning the tendon has popped out of its restraining sleeve, will present as swelling on the flexor (palmar) surface usually of the proximal phalanx. There are no orthopaedic tests in-office to perform. MRI is not very useful; however, diagnostic ultrasound is and has become the gold standard allowing dynamic evaluation of movement of the tendon.

Management

Injuries have been classified into a system of Grade I through Grade IV.[24] Following is a description of each with the associated recommended treatment approach:

- Grade I—a pulley strain with no dehiscence of the tendon from bone (< 2 mm). Circumferential wrapping (or an H-type taping) around the distal end of the proximal phalanx with gradual return to full climbing over six weeks although continued taping up to three months is recommended.
- Grade II—either a complete rupture of the A4 pulley or partial rupture of the A2 or A3 pulleys. The same management approach as Grade I injuries is recommended.
- Grade III—complete rupture of the A2 or A3 pulleys. Immobilization in a thermoplastic splint or soft-cast ring for 10–14 days. This is followed by mild mobilization and protective taping with a return to climbing in six to eight weeks after injury using protective taping for up to six months.
- Grade IV—complex injuries involving ruptures and associated lumbrical muscle or collateral ligament injury. These require surgical repair that either includes a palmaris tendon graft or extensor retinaculum grafts. The latter are more difficult to perform and there appears to be no difference in outcome.

METACARPAL PHALANGEAL JOINT
Collateral Ligament Sprain
Classic Presentation

The patient presents with a complaint of pain at the MCP joint after a fall on the hand that stretched the associated finger to the side. The patient initially may not have sought help. Persistent pain and swelling usually prompt the patient to seek advice.

Cause

Tearing of the radial collateral ligament of the ulnar three digits is most common. When the ligament is most taut, the finger is in flexion. The finger is deviated away from the side of injury.

Evaluation

The MCP joint is most lax in full extension. Tautness increases with flexion; therefore, stress testing of the collateral ligaments with a varus and a valgus force is best accomplished at 70° of flexion. Radiographs should be taken to determine any associated fractures at the base of the proximal phalanx.

Management

Because of the support provided by the intrinsic muscles of the hand, lateral instability is not a strong concern. Immobilization in flexion for three weeks is followed by buddy-taping to the adjacent fingers for an additional three weeks. It is important not to splint in extension, which would allow shortening of the collaterals and a residual functional deficit in active and passive flexion.

Dislocation

Classic Presentation

The patient presents with pain and deformity at the MCP joint and proximal phalanx (dorsally positioned) following a hyperextension accident, often a fall on an outstretched hand.

Cause

Dislocation usually involves volar displacement of the metacarpal head through a rent in the volar plate. The metacarpal head is caught between the lumbricals, long flexors, and other soft tissue structures. Reduction is usually impossible because of this soft tissue blockage.[25] The little finger and index finger are most often involved.

Evaluation

Because of the volar displacement of the metacarpal head, the proximal phalanx is dislocated dorsally. This deformity, coupled with a prominence at the MCP joint on the palmar surface of the hand, is indicative of dislocation. Radiographs may demonstrate widening of the joint space (volar plate caught in the joint) or articular fracture at the MCP.

Management

MCP subluxations may be converted to a dislocation by an attempt at reduction. This occurs when using the standard procedure for dislocation of a phalanx; distraction with increasing the deformity into hyperextension. MCP dislocations should be referred for reductions.

Metacarpal Fractures

Classic Presentation

The patient presents with pain and often swelling over a metacarpal joint following either a direct blow or an axial compression force such as punching a wall with an unprotected hand. (*Author's note:* Patients often are embarrassed by the mechanism and often will give a fictitious history. The fracture is sometimes the result of taking out anger on an inanimate object.)

Cause

Fractures may be transverse, spiral, or oblique and may involve the base, neck, or shaft. Direct blows or axial compression forces are most common. Fracture of the neck of the fifth metacarpal is called a boxer's fracture.[26] There is some disagreement about the definition of and distinction between a boxer's fracture and a bar-room fracture. The lines have blurred and they seem to be used interchangeably.

Evaluation

Observation should include a search for rotational deformity evident at the MCP joint and with finger flexion. This is determined by noting nail alignment. Additionally, percussion of the extended finger or of the metacarpal with the fingers flexed often will increase pain. Radiographs usually indicate the type and extent of injury.

Management

Depending on the scope of practice in a given state, management with casting or stock appliances may be acceptable if there is no fracture displacement. If not within the scope of practice and experience of a chiropractor or if there is displacement, referral for reduction and possible wire or screw fixation should be made. In general, third and fourth metacarpal fractures are inherently more stable than first and fifth. A 40° volar angulation is often considered an acceptable "functional" deformity.

Dupuytren's Contracture

Classic Presentation

The patient complains of stiffening in his or her hand so that the little and ring fingers are progressively kept in a flexed position. The patient may be a musician, often a guitarist.

Cause

The cause is unknown. However, nodular thickening occurs in the flexor tendon, usually the fourth or fifth fingers. Eventually, the fingers become flexed at the MCP and PIP joints with the DIP joint held in extension. One predisposition that has been suggested is alcoholism.[27]

Evaluation

Inspection and palpation reveal a flexion deformity with nodularity and flexor tendon/fascial thickening on the palmar aspect of the hand. Early in the course, passive stretch into extension is possible.

Management

Early management includes avoidance or modification of any possible inciting activity. Constant stretching may be of benefit. One easy stretch is to sit on the hands. If not effective, immobilization at night with a soft cast to hold the fingers in neutral has been reported to be helpful. Failure of conservative care may require surgery if the contracture is significantly affecting activities of daily living or occupation. The surgery is technically difficult, however, and should be performed by a specialist.

Trigger Finger or Thumb

Classic Presentation

The patient presents with a complaint of his or her fingers getting "stuck" when trying to extend from a flexed position. She or he often reports having to extend the involved finger or thumb passively. The patient may have a history of chronic occupational over-use, especially grasping maneuvers.[28]

Cause

The flexor tendons of the fingers or thumb pass through a soft-tissue pulley system at the base of the proximal phalanx of the thumb or finger. Through inflammation, trauma, or congenital variation, the tendon sheath enlarges proximal to the pulley system and is caught as the finger or thumb moves into extension.[29] This is a form of stenosing tenosynovitis.

Evaluation

A discrete nodule is palpated at the base of the proximal phalanx of the involved finger or thumb. The nodule may be tender to pressure or gripping. Active extension is blocked and when possible causes a snapping action. If active extension is not possible, passive movement can accomplish extension accompanied with a snap as the nodule clears under the pulley.

Management

Conservative approaches include underwater ultrasound with stretching, cross-friction massage, and avoidance of aggravating activities. Failure of conservative care (trial of several months) should result in a referral for cortisone injection. The cure rate with one to two injections is 91% according to one study.[30] Failure with cortisone injection requires a referral for surgical release under local anesthesia.

THUMB

Gamekeeper's Thumb

Classic Presentation

The patient presents with pain at the base of the thumb and reports having fallen on the thumb, bending it back.

Cause

Abduction or hyperextension causes tearing of the ulnar collateral ligament at the MCP joint of the thumb (medial side of the thumb). Common scenarios include a fall on the hand or a ski pole injury whereby the strap pulls the thumb back. Athletes who are hit on the thumb by a ball (such as in volleyball, basketball, or football) may have the thumb hyperextended.

Evaluation

Tenderness and swelling are often found at the inside web space of the thumb. Stressing the thumb into extension or abduction is painful. The pain may be too great to allow stability testing. If stability testing is possible, pull the thumb into abduction, with the thumb in extension and also with slight flexion. Then test extension again with the thumb in extension and flexion.[31] If a complete tear is present, pinch strength between the thumb and index finger is lost. Radiographs should be taken with stress applied. If stress views demonstrate more than 35° abduction (subtracting starting position of abduction from stress position of abduction), a rupture is likely.[32] With physical examination and radiographs, always compare with the uninjured side.

Management

First-degree and mild second-degree tears are managed with immobilization and stabilization with thumb taping, including a cinching between the thumb and index finger for a few days to a week.[33] Bad second-degree tears are immobilized with a thumb spica for two to three weeks. Complete tears are referred as soon as possible for surgery.

Bowler's Thumb
Classic Presentation

The patient complains of pain, numbness, or tingling on the palmar surface of the thumb. He or she is often a bowler.

Cause

Constant irritation of the ulnar digital nerve of the thumb leads to perineural fibrosis. The irritation is from the edge of the thumb hole in the bowling ball of bowlers, or any utensil or tool that chronically compresses the nerve. Other mechanisms include overstretch of the thumb into extension acutely or chronically.[34]

Evaluation

Tapping of the nerve causes pain and sensory symptoms in the distal thumb. Tenderness of the proximal joint is often found. Passive extension may increase symptoms.

Management

Padding of the volar thumb area will decrease any compressive force. Enlargement of the thumb hole on a bowling ball may help. Taping or bracing the thumb to prevent extension of the thumb may help if the underlying mechanism is stretch. Modification of any inciting activity is the main goal.

Dislocation
Classic Presentation

The patient presents with pain and deformity at the base of the thumb following a hyperextension injury.

Cause

Hyperextension tears the volar plate, allowing proximal phalanx dislocation dorsally.

Evaluation

Tenderness and deformity are found at the base of the thumb with posteriority of the proximal phalanx. Radiographs are necessary to determine any associated fracture.

Management

Reduction may be possible, avoiding straight traction, which may cause the volar plate to be caught in the joint. Push the dorsal aspect of the proximal phalanx in a volar direction while pushing the metacarpal dorsally to acquire reduction. If unsuccessful, refer for reduction under local block or open reduction. Postreduction, the joint is immobilized in a gutter splint or thumb spica for two to three weeks. Cautious range of motion exercises are then begun and progressively increased to resisted exercise for two to four weeks. Return to play may require a fiberglass cast for two weeks if allowed by the specific sport rules.

Bennett's Fracture
Classic Presentation

A patient presents in acute, severe pain following a fall or blow that caused axial compression to the thumb. There is deformity and rapid swelling.

Cause

Axial compression causes a transarticular fracture at the first metacarpal base. A triangular fragment of bone is held in place by the volar ligament while the shaft dislocates over it. The dislocated section is held out of place by the action of the abductor pollicis longus.

Evaluation

Deformity and swelling are usually severe, warranting immediate radiographic examination.

Management

Referral is required for open reduction and pinning.

ARTHRITIDES

Rheumatoid Arthritis

Classic Presentation

The patient is often a woman (aged 20 to 40 years) who complains of finger or wrist pain. She says that the joints are swollen and that in the morning it takes over an hour for her to be able to move her fingers comfortably. There is often an associated complaint of fatigue and possible weight loss.

Cause

RA is an autoimmune disorder causing an inflammatory arthritis characterized by bilateral distribution often beginning in the hand (PIP and MCP joints). At the joint a reactive pannus forms, causing swelling and eventual erosion. Genetic predisposition is based on the patient's possessing the class 2 human leukocyte antigen (HLA).

Evaluation

When the disease is active, the joints are often warm, swollen, and tender. Finding symmetric involvement adds weight to the suspicion of RA. Other joints commonly involved include the wrists, knees, ankles, and toes. Later changes include flexor contractures and ulnar deviation of the fingers. Laboratory findings include a positive rheumatoid factor (IgM antibody found in 75% of patients), elevated erythrocyte sedimentation rate (ESR), C-reactive protein, and an associated anemia (often hypochromic and normocytic). Radiographic findings usually confirm the diagnosis; however, these are not evident in the early stages of the disease. The early changes include soft tissue swelling and juxta-articular demineralization. Eventually, uniform loss of joint space and joint erosions become apparent. Particular concern for the chiropractor is involvement of the transverse ligament at the dens of C2. This may lead to instability and would be a contraindication to upper cervical adjusting. An evaluation of the atlantodental interspace is necessary to determine stability of the C2-C1 articulation visible on a lateral view.

Management

It is important to remember two factors regarding the natural course of RA in patients: (1) those with active disease have periods of exacerbation and remission that are usually unpredictable, and (2) 50% to 75% of patients presenting with RA will experience a remission within two years.[35] Various medical approaches are used during acute RA episodes, including aspirin and other nonsteroidal anti-inflammatory drugs (NSAIDs), methotrexate, sulfasalazine, antimalarial drugs (Plaquenil), and—in difficult cases—gold salts (chrysotherapy) (e.g., Aurolate). Injectable gold is now seldom used due to high toxicity potential. A short course of corticosteroid (prednisone) treatment often will dramatically improve the symptoms; however, it will not alter the course of the RA. A special class of medications used in the management of rheumatoid and rheumatoid-like inflammation are disease-modifying antirheumatic drugs (DMARDs). DMARDs are prescribed either as sequential monotherapy, step-up therapy, induction therapy, or a more individually targeted approach of tight control There are two classifications: biologics and nonbiologics. The older nonbiologics include drugs such as methotrexate, cyclosporine, and sulfasalazine. The biologics work off different principles. Delivery is either through self-injection subcutaneously (SQ) or through infusion therapy. Biologics are genetically engineered proteins used to address one of several aspects of immune regulation. The most common are anti-TNF inhibitors such as Cimzia, Enbrel, Humira, Remicade, and Simponi.

Conservative approaches involve passive mobilization of the joints through a pain-free range of motion. Avoidance of thrusting into inflamed joints is crucial in preventing aggravation of RA.

Psoriatic Arthritis

Classic Presentation

The patient complains of unilateral finger pain and swelling of nontraumatic origin. The patient may also complain of sacroiliac pain. The patient will have either a past diagnosis of psoriasis or a secondary complaint of skin lesions on the extensor surfaces of the arms and/or legs or scalp.

Cause

Psoriatic arthritis is a seronegative arthritis, meaning it is negative for rheumatoid factor (as are Reiter's syndrome and ankylosing spondylitis). There is a genetic predisposition associated with various HLA subtypes. Only 20% of patients with psoriasis have arthritis associated with their condition.[36] The arthritis can be mild or fulminant (arthritis mutilans).

Evaluation

A search for skin lesions should be made in patients with a new, nontraumatic arthritis. Eighty percent of psoriatic arthritis patients have skin lesions prior to the onset of arthritis. The skin lesions may be quite obvious as silvery scales on the extensor surfaces of the arms and legs or subtle patches in the gluteal cleft, scalp, or umbilicus. In general, the more pronounced or involved the skin lesions, the worse the arthritis (when associated with arthritis). Involvement of the fingers or toes may create a "sausage" appearance. Laboratory evaluation is negative for rheumatoid factor (seronegative). ESR and uric acid levels may be elevated during the active phase. HLA B-27 is found in almost half of patients; however, it is nonspecific, given that ankylosing spondylitis may coexist with psoriatic arthritis. HLA B-17, Bw38, and Bw39 are also found. Radiographically, marginal erosions, especially of the DIP and PIP joints, are common with tuft erosion causing a sharpened pencil appearance. Fluffy periosteal bone may be visible along the shafts of the metacarpals and phalanges. The sacroiliac involvement may be evident in 15% to 20% of patients. Atypical syndesmophytes appearing on the anterior vertebral body may be evident also.

Management

Medical treatment is similar to that for RA except that antimalarial agents may exacerbate psoriatic arthritis. Drugs used to treat both RA and the seronegative disorders like psoriatic arthritis are called DMARDs. If dermatologically more severe (measured by the Psoriasis Area Severity Index [PASI]) or when arthritis is present, cyclosporine, methotrexate, and acitretin are used with a 75% improvement in skin lesions. Methotrexate is associated with hepatic toxicity, cyclosporine with hypertension and nephrotoxicity, and acitretin with elevated serum lipids, mucocutaneous toxicity, and teratogenicity.[37] As a result, 40% of patients feel frustrated by the inadequacy of treatment, with 32% considering the treatment too aggressive.[38] Highly promising new drugs are being marketed, but they are extremely expensive, costing as much as $26,000 annually. These drugs are part of a new class of medications called immune modulators (also known as biological response modifiers or "biologics").[39] Their advantage may be the avoidance of adverse effects on organs or adverse drug reactions; however, their long-term effect on immunosuppression is unknown. Examples are alefacept and etanercept.[40] The ending of "-cept" is an indication of the drug's effect, which is fusion of a receptor to the Fc portion of human IgGI. Finally, drugs designed to prevent T-cell activation with CTLA4lg are being developed. Delivery is either through self-injection subcutaneously (SQ) or through infusion therapy. Biologics are genetically engineered proteins used to address one of several aspects of immune regulation:

- Anti-TNF inhibitors—Cimzia, Enbrel, Humira, Remicade, and Simponi
- T-cell inhibitors—Orencia
- IL-6 inhibitors—Actemra

There are no studies discussing the chiropractic management of this arthritis.

APPENDIX 10–1

References

1. Lampe EW. Surgical anatomy of the hand. *Clin Symp.* 1969;21:32–33.
2. Kapandji JA. *The Physiology of the Joints.* New York: Churchill Livingstone; 1970:1.
3. Posner MA, Kaplan EB. Osseous and ligamentous structures. In: Spinner M, ed. *Kaplan's Functional and Surgical Anatomy of the Hand.* Philadelphia: JB Lippincott; 1984:23–51.
4. Posner MA. Hand injuries. In: Nicholas JA, Hershman EB, Posner MA, eds. *The Upper Extremity in Sports Medicine.* St. Louis, MO: Mosby; 1990:495–594.
5. Eaton RG. Acute and chronic ligamentous injuries of the fingers and thumb. In: Tubiana R, ed. *The Hand.* Philadelphia: WB Saunders; 1985;2:877.
6. Gonzalez SM, Gonzalez RI. Dupuytren's disease. *West J Med.* 1990;152:430.
7. Gerstner DL, Omer GE. Hand injuries: evaluation and initial management. *J Musculoskeletal Med.* 1988;10:19–29.
8. Ruby LK. Common hand injuries in the athlete. Symposium on sports injuries. *Orthop Clin North Am.* 1980;11:819–839.
9. Corely FH. Commonly missed fractures in the hand and wrist. *J Musculoskeletal Med.* 1993;10:55–68.
10. McCue FC III, Mayer V, Moran DJ. Gamekeeper's thumb: ulnar collateral ligament rupture. *J Musculoskeletal Med.* 1988;12:53–63.
11. Peyron JG. Osteoarthritis: the epidemiologic viewpoint. *Clin Orthop Rel Res.* 1986;213:117–123.
12. American Society for Surgery of the Hand. *The Hand: Examination and Diagnosis.* 2nd ed. New York: Churchill Livingstone; 1983.
13. Katz WA. Hands and wrists. In: Katz WA, ed. *Rheumatic Diseases: Diagnosis and Management.* 2nd ed. Philadelphia: JB Lippincott; 1988.
14. McCue FC, Baugher WH, Bourland WL, et al. Hand injuries in athletes. *Surg Rounds.* 1978;1:8.
15. Stark HH, Boyes JH, Wilson JN. Mallet finger. *J Bone Joint Surg Am.* 1962;44:62.
16. Vetter WL. How I manage mallet finger. *Physician Sportsmed.* 1989;17:140.
17. McCue FC, Cabrera JM. Common athletic digital joint injuries of the hand. In: Strickland JW, Rettig AC, eds. *Hand Injuries in Athletes.* Philadelphia: W B Saunders; 1992:49–94.
18. Kahler DM, McCue FC III. Metacarpophalangeal and proximal interphalangeal joint injuries of the hand including the thumb. *Clin Sports Med.* 1992;11:57–76.
19. Boyes JH. *Bunnel's Surgery of the Hand.* 5th ed. Philadelphia: JB Lippincott; 1970:439.
20. McCue FC, Honner R, Gieck JH, et al. A pseudoboutonnière deformity. *J Br Soc Surg Hand.* 1975;7:166.
21. Ruby LK. Common hand injuries in the athlete. *Orthop Clin North Am.* 1980;33:819.
22. McCue FC, Andrews JR, Hakala M. The coach's finger. *J Sports Med.* 1974;2:270–275.
23. Rettig AC. Hand injuries in football players: soft tissue trauma. *Physician Sportsmed.* 1991;19:97–107.
24. Crowley TP. The flexor tendon pulley system and rock climbing. *J Hand Microsurg.* 2012;4(1):25-29.
25. Green DP, Terry GC. Complex dislocation of the metacarpophalangeal joint: correlative pathological anatomy. *J Bone Joint Surg Am.* 1973;55:1480–1486.
26. McKerrel J, Bowen V, Johnston G, et al. Boxer's fractures: conservative or operative management? *J Trauma.* 1987;(26)4:27–48.
27. Burgess RC, Watson HK. Stenosing tenosynovitis in Dupuytren's contracture. *J Hand Surg Am.* 1987;12:89.
28. Osterman AL, Moskow L, Low DW. Soft-tissue injuries of the hand and wrist in racquet sports. *Clin Sports Med.* 1988;7:329–348.
29. Hueston JT, Wilson WF. The etiology of trigger finger. *Hand.* 1972;4:257–260.
30. Marks MR, Gunther SF. Efficacy of cortisone injection in treatment of trigger finger and thumbs. *J Hand Surg Am.* 1989;14:722–727.
31. McCue F, Garroway R. Sports injuries to the hand and wrist. In: Schneider RC, Kennedy JC, Plant ML, eds. *Sports Injuries: Management, Prevention, and Treatment.* Baltimore: Williams & Wilkins; 1984:752–759.
32. Gerber C, Senn E, Matter P. Skier's thumb: surgical treatment of recent injuries in the ulnar collateral ligament of the thumb's metacarpophalangeal joint. *Am J Sports Med.* 1981;9:171.
33. Gieck JH, Mayer V. Protective splinting for the hand and wrist. *Clin Sports Med.* 1986;5:801.
34. Dobyn JH, O'Brien ET, Linschied RL, et al. Bowler's thumb: diagnosis and treatment: review of seventeen cases. *J Bone Joint Surg Am.* 1972;54:751–755.
35. Hellman DB. Arthritis and musculoskeletal disorders. In: Tierney LM Jr, McPhee SJ, Papadakis MA, eds. *Current Medical Diagnosis and Treatment.* 34th ed. Norwalk, CT: Appleton & Lange; 1995:711.

36. Espinoza LR. Psoriatic arthritis: clinical response and side-effects of methotrexate therapy. *J Rheumatol.* 1992;19:872.

37. Cather J, Menter A. Novel therapies for psoriasis. *Am J Clin Dermatol.* 2002;3:159–173.

38. Krueger GG, Koo J, Lebwohl M, et al. The impact of psoriasis on quality of life. *Arch Dermatol.* 2001;137:280–284.

39. Ellis CN, Krueger GG. Treatment of chronic plaque psoriasis by selective targeting of memory effector lymphocytes. *N Engl J Med.* 2001;345(4):248–255.

40. Krueger GG, Papp KA, Stough DB, et al. A randomized, double-blind, placebo-controlled phase III study evaluating efficacy and tolerability of 2 courses of alefacept in patients with chronic plaque psoriasis. *J Am Acad Dermatol.* 2002;47:821–833.

APPENDIX 10-2

Wrist and Hand Diagnosis Table

Diagnosis	Comments	History Findings	Positive Examination Findings	Radiography/Special Studies	Treatment Options
Subluxation or Fixation of: Carpometacarpal Joint Metacarpal/phalangeal Joint Interphalangeal Joint	• Should be used when chiropractic manipulation is used as Tx for any wrist/hand problem/Dx. • Can be primary Dx if patient is asymptomatic or mildly symptomatic (e.g., mild stiffness or pain level < 2/10). • Must indicate chiropractic exam findings to support Dx.	*Nonspecific*	*Palpation*—Local tenderness or other signs of subluxation. *Ortho*—None *Neuro*—None *Active ROM*—Variable restriction *Passive ROM*—End-range restriction *Motion palpation*—Specific articular restriction or symptoms produced on end-range	• Radiography not required for the diagnosis of subluxation. • Radiographic biomechanical analysis may assist in treatment decisions.	• Chiropractic adjustive technique • Decisions regarding specifically which technique(s) is/are applied and modifications to the given approach will be directed by the primary Dx and patient's ability to tolerate preadjustment stresses.
Carpal Sprain/Strain Carpalmetacarpal Joint Sprain Metacarpal/Phalangeal Joint Sprain Interphalangeal Joint Sprain Note: Sprain/strain is not synonymous with spasm or hypertonicity.	• Codes are used for either strain of a muscle/tendon or sprain of a ligament. • Note, however, that tendon overuse generally would fall under general tendinitis or insertional tendinitis.	*Mechanism*—Overstretch or over-contraction acute event; often a fall on hand/wrist or direct blow to area	*Ortho*—Each joint is tested by testing stability (often reproduces mechanism of injury); positives include pain and/or instability. Specific tests for carpal bones include Watson's, Ballotement, and shuck tests. *Active ROM*—Pain or weakness may be reported *Passive ROM*—Pain on end-range stretch of ligament	• Radiography generally recommended to rule out any associated fracture. • Stress radiographs may be needed. • CT, fluoroscopy, or MRI may be needed to detect degree of damage when instability or pain is persistent.	• With severe sprains, referral to orthopaedist may be required; for less severe, the following is applicable: —Orthotic support (taping or brace) —Ergonomic advice —Strengthening and preventive exercises —Myofascial therapy

Condition	Description	Clinical Findings	Diagnostic Testing	Treatment
Carpal Tunnel Syndrome	• Carpal tunnel is one site of compression of the median nerve. It is important to differentiate from other sites of entrapment.	*Onset*—Usually insidious onset of numbness and tingling on palmar surface of thumb and first 2½ digits; paresthesias are often worse with sleeping *Ortho*—Positives for reproduction of complaint with Tinel's or compression testing, Phalen's, reversed Phalen's; weakness of pinch and/or grip strength *Neuro*—Possible hypoesthesia in palmar area of thumb and first 2½ digits; thenar atrophy in chronic cases *Motion palpation*—Possible restriction of lunate or distal radioulnar joint	• Radiography not used for Dx unless traumatic in onset. • Electrodiagnostic testing will demonstrate a decrease in nerve conduction velocity with an increase in latency.	• Myofascial therapy may be helpful. • Nutrition advice may include B6. • Neutral or cock-up splint worn initially at night to relieve symptoms. • Address any ergonomic considerations such as keyboard or mouse usage.
Tendinitis of Wrist	• Usually a result of overuse.	*Mechanism*—Often no Hx of trauma; chronic repetitive microtrauma is most common cause; establish causative activity *Worse with specific ROM*—ROM that uses tendon action most is painful (e.g., active extension is painful with extensor carpi radialis tendinitis) *Palpation*—Tenderness found at insertion point or origin. *Active ROM*—Resisted testing of involved muscle/tendon pattern reproduces complaint *Passive ROM*—End-range stretch in opposite direction of contraction pattern may elicit pain	• Radiography not usually necessary initially except to rule out fracture/dislocation with acute trauma.	• Limited orthotic support. • Physiotherapy for pain and swelling control. • Herbal recommendations for pain and swelling. • Modify inciting activity. • Strengthen tendon with emphasis on eccentric movements.
de Quervain's Tenosynovitis	• May be confused with intersection syndrome with involvement of extensor tendons proximal to wrist.	*Mechanism*—Tenosynovitis of the abductor pollicis longus and extensor pollicis brevis; due to repetitive activities involving ulnar deviation of the wrist; also seen in pregnancy *Ortho*—Finkelstein's test is positive for pain at anatomical snuff-box	• Radiography not usually indicated.	• In early stages, ice, immobilization, and electrotherapy may be helpful. • In later stages when stenosis occurs, conservative care is less effective.

(continues)

Wrist and Hand Diagnosis Table (continued)

Diagnosis	Comments	History Findings	Positive Examination Findings	Radiography/Special Studies	Treatment Options
Trigger Finger	• May be secondary to a chronic tendinitis or develop insidiously. • Considered a form of stenosing tenosynovitis.	*Mechanism*—Nodule develops in flexor tendon and is caught in soft-tissue pulley on flexor surface *History*—Gradual development of difficult movement of finger, in particular into extension that may be blocked	*Palpation*—Often a tender nodule is palpable at base of proximal phalanx *Active ROM*—Flexion may be limited; however, extension is blocked or snapping occurs during movement	• Radiography not used for diagnosis.	• Mild, constant stretching. • Physiotherapy may assist in decreasing size of nodule. • Nodules that do not resolve may respond to a cortisone injection. • If an underlying mechanism can be established, modify or eliminate.
Extensor Tendon Rupture Mallet Finger	• It is important to not dismiss the problem as a simple sprain due to mallet finger complications associated with tendon rupture or fracture. • Also check for possible central slip tearing of PIP joint.	*Mechanism*—Compressive force on tip of extended finger forcing it into flexion causing avulsion of extensor digitorum tendon	*Observation*—Distal joint may be in a flexed or "dropped" position *Ortho*—Active extension of DIP joint is impossible	• Radiographs are required, with two planes of view to visualize any bony avulsion or epiphyseal fracture in younger patients; large bony avulsion usually is an indication of the need for surgical correction.	• Splinting of DIP joint in extension for up to six weeks. • Gradual active and passive ROM exercises may then begin. • Follow with six weeks of night and/or athletic splinting.
Central Slip Tear	• Avulsion of tendon at PIP will eventually result in Boutonnière's Deformity if not managed appropriately. • Caution that injury is not misdiagnosed as simple finger sprain.	*Mechanism*—Hyperflexion injury of PIP joint tears central slip of ED tendon as lateral bands drop anteriorly; the PIP joint is held in flexion with DIP joint extended	*Palpation*—Tenderness at PIP joint; possible swelling *Ortho*—Active extension of PIP not possible	• Radiographs should be ordered to rule out any bony avulsion or epiphyseal injury.	• PIP joint splinted in extension for six weeks. • Additional four to six weeks of night and/or athletic splinting.
Flexor Digitorum Tendon Rupture (Football or Jersey Finger)	• Caution that this injury results in tendon migration as far as into the hand.	*Mechanism*—Hyperextension of DIP joint resulting in rupture of the FDP rupture	*Ortho*—Patient unable to actively flex the DIP joint	• Radiographs should be ordered to rule out any bony avulsion.	• Refer for surgical reattachment (best results in three to four days post-injury).

Volar Plate Injury	*Mechanism*—Hyperextended finger causes tearing of volar plate on palmar surface of PIP joint	*Palpation*—Tenderness on volar plate of involved finger *Ortho*—No consistent finding; however, resisted flexion or passive extension may increase pain	• Radiographs should be ordered to rule out any bony avulsion or epiphyseal injury.	• PIP joint is splinted in 30° of flexion for four to five weeks. • If unsuccessful, surgical referral may be needed.
	• Caution that injury is not misdiagnosed as simple finger sprain and not properly splinted, leading to a pseudoboutonnière's deformity (flexion at PIP with normal DIP).			
Ganglion	*Cause*—It is thought that repetitive microtrauma causes ganglions to develop in either the capsule or tendons of the wrist or dorsal scapholunate ligament	*Palpation*—A tender nodule may be evident on palpation (most common on dorsum of wrist) *Ortho*—Passive dorsiflexion may make pain worse	• Radiographs not recommended.	• Attempts at compression to rupture the capsule of the ganglion should be applied cautiously. • Surgical excision if persistent or unresponsive.
	• Ganglions have a tendency to increase and decrease in size regardless of treatment approach.			
Raynaud's Syndrome	*Cause*—Abnormality of sympathetic NS affecting vascularity in fingers; exposure to cold leads to pain	*Signs/Symptoms*—Exposure to cold results in a triphasic response of pallor, cyanosis, and reactive redness (hyperemia) *Test*—Allen's test may show occlusion of radial artery if due to disease	• Radiographs not recommended.	• Treatment based on underlying cause; if due to a known disease, treatment of disease is recommended. • Avoidance of sympathetic stimulation and exposure to cold with appropriate protection are conservative options. • Failure to respond should result in medical referral.
	• May be associated with other disorders (Raynaud's disease) or may be idiopathic (Raynaud's phenomenon).			
Gamekeeper's Thumb	*Mechanism*—Hyperextension or hyperabduction of thumb may result in tearing of the ulnar collateral ligament	*Ortho*—Passive extension or abduction recreates pain on the medial aspect of the thumb and may indicate laxity	• Radiographs should be ordered to determine if there are any associated avulsion fragments; stress radiographs may also be ordered.	• Taping or splinting of mild to moderate injuries for two to three weeks will usually allow sufficient healing. • Injury associated with full rupture (laxity) or bony avulsion may require surgical consult.
	• Patients have pain on the inside of the thumb.			

(continues)

Wrist and Hand Diagnosis Table (continued)

Diagnosis	History Findings	Positive Examination Findings	Radiography/Special Studies	Comments	Treatment Options
Myofasciitis	Nonspecific	Trigger points are evident as localized tenderness in a muscle that corresponds to traditional (Travell/Simons) trigger point charts. These points may be local or refer pain when compressed.	• Not required or recommended.	• Used when specific trigger points are identified on physical examination. • Also may be used if a strain is not evident from the history but there are indications of muscle tenderness, stiffness, or pain.	• Myofascial approaches such as myofascial stripping, trigger point massage, or spray and stretch approaches are the standard. • Home stretching and modification of activity suggestions.
Laxity Hypermobility	A history of a single event, traumatic injury to the joint is not found; however, either overuse (microtrauma) or generalized inherent looseness is evident	Capsular or ligament testing reveals "looseness" that falls within the physiologic range of normal.	• Not usually recommended unless when differentiating pathological laxity from congenital or overuse acquisition.	• May represent inherent looseness in the joint or acquired secondary to injury.	• Strengthening program • Bracing or functional taping during rehabilitation or during strenuous activities.

Hip, Groin, and Thigh Complaints

Context

Although the hip and shoulder are the most proximal joints of their respective limbs, the hip is unique in several aspects. Unlike the shoulder, the hip is quite stable and requires a major force to cause a dislocation. Although common shoulder problems are often soft-tissue generated, the hip is more prone to bone or joint damage. As a weight-bearing joint it is commonly affected by degenerative changes and fracture in senior patients. Disorders of the hip are probably more age-related than any other joint. Many presentations fit an age-related categorization: congenital disorders in the infant, growth plate and vascular etiologies in the adolescent, trauma in the young adult, and fracture or arthritis in the elderly. The diagnosis of many of these disorders is dependent on radiographic confirmation.

Patients often claim hip pain when, in fact, the pain is in either the low back or buttocks. It is important, as with all pain, to have the patient localize the problem. Hip pain may be due to intrinsic pathology of the hip joint or referred from a number of geographically and neurally related structures. Associated pain in the lumbopelvic or abdominal areas often will identify the source, but not always. The overlap with groin pain extends the diagnostic list substantially. Pain in the groin also may be caused by local pathology or referred from the hip, pelvis, genitals, or abdomen. Associated signs or symptoms will usually help differentiate between mechanical and visceral sources.

A common traumatic history is a fall onto the hip. This often results in soft tissue injury such as a contusion or a trochanteric bursitis. Fracture should be ruled out, in particular in the senior patient. An insidious onset of hip pain is suggestive of osteoarthritic changes in the middle-aged or senior adult. In the child or adolescent, avascular necrosis, slipped epiphysis, or a reactive synovitis should be considered. With children it is important to remember that the knee is a common referral site for hip disorders.

Thigh pain is often differentiated on the basis of a history of either direct trauma (contusion) or sudden-movement onset (strain). When anterior numbness, paresthesias, or weakness are complaints, femoral nerve involvement should be evaluated. Lateral sensory complaints usually represent lateral femoral cutaneous nerve (meralgia paresthetica) involvement or trigger point referral. Posterior neurologic complaints suggest sciatic nerve irritation, referral from trigger points, or lumbar/sacral facet problems.

General Strategy

History

- Determine what the patient means by "hip" pain (groin, buttocks, hip, pelvis, etc.).
- Localize the pain to a quadrant of lateral, medial, anterior, or posterior pain.
- Determine whether any overt trauma occurred such as a fall on the hip (in younger patients, suspect a slipped epiphysis or an avascular process; in the elderly, a fracture).
- If there was trauma, determine whether the patient can bear weight; if not, radiographs including anteroposterior (AP) and lateral (frog-leg) views are essential.
- If there was a sudden onset with sporting activity, determine the mechanism (in younger patients consider an apophysitis).

- Determine whether there is a history of overuse (suspicion of a stress fracture in a high-level athlete; myofascial problems in all patients).
- Determine whether there are any associated visceral complaints (radiation of pain from the back to the groin is suggestive of renal disease; from the groin to the hip suggests genitourinary disease or hernia).

Evaluation

- Determine whether there is a range of motion (ROM) restriction suggestive of capsular involvement of the hip (internal rotation and extension), a positive FABER (flexion, abduction, external rotation) test, or increased pain by axial compression into the joint (found with synovitis of various causes and with osteoarthritis [OA]).
- Determine whether there is associated anteversion/ retroversion or asymmetric restrictions in either passive external or internal rotation.
- If groin pain is the complaint, test adductors and hip flexors to determine strain, palpate for tenderness at attachment sites of muscles, and palpate for hernias in patients with chronic pain made worse with straining; if pain is radiating to the groin from the back, perform a kidney punch test; palpate lymph nodes if genital complaints or lesions are present.
- If snapping around the hip is the complaint, determine the location and determine on which ROM the snapping or popping occurs (adduction for iliotibial band syndrome snapping, abduction for iliopectineal or psoas snapping).
- Determine whether there are other musculoskeletal complaints (may be a clue to hip pain being the result of accommodation to other lower extremity or low back problem).
- Radiographs of the hip should be ordered if an obvious soft tissue cause is not evident or if pain is trauma-induced; include AP and frog-leg (lateral) views.
- Determine whether further imaging techniques are appropriate (bone scan with suspicion of stress fracture or synovitis; magnetic resonance imaging [MRI] if there is a suspicion of tumor or infection; computed tomography [CT] scan if there is a suspicion of a pelvic fracture).

Management

- Refer cases to the appropriate medical specialist if any of the following are found: fracture, avascular necrosis, dislocation, tumor, infection, or hernia.
- Management of soft tissue problems involves stretching, myofascial release techniques, appropriate exercise, and preventive approaches through correction of any underlying biomechanical faults.
- OA is managed initially with physical therapy modalities and possibly manipulation; long-term management involves a strengthening program for the hip and thigh.

Relevant Anatomy

As essentially a ball-and-socket joint, the hip shares with the shoulder a great degree of movement capability. Unlike the shoulder, however, the hip is a primary weight bearer and as such is more prone to acute and chronic consequences of trauma such as degenerative changes, fractures, and synovitis. As a weight-bearing joint, the effect of femoral head fit and positioning is crucial to proper function. The angulation of the femoral head is referred to as *version*. When the hip is determined to be anteverted, the femoral head faces forward (with relative posterior positioning of the greater trochanter). With retroversion the angulation of the femoral head faces backward with positioning of the greater trochanter anteriorly. These angulations place a biomechanical demand on the bones and joints below. In growing children and adolescents, these demands may result in compensations that may cause torsion of the femur or tibia and foot compensations of pronation or supination. Another mechanical factor is the angulation of the neck of the femur. An increased angle (coxa valga) or decreased angle (coxa vara) is age-related or may be changed by fracture or pathology of the femoral neck. The angle normally decreases from birth (average of 160°) to adulthood (average of 120°).

The hip is inherently stable because of its articulation with the pelvis and the thick support of musculature. The capsule is supported by the iliofemoral and pubofemoral ligaments anteriorly and the iliofemoral and ischiofemoral ligaments posteriorly (**Figure 11–1**). Ligaments tighten on extension and are more relaxed in

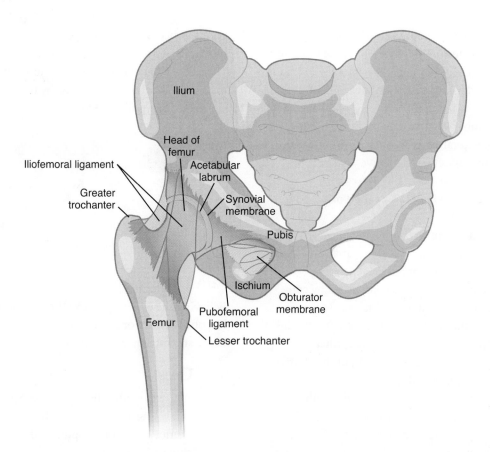

Figure 11–1 The ligamentous support of the hip. Anterior view showing main ligaments; coronal section showing articular cavity and capsule.

flexion. Specifically, the iliofemoral ligament tightens in hip external rotation and adduction, the ischiofemoral ligament tightens in hip internal rotation and abduction, and the pubofemoral ligament tightens in hip external rotation and abduction. Although these capsular ligaments are substantial enough to require macro trauma to damage them with a single traumatic event, it is becoming evident that repetitive hip external rotation as seen in such activities as ballet, golf, gymnastics, martial arts, and baseball may lead to capsular laxity through microtrauma.[1] This focal rotational laxity, as it is referred to, contrasts with the more global laxity seen with connective tissue disorders such as Down's, Marfan's, and Ehlers-Danlos syndromes among others.

The ligamentum teres is a unique structure that attaches at the fovea capitis of the femoral head and the acetabular notch. It tightens during adduction, flexion, and external rotation.[2] Damage to the ligamentum teres appears to be far more common than once thought, accounting for the third most common lesion in athletes when viewed arthroscopically.[3]

As with the shoulder, the acetabulum contains a labrum. The labrum helps provide stability to the hip joint. It deepens the acetabulum and acts as a seal to maintain negative intra-articular pressure. It also protects the articular cartilage and provides proprioceptive input.[4] A number of anatomical problems may contribute to labral damage, which can then predispose to degeneration and early osteoarthritis. Damage is also possible through trauma, often extreme external rotation. The articular cartilage of the hip is thicker anterosuperiorly. Although it was generally assumed that degeneration occurred primarily from osteoarthritis and rheumatoid arthritis, it appears that anterosuperior acetabulum chondral lesions are associated with a host of abnormalities such as labrum tears, anterior capsular laxity, and femoroacetabular impingement (FAI).[5] During standing the hips bear approximately one third of body weight. This increases to 2.4 to 2.6 times body weight when standing on one leg. During walking, the hip can bear as much as 1.3 to 5.8 times body weight. Use of a cane can reduce this load by as much as 40%.[6]

Function of the hip may be affected by pelvic motions such as anterior, posterior, or lateral tilt. These motions are affected by the cocontraction or relaxation of various muscle groups. Anterior tilt is caused by the contraction of the hip flexors. Posterior tilt can be accomplished by contraction of lumbar spine extensors, hip extensors, or trunk flexors. Lateral tilt is accomplished through contraction of hip abductors. Excessive weakness or tightness of these muscles may allow or cause abnormal mechanical function through the creation of a functionally short or long leg.

Flexion of the hip is controlled by the iliopsoas and rectus femoris (**Figure 11–2**). Assistance may be provided by the adductors, tensor fascia lata, and sartorius (L2-L4). Extension is primarily accomplished by contraction of the gluteus maximus, ischial portion of the adductor magnus, and hamstrings (L5-S2). The gluteus medius and piriformis may assist. Internal rotation and abduction are due to the contraction of the gluteus medius, gluteus minimus, and the tensor fascia lata (L4-S1). External rotation is accomplished mainly by the piriformis, gemellus, and obturator muscles (L5-S2), with some posture-dependent assistance from the iliopsoas and gluteus maximus. Adduction is primarily accomplished by the adductor group and the gracilis muscle (L3-L5). The strongest movements are extension, adduction, and external rotation. With walking, the unsupported pelvis is supported by the contralateral hip abductors (primarily gluteus medius).

Evaluation

History

Careful questioning of the patient during the history taking can point to the diagnosis (**Table 11–1**).

Pain Localization

By having the patient point to the area of pain and describe whether or not the onset was traumatic, the diagnostic list can be narrowed.

Iliac Crest

- Anterior superior iliac spine (ASIS)—sartorius strain or, in younger patients, apophysitis or avulsion
- Anterior inferior iliac spine (AIIS)—rectus femoris strain or, in younger patients, apophysitis or avulsion

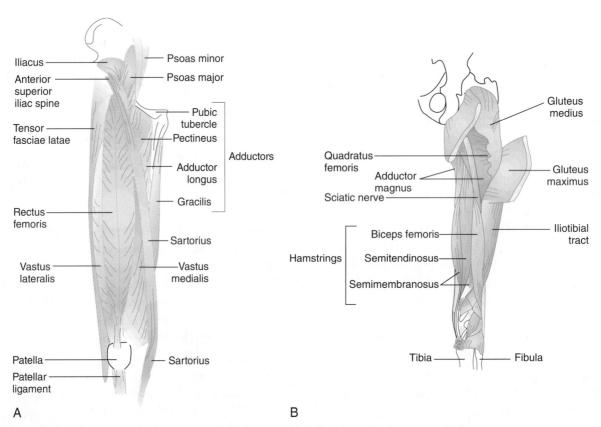

A   B

Figure 11–2 (A) Quadriceps muscles (anterior view); (B) hamstring and gluteal muscles (posterior view).

Table 11–1 History Questions for Hip, Groin, and Thigh Complaints

Primary Question	What Are You Thinking?	Secondary Questions	What Are You Thinking?
Did you fall on your hip?	Hip pointer, hip fracture, traumatic synovitis, slipped epiphysis	Are you able to bear weight and walk?	If yes, hip pointer or contusion is likely; unable to bear weight indicates the other possibilities
Was there a blow to your thigh?	Contusion of hamstrings or quadriceps	Were you hit in the front and do you have difficulty flexing your knee?	Quadriceps contusion
		Were you hit in the back of the thigh and does it hurt to bend forward?	Hamstring contusion
Did you feel a sharp pain in your thigh or groin while performing a sport or recreational activity?	Hamstring, adductor, or quadriceps pull; in younger patients apophysitis is possible	Does it hurt to flex the knee or fully straighten the knee?	Hamstring pull
		Does it hurt to lift the leg?	Iliopsoas or adductor strain (pull)
		Does it hurt to extend the knee?	Quadriceps strain (pull)
Do you have any associated signs and symptoms?	Referral from other joints, septic or aseptic synovitis, OA or other arthritides, tumor, Paget's disease	Did you have a previous respiratory infection (especially in children)?	Septic or aseptic synovitis (needs special imaging to differentiate)
		Do you have any menstrual irregularities?	Possibly gynecologic referral
		Is the pain worse at night, and have you lost any weight recently? Any previous history of cancer?	Metastasis or primary tumor
		Is the pain in both hips and do you have any hand or finger pain?	Rheumatoid arthritis is likely
		Have you noticed a change in hat size?	Paget's disease is possible
		Have you had previous trauma or previous disease of the hip?	OA
		Does the pain radiate from the back to groin?	Renal pathology
		Do you have pain in the groin with bearing down or lifting?	Inguinal hernia

- Lateral iliac crest—hip pointer (if due to a direct blow or fall); iliac crest apophysitis; oblique abdominal, tensor fascia lata, or gluteus medius strain
- Posterior iliac crest—Maigne's syndrome (from T12), strain of gluteus maximus or iliac fascia, or referral from the low back

Groin

- Pubic bone—osteitis pubis, adductor tendinitis
- Inguinal area—hernia, abdominal strain, lymphadenopathy, iliopsoas bursitis, or tendinitis

- Lateral hip—trochanteric bursitis, tensor fascia lata, or gluteus medius trigger points
- Ischial tuberosity—hamstring sprain, ischial bursitis, or avulsion injury
- Generalized deep pain—synovitis, fracture, OA, Paget's disease

It may be frustrating to have forgotten to clarify the location of the patient's complaint. Often patients have a larger target area in mind when they describe their pain as "hip" pain. Many patients mean buttock pain or thigh pain. After it is clear that hip pain is the chief complaint, it is important to distinguish among associated complaints of snapping, crepitus, and decreased ROM or stiffness. Pain is nonspecific; however, snapping suggests a bursa or tendon source. Decreased ROM is found with many conditions; however, the pattern of restriction may be quite revealing, as discussed earlier in the general strategy section. Also, when there is a chief complaint of stiffness without significant pain, the diagnostic list is narrowed.

Age and Onset

By approaching the history from the perspective of age and mode of onset, a high level of suspicion for a specific cause can be gained. Many of these suspicions are quickly confirmed or eliminated with a radiographic evaluation. The following are classic presentations based on age.

Pediatric/Childhood Onset

The earliest indicator of a congenital hip disorder may be a nonpainful limp that is of concern to the parents. This would be suggestive of an undetected hip dysplasia or a congenital hip dislocation.

Adolescent/Young Adult Onset

An insidious onset of pain in the adolescent should raise the suspicion of either a slipped femoral capital epiphysis (or preslip) or an avascular necrosis (Perthes' disease). When the onset is sudden and/or traumatic, a search for a slipped epiphysis should be followed. However, a similar presentation may be found with a transient synovitis, which is not clearly evident on radiographs. When the onset is insidious yet associated with a repetitive activity such as running, marching, dancing, or aerobics, suspicion of a stress fracture should be high.

Middle-Aged Adult Onset

Hip pain in the middle-aged adult is unusual unless the patient has had previous problems as a child or adolescent. The obvious exceptions are pregnancy, during which hip pain may be part of the mechanical discomfort associated with extra weight bearing, and trauma. If pain began subsequent to a physical activity, such as sports, or an unaccustomed activity, such as cleaning the yard, local muscle strain should be considered. Occasionally, the answer to questions regarding the use of orthotics or heel lifts is revealing. The altered mechanics may result in strain or reactive bursitis. In the middle-aged group of patients, it is always important to distinguish between a local joint problem and one that is part of a bigger complex of joint complaints. Arthritides such as rheumatoid arthritis (RA)

have their initial noticeable signs/symptoms in middle age, although they are less common in the hip. Crystalline deposition disorders, as well, may begin in middle age.

Although it may appear that the diagnosis of hip pain would be relatively straightforward based on common age-related disorders, insidious hip pain is often a dilemma. When none of the obvious causes are found, a decision as to which imaging tool is most appropriate (and cost effective) must be determined. The other complication is that the hip, more than many other joints, is dependent on proper alignment and functioning of the distal joints of the lower extremity kinematic chain. Disorders in any of these joints may cause adaptive compensation at the hip. Being the primary weight-bearing joint of the lower extremity, impact forces must be attenuated, especially in the straightened leg.

Weakness

Isolated weakness in the hips is usually a patient perception due to restricted ROM. OA or muscle contracture provides resistance to movement attempts. Further differentiation can be made by the findings of strong contractions in the midrange combined with restricted passive ROM findings upon examination. When muscle pathology is present, as in muscular dystrophy, the patient often will develop perceptible muscle weakness first in the proximal muscle around the hip and pelvis. There will be no associated complaints of pain or sensory aberrations. If weakness is associated with pain, it is important to ascertain the movement pattern to determine whether there is a specific muscle or tendon cause. Painless difficulty in standing up is suggestive of muscular dystrophy but is not specific for this disorder.

Restriction

If the patient feels that he or she has restricted movement, age and associated symptoms help distinguish the cause. In older patients, OA or perhaps Paget's disease is possible. In a younger patient, especially in males, ankylosing spondylitis is possible (due primarily to pelvic involvement). If the restriction is less discernible after moving around for a half hour or longer, OA is often the cause in older patients.

Snapping

Snapping at the hip is usually a benign problem. In addition to tendon snapping, there is often a suction effect that occurs at the hip joint, causing a pop similar to that caused by manipulation. On rarer occasions, a loose body may be present. Tendon snapping is usually evident with localization of the snapping coupled with the type of movement that creates the snapping.

- Anterior snapping with hip abduction or external rotation suggests that the psoas tendon is snapping over the lesser trochanter or iliopectineal eminence.
- Lateral snapping with hip adduction coupled with flexion or extension suggests that the iliotibial band is snapping over the greater trochanter.
- Posterior snapping with flexion or extension suggests that the biceps femoris tendon is snapping over the ischial tuberosity.
- Pubic bone snapping may occur during pregnancy or the postpartum period or, in rare cases, following a traumatic spread-eagle injury (indicates instability).

Further distinction can be made during the physical examination, palpating the area while the patient performs the provocative movement. It is important to remember that there are interposed bursae at these sites that may be inflamed and cause pain due to the constant snapping.

Groin Pain

The history is particularly important in differentiating the various causes of groin pain. When the pain follows a twisting, sudden, or forceful movement of the hip, adductor strain is often the cause. If the report is that pain occurred after a lifting incident and is made worse with bearing down (Valsalva maneuver), a hernia is likely. If the patient is a man who reports an associated testicular mass, then epididymitis, testicular cancer, a varicocele, or testicular torsion is possible. Testicular torsion usually causes pain severe enough to cause the patient to seek medical attention. Palpation of the testes must be performed to differentiate each. Groin pain in women that is not readily reproducible suggests a gynecologic cause. Questions regarding a relationship to the patient's menstrual period may reveal a connection.

Thigh Complaints

Thigh pain is usually due to direct trauma that results in a contusion or due to overcontraction that leads to either muscle tear or rupture. A history of a direct blow to the quadriceps or hamstrings is highly suggestive of a contusion with subsequent hematoma formation. It is

important to question the patient regarding the events following the trauma. If the patient returned to a strenuous activity or applied deep heat or massage, a concern for myositis ossificans is generated.

When sudden pain follows a strenuous activity such as running to first base or sprinting, location of the pain will usually isolate a quadriceps or hamstring strain. It is important to determine whether the patient stretches or warms up prior to activity.

When the complaint is more of numbness or paresthesia into the thigh, localization to the lateral thigh suggests meralgia paresthetica. Determining whether the patient is obese, pregnant, sits for long periods, or carries keys or other objects in his or her front pockets may unearth the underlying cause. When the numbness is more anterior, the femoral nerve is involved, and it is likely that the patient is a known diabetic or has signs indicating canal stenosis (claudication signs with walking). Subjective numbness may occur with various trigger-point referrals.

Examination

Given the context of patient presentation, the evaluation of the patient on physical exam extends from very brief to extended. For example, if the patient is unable to bear weight or comfortably move the hip, it would seem prudent to begin the examination with localization of the complaint with palpation. This should be followed immediately by radiographic examination.

Direct palpation of the hip joint is not possible, causing the examiner to rely on indirect, provocative maneuvers. Orthopaedic testing for the hip is rather limited. Many tests are used as a means of differentiating the hip from other causes through a localizing response by the patient. For example, the Patrick test or FABER test is accomplished by placing the ankle of the tested leg over the well-side knee and abducting and externally rotating the hip (**Figure 11–3**). This test may produce pain at the hip or the sacroiliac (SI) joint. Although the FABER test is a good test for intra-articular pathology with a sensitivity of 88%, it is nonspecific.[7] A more specific test involves applying an axial compression force through the femur into the hip joint with the knee flexed to 90° or more. This can be retested with the hip flexed and internally rotated. This is sometimes referred to as Laguerre's test. The quadrant test involves placing the hip in the same Laguerre's position while the patient is asked to resist the examiner's attempt at abduction. Most other

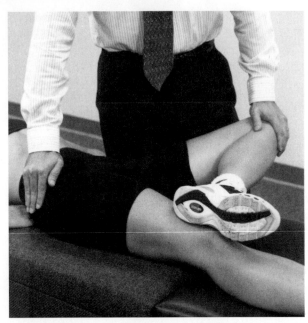

Figure 11–3 FABER test. The patient's hip is placed into flexion, abduction, and external rotation.

testing is based on an effort to distinguish between hip pain of low back or SI origin (see Chapter 6).

There are a number of femoroacetabular impingement (FAI) tests. The general test position involves passive hip flexion, internal rotation, and adduction (see **Figure 11–4**). The intention is to compress the anterior superior labrum and acetabular rim. Two variations include the Fitzgerald[8] provocative maneuver and the McCarthy[9] sign. The Fitzgerald provocative maneuver's positive finding for impingement is a sharp, catching pain, with or without a click, with the hip passively

brought into full flexion, external rotation, and full abduction, then extending with internal rotation and adduction. Fitzgerald suggests that this maneuver is more sensitive for anterior tear detection, while switching the initial external rotation to internal rotation and extending with external rotation is specific for posterior tears. The McCarthy sign has the examiner first flex the opposite hip while the affected hip is extended with internal rotation, then with external rotation in an attempt to reproduce a painful click. Some studies indicate a high degree of sensitivity when compared to surgical identification.[10,11] One study indicated a sensitivity of 75% and a specificity of 45% in detecting FAI compared to MRA.[12]

Instability is sometimes assessed clinically using long-axis traction. With the supine patient's hip placed in 30° flexion, 30° abduction, and 10° to 15° of external rotation, the examiner leans back using his body weight.[13] Patients with instability may feel movement or a sense of apprehension.

Various stretch maneuvers can be applied to the hip joint. The Thomas test requires the supine patient to draw one leg toward the chest while the examiner observes the position of the opposite leg. If the hip or knee flexes, tightness in the hip flexors is likely. A focus on the rectus femoris can be accomplished by having the patient repeat the test with the knee hanging over the edge of the examination table (see **Figure 11–5**). If the knee extends while the patient flexes the opposite hip to his or her chest, the rectus femoris is tight. A prone test for hip flexor tightness can be accomplished by passively extending the hip with the knee extended. If the hip is extended with the knee flexed, the rectus femoris is

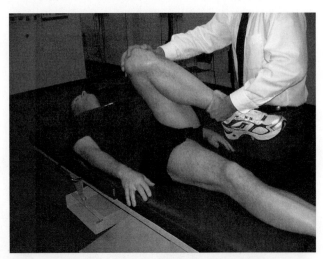

Figure 11–4 Acetabular impingement test. Hip flexion, internal rotation, and adduction.

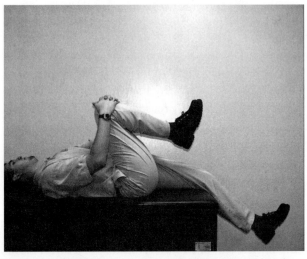

Figure 11–5 Modified Thomas test indicating tightness of left rectus femoris.

tested. This same test may stretch the femoral nerve and cause radiation of pain or other sensory complaints into the anterior thigh. Stretch testing of the abductors and adductors should also be performed. If the abductors are shortened due to contracture, a functional long leg with lowering of the ipsilateral pelvis will be created, associated with adduction of the opposite hip with a raised pelvis.[13] If the adductors are shortened, the ipsilateral leg is functionally shortened with a raised pelvis. On the opposite side, the hip abducts, lowering the pelvis.

Ober's test is often performed on patients complaining of lateral knee pain (Figure 12–11). For the hip, this test is less a provocative test and more a test of abductor flexibility. With the patient lying on his or her side and the bottom leg flexed to 90°, the examiner slowly lowers the top extended leg off the edge of the table while stabilizing at the iliac crest to avoid abdominal stretching. If the patella does not pass below the top edge of the table, tightness of the gluteus medius or the iliotibial band or its attachments (the gluteus maximus and the tensor fascia lata) is likely.

Another biomechanical factor that should be assessed is anteversion or retroversion of the femur. This refers to the angle the femoral neck forms with the femoral condyles. The degree of anteversion is based on the forward projection of the femoral neck into the acetabulum. With abnormal anteversion the femoral condyles are internally rotated with respect to the femoral neck; the reverse occurs with retroversion. Anteversion and retroversion are measured by using the Craig test. This test can be coupled with a measure of internal and external rotation of the hip. With the patient prone, the knee is bent to 90° and both active and passive internal and external rotation are measured. For the Craig test, palpation of the greater trochanter is necessary. As the patient's hip is passively internally and externally rotated, the examiner finds a point at which the greater trochanter feels parallel to the exam table (**Figure 11–6**). The angle formed by the lower leg and vertical is considered the angle of anteversion (if internally rotated) and retroversion (if externally rotated). See **Figure 11–7**. The average angle is considered to be between 12° and 25° of anteversion in the adult.[15] Excessive anteversion leads to internal rotation of the femur with potential valgus forces to the knee and possible hyperpronation.

Leg length measurement should be considered a gross but potentially valuable data source. The standard approach is to measure the supine patient from the ASIS to the medial malleolus on the same side (true or

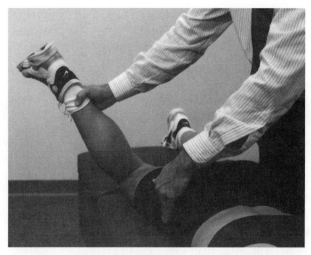

Figure 11–6 Craig test for anteversion/retroversion of the hip. While palpating the greater trochanter the patient's leg is internally or externally rotated until the greater trochanter is pointing parallel to the table. The angle formed by internal rotation with a vertical line indicates the degree of anteversion; the external rotation angle indicates retroversion.

anatomic leg length) and then to measure the opposite side and compare the measurements. The same approach is repeated, but this time using the umbilicus and the medial malleolus (apparent or functional leg length). If there is a difference in the "true" leg length, an anatomic short leg (often due to a previous fracture or deforming

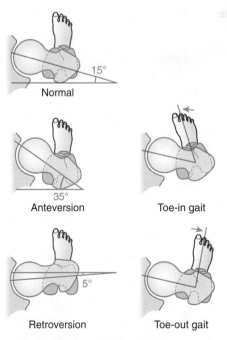

Figure 11–7 Torsion angles of the hip. (A) Positions of femoral neck. (B) Different foot positions with anteversion and retroversion at the hip (coronal views).

process at the hip) is present. If the leg length deficiency is in the apparent measurement, a variety of soft tissue factors are likely involved. The interexaminer agreement is only about 40% when examiners had to be within 6 mm of each other to be considered in agreement.[16] When this was extended to 12.5 mm, the agreement increased to 86%. Also, Beattie[17] found that the reliability was high when the mean of two measurements was used. The large literature review published by Manello[18] demonstrates the continuing controversy regarding the contribution of leg length discrepancy to an increase in or predisposition to low back, pelvic, or hip pain. Generally, however, to be clinically significant, the leg length discrepancy needs to be equal to or greater than 0.5 in. This means that discrepancies beyond this range have been shown to predispose individuals to conditions such as subtrochanteric bursitis or SI dysfunction.[19] With a functionally short or long leg, recheck findings with regard to abductor, adductor, or hip flexor/extensor tightness or weakness. If the leg length appears only on weight-bearing, check for unilateral pronation or supination as potential causes.

There is a new interest in determining hip pain in athletes given it is a common cause of disability in high-level performers, in particular in soccer.[20] This has led to sophisticated approaches to analysis of hip and pelvis loading for running, jumping, and landing. There is an emphasis now on correcting these faults prior to a surgical solution. Some elements that have been evaluated include:

- The 3G approach (groin, gluteal, and greater trochanter triangles) is a systematic approach to looking at the muscular/fascial triangle as integrated and supplementary to one another.[21]
- An increased alpha angle on radiographs to predict groin injury.[22]
- Hernias are being re-evaluated as a "groin disruption injury," the result of functional instability of the pelvis.[23] The approach to management can be focused rehabilitation based on high-speed analysis of movement or, if unsuccessful, surgical stabilization.

Radiographs may include the standard AP lumbo-pelvic film or localize for better quality with an AP hip view complemented by a lateral (frog-leg) view. Most osseous and some soft tissue abnormalities may be evident. If avulsion fractures are suspected, the AP view may require some internal or external rotation in order to view the fragment clearly. Following are some radiographic findings associated with some selected disorders:[24]

- OA—The superior acetabular joint space shows narrowing with osteophyte formation at the head/neck junction; there is subchondral sclerosis.
- RA—Early phase changes are uniform, symmetric loss of joint space with associated periarticular osteoporosis. Later changes may include subchondral cyst formation and destruction of the femoral head or acetabular roof even to the point of protrusio acetabuli (protrusion of the femoral head axially through the acetabulum into the pelvis).
- Paget's disease—The bone is thickened, with more apparent trabeculae (cross-hatching) with eventual distortion of the femoral neck or shaft shape.
- Legg-Calvé-Perthes disease (ages 4 to 8 years)—Initial changes include fissuring, flattening, and sclerosis of the epiphysis with a secondary phase of remodeling leading to the classic mushroom deformity; a varus deformity usually results.
- Slipped capital epiphysis (ages 8 to 17 years)—This is a Salter-Harris type I injury characterized by posterior-inferior displacement of the epiphysis best seen on the lateral view.
- Acetabular dysplasia—The center wedge angle of Wiberg is measured.
- Femoral acetabular impingement—Anterior asphericity of the femoral head, lack of femoral head–neck offset, and retroversion of the acetabulum.[25]
- Fractures may be due to osteoporosis, Paget's disease, metastasis, and other pathologic processes, or trauma. Femoral neck fractures are intracapsular (subcapital and transcervical regions) or extra-capsular (trochanteric, subtrochanteric, and basicervical); intracapsular fractures are more serious and twice as common.[26]

Magnetic resonance imaging (MRI) is valuable for a host of intra-articular disorders, specifically the early phase of avascular necrosis. Magnetic resonance arthrography (MRA) is particularly valuable for identifying acetabular labrum tears with a reported sensitivity range of between 66% to 95% and a specificity range of 71% to 88%.[27]

Groin

- With trauma or pain following a sudden forceful maneuver of the hip, palpate for sites of tenderness (e.g., adductor origin); if the history indicates a blow to the region, radiograph for possible fracture.
- If pain was insidious or due to overuse, palpate for adductor tenderness and local lymphadenopathy.
- If pain followed a lifting injury or increases with bearing down, perform a hernia evaluation.
- When a gynecologic or genital source is suspected, perform or refer for a thorough examination.

When groin pain is traumatic or due to a sudden forceful movement, palpate for tenderness at the pubic bone and adductor origin. Have the patient attempt adduction, flexion, and extension against resistance to isolate specific muscle/tendon involvement. Pain with resisted hip flexion suggests iliopsoas or possibly rectus femoris strain. Pain with resisted adduction suggests adductor tendinitis. If tenderness is severe, consider radiographs to determine possible fracture. For patients with a history of pain following lifting or those who experience pain with bearing down, perform a hernia examination. This includes palpation for direct, indirect, and femoral hernias.

Reproduction of the pain with SI or hip testing indicates referral to the groin from these areas. If pain originates in the thoracolumbar area, perform a kidney punch test. A search for skin lesions or discharge may suggest a venereal cause.

Thigh

Trauma to the thigh requires a search for contusions. In the anterior thigh, a quadriceps contusion is likely. Palpation is important with injuries that are a few weeks old to determine the development of myositis ossificans. Posterior involvement indicates hamstring contusion. When pain follows sudden or forceful contraction of the legs such as with running, palpation for sites of tenderness is important. If the pain is posterior at the middle to distal thigh, a hamstring sprain has occurred. Occasionally a defect in the muscle can be palpated. The degree of tearing is often reflected in the patient's ability to flex the knee against resistance. The same principles apply to a quadriceps strain, with the severity based on the patient's ability to extend the knee against resistance or perform a quadriceps isometric contraction.

When thigh complaints include numbness or paresthesia, it is important to determine whether the symptoms are subjective or objective. Objective numbness in the anterolateral thigh implicates the lateral femoral cutaneous nerve, suggesting meralgia paresthetica. If numbness is objectifiable in the anterior thigh, femoral nerve involvement is likely, especially if associated with weakness of knee extension.

Management

For more detail on management of individual disorders see the later section, "Selected Disorders of the Hip, Groin, and Thigh."

Medical referral is necessary when fracture, dislocation, avascular necrosis, infection, tumor, or visceral pathology is suspected or found. Acute pain is managed with physical therapy and support. With muscle strains, a compressive bandage or taping or a substituting type of elastic wrap may help decrease continued strain to the muscle. These include neoprene sleeves for hamstring and quadriceps strains and hip spica wraps for adductor or iliopsoas strains.

Management of most other complaints focuses on restoring normal mobility to the hip joint and pelvis, from both a gross ROM perspective (voluntary muscular component) and an accessory motion perspective (involuntary component). OA often results in hip joint contractures. A combination of stretching and general hip stabilization exercises coupled with hip manipulation is often effective.

Prevention of further soft tissue injury at the hip and thigh involves a routine of stretching and warming up prior to activity. For patients who have had or are at potential risk for hip fracture, evaluation of common environmental obstacles should be performed with recommendations for avoidance of falls. This would include taping down of rugs, placing nonslip strips on steps or stairs, ensuring proper lighting at night, and strategically placing balance points for use of a walker or cane.

Algorithm

An algorithm for evaluation and management of hip pain is presented in **Figure 11–8**.

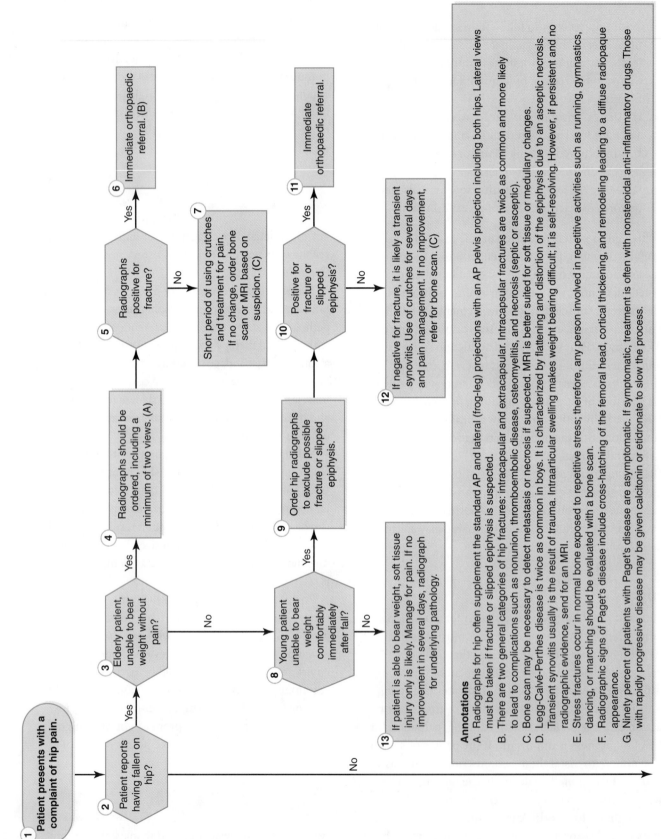

1 Patient presents with a complaint of hip pain.

2 Patient reports having fallen on hip?

3 Elderly patient, unable to bear weight without pain?

Yes → **4** Radiographs should be ordered, including a minimum of two views. (A)

→ **5** Radiographs positive for fracture?

Yes → **6** Immediate orthopaedic referral. (B)

No → **7** Short period of using crutches and treatment for pain. If no change, order bone scan or MRI based on suspicion. (C)

No (from 3) → **8** Young patient unable to bear weight comfortably immediately after fall?

Yes → **9** Order hip radiographs to exclude possible fracture or slipped epiphysis.

→ **10** Positive for fracture or slipped epiphysis?

Yes → **11** Immediate orthopaedic referral.

No → **12** If negative for fracture, it is likely a transient synovitis. Use of crutches for several days and pain management. If no improvement, refer for bone scan. (C)

No (from 8) → **13** If patient is able to bear weight, soft tissue injury only is likely. Manage for pain. If no improvement in several days, radiograph for underlying pathology.

No (from 2) →

Annotations

A. Radiographs for hip often supplement the standard AP and lateral (frog-leg) projections with an AP pelvis projection including both hips. Lateral views must be taken if fracture or slipped epiphysis is suspected.

B. There are two general categories of hip fractures: intracapsular and extracapsular. Intracapsular fractures are twice as common and more likely to lead to complications such as nonunion, thromboembolic disease, osteomyelitis, and necrosis (septic or aseptic).

C. Bone scan may be necessary to detect metastasis or necrosis if suspected. MRI is better suited for soft tissue or medullary changes.

D. Legg-Calvé-Perthes disease is twice as common in boys. It is characterized by flattening and distortion of the epiphysis due to an asceptic necrosis. Transient synovitis usually is the result of trauma. Intraarticular swelling makes weight bearing difficult; it is self-resolving. However, if persistent and no radiographic evidence, send for an MRI.

E. Stress fractures occur in normal bone exposed to repetitive stress; therefore, any person involved in repetitive activities such as running, gymnastics, dancing, or marching should be evaluated with a bone scan.

F. Radiographic signs of Paget's disease include cross-hatching of the femoral head, cortical thickening, and remodeling leading to a diffuse radiopaque appearance.

G. Ninety percent of patients with Paget's disease are asymptomatic. If symptomatic, treatment is often with nonsteroidal anti-inflammatory drugs. Those with rapidly progressive disease may be given calcitonin or etidronate to slow the process.

Figure 11-8 Hip Pain—Algorithm

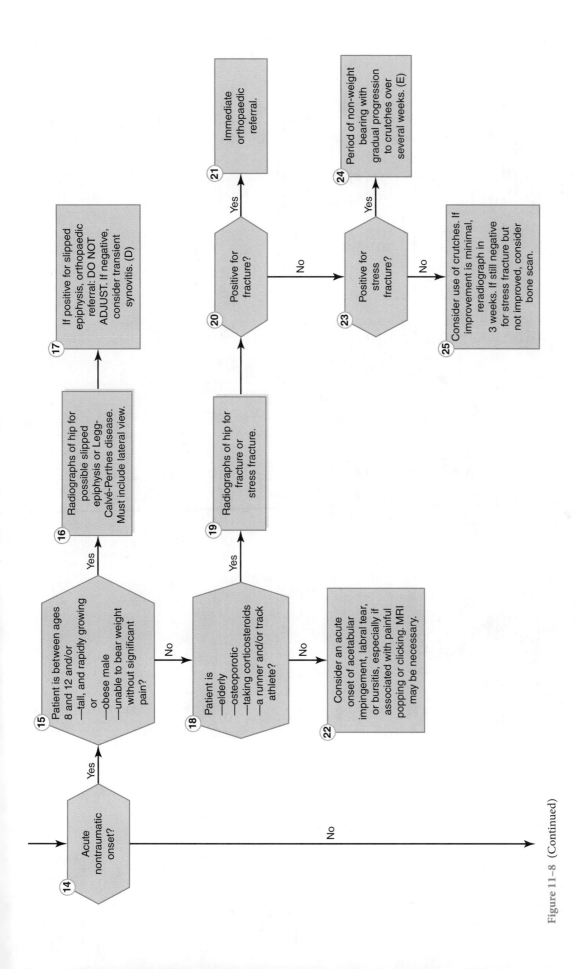

14 Acute nontraumatic onset?

Yes →

No →

15 Patient is between ages 8 and 12 and/or
—tall, and rapidly growing
or
—obese male
—unable to bear weight without significant pain?

Yes →

No →

16 Radiographs of hip for possible slipped epiphysis or Legg-Calvé-Perthes disease. Must include lateral view.

17 If positive for slipped epiphysis, orthopaedic referral: DO NOT ADJUST. If negative, consider transient synovitis. (D)

18 Patient is
—elderly
—osteoporotic
—taking corticosteroids
—a runner and/or track athlete?

Yes →

No →

19 Radiographs of hip for fracture or stress fracture.

20 Positive for fracture?

Yes →

No →

21 Immediate orthopaedic referral.

22 Consider an acute onset of acetabular impingement, labral tear, or bursitis, especially if associated with painful popping or clicking. MRI may be necessary.

23 Positive for stress fracture?

Yes →

No →

24 Period of non-weight bearing with gradual progression to crutches over several weeks. (E)

25 Consider use of crutches. If improvement is minimal, reradiograph in 3 weeks. If still negative for stress fracture but not improved, consider bone scan.

Figure 11-8 (Continued)

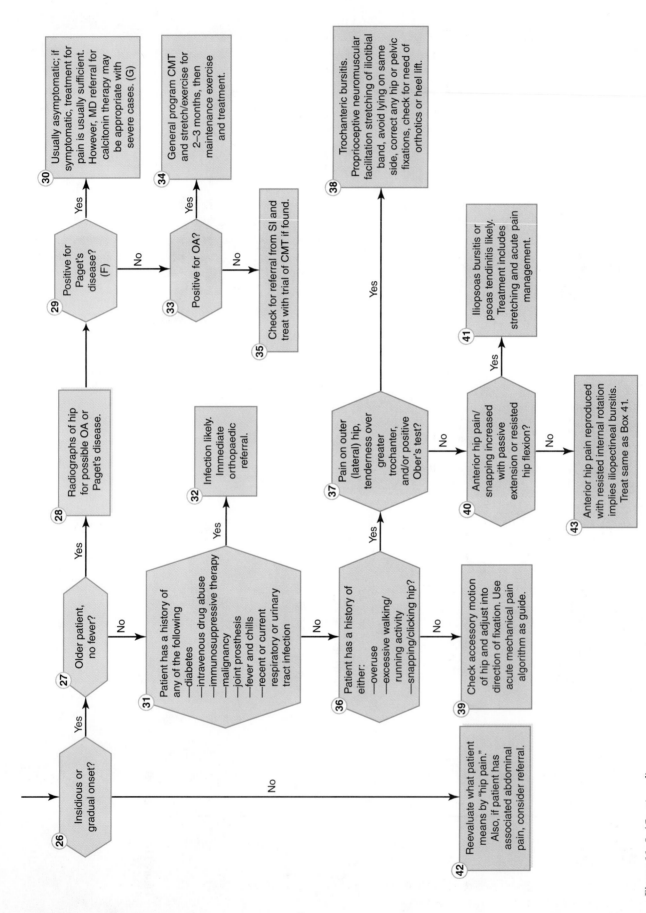

Figure 11-8 (Continued)

Selected Disorders of the Hip, Groin, and Thigh

HIP

Hip Fractures

Classic Presentation

An elderly patient presents with hip pain, unable to bear weight, and a history of a fall onto the hip.

Causes

In the elderly, the most common cause or predisposition of hip fracture is osteoporosis and therefore it is seen more frequently in women. One study suggests that the fracture is due to a combination of bone fatigue and axial muscular compressive forces, which then leads to falling.[28] Obviously, falls can result in fracture also. Other considerations are Paget's disease, endocrinopathies, multiple myeloma, and renal osteodystrophy.[29] In the young patient, other than a major traumatic event, pathologic fracture may be due to benign and malignant tumors. Benign tumors include a unicameral bone cyst and fibrous dysplasia. Malignant causes include osteogenic sarcoma and Ewing's sarcoma.[30]

Evaluation

In the event of trauma, beyond palpation, the next step is radiographic evaluation. A search for fractures must include both an AP view and a lateral view. Fractures are divided into intracapsular (subcapital and transcervical) and extracapsular (basicervical, trochanteric, and subtrochanteric). Intracapsular fractures are twice as common as extracapsular fractures and, unfortunately, are more likely to result in serious complications such as osteonecrosis, nonunion, thromboembolic disease, and osteomyelitis.[31]

Management

Advances in orthopaedic stabilization techniques and new advances in bone healing have helped increase the success rate of surgery. Unfortunately, the death rate following hip fracture is still approximately 15% (due to the above-mentioned complications).

Stress Fractures

Classic Presentation

The patient is young and active, often participating in activities such as long-distance running, gymnastics and, less often, dancing or marching. The pain is insidious and is worse with weight-bearing. The pain is often anterior and deep.

Mechanism

With repetitive stress to the femoral neck, microfractures appear. Cellular damage leads to increased remodeling. When osteoclastic activity exceeds osteoblastic activity, the bone is weakened.

Evaluation

Little is found on the examination except for perhaps end-range restriction and pain with flexion and internal rotation. Radiographs often are unrevealing. When the index of suspicion is high, a bone scan is highly sensitive.[32] If a tumor is included in the differential, MRI is valuable.

Management

There are two different types of femoral neck stress fractures. Management is different for each.
1. Transverse—Begins in the superior cortex and continues across the neck. These fractures are potentially unstable and may lead to serious complications. Therefore, percutaneous pinning is the recommended treatment.
2. Compression—Begins along the inferior cortex and may progress to sclerosis; however, it is stable. Rest and elastic support are necessary for two weeks, followed by non-weight-bearing exercises such as bicycling or swimming. It takes on average four to six weeks for a stress fracture to heal.

Congenital Hip Dislocation and Hip Dysplasia

Classic Presentation

Congenital hip dislocation is usually diagnosed on physical exam of the neonate; if undetected, the child would, upon weight-bearing, have a limp and diminished active abduction.

Causes

Dislocation is due to acetabular deformities. Inversion of the limbus combined with capsular tightness causes dislocation and prevents a stable relocation.[33]

Evaluation

The classic tests used for early detection are Ortolani's click test and Barlow's maneuver. Radiographs may appear normal until the infant is four to six weeks of age. Radiographic identification of dysplasia is based on a triad of an underdeveloped proximal femoral epiphysis, lateral displacement of the femur, and an increased inclination of the acetabular roof (Putti's triad).[34] Severe degenerative changes are visible in chronic dislocators. MRI and diagnostic ultrasound are used to detect early dysplastic changes.[35]

Management

Management is dependent on age. In infants up to six months, a harness (e.g., Pavlik) is used to hold the hip in flexion and prevent adduction. From ages 6 to 15 months (before walking), two to three months in a spica cast is recommended. In toddlers or in children who have not responded to closed reduction, open reduction is necessary.

Traumatic Hip Dislocations

Classic Presentation

Based on whether anterior or posterior; posterior dislocations account for 90% of sports-related hip dislocations.
- Posterior—An acute injury is reported with a major force applied to a flexed, adducted hip. After the injury, the hip is held in flexion, adduction, and internal rotation. The pain is severe. Pain down the back of the leg may indicate sciatic nerve damage.
- Anterior—Patient reports a force/blow to an extended, externally rotated leg. Immediately after injury, the leg is held in flexion, abduction, and internal rotation.

Evaluation

Visual observation and history are usually enough to raise the suspicion. Radiographs to determine the extent of damage are needed. However, these would be performed in an emergency department setting.

Management

Relocation is not possible without anesthesia. This is followed by rest and a period of non-weight-bearing with gradual return to supported walking with crutches.

Slipped Capital Epiphysis (Adolescent Coxa Vara)

Classic Presentation

An overweight child or a young, rapidly growing adolescent (age 8 to 17 years) presents with a traumatic (50% of the time) history, although sometimes relatively minor. Acute slippage may occur. Chronic slippage presents as a gradual hip pain with antalgia. Children may have only knee pain. This is the most common hip condition in adolescents, affecting between 0.7 and 3.4/100,000.[36]

Causes

Although trauma is reported in 50% of cases, half of cases have no obvious traumatic history. An acute slippage is a Salter-Harris type I epiphyseal fracture. Hormonal influences may play a role in obese individuals[37] (Fröhlich syndrome-like appearance) or in tall, fast-growing adolescents.

Evaluation

The physical examination may be generally unremarkable; however, sometimes when the hip is taken passively into flexion, it rotates externally.[38] The definitive diagnosis is with hip radiographs. It is essential to understand that the slippage may not be visible on the anterior view. The lateral view gives a clearer picture of the typical posterior/inferior slippage of the femoral epiphysis.[39] Bilateral views should be taken because of occurrence in the opposite hip in 10% to 20% of cases.

Management

Surgical pinning is often used. Acute slipped capital femoral epiphysis is managed with a short period of traction, followed by internal rotation to accomplish reduction, followed by pinning or screw fixation. It is imperative that there is no attempt to reduce the slippage with manipulation. The consequences can be disastrous, including avascular necrosis.

Avascular Necrosis

Classic Presentation

Legg-Calvé-Perthes disease is a form of avascular necrosis. The patient is usually male (four or five times more commonly) between the ages of 4 and 9 years (80%) presenting with a complaint of mild hip pain and an associated limp of insidious onset. Symptoms are bilateral 10% of the time;[40] 17% of patients have a traumatic history.[41] Fifteen percent of patients present with knee pain only. Avascular necrosis may be due to a multitude of other factors. The patient is more likely though, to present with a history of past trauma or metabolic disease.

Causes

Legg-Calvé-Perthes disease is believed to be due to an undetermined disruption of the vascular supply to the femoral head.[42] Other than Legg-Calvé-Perthes disease, avascular necrosis is secondary to subcapital fractures (20%), posterior hip dislocations (8%), long-term steroid use, hyperlipidemia, alcoholism, pancreatitis, and hemoglobinopathies.[43]

Evaluation

Usually there is limitation of hip abduction and internal rotation (secondary to muscle spasm). The Trendelenburg test is often positive. Over time, atrophy and limb length inequality may be evident. The definitive diagnosis is radiographic. In progression the changes begin with a small radiopaque femoral nucleus, followed by a crescent sign, fragmentation, reossification with remodeling, and deformity of the femoral head.

Management

Management is often conservative. It is generally agreed that children younger than 4 years of age or those with minor involvement (less than half of the femoral head) usually require no treatment. Children older than 4 to 5 years old who have good motion (abduction greater than 30°) may not require bracing or surgery.[44] Referral for medical consultation is required. There is no apparent evidence to support the use of crutches or non-weight-bearing in most cases. When subluxation occurs due to femoral head deformation, use of a Petrie cast or ambulatory brace may help maintain needed abduction. Surgical options are rarely required but include osteotomy. Healing takes about 18 months.

Femoroacetabular Impingement

Classic Presentation

A patient complains of sharp, deep hip pain with squatting. Running, stopping and starting or changing direction may also cause pain. The pain is felt anteriorly.

Cause

Femoroacetabular impingement (FAI) is a relatively recently recognized condition resulting from a number of hip abnormalities that limit motion, in particular, flexion and internal rotation. There are two types. The cam type is due to abnormalities of the femur with a decreased offset between the femoral head and neck. The pincer type is due to acetabular abnormalities that lead to excessive coverage by the anterior acetabular rim. There is also a mixed type.

Evaluation

There is a significant decrease in flexion and internal rotation. External rotation may also be affected.[45] For the more common anterior impingement, the anterior impingement test is performed. With the hip passively flexed to 90°, forced internal rotation causes anterior pain. For the less common posterior impingement, the posterior impingement test is performed with the patient supine and the hip flexed. By extending the hip and externally rotating the posterior hip, pain is elicited with a positive test. The FABER test may cause lateral hip pain in patients with FAI. Radiographic evaluation focuses on the standard AP and frog-leg with a measurement and search for:

Pincer lesions

- Acetabular retroversion—acetabular wall is more lateral than the posterior wall; "posterior wall sign" is when the AP view shows that the wall is more medial than the center of the femoral head.
- Coax profunda—when the floor of the acetabular fossa contacts or overlaps the ilioischial line on the AP view.
- Protrusio acetabuli—femoral heads protrude through the acetabulum.

Cam lesions

- Pistol grip deformity.
- The alpha angle—measured on a cross-table view to determine asphericity and cam impingement on the anterior aspect of the femoral head–neck junction.

MRI is also used and can determine associated pathologies.

Management

There are no reports of conservative management of FAI. Surgical approaches include dislocation of the hip and femoroacetabular osteoplasty.[10, 46] Arthroscopic treatment with either rim trimming, labral refixation, or debridement, dependent on the degree of damage has also demonstrated good short-term results.[47]

Acetabular Labrum Tears

Classic Presentation

A patient presents with moderate to severe pain with groin pain predominant. The patient has night pain. The pain is worse with activity and causes the patient to limp. Clicking and occasional giving-way of the hip occur. (*Note:* There is a wide variation in report of onset from no trauma to severe trauma.)

Causes

There are many suggested causes including macro- to micro- (repetitive) trauma. Predispositions could include FAI, capsular laxity, or hip dysplasia. Labral damage may cause chondral lesions (in 73% of patients with labrum tears)[5] and early degeneration.[48] A lesion that can mimic labrum tears is a ligamentum teres (LT) tear; the connecting ligament between the top of the humeral head to the acetabulum.

Evaluation

The history clues most often reported, in addition to those in the classic presentation above, include hip locking or catching. It should be noted that groin pain is a common referral area for intra-articular hip pathology (visceral pathology [genitourinary] generally radiates from the flank to the groin). The report of clicking and giving way has a relatively high likelihood ratio (6.67). The cluster of these complaints would help identify the likely labrum tear cause. However, it appears that the diagnosis is elusive; one study indicates a time from the onset of symptoms to diagnosis of 21 months and a mean of 3.3 healthcare providers prior to receiving the correct diagnosis.[49] There are different classifications of labrum tears. One classification identifies four types: radial, radial fibrillated, longitudinal peripheral, and abnormally mobile.[51] Radial are the most common and usually occur in the anterosuperior location. Other classifications define the type of tear by a clock face descriptor (e.g., 6 o'clock position) or ranked based on the size of any associated articular cartilage damage.

Physical examination, although sensitive to labrum tears, is not very specific. A number of tests can be used to indirectly assess labrum tears including FABER, FAI tests, long-axis distraction, and ROM findings. The impingement test (see Figure 11–4) has the highest sensitivity (as high as 95%).[49] Radiographs are not helpful in making the diagnosis; however, they may provide indirect evidence of cause or effect from a labrum tear. The findings may include hip dysplasia, osteoarthritis, a lack of femoral head/neck offset or other congenital, developmental, or acquired structural abnormalities. MRI may be valuable in the diagnosis of labrum tears, but MRA has been demonstrated to be far superior, although both have limitations. Anterior labrum tears (the most common) are visualized well with MRI and MRA, whereas posterior tears are not. Studies indicate a sensitivity range of 75% to 90%, an accuracy of about the same, and a specificity of about 83% for anterior tears, whereas the detection of posterior tears was as low as 20% and lateral tears as low as 11%. Arthroscopy is, by default, the "gold standard" for diagnosis and treatment. Evaluation should also include a check for a ligamentum teres (LT) tear. There is a new test for this previously underappreciated cause of hip pain and disability.[50] Tears of the LT are a common cause of chronic groin and thigh pain found in 8% to 51% of patients undergoing hip arthroscopy. These tears are not easily seen on MRI, with only about 2% being visible. A new clinical test makes an attempt at increasing the clinical suspicion of an underlying tear of the LT with arthroscopy being the gold standard with direct visualization (**Figure 11–9**). The test is performed with the patient supine and the knee flexed 90°. The hip is fully passively flexed and then backed-off by 20° to 30° leaving the hip at about 70° flexion. The hip is then abducted fully and again backed-off into adduction by about 30° leaving the hip at around 30° hip abduction. At the knee, the leg is rotated internally and externally noting if either produces pain. This would indicate a positive test for a torn LT.

Management

Generally, the literature is sparse on conservative management with no data on manipulative management of acetabular labrum tears.

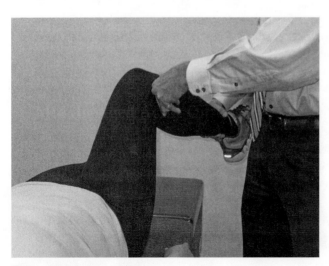

Figure 11–9 Ligamentum teres test.

Two small studies indicate that the use of NSAIDs and partial weight-bearing for two to four weeks may help some patients.[8,52] The standard medical approach is labral debridement using arthroscopy. Short-term success is quite high, especially for minor labral lesions, and in those without other hip pathology such as osteoarthritis or other involvement of the cartilage.[53–55] If surgery is to be performed, the data indicate early intervention may prevent further damage.

Trochanteric Pain Syndrome

Classic Presentation

Several bursae are capable of producing symptoms. The two major bursae are the subgluteus medius and subgluteus maximus. A smaller bursa with the gluteus minimus is less often involved. The patient presents with well-localized lateral hip pain usually with only a minor degree of limp. The patient is often between 40 and 60 years of age. Less commonly subtrochanteric bursitis may cause pain radiating to the low back, the lateral thigh, and the knee.[56–58] The patient often will not be able to sleep on the involved side.

Cause

Any condition that leads to altered hip mechanics, including low back pain, leg length discrepancy, arthritic conditions, surgery, and neurologic conditions with paresis, may cause subtrochanteric bursitis. The result is some loss of internal rotation. The degree of discomfort is often proportional to the degree of activity. Repetitive activity can be a major cause in the younger population because the friction over the bursa causes it to be inflamed.

Evaluation

Tenderness and sometimes swelling are found over the greater trochanter. Palpation may cause a "jump" sign when localized to the lower portion of the trochanter with the knee and hip flexed. Pain may be increased with hip motion and maneuvers such as the Patrick test or Ober's test. The distinction between trochanteric pain syndrome and osteoarthritis has not been fully differentiated; however, a 2013 study attempts to find the unique features.[59] Patients with lateral hip pain with tenderness on palpation of the greater trochanter and with a FABER test are likely to have trochanteric pain syndrome if there is an absence of difficulty with putting on their shoes and socks.

Management

Management includes correction of abnormal biomechanics such as leg length discrepancies combined with indicated adjustment of the pelvis or hip. Additionally, stretching of the hip abductors using proprioceptive neuromuscular facilitation (PNF) techniques should be prescribed and performed in office. Ultrasound has little applicability unless a chronic bursitis is suspected or perhaps in assisting stretching of any tight contributing muscles. Side-posture adjusting may aggravate and in rare cases cause a trochanteric bursitis. Therefore, side-posture adjusting is contraindicated for one to two weeks during acute-care treatment. Alternative techniques should be employed during this time. In runners, pay particular attention to running technique and surface. They should be advised to avoid both banked surfaces and allowing the feet to cross the midline when running. A randomized controlled trial[60] comparing a corticosteroid injection, home training, and shockwave therapy found that although there was clear superiority with corticosteroid injection, this was lost at one month, with radial shockwave therapy performing the best at one month and four months. A review[61] published in 2011 concluded that most conservative approaches work with a special mention to shockwave therapy. For recalcitrant cases, a corticosteroid injection is suggested and then, if ineffective, surgery is recommended.

Iliopectineal and Iliopsoas Bursitis

Classic Presentation

The patient often presents with a severe, acute anterior hip pain with an antalgic gait. He or she may also report pain radiating down the anterior aspect of the leg. This is due to pressure on the neighboring femoral nerve. The patient often will assume a position of flexion and external rotation of the hip to relieve the pain.

Cause

These anterior bursitises are possibly due to hip flexor tightness coupled with repetitive activity.

Evaluation

There is often deep anterior tenderness at the hip. Specifically, the bursa is located about 1 to 2 cm below the middle third of the inguinal ligament. The iliopsoas bursa may be palpated with the supine patient's hip flexed to 90° while palpating over the lesser trochanter. Resisted hip flexion or more specific iliopsoas testing will reproduce the pain.[62]

Management

Rest and stretching of the hip flexors often will resolve the problem. Myofascial release of the iliopsoas must be performed cautiously.

Ischial Bursitis

Classic Presentation

Often the patient reports sitting for long periods of time on hard surfaces (benchwarmer's bursitis) or during horseback riding. She or he may have referral down the back of the leg mimicking sciatica. The patient may notice that pressing the foot down on the brake pedal (or gas pedal) of a car may relieve the pain. This is due to accompanying extension of the knee, which rotates the ischial tuberosity away from the sitting surface. In the younger athletic patient, speed work (sprinting) may cause a bursitis due to excessive hamstring contraction. This must be differentiated from an apophysitis.

Cause

Ischial bursitis is caused by a direct blow to the bursa, acute or chronic trauma (as in horseback riding), or prolonged irritation from hard-surface sitting. Chronic hamstring strains and occasionally prolonged standing may also cause irritation.[63]

Evaluation

The patient may list toward the affected side with an accompanying shortened stride length. Toe standing may be painful. There is well-localized tenderness over the ischial tuberosity. Straight leg raising and Patrick's test may also reproduce pain.

Management

Padding such as a small inflatable pillow may help in the acute phase. Avoidance of the inciting activity is necessary for long-term management.

Snapping Hip Syndrome

Classic Presentation

Other than snapping, many patients do not have pain. The location of the snapping is a good indicator of the offending structure. If traumatic, consider an acetabular labrum tear.

Cause

Snapping at the hip is often due to tendons that snap over bony prominences or bursae. Occasionally, abduction may cause a suction effect similar to joint gapping with manipulation. Even more rarely, a loose body may be found in the joint. However, with loose bodies, there are accompanying signs of mechanical blockage of movement.

Evaluation

The location and movement pattern are often helpful. Lateral hip snapping usually occurring on hip flexion with the hip in adduction is most often due to the iliotibial band's snapping at the greater trochanter. Anterior snapping or popping occurring with active extension of the flexed, abducted, and externally rotated hip often indicates iliopsoas tendon involvement or occasionally snapping of the iliofemoral ligaments over the anterior joint capsule. Posterior snapping in the buttocks region is probably due to the biceps femoris tendon's snapping over the ischial tuberosity.

Management

Usually these are benign and position-dependent. If painful or irritating to the patient, strengthening rather than stretching the involved muscle is often helpful. Stabilization seems to reduce occurrence. If unsuccessful, stretching may be employed as a second treatment option. For recalcitrant cases of a snapping iliopsoas tendon, arthroscopic surgery with tendon release may be of benefit.[64] In these cases, it has been found that intra-articular pathology often exists.

Transient Synovitis

Classic Presentation

A child less than 10 years of age complains of an acute or gradual onset of pain in the inguinal area with difficulty bearing weight. The child will often hold the hip in external rotation, abduction, and flexion. Trauma is not often part of the history; however, a prior viral infection is often elicited.

Cause

The cause is unknown in many cases; however, it may be a portent of either rheumatoid disease or ensuing Legg-Calvé-Perthes disease (1.5% to 10% of cases).[65]

Evaluation

Findings of a decrease in internal rotation and some restriction of other movements with some general tenderness to palpation are commonly found; however, they are nonspecific. Radiographs are not revealing. A bone scan is often diagnostic, but the specificity is low. Ultrasound may demonstrate fluid in the joint. The primary differential is a septic hip. However, the initial history is similar, with a preceding respiratory infection. Aspiration may be needed to make the diagnosis. Septic arthritis is a medical emergency. MRI may help differentiate.

Management

In the idiopathic benign form, resolution over several weeks occurs with a non-weight-bearing period followed by crutch use over several weeks. One review[66] indicated that resolution should occur in two weeks on average with recurrence rates anywhere from 0% to 26%. The caution is to recheck all cases over six months to avoid missing the start of Legg-Calvé-Perthes disease.

Osteoarthritis

Classic Presentation

In primary OA a middle-aged or elderly patient presents with hip and possibly buttock, groin, or knee pain that was insidious in onset. Additionally, the patient notes a slow stiffening (specifically internal rotation). This often results in the patient's walking with the hip held in external rotation. The patient may complain of low back pain due to excessive extension with weight-bearing to compensate for limited hip extension.

In secondary OA, the presentation may be similar; however, there may be a history of trauma to the hip, or the patient may have other joint involvement if crystal deposition (i.e., gout) is a factor.

Cause

Primary OA is due to progressive degeneration of femoral and acetabular articular cartilage. This is presumably caused by the accumulation of microtrauma. However, primary OA of the hip is not common. It is considered when there are preexisting abnormalities of the acetabulum or femoral head (congenital or acquired).[67] Secondary OA may be due to calcium pyrophosphate dihydrate crystal deposition disease, acromegaly, hemochromatosis, neuroarthropathy, and other articular problems.

Evaluation

There is restriction to passive internal rotation and extension of the hip. Eventually, abductor or adductor contracture may develop. Pain may be produced by axially compressing the femur into the acetabulum. Nonuniform loss of joint space is found radiographically. Superior joint space narrowing with associated findings of subchondral cysts and osteophytes is the hallmark of OA. It is important to note that many patients receive the diagnosis of OA when in fact there are no radiographic findings to support this diagnosis.

Although more common in the shoulder, there are reports of adhesive capsulitis of the hip.[68, 69] It appears from the few reports in the literature that there is always a precipitating traumatic event. There is little to suggest how to approach this entity diagnostically given that the literature speaks only to radiographic and arthroscopic evaluation. It would appear that in patients with severely restricted hip rotation following trauma with no evidence of fracture, adhesive capsulitis should be considered.

Management

If appropriate, reduction of weight will be of benefit. Non-weight-bearing exercise is often quite beneficial, including pool exercises and bicycle riding. Strengthening of the joint often will relieve constant pain. Stretching of hip contractures may be accomplished with gentle PNF stretching or deeper myofascial release techniques. Use of a cane should be limited to those with severe pain. A recent review of the literature by Brantingham et al. concluded that there is good evidence for short- and long-term success using manipulation for patients with OA of the hip.[70]

Rheumatoid Arthritis

Classic Presentation

A woman between ages 25 and 55 years presents with hip pain and associated periarticular soft tissue swelling, stiffness, and ROM restriction. At some point in the presentation the pain is bilateral.

Cause

The cause is a synovial inflammatory process that creates a destructive pannus.

Evaluation

Radiographically there is uniform, symmetric joint space diminution superiorly. Eventually this is bilateral. Associated findings are periarticular osteoporosis, subchondral cysts, and osseous destruction. In later stages, ankylosis and protrusio acetabuli (femoral head protrudes through the acetabulum) may occur. Similar findings are seen in other joints such as the hands, knees, ankles, and cervical spine. Positive laboratory findings include an elevated erythrocyte sedimentation rate (ESR) and a positive rheumatoid factor.

Management

Comanagement is often necessary. For acute periods, the use of nonsteroid anti-inflammatory drugs is often helpful. Mild, passive movements may be helped by maintaining hip motion and help reduce swelling. The RA hip should not be aggressively manipulated.

Tumors

Classic Presentation

A patient aged 50 years or older presents with a complaint of deep bone pain (66% to 80% of cases).[71] There was an insidious onset and the pain is not relieved by rest; it is worse at night. Past history may include a previous diagnosis of lung, breast, kidney, prostate, or thyroid cancer (if metastatic).[72]

Causes

The causes are metastasis and multiple myeloma.

Evaluation

Laboratory may reveal an increase in ESR, serum calcium, alkaline phosphatase, and, if from a prostate tumor, prostate-specific antigen. Multiple myeloma has characteristic findings of Bence-Jones proteinuria, increased ESR, monoclonal spiking on electrophoresis, and an M spike on immunoelectrophoresis. Radiographic changes may be lytic or blastic, depending on the type of tumor. Breast and kidney tumors tend to be lytic, whereas a prostate tumor tends to be blastic. Multiple myeloma has a lytic presentation.

Management

Referral for oncologic consultation is needed.

Paget's Disease

Classic Presentation

Ninety percent of patients are asymptomatic. They may notice an increase in hat size or develop an insidious onset of low back and/or hip pain if symptomatic. Usually Paget's disease is found inadvertently on radiographs of middle-aged or elderly patients.

Cause

The cause is unknown; however, a viral etiology is suspected. In less than 2% of cases sarcomatous degeneration is a complication.[73]

Evaluation

Radiographic evaluation will demonstrate a cross-hatched appearance of the femoral head trabeculae. Later changes include remodeling, with increased opacity and deformation, and later bowing.

Management

There is no medical treatment that prevents or cures Paget's disease. Asymptomatic patients are not treated. Those who are symptomatic are treated with a choice of various drugs. The most common drug used with pagetic pain is calcitonin, now available in a nasal spray. Other drugs include the diphosphonates, which inhibit osteoclast activity.

GROIN

Osteitis Pubis

Classic Presentation

The patient often will report either a sudden, forced adduction injury or a repetitive minor trauma seen with kicking or running. Pregnant women may be prone to irritation also.

Cause

Direct compressive or distractive injury may cause pain at the pubic joint.

Evaluation

There is tenderness at the pubic joint with compression and sometimes with compression of the two ASISs toward each other. Resisted adduction is also provocative in many cases. Occasionally a bone scan is necessary to diagnose because of the lack of sensitivity on radiographs.

Management

Management includes rest with a slow return to activity and gradual increase in flexibility; avoidance of the inciting activity, especially side-foot kicking or bilateral adduction maneuvers. Gross instability at the joint may require surgical stabilization.

Adductor Sprain

Classic Presentation

The patient is usually an athlete who is involved in kicking, sprinting, water skiing, or jumping (high jumps or hurdles). He or she reports a sudden pulling sensation in the groin that was incapacitating.

Cause

The cause of an adductor sprain is sudden contraction of the adductors from a stretched position of hip abduction or flexion. The most common site is at the myofascial junction of the adductor magnus.

Evaluation

The patient has a discrete site of tenderness in the adductor muscle group or at the pubic attachment. Resisted adduction sharply increases the pain or discomfort.

Management

Elastic figure-of-eight strapping is applied with the hip in slight extension and internal rotation. This will assist the adductor in normal walking for a week or so. Gentle stretching and a slow return to activity are suggested.

THIGH

Hamstring Strain

Classic Presentation

The patient is often an athlete or "weekend warrior" who feels a sudden pull or pop at the back of the thigh following a forceful knee extension maneuver.

Cause

The mechanism is an overcontraction of the hamstrings while in a position of stretch. Tearing occurs most often at the junction of the muscle and aponeurosis. Avulsion of the ischial apophysis is possible in younger athletes.

Evaluation

Palpation of a site of tenderness at the distal muscle belly associated with increased pain on resisted knee flexion is diagnostic. Pain is correlated to the degree of injury. Full ruptures are quite painful.

Management

Treatment includes rest, ice, use of crutches for several days, gentle stretching when tolerable, and a long-term goal of restrengthening beginning when 75% of the normal ROM is available. For first-degree strains, return to normal activity is often within a couple of weeks; for second-degree, four to six weeks; for full ruptures, it often takes three to four months to return to a normal level of activity. A focus on prevention includes pre-event stretching, maintaining a proper strength ratio between the hamstrings and quadriceps (0.6:1), and proper strength balance between hamstrings.

Quadriceps Strain

Classic Presentation

The patient reports feeling a sudden pulling pain in the anterior thigh after attempting to sprint, "missing" a kick, or suddenly stopping.

Cause

Sudden contraction of the quadriceps may result in a simple pull or a full rupture. Some predispositions include tight quadriceps (or not stretching prior to a sport activity), imbalance between the quadriceps of the opposite leg, or a short leg.

Evaluation

Actively extending the knee causes pain. Inability to perform a simple quadriceps isometric contraction with the leg extended indicates moderate to severe damage. A palpable defect or muscle mass on resisted extension indicates possible rupture.

Management

Management includes ice coupled with a neoprene or elastic support wrap. Crutches may be needed for several days, depending on the degree of injury. Stretching should be initiated as early as possible but with caution. Complete ruptures require surgical repair.

Contusions and Myositis Ossificans

Classic Presentation

The most common area is the quadriceps. The patient will report a direct blow to the knee followed by swelling and decreased ability to flex the knee.

Cause

A direct blow causes damage to the underlying muscle with subsequent hematoma formation. When the hematoma is encouraged to remain, myositis ossificans may occur. The contributing factors for myositis ossificans are forcefully stretching after injury, deep massage to the area of injury, and the use of deep heat such as ultrasound.

Evaluation

There is an obvious area of swelling and often discoloration. The patient's active and passive ability to flex the knee is limited. If the injury occurred several weeks before, a painful lump may be palpable, indicating possible myositis ossificans. Radiographs often will demonstrate the degree of maturation of this calcification response.

Management

Application of a tensor bandage with an ice pack in a flexed knee position for several hours (alternating icing for 20 minutes, no ice for 10 to 20 minutes) is helpful in preventing accumulation of blood into the area. With moderate to severe contusions, use of crutches for two to three days may be helpful. Mild stretching may begin after two to three days. Treatment decisions regarding myositis ossificans development are made after several weeks, based on the deformity and degree of knee flexion restriction. Surgical excision may then be performed if deemed desirable.

Meralgia Paresthetica

Classic Presentation

The patient complains of numbness or tingling in the lateral thigh.

Cause

Compression of the lateral femoral cutaneous nerve may occur at the inguinal ligament, or slightly below, due to prolonged sitting. The patient is often either overweight or carries keys or other objects in the front pockets.

Evaluation

The symptoms may be made worse with direct pressure on the nerve where it is most superficial, about 1 inch inferior to the ASIS. Maneuvers that increase symptoms include passive hip extension or forced hip flexion causing traction and compression, respectively. An area of sensory deficit or hyperesthesia may be found at a lateral patch of skin on the anterolateral thigh.

Management

Treatment and prevention include avoiding prolonged sitting, losing weight if necessary, and avoidance of carrying objects in the pockets. In the acute phase, physical therapy modalities such as interferential techniques may be helpful.

The Evidence—Hip

Translation Into Practice Summary (TIPS)

The literature on history and examination of the hip is focused on identifying osteoarthritis, instability, labrum tears/impingement, and fracture. The age of the patient and the relationship to trauma or no trauma is a useful indication of specific problems. For many conditions, the diagnosis is primarily radiographic (i.e., x-ray or special imaging) with no specific tests designed or tested for the physical examination. For example, for hip joint infection, Legg-Calvé-Perthes, slipped-epiphysis, avascular necrosis, stress fracture, and tumor, there are no helpful physical examination indicators.

The Literature-Based Clinical Core

- Age gives a helpful starting point in determining the risk of specific disorders.
- For most age-related conditions other than osteoarthritis, there are no specific literature-based tests and diagnosis is reliant on radiography/special imaging.
- The combination of findings on history and examination are useful in ruling-in or out osteoarthritis. Four or five of the following: squatting-aggravates symptoms, lateral pain with active hip flexion, scour test with adduction causing lateral hip or groin pain, pain with active hip extension, and passive internal rotation of less than or equal to 25°. Limitation in the planes of movement is helpful in identifying osteoarthritis.
- The patellar-pubic percussion test is good at ruling-in or out hip fractures but is of questionable practical value except on-field.
- Clicking of the hip associated with pain is suggestive of labrum pathology.
- Hip dysplasia or instability in infants may be indicated by limited hip abduction.
- Flexion-abduction, external rotation (FABER) testing and flexion-internal rotation-adduction (FAIR) are sensitive for hip pathology but entirely nonspecific.

- Trendelenburg's test is moderately good at detecting lateral tendon pathologies and gluteus medius tears.
- Although hip ROM testing is reliable, pain with resistance is more valuable in detecting lateral tendon pathologies such as gluteus minimus or medius problems.
- The tests for labrum tears and impingement have not been evaluated in the literature.

The Expert Opinion-Based Clinical Core

- A history of recent infection and the insidious onset of hip pain warrant investigation of hip joint infection, especially if the pain prevents weight bearing.
- The sudden insidious onset of hip pain and inability to bear weight in a young patient warrant the investigation for slipped epiphysis.
- A limp and/or knee pain in a child warrants the investigation of Legg-Calvé-Perthes.
- Persistent hip or groin pain in an athlete, in particular a female athlete, is highly suspicious for stress fracture.
- Lateral hip pain, worse when lying on that side with greater trochanter tenderness, is likely trochanteric bursitis. However, the newest general designation when the bursa is not found to be involved is trochanteric pain syndrome.

APPENDIX 11-1

References

1. Philippon MJ. The role of arthroscopic thermal capsulorrhaphy in the hip. *Clin Sports Med.* 2001;20(4):817–829.
2. Wenger D, Miyanji F, Mahar A, Oka R. The mechanical properties of the ligamentum teres: a pilot study to assess its potential for improving stability in children's hip surgery. *J Pediatr Orthop.* 2007;27(4):408–410.
3. Byrd JW, Jones KS. Hip arthroscopy in athletes. *Clin Sports Med.* 2001;20(4):749–761.
4. Kim YT, Azuma H. The nerve endings of the acetabular labrum. *Clin Orthop Relat Res.* 1995(320):176–181.

5. McCarthy JC, Noble PC, Schuck MR, Wright J, Lee J. The Otto E. Aufranc Award: The role of labral lesions to development of early degenerative hip disease. *Clin Orthop Relat Res.* 2001(393):25–37.

6. Brand RA, Crowninshield RD. The effect of cane use on hip contraction force. *Clin Orthop.* 1980;147:181–184.

7. Mitchell B, McCrory P, Brukner P, O'Donnell J, Colson E, Howells R. Hip joint pathology: clinical presentation and correlation between magnetic resonance arthrography, ultrasound, and arthroscopic findings in 25 consecutive cases. *Clin J Sport Med.* 2003;13(3):152–156.

8. Fitzgerald RH, Jr. Acetabular labrum tears. Diagnosis and treatment. *Clin Orthop Relat Res.* 1995(311):60–68.

9. McCarthy JC. The diagnosis and treatment of labral and chondral injuries. *Instr Course Lect.* 2004;53:573–577.

10. Beck M, Leunig M, Parvizi J, Boutier V, Wyss D, Ganz R. Anterior femoroacetabular impingement: part II. Midterm results of surgical treatment. *Clin Orthop Relat Res.* 2004(418):67–73.

11. Ito K, Leunig M, Ganz R. Histopathologic features of the acetabular labrum in femoroacetabular impingement. *Clin Orthop Relat Res.* 2004(429):262–271.

12. Narvani AA, Tsiridis E, Kendall S, Chaudhuri R, Thomas P. A preliminary report on prevalence of acetabular labrum tears in sports patients with groin pain. *Knee Surg Sports Traumatol Arthrosc.* 2003;11(6):403–408.

13. Martin RL, Enseki KR, Draovitch P, Trapuzzano T, Philippon MJ. Acetabular labral tears of the hip: examination and diagnostic challenges. *J Orthop Sports Phys Ther.* 2006;36(7):503–515.

14. Steindler A. *Kinesiology of the Human Body.* Springfield, IL: Charles C Thomas; 1977.

15. Frankel VH, Nordin M. Biomechanics of the hip. In: *Basic Biomechanics of the Musculoskeletal System.* Philadelphia: Lea & Febiger; 1980.

16. Nicholas PJR, Bailey NTJ. The accuracy of measuring leg length difference. *Br Med J.* 1955;29:1247–1248.

17. Beattie P. Validity of derived measurements of leg length difference obtained by use of a tape measure. *Phys Ther.* 1990;70:150–157.

18. Manello DM. Leg length inequality. *J Manipulative Physiol Ther.* 1992;15:576–580.

19. Mondel DL, Garrison SJ, Geiringer SR, et al. Rehabilitation of musculoskeletal and soft tissue disorders. *Arch Phys Med Rehabil.* 1988;69S:130–138.

20. Bedi A, Dolan M, Leunig M, Kelly BT. Static and dynamic mechanical causes of hip pain. *Arthroscopy.* 2011;27(2):235–251.

21. Franklyn-Miller A, Falvey E, McCrory P. The gluteal triangle: a clinical patho-anatomical approach to the diagnosis of gluteal pain in athletes. *Br J Sports Med.* 2009;43(6):460–466.

22. Larson CM, Sikka RS, Sardelli MC, et al. Increasing alpha angle is predictive of athletic-related "hip" and "groin" pain in collegiate National Football League prospects. *Arthroscopy.* 2013;29(3):405–410.

23. Garvey JF, Hazard H. Sports hernia or groin disruption injury? Chronic athletic groin pain: a retrospective study of 100 patients with long-term follow-up. *Hernia.* 2013. [Epub ahead of print]

24. Taylor JAM, Harger BL, Resnick D. Diagnostic imaging of common hip disorders: a pictorial review. *Top Clin Chirop.* 1994;1(2):8–23.

25. Wenger DE, Kendell KR, Miner MR, Trousdale RT. Acetabular labral tears rarely occur in the absence of bony abnormalities. *Clin Orthop Relat Res.* 2004(426):145–150.

26. Yochum TR, Rowe LJ. *Essentials of Skeletal Radiology.* 2nd ed. Baltimore: Williams & Wilkins; 1996:714.

27. Byrd JW, Jones KS. Diagnostic accuracy of clinical assessment, magnetic resonance imaging, magnetic resonance arthrography, and intra-articular injection in hip arthroscopy patients. *Am J Sports Med.* 2004;32(7):1668–1674.

28. Cotton DW, Whitehead CL, Vyas S, et al. Are hip fractures caused by falling and breaking or breaking and falling? Photoelastic stress analysis. *Forensic Sci Int.* 1994;65:105–112.

29. DeLee JC. Fractures and dislocations of the hip. In: Rockwood CA Jr, Green DP, eds. *Fractures in Adults.* 2nd ed. Philadelphia: JB Lippincott; 1984:1211–1356.

30. Waters PM, Millis MB. Hip and pelvis injuries in the young athlete. *Clin Sports Med.* 1988;7:513–526.

31. Garden RS. Malreduction and avascular necrosis in sub-capital fractures of the femur. *J Bone Joint Surg Br.* 1967;63:183–197.

32. Meaney JE, Carty H. Femoral stress fractures in children. *Skeletal Radiol.* 1992;21:173–176.

33. Resnick D, Niwayana G. *Diagnosis of Bone Disorders.* Philadelphia: WB Saunders; 1995.

34. Putti V. Early treatment of congenital dislocation of the hip. *J Bone Joint Surg Am.* 1929;11:798.

35. Miralles M, Gonzales G, Pulpeiro JR, et al. Sonography of the painful hip in children: 500 consecutive cases. *Amer J Radiol.* 1989;152:579–582.

36. Stanitski CL. Acute slipped capital femoral epiphysis. *J Am Acad Orthop Surg.* 1994;2:96–106.

37. Kelsey JL, Acheson DM, Keggi KJ. The body build of patients with slipped capital femoral epiphysis. *Am J Dis Child.* 1972;124:276.

38. MacEwen GD, Bunnell WP, Ramsey PL. The hip. In: Lowell WW, Winter RB, eds. *Pediatric Orthopedics.* Philadelphia: JB Lippincott; 1986.

39. Wilson PD, Jacobs B, Schecter L. Slipped capital femoral epiphysis: an end-result study. *J Bone Joint Surg Am.* 1965; 47:1128–1145.

40. Barker DJP, Hall AJ. The epidemiology of Perthes disease. *Clin Orthop.* 1986;209:89.

41. Fisher RI. An epidemiologic study of Legg-Perthes disease. *J Bone Joint Surg Am.* 1972;54:769.

42. Pires de Camago F, Maciel de Gidoy R, Tovo R. Angiography in Perthes disease. *Clin Orthop.* 1984;191:216.

43. Turek SL. *Orthopedic Principles and Their Application.* Philadelphia: JB Lippincott; 1984:1109–1268.

44. McAndrew MP, Weinstein SL. A long-term follow-up of Legg-Calvé-Perthes disease. *J Bone Joint Surg Am.* 1984;66:860.

45. Philippon MJ, Maxwell RB, Johnston TL, Schenker M, Briggs KK. Clinical presentation of femoroacetabular impingement. *Knee Surg Sports Traumatol Arthrosc.* 2007;15(8):1041–1047.

46. Parvizi J, Leunig M, Ganz R. Femoroacetabular impingement. *J Am Acad Orthop Surg.* 2007;15(9):561–570.

47. Philippon MJ, Stubbs AJ, Schenker ML, Maxwell RB, Ganz R, Leunig M. Arthroscopic management of femoroacetabular impingement: osteoplasty technique and literature review. *Am J Sports Med.* 2007;35(9):1571–1580.

48. McCarthy JC, Noble PC, Schuck MR, Wright J, Lee J. The watershed labral lesion: its relationship to early arthritis of the hip. *J Arthroplasty.* 2001;16(8 Suppl 1):81–87.

49. Burnett RS, Della Rocca GJ, Prather H, Curry M, Maloney WJ, Clohisy JC. Clinical presentation of patients with tears of the acetabular labrum. *J Bone Joint Surg Am.* 2006;88(7):1448–1457.

50. O'Donnell J, Economopoulos K, Singh P, Bates D, Pritchard M. The Ligamentum Teres Test: A Novel and Effective Test in Diagnosing Tears of the Ligamentum Teres. *Am J Sports Med.* 2014;42:138–143.

51. Lage LA, Patel JV, Villar RN. The acetabular labral tear: an arthroscopic classification. *Arthroscopy.* 1996;12(3):269–272.

52. Ikeda T, Awaya G, Suzuki S, Okada Y, Tada H. Torn acetabular labrum in young patients. Arthroscopic diagnosis and management. *J Bone Joint Surg Br.* 1988;70(1):13–16.

53. Byrd JW, Jones KS. Prospective analysis of hip arthroscopy with 2-year follow-up. *Arthroscopy.* 2000;16(6):578–587.

54. O'Leary J A, Berend K, Vail TP. The relationship between diagnosis and outcome in arthroscopy of the hip. *Arthroscopy.* 2001;17(2):181–188.

55. Santori N, Villar RN. Acetabular labral tears: result of arthroscopic partial limbectomy. *Arthroscopy.* 2000;16(1):11–15.

56. Swezey R. Pseudo-radiculopathy in subacute trochanteric bursitis of the subgluteus maximus bursa. *Arch Phys Med Rehabil.* 1976;57:387–390.

57. Troycoff RB. "Pseudotrochanteric bursitis": the differential diagnosis of lateral hip pain. *J Rheumatol.* 1992;18:1810–1812.

58. Baum J. Joint pain: it isn't always arthritis. *Postgrad Med.* 1989;85:311–321.

59. Fearon AM, Scarvell JM, Neeman T, Cook JL, Cormick W, Smith PN. Greater trochanteric pain syndrome: defining the clinical syndrome. *Br J Sports Med.* 2013;47(10):649–653.

60. Rompe JD, Segal NA, Cacchio A, Furia JP, Morral A, Maffulli N. Home training, local corticosteroid injection, or radial shock wave therapy for greater trochanter pain syndrome. *Am J Sports Med.* 2009. 2009 as doi:10.1177/0363546509334374.

61. Lustenberger DP, Ng VY, Best TM, Ellis TJ. Efficacy of treatment of trochanteric bursitis: a systematic review. *Clin J Sport Med.* 2011;21(5):447–453.

62. Rotini R, Sinozzi C, Ferrari A. Snapping hip: a rare form with internal etiology. *Ital J Orthop Traumatol.* 1991;17:283–288.

63. Swartout R, Compere EL. Ischiogluteal bursitis. *JAMA.* 1974;227:551–552.

64. Byrd JW. Evaluation and management of the snapping iliopsoas tendon. *Instr Course Lect.* 2006;55:347–355.

65. Haueisen DC. The characterization of transient synovitis of the hip in children. *J Pediatr Orthop.* 1986;6:11.

66. Asche SS, van Rijn RM, Bessems MK, Bierma-Zeinstra S. What is the clinical course of transient synovitis in children? A systematic review of the literature. *Chiropr Man Therap.* 2013;21:39.

67. Harris WH. Etiology of osteoarthritis of the hip. *Clin Orthop.* 1988;213:20–38.

68. Byrd JW, Jones KS. Adhesive capsulitis of the hip. *Arthroscopy.* 2006;22(1):89–94.

69. Griffiths HJ, Utz R, Burke J, Bonfiglio T. Adhesive capsulitis of the hip and ankle. *AJR Am J Roentgenol.* 1985;144(1):101–105.

70. Brantingham JW, Bonnefin D, Perle SM, et al. Manipulative therapy for lower extremity conditions: update of a literature review. *J Manipulative Physiol Ther.* 2012;35(2):127–166.

71. Palmer E, Henrikson B, McKusick K, et al. Pain as an indicator of bone metastasis. *Acta Radiol.* 1988;24:445–450.

72. Resnick D. *Bone and Joint Imaging.* Philadelphia: WB Saunders; 1989.

73. Gallacher SJ. Paget's disease of bone. *Curr Opin Rheumatol.* 1993;5:351.

APPENDIX 11–2

Hip Pain Diagnosis Table

Diagnosis	Comments	History Findings	Positive Examination Findings	Radiography/Special Studies	Treatment Options
Hip Subluxation/Fixation	• Can be primary Dx if patient is asymptomatic or mildly symptomatic (e.g., mild stiffness or pain level < 2/10). • Must indicate chiropractic exam findings to support Dx.	*Nonspecific*	*Palpation*—Local tenderness or other signs of subluxation *Ortho*—None *Neuro*—None *Active ROM*—Variable restriction *Passive ROM*—End-range restriction *Motion palpation*—Specific articular restriction or symptoms produced on end-range	• Radiography not required for the diagnosis of subluxation. • Radiographic biomechanical analysis may assist in treatment decisions.	• Chiropractic adjustive technique. • Decisions regarding specifically which technique(s) is/are applied and modifications to the given approach will be directed by the primary Dx and patient's ability to tolerate pre-adjustment stresses.
Hip/Thigh Sprain/Strain *Note: Sprain/strain is not synonymous with spasm or hypertonicity.*		*Mechanism*—Overstretch or overcontraction Hx as acute event *Worse with Specific ROM*—Contraction of muscle or stretch of muscle or joint	*Ortho*—Specific tests for each muscle including tenderness at muscle/tendon *Neuro*—None *Active ROM*—Pain on active ROM that contracts involved muscles *Passive ROM*—Pain on end-range stretch of involved muscle or ligament	• Radiography not required for diagnosis unless significant trauma implies fracture or eiphyseal injury.	• Myofascial therapy. • Limited orthotic support (taping or brace). • Ergonomic advice. • Strengthening and preventive exercises.

(continues)

Hip Pain Diagnosis Table (continued)

Diagnosis	Comments	History Findings	Positive Examination Findings	Radiography/Special Studies	Treatment Options
Meralgia Paresthetica	• Must be differentiated from nerve root source.	*Mechanism*—Entrapment of the lateral femoral cutaneous nerve is often due to pressure from obesity/pregnancy or external objects such as keys, etc. pressing on nerve distal to the inguinal ligament *Symptoms*—Complaint is mainly hypersensitivity and/or numbness and tingling; no weakness reported	*Palpation*—Direct pressure one-inch distal to ASIS may reproduce complaint *Ortho*—Forced passive, full flexion of hip or passive extension may reproduce complaint *Neuro*—Hyperesthesia over lateral anterior thigh; no motor deficits	• Radiographs not required. • Electrodiagnostic studies rarely needed unless to differentiate from nerve root.	• Eliminate any pressure causes, including recommendations to loosen belt, lose weight, and avoid wearing objects that press on nerve. • Physiotherapy may be beneficial in acute stages.
Gluteal or Iliopsoas Tendinitis, Trochanteric or Ischial Bursitis	• Patient may complain of snapping in addition to specific areas of pain. • Snapping may be painless and not represent an active acute condition.	*Mechanism*—Often no Hx of overt trauma; however, overuse may cause a friction effect resulting in a chronic bursitis	*Palpation*—Tenderness at specific bursal or tendon insertion site *Ortho*—Stretch or stretch/contraction of involved muscle/tendon may increase pain for tendinitis	• Radiography not usually necessary initially except to rule out fracture with acute trauma.	• Myofascial therapy for muscle/ tendon problems. • Physiotherapy for pain and swelling control for bursitis. • Padded protection for superficial bursa. • Stretching and strengthening of involved muscle/tendon. • Ergonomic advice to avoid irritation of involved bursa.

Myofasciitis	• Used when specific trigger points are identified on physical examination. • Also may be used if a strain is not evident from the history but there are indicators of muscle tenderness, stiffness, or pain.	*Onset:* Nonspecific regarding onset *Symptoms:* Patient usually complains of pain, aching, and/or tenderness in specific muscle or tendon areas that may radiate pain in non-dermatomal pattern	Trigger points are evident as localized tenderness in a muscle that corresponds to traditional (Travell/Simons) trigger point charts. These points may be local or refer pain when compressed	• Not required or recommended.	• Myofascial approaches such as myofascial stripping, trigger point massage, or spray and stretch approaches are the standard. • Home stretching and modification of activity suggestions.
Laxity Hypermobility	• The hip is an inherently stable joint and if laxity is present it is difficult to demonstrate clinically.	A history of a single-event traumatic injury to the joint is not found; however, either overuse (microtrauma) or generalized inherent looseness is/are evident	Capsular or ligament testing reveals "looseness" that falls within the physiologic range of normal	• Not usually recommended unless when differentiating pathological laxity from congenital or overuse acquisition.	• Strengthening program. • Bracing or functional taping during rehabilitation or during strenuous activities.

Knee Complaints

Context

Knee complaints are common in an orthopaedic setting.[1] In a general community setting, 10% to 15% of adults report knee symptoms.[2] Knee pain accounts for approximately 3% to 5% of all visits to medical physicians.[3] Statistics for chiropractic visits are less clear. Generally, the Job Analysis of Chiropractic[4] reports that 9.4% of patients who seek chiropractic care have lower-extremity complaints. It is unclear which percentage is attributable to knee complaints. Although there are no available statistics on the frequency of presentation in chiropractic offices, chiropractors often serve a role as a conservative management alternative to orthopaedic consultation. In this context, the chiropractor's approach includes an evaluation of possible spinal or pelvic contributions in addition to local knee dysfunction or pathologic conditions. The distinction between referred or radiating pain and local knee problems may be as obvious as a direct radiation of pain from the low back, pelvis, or hip to the knee; however, the biomechanical contribution may not be quite as evident. Inherent in the evaluation process is the need to determine any neurologic connection between a knee complaint that is associated with a low back or pelvic complaint. When knee pain is due to an obvious direct trauma, the evaluation process focuses on a regional evaluation. If, however, the knee pain is local and either insidious or due to an overuse phenomenon, biomechanical evaluation of the lower extremity and lumbopelvic region must be included to determine contributing factors.

The knee may be the site of pain originating from or caused by a variety of sources, including the following:

- Referred pain from pain-sensitive structures in the low back, pelvis, and lower extremity (including facet joints, the sacroiliac and hip joints, and trigger points)
- Radiating pain from nerve root compression
- Peripheral nerve root entrapment (sciatic, peroneal, saphenous, etc.)
- Generalized dysfunction of the lower extremity (femoral anteversion/retroversion, genu varum/valgus/recurvatum, tibial torsion, pronation/supination, etc.)
- Local causes of pain
  1. Trauma
  2. Overuse
  3. Other (tumor, aneurysm, infection, etc.)

The knee is frequently injured based in part on its position of exposure to outside trauma. Virtually unprotected from outside forces, the knee is vulnerable to any number of impact injuries, including blows from the outside (valgus forces), dashboard injuries, and direct impact falls. Superficial damage may be readily accessible via palpation and stress testing. Internal damage is more often disguised, yielding only indirect and often delayed clues to the degree of injury. When intra-articular swelling is present, orthopaedic assessment is often delayed or the results of testing minimized because of the positional restrictions imposed on testing and reactive muscle spasm. The stability provided by joint effusion may delay the appreciation of an unstable knee. The true residual integrity of the knee may take several weeks to become apparent following the resolution of swelling.

Soft tissue injuries are usually the result of either overuse or disuse. Overuse is usually detected through careful questioning regarding activities that require repetitive movement or prolonged or awkward positioning. This may also require an evaluation of the patient performing or acquiring the suspected inciting activity. A suspicion of disuse requires an evaluation of any biomechanical predispositions such as pronation/supination, lower extremity torsion, or patellar tracking abnormalities. If a patient presents with an insidious onset of pain with accompanying swelling, a radiographic and possibly a laboratory search for arthritides, neoplasm, or infection should be instituted. With children it is particularly important to include an evaluation of the hip. The knee is often a site of pain referral with intrinsic hip abnormalities in children.

Some common clinical presentations are as follows:

- The athlete with anterior knee pain (patellofemoral arthralgia and/or patellar tracking disorders)
- The elderly patient with a complaint of knee pain and stiffness (osteoarthritis)
- The younger athlete with a complaint of tibial tuberosity pain (Osgood-Schlatter disease)
- The patient with the complaint of instability (chronic anterior cruciate ligament [ACL] damage)
- The patient with a complaint of painful locking (meniscus tear)

General Strategy

History

Clarify the Chief Complaint

- Determine whether the complaint is one of pain, stiffness, locking, swelling, instability, crepitus, or numbness and tingling.
- Localize the complaint to anterior, posterior, lateral, or medial.

Clarify the Mechanism If Traumatic

- Hyperextension: consider an isolated ACL tear or patellar dislocation.
- Hyperflexion: consider a posterior cruciate ligament (PCL) tear (if associated with major trauma, an associated ACL tear).
- Sudden deceleration (stopping or cutting): consider an isolated ACL tear.
- Valgus force (no rotation): consider medial collateral ligament (MCL) tear.
- Valgus force with rotation (foot fixed on the ground): consider multiple tissue damage including ACL, MCL, and menisci.

- Blow to a flexed knee (local damage can include contusion, fat pad irritation, or patellar fracture): consider a PCL tear if significant force is applied.
- Determine the timing, location (intra-articular or extra-articular) and degree of any accompanying swelling.
- Determine whether there was or is locking, instability, or weakness associated with the injury or postinjury.

Determine Whether the Mechanism Might Be One of Overuse or Misuse

- Repetitive flexion and extension in midrange (e.g., running): consider iliotibial band (ITB) syndrome or popliteus tendinitis with lateral knee pain.
- Repetitive jumping or sprinting: consider patellar tendinitis (jumper's knee); in adolescents consider apophyseal injury such as Osgood-Schlatter disease with anterior knee pain.
- Constant valgus stress applied directly or indirectly: consider chronic MCL strain or pes anserinus tendinitis with medial knee pain.
- Constant squatting: consider meniscus injury.

If insidious, determine the following:

- Are there associated systemic signs of fever, malaise/fatigue, lymphadenopathy, multiple affected areas, etc.?
- Are there local signs of inflammation, including swelling, heat, or redness?
- Is there local deformity?
- Is there associated weakness, numbness, tingling, or other associated neurologic dysfunction?

Determine Whether the Patient Has a Current or Past History/Diagnosis of the Knee Complaint or Other Related Disorders

- Determine whether there are any past traumas, surgeries, or diagnoses.
- Determine whether there have been any studies such as radiography or magnetic resonance imaging (MRI) performed on the patient.
- Determine whether there are any associated low back, hip, or lower leg/foot/ankle complaints.

Evaluation

- Based on the history and presentation, perform either a region-specific or a condition-specific examination (e.g., examine the medial knee region versus perform meniscus tests).
- Determine whether radiographic views should be obtained; based on condition, determine whether specific views should be ordered.
- Avoid the initial use of MRI unless severe damage is suspected or a delayed diagnosis will affect future function; if the patient is unresponsive to conservative care, MRI may play a valuable role in determining the degree of damage and the need for surgery.

Management

- Infection, tumor, and fracture require medical referral.
- Nonisolated ACL tears require a surgical consultation.
- Isolated ACL and MCL tears may respond to conservative management, including a period of bracing and cautious rehabilitation; the decision to manage conservatively is based on age, activity level, and functional requirements of the individual and the experience of the doctor.
- Meniscus tears that are the source of unresolving signs and symptoms or are demonstrated as large tears on MRI are best managed with minimal surgical intervention.
- Most other conditions can be managed with a combination of manipulation/mobilization, rehabilitation, and activity modification.

Relevant Anatomy and Biomechanics

There are three "articulations" at the knee: (1) tibiofemoral, (2) tibiofibular, and (3) patellofemoral. The first two are synovial articulations. The patellofemoral articulation is a functional joint in which many of the same pathologic conditions found in true joints must be considered. The knee is statically supported by a peripheral system made up of the capsule, its thickenings, and the collateral ligamentous

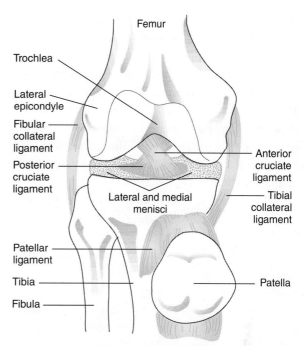

Figure 12–1 Major ligaments of the knee joint.

system (**Figure 12–1**). Internally, stability, and control of rotation are provided by the meniscal cruciate system. The cruciates, capsule, and collateral ligaments connect the femur to the tibia. The unique orientation of the cruciates allows tension to develop through most ranges of motion. The cruciates are named according to their tibial attachment. The ACL is smaller (about the size of the little finger) and more vulnerable than the PCL (about the size of the thumb). The middle genicular artery runs along the length of the ACL and is often torn with midsubstance tears of the ACL. The ACL acts as the primary restraint to forward movement of the tibia on the femur non-weight-bearing and posterior movement of the femur on the tibia with weight-bearing. The PCL serves a synergistic role in providing restraint to backward movement of the tibia on the femur non-weight-bearing and resisting forward movement of the femur on the tibia with weight-bearing. The MCL is longer than the lateral collateral ligament (LCL) and has a more direct connection to the capsule. The LCL connects the distal femur to the fibular head and is separated from the joint by the tendon of the popliteus muscle. The popliteus acts as the primary lateral protection to valgus forces. It also acts as a secondary support for the PCL. The MCL acts as the primary protection to varus forces and acts as a secondary support for the ACL.

The menisci act to deepen the joint, adding static stability. They aid in shock absorption and help govern rotational movement at the knee. Neural reflexes are activated by stimulation or stretching of the knee ligaments.[5] These are important protective reflexes that cause contraction of muscles in response to a perceived stress. One study incorporated nine patients who volunteered to have their ACLs electrically stimulated using an arthroscopic technique.[6] Surface EMG was used to record hamstring activity. The activity was measured first with no local anesthesia and then with local anesthesia. A marked increase in hamstring activity occurred without anesthesia, but there was no increased activity with anesthesia, indicating a reflex arc between the ACL and hamstrings.

The patella is the largest sesamoid bone in the body. It functionally extends the lever arm for the quadriceps muscle, making extension of the knee much more effective. Stabilization of the patella is provided by the quadriceps muscles, their fascial extensions (retinacula), and the distal attachment to the tibial tuberosity via the patellar tendon (**Figure 12–2**). The spaces between the femur and the patella and the tibia and the patella are cushioned by the suprapatellar pouch and the infrapatellar fat pad, respectively. When the patella is not stable because of a high-riding position (patella alta) or underdevelopment of the lateral femoral condyle or posterior surface of the patella, abnormal motion occurs that may damage or irritate ligaments, muscles, and cartilage.

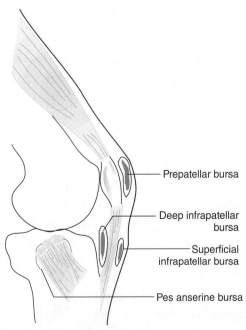

Prepatellar bursa

Deep infrapatellar bursa

Superficial infrapatellar bursa

Pes anserine bursa

Figure 12–2 Commonly irritated bursae of the knee.

It has been assumed that certain knee structures are more sensitive than others if sensitivity is defined as conscious perception of pain. Yet, most of the research has focused on mapping responses with sensory evoked potential in anesthetized patients or summarizing neurosensory output from the entire joint with respect to perception of knee position (i.e., proprioception). A recent study[7] focuses on the conscious perception of pain in an unanesthetized patient. A list of pain-sensitive structures based on this study follows.

- Probing/palpation of the central ridge and medial and lateral facets of the patella resulted in no pain.
- Probing/palpation of the odd facet of the patella resulted in a nonpainful awareness that was poorly localized by the patient.
- Probing/palpation of the suprapatellar pouch, the joint capsule, and the medial and lateral retinaculum resulted in a moderate to severe pain that was well localized.
- Probing/palpation of the femoral insertions of the ACL and PCL resulted in a nonpainful awareness that was poorly localized.
- Probing/palpation of the tibial insertion and femoral origin of the ACL/PCL resulted in a moderate to severe, poorly localized pain.
- Probing/palpation of the menisci resulted in nonpainful awareness that was poorly localized for the inner rim and slight to moderate, poorly localized pain at the capsular margins and anterior and posterior horns.
- Probing/palpation of the articular surfaces of the femoral condyles, trochlea, and tibial plateaus produced a nonpainful awareness or slight pain that was poorly localized.

These findings support some of the commonly held beliefs that follow:

- Damage to the points of origin of the cruciates and peripheral attachment points for the menisci is painful; however, internal derangements (midsubstance tears of the cruciates and deeper meniscal tears) are not in and of themselves extremely painful (subsequent to injury). The pain is probably more due to the associated effusion (bloody or synovial).
- Damage to articular cartilage and hyaline cartilage on the posterior patellae is virtually painless.
- Irritation or damage to the suprapatellar pouch, retinaculi, and joint capsule causes moderate to

severe pain and is often the source of pain when deeper structures are torn (e.g., capsular tearing or distension with internal derangement).

The primary movements of flexion and extension predominate in most functional activities. The other four movement patterns of internal/external rotation and abduction/adduction are less often voluntarily (actively) acquired or needed. Rotation and abduction/adduction at the knee are more often the consequence of voluntary hip movement. Passive abduction/adduction at the knee is not possible with the knee in full extension. As the knee flexes, these movements increase; however, they are still passively acquired. Rotation range of motion increases as the knee flexes because of the increasing mechanical advantage of the hamstrings and other secondary rotators. Flexion is primarily due to the hamstring muscles. Assistance is given by the ITB when the knee is flexed beyond 30° to 40°. Extension of the knee is performed by the quadriceps muscles with some assistance by the ITB through the last 30° to 40°. Extension is a stronger movement pattern than flexion. In the non-weight-bearing knee, internal rotation is due to the popliteus, semimembranosus, and semitendinosus muscles with some minor assistance from the sartorius and gracilis muscles. External rotation is mainly accomplished by the biceps femoris with assistance from the ITB.

Starting with the knee in extension, the bony and soft tissue components involved in stability and movement are sequenced. The knee is locked into external rotation when in full extension due in part to the lateral femoral condyle being shorter than the medial condyle. In full extension, this externally rotated position uncrosses the cruciates to some degree and places slightly more stress on the peripherally placed collateral ligaments. The tendons of the pes anserinus muscles, hamstrings, and ITB act as static stabilizers when the knee is in full extension. As the knee flexes, it rotates internally. This rotation crosses the cruciates and takes some tension off the collaterals. Through the first 20° to 30° a rolling motion occurs between the tibia and the femur. Past 30° a sliding (gliding) motion occurs.

Restriction to extension is provided by tension in the posterior capsule and by the cruciates and the bony "lock" of the screw-home mechanism. Flexion is limited by approximation with the calf to the hamstring muscle group. Additional restriction may be provided by tension in the anterior capsule or tightness in the quadriceps. Rotation is limited (and governed) by the cruciates and menisci.

Evaluation

History

Careful questioning of the patient during the history taking can point to the diagnosis (**Table 12-1**).

Pain Localization

Possible causes of pain based on localization (**Figure 12-3**, A through D, and **Table 12-2**) follow:

- Anterior
  1. Traumatic—patellar fracture, fat pad irritation, contusion of other soft tissue structures, meniscus tear, pes anserinus bursitis (anteromedial)
  2. Nontraumatic—extensor disorders (patellar tendinitis or Osgood-Schlatter disease), patellofemoral disorders (patellofemoral arthralgia or chondromalacia)
- Posterior
  1. Traumatic—PCL tears, meniscus tears, gastrocnemius soleus tears (tennis leg), semimembranosus bursitis
  2. Nontraumatic—strain of gastrocnemius or soleus, semimembranosus insertion tendinitis, bursitis, Baker's cyst, popliteal thrombus, referral from other disorders
- Lateral
  1. Traumatic—LCL tear, ACL tear with associated fracture, meniscus tear, fibular head subluxation
  2. Nontraumatic—ITB syndrome, popliteus tendinitis
- Medial
  1. Traumatic—MCL tear or rupture, medial meniscus tear
  2. Nontraumatic—MCL sprain, pes anserinus tendinitis, bursitis

Traumatic and Overuse Injuries

When the patient reports trauma, several clues taken together may indicate a specific damaged structure. The mechanism of injury, coupled with the associated signs or symptoms at the time of injury, may be suggestive of a characteristic pattern for a specific problem. There are four helpful questions:

1. Was there any swelling following the injury? Swelling that occurs immediately or within the first few hours is suggestive of hemarthrosis. Blood in

Table 12–1 History Questions for Knee Pain

Primary Question	What Are You Thinking?	Secondary Question	What Are You Thinking?
Was there trauma? (Did you hurt your knee in an accident or sports injury?)	Fracture, meniscal, cruciate, or collateral ligament tear	**Hyperextended knee?**	ACL injury
		Knee hit from outside?	MCL, ACL, or meniscus
		Weight on knee, twisted it (with or without contact)?	Meniscus
		With bent knee, fell on or hit front of knee?	PCL
		Pop at time of injury?	ACL, meniscus, or fracture
		Immediate joint swelling?	ACL or fracture
		Delayed swelling?	Meniscus or other joint irritation
		Knee painfully locks in one position?	Meniscus or flap of ACL
		Knee is held at 20° to 30° flexion to avoid pain?	General indicator of fluid in the joint
		Knee painfully gives way?	Nonspecific; pain inhibits quadriceps
Did the pain begin after a repetitive activity?	Overuse syndromes; patellofemoral, patellar or popliteal tendinitis, ITB syndrome, mild sprain or strain	**Is the pain in the front of your knee and worse with jumping?**	Patellar tendinitis or Osgood-Schlatter disease
		Is the pain on the outside of your knee and worse with downhill walking?	Popliteus tendinitis or ITB syndrome
		Is the pain on the inside of your knee and worse with breast-stroke kick, bicycling, or skiing?	MCL sprain; possible pes anserinus strain
Is the complaint more of stiffness?	Osteoarthritis, posttraumatic adhesions, subluxation	**Do you have a past history of trauma or surgery?**	Post-meniscectomy likely; trauma, adhesions from poor rehabilitation
		Age and weight of patient?	Osteoarthritis (confirm with weight-bearing films)
Is there a sense of weakness or instability?	Capsular instability, neurologic weakness	**Past injury of painful swelling resolving with increasing instability?**	ACL insufficiency due to past tear
		Past/current history of low back pain?	Neurologic weakness, especially if low back pain improved
Are there other problems that seemed to occur at or slightly before the beginning of your knee pain?	Arthritides, connective tissue disease, visceral referred pain	**Other joints that hurt?**	Check for arthritides (gout, rheumatoid arthritis, osteoarthritis, pseudogout, etc.)
		Sore throat several weeks before?	Rheumatic fever (check for murmurs)
		Abdominal pain or chronic diarrhea?	Inflammatory bowel disease arthropathy

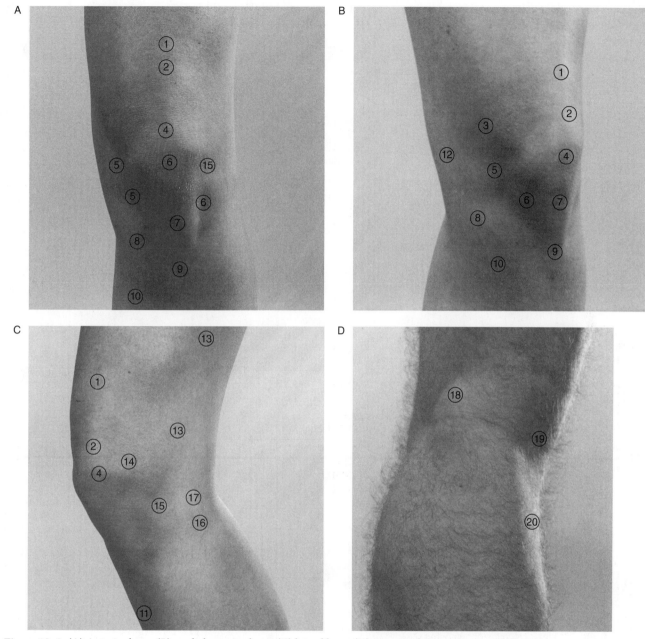

Figure 12–3 (A) Anterior knee; (B) medial anterior knee; (C) lateral knee; (D) posterior knee.

Table 12–2 Knee Pain Localization

#	Structures	Overt Trauma	Insidious or Overuse
1	Quadriceps (rectus femoris)	Strain or rupture, contusion	Strain
2	Quadriceps tendon, suprapatellar pouch (deep)	Avulsion of quadriceps tendon, suprapatellar bursitis	Tendinitis, apophysitis in younger individuals
3	Vastus medialis obliquus (VMO) insertion, medial retinaculum	Sprain of medial retinaculum or strain of VMO due to patellar dislocation	Patellar tracking disorder with chronic sprain/strain of medical retinaculum or VMO
4	Patella, patellar bursa	Fracture, dislocation, bursitis	Bipartite patella, chondromalacia patella

(continues)

Table 12–2 Knee Pain Localization (continued)

#	Structures	Overt Trauma	Insidious or Overuse
5	Medial tibiofemoral joint, meniscus, coronary ligament, medial patello-femoral ligament, medial plica	Fracture, medial meniscus tear, traumatic plica irritation	Sprain of either coronary ligament or patellofemoral ligament, or medial plica syndrome
6	Infrapatellar fat pad	Fat pad irritation	Fat pad irritation
7	Patellar tendon, infrapatellar bursa	Bursitis	Patellar tendinitis
8	Medial proximal tibia, pes anserinus insertion	Fracture, pes anserinus bursitis	Pes anserinus bursitis
9	Tibial tuberosity, patellar tendon insertion	Fracture, avulsion fracture	Osgood-Schlatter disease in youngsters; patellar insertional tendinitis in adults
10	Tibialis anterior, extensor tendons	Contusion	Anterior shin splints, extensor strain
11	Tibia	Fracture	Stress fracture
12	MCL, medial meniscus	Medial collateral sprain or rupture, medial meniscus tear	Mild MCL sprain, osteoarthritis
13	ITB	Contusion	ITB syndrome
14	Vastus lateralis, lateral retinaculum	Contusion	Vastus lateralis strain, lateral retinaculum sprain or fibrosis
15	Lateral tibiofemoral joint, lateral meniscus	Meniscus tear, fracture	Meniscus tear, capsular sprain
16	Fibular head, LCL insertion	Subluxation, dislocation, LCL sprain	Subluxation
17	Insertion of biceps femoris onto fibular head, peroneal nerve	Direct trauma to peroneal nerve	Biceps femoris insertional tendinitis, peroneal nerve entrapment
18	Lateral meniscus, popliteus tendon, lateral gastrocnemius	Lateral meniscus tear	Popliteus tendinitis, lateral gastrocnemius strain, lateral meniscus tear
19	Semimembranosus insertion, medial meniscus, semimembranosus bursa	Medial meniscus tear	Bursitis, insertional tendinitis, medial meniscus tear
20	Medial head of gastrocnemius	Tennis leg	Strain of medial gastrocnemius

Note: See Figure 12–3 for localization of numbered areas.

the joint causes irritation and is usually more painful and tense than with synovial swelling. There are two strong possibilities with hemarthrosis: an ACL tear and a fracture. If swelling is delayed, taking more than several hours, and is not especially painful (unless the patient moves the knee), synovial swelling is likely. Anything that acts to irritate the synovium can cause increased synovial fluid production. Common causes include meniscus tears, ACL flaps, and loose bodies.

2. Did the knee give way at the time of injury? Giving way is a potentially helpful clue when not painful.

Painful giving way often represents a reflex inhibition of the quadriceps that occurs with many painful knee conditions. However, if there was no pain at the time of giving way, instability (often ACL related) is likely the cause.

3. Was there a pop at the time of injury? A pop at the time of injury is indicative of an ACL tear, especially if the pop was accompanied by immediate pain and swelling. Other causes include a dislocated patella and, more rarely, a meniscus tear.

4. Does the knee lock? Locking of the knee can be divided into pseudolocking and true locking.

Pseudolocking occurs when the knee is held at approximately 30° of flexion in an attempt to accommodate joint effusion. The knee joint has the largest volume capacity at 30°. Therefore, when intra-articular swelling is present, less tension is developed with the knee in this position. Although it may be painful to move the knee, it is usually possible to move a few degrees into flexion or extension. True locking occurs with mechanical blockage. The knee is often in flexion and is rigidly, painfully locked in one position. No movement is possible until the knee is unlocked (often with a forced extension attempt). True locking is indicative of a meniscus tear or, less often, osteochondritis dissecans.

The mechanism of injury may be helpful when a contact injury is reported. Outside blows to the knee in a valgus direction are likely to damage medial structures. With the knee flexed, the MCL is most vulnerable. When the knee is in extension, the pes anserinus group is also vulnerable. Rotational injuries with a fixed foot often result in a sequence of damage beginning with a meniscus tear. If combined with an outside valgus force, the MCL, ACL, and meniscus may be damaged (terrible triad/O'Donoghue triad). Hyperextension injuries are often noncontact, but they may damage the ACL as a result of simultaneous contraction of the quadriceps. ACL damage also may occur with sudden deceleration or cutting maneuvers. One study[8] seems to indicate that perhaps there is another explanation (in particular with skiing injuries) because it appears that the quadriceps contraction actually acts to stabilize the knee. When performing open-chain exercises (e.g., seated knee extensions), the quadriceps may in fact provide some stability in the range of 70° to 80° of flexion or more. The authors feel that ACL injury with skiing is probably due more to rotations and translations that are imposed by a large moment arm created by the ski–boot complex.

Overuse injuries are most often sports related. Running may predispose the individual to ITB syndrome. If the patient is running or walking downhill, popliteus and ITB syndrome are possible if the patient presents with lateral pain. Pronation is believed to predispose the individual to several conditions, including chronic first-degree MCL tears, patellofemoral tracking problems, ITB syndrome, and popliteus tendinitis. Jumping and sprinting activities will predispose the patient to one of several extensor disorders, including patellar tendinitis and several age-related apophyseal problems including Osgood-Schlatter disease and Sinding-Larsen disease. Pain is felt more at the tibial tuberosity with Osgood-Schlatter disease, more at the patellar tendon with patellar tendinitis, and more at the inferior pole of the patella with Sinding-Larsen disease. If pain is felt going up or down steps, patellofemoral problems such as patellofemoral arthralgia or chondromalacia should be suspected.

Weakness

The complaint of weakness must always be clarified. It is important to determine whether the patient has pain associated with the sense of weakness, or stiffness that might be misinterpreted as weakness. True motor weakness at the knee is unusual unless found bilaterally with central nervous system/spinal cord disorders. Unilateral weakness may occur in diabetics with amyotrophy. Most lumbar disc lesions occur at the lower lumbar segments affecting more distal movement patterns; however, with L5 nerve root lesions, some patients have weakness of the hamstrings. When the knee is stiff from osteoarthritis (OA) or the patient is very inflexible, the patient must work against this restriction. This may be perceived as weakness. When pain accompanies weakness, testing should focus on contractile structures about the knee. Researchers evaluating the selective tension approach developed by Cyriax found that although intraexaminer reliability was acceptable after a training session, interexaminer reliability was not acceptable.[9] The study may have had limits due to the limited number of examiners and type of patient.

Instability

Instability is most often due to ACL injury. Meniscus injuries may also cause a giving way. The degree of instability may be a helpful guide. ACL instability is often nonpainful and felt with rotational movement patterns. Patients often report having to walk a particular way to lock the knee prior to placing weight on it. Instability with meniscus tears is more often painful due to mechanical interference with normal movement. Instability may also be felt with a proximal tibiofibular subluxation. This occurs at approximately 30° of flexion.

Restricted Motion

Restricted motion may be indicative of intra-articular swelling, joint mice, joint contracture, or tight musculature. Contractile causes of restricted motion are often uniplanar (i.e., flexion/extension). Joint effusion causes a restricted pattern whereby full extension is not possible and flexion beyond 90° is often difficult. The historical distinction is often the difference between acute traumatic onset, acute nontraumatic onset, and insidious onset. Acute traumatic internal damage will almost always cause joint effusion. Acute nontraumatic onset is also likely to be joint effusion but due to different causes, such as inflammatory arthritides or infection. Chronic or insidious onset is more likely due to soft tissue contracture, especially when associated with a history of immobilization or lack of activity. If the patient reports stiffness after sitting for long periods of time that resolves with 15 to 30 minutes of activity, two common possibilities are patellofemoral problems and OA. Patellofemoral disorders are more common in the younger patient; OA is more common in the older patient (unless there is a previous history of trauma).

Superficial Complaints

Superficial complaints include numbness and tingling and localized swellings. Numbness and tingling local to the medial knee are often due to saphenous nerve irritation. If extending into a longer area of numbness, a nerve root lesion is possible. Localized swellings are caused by inflamed bursae, ganglions, meniscal cysts,

lipomas, or, on rare occasions, villonodular synovitis (visible as calcified masses on x-ray). When deformity is present at the joint line, especially in an older patient, OA is the likely cause. Localized swelling at the tibial tuberosity in an adolescent is highly indicative of Osgood-Schlatter disease.

Examination

The physical examination may be restricted, and findings may be obscured by swelling or decreased range of motion. This may result in frustration on the part of the chiropractor or the patient and lead to a desire for more expedient evaluation tools. The important contribution of the clinical examination is often undermined by the premature use of more expensive technologies such as magnetic resonance imaging (MRI) and arthrography. A recent study[10] indicated that with traumatic knee pain, the correct diagnosis was arrived at 83% of the time when the history, clinical examination, and routine radiographs were used to make the diagnosis. The diagnoses were later confirmed by arthroscopy (see **Table 12-3**). A small study[11] of children and adolescents confirmed a similar finding. The results indicated that the positive correlation between clinical examination and arthroscopic findings was 78.5%. When judging the

Table 12-3 Some Neoplasms of the Knee

Type	Summary Information
Osteosarcoma	• The most common malignancy of the knee • Second most common primary bone tumor; most common, though, in ages 10–25 years; male/female ratio is 2:1 • 60% of all osteosarcomas are found in the knee; 40% in the distal femur • Usually >5 cm, metaphyseal location, sclerotic, disruption of cortex with Codman's triangle, hair-on-end or onion-skin periosteal response
Chondrosarcoma	• Third most common primary bone tumor • Only 7% involve the knee • May be secondary to osteochondroma, enchondroma, Paget's, fibrous dysplasia, or irradiation • May be asymptomatic with little swelling; found in ages 40–60 years; male/female ratio is 2:1 • Central or peripheral location • Central are osteolytic with endosteal scalloping, and popcorn sign
Synovial sarcoma (synovioma)	• Rare malignant tumor arising from synovium of joint capsules, bursae, or tendon sheaths • 50% occur in the knee; usually found in ages 20–40 years • May be rapidly fatal • A painful tender lump may be palpable • A spherical soft tissue mass >7 cm is commonly found

Table 12–3 Some Neoplasms of the Knee (continued)

Type	Summary Information
Ewing's sarcoma	• Rare malignant bone tumor found usually in the first two decades of life • Usually in long bone diaphysis; about half around the knee • Gradually increasing pain, soft tissue mass, possible fever, anemia and leukocytosis • Great variation, however, diaphyseal moth-eaten appearance (cracked-ice) and a laminated periosteal response are often seen
Metastatic carcinoma	Knee accounts for <1.5% of skeletal metastasis sites • Most commonly from the lungs • Other sites may be thyroid, breast, prostate, and melanoma • Most are osteolytic • Blown-out, soap-bubble appearance is associated with renal and thyroid tumors
Osteochondroma (exostosis)	• A benign developmental defect following lateral herniation of an epiphyseal plate • Most common tumor of the entire skeleton; 50% around the knee • Growth stops with skeletal maturity; 1% may undergo malignant transformation • May be either pedunculated or sessile • Hereditary multiple exostosis is male dominant with a 10% chance of malignant transformation
Nonossifying fibroma (fibrous cortical defect)	• Very common in the first two decades, with 40% of children having one or more: 95% found in those <20 years of age • 75% occur at the knee; mainly distal femur • Flame-shaped lesion, eccentrically placed in the long-bone metaphysis • Usually active on bone scan
Aneurysmal bone cyst	• Metaphyseal, expansile lesion, usually with a calcified eggshell rim • Usually occurs in the first three decades • Trauma may be initiating factor • Active on bone scan; it may be necessary to differentiate from a malignant expansile tumor
Giant cell tumor (osteoclastoma)	• 60% occur at the knee, with 80% benign and 20% malignant; malignant transformation usually occurring within the first 5 years • Involves both the metaphysis and epiphysis to the subarticular plate • Scalloping and thinning of cortex; eccentric location often at distal femur
Pigmented villo-nodular synovitis (benign synovioma)	• Benign disorder with synovial hyperplasia and hemosiderin deposition • Most common site is the knee • Usually young adults with swelling; however, little pain • Plain films may demonstrate a soft tissue swelling • MRI demonstrates lesion

positive predictive value for ACL or meniscal injuries, the clinical examination values were 96.2% and the negative predictive value was 93.3%. Compare this to the MRI values, which had a positive predictive value of 71.4% and a negative predictive value of 72.4%. Although a small study, it supports previous studies that suggest a premature referral for MRI may result in no added diagnostic value above the clinical examination, yet increase healthcare costs. Therefore, focus should be on a

thorough history and examination, even if delayed, prior to resorting to or relying on the "definitive" answer of MRI. Exceptions are made when the clinical examination is not clear or there is an immediate need to determine the extent of damage.

The acute injury evaluation on the field follows a sequential approach. The first step is a search for neurologic and vascular integrity through palpation, observation, and active movement testing distal to the knee. If neurovascular function is intact and no obvious fracture is evident, the next step in the evaluation is testing for collateral ligament damage. This is performed, if possible, in full extension first, then at 30° flexion if negative for laxity. If the integrity of the collaterals is intact, the cruciates are next challenged using the Lachman's test (or an anterior drawer test if the patient cannot extend the knee to 10° to 20° of flexion). Further evaluation includes meniscus testing and testing of the integrity of the patellar restraint system. If the athlete can bear weight, he or she should be tested sequentially through two-legged balance and squatting movements to single-legged balance with an attempt at 20° to 30° of squat. If the patient passes this evaluation, more complex skills, such as running, then stopping, are evaluated.

The in-office evaluation of the knee is first begun with palpation for specific sites of tenderness in an attempt to localize, primarily, superficial tissue. This is directed by whether the history is one of trauma or overuse. With traumatic injury, palpation of the collateral ligaments at the joint line often will indicate tenderness with sprains. Palpation of the joint line anteriorly, medially, and posteromedially may reveal tenderness with meniscus tears. In addition, anterior joint line tenderness at the medial joint line may indicate damage to the coronary ligament (capsular ligament at the joint). Tenderness on either side of the patella may indicate retinacular tearing. Tenderness on either side of the patellar tendon with the knee flexed is a strong indicator of fat pad irritation. Palpation is aided by placing the patient's knee in the Hardy or figure-four position with the involved side ankle resting on the well leg in a seated position. This position opens up the joint space and places tension on the collateral ligaments, making them more accessible.

When the history indicates no obvious trauma, palpation may focus on the insertion sites for various muscle/tendon possibilities.

- Tenderness at the lateral epicondyle of the femur or anterolateral tibia is found with ITB syndrome.
- Tenderness behind the LCL or in front of the femoral insertion of the LCL is indicative of popliteus tendinitis.
- Tenderness at the insertion of the vastus medialis oblique (VMO) indicates a tracking abnormality; this may also be evident at the adductor tubercle.
- Tenderness at the posterior knee superior to the joint line with the knee bent may be found with gastrocnemius strain; below the joint line, with soleus strain.

The strategy for evaluation of superficial soft tissue damage (in addition to palpation) is to compress, stretch, or contract the tissue. Testing for less accessible, deep intra-articular damage requires indirect tests such as compression testing for the menisci and stability testing for the cruciates. Although there are numerous variations of standardized testing, the primary tests are addressed here.

Anterior Cruciate

ACL testing is based on challenging the posterior-to-anterior stability of the tibia. The position of testing varies. If an anterior pull on the tibia is applied at 10° to 20° of knee flexion, it is called the Lachman test (**Figure 12–4**); at 90° it is called the anterior drawer test (**Figure 12–5**). The difference is in the sensitivity. For acute injuries, Lachman's test is more sensitive.[12] This is primarily due to the position of slight flexion that places the hamstrings at a disadvantage. If the hamstrings are in spasm, the direct line of pull with the knee at 90° is an additional force to pull against with the anterior drawer test. Rotational testing refers to testing for damage to the ACL and other structures. When medial or lateral stabilizing structures are damaged along with the ACL, a rotational instability is created. The first evaluation for this is a modification of the anterior drawer test. By pulling forward with the knee in internal and then external rotation, the lateral and medial supporting structures, respectively, are tested (Slocum's test).

The prototype rotational test is referred to as the pivot shift test (**Figure 12–6**). This test takes advantage of the

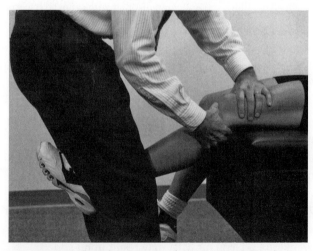

Figure 12–4 Lachman's test. To test for anterior stability, the knee is flexed about 10° to 20°. The femur is stabilized while the examiner pulls forward on the tibia.

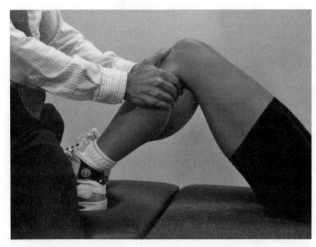

Figure 12–5 Anterior drawer test. The patient's hip is flexed to 45° and the knee is flexed to 90°. The examiner stabilizes the foot while pulling forward on the tibia. The posterior drawer test uses the same position but pushes the tibia back.

passive tension of the ITB.[13] This tension will pull the tibia forward into medial subluxation when an ACL tear is present along with medial or lateral damage. As the knee approaches 30° to 40° of flexion, the ITB crosses the

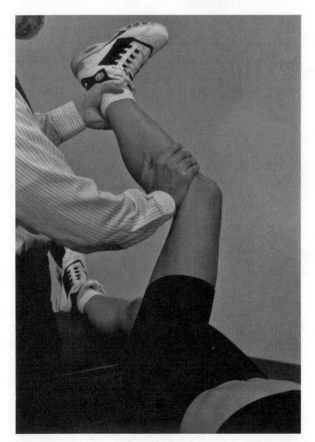

Figure 12–6 The pivot shift test for rotary instability. The patient's knee is held in 10°of flexion.While applying a valgus force at the fibular head with the knee internally rotated, the knee is passively flexed.

axis of rotation (the lateral epicondyle) and now acts as a flexor. This will passively pull the tibia back into neutral. Although there are many variations of this test, this is the basic mechanism by which most of these tests function.

A meta-analysis by Benjaminse et al.[14] agrees with past reviews that indicate that:

- The Lachman test has a pooled sensitivity of 85% and a pooled specificity of 94%.
- The pivot-shift test is very specific with a pooled specificity of 98% but only 24% sensitivity.
- The anterior drawer test is poor in acute settings, but in chronic ACL conditions it has very good pooled sensitivity (92%) and specificity (91%).

Meniscus

Testing for the meniscus is essentially a compressive challenge. The two most widely used tests (other than joint line tenderness) are McMurray's and Thessaly's.[15] McMurray's test applies compression to the posterior and middle third of the meniscus (**Figure 12–7**, A and B). The first part of the test is a full-compression maneuver accomplished by passively flexing the patient's heel to the buttock. While in this end-range position, the tibia is internally and externally rotated while the examiner palpates the joint line for clicking or popping. A positive test is signaled by clicking and popping with accompanying pain. Soft positives may include clicking, popping, or pain only. The next portion of the test is to apply a combination of valgus/varus and internal/external rotation while extending the leg passively to 90°. Although it is often suggested that a specific combination of forces tests a specific meniscus (medial versus lateral), this is not borne out by studies.[16] When a positive McMurray's test is found, it more often represents a medial meniscus tear.

The Thessaly test involves the patient bearing weight on the involved side (with the examiner's support) and bending the knee into partial flexion of 20°.[17] The patient then rotates in each direction several times to determine if this elicits pain, joint line discomfort, or locking/catching (**Figure 12–8**).

Apley's is a compression and distraction test combination.[18] The advantage of Apley's test is that the anterior meniscus can be compressed because of the direct axial compression directed through the tibia. With the patient prone, the tibia is internally and externally rotated as the examiner continues to apply a compressive force while passively extending the leg. A positive test is the production of joint line or deep pain. A confirmation of this

A
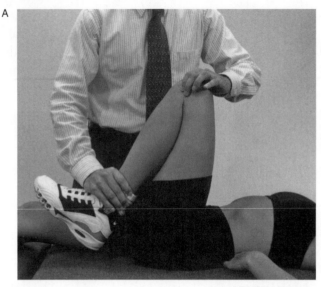

B
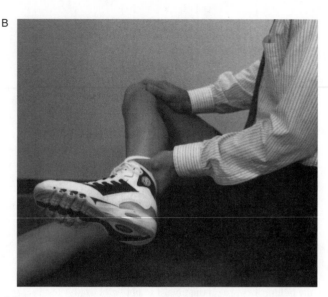

Figure 12–7 McMurray's test for the meniscus. (A) The first position is full flexion. While the examiner internally and externally rotates the knee, the joint line is palpated for clicking or popping. (B) If the first position is unrevealing, the knee is extended while applying combinations of varus, valgus, internal rotation, and external rotation.

finding may be evident with a relief of pain with distraction of the tibia in this same position.

A relatively new test has been proposed for evaluating the lateral meniscus.[19] The authors call it the dynamic test. The patient is positioned with the hip in 60°

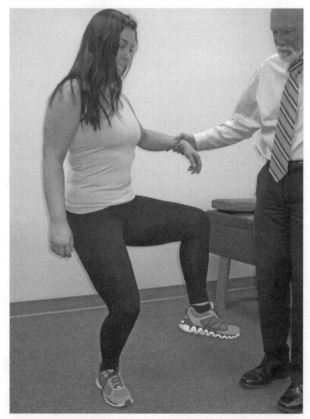

Figure 12–8 Thessaly test.

abduction, flexed and rotated externally about 45°. The knee is flexed 90°. The examiner palpates the lateral joint line and keeps pressure at the outer rim while adducting the hip, keeping the knee flexed. The test is considered positive if (1) pain is felt and increased at the point of finger pressure during the maneuver, or (2) a sharp pain is felt in the final position (**Figure 12–9**, A and B). The reported sensitivity was 85%, specificity 90.3%, positive predictive value 73.2%, and negative predictive value 95%.

Shellbourne et al.[20] attempted to find the correlation of joint line tenderness to meniscal lesions in patients with acute ACL tears determined by surgery. Of the patients involved, 51% had medial joint line tenderness (JLT); of those patients, 45% had a medial meniscus tear, 49% had no medial JLT, and 35% of these had a medial meniscus tear. Furthermore, 34% had lateral JLT and 58% had a lateral meniscus tear; 66% had no lateral JLT, but 49% had a lateral meniscus tear. Medial JLT was 45% sensitive, 35% specific for a medial meniscus injury. Lateral JLT was 58% sensitive and 49% specific for a lateral meniscus injury. This study suggests that joint line tenderness is often not likely a predictor of an associated meniscal tear with an acute ACL tear.

McMurray's test is very specific but has a very low sensitivity for meniscal tears. Palpation for JLT has fairly good sensitivity but lacks good specificity. There do not appear any well-designed tests that determine the stability of the collateral ligaments that are scientifically validated for specificity and sensitivity. **Exhibit 12–1** is

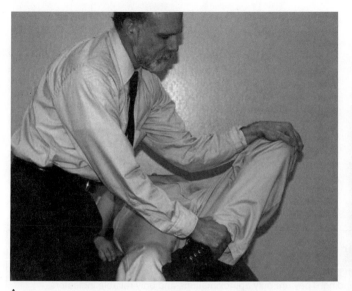 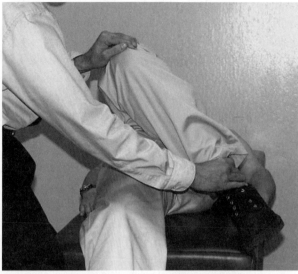

A   B

Figure 12–9 The Dynamic test for lateral meniscus tears. (A) The patient is positioned with the hip in 60° abduction, flexed and rotated externally about 45°. The knee is flexed 90°. (B) The examiner palpates the lateral joint line and keeps pressure at the outer rim while adducting the hip, keeping the knee flexed.

a graphical representation of determining the likelihood of a meniscus tear. The use of MRI in detecting meniscal tears is moderately reliable. In 106 patients (115 menisci) who were subjected to MRI and arthroscopy for evaluation of meniscal tear, reparability showed only a fair success rate (67%) in correctly identifying the tear type, side of the tear, and type of tear.[21] The averages for predicting meniscectomy were accuracy (69%), sensitivity (68%), specificity (75%), positive predictive value (90%), and negative predictive value (43%). The following criteria were used to judge whether a meniscal tear would possibly heal, and whether it was surgically reparable:

- At least 1 cm in length
- Displaceable with a probe
- Located within 3 mm of the meniscosynovial junction
- Seen to extend through at least 51% of the meniscal thickness
- Associated with minimal damage to the inner meniscal fragment or meniscal peripheral body

Collateral Ligaments

The MCL is by far the most frequently injured collateral ligament. The principles used to test the MCL can easily be applied to the LCL when damage is suspected. Testing begins with the knee in full extension. A valgus force is applied through leverage against the lower leg. If the knee is unstable, there will be a palpable and visible increase in opening on the medial side of the knee. In children, opening in this position more often represents epiphyseal damage and indicates the need for a stress radiograph. If no opening occurs in full extension, the examiner proceeds and positions the knee at 30° of flexion and reapplies the same valgus force. At 30°, if the knee opens medially and feels as though no end-point was reached, a third-degree rupture of the MCL has occurred. If there is opening with an end-point reached, a second-degree tear is present. If there is no opening but pain is produced, it is likely that there is a first-degree sprain. Cross-checking with contraction of the medial musculature will differentiate ligament pain from muscle pain in most cases. Only one study[22] has tested the reliability of collateral ligament stability testing, and it does not appear to have a high interexaminer reliability.

Patellofemoral Disorders

There are basically three approaches to patellofemoral testing: (1) compression, (2) stability, and (3) tracking. Compression testing involves direct compression of the patella with the knee flexed 5° to 10°. If pain is produced, chondromalacia patellae is suspected. The extension of this test is to ask the patient to contract the quadriceps while the examiner holds the patella down with a superior-to-inferior force (patellar inhibition test).

Stability testing for the patella is the reverse order of positions used for collateral ligament testing. The patient's knee is placed in 30° of flexion first while the examiner cautiously applies a lateral force to the medial patella. If this does not produce pain or apprehension, the test is cautiously repeated in full extension.

Tracking is tested by having the patient go through a full squat. The patella is palpated throughout the movement, and the patient is asked to identify any specific range where pain is felt. In general, if the pain is felt only at the bottom of the squat, patellar problems are less likely; meniscus problems are more likely. Tracking can also be evaluated indirectly by examining postural abnormalities that may contribute to tracking

predisposition. For example, the combination of anteversion of the hip combined with external tibial torsion causes an increase in the Q (quadriceps) angle, leading to strain at the patella and medial knee. Version of the hip is discussed in Chapter 11.

Internal or external tibial torsion is often determined by simple observation. With the patient seated, the examiner can obtain an axial view of the knee and foot (**Figure 12–10**). If the foot is turned out more than 20°, external tibial torsion is likely; if internally rotated more than 15°, internal tibial torsion is likely. Although the

Exhibit 12–1 Likelihood Patient Has a Meniscus Tear

Approximating Probability: The likelihood ratios (LRs) in this graphical representation represent estimates of probability based on the aggregate of multiple reviews of each test finding. They are only approximations and only reliable indicators of a change in the context of a patient having an intermediate pre-test probability of between 20% to 80%. If the pre-test probability is very high or very low, the LR has little effect on changing the probability.

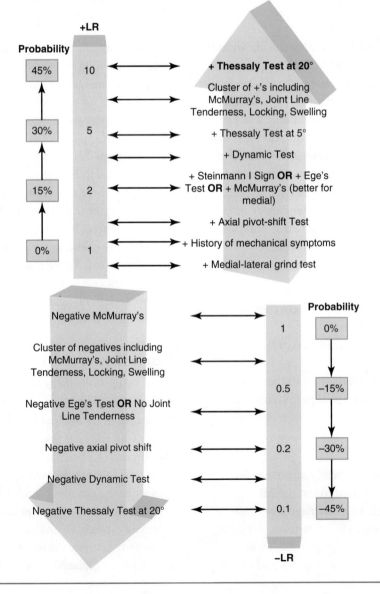

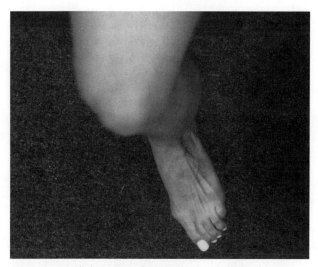

Figure 12–10 Skyline view of external torsion of the tibia.

Q angle is often given significant weight in the diagnosis and management of patellofemoral disorders, a recent review[23] challenges these assumptions. This review of the literature on Q angle measurements indicates the following:

- There is very little evidence to suggest that a Q angle greater than 15° to 20° will, as a single factor, predispose the knee to tracking problems.
- Although women display a larger mean Q angle than men, the underlying reasons are not apparent at this time; the assumption that women have wider hips than men is not supported by the literature.

One final strategy in evaluating for patellofemoral tracking causes is to palpate and test for the presence of a plica, which might contribute to tracking abnormalities. There are various approaches, but the basic idea is to press the patella from lateral to medial while the leg is either actively or passively extended. Stuttering or snapping at the medial, inferior patella suggests the presence of plica.

The functional portion of the knee examination focuses on tightness of lateral structures with emphasis on the ITB and weakness of medial structures with focus on the VMO. The primary ITB test is the modified Ober's test, which is designed to evaluate ITB or hip abductor tightness. VMO testing is nonspecific, but an evaluation of tracking through the last 20° may identify a functionally "weak" VMO. This is an indirect finding indicated by stuttering of extension or inability to extend while keeping the knee in the same position (without pressing down or lifting up at the knee).

Extensor Disorders

Extensor disorders refer to damage or irritation to the quadriceps muscle and its attachment points at the patella and the patellar tendon and its attachment into the tibial tuberosity. By simply having the patient extend the knee from a flexed position against the examiner's resistance, pain is often produced at the site of the pathologic process. Pain at the tibial tuberosity in an adolescent indicates Osgood-Schlatter disease, whereas in an adult pain suggests patellar tendinitis. Pain at the patellar tendon is strong evidence for patellar tendinitis; on occasion, however, a deep infrapatellar bursitis or fat pad syndrome may cause pain. Pain at the inferior pole of the patella in an adolescent is suggestive of a process similar to Osgood-Schlatter disease called Sinding-Larsen disease.

Specific Soft Tissue or Muscle/Tendon Tests

- ITB: The ITB is tested in two ways: direct pressure over the lateral epicondyle and stretching of the ITB in an attempt to determine predisposition. Direct pressure over the lateral epicondyle is performed with the knee flexed to 30° to 40° and is referred to as Noble's test. Stretching of the ITB is accomplished through passive adduction of the hip. This is referred to as Ober's test (**Figure 12–11**). A modification of this test is to stretch the hip with the knee extended over the side of the table. Although this maneuver may not reproduce the pain, it often indicates tightness when the patella fails to lower below the level of the top of the examination table. It is important to stabilize the iliac crest to prevent stretch above this point.
- Popliteus: The popliteus is evaluated through resisted internal rotation. This may increase the

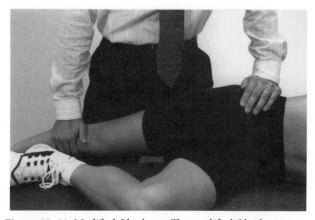

Figure 12–11 Modified Ober's test. The modified Ober's test involves extending the leg off the back of the table while stabilizing the ilium in an attempt to stretch the ITB and hip abductors.

lateral knee pain found with popliteus tendinitis. Palpation points of tenderness are found in front of the LCL on the distal femur or directly behind the LCL. Another approach is to have the patient bear all the body weight onto the affected side and bend the knee to 30°. If the femur is internally rotated, pain may increase with popliteus tendinitis.

- Semimembranosus: The semimembranosus may be involved in an insertional tendinitis. There is tenderness at the posterior attachment of the muscle or resisted knee flexion may increase pain at the posterior medial knee.
- Biceps femoris: Pain at the posterior fibular head may be increased with resisted knee flexion.

Evaluation for Stiffness

When there is restricted range of motion (ROM) at the knee, an attempt at distinguishing between soft tissue involvement and an internal pathologic process is necessary. When there is tightness in the capsule, gentle stretching of the knee in the direction of restriction will usually increase the range without a significant increase in pain. Mild contraction of an antagonist muscle followed by passive movement into the restricted movement pattern will usually increase ROM when that muscle is the cause.

When neither approach helps or when the attempts at increased movement are met with pain, an intra-articular process is most likely.

Radiographs/Special Studies

Diagnostic imaging guidelines were recently released in 2008.[24] These practice guidelines for musculoskeletal complaints in adults are an evidence-based approach developed through a rigorous process involving an international team of chiropractic experts. These provide an excellent source for determining the need for imaging, the types of imaging recommended, and physical examination and history indicators that will help direct decision making. Standard radiographs of the knee include an anterior-to-posterior (AP) non-weight-bearing view and a lateral non-weight-bearing view with the knee flexed to 30°. Based on the Ottawa rules,[25] radiographs should be ordered after acute knee injury if any of the following are true:

- The patient is over the age of 55 years.
- There is isolated tenderness at the patella.

- There is isolated tenderness at the fibular head.
- The patient is unable to flex the knee 90°.
- The patient is unable to bear weight immediately after the injury or take four steps in the emergency department.

In this landmark study, patients who were not initially radiographed were told to return if the pain did not improve or progressively worsened. Approximately 4,000 patients were followed for two 12-month periods (one year before and one year after the intervention). There was a reduction of 26% in the referral rate for knee radiographs compared to a reduction of only 1% in the control group. On average, the time spent in the ED was reduced by about 30 minutes and the cost was reduced to less than half ($80 versus $118). No significant fractures were missed. With suspected ACL damage, indirect indicators include the lateral capsular sign (Segond's fracture) indicated by a lateral tibial plateau fracture seen on the AP view, a tibial spine fracture seen on the tunnel view, and the lateral notch sign (depression fracture of the lateral femoral condyle) best seen on the lateral view.[26] Evaluation of the osteoarthritic knee is via a posterior-to-anterior (PA) view that is taken bearing weight with the knees bent to 45° and a 10° caudal tube tilt. When osteochondritis dissecans is suspected, a tunnel view is required. Osteochondritis is indicated most often by a divot of bone on the distal, lateral portion of the medial femoral condyle. Patellofemoral evaluation may be performed via several tangential views. The standard sunrise view provides little information unless OA of the patella or fracture is being evaluated. Other views such as the Merchant and Lauren view are variations on this theme that are used to evaluate tracking abnormalities. Two measurements, the congruence angle and the patellar tilt, are respective lines of mensuration used with these views. For patients with suspected past subluxation or dislocation of the patella, a combined approach using an axial (i.e., tangential) view coupled with a flexed and extended lateral view is sensitive for detecting malalignment and indicators of trochlear insufficiency.[27] For an accurate interpretation, the lateral view must line up the femoral condyles without any rotation effects causing misinterpretation of patellar tilting. MRI of the knee should be reserved for suspicion of major ACL or meniscal pathology or when the patient is unresponsive to conservative care. Magnetic resonance imaging (MRI) can be used to detect a number of knee lesions including the following:

1. Meniscus tears
2. Cruciate tears

3. Collateral ligament tears
4. Infection
5. Bone infarct
6. Bone marrow infiltration
7. Patellar tendinosis
8. Soft tissue tumors

The patient is supine with the leg externally rotated between 10° and 15°. A surface quadrature coil is necessary to increase the signal-to-noise ratio. Both sagittal and coronal images are considered routine with thickness slices between 3 and 5 mm. Slice thicknesses as small as 1.5 mm are obtainable with two new techniques: fast low angle shot (FLASH) and gradient recalled acquisition in the steady state (GRASS).

For meniscus tears a sagittal, spin-echo, T1-weighted image is commonly used. Coronal views are also used and may identify common tears such as the bucket handle, parrot-beak, and the variant, discoid meniscus. The meniscus usually has a low-intensity (dark) image on MRI. It appears as a bowtie-like structure on sagittal images. Tears usually have a higher signal intensity (lighter), probably due to fluid content. Care must be taken to avoid misinterpreting several normal structures as pathology, including the transverse ligament, popliteus tendon, lateral inferior geniculate artery, and concavity of the outer portion of the meniscus.

The cruciate ligaments are also low-signal diagonal images. If, upon viewing several sagittal, 3 mm sliced images, the ACL is not seen, it is assumed that it is torn. The posterior cruciate is assumed to be torn when its diagonal, low-intensity image is interrupted. If the image is widened, or the intensity is increased, swelling is likely indicating damage. On coronal images, the ACL appears as a diagonal low-signal structure, while the PCL appears as a vertical low-signal structure.

Researchers in one study[28] evaluated the relevance of abnormal findings on MRI of the anterior horn of the meniscus and existence of actual pathology. There was a 74% false-positive rate (26% true-positive rate). The authors recommend clinical correlation with MRI findings because some of the false-positive patients were asymptomatic and some had other pathologies.

An interesting study by LaPrade et al.[29] examined the prevalence of abnormal MRI findings in asymptomatic knees. This study indicates that there is a 5.6% prevalence of meniscal tears in an asymptomatic population. There was also an unexplained prevalence of 24.1% of Grade II signal changes of the posterior horn of the medial meniscus. There was approximately a 15% overall prevalence of other abnormal findings. They conclude that magnetic resonance findings are significant only when correlated with clinical findings.

Management

- Patients with fracture, tumor, or infection should be referred for medical management.
- Patients with isolated ACL tears with resolved swelling may be managed conservatively if they are not serious amateur or professional athletes. This includes hamstring training, proprioceptive neuromuscular facilitation (PNF) training, and bracing.
- Patients with small, peripheral meniscus tears or those that are demonstrated via MRI to be vertical, stable tears may initially be managed conservatively. If nonresponsive, it is important to recommend repair; when possible, it should be without meniscectomy.
- All soft tissue disorders, such as tracking disorders, first- and second-degree muscle/tendon problems, and first- and second-degree ligament disorders, can be managed conservatively. Isolated rupture of the MCL may be managed conservatively with casting and rehabilitation by experienced doctors; for those with less experience, comanagement or referral for surgery is recommended.
- When restrictions to accessory movement are found, short-arc, quick-impulse adjusting should be attempted with the knee in a distracted position. If not distracted, the knee should not be adjusted into flexion or in full extension. Recent evidence[30] supports the need to evaluate the low back and sacroiliac (SI) joint for subluxation. Manipulation of the SI joint was found to reduce inhibition of knee extensors.

There is a new focus on hip exercises as preventive for patellofemoral and other knee problems. The EMG evidence suggests that minimizing TFL activation is important and can be accomplished using the following: the clam, sidestep, unilateral bridge, and both quadruped hip extension exercises.[31]

Manipulation

An interesting descriptive study evaluated the effect of sacroiliac manipulation (adjusting) on knee muscle inhibition in patients with anterior knee pain.[32] The results of this pilot study indicated that using Cybex muscle testing, SI manipulation may benefit patients with anterior knee pain by decreasing muscle inhibition. A follow-up randomized controlled trial[33] also confirmed an immediate effect on reducing knee extensor muscle inhibition. Certainly, larger controlled studies are needed.

As indicated in a review of chiropractic treatment of lower extremity problems,[34, 35] there are few large studies, but the preponderance of studies indicate benefit for those with osteoarthritis and patellofemoral arthralgia when manipulation is incorporated. Primarily, there are single case reports of chiropractic manipulation being effective for patients with knee pain.[36, 37] Knee joint mobilization does have some literature support. The results of a study by Moss et al.[38] indicate that using accessory motion mobilization on osteoarthritic knees produces some immediate decrease in pain and a reduction in the "up and go" test of knee function.

A separate review by Crossley et al.[39] on management of patellofemoral pain seemed to indicate that there was some improvement with corrective foot orthosis and a progressive resistance brace. There is no literature for or against the use of patellofemoral orthoses, acupuncture, low-level laser, chiropractic patellar mobilization, or patellar taping. A possible value for manipulation under anesthesia is for patients with total knee arthroplasty. Some studies[40, 41] indicate improvement in range of motion following MUA.

Rehabilitation

In early electromyographic (EMG) studies conducted in the 1980s, Soderberg et al.,[42, 43] using surface electrodes, determined that more muscle activity was detected in the vastus medialis, biceps femoris, and gluteus medius using quadriceps isometric "setting" exercises than with a straight leg raise (SLR). The rectus femoris, on the other hand, was more active during the SLR. Skurja et al.[44] also found similar types of activity when comparing isometric knee extension with the SLR. These findings went unchallenged for more than a decade. Another assumption, partially based on these studies, was that the vastus medialis oblique was isolated in its increased activity through the last 10° to 15° of knee extension.

More recently, researchers have attempted to test some of these old concepts and to go beyond testing only the SLR or isometric exercise. Newer motivations are the need to find low-tech approaches to exercising complaints with specific problems such as patellofemoral disorders

and anterior cruciate deficiency. Each presents unique problems to prescribing the type of exercise, and more importantly the range of motion least harmful to each group. The "paradox" has been that patients with ACL deficiency might do better with closed-chain (i.e., foot in contact with a surface) exercise in moderate degrees of flexion whereas patients with patellofemoral problems would suffer from the increases in joint reaction and compression forces. Patients with patellofemoral problems do better with exercises close to full extension, but this is a range considered functionally dangerous for patients with ACL injury or deficiency (especially if performed as an open-chain exercise) due to the imbalance of quadriceps contraction pulling the tibia forward without concomitant hamstring protection.

In 1994 Cryzlo et al.[45] measured the EMG activity about the knee using indwelling wire electrodes during the performance of a number of exercises. These exercises included the following:

- The SLR—subject supine, raises leg with knee straight until 75° of hip flexion is reached
- Short-arc knee extension (SAEX)—subject seated with knee flexed to 45° off the end of the table; subject extended from 45° to full extension using a 12.5-lb weight
- Short-arc knee extension with hamstring co-contraction (SAEHS)—same as the SAEX; however, subjects asked to press back against thigh roll (to elicit hamstring contraction) as they extended through 45° to full extension
- The squat—subjects were asked to perform a two-legged squat to 90° of knee flexion, hold for three seconds, and return to original position
- Isometric knee co-contraction (ICO)—"setting" exercises were performed at 15°, 30°, and 45° of knee flexion with the subject contracting isometrically both the hamstrings and quadriceps

A summary of the results follows:

- Although during the SLR there was more rectus femoris activity than with the vasti muscles, it was not statistically significant. Also, activity of the VMO and vastus lateralis oblique (VLO) was essentially equal; there was no predominance of VMO activity. Activity of both the VMO and VLO was highest during the first 15° of the SLR. Basically the same was found for the SAEX and SAEHS exercises with significant increases in activity through the last 15° of knee extension.

Although the SAEHS was designed to increase hamstring contraction, the activity level was quite low (highest activity between 30° and 45°).

- With the squat, the VMO/VLO and rectus activity was generally higher than the hamstring activity. The VMO/VLO activity was more than the rectus femoris during the ascend phase and highest during the hold phase. For the rectus femoris, the highest activity was also during the hold phase. Hamstring activity was highest during the ascend phase (although extremely low activity in general).
- Isometric knee co-contraction was the only exercise to provide a balanced activity between flexors and extensors. It was the only exercise tested that demonstrated any significant activity for the hamstrings.

Clinically, the usefulness of these data is interpreted as follows:

- Although the squat exercise may be a valuable alternative to knee extension in the patient with ACL deficiency, it does little to activate (strengthen) the hamstrings. The hamstrings are necessary for a stable joint with patients with ACL deficiency. A balanced exercise might be SAEHS or the ICO in all ranges except 15° of flexion to full extension. In this terminal range of knee extension there is an overbalance of quadriceps activity over hamstring activity.
- The final arc of 15° of extension is suggested for strengthening the quadriceps; however, there is very little to suggest selected contraction of any of the quadriceps group (i.e., VMO over VLO or rectus).

Elastic Tubing Exercise

A recent study by Hintermeister et al.[46] evaluated EMG activity (surface electrodes) of five exercises that utilized elastic tubing. These exercises included the following:

- Single knee dip—subject stood on elastic tubing with involved side only; holding end of tubing in hand (on involved side), other end attached to chair (which the subject used to stabilize with); the subject performed partial squats on the involved side only at a rate of 30 knee dips/minute while balancing with the chair.
- Double knee dip—subject stood on tubing and grasped end of tubing with hands (held at waist level) and performed squats.

- Leg press—subject was seated with tubing around heel and other end attached behind the subject; with the hip in maximum flexion there was some tautness in the tubing; the subject then pressed the leg into extension against the resistance of the tubing.
- Hamstring pull—subject was seated with the tubing anchored around the ankle with the other end anchored in front; with the knee flexed to approximately 20° there was some tautness in the tubing; subject was instructed to drag the foot across the floor as far as possible and lift slightly while returning to the initial position.
- Side-to-side jump—subject had the tubing secured around her or his waist and anchored away from her or him to the side; subject then jumped laterally (to her or his side) in the opposite direction of the tubing attachment.

The results suggested a progression of demand on the knee musculature. A summary of the EMG findings and the sequence of demand on knee musculature follows:

- Double knee dip—demand on the vasti muscles was over 50% of a maximum voluntary contraction (MVC). There was more activity of the VMO over the VLO; however, this may not be clinically significant.
- The leg press—not a very powerful exercise; however, there seemed to be preferential recruitment of the rectus femoris over the vasti muscles and some activation of the tibialis anterior muscle.
- Hamstring pull—it was no surprise that the hamstring activity was significant (more for the medial hamstrings) and, in addition, there was significant adductor firing that occurred with the hamstring activity.
- Single knee dip—similar results to the double knee dip; however, significant increases in activity of the vasti muscles and rectus femoris with some preferential recruitment of the VMO (VMO, 103%; VLO, 83%; rectus femoris, 73% MVC).
- Side-to-side jump—as might be guessed, the most demanding exercise was the jump with approximately 10% increases in all quad muscle activity over the single knee dip. Also the medial gastrocnemius demonstrated significant activity.

Recommendations by the authors suggest using the less stressful exercises first based on the needs of a specific rehabilitation program (e.g., ACL problem versus patello-femoral problem). For example, for patients with an ACL deficiency, a hamstring pull and leg press might be good starting exercises. Progression to more challenging exercises should be based on the ability to perform the less stressful exercises first. It should be noted that most of the exercises demonstrated a slight increase in VMO activity compared with VLO activity; however, most researchers do not believe that this is clinically significant.

VMO Recruitment

It is generally accepted that the VMO is important for patellar stabilization, in particular through the last 15° or so of extension. As a result, many studies have attempted to determine if any particular exercise was significantly better at isolating the VMO. It has been almost unanimously agreed based on numerous EMG studies that most exercises do not show a clinically significant increase in VMO activity over VLO activity. A study by Laprade et al.[29] reemphasizes this point and in addition calls into question a commonly reported claim that adding adduction to knee extension increases VMO activity over extension alone. In the past it was assumed that because the VMO originates primarily from the adductor longus and magnus tendons and the medial intramuscular septum adding adduction would increase or preferentially stimulate the VMO. This is a logical assumption not borne out by this study. Although one study (upon which most of this connection between adduction and VMO activity was based) indicated significant increases, it is clear that the study's EMG values were not normalized, and therefore the conclusions must be questioned. It also has been suggested that the VMO might have some medial (internal) rotation effect on the tibia. This is based on the observation that the lowermost fibers of the VMO attach to the anteromedial aspect of the tibia. The study by Laprade et al. tests this hypothesis. This study also addresses whether there are any significant differences in VMO or VLO recruitment between patients with and without patellofemoral pain syndrome.

In this current study by Laprade et al.[47] subjects were asked to perform four isometric exercises while surface EMG readings were taken:

1. Adduction—subjects adducted their thighs against two rubber cups with their knees flexed to 50° and hips flexed to 80°.
2. Adduction with knee extension—subjects performed simultaneous adduction and knee extension; subjects were instructed to squeeze their knees together and lift against an ankle strap.
3. Medial tibial rotation—the subject's knee was at 70° flexion/30° lateral rotation and hip at 80°

flexion; a footplate that was padded provided resistance to medial rotation.
4. Medial tibial rotation with knee extension—similar to the positioning for medial rotation; the subjects were asked to simultaneously medially rotate and extend the knee.

The results did not demonstrate any difference in the activity of VMO or VLO muscles or ratio of activity between the VMO/VLO between the symptomatic and asymptomatic groups. The results also indicated no preferential recruitment of the VMO over the VLO for most exercises including adduction with extension. There was some increase in VMO over VLO contraction using medial rotation with extension. Still, the difference between VMO and VLO activity would in no way isolate the VMO over the VLO. This exercise would, however, guarantee a good strengthening effect for both muscles with some degree of VMO focus.

Graded Treadmill Walking

Treadmill walking is often prescribed during the early phases of rehabilitation after significant injury or surgery. One study[48] measured the EMG activity of leg muscles at 0% to 24% grade (incline). As the grade increased, there were significant increases in VMO, vastus lateralis, and biceps femoris activity. The increases in the vasti muscles were about double those of the biceps femoris. Interestingly, there was no such increase in the peak amplitude of the medial hamstrings. Although there were increases for the quads and biceps femoris, it is not known whether this amount of increase contributes to a strengthening effect. The average amplitude was less than 25% of a maximum voluntary contraction for all the muscles regardless of grade.

As the grade was increased, the ankle and hip ROM increased while the knee ROM decreased. The decrease in knee ROM was due to a specific decrease in knee extension with an increase in grade. So, although the knee flexion angles remained similar through different grades, the amount of extension achieved decreased with increasing grade. The authors suggest that a balance between the needs of an anterior cruciate-deficient patient and a patient with patellofemoral pain may be met by having the patient use a grade of just greater than 12%. They suggest that at this grade, the knee remains bent around 30° and therefore avoids extension, which is detrimental to the ACL patient. This amount of grade also avoids the middle to extreme flexion positions that may be detrimental to the patient with patellofemoral pain.

Stair-Stepping

Stair-steppers have become quite popular as an aerobic alternative to treadmills. Little research has been performed for stair-steppers; therefore, most of the claims are anecdotal or promotional. One study[49] evaluated the EMG activity of muscles about the knee and hip. The researchers monitored the activity of these muscles with increasing cadence and also measured again with retrograde stepping. Their results indicated increases in muscle activation for the gluteus maximus, rectus femoris, vastus medialis, and gastrocnemius with increases in stepping cadence. There were no significant increases for the semimembranosus and semitendinosus except for the extremes of 35 to 95 steps/minute. However, with retrograde stepping at a cadence of 60 steps/minute, there was an increase in the medial hamstring activity. Interestingly, there was no increase in gluteus maximus activity as predicted by many stair-stepper enthusiasts and manufacturers.

Placed in the context of rehabilitation for an ACL-deficient knee, it was observed by the authors that the increase in hamstring activity was minimal whereas the quadriceps increase was greater with stair-stepping. To achieve a balance so that there is less strain on the ACL and more stability from the hamstrings, it was recommended that stepping at a slower cadence was probably safest. There was no particular advantage to faster stepping given the lack of hamstring activity increases. They also felt that although there was an increase in medial hamstring activity with retrograde stepping, it was rather minimal and the awkwardness of the activity did not justify using this method as

an alternative to forward stepping. It should be noted that retrograde stepping is more aerobically demanding.

Bicycle Riding

It is generally accepted that bicycle riding is a good approach to rehabilitation of ACL injury whether surgically managed or not. The concerns, as always with ACL deficiency, are extension of the knee and quadriceps contraction pulling the tibia forward on the femur. A recent study[50] measured the strain behavior for the ACL with bicycle riding using different power levels and cadences (60 and 90 rpm) and found no significant differences among them. This finding suggests that there is enough muscular control to compensate for increases in either resistance or cadence. In fact, the quadriceps were most active when the knee was in flexion, which would act as a stabilizer through a posteriorly directed pull. Although this may seem contradictory to visual judgment, due to an angle of pull change at around 60° to 70° of knee flexion, the quadriceps produce a posteriorly directed force. ACL strain was greatest between about 120° to 200° (0° with pedal at top; 180° with pedal at bottom). This correlates with a high EMG activity of the gastrocnemius.

Summary Approach to Knee Rehabilitation

A general exercise approach begins with isometric setting exercises (**Tables 12–4** and **12–5**). These are performed both in full extension (if possible) and at 20° to 30°. In this minimally flexed position, the patient pushes the

Table 12–4 General Knee Rehabilitation*

Type	Muscles	Sets	Repetitions	Contractions	Rest Period
Quad setting (isometrics)	Quadriceps/hamstrings	1 or 2	10–12	8 seconds	3–5 seconds
Straight leg raises	Quadriceps/psoas	2 or 3	10–12	3–5 seconds	3–5 seconds
Supine (with setting)	Vastus medialis / Biceps femoris				
Vastus medialis	Vastus medialis				
Biceps femoris	Biceps femoris				
Stretching (use proprioceptive neuromuscular facilitation [PNF] hold-relax approach)	Gastrocnemius/soleus / Hamstrings / Tensor fasciae latae / Quadriceps / Adductors	5	10–20	8–10 seconds	5 seconds

*Initial phase, performed three times daily. A rest period of 1 to 3 minutes between sets is recommended.

Table 12–5 General Knee Exercise Program

Exercise/Stretch	Activity	Amount
Beginning Phase—Begin When Patient Has 90% ROM; No Joint Irritation		
Stretch	PNF stretch for hamstrings, ITB, and gastrocnemius	3–5 sets; 10–20 reps
Isometrics	Performed every 20°	1–2 sets; 10–20 reps
Straight leg raise with weights	Supine, prone, and side-lying (5–10 lb)	2–3 sets; 10–20 reps
Functional work	Shallow knee bends, lunges, and step-downs	2–3 sets; 10–12 reps
Isotonic exercise (with elastic tubing)	All knee motions	Base on PRE or DAPRE approach
Aerobic exercise	Well-leg bicycling and rowing, upper body work	30 minutes; three times weekly at target heart rate
Intermediate Phase—Begin When Patient Has 75% Strength and Endurance of Well Leg. Continue the stretch, functional work, and aerobic exercise and add the following:		
Isotonics	Knee and hip work (emphasize eccentrics)	Base on PRE or DAPRE approach
Sport cord training	1/3 knee bends, leg presses, and forward-backward run	Average of 3 sets; 20 reps
PNF diagonals	D1 and D2 hip flexion/extension first; knee straight, progressing to same patterns incorporating knee flexion/extension	Several sets to fatigue
Proprioceptive work	Wobble or balance boards using both legs, progressing to one-legged balance if possible	Average of 5 sets; 3–5 minutes
Advanced Phase—Begin When Patient Has 90% Strength and Endurance of Well Leg. Continue stretch and proprioceptive work; continue above isotonic work if isokinetic machines are not available.		
Isokinetics	Knee flexion/extension patterns	10–20 reps at multiple speeds (emphasize faster speeds to decrease load)
PNF sport or activity specific	Patterns imitate patient's sport patterns	Several sets to fatigue
Agility drills	Figure-eights, cutting maneuvers, cariocas, rope jumping, side-to-side jumping sliders	5–10 sets for total of 45 minutes
Plyometrics	Progress from two-legged to one-legged jumping; progress from straight-line to side-to-side jumping	Several sets to fatigue

Key: ROM, range of motion; PNF, proprioceptive neuromuscular facilitation; PRE, progressive resistance exercise; DAPRE, daily adjustable progressive resistance exercise.

heel into the ground or table to achieve a co-contraction of the hamstrings and quadriceps. When the knee is prepared with a facilitation phase of isometrics, progression to isotonics within the pain-free range is then begun, starting with a weight that allows pain-free performance of three sets of ten repetitions. Increases in weight are dictated by the progressive resistance exercise (PRE) or daily adjustable progressive resistance exercise (DAPRE) protocols (**Table 1–8**). When patellofemoral problems are found, terminal extension exercises through the last

20° may be helpful. If there is instability in the knee, however, open-chain knee extension exercises should be avoided and substituted with closed-chain exercises such as partial squats or leg presses.

When using a bicycle for rehabilitation it is important to keep the seat height at a level that prevents full knee extension if there is underlying ACL insufficiency (**Table 12–6**). For patellofemoral problems, avoid a low-seat position that adds compressive forces to the patella. Pool or aquatic exercise is a useful approach

Table 12–6 Exercise Program for Specific Conditions: Specific Emphasis on Modifications to the General Program

Condition	Emphasize	Avoidance/Contraindication
ITB syndrome	ITB stretching	Initially, downhill running Initially, side-posture adjusting (same side)
Patellofemoral arthralgia and chondromalacia	VMO strengthening Vastus lateralis and ITB stretching Orthotics (if pronation found) Bracing or taping initially to allow pain-free exercise	Initially knee extension between 20° and 90° Low-seat position on bicycle
Meniscus tears	General rehabilitation	Full flexion (full squat) positions Full extension with rotation
ACL tears	Hamstring training Specific focus on vastus lateralis, biceps femoris, and tibialis anterior muscles Functional bracing Proprioceptive training PNF diagonal flexion patterns	Isometric (open-chain) exercise against resistance at 20° Isotonic exercise (open-chain) from 20° to 70° Leg extensions with heavy weight
PCL tears	Quadriceps training PNF knee extension patterns	Open-chain hamstring exercises
MCL tears	Strengthening of both abductors and adductors Strengthening of internal rotators Hinged-knee support for 1–3 weeks	Resisted knee extension from 45° to full extension initially
Patellar tendinitis	Eccentric training of quads Patellar strap or taping may have limited usefulness initially	Initially avoid jumping activities Initially avoid high-weight extensions
Osgood-Schlatter disease	Stretching of quadriceps, hamstrings, and gastrocnemius Bracing	Jumping and running activities should be decreased to reduce pain

for patients with osteoarthritis of the knee, progressing to bicycle riding and finally full weight-bearing exercise.

Stretching of the hamstrings, quadriceps, gastrocnemius, and ITB (and attachments) is important to maintain proper flexibility at the knee. It is particularly important for patellofemoral tracking problems.

Bracing is used for three purposes: (1) for those patients with ACL-deficient knees (functional brace), (2) for those in need of support during rehabilitative training, and (3) for prophylactic purposes to protect against further injury. Functional braces are quite expensive. They represent a variety of custom-fitted supports that provide a block to full knee extension and various hinge supports for both protection from further injury and control of rotational movement. Examples include the CTi and Townsend.[51] Prophylactic bracing provides metal bars to prevent valgus or varus forces from causing further damage. Examples include the Anderson Knee Stabler and McDavid Knee Guard. Used with sporting activities,

these braces may help or ironically may increase the injury rate, possibly due to an early fatigue of the involved leg or prestressing of the knee due to poor fitting.[52, 53]

Rehabilitative support may be provided by taping or brace support. Patellofemoral tracking problems are in need of patellar stability and tracking control. Various braces with patella holes and strapping support or taping applying a strapping approach (McConnell taping) are used.[54] Braces for patients with Osgood-Schlatter disease incorporate a reverse horseshoe design to provide a restraint to superior pull on the tibial tuberosity. Many of these devices probably function more from a proprioceptive mechanism than from the support they are purported to provide.[55]

Algorithms

Algorithms for traumatic knee pain and nontraumatic knee complaints are presented in **Figures 12–12** and **12–13**.

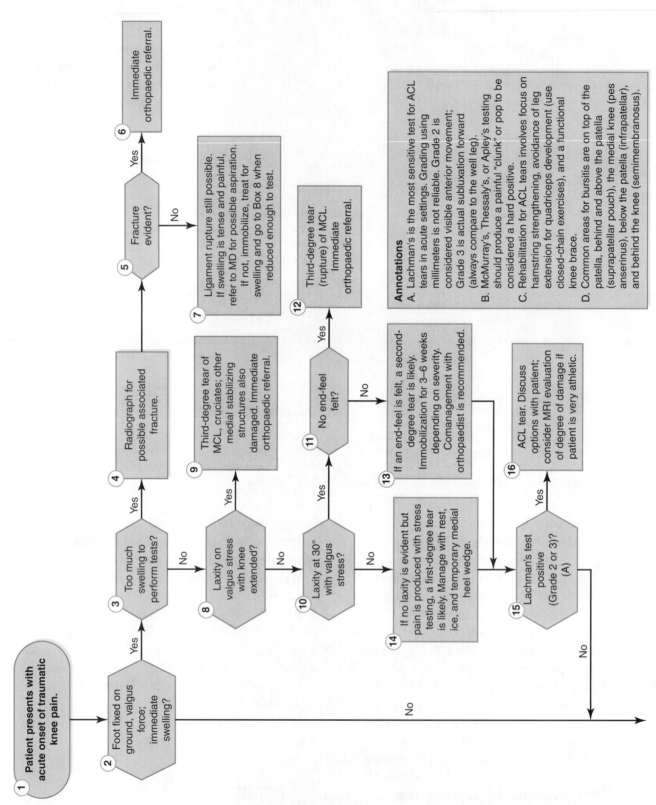

1 Patient presents with acute onset of traumatic knee pain.

2 Foot fixed on ground, valgus force; immediate swelling? — No ⟶

2 Yes

3 Too much swelling to perform tests? — Yes ⟶ **4** Radiograph for possible associated fracture.

3 No

4 ⟶ **5** Fracture evident? — Yes ⟶ **6** Immediate orthopaedic referral.

5 No ⟶ **7** Ligament rupture still possible. If swelling is tense and painful, refer to MD for possible aspiration. If not, immobilize, treat for swelling and go to Box 8 when reduced enough to test.

8 Laxity on valgus stress with knee extended? — Yes ⟶ **9** Third-degree tear of MCL, cruciates; other medial stabilizing structures also damaged. Immediate orthopaedic referral.

8 No

10 Laxity at 30° with valgus stress? — Yes ⟶ **11** No end-feel felt? — Yes ⟶ **12** Third-degree tear (rupture) of MCL. Immediate orthopaedic referral.

11 No ⟶ **13** If an end-feel is felt, a second-degree tear is likely. Immobilization for 3–6 weeks depending on severity. Comanagement with orthopaedist is recommended.

10 No ⟶ **14** If no laxity is evident but pain is produced with stress testing, a first-degree tear is likely. Manage with rest, ice, and temporary medial heel wedge.

15 Lachman's test positive (Grade 2 or 3)? (A) — Yes ⟶ **16** ACL tear. Discuss options with patient; consider MRI evaluation of degree of damage if patient is very athletic.

15 No

Annotations

A. Lachman's is the most sensitive test for ACL tears in acute settings. Grading using millimeters is not reliable. Grade 2 is considered visible anterior movement; Grade 3 is actual subluxation forward (always compare to the well leg).

B. McMurray's, Thessaly's, or Apley's testing should produce a painful "clunk" or pop to be considered a hard positive.

C. Rehabilitation for ACL tears involves focus on hamstring strengthening, avoidance of leg extension for quadriceps development (use closed-chain exercises), and a functional knee brace.

D. Common areas for bursitis are on top of the patella, behind and above the patella (suprapatellar pouch), the medial knee (pes anserinus), below the patella (infrapatellar), and behind the knee (semimembranosus).

Figure 12–12 Traumatic Knee Pain—Algorithm

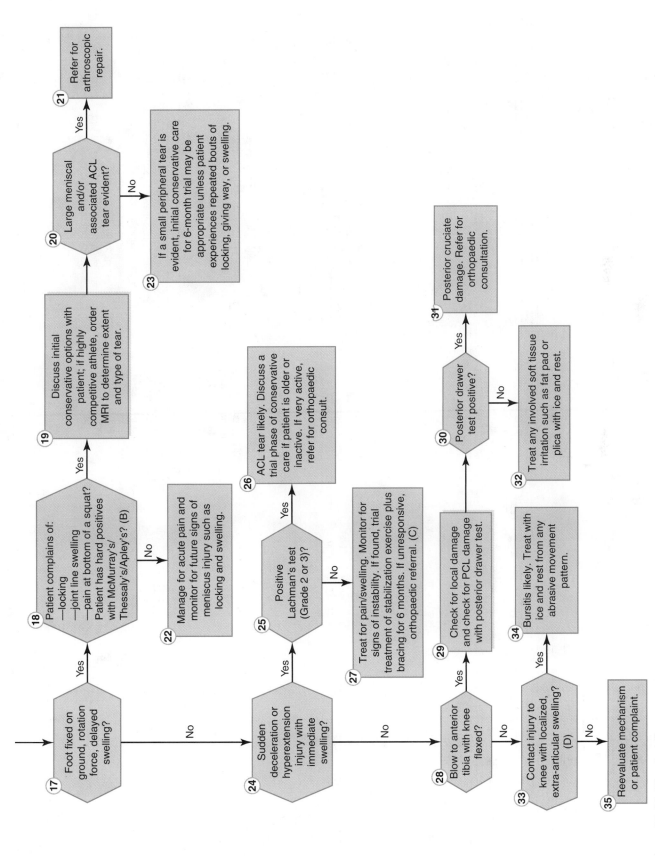

17 Foot fixed on ground, rotation force, delayed swelling?

18 Patient complains of:
—locking
—joint line swelling
—pain at bottom of a squat?
Patient has hard positives with McMurray's/Thessaly's/Apley's? (B)

19 Discuss initial conservative options with patient; if highly competitive athlete, order MRI to determine extent and type of tear.

20 Large meniscal and/or associated ACL tear evident?

21 Refer for arthroscopic repair.

22 Manage for acute pain and monitor for future signs of meniscus injury such as locking and swelling.

23 If a small peripheral tear is evident, initial conservative care for 6-month trial may be appropriate unless patient experiences repeated bouts of locking, giving way, or swelling.

24 Sudden deceleration or hyperextension injury with immediate swelling?

25 Positive Lachman's test (Grade 2 or 3)?

26 ACL tear likely. Discuss a trial phase of conservative care if patient is older or inactive. If very active, refer for orthopaedic consult.

27 Treat for pain/swelling. Monitor for signs of instability. If found, trial treatment of stabilization exercise plus bracing for 6 months. If unresponsive, orthopaedic referral. (C)

28 Blow to anterior tibia with knee flexed?

29 Check for local damage and check for PCL damage with posterior drawer test.

30 Posterior drawer test positive?

31 Posterior cruciate damage. Refer for orthopaedic consultation.

32 Treat any involved soft tissue irritation such as fat pad or plica with ice and rest.

33 Contact injury to knee with localized, extra-articular swelling? (D)

34 Bursitis likely. Treat with ice and rest from any abrasive movement pattern.

35 Reevaluate mechanism or patient complaint.

Figure 12–12 (Continued)

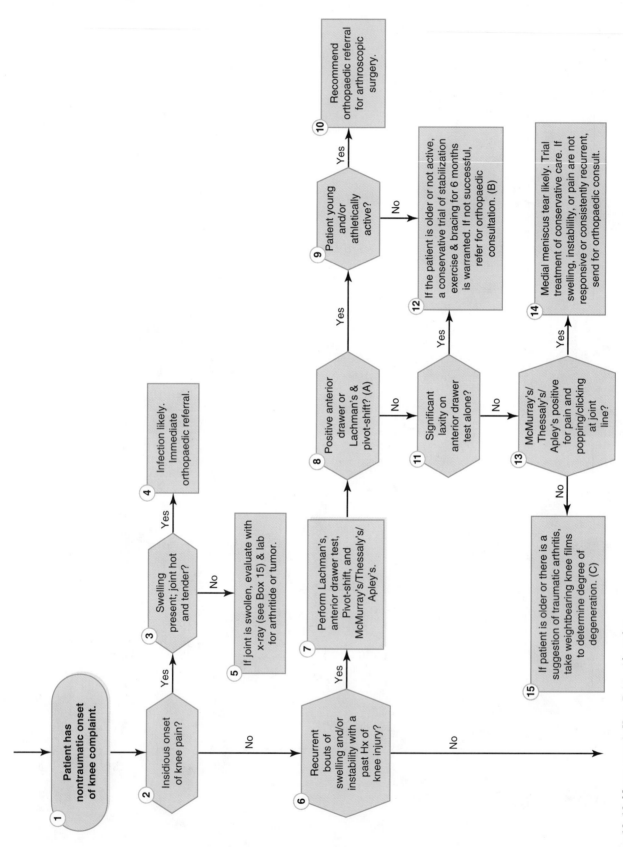

Figure 12–13 Nontraumatic Knee Pain—Algorithm

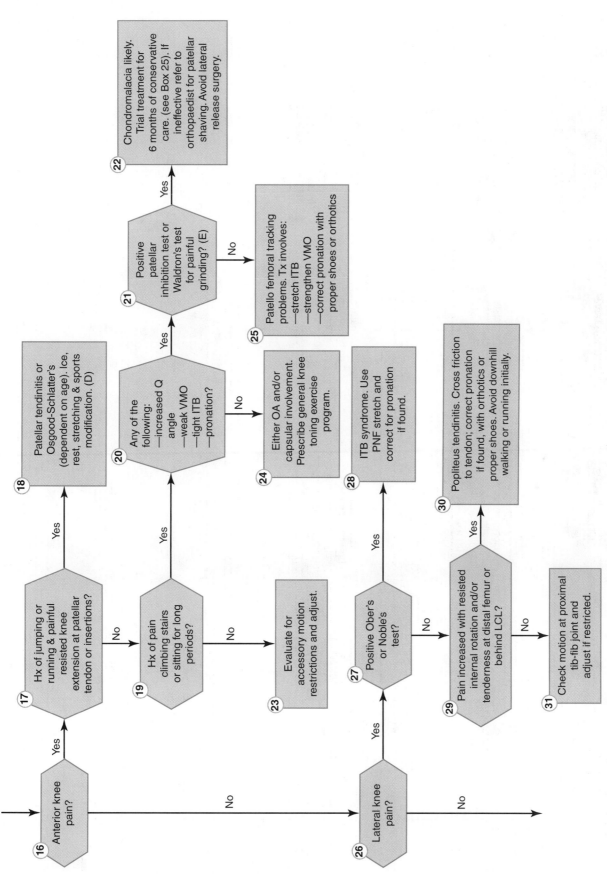

Figure 12–13 (Continued)

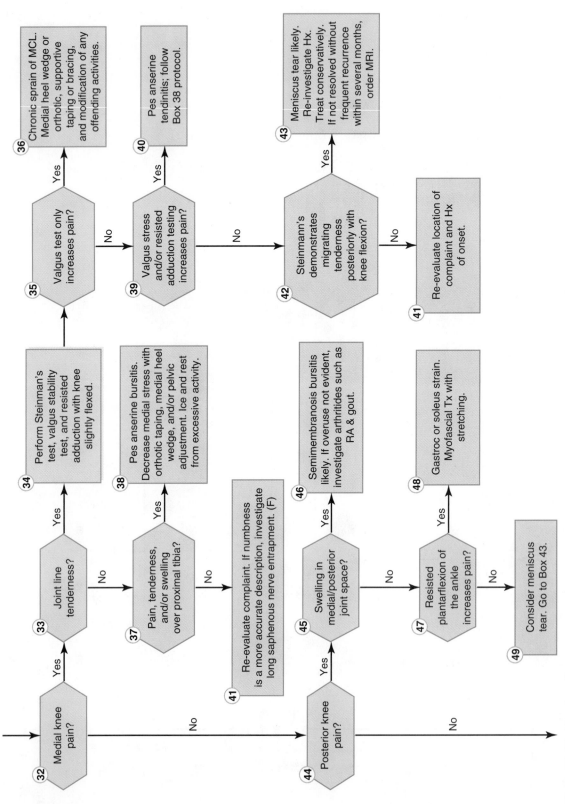

Figure 12–13 (Continued)

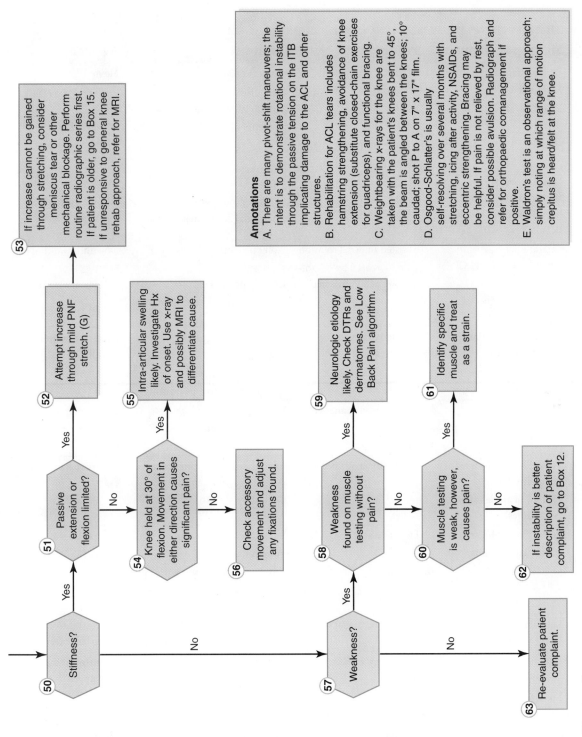

Figure 12–13 (Continued)

Selected Disorders of the Knee

A summary of most of the disorders discussed on the following pages is presented in **Table 12–7**.

Table 12–7 Summary of Knee Disorders

Disorder	Signs and Symptoms	Positive Tests	Treatment	Avoidance
Patellofemoral arthralgia and chondromalacia patellae	Peripatellar pain Movie sign Painful crepitus	Clarke's Waldron's Retinacular test VMO Coordination test Modified Ober's	Correct pronation Strengthen VMO Stretch lateral structures (ITB) Brace/tape for stability	Flexion/extension through crepitus range Low-seat position for bicycling
ITB syndrome	Lateral knee pain at insertion or more commonly lateral epicondyle at 30° flexion	Modified Ober's Noble's	Stretch ITB Correct pronation Rotational adjustment of knee	Downhill running Side-posture adjusting on same side
Popliteus tendinitis	Lateral knee pain with tenderness behind LCL	Resisted internal rotation Pain increased by weight-bearing at 30°; internal rotation of femur	Isometric internal rotation exercises Correct pronation Cross-friction of tendon in front of or behind LCL	Downhill walking or running
Osgood-Schlatter disease	Tender and/or enlarged tibial tuberosity Tight quadriceps	Resisted extension increases pain	Stretch quadriceps Bracing Icing after activity Eccentric quadriceps training	Excessive jumping or running
Bursitis	Localized swelling/tenderness	Compressive maneuvers	Ice Pulsed ultrasound	Pressure Direct trauma Overuse
Superior tibial fibular subluxation	Lateral knee pain with instability History of ankle injury (sometimes)	Instability at 30° full weight-bearing	Fibular head adjustment (support or crutches may be needed for 1 or 2 days post-adjustment)	Excessive hamstring exercises
ACL tear	Pop at time of injury Immediate swelling Gradual instability	Lachman's Drawer Pivot shift	Strengthen hamstrings Functional bracing Proprioceptive training Surgery (often needed for active individuals)	Knee extension exercises
MCL tear	Ligament tenderness Possible sense of instability	Stability testing at 0° or 30°	General strengthening Hinged brace for several weeks	Knee extension from 60° to full extension
Meniscus tear	Joint line tenderness Swelling Locking Giving way	McMurray's Apley's MRI	Acute pain relief Adjust with distraction Refer if signs/symptoms continue	Squatting and rotation stress
Osteochondritis dissecans	Anterior knee pain Possible locking	Wilson's test Tunnel view radiograph	Surgery if loose fragment	Manipulation

TRAUMATIC
Anterior Cruciate Ligament Tears
Classic Presentation

Patients present in either an acute or a chronic phase. In an acute presentation, the patient will report a sudden onset of knee pain following either a hyperextension maneuver or a contact injury with the knee being hit from the side. He or she may remember a "pop" heard at the time of injury. Joint swelling appears quickly. The patient is unable to bear weight.

In the chronic presentation, the patient will have a past history of the above presentation with a follow-up history of gradual resolution of swelling and pain. The presenting complaint is usually more one of instability rather than pain. There may also be reported occurrences of nontraumatic joint line swelling.

Cause

ACL damage can be isolated (often a noncontact injury) usually due to hyperextension and/or sudden contraction of the quadriceps as occurs with sudden stopping or cutting. In a recent study, electromyography and knee flexion analysis were performed for cutting, stopping, and landing.[56] The maximum quadriceps contraction was 161% of maximum voluntary contraction (MVC) occurring just before heel strike and peaking in mid-eccentric motion. At foot strike, the average angle of knee flexion was only 22°. Hamstring activity (protective) was very low—as low as 14%. The combination of knee angle, high quadriceps activity and low protective hamstring activity may indicate why these maneuvers are commonly involved with isolated ACL tears. Contact injury with a rotary component is more likely to damage the ACL and other structures such as the menisci or MCL. When the ACL tears, it usually occurs in the midsubstance of the ligament. Because of the paralleling vascular supply, vascular rupture often occurs, leading to a quickly developing joint swelling that is tense and painful.

Evaluation

In an acute setting, the most helpful indicators are historical, including the mechanisms described above plus immediate swelling, and a "pop" heard at the time of injury. Evaluation in the acute setting is with Lachman's test.[57] The test is applied by stabilizing the distal femur while the examiner attempts to pull the proximal tibia forward with the knee held at 10° to 20° of flexion (Figure 12–4). In more chronic settings, the anterior drawer test may be used. It is the same approach of pulling the tibia forward; however, the hip is flexed to 45°, knee at 90° (Figure 12–5). The disadvantage of this test is that contracted or spasmed hamstrings are in a biomechanically advantaged position, resisting the examiner's attempt at forward displacement of the tibia. It is probably not possible to detect partial tears clinically with these tests.[58] If multiple tissue damage is suspected, the examiner uses a rotary test, "pivot shift" approach (Figure 12–6). There are many variations, but each relies on the passive tension of the ITB to pull the tibia forward when approaching extension, and to pull it back into neutral as more flexion is acquired.[8] In general, the examiner applies a valgus force at the fibular head with rotation at the tibia while flexing and extending the knee, attempting to detect not only anterior-to-posterior movement but also rotation of the tibia. Radiographs may demonstrate a small fracture referred to as the lateral capsular sign at the lateral tibial plateau (Segond's fracture). Also, tibial spine fractures (seen on a tunnel view) and the lateral notch sign (lateral femoral compression fracture seen on the lateral view) are indirect indicators of ACL rupture. Articular cartilage damage is also quite common with ACL tears. MRI is useful in determining the integrity of the ACL.

Management

Treatment of ACL tears is dependent on several factors.
1. Isolated tears are more responsive to conservative care than complicated tears.
2. Complicated tears (acute rotary instability) deserve orthopaedic consult with possible surgical consequences.
3. Age- and activity-related criteria are used to determine need and quality of stability.

Conservative treatment should be reserved for chronic ACL deficiency (in particular, in the older, less athletic individual) and acute tears with resolved swelling. Treatment is directed at substituting other structures for the laxity created by the loss of the ACL.

Attempting to develop a clinical decision approach regarding surgical management, authors in one study[59] reached several suggestions.
1. Measures of anterior tibiofemoral laxity, while indicative of ACL rupture, cannot be used to predict degree of dysfunction resulting from an ACL rupture.
2. Simple clinical outcome scales based on patient self-report are better indicators of the degree of dysfunction associated with ACL rupture than laxity measures, or scales such as the International Knee Documentation Committee (IKDC) that combine physical examination findings and patient self-report of function.
3. Noncopers can be accurately identified and discriminated from the small, unique subset of copers based on tests early after injury.

Copers were defined as those subjects who were able to return to function at a high level (Level I) at least weekly after injury without complaint of instability. Noncopers are defined as those who are unable to return to their premorbid level of sports play or activity because of repeated episodes of giving way.

A 10-year prospective trial[60] tested the outcome of using a patient management algorithm and screening examination for highly active individuals with ACL injury. A summary follows:

- As seen in many other trials, with highly active individuals the most discriminating factor for needing surgery was concomitant injury of the meniscus in particular, or a Grade II or III collateral ligament injury.
- Patients were classified as copers (good potential for nonsurgical management) or noncopers (surgical candidates) based on concomitant injury, unresolved impairments, and results from a screening examination that relied heavily on function testing (primarily a timed hop test).
- Out of 345 patients who met the study criteria, 198 were classified as noncopers (58%). The remaining 146 were classified as copers (42%).
- Sixty-three of 88 potential copers returned to preinjury activities without surgery (72% of copers and 18% of all subjects).
- At 10-year follow-up, only 25 of the original 63 who returned to full activity did not have surgery (7% of total group of ACL injured patients and 28% of copers).
- By using the strategy developed by the University of Delaware, it appears that about 18% of a group of ACL injured patients might be identified as those not initially needing surgery.
- The primary rehabilitation strategy was a perturbation training approach where a platform is used to challenge an individual by constantly shifting the stability of the platform, thus demanding accommodation by the patient.

If the patient is an athlete, surgery is often the only option.[61] In less active individuals, a stabilization program coupled with bracing may be sufficient (**Table 12–8**). The stabilization program focuses on hamstring strengthening, closed-chain quadriceps exercises (avoiding seated knee extensions), and proprioceptive training with balance devices.[62] It is generally recommended to avoid open kinetic chain (OKC) exercises to avoid displacement of the tibia and further stretching of the joint capsule and soft tissue. However, a recent study[63] indicated that when athletes with ACL tears were randomized into either an OKC exercise group or a closed kinetic chain (CKC) exercise group there was a greater degree of quadriceps strength development in the OKC with no indication of increased translation or laxity. Bracing is usually custom-fitted with a functional brace that should offer some degree of protection against hyperextension and rotational forces. Surgical options include stabilization with local tendons or synthetic materials. In a recent study, researchers tested the Legend brace, a functional brace for ACL deficiency or reconstruction for patients with ACL deficiency.[64] The individuals were tested weight-bearing and non-weight-bearing for anterior-to-posterior (AP) shear, internal/external torque, and varus/valgus moments. The brace effectively diminished AP shear and internal torque; however, it did not reduce strain from external torque or varus/valgus moments.

In another study, college football players in full gear ran a 40-yard dash and a four-cone agility drill wearing braces on both knees or no brace at all.[65] The braces tested were the DonJoy Legend, the Breg Tradition, the OMNI-AKS 101W, the McDavid Knee Guard, and the Air Armor Knee (models 1 and 2). The results were that with the 40-yard dash, the Air Armor 1 and Omni did not affect speed; and the Air Armor 1 and the McDavid Knee Guard showed the least amount of migration. With the four-cone drill, only the Breg caused a slower speed performance compared to the control; the Air Armor 1 and 2 showed the least amount of migration.

Prolotherapy is an alternative treatment that incorporates injection, usually of dextrose, into a joint to assist in healing and perhaps increase stability through a proposed mechanism or increasing growth of normal cells or tissue. In a recent prospective study, researchers evaluated the effect of prolotherapy that consisted of dextrose injection every two to four months over a one- to

Table 12–8 Conservative Management of ACL Tears

Parameter	Acute Stage	Subacute Stage	Chronic Stage
Criteria for diagnosis of staging	Positive Lachman's with associated intra-articular swelling, pain; unable to bear weight; in select patients, MRI confirmation.	Positive Lachman's with reduced intra-articular swelling; able to bear weight; ROM limited.	Positive Lachman's or drawer sign; minimal or no swelling; knee feels unstable with rotation maneuvers; full or close to full ROM.
Goals	Reduce swelling, control pain, determine patient's functional needs for future planning of management.	Continue to reduce swelling and control pain; increase ROM, and develop basic strength and proprioception.	Strengthen the hamstrings to 80% of well leg quadriceps; proprioceptively train the lower extremity to react to quick changes in ground surfaces.

Table 12–8 Conservative Management of ACL Tears (continued)

Parameter	Acute Stage	Subacute Stage	Chronic Stage
Concerns	The swelling is a hemarthrosis, making it painful and potentially destructive; associated damage to meniscus, capsule, and fracture must be considered and/or evaluated.	As swelling decreases, more instability than originally suspected may become evident; if unacceptable to patient or indicators of gross laxity, order MRI or refer for orthopaedic consultation.	Patient may become overaggressive in rehabilitation phase and reinjure leg through overcontraction of quadriceps or hyperextension.
Requirements for progression to next stage	Pain and swelling reduced enough to allow 50% ROM; isometric strength evident in available range.	90% ROM available; isotonic contraction through available range if capable of achieving 3 sets of 10 repetitions with minimal weight.	Full ROM; 80% strength of well leg quadriceps; able to perform complex movements such as side stepping and cuts without pain or instability.
Manipulation/ mobilization	Contraindicated in the knee at this time.	Mild mobilization may assist in reducing remaining swelling and increase ROM.	Manipulation of any associated foot/ ankle, hip, pelvic, or lumbar fixations; mild mobilization to the knee.
Modalities	Ice, elevation, TENS, or high-volt galvanic (80–120 Hz/20 min 3 times daily).	Ice and high-volt galvanic (1–150 Hz/20 min/day).	None needed; however, ice after activity if mild swelling still occurs.
External brace, support, etc.	Immobilization should be kept to a minimum; a long cylindrical knee immobilization device may be helpful for up to 5 days.	Protective hinge-brace allowing ROM with an extension block.	Functional knee brace is needed when performing sports activities (includes stabilization in rotation, anteroposterior glide, protection from hyperextension and valgus forces).
ROM/flexibility	Passive ROM within available range; elevation when possible.	Gradual increase in ROM with postisometric and mild PNF techniques.	Maintain flexibility of quadriceps, hamstrings, and triceps surae groups.
Open-chain exercise	Isometrics within available range.	Isotonics within available range performed as straight-leg exercises first; bicycle riding okay if well leg is used for pedaling (bad leg along for the ride); avoid high seat position.	Progressive strengthening using DAPRE or PRE approach.
Closed-chain exercise	None.	Mild quarter squats with weight on both feet with brace worn.	Three-quarter squats with resistance from weight or elastic tubing; leg presses also good.
Proprioceptive training	Electrical stimulation at quadriceps and hamstrings with minimal contraction.	Seated wobble board training; begin mild PNF diagonal training; PNF rhythmic stabilization at 30° for hamstrings.	BAPS or wobble board training; balance jumps on minitrampoline; train with full-resistance PNF diagonal patterns.
Associated biomechanical items	Avoid hyperextension or active extension through the last 60°.	Avoid hyperextension.	Continue to avoid hyperextension on bicycle; avoid knee extension machines through the last 60°.
Lifestyle/activity modifications	No weight-bearing, bed rest for 3–5 days with gradual attempts at partial weight-bearing with crutches.	Use crutches for any stair climbing; avoid activities that cause extension of the knee, especially while standing.	Use the functional brace with sporting activities.

Key: TENS, transcutaneous electrical nerve stimulation; BAPS, biomechanical ankle platform system (Medipedic [Jackson, Michigan]).

three-year period.[66] The results indicate that those patients with symptomatic ACL laxity had both clinically and statistically significant improvement in ACL laxity.

In a recent study, researchers compared three groups of patients over a period of about one year who had received surgery for their ACL deficient knees.[67] These groups were: Group 1–bone-patellar tendon-bone graft, Group 2–semitendinosus and gracilis graft with iliotibial band augmentation, and Group 3–semitendinosus and gracilis only. Outcomes were based on a subjective survey and testing with a KT-1000. Reconstruction with a semitendinosus and gracilis or a patellar graft yielded similar subjective results. The patellar autograph gave better objective results (stability measured by the KT-1000). There was no benefit to the addition of the ITB tenodesis. Previous studies have indicated that AP translation of the knee increases after 30 minutes of running. In one study, researchers evaluated and compared normal knees, ACL deficient knees, and reconstructed ACL ligament knees after exercise.[68] All demonstrated increased laxity using a single-examiner testing with a KT-1000. The normal knee demonstrated a mean of 0.75 mm; the ACL-deficient knee demonstrated a mean of 0.62 mm; and the reconstructed knee demonstrated a mean of only 0.25 mm.

Damage to the articular surface appears to lead to degenerative osteoarthritis and, with time, can lead to full knee replacements. ACL tears have been shown to cause chondral lesions. Pain, catching, and swelling have been noted with these lesions in those patients participating in impact loading activities. In one study,[69] researchers looking at 31,516 arthroscopies provided by 136 surgeons from June 1991–October 1995, 63% demonstrated chondral defects. These defects were 41% Grade III (partial thickness involvement greater than 50% of the depth of cartilage) and 19.2% Grade IV (full thickness lesions, down to the bone). The average age was 43 years. While this procedure appears to be promising, ongoing research and long-term follow-up is necessary before final conclusions can be reached.

Indications for autologous chondrocyte implantation (ACI) are focal full-thickness chondral defects of the femoral condyles, trochlea, and osteochondral defects (OCD). OCD of the patella, tibia, and multiple defects are relative indications for the procedure. Contraindications include inflammatory arthritis, moderate-to-severe degenerative joint disease, and osteoarthritis. Preventing a symptomatic cartilage defect from progressing to advanced degenerative arthritis and providing long-term relief while allowing patients to return to physical activities is the goal when considering autologous chondrocyte replacement (ACR). A recent review[29] concluded that there is insufficient evidence that ACR is cost effective compared with two other approaches that include microfracture or mosaicplasty.

Posterior Cruciate Injury

Classic Presentation

A young athlete complains of knee pain following a blow to the front of his tibia with the knee in a flexed position. Although the swelling was minimal, he noticed discoloration down the back of his lower leg after a couple of days.

Cause

A posterior cruciate tear is less common than an ACL tear. It is usually caused by an anterior blow to the tibia with the knee in a flexed position or by forced hyperflexion. The incidence of PCL injury is between 1% to 44% of acute knee injuries.[22] This large variation in reported incidence is due to the setting (e.g., motor vehicle versus sports or other injury). It is likely that PCL injury occurs more commonly in contact sports.

Evaluation

Swelling is usually less severe due to rupture of the capsule with drainage down the fascial plain of the lower leg. In many cases this will, over days, lead to discoloration of the back of the calf. Testing should begin with observation with the patient supine and the knee flexed to 90°. Depression of the tibial tubercle compared with the healthy leg is a common finding. As mentioned above, damage to the cruciates may occur in isolation, or with other structures. When there is isolated damage, straight instability may be evident on stress testing. The standard test for the PCL is the posterior drawer test. The patient set-up is the same as for the anterior drawer test with the patient supine, hips flexed to 45°, and knees flexed to 90°. The examiner first observes for a "sag" sign where the tibial tuberosity of the involved leg is posterior in relationship to the well leg. If so, grasping the calf and pulling toward neutral would be necessary to establish the "start" position. With the patient relaxed, the examiner exerts a posteriorly directed force on the tibia, observing and palpating for posterior displacement. The same standard of measure is used as for the ACL with Grade I being in the range of 5 mm, Grade II in the range of 6–10 mm, and Grade III greater than 10 mm (1 cm). By using a combination of the drawer test coupled with internal and external rotation (such as the Slocum test used for anterior rotary instability), the examiner may detect the posterior instability that has a rotary component. With an internal rotation/posterior force, the examiner may detect excessive movement indicative of posteromedial instability. Posterolateral instability is detectable with an external rotation/posterior force coupling. This test may be performed in either the supine or seated position. Another valuable test is the dynamic posterior shift test. The patient's hip is flexed to almost 90° and maintained in this position while the examiner passively extends the knee. Gravity, plus the tightening effect of the hamstrings, will cause the tibia to subluxate posteriorly in knees with posterior laxity.

Continuing to extend the knee to near full extension, the knee will suddenly jerk, or clunk, into reduction. The patient may feel a reproduction of the instability sensation during the maneuver. Finally, a simple active test is to have the patient sit with the knees off the end of the table. The examiner resists knee flexion and observes for posterior movement at the tibia.

Management

It appears that many individuals with PCL damage are able to continue participating in sports. Rehabilitation focuses on strengthening the quadriceps with initial de-emphasis on the hamstrings. Surgical repair is usually not as successful as for ACL injury and normally has some degree of residual laxity.

Both a prospective study and a more recent study in 2002[70, 71] followed 133 patients from the time of injury to an average of 5.4 years follow-up. The intention was to determine the natural history of acute, isolated PCL tears over time. Sixty-eight patients returned for long-term follow-up. Evaluation included stability testing and several functional questionnaires including the Noyes knee score, Lysholm score, and Tegner activity score. A summary of their findings follows:

- Patients with greater laxity did not have the worst subjective scores.
- Half of all patients returned to the same sport at the same, or higher, level (regardless of the severity of laxity).
- One-third returned to the same sport at a lower level.
- One-sixth did not return to the same sport.
- There was no change in laxity from time of injury to follow-up.
- There was no relationship between the amount of pain and the degree of laxity.
- There was no radiographic indication of an increase in osteoarthritis.
- There were few associated meniscal tears with isolated PCL tears (probably due to the fact that the injury occurs on an unloaded knee).
- Although there were differences in the athlete's ability to perform tests of quadriceps strength, it was not felt that there was an obvious deficiency in quadriceps strength in patients with PCL injury. Patients with low subjective scores on knee questionnaires may need more focus on quadriceps training.

In the second study, there was no relationship between subjective scoring and degree of instability and no specific indicators of who will deteriorate.

Meniscus Tears

Classic Presentation

The patient presents with a complaint of knee pain usually following a rotational injury to the knee. Injury of the knee involving flexion and internal rotation of the tibia may cause traction, pulling the posterior horn of the medial meniscus toward the center of the joint, resulting in a peripheral tear at the attachment site and a longitudinal tear of the meniscus substance. With posterior horn tears, the meniscus will often return to its normal anatomic position with extension of the knee; however, if the tear extends beyond the MCL (creating a bucket-handle tear), a problem with locking may occur when the knee is in a flexed position. The patient noticed that swelling in the knee developed over a number of hours. Since the injury, the patient may have episodes of knee locking wherein he or she experiences significant pain and is unable to move the leg for a few seconds until the involved knee is forcefully extended. Knee swelling or giving way may be the main complaint. A study evaluating MRI findings in asymptomatic patients revealed that 16% of asymptomatic patients have meniscal tears. For patients 45 years or older, the prevalence increased to 36%.[72]

One study attempting to determine the relative value of adding MR to the evaluation of younger patients with suspected meniscal injury had interesting results.[73] The clinical exam and MRI had similar diagnostic performances, questioning the need for MRI in most cases. There was lower sensitivity for patients younger than 12 years of age. Some differences between the clinical exam and MRI were based on specific pathologies:

- Lateral discoid meniscus: CE = 89%, MRI = 39% sensitivity
- Medial meniscus tear: CE = 81%, MRI = 90% sensitivity

Researchers in one study evaluated the relevance of abnormal findings on MRI of the anterior horn of the meniscus and existence of actual pathology.[74] There was a 74% false-positive rate (26% true-positive rate). The authors recommend clinical correlation with MRI findings because some of the false-positive patients were asymptomatic and some had other pathologies.

Cause

Most meniscus injuries are due to combined compression with rotation at the knee. There are many types of tears; however, they are generally divided into horizontal and vertical tears. Because of the minor blood supply, meniscus tears do not usually bleed much into the joint. The free edge of the tear, however, may cause irritation with a reactant synovial fluid production. The meniscus is often involved when the ACL is torn, in which case the predominance of signs and symptoms will come from the cruciate damage.

Evaluation

In addition to the history, it is important to challenge the knee with compression and rotation. The two primary tests are McMurray's and Thessaly's.[15, 75] The combination of joint line tenderness with a positive McMurray's or Thessaly's test is a strong indicator of meniscal involvement. The McMurray test begins with forced, passive flexion of the knee coupled with rotation as the examiner palpates the joint line for popping (clunking) and pain (Figure 12–7). If negative, the knee is passively extended with combined forces of internal or external rotation coupled with varus and valgus forces. Thessaly's test involves the patient weight-bearing on the involved foot and rotating on the knee to elicit pain, joint line discomfort, or locking or catching. (Figure 12–8). Apley's compression test is performed with the patient prone. An axial force is applied through the tibia to the knee as it is passively rotated. This is performed in all degrees of flexion and extension. A lateral meniscus test called the dynamic test may also be useful (Figure 12–9). Further evaluation with MRI may be helpful in determining the type and extent of tear and assisting in the decision whether or not to treat surgically.

Management

There are a number of tears that can be treated conservatively while others may require surgical repair. Radial type tears seem less easily reparable, although some complete tears do warrant attempts at repair. Radial tears in the inner one-third (nonvascular zone) of less than 5 mm may not heal but can be left alone. Healing of chronic bucket-handle tears requiring partial meniscectomy are unlikely to occur often, while acute bucket-handle tears seem to respond better to repair. Radial tears in the posterior horn seem to heal better than those occurring in the middle portion due to greater vascularity.

Longitudinal (vertical) tears in the periphery are most amenable to repair, and it has been stated that stable tears less than 1 cm in length can be left alone. Stable tears are defined as:

- Those in which the central portion cannot be displaced more than 3 mm.
- Longitudinal tears that are stable in the peripheral two-thirds can generally be left alone, especially if they do not exceed 5 mm.
- Tears that are partial thickness tears can be left alone if they do not exceed 5 mm in length.
- Oblique and horizontal tears show greater difficulty healing and may require surgical intervention. In patients with degenerative menisci or discoid menisci, surgical repair is ill-advised.

Studies[76, 77] have examined factors that affect healing for meniscal repair. The authors conclude that the ideal patient profile for meniscal repair is a patient younger than 30 years of age who has a tear within 3 mm of the meniscosynovial junction. The injury should be repaired relatively soon and in conjunction with an ACL reconstruction.

A "conservative" rehabilitation protocol demonstrated a higher rate of complete healing. This consisted of protected weight-bearing (crutches with partial touching of the ground) and protected range of motion from 20° to 90° for the first six weeks.

Given the concern of osteoarthritis in patients treated with partial meniscectomy, one review of the literature investigated the likelihood of osteoarthritic progression.[78] Osteoarthritis progressed more often after medial partial meniscectomy in patients older than 40 years of age. For those with medial meniscectomy the best radiographic results were in patients with valgus knees (compared to varus).

Although chiropractors do not perform surgery, we are often asked whether surgery should be considered for meniscus injury and what type of surgery is best. One study[79] helps define some differences between two common arthroscopic approaches to meniscus repair. It is well known that total meniscectomy leads to early degenerative changes in the knee. Unfortunately, even partial meniscectomy will often lead to advanced degenerative changes. Therefore, when possible, meniscal repair is recommended. Unfortunately, healing rates are reported between 50% and 89%. The two common approaches used are the outside-in and the inside-out techniques. The advantage of the inside-out technique is that it allows for more consistent suture placement perpendicular to the tear. However, it requires a larger incision and more risk of neurovascular damage. The outside-in technique reduces this risk and does not require a large incision; unfortunately, it can address only anterior and middle-third tears.[80] This is due mainly to the anterior placement of the needles. This study confirmed that posterior horn tears of the medial meniscus did not heal well, if at all, with the outside-in technique. The authors recommend the outside-in technique for all lateral meniscus tears, and for anterior and middle tears of the medial meniscus. The inside-out technique should be reserved for posterior tears of the medial meniscus. A newer technique, an "all-inside" repair device, has not demonstrated a higher success rate, with greater than one-third failure rate reported.[81]

Vertical, stable tears in the peripheral meniscus often will heal, especially in the younger patient.[82] Most other tears will usually progress to recurrent bouts of swelling and pain with decreasing asymptomatic periods. Arthroscopic repair or partial meniscectomy is the most common surgical approach with isolated meniscal damage. In the 1980s, patients were entered into a long-term study of meniscal allograft transplantation with ACL reconstruction.[83] Two types of allografts were used: lyophilized and deep-frozen. At almost 15 years (and previously after 3 years) patients were reevaluated with knee questionnaires (Lysholm), radiographs, MRI, and in some cases arthroscopy. The deep-frozen were far more successful and served the function of a real meniscus compared with the lyophilized. The latter carries an increased risk of early degenerative changes in the knee.[84] Chiropractic manipulation may be helpful in reducing meniscus symptoms. Whether it affects the long-term course of meniscus tears remains to be seen. Manual reduction of a meniscus lock is also an important management tool.

Medial Collateral Ligament Tear

Classic Presentation

When the tear is second- or third-degree, the patient will report a history of contact or noncontact injury that forced the knee into valgus. There is often sharp medial pain with associated swelling at the time of injury. With first-degree tears, the patient frequently will have no history of trauma; however, he or she will report a history of an overuse activity with more mild to moderate pain at the medial knee.

Cause

Either traumatic outside-to-inside forces (valgus stress) will lead to partial or total disruption of the MCL fibers or chronic strain through valgus-loading biomechanical factors (e.g., pronation) will lead to chronic stress resulting in a first-degree sprain.

Evaluation

With trauma, it is important to test for MCL integrity. The examiner applies a valgus force to the extended knee. If there is significant opening (compared with the opposite, well leg), a third-degree tear (rupture) of the MCL has occurred in addition to other medial stabilizers such as the meniscus or cruciates. (*Note:* In children a positive finding likely represents epiphyseal damage and warrants stress radiography.) If the test is negative for instability in extension, the patient is evaluated in 20° to 30° of flexion (with the hip stabilized to prevent rotation). If the knee opens in this position without an end-feel, an isolated third-degree tear has occurred. If there is opening with a definite end-point (compared with the opposite side) a second-degree tear is likely. If there is no instability but the test produces medial joint pain, a first-degree sprain or pes anserinus tendinitis is possible. Adding an active contraction into knee flexion or medial rotation may cause pain with a pes anserinus strain.

Management

Third-degree sprains with associated meniscal or cruciate involvement should be referred for orthopaedic surgical management. Isolated third-degree tears are occasionally managed with two to three weeks of restricted bracing followed by gradual weight-bearing and rehabilitation.[85] Second-degree tears are managed with two weeks of hinge-cast immobilization followed by rehabilitation. First-degree tears involve correcting any biomechanical predispositions such as orthotics for pronation, modification of sporting or recreational activity, and strengthening of the medial and lateral stabilizers. In an animal study by Warden et al.[86] standard low-intensity pulsed ultrasound was compared to pulsed ultrasound delivered NSAID (celecoxib; COX-2 inhibitor) in knee ligament healing. At two weeks, those treated with the standard pulsed ultrasound were about 30% stronger, stiffer, and about 50% more able to absorb energy before failure. Those treated with the NSAID could absorb about 33% less energy than those in the standardized group. However, there were no difference between groups after 4 and 12 weeks. The authors conclude that low-intensity pulsed ultrasound accelerated but did not improve healing, and that the NSAID treatment caused a delay but did not affect healing over time. Their clinical concern is that there might be a window of time for patients treated with pulsed ultrasound delivering an NSAID where re-injury is more likely to occur.

There is some evidence that conventional therapeutic ultrasound may be beneficial in accelerating fracture repair.[87] Animal studies have produced some interesting results. Although at 25 days after active treatment with ultrasound did not demonstrate any benefit over inactive ultrasound (control group), at 40 days there was a demonstrated benefit compared to those not treated with continuous ultrasound: a 17% increase in bone mineral content at the fracture site in those treated with the active ultrasound. The ultrasound treated group had an 81% greater mechanical strength when compared to the nontreatment group.

NONTRAUMATIC

Patellofemoral Arthralgia and Chondromalacia

Classic Presentation

The patient complains of anterior knee pain. The pain is worse with going up and down steps and sitting for long periods of time. There is often associated crepitus and pain going through any squatting maneuver.

Cause

Patellofemoral arthralgia is thought to be primarily a soft tissue disorder associated with the consequences of a patellar tracking disorder. Researchers in a two-year prospective study evaluated 282 athletes, 24 of whom developed anterior knee pain.[88]

Anthropometric measurements, functional tests, EMG measure of reaction time, and mobility of the patella were measured as a baseline. For those who developed anterior pain, there were only four possible predictors:

1. A slowed vastus medialis/lateralis response time
2. A decrease in explosive strength
3. A shortened quadriceps
4. A hypermobile patella

Stress on stabilizing structures such as the VMO and medial or lateral retinaculum may be the primary cause. Other possible involvement occurs with pinching or irritation of the infrapatellar fat pad. Chondromalacia patellae is due to degeneration of the hyaline cartilage on the back surface of the patella. A gradual deterioration occurs, often related to maltracking or instability of the patella. Underlying predispositions appear to be an increased Q angle, underdevelopment of the femoral condyles or the patella, patella alta (high riding), and, more functionally, weak medial stabilizers (VMO) and tight lateral structures such as the vastus lateralis and ITB.

Evaluation

Waldron's test is performed by having the examiner listen to and feel the patella as the patient goes through a squatting maneuver. If pain and crepitus are felt during a specific range, patellar involvement is likely. If the pain is felt only at the bottom of the squat, it is more likely to be due to meniscal pathology. The patellar inhibition test attempts to hold the patella down stationary with the knee at 10° to 15° extension while the patient contracts the quadriceps. Pain with grinding is indicative of chondromalacia patella. Other tests include the VMO coordination test, which tests the ability of the VMO to stabilize the patella through the last 15° of knee extension; Ober's test, designed to stretch the leg into adduction, thereby stretching the ITB (see below); and patellar stability tests. Palpation around the patella may reveal tenderness at the vastus insertions, retinacula, patellar meniscal ligaments, or a plica. Determination of biomechanical factors contributing to tracking problems includes measurement of the Q angle, checking for femoral anteversion and tibial torsion, and checking for pronation. Radiographs to detect patellar tilt incorporate the tangential (i.e., axial) view. They include the sunrise view, Merchant view, and Lauren view. Also, detection of past subluxation or dislocation may be visible on the flexed or extended lateral view.

Management

The primary goal is to correct maltracking of the patella. This is usually accomplished through general knee-stabilizing exercises coupled with orthotic support (**Table 12–9**). Knee bracing at the patellar tendon may relieve some of the acute discomfort. Various patellar braces are available, based primarily on the principle of providing a support for the patella via a hole cut in the brace and/or strapping or internal padding. Taping involves the use of a strapping tape to pull the patella in the desired direction. Although this may not provide the stability intended, it does seem to provide a strong proprioceptive support to proper tracking.[48] McConnell and other taping approaches have been used successfully to decrease pain in patients with patellofemoral knee pain. There is some question though as to the mechanism by which this occurs. Does pain decrease due to mechanical stabilization of the patella or realignment? A study using computed tomography (CT) evaluated sixteen female patients with anterior knee pain and patellofemoral incongruence.[89] An axial CT of knee was taken prior to taping and after taping without quadriceps contraction and then with contraction. Patellar alignment was measured as patellar lateralization and patellar tilt. Although there was initial partial correction with

Table 12–9 Rehabilitation of Patellofemoral Disorders

Parameter	Initial	Intermediate	Advanced
Criteria	Anterior knee pain with going up and down stairs or after sitting for extended periods; positive tests for ITB tightness and/or VMO coordination; possible positive patellar inhibition test or pain/crepitus while squatting.	Anterior knee pain reduced, ITB tightness improved, VMO facilitated.	No pain with activity.
Goals	Reduce pain and any associated retinacular tenderness; evaluate for need of foot orthotic support.	Continue to strengthen VMO; strengthen the knee with general knee-toning exercises; train patient in stair climbing.	Functionally train individual for specific sport activity.

Table 12–9 Rehabilitation of Patellofemoral Disorders (continued)

Parameter	Initial	Intermediate	Advanced
Concerns	Possible chondromalacia, not visible on radiograph; failure to respond is suggestive.	Patient feels better and is not compliant or not able to be compliant with stair and squat restriction.	Overenthusiastic training.
Requirements for progression to next stage	Decrease in pain with ascending/descending steps; VMO strength increasing; ITB more flexible.	Accomplished intermediate stage of knee strengthening; able to ascend/descend steps properly without discomfort; VMO coordination test is negative.	
Manipulation/mobilization	Manipulation/mobilization of the patella into restricted ranges; manipulation of any corresponding lower extremity or lumbopelvic fixations.	Manipulation/mobilization of the patella into restricted ranges; manipulation of any corresponding lower extremity or lumbopelvic fixations.	Manipulation/mobilization of the patella into restricted ranges; manipulation of any corresponding lower extremity or lumbopelvic fixations.
Modalities	Ice, rest, EMS for VMO.	Ice after activity.	None.
External brace, support, etc.	Patellar stabilizing brace or McConnell taping; cast for orthotics if necessary or use temporary trial of medial heel wedge.	Patellar stabilizing brace or McConnell taping.	Wean patient off support.
ROM/flexibility	Stretch quadriceps, hamstrings, ITB, and triceps surae group.	Stretch quadriceps, hamstrings, ITB, and triceps surae group.	Stretch quadriceps, hamstrings, ITB, and triceps surae group.
Open-chain exercise	Extension through last 10° to 15° if tolerable; combine with adduction for better facilitation of VMO.	Extension through full range of pain and crepitus free; for additional support, strengthen abductors, adductors, and flexors using PRE or DAPRE approach.	Isokinetic exercises are added if appropriate.
Closed-chain exercise	Mini squats through crepitus/pain-free range (knee over toe).	Squats continue through an increased crepitus/pain-free range with elastic tubing resistance; perform lateral step-ups; train in single-stair-climbing technique.	Plyometrics may begin if patient passes test with single leg squats and hops.
Proprioceptive training	Begin wobble board (BAPS board) training; have patient cocontract with ramped EMS.	Progress with BAPS training and minitrampoline jumping; PNF diagonal training if patient is athletic.	Sports-specific PNF patterns.
Associated biomechanical items	Avoid low-seat position with bicycling; avoid knee extension or squats in crepitus/pain range.	Avoid low-seat position with bicycling; avoid knee extension or squats in crepitus/pain range.	Avoid low-seat bicycle positions.
Lifestyle/activity modifications	Avoid stair climbing, squatting, and prolonged sitting.	Minimal stair climbing, mini squats; take frequent breaks when having to sit for long periods (e.g., driving movies).	None.

Key: EMS, electrical muscle stimulation; BAPS, biomechanical ankle platform system (Medipedic [Jackson, Michigan]).

Note: Any time a chiropractic adjustive technique is used as treatment, an associated subluxation/segmental dysfunction code will be used.

taping, this was lost with quadriceps contraction. These findings indicate that mechanical stabilization or realignment of the patella likely is not the reason why pain relief occurs with this type of taping. It is more likely that a proprioceptive effect occurs as indicated in similar studies of ankle taping. In one study, researchers attempted to determine whether a standardized treatment program would make a difference in pain levels for patients with patellofemoral pain.[90] Seventy-one subjects, 40 years of age or younger with patellofemoral pain of one month or longer, were randomized into two groups. The treatment group received a standardized program of six treatment sessions including quad training, patellofemoral mobilization, patellar taping, and home exercises. The placebo group received sham ultrasound, light application of gel, and placebo taping. The trained group scored significantly higher on measures of pain reduction and disability. Orthotic support may also be needed in pronated patients. Chiropractic manipulations of the foot, ankle, hip, and knee are often used to guarantee a more fully functioning integrated lower extremity. Patients with true chondromalacia who fail a conservative approach for six months should be referred for surgical consultation. The primary surgical procedures include shaving of the posterior patella arthroscopically and a lateral release.

Iliotibial Band Syndrome

Classic Presentation

The patient complains of lateral knee pain that gradually increased over a few days to weeks. The pain seems to be related to running (although sedentary individuals may develop similar pain). Specifically, downhill running seems to be aggravating and pain occurs when extending the leg just before heel strike. Some patients may hear a squeaking sound with flexion-extension of the knee.

Cause

The cause of this syndrome is believed to be a tight ITB that rubs against the lateral epicondyle of the femur at approximately 30° to 40° of knee flexion. Predispositions included hyperpronation and downhill running. Recent evidence suggests the possibility that either a thicker or wider band predisposes patients to this syndrome. In addition, it appears that not all repetitive activity is predisposing. It appears that the longer one performs a repetitive activity with the knee flexed to 30° to 40°, the more likely ITB syndrome will develop. Therefore, downhill running or slower running (jogging) may be the major factor because these activities occur primarily with the knee in the "impingement" range. Running at faster speeds seems less likely a cause.

Evaluation

Palpation for tenderness is targeted to the lateral epicondyle (approximately 3 cm proximal to the lateral joint line). Tenderness may be increased if pressure is applied at the lateral epicondyle while flexing and extending the knee. Tenderness increases in the "painful arc" of 30° to 40°. This is often referred to as Noble's test. Ober's test is designed mainly to detect tightness in the muscular attachments into the ITB, including the gluteus maximus and tensor fasciae latae or the band itself (**Figure 12–11**). The patient lies on his or her unaffected side. The examiner moves the bottom limb into flexion to avoid blocking of the following adduction movement. The top leg is then passively lowered over the back of the table to determine available adduction and any associated pain. It is crucial to stabilize the patient's iliac crest to avoid stretching above the pelvis (isolate the stretch to the ITB). Pain may also be increased by bearing full weight onto the involved side with the knee bent to 30° to 45°. Wang et al.[91] used diagnostic ultrasonography to demonstrate that the modified Ober position is likely more effective at stretching the ITB. In another study Wang et al.[92] evaluated the benefit of using ultrasonography to measure the effects of stretching and found, for the width of the ITB, the examiner reliability was high.

Management

The primary approach is to stretch the ITB and its muscular attachments using a postisometric relaxation technique. Modification of running/jogging activities is necessary during the acute phase. Sudden stretching of the ITB with side-posture adjusting should be avoided for one to two weeks. Because of the pelvic attachments of the ITB, tensor fasciae latae, and gluteus maximus, pelvic manipulation should be considered if consistent with chiropractic evaluation findings.

Popliteus Tendinitis

Classic Presentation

The patient presents with complaints similar to those of the patient with ITB syndrome, with a report of lateral knee pain following downhill running or walking.

Cause

The popliteus functions as an internal rotator when the knee is non-weight-bearing. In addition, it plays a supportive role for both the posterior PCL and the LCL, preventing forward movement of the femur on the tibia and varus angulation, respectively. Finally, the popliteus acts to pull the posterior lateral meniscus posteriorly during knee flexion. The popliteus muscle takes its origin off the back of the tibia, spiraling around as a tendon under the LCL and inserting into the distal femur just in front of the LCL.

Evaluation

A history of downhill walking or running is often found. Tenderness is found at the insertion point on the distal femur just anterior to the LCL attachment. Tenderness also may be found directly behind the LCL. Resisted internal rotation may cause pain at the lateral knee. Bearing full weight on the involved side with the knee bent 30° and then internally rotating the femur may increase the discomfort in some patients. Ancillary findings may include hyperpronation on the involved side.

Management

In addition to ice and rest, cross-friction over the tendon section of the popliteus just in front of and just behind the LCL is often effective. Orthotic support may be needed for the hyperpronated foot and adjusting of any lower extremity fixations.

Proximal Tibial-Fibular Subluxation

Classic Presentation

The patient reports the sudden onset of lateral knee pain following a sudden dorsiflexion or plantarflexion injury at the ankle. Another presentation may be a patient who experiences pain less abruptly while performing leg curls (for hamstrings). The patient may have added complaints of instability or pain radiating down the side of the lower leg.

Cause

The proximal tibial-fibular articulation is a synovial joint. Movement at this joint is influenced by movement at the ankle. When the ankle dorsiflexes, the proximal fibula moves superiorly and rotates outward; with plantarflexion, the fibula moves inferior and rotates inward. Sudden forced movements (in particular dorsiflexion) may force the fibula into a fixed position. With hamstring curls, the biceps femoris may draw the fibular head posteriorly, leading to fixation or, in some patients, chronic hypermobility. Due to the proximity of the peroneal nerve to the fibular head, compression or entrapment may occur with the result of radiating pain down the outside lower leg.

Evaluation

Joint play assessment in the supine position is accomplished with the knee extended. Palpation at the fibular head should reveal normal movement with passive dorsiflexion and plantarflexion of the ankle. With the knee bent to 90°, the examiner may pull and push the fibular head to determine any sense of fixation or hypermobility.

Management

The standard approach is to adjust the fibular head. In hypermobile joints, it may be necessary to impose one or two days of non-weight-bearing. Decreasing the amount of resistance on the leg curl may also be beneficial as a preventive approach.

Patellar Tendinitis (Jumper's Knee)

Classic Presentation

The patient is often an athlete complaining of anterior knee pain with activities that involve jumping or sprinting.

Cause

Repetitive stress to the patellar tendon (ligament) is common with jumping and running sports. It appears that this is often an eccentric injury. The prevalence of jumper's knee in elite volleyball players is as high as 40%–50%.[93] Chronic patellar tendinosis may be due to increased spouting of nonvascular, sensory, substance P-positive nerve fibers, and a decrease in vascular sympathetic nerve fibers.[94]

Evaluation

Pain is felt at the patellar tendon or at the attachments to the patella or tibial tuberosity. Resisted extension starting with the knee bent beyond 90° usually will increase pain at the tendon. Researchers, using diagnostic ultrasonography, evaluated 58 soccer players' patellar and Achilles tendons pre- and postseason.[95] Those with abnormal findings for the patellar tendon on preseason evaluation had a 17% risk of developing symptoms compared to those without abnormal findings. Computed tomography (CT) and magnetic resonance imaging (MRI) are also helpful in diagnosing this condition.

Management

The mainstays of treatment are rest, ice, and stretch. After acute symptoms have been resolved, gradual eccentric training (avoidance of plyometrics) should be initiated. Patellar tendinosis can be a very difficult condition to deal with given that it occurs in athletes who are high performers. Rest or major modification to activity is often a difficult prescription. As a result, those who try to maintain their level may find themselves in a surgical scenario. One study[96] grouped patients according to a classification system similar to that used by Ferretti et al.[97] and Lian et al.[98]

Stage I designates those individuals who have pain only with activity and have no apparent functional impairment. Stage II designates those with discomfort with activity and after activity, although the individual can still perform at a satisfactory level. Stage III designates those individuals who have pain with activity and pain after activity is more prolonged. Stage III individuals cannot perform at a satisfactory level due to the pain. There were a total of 42 athletes; all were managed with NSAIDs, physical therapy, and exercise. Exercise was initiated with isometric quadriceps contractions and stretching of the quads, hamstrings, and adductors/abductors of the hip. There was also a focus on eccentric training of the quadriceps. At six months, 33 out of the 42 were asymptomatic and able to return to sports. Nine Stage III patients required surgery. At a mean follow-up of 4.8 years, all patients were doing well. Those with Stage II involvement fared better than those with Stage III. This may indicate that the earlier the athlete is managed in the course of involvement based on symptoms, the better the outcome. Shockwave treatment for tendon and fascial problems has gained momentum. A long-term follow-up by Vulpiani et al.[99] indicated that at two-year follow-up, satisfactory results were found with the majority of participants (specifically performing athletes), with an average return-to-sport time of about six weeks. The protocol involved an average of four sessions at a 2/7–day intervals. Impulses were between 1,500–2,500 with energy varying between 0.08 and 0.44 mJ/mm^2.

A Cho-Pat brace may provide some relief of symptoms, especially in the early stages. Cross-friction massage, active release technique, and Graston technique may also be beneficial alternative conservative treatments. Other conservative forms of treatment recommended include eccentric exercise, decline squat, therapeutic ultrasonography and iontophoresis. Surgical repair should only be performed in the Stage III athlete in which periods of conservative care have failed, and in Stage IV with complete rupture.

Another approach for tendinosis that is not responsive to eccentric training is sclerosing of neovessels that develop in the involved area of the tendon. Research thus far indicates promise in the short term.[100]

Surgery should be reserved for recalcitrant cases. Conservative approaches that have demonstrated some value in the literature include eccentric training and extracorporeal shockwave therapy. In one small study,[101] concentric training versus eccentric training was compared in active athletes with symptoms of patellar tendinosis. At 32-month follow-up, those in the eccentric group were satisfied with their results. The protocol consisted of a 12-week daily program that included a six-week cessation of all sporting activity. Eccentric training was on a decline board. All patients in the concentric trained group proceeded to either surgery or sclerosing injections. Another study[102] demonstrating improvement using a 25° decline board over a standard step protocol found that at a 12-month follow-up, although both groups improved, the decline-board group had greater clinical gains. The decline eccentric protocol required a 12-week intervention performed daily. The group performed single-leg squats on a 25° decline board utilizing a typical Curwin Stanish[103] protocol of three sets, 10–15 repetition approach with moderate pain occurring in the last set. The downward, or eccentric, component was performed using the symptomatic leg with the upward, or concentric, component performed by the well leg.

Other approaches include shockwave therapy and injection of platelet-rich plasma (PRP) (see Chapter 1 for a broader discussion). Two recent studies indicated that both had value in the management of chronic patellar tendinitis, but PRP is still controversial, being banned in some countries and the International Olympic Committee at the time of this publication.[104–106]

Patellar Dislocation and Subluxation

Classic Presentation

A young female attempts to cut to the opposite direction while playing soccer. She falls, grabbing her knee. She says that she felt her knee "go out." There is a large lateral mass (with dislocation).

Cause

Patellar dislocation is not always due to malalignment. It is possible for the athlete to dislocate the patella by planting the foot in a flexed position while attempting to cut to the opposite direction. A valgus force is then created while the quadriceps is contracting strongly. Complications are common and numerous. Many of the soft tissue stabilizing structures for the patella are torn, such as the medial retinaculum, VMO, or even the quadriceps tendon. Other damage includes articular cartilage damage to the patella or femoral condyle (this often occurs when the patella relocates, hitting the lateral femoral condyle). Osteochondral fractures may also occur in the same setting, particularly in younger athletes.

Patellar dislocation is a common event in sports. Over the years a profile of a young, overweight, sedentary, adolescent girl as the prime victim has been developed. Researchers in one study[107] evaluated and followed 74 patients with acute lateral patellar dislocation. The results seem to indicate a profile that has some common characteristics but does not fit with the stereotype once assumed. The findings are summarized as follows:

- 69% of patients were under 20 years of age.
- 72% of patients had their dislocation occur with sports; 21% with activities of daily living, and 7% due to a direct blow.

- There was a 50% incidence of patella alta (a high-riding patella).
- All patients demonstrated a lateral hanging patella (patella laterally displaced as seen on a tangential view of the patella).
- There were no statistically significant relationships with a history of lower extremity problems as an infant or child, and no apparent relationship to a family history of dislocation.
- At 6 months, 68% of patients noted limitation with strenuous activities.

Evaluation

Historical description by the patient normally reveals that the patient felt the knee go out of place (or back in place during reduction). Other signs and symptoms are variable depending on the number of damaged structures; however, medial knee pain and swelling are common. If there is sufficient swelling to disguise that the displaced patella and/or reduction has occurred, the examiner may initially miss the diagnosis. Patellar subluxation is similar in presentation and is often impossible to differentiate from spontaneous reduction of a dislocated patella. With spontaneous reduction there is usually an immediate hemarthrosis. Subluxation is common in those who have had dislocation in the past and in those who have damaged patellar restructuring tissues and allowed them to heal elongated. Testing should include the apprehension test first at 30°, then at full extension if negative.

Management

In the acute setting, the displacement is readily apparent. Reduction is accomplished by carefully extending the knee. If unsuccessful, mild medial directed pressure is added. No other attempts should be made if the above maneuvers do not succeed. In all of the preceding scenarios, whether reduction has occurred or not, the knee should be packed in ice, splinted, and the patient sent for radiographs and treatment.

Treatment involves immobilization in a cylinder cast for four to six weeks. Patellar stabilization braces should be worn during activity. The vastus medialis obliques should be facilitated and strengthened.

Osgood-Schlatter Disease

Classic Presentation

The patient is often a young athlete complaining of pain and swelling at the tibial tuberosity.

Cause

The tibial apophysis is susceptible to repetitive stresses. When adolescents are performing demanding activities such as running and jumping, the apophysis may undergo an inflammatory reaction. It is rare for the tendon to avulse the apophysis.

Evaluation

The characteristic findings of a young athlete with tibial tuberosity pain, tenderness, and swelling are almost pathognomonic. Added testing may include resisted extension in an attempt to increase pain. It is not uncommon to develop Osgood-Schlatter disease bilaterally.

Management

Rest, ice, modification of the inciting sport activity, and gradual quadriceps stretching are the primary approaches. It is often helpful to use an Osgood-Schlatter brace or taping at the patellar tendon during activity. The general rule of thumb is that if the athlete is able to reduce the discomfort with rest, the injury will be self-resolving, and further evaluation with a radiograph is not necessary. However, if the athlete is experiencing pain that is unrelieved by rest, radiographs should be taken in an effort to determine whether there is an avulsion. A chiropractic or medical radiologist must review the radiographs because of the subtleties and variations of the apophyses.

Tennis Leg

Classic Presentation

The patient is often a middle-aged athlete playing tennis when she or he feels a sudden pain in the back of the upper calf followed by an inability to walk on the toes. The pain is often described as that of having been shot or hit on the back of the knee.

Cause

Tearing of the musculotendinous junction of the medial head of the gastrocnemius is the most common cause.[108] This occurs when the knee is suddenly extended while the foot is dorsiflexed. Another mechanism may be sudden dorsiflexion of the foot/ankle with the knee already extended.

Evaluation

Tenderness and some swelling are usually evident at the upper medial calf. The patient has increased pain on resisted plantarflexion of the foot or is unable to raise up on the sole and toes of the foot on the involved side.

Management

Management depends on the degree of damage. A full tear may require a long leg cast with the knee in 60° of flexion and the foot in 10° to 15° of plantarflexion for several weeks. More mild injuries can be managed with crutch-supported walking with gradual return to weight-bearing with a temporary heel lift (6 to 12 mm) to take the stretch off the torn muscle. Gradual stretching after one week should progress to mild plantarflexion isometrics progressing to toe raises when tolerated.

Osteoarthritis

Classic Presentation

The patient with osteoarthritis (OA) complains of stiffness and knee pain that is worse with prolonged sitting or walking. She or he is generally older or has a past history of trauma or surgery to the knee. Recurrent bouts of mild swelling and a progressive bowlegged appearance may be accompanying complaints.

Cause

Degeneration of articular cartilage is often secondary to meniscal tearing or degeneration. This occurs with age. Often significant, single trauma events or a past knee surgery (including ACL or meniscal surgeries) predispose the individual to early degeneration.

Evaluation

A varus angulation of the involved knee may be apparent. Palpation may uncover osteophytic development at the joint line. Joint line swelling may also be palpable. Laxity testing with an anterior drawer maneuver will often demonstrate a loose joint with early OA. Laxity in neutral is due to joint capsular laxity. Tightening on internal rotation indicates an intact ACL. In advanced OA less movement than normal is found on drawer testing. Radiographic evaluation must include a bilateral, PA, weight-bearing view usually taken with a 7 × 17 cassette. The patient faces the bucky with the knees bent 45° and the tube is angled caudad 10° to 15° with the central ray between the knees. Characteristic findings are varying degrees of decreased medial joint space, subchondral cysts, and osteophyte formation.

Management

One study indicated that at an 11-year follow-up evaluation, most patients did not show significant progression of OA radiographically.[109] Those patients with radiographic evidence of OA and knee pain or OA of the contralateral side had the worse prognosis. Numerous studies[110-113] indicate the value of exercise for long-term management of OA of the knee. However, some studies indicate that the degree of varus/valgus laxity may decrease this strengthening effect.[114] Specifically, it has been found that low-intensity cycling is just as effective as high-intensity cycling for improving function and decreasing pain.[115] Aquatic exercise is a good initial approach that improves strength without the risk of weight-bearing exacerbation.

Three alternative approaches to managing OA of the knee include acupuncture, pulsed electrical stimulation, and prolotherapy (injection of growth factors or growth factor stimulators such as dextrose). All have been evaluated in a randomized trial and were shown to be of benefit.[116-118] A recent study seemed to indicate that those treated with platelet-rich plasma (PRP), one approach to delivering growth factors, demonstrated a slowing of degenerative changes as measured on MRI.[119] More studies are necessary given this is only one small study.

Towheed et al.[120] in a Cochrane review and other publications,[121] emphasize that using the Rotta formulation for glucosamine likely has benefit for osteoarthritis of the knee. However, many studies are of poor quality and five randomized controlled trials failed to demonstrate a positive change in pain, function, and stiffness using the Western Ontario and McMaster Universities Osteoarthritis Index (WOMAC). They speculate that either the Rotta product may be more standardized or that there is a difference in the type of glucosamine used. Finally, they remind the clinician that in a study by Clegg et al.,[122] the placebo effect evaluating pharmacotherapeutics with osteoarthritis has shown as high as a 60% positive response rate (this includes medications). Gregory et al.[123] reviewed the literature to date on dietary supplements for osteoarthritis in 2008 and concluded that there was only literature to support glucosamine and chondroitin sulfate. There was also some support for S-adenosylmethionine; however, the high cost and product quality may limit use. Another study reported improvement beyond placebo and also indicated more preservation of joint space radiographically.[124] It appears that bone marrow edema may be a risk factor for structural deterioration with OA of the knee.[125] This may be visualized on MRI.

Knee replacement surgery should be reserved for those unresponsive to a conservative regimen that includes exercise.

Some recent studies have attempted to determine the effectiveness of medical management of knee osteoarthritis. The results tend to question the value of the standard approaches. One study evaluated the effectiveness of corticosteroid injections versus hyaluronic acid injection.[126] There appeared to be no difference between the two groups with regard to pain relief or function at six months. Interestingly there was no control group of patients who were no-treatment or received a sham or placebo treatment. A more recent study using a placebo (saline) seems to confirm the same results; however, it indicated that those patients with radiologically milder disease at baseline may have had less progression of joint space narrowing when treated with hyaluronic acid.[127] Researchers in another study produced results that were somewhat controversial because this was a surgical study that incorporated a placebo of a "sham" surgery for osteoarthritis.[128] Patients were randomly assigned to receive arthroscopic debridement, arthroscopic lavage, or placebo surgery. Those undergoing placebo surgery received simulated debridement without having the arthroscope inserted. The results were that arthroscopic lavage or debridement was no better than placebo after a 24-month period follow-up. As evidenced in past studies, a Cochrane review[129] evaluated the benefit of arthroscopic debridement for knee OA and found that there was no value, especially over the long term.

Many studies have been conducted to determine the host of therapeutic options for osteoarthritis of the knee. A summary of some of these therapies and literature conclusions follows.

- Exercise is an effective management approach to OA of the knee with significant reductions in pain and improvements in function.[130] Specifically, researchers in one study evaluated the type of exercise and its sequence of prescription.[131] Their conclusion was that isotonic exercise was preferable as the initial strengthening approach due to decreased drop-out rate due to an increase in pain that was found with isokinetic exercise. They also conclude that isokinetic should follow an initial isotonic approach to increase joint stability and walking endurance. A meta-analysis, published in the Cochrane Database, concluded that there was no difference between the effect of high-intensity exercise versus low-intensity exercise.[132] When OA of the patellofemoral joint is the primary site of involvement, it appears from the results of one study that only small improvements occur in knee pain scores and quadriceps muscle strength after 10 weeks.[133]
- Taping and bracing may also be effective management approaches. A recent blinded, randomized controlled trial was conducted to evaluate the effectiveness of knee tape.[134] Those who were given therapeutic taping had significant improvement in pain compared to the control tape and no-tape groups. These effects were maintained after three weeks. Another study designed to evaluate the effectiveness of an elastic knee brace produced results that indicate small, short-term beneficial effects with acute exacerbations.[135]
- Use of glucosamine and chondroitin appears to have both an effect on symptoms and structural changes in the knee. The results from a recent meta-analysis indicate that both glucosamine and chondroitin improved both WOMAC scores, and it demonstrated improvements in joint space narrowing.[136]
- Low-level laser therapy is still a controversial approach that has been used for over 10 years. A recent Cochrane meta-analysis reported that because there are different types of lasers (Classes I, II, and III), there was lack of standardized outcome measures and different methods of application, so no conclusions could be drawn.[137] Despite some positive findings, there were no data on the effect of wavelength, treatment duration, dose, and site of application (over nerves or joints). The recommendation was to conduct more controlled studies with these variables in mind.

Osteochondritis Dissecans (OD)

Classic Presentation

A 14-year-old male athlete complains of an insidious onset of anterior knee pain that is now causing him to limp. He says that occasionally his knee locks and swells.

Cause

OD is a defect in osteochondral bone and articular cartilage that usually affects the lateral portion of the medial femoral condyle. It may occur bilaterally in 20% of cases. Probably due to an inadequate or disturbed vascular supply, a divot of bone will separate and in some cases dislodge into the joint. Although mainly seen in young athletic boys, there is a secondary onset that happens in adults. The adult version is more likely to progress to surgical excision.

Evaluation

Patients will complain of an insidious onset of pain. Later effects are mechanical from the dislodged area (if this occurs) and will include locking and swelling. A clinical test for osteochondritis dissecans (OD) is Wilson's test. Introduced in 1967, Wilson noted that children with OD walked with external rotation. He assumed this was due to condyle impingement with internal rotation that was relieved by external rotation. Based on these observations, he developed a test that was positive when the patient's knee was extended with internal tibial rotation, and somewhere between 90° and 30° pain occurs. The pain is then relieved by external tibial rotation. Until recently, this test was untested. Researchers in a recent study evaluated the clinical significance of Wilson's test comparing positive and negative results for patients with radiographically documented OD.[138] Seventy-five percent of individuals with radiographically positive OD had a negative Wilson's test, calling into question the value of this testing procedure. The radiographic diagnosis is usually apparent on a tunnel view of the knee.

A similar process in older patients is referred to as spontaneous osteonecrosis (SONC) of the medial tibial plateau. This exclusively senior patient condition has varying outcomes, but most patients progress to significant degenerative disease.[139]

Management

Rest and protection are the initial approaches. If no healing occurs, surgical excision may be necessary. A study by Jurgensen et al.[140] evaluated the rates of remission of arthroscopically versus nonsurgically treated osteochondritis (as noted on MRI). They found partial or complete remission in 30% of lesions and no change in 63% of lesions managed nonsurgically, while in those treated arthroscopically there was a remission of 37% and no change in 57%.

The Evidence—Knee

Translation into Practice Summary (TIPS)

The literature on history and examination of the knee is extensive. The literature points clearly to some valuable findings indicating the need for x-ray to determine if fracture is present posttrauma, and for the clinical examination, cruciate ligament injury, and to a lesser degree for meniscus tears and collateral ligament tears. The literature on patellofemoral tracking problems/dysfunction is mixed with good reliability of tests, but the clinical utility has yet to be determined. There is no literature on the history and examination for extensor disorders (e.g., Osgood-Schlatter's) regarding reliability or validity.

The Literature-Based Clinical Core

- The Ottawa Knee Rule and Philadelphia Rule are good for determining the need for x-ray in detecting knee fractures.
- The American College of Radiology Criteria are a good prediction rule for ruling-in and potentially ruling-out osteoarthritis.
- The anterior-drawer test, pivot shift, and Lachman's are good for ruling in anterior cruciate ligament tears; however, the best test for ruling-out an ACL tear is Lachman's (best under anesthesia).
- Joint line tenderness and McMurray's, and the Thessaly test (although the CIs are wide) are reasonably good at ruling-in or ruling-out meniscus tears.
- The literature for end-feel evaluation (Cyriax approach) indicates poor reliability.
- The moving patellar apprehension test is good at ruling-in and ruling-out patellar instability.
- The combination of findings which include standard tests plus a history of trauma, difficulty bearing weight, and being over the age of 40 years is good at ruling-in but not ruling-out meniscus tears.
- Indicators of potential medial plica such as a palpable plica or medial patellar pain are not sensitive or specific for plica.
- Valgus testing for MCL tears is not good at ruling-in or ruling-out.

- Patellar alignment evaluation is poor, Q-angle testing is reliable; however, there is no proven clinical value to these findings.

The Expert-Opinion-Based Clinical Core

- A history of popping heard at the time of injury with immediate joint swelling is a strong indicator of an acute anterior cruciate ligament tear.
- Knee trauma with effusion coupled with mechanical signs of catching or locking indicate a meniscus tear.
- Pain and tenderness at the tibial tuberosity with swelling in an adolescent are strong indicators of Osgood-Schlatter's.
- A Clark's or grind test performed at 15° to 20° of knee flexion may help eliminate false positives for chondromalacia.
- Popping and clicking at the hip may introduce false positives into McMurray's and other tests.

APPENDIX 12–1

References

1. Ellison AE. *Athletic Training and Sports Medicine.* Chicago: American Academy of Orthopedic Surgeons; 1985.
2. Praemer A, Furner S, Rice DP. *Musculoskeletal Conditions in the United States.* Rosemont, IL: American Academy of Orthopedic Surgeons, 1999.
3. Katz JN, Solomon DH, Schaffer JL, et al. Outcomes of care and resource utilization among patients with knee and shoulder disorders treated by general internists, rheumatologists, orthopedic surgeons. *Am J Med.* 2000;108:28–35.
4. National Board of Chiropractic Examiners. *Job Analysis of Chiropractic: A project report, survey analysis and summary of the practice of chiropractic within the United States, 2000.* Greeley, CO: National Board of Chiropractic Examiners, 2000, p. 79.
5. Solomono M, Barata R, Zhou BH, et al. The synergistic action of the anterior cruciate ligament and thigh muscles in maintaining joint stability. *Am J Sports Med.* 1987;15:207.
6. Tsuda E, Okamura Y, Otsuka H, et al. Direct evidence of the anterior cruciate ligament-hamstring reflex arc in humans. *Am J Sports Med.* 2001;29(1):83–87.

7. Dye SF, Vaupel GL, Dye CC. Conscious neurosensory mapping of the internal structures of the human knee without intraarticular anesthesia. *Am J Sports Med.* 1998;26(6):773–777.

8. Aune AK, Cawley PW, Ekeland A. Quadriceps muscle contraction protects the anterior cruciate ligament during anterior tibial translation. *Am J Sports Med.* 1997;25(2):187.

9. Hayes KW, Petersen CM. Reliability of classifications derived from Cyriax's resisted testing in subjects with painful shoulders and knees. *J Orthop Sports Phys Ther.* 2003;33:235–246.

10. O'Shea KJ, Murphy KP, Heekin D, Herzwum PJ. The diagnostic accuracy of history, physical examination and radiographs in the evaluation of traumatic knee disorders. *Am J Sports Med.* 1996;24:164–167.

11. Stanitski CL. Correlation of arthroscopic and clinical examinations with magnetic resonance imaging findings of injured knees in children and adolescents. *Am J Sports Med.* 1998;26(1):2–6.

12. Johnson T, Althoff L. Clinical diagnosis of ruptures of the anterior cruciate ligament: a comparison study of the Lachman test and the anterior drawer sign. *Am J Sports Med.* 1982;10:100–102.

13. Bach BR, Warren RF, Wickiewics TL. The pivot shift phenomenon: results and description of a modified clinical test for anterior cruciate ligament insufficiency. *Am J Sports Med.* 1988;16:571–576.

14. Benjaminse A, Gokeler A, van der Schans CP. Clinical diagnosis of an anterior cruciate ligament rupture: a meta-analysis. *J Orthop Sports Phys Ther.* 2006;36(5):267–288.

15. Konan S, Rayan F, Haddad FS. Do physical diagnostic tests accurately detect meniscal tears? *Knee Surg Sports Traumatol Arthrosc.* 2009;17(7):806–811.

16. Evans PJ, Bell GD, Frank C. Prospective evaluation of the McMurray test. *Am J Sports Med.* 1993;21:604–608.

17. Karachalios T, Hantes M, Zibis AH, Zachos V, Karantanas AH, Malizos KN. Diagnostic accuracy of a new clinical test (the Thessaly test) for early detection of meniscal tears. *J Bone Joint Surg Am.* May 2005;87(5):955–962.

18. Apley AG. The diagnosis of meniscus injuries. *J Bone Joint Surg.* 1947;29:78–84.

19. Mariani PP, Adriani E, Maresca G, Mazzola CG. A prospective evaluation of a test for lateral meniscus tears. *Knee Surg Sports Traumatol Arthrosc.* 1996;4:22–26.

20. Shelbourne KD, Martini DJ, McCarroll JR, VanMeter CD. Correlation of joint line tenderness and meniscal lesions in patients with acute anterior cruciate ligament tears. *Am J Sports Med.* 1995;23(2):166–169.

21. Matava MJ, Eck K, Totty W, Wright RW, Shively RA. Magnetic resonance imaging as a tool to predict meniscal reparability. *Am J Sports Med.* 1999;27(4):436–443.

22. McClure PW, Rothstein JM, Riddle DL. Intertester reliability of clinical judgments of medial knee ligament integrity. *Phys Ther.* 1989;69:268–275.

23. Livingston LA. The quadriceps angle: a review of the literature. *J Orthop Sports Phys Ther.* 1998;28:105–109.

24. Bussieres AE, Taylor JA, Peterson C. Diagnostic imaging practice guidelines for musculoskeletal complaints in adults—an evidence-based approach. Part 1. Lower extremity disorders. *J Manipulative Physiol Ther.* 2007;30(9):684–717.

25. Stiell IG, Wells GA, Hoag RH et al. Implementation of the Ottawa Knee Rule for the use of radiography in acute knee injuries. *JAMA.* 1997;278:2075–2079.

26. Garth WP, Jr, Greco J, House MA. The lateral notch sign associated with acute anterior cruciate ligament disruption. *Am J Sports Med.* 2000;28(1):68–73.

27. Murray TF, Dupont JY, Fulkerson JP. Axial and lateral radiographs in evaluating patellofemoral malalignment. *Am J Sports Med.* 1999;27(5):580–584.

28. Shepard MF, Hunter DM, Davies MR, Shapiro MS, Seeger LL. The clinical significance of anterior horn meniscal tears diagnosed on magnetic resonance images. *Am J Sports Med.* 2002;30(2):189–192.

29. LaPrade RF, Burnett QM, 2nd, Veenstra MA, Hodgman CG. The prevalence of abnormal magnetic resonance imaging findings in asymptomatic knees. With correlation of magnetic resonance imaging to arthroscopic findings in symptomatic knees. *Am J Sports Med.* 1994;22(6):739–745.

30. Suter E, McMorland GM, Herzog W, Bray R. Conservative lower back treatment reduces inhibition in knee-extensor muscles: a randomized controlled trial. *J Manipulative Physiol Ther.* 2000;23:76–80.

31. Neneck GJ, Powers CM. Which exercises target the gluteal muscles while minimizing activation of the tensor fascia lata? Electromyographic assessment using fine-wire electrodes. *J Orthop Sports Phys Ther.* 2013;43(2):54–64.

32. Suter E, McMorland G, Herzog W, Bray R. Decrease in quadriceps inhibition after sacroiliac joint manipulation in patients with anterior knee pain. *J Manipulative Physiol Ther.* 1999;22(3):149–153.

33. Suter E, McMorland G, Herzog W, Bray R. Conservative lower back treatment reduces inhibition in knee-extensor muscles: a randomized controlled trial. *J Manipulative Physiol Ther*. 2000;23(2):76–80.

34. Hoskins W, McHardy A, Pollard H, Windsham R, Onley R. Chiropractic treatment of lower extremity conditions: a literature review. *J Manipulative Physiol Ther*. 2006;29(8):658–671.

35. Brantingham JW, Bonnefin D, Perle SM, et al. Manipulative therapy for lower extremity conditions: update of a literature review. *J Manipulative Physiol Ther*. 2012;35(2):127–166.

36. Polkinghorn BS. Conservative treatment of torn medial meniscus via mechanical force, manually assisted short lever chiropractic adjusting procedures. *J Manipulative Physiol Ther*. 1994;17(7):474–484.

37. Meyer JJ, Zachman ZJ, Keating JC, Jr., Traina AD. Effectiveness of chiropractic management for patellofemoral pain syndrome's symptomatic control phase: a single subject experiment. *J Manipulative Physiol Ther*. 1990;13(9):539–549.

38. Moss P, Sluka K, Wright A. The initial effects of knee joint mobilization on osteoarthritic hyperalgesia. *Man Ther*. 2007;12(2):109–118.

39. Crossley K, Bennell K, Green S, McConnell J. A systematic review of physical interventions for patellofemoral pain syndrome. *Clin J Sport Med*. 2001;11(2):103–110.

40. Keating EM, Ritter MA, Harty LD, et al. Manipulation after total knee arthroplasty. *J Bone Joint Surg Am*. 2007;89(2):282–286.

41. Namba RS, Inacio M. Early and late manipulation improve flexion after total knee arthroplasty. *J Arthroplasty*. 2007;22(6 Suppl 2):58–61.

42. Soderberg GL, Cook TM. An electromyographic analysis of quadriceps femoris muscle setting and straight leg raising. *Phys Ther*. 1983;63:1434–1438.

43. Soderberg GL, Miner SD, Arnold K, et al. Electromyographic analysis of knee exercises in healthy subjects and in patients with knee pathologies. *Phys Ther*. 1998;76:1691–1696.

44. Skurja M, Perry J, Cromley J, Hislop H. Quadriceps action in straight leg raise versus isolated knee extension. *Phys Ther*. 1980;60:582.

45. Cryzlo SM, Patek RM, Pink M, Perry J. Electromyographic analysis of knee rehabilitation exercises. *J Orthop Sports Phy Ther*. 1994;20:36–43.

46. Hintermeister R, Bey M, Lange G, et al. Quantification of elastic knee rehabilitation exercises. *J Orthop Sports Phys Ther*. 1998;28:40–50.

47. Laprade J, Sulham E, Brouwer B. Comparison of five isometric exercises in the recruitment of the vastus medialis oblique in persons with and without patellofemoral pain syndrome. *J Orthop Sports Phys Ther*. 1998;27:197–204.

48. Lange GW, Hintermeister R, Schlegel T, et al. Electromyographic and kinematic analysis of graded treadmill walking and the implications for knee rehabilitation. *J Orthop Sports Phys Ther*. 1996;25:294–301.

49. Zimmerman CL, Cook TM, Bravand MS, et al. Effects of stair-stepping exercise direction and cadence on EMG activity of selected lower extremity muscle groups. *J Orthop Sports Phys Ther*. 1994;19:173–180.

50. Fleming BC, Beynnon BD, Renstrom PA. The strain behavior of the anterior cruciate ligament during bicycling: An in vivo study. *Am J Sports Med*. 1999;26(1):109–118.

51. France EP, Cawley PW, Paulos LE. Choosing functional knee braces. *Clin Sports Med*. 1990;9:743–750.

52. Styf JR, Lundin O, Gershuni DH. Effects of a functional knee brace on leg muscle function. *Am J Sports Med*. 1994;22:6.

53. Paulos LE, France EP, Rosenberg TD, et al. The biomechanics of lateral knee bracing, I: response of the valgus restraints to loading. *Am J Sports Med*. 1987;15:419.

54. McConnell J. The management of chondromalacia patellae: a long term solution. *Aust J Phys Ther*. 1986;32:215.

55. Penau R, Frank C, Fick G. The effect of elastic bandages on human knee proprioception in the uninjured population. *Am J Sports Med*. 1995;23:2.

56. Colby S, Francisco CS, Yu B, et al. Electromyographic and kinematic analysis of cutting maneuvers: implications for anterior cruciate ligament injury. *Am J Sports Med*. 2000;28(2):234–240.

57. Cooperman JM, Riddle DL, Rothstein JM. Reliability and judgments of the integrity of the anterior cruciate of the knee using the Lachman's test. *Phys Ther*. 1990;70:225–233.

58. Lintner DM, Kamaric E, Mosely B, Noble PC. Partial tears of the anterior cruciate ligament: are they clinically detectable? *Am J Sports Med*. 1995;23:1.

59. Hurd WJ, Axe MJ, Snyder-Mackler L. A 10-year prospective trial of a patient management algorithm and screening examination for highly active individuals with anterior cruciate ligament injury: part 2, determinants of dynamic knee stability. *Am J Sports Med*. 2008;36(1):48–56.

60. Hurd WJ, Axe MJ, Snyder-Mackler L. A 10-year prospective trial of a patient management algorithm and screening examination for highly active individuals with anterior cruciate ligament injury: part 1, outcomes. *Am J Sports Med.* 2008;36(1):40–47.

61. Buss DD, Min R, Skyhar M, et al. Nonoperative treatment of acute ACL injuries in a selected group of patients. *Am J Sports Med.* 1995;23:2.

62. Ihara H, Nakayama A. Dynamic joint control training for knee ligament injuries. *Am J Sports Med.* 1988;14:309–315.

63. Tagesson S, Oberg B, Good L, Kvist J. A comprehensive rehabilitation program with quadriceps strengthening in closed versus open kinetic chain exercise in patients with anterior cruciate ligament deficiency: a randomized clinical trial evaluating dynamic tibial translation and muscle function. *Am J Sports Med.* 2008;36(2):298–307.

64. Felming BC, Renstrom PA, Beynnon BD, et al. The influence of functional knee bracing on the anterior cruciate ligament strain biomechanics in weightbearing and non-weightbearing knees. *Am J Sports Med.* 2000;28(6):815–824.

65. Greene DL, Hamson KR, Bay RC, Bryce CD. Effects of protective knee bracing on speed and agility. *Am J Sports Med.* 2000;28(4):453–459.

66. Reeves KD, Hassanein KM. Long-term effects of dextrose prolotherapy for anterior cruciate ligament laxity. *Altern Ther Health Med.* 2003;9(3):58–62.

67. Anderson AF, Snyder RB, Lipscomb Jr. AB. Anterior cruciate ligament reconstruction: a prospective randomized study of three surgical methods. *Am J Sports Med.* 2001;29(3):272–279.

68. Kirkley A, Mohtadi N, Ogilivie R. The effect of exercise on anterior-posterior translation of the normal knee and knees with deficient or reconstructed anterior cruciate ligaments. *Am J Sports Med.* 2001;29(3):311–314.

69. Gillogly SD, Voight M, Blackburn T. Treatment of articular cartilage defects of the knee with autologous chondrocyte implantation. *J Orthop Sports Phys Ther.* 1998;28(4): 241–251.

70. Shelbourne KD, Davis TJ, Patel DV. The natural history of acute, isolated, nonoperatively treated posterior cruciate ligament injuries. A prospective study. *Am J Sports Med.* 1999;27(3):276–283.

71. Shelbourne KD, Muthukaruppan Y. Subjective results of nonoperatively treated, acute, isolated posterior cruciate ligament injuries. *Arthroscopy.* 2005;21(4):457–461.

72. Boden SD, Davis DO, Dina TS, et al. A prospective and blinded investigation of magnetic resonance imaging of the knee: abnormal findings in asymptomatic patients. *Clin Orthop.* 1992;282:177–185.

73. Kocher MS, DiCanzio J, Zurakowski D, Micheli LJ. Diagnostic performance of clinical examination and selective magnetic resonance imaging in the evaluation of intraarticular knee disorders in children and adolescents. *Am J Sports Med.* 2001;29(3):292–296.

74. Shepard MF, Hunter DM, Davies MR, et al. The clinical significance of anterior horn meniscal tears diagnosed on magnetic resonance images. *Am J Sports Med.* 2002; 30(2):189–192.

75. Souza TA. Which orthopedic tests are really necessary? In: Lawrence DJ, Cassidy JD, McGregor M, et al., eds. *Advances in Chiropractic.* St. Louis, MO: Mosby-Year Book; 1994;1:101–154.

76. Eggli S, Wegmuller H, Kosina J, Huckell C, Jakob RP. Long-term results of arthroscopic meniscal repair. An analysis of isolated tears. *Am J Sports Med.* 1995;23(6):715–720.

77. Tenuta JJ, Arciero RA. Arthroscopic evaluation of meniscal repairs. Factors that effect healing. *Am J Sports Med.* 1994;22(6):797–802.

78. Fabricant PD, Jokl P. Surgical outcomes after arthroscopic partial meniscectomy. *J Am Acad Orthop Surg.* 2007;15(11):647–653.

79. van Trommel MF, Simonian PT, Potter HG, Wickiewicz TL. Different regional healing rates with the outside-in technique for meniscal repair. *Am J Sports Med.* 1998;26(3):446–452.

80. Abdelkafy A, Aigner N, Zada M, Elghoul Y, Abdelsadek H, Landsiedl F. Two to nineteen years follow-up of arthroscopic meniscal repair using the outside-in technique: a retrospective study. *Arch Orthop Trauma Surg.* 2007;127(4): 245–252.

81. Tuckman DV, Bravman JT, Lee SS, Rosen JE, Sherman OH. Outcomes of meniscal repair: minimum of 2-year follow-up. *Bull Hosp Jt Dis.* 2006;63(34):100–104.

82. Weiss C, Lundberg M, Maberg P, et al. Non-operative treatment of meniscal tears. *J Bone Joint Surg Am.* 1989;71:811–822.

83. Wirth CJ, Peters G, Milachowski KA, et al. Long-term results of meniscal allograft transplantation. *Am J Sports Med.* 2002;30(2):174–181.

84. Ranger C, Klestill T, Gloetzer W, et al. Osteoarthritis after arthroscopic partial meniscectomy. *Am J Sports Med.* 1995;23:2.

85. Reider B, Sathy MR, Talkington J, et al. Treatment of isolated medial collateral ligament injuries in athletes with early functional rehabilitation: a five-year follow-up study. *Am J Sports Med.* 1993;22:4.

86. Warden SJ, Avin KG, Beck EM, DeWolf ME, Hagemeier MA, Martin KM. Low-intensity pulsed ultrasound accelerates and a nonsteroidal anti-inflammatory drug delays knee ligament healing. *Am J Sports Med.* 2006;34(7):1094–1102.

87. Warden SJ, Fuchs RK, Kessler CK, Avin KG, Cardinal RE, Stewart RL. Ultrasound produced by a conventional therapeutic ultrasound unit accelerates fracture repair. *Phys Ther.* 2006;86(8):1118–1127.

88. Witvrouw E, Lysens R, Bellemans J, et al. Intrinsic risk factors for the development of anterior knee pain in an athletic population. *Am J Sports Med.* 2000;28(4):480–489.

89. Gigante A, Pasquinelli FM, Paladini P, et al. The effects of patellar taping on patellofemoral incongruence: a computed tomography study. *Am J Sports Med.* 2001;29(1):88–92.

90. Crossley K, Bennell K, Green S, et al. Physical therapy for patellofemoral pain: a randomized, double-blinded, placebo-controlled trial. *Am J Sports Med.* 2002;30(6):857–865.

91. Wang TG, Jan MH, Lin KH, Wang HK. Assessment of stretching of the iliotibial tract with Ober and modified Ober tests: an ultrasonographic study. *Arch Phys Med Rehabil.* 2006;87(10):1407–1411.

92. Wang HK, Ting-Fang Shih T, Lin KH, Wang TG. Real-time morphologic changes of the iliotibial band during therapeutic stretching; an ultrasonographic study. *Man Ther.* Aug. 2007.

93. Ferretti A, Papandrea P, Conteduca F. Knee injuries in volleyball. *Sports Med.* 1990;10(2):132–138.

94. Lian O, Dahl J, Ackermann PW, Frihagen F, Engebretsen L, Bahr R. Pronociceptive and antinociceptive neuromediators in patellar tendinopathy. *Am J Sports Med.* 2006;34(11):1801–1808.

95. Fredberg U, Bolvig L. Significance of ultrasonographically detected asymptomatic tendinosis in the patellar and Achilles tendons of elite soccer players. A longitudinal study. *Am J Sports Med.* 2002;30(4):488–491.

96. Panni AS, Tartarone M, Maffulli N. Patellar tendinopathy in athletes. Outcome of nonoperative and operative management. *Am J Sports Med.* 2000;28(3):392–397.

97. Ferretti A, Papandrea P, Conteduca F, Mariani PP. Knee ligament injuries in volleyball players. *Am J Sports Med.* 1992;20(2):203–207.

98. Lian O, Refsnes PE, Engebretsen L, Bahr R. Performance characteristics of volleyball players with patellar tendinopathy. *Am J Sports Med.* 2003;31(3):408–413.

99. Vulpiani MC, Vetrano M, Savoia V, Di Pangrazio E, Trischitta D, Ferretti A. Jumper's knee treatment with extracorporeal shock wave therapy: a long-term follow-up observational study. *J Sports Med Phys Fitness.* 2007;47(3):323–328.

100. Hoksrud A, Ohberg L, Alfredson H, Bahr R. Ultrasound-guided sclerosis of neovessels in painful chronic patellar tendinopathy: a randomized controlled trial. *Am J Sports Med.* 2006;34(11):1738–1746.

101. Jonsson P, Alfredson H. Superior results with eccentric compared to concentric quadriceps training in patients with jumper's knee: a prospective randomised study. *Br J Sports Med.* 2005;39(11):847–850.

102. Young MA, Cook JL, Purdam CR, Kiss ZS, Alfredson H. Eccentric decline squat protocol offers superior results at 12 months compared with traditional eccentric protocol for patellar tendinopathy in volleyball players. *Br J Sports Med.* 2005;39(2):102–105.

103. Stanish WD, Rubinovich RM, Curwin S. Eccentric exercise in chronic tendinitis. *Clin Orthop Relat Res.* 1986(208):65–68.

104. Vetrano M, Castorina A, Vulpiani MC, Baldini R, Pavan A, Ferretti A. Platelet-rich plasma versus focused shock waves in the treatment of jumper's knee in athletes. *Am J Sports Med.* 2013;41(4):795–803.

105. Smith J, Sellon JL. Comparing PRP injections with ESWT for athletes with chronic patellar tendinopathy. *Clin J Sport Med.* 2014;24(1):88–89.

106. Park YG, Han SB, Song SJ, Kim TJ, Ha CW. Platelet-rich plasma therapy for knee joint problems: review of the literature, current practice and legal perspectives in Korea. *Knee Surg Relat Res.* 2012;24(2):70–78.

107. Atkin DM, Fithian DC, Marangi KS, Stone ML, Dobson BE, Mendelsohn C. Characteristics of patients with primary acute lateral patellar dislocation and their recovery within the first 6 months of injury. *Am J Sports Med.* 2000;28(4):472–479.

108. Miller WA. Rupture of the musculotendinous junction of the medial head of gastrocnemius muscle. *Am J Sports Med.* 1977;5:191–193.

109. Spector TD, Dacre JE, Harris PA, Huskisson EC. Radiological progression of osteoarthritis: an 11-year follow-up study of the knee. *Am Rheum Dis.* 1992;51(10):1107–1110.

110. Rogind H, Bibbow-Nelsen B, Jensen B, et al. The effects of a physical training program on patients with osteoarthritis of the knees. *Arch Phys Med Rehabil.* 1998;79(11):1421–1427.

111. Deyle GD, Henderson NE, Matckl RL, et al. Effectiveness of manual physical therapy and exercise in osteoarthritis of the knee: a randomized, controlled trial. *Ann Intern Med.* 2000;132(3):173–181.

112. O'Reilly SC, Muir KR, Doherty M. Effectiveness of home exercise on pain and disability from osteoarthritis of the knee: a randomized controlled trial. *Am Rheum Dis.* 1999;58(1):15–19.

113. Maurer BT, Stern AG, Kinossian B, et al. Osteoarthritis of the knee: isokinetic quadriceps exercise versus an educational intervention. *Arch Phys Med Rehabil.* 1999;80(10):1293–1299.

114. Sharma L, Hayes KW, Felson DT, et al. Does laxity alter the relationship between strength and physical function in knee osteoarthritis? *Arthritis Rheum.* 1999;42(1):25–32.

115. Mangione KK, McCully K, Gloviak A, et al. The effects of high-intensity and low-intensity cycle ergometry in older adults with knee osteoarthritis. *J Gerontol A Biol Sci Med Sci.* 1999;54(4):M184–M190.

116. Berman BM, Singh BB, Lao L, et al. A randomized trial of acupuncture as an adjunctive therapy in osteoarthritis of the knee. *Rheumatology (Oxford).* 1999;38(4):346–354.

117. Zizic TM, Hoffman KC, Holt PA, et al. The treatment of osteoarthritis of the knee with pulsed stimulation. *J Rheumatol.* 1995;22(9):1757–1761.

118. Reeves K D, Hassanein K. Randomized, prospective double-blind placebo-controlled study of dextrose prolotherapy for knee osteoarthritis with or without ACL laxity. *Altern Ther Health Med.* 2000;6(2):68–74, 77–80.

119. Halpern B, Chaudhury S, Rodeo SA, et al. Clinical and MRI outcomes after platelet-rich plasma treatment for knee osteoarthritis. *Clin J Sport Med.* 2012;23(3):238–239.

120. Towheed TE, Anastassiades T. Glucosamine therapy for osteoarthritis: an update. *J Rheumatol.* 2007;34(9):1787–1790.

121. Towheed TE, Maxwell L, Anastassiades TP, et al. Glucosamine therapy for treating osteoarthritis. *Cochrane Database Syst Rev.* 2005 (2): CD002946.

122. Clegg DO, Reda DJ, Harris CL, et al. Glucosamine, chondroitin sulfate, and the two in combination for painful knee osteoarthritis. *N Engl J Med.* 2006;354(8):795–808.

123. Gregory P, Sperry M, Freidman-Wilson A. Dietary supplements for osteoarthritis. *Am Fam Physician.* 2008;77(2):177–184.

124. Reginster JY, Deroisy R, Paul I, et al. Glucosamine sulfate significantly reduces progression of knee osteoarthritis over 3 years: a large, randomised, placebo-controlled, double-blind, prospective trial. Presented at the 63rd Annual Scientific Meeting, American College of Rheumatology; Nov. 13–17, 1999; Boston, MA.

125. Felson DT, McLaughlin S, Goggins J, et al. Bone marrow edema and its relation to progression of knee osteoarthritis. *Ann Intern Med.* 2003;139:330–336.

126. Leopold SS, Redd BB, Warme WJ, et al. Corticosteroid compared with hyaluronic acid injections for the treatment of osteoarthritis of the knee: a prospective, randomized trial. *J Bone Joint Surg.* (Am). 2003;85:1197–1203.

127. Jubb RW, Piva S, Beinat L, et al. A one-year, randomized, placebo (saline) controlled clinical trial of 500–730 kDa sodium hyaluronate (Hyalgan) on the radiological change in osteoarthritis of the knee. *Int J Clin Pract.* 2003;57(6):467–474.

128. Mosseley JB, O'Malley K, Petersen NJ, et al. A controlled trial of arthroscopic surgery for osteoarthritis of the knee. *N Engl J Med.* 2002;347:81–88.

129. Laupattarakasem W, Laopaiboon M, Laupattarakasem P, Sumananont C. Arthroscopic debridement for knee osteoarthritis. *Cochrane Database Syst Rev.* 2008 (1): CD005118.

130. Fransen M, McConnel S, Bell M. Exercise for osteoarthritis of the hip or knee. *Cochrane Database Syst Rev.* 2003; (3): CD004286.

131. Huang MH, Lin YS, Yang RC, Lee CL. A comparison of various therapeutic exercises on the functional status of patients with knee osteoarthritis. *Semin Arthritis Rheum.* 2003;32(6):398–406.

132. Brosseau L, MacLeay L, Robinson V, et al. Intensity of exercise for the treatment of osteoarthritis. *Cochrane Database Syst Rev.* 2003; (2): CD004259.

133. Quilty B, Tucker M, Campbell R, Dieppe P. Physiotherapy, including quadriceps exercises and patellar taping for knee osteoarthritis with predominant patello-femoral joint involvement: a randomized controlled trial. *J Rheumatol.* 2003;30(6):1311–1317.

134. Hinman RS, Crossley KM, McConnell J, Benell KL. Efficacy of knee tape in the management of osteoarthritis of the knee: blinded randomized controlled trial. *BMJ.* 2003;327:135–141.

135. Pajareya K, Chadchavalpanichaya N, Timdang S. Effectiveness of an elastic knee sleeve for patients with knee osteoarthritis: a randomized single-blinded controlled trial. *J Med Assoc Thai*. 2003;86(6):535–542.

136. Richy F, Bruyere O, Ethgen O, et al. Structural and symptomatic efficacy of glucosamine and chondroitin in knee osteoarthritis: a comprehensive meta-analysis. *Arch Intern Med*. 2003;163:1514–1522.

137. Brosseau L, Welch V, Wells G, et al. Low level laser therapy (Classes I, II, and III) for treating osteoarthritis. *Cochrane Database Syst Rev*. 2003; (2): CD002046.

138. Conrad JM, Stanitski CL. Osteochondritis dissecans: Wilson's sign revisited. *Am J Sports Med*. 2003; 31(5):777–778.

139. Satku K, Kumar YP, Chang SM, Thambyah A. The natural history of spontaneous nosteonecrosis of the medial tibial plateau. *J Bone Joint Surg Br*. 2003;85(7):983–988.

140. Jurgensen I, Bachmann G, Schleicher I, Haas H. Arthroscopic versus conservative treatment of osteochondritis dissecans of the knee: value of magnetic resonance imaging in therapy planning and follow-up. *Arthroscopy*. 2002;18(4):378–386.

Appendix 12-2

Knee Diagnosis Table

Diagnosis	Comments	History Findings	Positive Examination Findings	Radiography/Special Studies	Treatment Options
Subluxation or Fixation of: **Tibiofemoral Joint** **Tibiofibular Joint** **Patellofemoral Joint (functional)**	• Should be used when chiropractic manipulation is used as Tx for any knee problem/Dx. • Can be primary Dx if patient is asymptomatic or mildly symptomatic (eg, mild stiffness or pain level < 2/10). • Must indicate chiropractic exam findings to support Dx.	*Nonspecific*	*Palpation*—Local tenderness or other signs of subluxation *Ortho*—None *Neuro*—None *Active ROM*—Variable restriction *Passive ROM*—End-range restriction *Motion palpation*—Specific articular restriction or symptoms produced on end-range	• Radiography not required for the diagnosis of subluxation. • Radiographic biomechanical analysis may assist in treatment decisions.	• Chiropractic adjustive technique. • Decisions regarding specifically which technique(s) is/are applied and modifications to the given approach will be directed by the primary Dx and patient's ability to tolerate pre-adjustment stresses.
Medial Collateral Ligament (MCL) Strain (specify degree) **Lateral Collateral Ligament (LCL) Strain (specify degree)**	The vast majority of collateral ligament strains are the medial; the lateral is rarely involved.	*Mechanism*—Overstretch due either to a single acute event (valgus strain for MCL; varus for LCL) or chronic stretch due to biomechanical predisposition or repetition strain (e.g., over-pronation)	*Ortho*—Stability testing in full extension and at 20°–30° reveals either laxity or pain; instability in extension indicates full rupture; instability with no end-feel at 20°–30° = 3rd degree tear; instability with end-feel = 2nd degree; no instability but pain indicates 1st degree *Neuro*—None unless full rupture occurs, then variable sensory deficits may occur	• Radiography recommended to determine fracture or with children/adolescents where a distinction between epiphyseal plate injury at ligament rupture is accomplished through stress radiographs. • When chronic, calcific deposition may indicate Pellegrini-Steida syndrome	• Refer for surgery if instability is found at extension. • Limited orthotic support (taping or brace) based on degree of injury; generally cylinder cast for 2nd degree, taping for 1st degree. • Myofascial therapy. • Biomechanical advice with regard to sports; possible recommendation of protective brace. • Strengthening and preventive exercises.

Cruciate Ligament Tear **Specify Anterior (ACL) or** **Posterior (PCL)**	• The vast majority of cruciate tears are anterior. • Patients may appear with acute injury or chronic complaints of instability.	*Mechanism*—ACL tears usually due to hyperextension or forced rotation with foot fixed and hit from outside; PCL tears usually due to hyperflexion or blow to flexed knee (anterior tibia) *Symptoms/Signs*—Often, pop heard at time of injury followed by immediate tense swelling and eventually a sense of instability	*Ortho*—Lachman's, drawer sign for straight instability (reverse tests for PCL), rotary stability tests such as pivot shift maneuver for multiple tissue damage In acute phase, testing may not be possible due to swelling	• Radiography necessary to rule out associated fractures (which are common). • MRI may be needed at some point to determine degree of injury and associated injury to other structures such as meniscus.	• In acute injury, non-weight-bearing and leg elevation to decrease swelling; if prolonged or if pain is severe, refer for aspiration and/or pain meds. • Rehabilitation acceptable for less active or older individuals, focusing on hamstring strengthening; avoidance of leg extension exercises (open chain), substitute squats or leg presses.
Medial Meniscus Tear **Lateral Meniscus Tear**	• Medial meniscus tears are most common and often associated with ACL tears. • Generally tears are horizontal (often degenerative) or vertical (single trauma induced).	*Mechanism*—Usually due to compression/rotation injury with foot fixed on ground *Symptoms/Signs*—Complaints of locking and swelling are common *Worse with specific ROM*—Terminal knee extension and flexion beyond 90° is painful	*Palpation*—Tenderness found anterior or as far as medial-posterior joint line *Ortho*—McMurray's and Apley's are primary tests *Passive ROM*—Flexion and end-range extension are limited and painful	• Radiography not usually necessary initially except to rule out fracture with acute trauma. • Degenerative meniscus tears are indirectly determined through weight-bearing PA views. • MRI may be necessary to determine the type and extent of tear and may help in surgical decision making.	• If locked, distraction adjusting may be helpful. • Limited orthotic support may provide some pain relief. • Physiotherapy for pain and swelling control. • Herbal recommendations for pain and swelling. • If mechanical symptoms become more frequent, referral for surgical repair is recommended.

(continues)

Knee Diagnosis Table (continued)

Diagnosis	Comments	History Findings	Positive Examination Findings	Radiography/Special Studies	Treatment Options
Osgood-Schlatter's or Sinding-Larsen	• Diagnosis is primarily through observation and palpation. • Remember that this does not represent an avulsion fracture. • Same process may affect distal or proximal pole of patella, called Sinding-Larsen's.	*Mechanism*—Tension at the tibial tuberosity apophysis leads to inflammation; inciting activities are jumping and sprinting	*Observation/Palpation*—Swelling at the tibial tuberosity with point tenderness (may be bilateral) *Ortho*—Resisted extension increases pain at tibial tuberosity (or patella with Sinding-Larsen's *Neuro*—None	• Radiography may be used, but mainly to rule out other causes such as tumor or fracture (if trauma occurred). • Remember that there is great variation at the apophysis and that radiolucent areas are filled with cartilage (does not represent an avulsion fracture).	• Ice/stretch quads and hams; decrease inciting activity if possible. • Modify activity to decrease stress to tibial tuberosity. • Limited orthotic support with Osgood-Schlatter's brace, Cho-Pat or McConnell taping. • Preventive and strengthening exercises and stretches, including eccentric quad exercises. • Refer if pain is felt at rest in addition to activity (possible impending avulsion).
Iliotibial Band (ITB) Syndrome	• As a pure entity, most common cause of lateral knee pain (nontraumatic). • May also be involved with patellar tracking problems.	*Mechanism*—Usually due to overuse (e.g., runner) due to a thick ITB (A to P and/or lateral to medial); band rubs lateral epicondyle at about 30°–40° of knee flexion; may be found in sedentary individuals who sit for long periods, functionally shortening ITB	*Ortho*—Compression with Noble's test for pain and stretch with modified Ober's test are often positive	• Radiography not recommended.	• Stretch of ITB using post-isometric relaxation approaches. • Correct any suspected biomechanical faults such as overpronation.

Patellar Tendinitis (Jumper's Knee) Tendinosis is a newer term used to indicate intra-tendinous degeneration due to atrophy (aging, microtrauma, vascular compromise, etc.). This is considered noninflammatory with hypocellularity, variable vascular ingrowth, local necrosis, and/or calcification, with accompanying fiber disorientation.	*Mechanism*—Primarily due to eccentric strain of patellar tendon with repetitive activities	• Found mainly in athletes who sprint or jump as main component of sport.	*Ortho*—Resisted extension causes pain at quadriceps tendon *Neuro*—None *Active ROM*—Jumping aggravates	• Radiography not recommended.	• Ice and stretch after activity. • Counterforce brace or taping such as Cho-Pat or McConnell taping. • Preventive and strengthening exercises with focus on eccentric training (avoid plyometrics though).
Pes Anserine Tendinitis or Bursitis	*Mechanism*—Either due to a direct blow to the medial proximal tibia or due to chronic stretching such as occurs in a hyperpronated individual	• Often tender area, always check bilaterally.	*Observation/Palpation*—Swelling at proximal/medial tibia with associated tenderness *Ortho*—Resisted challenge for gracilis, sartorius, or semitendinosis may increase pain	• Radiography not recommended.	• Conservative trial of ice and stretching. • Reduce swelling with pulsed ultrasound or comparable physiotherapy. • Correct any biomechanical contributors with heel lifts, medial heel wedges, or taping.
Chondromalacia Patella Patellofemoral Arthralgia (PFA)	*Mechanism*—Patellar maltracking causes damage to posterior patellar cartilage leading to degeneration *Signs/symptoms*—Patient complains of pain on ascending/descending steps or sitting for long periods (movie sign)	• Chondromalacia must be distinguished from patellofemoral arthralgia (PFA): chondromalacia represents actual patellar pathology, whereas PFA represents a soft tissue of pain such as occurs with medial retinacular or fat pad irritation.	*Ortho*—Pain with crepitus going through a squat; may be indirect indicators, such as an increased Q angle or other indicators of maltracking	• Radiography not usually indicated; there are many investigational approaches to determine patellar tracking using modified tangential views; not generally necessary. • Definitive Dx requires CT or MRI.	• Conservative trial of ice and quad, ham, and tibialis anterior stretching. • Bracing or taping may help temporarily, while patellar stability and tracking are improved through training and strengthening. • Correct any biomechanical contributors with heel lifts, medial heel wedges, or taping.

(continues)

Knee Diagnosis Table (continued)

Diagnosis	Comments	History Findings	Positive Examination Findings	Radiography/Special Studies	Treatment Options
Myofascitis	• Used when specific trigger points are identified on physical examination. • Also may be used if a strain is not evident from the history but there are indicators of muscle tenderness, stiffness, or pain.	*Onset:* Nonspecific regarding onset *Symptoms:* Patient usually complains of pain, aching, and/or tenderness in specific muscle or tendon areas that may radiate pain in non-dermatomal pattern	• Trigger points are evident as localized tenderness in a muscle that corresponds to traditional (Travell/Simons) trigger point charts; these points may be local or refer pain when compressed	• Not required or recommended.	• Mysofascial approaches such as myofascial stripping, trigger point massage, or spray and stretch approaches are the standard. • Home stretching and modification of activity suggestions.
Laxity Hypermobility		A history of a single event, traumatic injury to the joint is not found; however, overuse (microtrauma) or generalized inherent looseness is evident	• Capsular or ligament testing reveals "looseness" that falls within the physiologic range of normal	• Not usually recommended unless when differentiating pathological laxity from congenital or overuse acquisition.	• Strengthening program. • Bracing or functional taping during rehabilitation or during strenuous activities.

Lower Leg Complaints

Context

Lower leg disorders range from benign to life threatening. A history that includes any apparent trigger such as trauma, overuse, or disuse will usually narrow down the limited list of disorders affecting the lower leg. In older patients, calf pain should always suggest the possibility of deep vein thrombosis (DVT). This potentially life-threatening disorder is not always easily differentiated from a minor traumatic swelling or muscle strain.

Exercise-induced lower leg pain is common among athletes. Unfortunately, the terminology is confusing because of the clinical overlap and lack of identification of specific pathologic lesions in many cases. *Shin splint* is a commonly used term; however, some clinicians will include this diagnosis under the broader category of compartment syndromes or subdivide shin splints (i.e., medial stress syndrome).[1] Biomechanical imbalances at the foot will often strain the calf musculature; therefore, an evaluation of excessive pronation or supination should be included in the evaluation.

In addition to pain, patients also complain of leg cramps and lower leg edema. Lower leg edema is discussed in more depth in Chapter 25. Cramps are often the result of excessive diuretic use, lack of hydration, or need for electrolytes.

General Strategy

History

- Determine the type of complaint: pain and/or swelling, numbness/tingling, cramping, cosmetic concern, or skin lesions.

- Distinguish between a traumatic onset and a nontraumatic onset.
- Determine whether the pain is diffuse or well localized.
- With a traumatic onset, determine whether there was minor trauma—mild sprain or DVT—or major trauma—fracture or compartment syndrome. Sudden onset without trauma would suggest muscle or tendon rupture (posteromedial knee—tennis leg; heel—Achilles rupture).
- Evaluate for vascular claudication when pain occurs in the leg with walking after 10 minutes in an older patient.
- With an overuse history determine whether the pain is felt only with activity (muscle/tendon strain or compartment syndrome) or initially with activity but now also at rest (stress fracture).
- With women ask about menstrual irregularities (stress fracture) or chronic use of birth control pills (DVT).
- With athletes determine whether there was a sudden change in training (i.e., increased mileage, change in running surface, hill training).
- When swelling is the chief complaint (see Chapter 25) determine whether the onset was traumatic or nontraumatic.

Evaluation

- Attempt to pinpoint an area of tenderness or swelling.
- Test with stretch and contraction to detect a specific muscle or tendon.
- When a stress fracture is suspected, obtain a radiograph first and proceed to a bone scan if

necessary; for DVT refer for Doppler ultrasound; for Achilles tendon rupture or possible partial rupture, diagnostic ultrasound or magnetic resonance imaging (MRI) is appropriate; for compartment syndrome, refer for measurement of compartment pressure.

Management

- Refer cases of DVT, Achilles rupture, or acute compartment syndrome.
- Manage stress fractures with rest, increased calcium intake, and modification of inciting activity; nonhealing fractures require referral for orthopaedic consultation.
- Achilles tendinitis may be helped with temporary taping, strengthening, and activity modification.

Relevant Anatomy

The lower leg is often discussed in reference to four fascial compartments:

1. Anterior—tibialis anterior, extensor digitorum longus, extensor hallucis, the deep peroneal nerve, and the anterior tibial artery and vein
2. Lateral—peroneus longus and brevis, and superficial peroneal nerve
3. Superficial posterior—soleus muscle, and tendons of the plantaris and gastrocnemius
4. Deep posterior—flexor digitorum and flexor hallucis longus, tibialis posterior, the peroneal and posterior tibial artery and vein, and the tibial nerve

Exercise and trauma-related pain may be confined to one of these compartments.[2] When hypertrophy or inflammation exceeds the accommodations of the compartment, a compartment syndrome may result. Muscle function can also be related to the compartments. The anterior compartment muscles are the extensors, the lateral evertors; superficial posterior compartment muscles cause plantarflexion; and the deep posterior compartment muscles are the primary invertors and stabilizers against overpronation (**Figure 13–1**).

The anterior compartment muscles contribute to shock absorption; when they are eccentrically weak they may cause anterior shin splints.[3] The muscles in the deep posterior compartment are stabilizers; when they are eccentrically weak they may cause posterior (medial) shin splints.

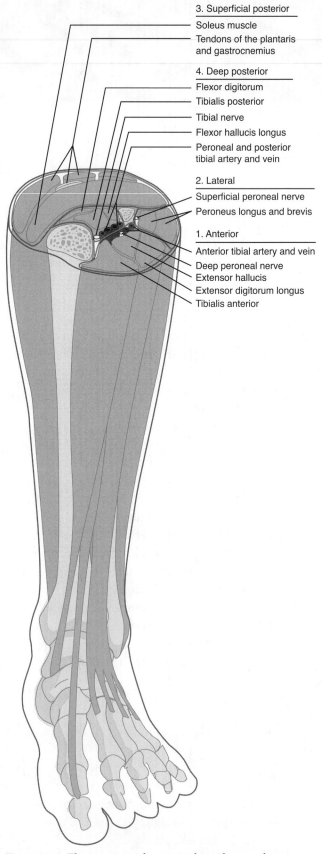

3. Superficial posterior
Soleus muscle
Tendons of the plantaris and gastrocnemius

4. Deep posterior
Flexor digitorum
Tibialis posterior
Tibial nerve
Flexor hallucis longus
Peroneal and posterior tibial artery and vein

2. Lateral
Superficial peroneal nerve
Peroneus longus and brevis

1. Anterior
Anterior tibial artery and vein
Deep peroneal nerve
Extensor hallucis
Extensor digitorum longus
Tibialis anterior

Figure 13–1 The anterior and posterior lower leg muscles.

Evaluation

History

Careful questioning of the patient during the history taking can point to the diagnosis (**Table 13–1**).

Pain Localization

Anterior.

- Proximal tibia—pes anserinus bursitis (medially), stress fracture, tumor
- Middle and distal tibia—stress fracture, periostitis
- Anterolateral—anterior shin splints

Posterior.

- Upper medial tibia—tennis leg (medial gastrocnemius tear), flexor digitorum longus tendinitis
- Middle and lower third of tibia—stress fracture, posterior shin splints
- Calf muscle belly—muscle tear, DVT
- Achilles tendon—Achilles tendinitis
- Insertion of Achilles into calcaneus—retrocalcaneal bursitis, exostosis, Achilles tendinitis

When the patient reports a sudden onset of pain in the calf, it is important to identify whether there was direct trauma or a sudden movement. Direct trauma may result

Table 13–1 History Questions for Lower Leg Complaints

Primary Question	What Are You Thinking?	Secondary Questions	What Are You Thinking?
Did the pain occur suddenly?	Tennis leg, DVT, fracture	Did you fall on or hit your leg?	Fracture, DVT
		Did you hear or feel a pop on the back of your leg while running or playing tennis?	Tennis leg (tear of medial gastrocnemius)
Did the pain appear without any particular trauma or activity?	DVT, shin splints	Are you taking birth control pills (for females) or have you been immobilized for a long time?	DVT
		Do you stand or walk on hard surfaces?	Shin splints
Does the pain occur mainly with activity?	Shin splints, stress fracture, Achilles tendinitis, chronic compartment syndrome, claudication	Did this occur with running? A sudden increase in speed, distance or duration?	Stress fracture, shin splints
		Do you work, walk, or run on hard surfaces?	Shin splints
		(For runners) Does the pain occur at a consistent distance or timing?	Compartment syndrome
		Is it worse with walking small distance; does it improve with rest?	Claudication (differentiate vascular from neurogenic causes)
		Is the pain close to your heel and worse when you go up on your toes?	Achilles tendinitis
Is the complaint one more of swelling?	Compartment syndrome, DVT, stress fracture, congestive heart failure (CHF)	Is the swelling localized to an inch or two?	Stress fracture; maybe DVT
		Is the swelling localized to one side of the lower leg?	Compartment syndrome
		Does the swelling improve with leg elevation?	Yes—vascular No—lymph
		Does the swelling involve the entire lower leg in both legs?	CHF, fluid retention due to renal problems, salt retention, liver disease

from a blow to the leg or accidentally bumping the leg against an object (e.g., coffee table). Minor trauma in an older patient may initiate a DVT. A strong blow to the lower leg in any patient may result in fracture and/or initiate enough swelling to produce a compartment syndrome. Tearing of the medial gastrocnemius may occur with extension of the knee coupled with dorsiflexion of the ankle. The patient often reports a "pop" associated with a severe stabbing pain.

Overuse injuries cause varying degrees of tendon irritation, bone irritation, and swelling or hypertrophy in the corresponding compartment. Patients who have just begun an exercise routine or work standing or walking on a hard surface may develop shin splints. Athletic patients who suddenly increase duration, intensity, or speed are prone to stress fractures.[4] With female athletes, it is important to determine menstrual status. Amenorrhea coupled with endurance-type training suggests stress fracture as a cause of tibial pain. Runners who complain of aching, cramping pain always occurring at a specific distance or timing is suggestive of chronic compartment syndrome. All of the above exercise-induced problems gradually will become worse. Distinction is based more on palpation findings; in some cases radiographic imaging (stress fracture), bone scans (stress fracture), or measurements of compartment pressure (compartment syndrome) are needed.

Claudication

Patients who complain of leg pain that occurs with walking and is relieved with rest likely have a form of claudication. The distinction clinically is between vascular and neurogenic claudication. Neurogenic claudication is secondary to spinal stenosis. Compression of nerves and/or the blood supply to nerves causes leg symptoms that are related to exertion. Patients will often have associated low back pain or radiation into the leg(s). The distinction between vascular and neurogenic claudication is not always clear; however, in general, it is related to posture. Patients with neurogenic claudication are more likely to be able to walk or ride a bicycle farther before the onset of leg pain when in a flexed position. Vascular claudication involves stenosis of peripheral blood vessels compromising the blood supply to muscles. This is most evident with increased demand as occurs with walking. Atherosclerotic blockage is most common. Risk factors include smoking, diabetes, hypertension, and hypercholesterolemia. The patient may be found to have diminished pulses, pallor, reduced capillary fill, trophic skin

changes and hair loss, and in severe cases, nonhealing ulcers or gangrene. Continuous-wave Doppler is used to measure arterial pressures, determine the ankle-brachial index (ABI) and segmental systolic pressures, and assess specific Doppler waveforms. The ABI is a ratio comparing the brachial pressure to the ankle pressure. This ratio is normally 1. Ratios in patients with vascular claudication are often between 0.5 and 0.8. Segmental systolic pressures should remain generally the same in the leg. A difference of > 20 mm Hg indicates blockage. Management strategies include controlling risk factors such as smoking cessation and control of diabetes, hypertension, and hypercholesterolemia. Ironically, a crucial factor to management is exercise. Walking should be gradually increased to a goal of 30 to 90 minutes per day for five days at a rate of about 2 miles/hour.

Examination

The examination focuses on palpation of the tender or swollen area. A general rule of thumb is that stress fractures, although causing a diffuse tenderness, often have a discrete localized area that is extremely tender. Percussion distal or proximal to this site often will cause pain at the site of the stress fracture.

When swelling is present, the distinction between localized and diffuse swelling may be helpful. A diffuse pattern of swelling that resolves with leg elevation is indicative of a vascular cause (venous drainage). Swelling localized to a specific compartment of the leg is suggestive of compartment syndrome. Localized swelling is suggestive of DVT if found more in the belly of the triceps surae group. Localized swelling on the tibia or fibula may represent a stress fracture. Defects are occasionally visible or palpable at the medial leg with tennis leg and several centimeters proximal to the insertion of the Achilles tendon with rupture. With Achilles rupture, squeezing of the calf muscle fails to produce passive plantarflexion (Thompson test).[5]

Passive dorsiflexion of the ankle may increase pain in the calf with DVT or calf strain. Adding resistance may increase the pain with muscle involvement, less with DVT. Further functional testing may indicate an involved muscle. For example, placing stretch on a tendon/muscle and then asking the patient to contract against the examiner's resistance may localize the problem.

When passive dorsiflexion causes severe posteromedial pain or when plantarflexion produces severe anterior pain, a related compartment syndrome is likely.

Further evaluation is strongly based on the suspected disorder. If a stress fracture is suspected, radiographs may demonstrate a healing callus or a periosteal reaction. However, it will often take two to three weeks for the callus to appear, if at all. Oblique views of the area may be needed to visualize the healing process. The definitive tool is a bone scan. If the suspicion is DVT, Doppler ultrasound is a decent alternative to venography, the gold standard.[6] When Achilles tendon pathology is suspected, soft tissue ultrasonography may be valuable but is operator-dependent. When Achilles rupture is suspected, disruption of Kager's triangle (a radiolucent area composed of the posterior flexors, tibia, and Achilles tendon) on a lateral radiographic view may be visible.[7]

Management

- Suspicion of DVT requires medical referral for further evaluation and possible anticoagulant therapy.
- If compartment syndrome is suspected, referral for compartment pressure measurement is suggested.
- Achilles tendon rupture requires surgical management in most cases; if the patient is older and not active, nonsurgical management, including a period of casting and non-weight-bearing may be sufficient; however, the re-tear rate is high in active or athletic individuals.[8]
- Achilles tendinitis can be managed with modification of activity, gentle stretching, ice after activity, and an elastic strapping support with the foot in plantarflexion; a graduated eccentric training program is often helpful.
- Stress fractures of the tibia usually will heal well with avoidance of impact loading from running or jumping for a period of a few weeks followed by low-impact conditioning for four to six weeks before returning to the full sport activity. Calcium intake should be increased to 1 g daily during the healing process and maintained at 800 mg daily during training.[9] Shock-absorption materials in the shoes may help dissipate impact forces.

Algorithm

An algorithm for evaluation and management of calf/heel pain is presented in **Figure 13–2**.

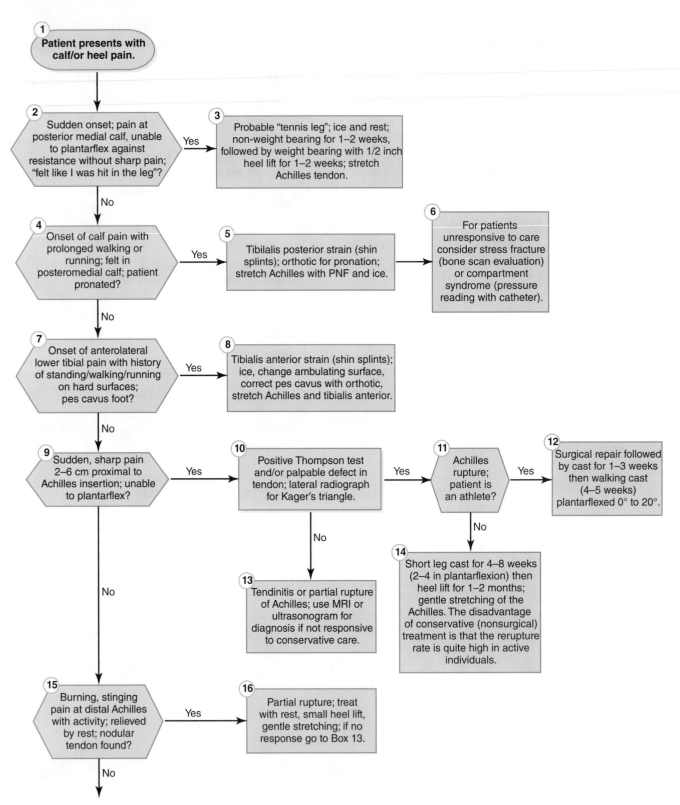

Figure 13–2 Calf/Heel Pain—Algorithm

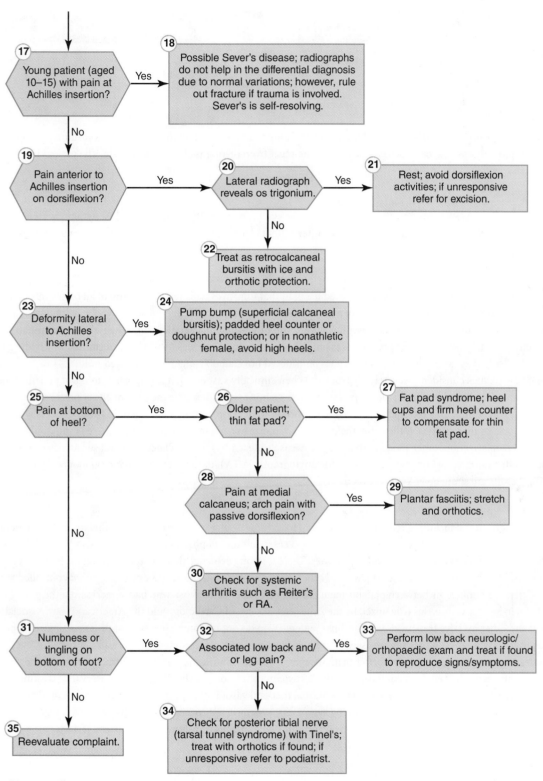

17 Young patient (aged 10–15) with pain at Achilles insertion? — Yes → **18** Possible Sever's disease; radiographs do not help in the differential diagnosis due to normal variations; however, rule out fracture if trauma is involved. Sever's is self-resolving.

No ↓

19 Pain anterior to Achilles insertion on dorsiflexion? — Yes → **20** Lateral radiograph reveals os trigonium. — Yes → **21** Rest; avoid dorsiflexion activities; if unresponsive refer for excision.

No ↓ (from 20)

22 Treat as retrocalcaneal bursitis with ice and orthotic protection.

No ↓ (from 19)

23 Deformity lateral to Achilles insertion? — Yes → **24** Pump bump (superficial calcaneal bursitis); padded heel counter or doughnut protection; or in nonathletic female, avoid high heels.

No ↓

25 Pain at bottom of heel? — Yes → **26** Older patient; thin fat pad? — Yes → **27** Fat pad syndrome; heel cups and firm heel counter to compensate for thin fat pad.

No ↓ (from 26)

28 Pain at medial calcaneus; arch pain with passive dorsiflexion? — Yes → **29** Plantar fasciitis; stretch and orthotics.

No ↓ (from 28)

30 Check for systemic arthritis such as Reiter's or RA.

No ↓ (from 25)

31 Numbness or tingling on bottom of foot? — Yes → **32** Associated low back and/or leg pain? — Yes → **33** Perform low back neurologic/orthopaedic exam and treat if found to reproduce signs/symptoms.

No ↓ (from 32)

34 Check for posterior tibial nerve (tarsal tunnel syndrome) with Tinel's; treat with orthotics if found; if unresponsive refer to podiatrist.

No ↓ (from 31)

35 Reevaluate complaint.

Figure 13–2 (Continued)

Selected Disorders of the Lower Leg and Posterior Heel*

Intermittent Claudication

Classic Presentation

An older patient complains of leg pain after walking for a few minutes, and must stop and rest before continuing. The description may be of a cramping, tightening, or tiredness in the legs. The relief from resting is almost immediate. The patient has indications of cardiovascular risk factors.

Cause

Peripheral vascular disease (PVD) due to atherosclerosis may be symptomatic or asymptomatic. Most patients with PVD are asymptomatic. Only about 20% of patients report symptoms of intermittent claudication.[10] The most common area affected is the superficial femoral artery demonstrating either stenosis or occlusion.

Evaluation

In older patients with a presentation of walking-induced leg pain that improves with rest, a measure of all cardiovascular risk factors is important for long-term management. Use of a bicycle test with patient in a flexed position may be helpful in distinguishing between spinal stenosis caused symptoms (i.e., pseudoclaudication or neurogenic claudication). The physical examination must include the ankle–brachial index.[11] Blood pressure is taken in both arms and both legs. A ratio is determined by dividing the highest ankle pressure by the highest arm pressure. Above 0.90 is considered normal; 0.71–0.90 is considered mild; 0.41–0.70 is considered moderate; and 0.00–0.40 is considered severely obstructed. When clinically suspected, it is important to retest patients who appear to have a normal index. The blood pressure is again measured to determine the index after the patient either performs a number of toe raises or walks on a treadmill. This retest after exercise is important to develop a pressure gradient in those patients who have blockage of the distal aorta or iliac arteries. Otherwise, the index may appear normal in these patients. If there is still doubt, or if a surgeon is considering revascularization, other imaging that may prove useful (each has its associated cost and sensitivity characteristics) includes duplex ultrasonography, computed tomographic angiography (CTA), or magnetic resonance angiography (MRA). Although CTA and MRA results are similar, CTA is less expensive.

Management

Management is multifactorial including reducing, or attending to, cardiovascular risk factors, exercise therapy, recommendations for aspirin use at 75 mg for the antiplatelet effect, and in selected cases, additional pharmacological treatment (e.g., cilostazol), and revascularization using endovascular or surgical approaches. There is strong evidence that an exercise program is an effective approach for many patients. This includes a Cochrane review[12] and other meta-analyses.[13] Additionally, one randomized controlled study indicated no difference in outcome between patients managed with exercise versus those who had surgery. Even the guidelines of the TransAtlantic Inter-Society Consensus (organized by the American College of Cardiology and the American Heart Association) recommend surgical and other invasive treatment only for those patients who do not respond to exercise or pharmacological approaches.[14] The exercise program works best if patients are asked to walk until pain is near maximum, and with walking sessions that last longer than 30 minutes. Supervised programs work better than unsupervised. This approach must be performed three or more times per week for at least six months with the benefits taking between one to two months to be noticed. Regarding conservative treatment through nutritional and other oral supplementation, one study indicated that oral vasodilating prostaglandins, vitamin E, and chelation therapy with EDTA did not appear to have an effect on reducing symptoms.[15] Medical approaches are controversial with regard to effectiveness but include implantation of stents or revascularization (surgery or percutaneous transluminal angioplasty [PTA]).[16]

Shin Splints

Classic Presentation

The patient complains of anterior or posterior lower leg pain that is often insidious in onset. If asked, the patient may remember walking or running on a hard surface. The pain is a deep ache that is often worse with weight-bearing.

Cause

Shin splints are ill defined. It appears that tendinitis, periostitis, muscle strain, or interosseous membrane strain have all been implicated. There are generally two types. The anterior shin splint involves the tibialis anterior, extensor hallucis longus, and digitorum

---

*See also Chapter 14, Foot and Ankle Complaints, and Chapter 25, Lower Leg Swelling.

longus. These muscles are used for shock absorption; when they are weak or placed under increased demand as in walking or running on hard surfaces or when the shoe has no shock-absorbing quality, the force is transmitted to the tibia and its attachments. The posterior type of shin splint involves the tibialis posterior, flexor hallucis longus, and flexor digitorum longus muscles. The soleus has also been implicated. These muscles act as ankle stabilizers and appear to be overstrained when the patient is hyperpronated.[3]

Evaluation

The pain is often at the middle or lower third of the tibia. Anterior shin splints are tender just lateral to the middle tibia. Pain and tenderness for posterior shin splints is posteromedial to the middle or lower tibia. Pain may be increased by stretch or contraction of the involved muscles. It is important to check the patient's shoes for proper shock-absorption capabilities. Stress fractures may appear similarly, yet the pain is usually more localized and on the tibia itself. With shin splints, the radiographs are usually normal. If the patient does not respond to treatment or there are enough historical clues to suggest stress fracture, such as endurance training in a young athlete or menstrual irregularities in a female athlete, referral for a bone scan is warranted.

Management

The acute care of shin splints involves rest from the inciting activity, ice, and support provided by elastic tape that is applied in an upward spiral pattern toward the area of tenderness. Support at the foot is also important and can be given temporarily by foot taping and/or medial heel wedges. Orthotics will often be needed if shin splints are recurrent (**Table 13–2**). Simply throwing away worn-out shoes and replacing them with a good shock-absorbing pair is often all that is needed. One study indicated that dietary calcium intake should be increased in those individuals with shin splints.[9]

Table 13–2 Shin Splint Management

Parameter	Acute	Subacute	Symptom-Free Stage
Criteria for diagnosis of staging	Anterior shin splints—pain/tender just lateral to middle tibia; posterior shin splints—pain/tender at posteromedial middle or lower tibia.	Pain is not constant, able to bear weight without pain; prolonged standing or walking may still cause pain.	No pain with walking and standing.
Goals and timing within each stage	Decrease pain and inflammation; approximately 1–3 days.	Strengthen and stretch lower leg muscles; increase shock absorption of shoe with anterior shin splints; support foot with posterior shin splints; about 1 week.	Emphasis on eccentric training, orthotics support, endurance training begins; 3–4 weeks.
Concerns	Pain may be due to stress fracture; consider bone scan if unresponsive.	Pain may be due to stress fracture; consider bone scan if unresponsive.	Overperformance of eccentrics.
Requirements for progression to next stage	Pain and tenderness decrease; isometric contraction not painful.	Proper shoe is chosen; concentric strength is present without pain.	No pain with eccentric training.
Manipulation/mobilization	Emphasis on tibial, calcaneal, and foot manipulation/mobilization.	Emphasis on tibial, calcaneal, and foot manipulation/mobilization.	As needed.
Modalities	Ice, compression, TENS, or high-volt galvanic (80–120 Hz/20 min/2–3×'s/1–2 days).	Ultrasound for 5–6 min/1.5 wt/cm² for 2–3 days; ice after any prolonged standing or walking.	Ice after activity.
External brace, support, etc.	Elastic taping from opposite side drawing around and up to painful area.	Elastic support as before; extra support with weight-bearing using strapping tape for arch support.	Wean patient off support.
ROM/flexibility/massage	Mild stretching of involved muscles; gentle stripping massage of involved muscles.	Stage 3 or 4 MRT to gastrocnemius; continue postisometric stretching of all lower leg muscles.	Maintain flexibility.

(continues)

Table 13–2 Shin Splint Management (continued)

Parameter	Acute	Subacute	Symptom-Free Stage
Open-chain exercise	Mild isometrics.	Isometrics at every 20°–30° arcs against resistance of wall or opposite leg progressing to elastic tubing training.	Continue through endurance phase of elastic tubing training.
Closed-chain exercise	None.	Standing toe raises (emphasize eccentric phase).	Continue eccentric training using three sets of 10.
Proprioceptive training	Diagonal PNF patterns without resistance.	Diagonal PNF patterns with resistance from examiner or elastic tubing; wobble board training begins; minitrampoline two-legged jumping.	Wobble board while bouncing a ball; minitrampoline, single-leg jumps for balance and strength.
Associated biomechanical items	Look at shoes to determine shock absorption and wear pattern.	Cast for orthotics if deemed necessary; temporarily support with taping or heel wedges.	Fit orthotics.
Lifestyle/activity modifications	Avoid running and standing for long periods on hard surfaces.	Progress to jogging or minitrampoline running; avoid prolonged standing.	Avoid prolonged standing on hard surfaces; educate patient regarding shoe wear and need for buying a new pair of shock-absorbing shoes at the appropriate time.

Key: TENS, transcutaneous electrical nerve stimulation; PNF, proprioceptive neuromuscular facilitation; MRT, myofascial release technique.

Tibial Stress Fracture

Classic Presentation

The patient is usually an active individual who develops insidious onset of tibial pain. Overuse from running or prolonged activity on hard surfaces may be evident in the history.

Cause

If a repetitive stress is applied to bone such as with running, the ability to remodel may be overwhelmed because of inadequate healing time. There is still debate as to whether stress to bone is due to weak muscles or fatigue that causes increased bone loading or more to the forceful repetitive contraction of muscles and the imposed stress at their origins onto bone. A recent study evaluated risk for recurrent stress fractures and found that for men, the most common fracture sites were the tibia and fibula (70%), and for females the foot and ankle (50%) were the most common fracture sites.[17] Sixty-one percent were runners. Forty percent of females reported menstrual irregularities. Biomechanical risk factors included high arch (pes cavus), leg-length inequality, and forefoot varus. An early stage of this microtrauma event has been called the medial tibial stress syndrome; when a fracture has not occurred, however, there is enough of an inflammatory and remodeling process to cause pain.[18] Tibial stress fractures account for half of all stress fractures occurring in athletes.[19] The location varies depending on the underlying inciting activity. Runners are more likely to have middle and distal third tibial fractures; ballet dancers, the middle third; and military recruits, the proximal tibia. Middle shaft fractures as seen in dancers have a reputation for delayed union or continuing on to full fractures (sometimes called the "dreaded black line" radiographically).[20]

Evaluation

The clinical presentation of an athlete who first notices shin pain at the end of a run that gradually becomes incapacitating over several days of running is highly suggestive. Additionally, menstrual irregularities in a patient complaining of shin pain is a clue to possible underlying osteopenia. Pain is often better initially with rest, but returns with any impact loading. Tenderness is often found at a discrete area on the tibial shaft. Percussion or tuning-fork testing at a distance either proximal or distal to the site may cause reproduction or worsening of the pain at the fracture site. Although stress fractures are difficult to diagnose in the early stages, attempts at using in-office approaches such as therapeutic ultrasound have not been shown to be helpful. In one recent study, therapeutic ultrasound was tested for its ability to detect stress fractures.[21] Continuous 1 Mhz ultrasound application was used on both the involved and uninvolved tibias at seven increasing intensities for 30 seconds each. Coupled with this approach was the use of a visual analog scale. None of the subjects found to have a stress fracture on MRI was diagnosed by the ultrasound approach. Radiographically, a small radiolucent line may be seen, or a localized periosteal new bone formation may be evident. Oblique films are often necessary. Definitive diagnosis may require a triphasic bone scan when radiographs are equivocal but the presentation suggests stress fracture.

Management

Most stress fractures can be managed conservatively with restriction of impact loading for several weeks. Immobilization usually is not necessary unless the athlete or patient refuses to stop the inciting activity. Crutches may be necessary in some patients who are symptomatic with walking. For the elite athlete, conditioning with bicycle riding or pool training with a water vest are good alternatives for maintaining aerobic fitness. Gradual return to activity begins with low-impact training over several weeks prior to full return.

Orthotic support, nutritional recommendations (especially calcium), and modification of activity are important for prevention. Ultrasonography and pulsed electromagnetic field therapy to accelerate healing time have been suggested but are unproven at this time.

Compartment Syndrome

Classic Presentation

The presentation varies depending on the compartment involved and whether it is acute or chronic. Typically, the patient often is an athlete complaining of aching or cramping of the leg following exercise. Pain is relieved by rest initially. There may be complaints of numbness/tingling into various parts of the foot.

Cause

The lower leg is divided into four compartments: (1) anterior, containing the tibialis anterior, extensors of the toes, anterior tibial artery and vein, and deep peroneal nerve; (2) deep posterior, containing the posterior tibialis and toe flexors and the posterior tibial artery and vein; (3) superficial posterior, containing the soleus, gastrocnemius, and plantaris; and (4) lateral, containing the peroneal muscles and nerve. Increased pressure in any of these fascial compartments may lead to damage to the muscles. Increased pressure also may cause numbness and paresthesia into the distribution of the corresponding nerve due to ischemia.[22] The most common cause is exercise induced; however, in acute situations, compartment syndrome may develop secondary to local trauma or fracture.

Evaluation

In athletes, the symptoms usually occur within 10 to 30 minutes of exercise. The pain will subside over minutes or hours following activity; initially the patient will remain pain-free until the next exercise session. The examination is often normal between exacerbations. Tenderness and swelling may be evident over the involved compartment. Pulses are often normal distally; however, some sensory changes may be evident in the distal distribution of the involved nerves. Fascial defects with muscle herniation are evident in approximately 40% of patients, but they may not be evident unless the athlete runs for several minutes. The definitive tool is measurement of compartmental pressure while resting and after exercise. Elevated levels reach 80 mm Hg, compared with the normal of 30 to 40 mm Hg following exercise. Levels above 40 mm Hg that remain elevated for 15 to 30 minutes or longer indicate compartment syndrome.[2]

Management

For chronic compartment syndrome a period of rest for four to eight weeks may be successful. For acute syndrome and patients who do not respond to conservative care, fasciotomy is the treatment of choice.

Achilles Tendinitis

Classic Presentation

The patient is often an athlete who complains of pain in the Achilles tendon following jumping or running activities.

Cause

The Achilles tendon is covered by a peritenon composed of mainly fatty areolar tissue. The area most affected is approximately 2 cm proximal to the calcaneal insertion. The demands on the tendon are high in running and jumping sports. Interestingly, the tendon has been shown to function with as little as 25% fiber continuity. Insertional problems include irritation of the retrocalcaneal bursa and irritation leading to a Haglund's deformity. Additionally, seronegative arthritides such as Reiter's syndrome and ankylosing spondylitis cause an enthesopathy at this site. Pain and tenderness at the calcaneus may indicate Sever's apophysitis in a younger athlete.

Evaluation

Chronic degeneration (tendinosis) may be evident as a knotty swelling, with more acute damage evident by local tenderness made worse by stretch and/or stretch and contraction. Palpable defects in the tendon may indicate impending rupture in an athlete complaining of sharp stabbing or burning pains at the site. Researchers using diagnostic ultrasonography evaluated the patellar and Achilles tendons of 58 soccer players at pre- and post-season.[23] Those with abnormal findings for the Achilles at pre-season had a 45% risk of developing symptoms. Triceps surae tightness may be a contributing factor. Passively dorsiflexing the ankle with the knee extended should demonstrate a normal angle of 20° to 30°. This is a measure of gastrocnemius tightness. To test the soleus, the knee is flexed and the ankle is dorsiflexed. For dorsiflexion of the ankle, 30° to 35° should be available. The Thompson test is performed on patients suspected of having a rupture. This would occur in an on-the-field scenario. If squeezing the calf in the prone relaxed patient does not produce passive plantarflexion of the foot, Achilles rupture is likely. When partial ruptures are suspected, MRI can help differentiate between tendinitis and partial rupture.[25]

Management

Achilles tendinitis is managed with rest, ice, and modification of the inciting activity. Taping the ankle in plantarflexion with an elastic support is helpful in the early stages. Heel lifts may also decrease the stretch effect on the injured Achilles. Long-term goals are to modify faulty training activity and to gradually and consistently stretch the triceps surae group. Orthotics may be necessary in those individuals with hyperpronation. Training should consist of a graduated eccentric loading program. An example would be to begin initially with toe raises with emphasis on slowly lowering the body weight. Additional weight can be carried to increase the training effect over time.

One RCT[24] demonstrated that the combination of low-energy shockwave therapy with eccentric exercise was better than eccentric exercise alone at four months follow-up. Two reviews[26,27] of eccentric exercise for Achilles tendinosis come to the conclusion that more studies using larger patient populations are needed. There is also the implication in one review that the effects are simply due to time. However, this is contradicted by most studies demonstrating that a "wait-watch-and-see" approach is less effective than eccentric exercise or shockwave therapy.[28] One study,[29] though, did indicate that at one year, patients performing a stretching regimen had similar success to those doing the eccentric approach. Fahlstrom et al.[30] found that a 12-week eccentric training protocol based on the Curwin–Stanish protocol resulted in a satisfactory result in 89% of participants with mid-portion Achilles tendinosis, whereas only 32% of participants with chronic insertional tendinosis had a satisfactory result. One study[31] indicates that nonathletes do not enjoy the same benefits as athletes with an eccentric training approach. This difference in effect may be due to the finding that healthy control tendons do not seem to have any change in collagen metabolism with eccentric training versus a noted increase in collagen synthesis rate in symptomatic athletes.[32] A novel approach being used in tendinosis throughout the body is a locally placed transdermal patch of nitric oxide.[33] This approach offers a conservative option that may be effective. Another approach involves the injection of a sclerosing agent into neovessels in the involved section of the tendon. The studies[34] performed to date indicate a good result, especially for those nonrespondents to eccentric training. An eight-year follow-up study of 83 of 107 patients diagnosed with acute or subchronic tendinopathy determined what happens to these patients over time.[35] Twenty-nine percent needed surgery; 84% of the total group recovered to previous activity levels; 93% were asymptomatic on the involved side even with strenuous exercise, although 41% started to suffer from problems on the noninvolved side. Injectable treatments include a host of components and techniques that include platelet rich plasma (PRP), sclerosing agents, protease inhibitors, and corticosteroids. A recent review judged the evidence for each still wanting.[36]

Yet not all agree. A review from 2013 suggests there may be some value without much risk.[37] More high-quality studies with comparison to control groups need to be performed.

Achilles ruptures may be managed with cast immobilization in nonathletic or older individuals. However, in athletes the re-rupture rate is quite high; therefore, surgery is the recommended treatment.[22] Recovery from surgery involves a walking cast, with full return taking several months.

APPENDIX 13–1

References

1. Clemens DB. Tibial stress syndrome in athletes. *J Sports Med*. 1974;2:81.

2. Black KP, Schultz TK, Cheung NL. Compartment syndromes in athletes. *Clin Sports Med*. 1990;9:471–487.

3. Reber L, Perry J, Pink M. Muscular control of the ankle in running. *Am J Sports Med*. 1993;21:805–810.

4. Hershman EB, Mailly T. Stress fractures. *Clin Sports Med*. 1990;9:183–214.

5. Thompson T, Doherty J. Spontaneous rupture of the tendon of Achilles: a new clinical diagnostic test. *Anat Res*. 1967;158:126.

6. Richlie DL. Noninvasive imaging of the lower extremity for deep venous thrombosis. *J Gen Intern Med*. 1993;8:271.

7. DiStefano VJ, Nixon JE. Ruptures of the Achilles tendon. *J Sports Med*. 1973;1:34.

8. Cetti R, Christensen SE, Ejsted R, et al. Operative versus nonoperative treatment of Achilles tendon rupture: a prospective randomized study and review of the literature. *Am J Sports Med*. 1993;21:791–799.

9. Myburgh KH, Srobler N, Nosakes TD. Factors associated with shin soreness in athletes. *Physician Sportsmed*. 1988;16:129.

10. Dolan NC, Liu K, Criqui MH, et al. Peripheral artery disease, diabetes, and reduced lower extremity functioning. *Diabetes Care*. 2002;25(1):113–120.

11. McDermott MM, Liu K, Guralnik JM, et al. The ankle brachial index independently predicts walking velocity and walking endurance in peripheral arterial disease. *J Am Geriatr Soc*. 1998;46(11):1355–1362.

12. Leng GC, Fowler B, Ernst E. Exercise for intermittent claudication. *Cochrane Database Syst Rev*. 2000(2): CD000990.

13. Bendermacher BL, Willigendael EM, Teijink JA, Prins MH. Supervised exercise therapy versus non-supervised exercise therapy for intermittent claudication. *Cochrane Database Syst Rev*. 2006(2):CD005263.

14. Norgren L, Hiatt WR, Dormandy JA, et al. Inter-Society Consensus for the Management of Peripheral Arterial Disease. *Int Angiol*. 2007;26(2):81–157.

15. Hirsch AT, Haskal ZJ, Hertzer NR, et al. ACC/AHA Guidelines for the Management of Patients with Peripheral Arterial Disease (lower extremity, renal, mesenteric, and abdominal aortic): a collaborative report from the American Associations for Vascular Surgery/Society for Vascular Surgery, Society for Cardiovascular Angiography and Interventions, Society for Vascular Medicine and Biology, Society of Interventional Radiology, and the ACC/AHA Task Force on Practice Guidelines (writing committee to develop guidelines for the management of patients with peripheral arterial disease)—summary of recommendations. *J Vasc Interv Radiol*. 2006;17(9):1383–1397; quiz 1398.

16. White C. Clinical practice. Intermittent claudication. *N Engl J Med*. 2007;356(12):1241–1250.

17. Korpelainen R, Orava S, Karpakka J, Sira P, Hulkko A. Risk factors for recurrent stress fractures in athletes. *Am J Sports Med*. 2001;29(3):304–310.

18. Mubarak SJ, Gould RN, Lee YF, et al. The medial tibial stress syndrome. *Am J Sports Med*. 1982;10:201–205.

19. Matheson GO, Clement DB, McKenzie DC, et al. Stress fractures in athletes: a study of 320 cases. *Am J Sports Med*. 1987;15:46–58.

20. Green NE, Rogers RA, Lipscomb AB. Nonunion of stress fractures of the tibia. *Am J Sports Med*. 1985;13:171–176.

21. Romani WA, Perrin DH, Dussault RG, et al. Identification of tibial stress fractures using therapeutic continuous ultrasound. *J Orthop Sports Phys Ther*. 2000;30(8):444–452.

22. Martens MA, Backaert M, Vermaut G, et al. Chronic leg pain in athletes due to recurrent compartment syndrome. *Am J Sports Med*. 1984;12:148.

23. Fredberg U, Bolvig, L. Significance of ultrasonographically detected asymptomatic tendinosis in the patellar and Achilles tendons of elite soccer players: a longitudinal study. *Am J Sports Med*. 2002;30(4):488–451.

24. Rompe JD, Furia J. Maffulli N. Eccentric loading versus eccentric loading plus shock-wave treatment for midportion Achilles tendinopathy: a randomized controlled trial. *Am J Sports Med*. 2009;37(3):463–470.

25. Clemens DB, Taunton JE, Smart GW. Achilles tendonitis and peritendinitis: etiology and treatment. *Am J Sports Med*. 1984;12:179.

26. Woodley BL, Newsham-West RJ, Baxter GD. Chronic tendinopathy: effectiveness of eccentric exercise. *Br J Sports Med*. 2007;41(4):188–198;discussion 199.

27. Kingma JJ, de Knikker R, Wittink HM, Takken T. Eccentric overload training in patients with chronic Achilles tendinopathy: a systematic review. *Br J Sports Med*. 2007;41(6):e3.

28. Rompe JD, Nafe B, Furia JP, Maffulli N. Eccentric loading, shock-wave treatment, or a wait-and-see

policy for tendinopathy of the main body of tendo Achillis: a randomized controlled trial. *Am J Sports Med.* 2007;35(3):374–383.

29. Norregaard J, Larsen CC, Bieler T, Langberg H. Eccentric exercise in treatment of Achilles tendinopathy. *Scand J Med Sci Sports.* 2007;17(2):133–138.

30. Fahlstrom M, Jonsson P, Lorentzon R, Alfredson H. Chronic Achilles tendon pain treated with eccentric calf-muscle training. *Knee Surg Sports Traumatol Arthrosc.* 2003;11(5):327–333.

31. Sayana MK, Maffulli N. Eccentric calf muscle training in non-athletic patients with Achilles tendinopathy. *J Sci Med Sport.* 2007;10(1):52–58.

32. Langberg H, Ellingsgaard H, Madsen T, et al. Eccentric rehabilitation exercise increases peritendinous type I collagen synthesis in humans with Achilles tendinosis. *Scand J Med Sci Sports.* 2007;17(1):61–66.

33. Murrell GA. Using nitric oxide to treat tendinopathy. *Br J Sports Med.* 2007;41(4):227–231.

34. Lind B, Ohberg L, Alfredson H. Sclerosing polidocanol injections in mid-portion Achilles tendinosis: remaining good clinical results and decreased tendon thickness at 2-year follow-up. *Knee Surg Sports Traumatol Arthrosc.* 2006;14(12):1327–1332.

35. Paavola M, Kammus P, Paakkala T, et al. Long-term prognosis of patients with Achilles tendinopathy: an observational 8-year follow-up study. *Am J Sports Med.* 2000;28(5):634–642.

36. Gross CE, Hsu AR, Chahal J, Holmes GB, Jr. Injectable treatments for noninsertional Achilles tendinosis: a systematic review. *Foot Ankle Int.* 2013;34(5):619–628.

37. Kumar V, Millar T, Murphy PN, Clough T. The treatment of intractable plantar fasciitis with platelet-rich plasma injection. *Foot (Edinb).* 2013;23(2-3):74–77.

Foot and Ankle Complaints

Context

The foot and ankle must provide support and shock absorption while at the same time balancing the body. This requires both mobility to adapt to varying terrain and stability to allow supported contact and push-off from the ground. Shock absorption occurs as a result of the dissipation of forces through complex movements at the foot and ankle and imposed adaptation through mainly rotation in the lower extremity at the knee, hip, and pelvis. Therefore, dysfunction at the feet may have consequences throughout the entire body. Foot problems may be local or referred; however, the need for lower-extremity compensation may result in more proximal pain, including low back pain.

As the most distal site of the body, the foot is also commonly affected by vascular disorders. Arterial occlusive disorders block blood flow. Valvular insufficiency in veins, coupled with gravity, may lead to a pooling effect and vascular stasis. Neurologic dysfunction associated with metabolic neuropathies such as seen with diabetes is often felt first distally in the feet. The bare foot is exposed to possible trauma and infection. The supported foot is vulnerable to the pressure effects and biomechanical alterations of footwear. When compromised by vascular and/or sensory deficits, a patient is more prone to the long-term consequences of unnoticed or unattended lesions. This is most often seen with the diabetic patient.

The most common conditions involving the foot and ankle are biomechanical in nature and include the following:

- First toe—hallux valgus/rigidus, turf toe, gout, and sesamoiditis
- Metatarsals—Morton's neuroma, metatarsalgia, "dropped metatarsal," and stress fractures
- Medical longitudinal arch—pronation/supination effects, navicular subluxation, and plantar fasciitis
- Lateral foot—cuboid subluxation, peroneal tendinitis, and fracture of the base of the fifth metatarsal
- Ankle—inversion and eversion sprains
- Achilles tendon/heel—tendinitis, bursitis, and fat pad syndrome

The majority of foot complaints are due to lack of proper support or inappropriate footwear. Points of overpressure or irritation from shoes may result in corns or calluses, sesamoiditis or aggravation of hallux valgus at the first toe, or fat pad syndrome at the heel. Tight-fitting shoes may also cause compression of metatarsals or cause damage to toenails (i.e., black toenails). If the foot is too mobile (i.e., hyperpronated), lack of support may cause plantar fasciitis and strain of the tibialis posterior and other tendons. Therefore it is requisite that shoes be examined and that the foot be evaluated for any predisposition to overstrain due to forefoot or hindfoot abnormalities (i.e., varus or valgus).

Ankle sprains are common. The most common are plantar flexion/inversion sprains. Although most injuries are dismissed as a simple sprain, it is important to rule out associated injury, including various fractures and ligament ruptures. Chronic ankle pain or instability (or both) is not uncommon following repeated ankle sprains. Therefore, it is important not only to manage the acute injury but also to attempt to prevent future occurrences. This often requires a determination of the needs of the associated activity or sport coupled with strict adherence to a postinjury rehabilitation program.

General Strategy

History

- Determine whether the complaint is one of pain, stiffness, popping/snapping, crepitus, locking, weakness, or numbness and tingling.
- Determine whether the patient had a traumatic onset or whether there is an obvious overuse history.
- With overuse, determine the type of activity, the types of shoes worn, and the type of surface on which the patient works or exercises.

Evaluation

- With trauma, palpate for points of tenderness and obtain radiographs for the possibility of fracture/dislocation if the patient is unable to bear weight or bony tenderness is found.
- With ankle sprain, challenge for stability posterior to anterior (drawer test), into inversion (lateral ankle), and into eversion (medial ankle).
- Examine the patient's shoes and feet for signs of excessive wear on the soles of both shoes and feet.
- When the onset is nontraumatic, challenge the musculotendinous attachments with stretch, contraction, and a combination of contraction in a stretched position.
- When trauma or overuse is not present, evaluate the patient's foot and ankle for swelling and deformity (bursitis, gouty tophi, osteoarthritis [OA], etc.).

Management

- Displaced or nonhealing fractures must be referred for medical management.
- Ankle sprains can be managed with mobilization/manipulation, use of a stabilizing brace or taping, and gradual return to weight-bearing with emphasis on prevention.
- Tendinitis and muscle strain can be managed conservatively with taping support, gradual stretching, ice, and activity modification.
- The patient should be educated regarding proper fitting of shoes and the special needs for specific sports requirements and type of foot (pes planus versus pes cavus).
- Orthotics may be a helpful preventive measure when biomechanical abnormalities are found, such as hindfoot or forefoot varus or valgus.
- Diabetic foot problems should be referred to the primary treating physician.

Relevant Anatomy and Biomechanics

Terminology used to describe foot architecture and deformity can be confusing. Basically, the foot is divided into a hindfoot, a midfoot (midtarsal), and a forefoot. Dysfunction in one part of the foot is often accommodated or compensated by movement in another portion of the foot. Following is a brief description of the joints in each section of the foot and definitions of functional or structural deviations that may occur:

- Hindfoot—The hindfoot includes the distal tibiofibular joint. In addition to several ligaments, the two bones are joined by a flexible interosseous membrane. The distance between the bones may widen with dorsiflexion of the ankle, as the talus wedges between the malleoli. With this movement the interosseous membrane is stretched, causing superior movement of the proximal tibiofibular joint with accompanying external rotation; the opposite occurs with plantarflexion. The talar/malleolar joint is referred to as the talocrural joint. The subtalar joint consists of the talus and calcaneus. Stability of this area is provided in part by the ligamentous support of the tibia and fibula, dorsiflexion of the ankle, or supination of the subtalar joint. Ligamentous support at the ankle is provided laterally by three ligaments: (1) the anterior talofibular ligament (supports the ankle against inversion and anterior-to-posterior movement), (2) the posterior talofibular ligament (prevents mainly excessive ankle dorsiflexion and adduction), and (3) the calcaneofibular ligament (a major stabilizer for inversion). The medial side of the ankle is supported by the deltoid ligament, which consists of the tibionavicular, tibiocalcaneal, and anterior and posterior tibiotalar ligaments. These ligaments act together to prevent excessive eversion of the ankle (**Figure 14–1**).
- Midfoot—The midtarsal joints are the interconnections between the talus and calcaneus

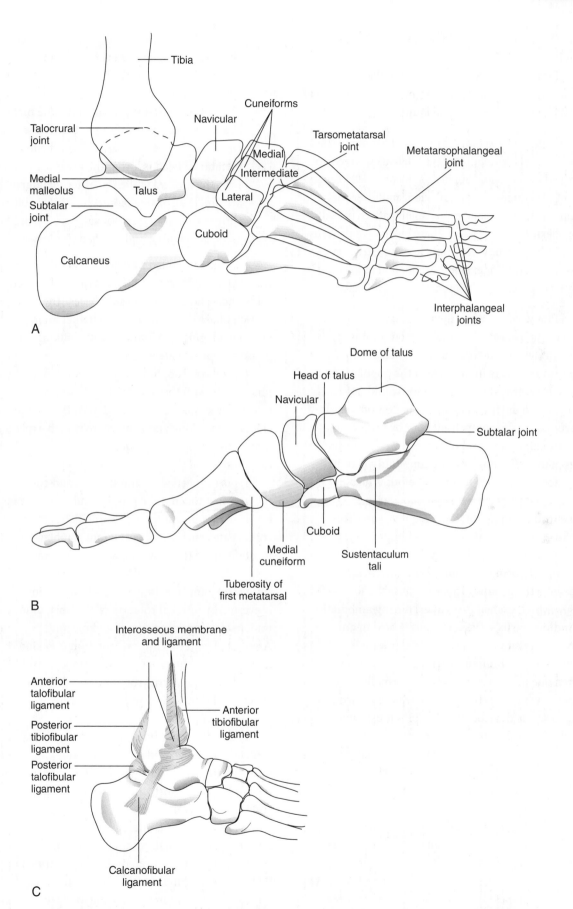

Figure 14–1 (A) Major bones and joints of the foot (lateral view); (B) major bones and joints of the foot (medial view); (C) major ligaments of the ankle joint (lateral view).

and the midtarsal bones, including the cuboid, navicular, and cuneiforms.

- Forefoot—The forefoot is made up of the distal articulations of the metatarsal, metatarsophalangeal (MTP), and interphalangeal joints.

The close-packed position for most of the foot is supination with the exception of the phalanges, which are close-packed in extension. Supination involves a triplanar movement of adduction, plantarflexion, and inversion. Pronation involves a triplanar movement pattern of abduction, dorsiflexion, and eversion. These movement patterns can occur independently in the foot and are often compensatory to each other. For example, supination in the hindfoot may be compensated by pronation in the forefoot.

- Forefoot varus—When the forefoot is held in an inverted position while the subtalar joint is in a neutral position, forefoot varus occurs. This deformity occurs in only 9% of the population.[1] If not compensated for, the first toe would not reach the ground during midstance and toe-off. Forefoot varus is usually compensated for by pronation of the subtalar joint, making this clinically similar to pes planus (flattened medial longitudinal arch).
- Forefoot valgus—When the forefoot is held in an everted position while the subtalar joint is in a neutral position, forefoot valgus occurs. This deformity occurs in 44.8% of a symptomatic population.[2] The midtarsal joint must supinate in an effort to bring the fourth and fifth metatarsal heads to the ground. This will cause the foot to appear high arched (pes cavus) during ambulation.
- Hindfoot varus—The calcaneus is held in an inverted position while the subtalar joint is in neutral with hindfoot (rearfoot) varus. This is often due to a developmental abnormality of the tibia in which it is bowed outward (tibia varum). The result is that the subtalar joint must rapidly pronate through an inordinate range of motion (ROM) in an effort to bring the medial condyle of the calcaneus toward the ground during ground contact. This produces excessive torque in the foot and lower extremity.
- Hindfoot valgus—The calcaneus is held in an everted position while the subtalar joint is in neutral with hindfoot (rearfoot) valgus. The major difficulty with this position is lack of stability at heel contact.
- Equinus (talipes equinus)—Simply put, this is a restriction to dorsiflexion at the talocrural joint.

Most often this is due to contracture of the soleus or gastrocnemius; however, developmental or acquired damage to the talus may also create this problem.

- Plantarflexed first ray—Normally the metatarsal heads are in alignment in the transverse plane when they are dorsiflexed. When the first metatarsal head is lower, the great toe is in contact with the ground while the other metatarsal heads are not, leading to a biomechanical problem similar to that in forefoot valgus. This problem is associated with a high-arched (pes cavus) foot.

Gait is often divided into an ipsilateral swing and a stance phase. The stance phase is divided into contact, midstance, and propulsion subphases. The time spent in each phase is dependent on whether an individual is walking, jogging, or running. With walking, the stance phase is approximately 62% of the total cycle. The contact and propulsion subphases account for 25% of the stance phase each, with the remaining 50% of time spent in the midstance subphase.[3] A basic description of the biomechanics of walking and running may help explain the impact that properly functioning feet have on the lower extremities and the rest of the body.

Support is needed for the split-second contact when the heel first touches the ground and when the foot leaves the ground at toe-off. Immediately after heel contact and during half of the foot-flat phase, the foot must dissipate the ground reaction force and accommodate to different terrain. This is accomplished through a "universal joint" reaction at the subtalar joint. The talus is everted by internal rotation of the tibia, unlocking the midtarsal, talocalcaneal joint and creating pronation. Associated with this internal rotation is flexion of the knee. The combination of these actions helps to dissipate ground forces. External rotation causes the opposite effect of talar inversion and the consequent rigid, locked position of supination.

The subtalar and midtalar joint complex (talocalcaneal, talonavicular, and calcaneocuboid joints) determines movement of most of the foot. However, the medial segment consisting of the first metatarsal and first cuneiform generally moves in a direction opposite that of the rest of the foot. Therefore, even when the hindfoot is structurally normal, compensations may result from abnormalities of the forefoot. Forefoot varus implies that the medial forefoot (the first toe in particular) does not contact the ground unless the foot pronates to bring it down. This is called a compensated forefoot varus.

Forefoot valgus has the opposite effect, with the first metatarsal in contact with the ground without contact of the fifth and fourth metatarsals.

Muscle function across the foot and ankle is quite complex during ambulation. Without reference to weight-bearing, the dorsiflexors of the foot/ankle are the tibialis anterior and peroneus tertius (see **Figure 13–1**). The plantarflexors are the peroneus longus and brevis and the tibialis posterior. Eversion of the foot/ankle is primarily due to the peroneals; inversion, primarily the tibialis anterior and posterior. These are simple uniplanar movement patterns; however, the foot functions more in a triplanar mode. From the standpoint of subtalar joint pronation and supination, tendons that pass medially to the subtalar joint axis are supinators, including the extensor hallucis longus, extensor digitorum longus, tibialis anterior and posterior, and flexors hallucis longus and digitorum longus. Those muscle tendons that pass laterally to the subtalar joint axis are pronators, including the three peroneal muscles. The peroneus longus may act as either a pronator or a supinator based on the position of the first metatarsal.

At heel contact, most lower leg muscles function eccentrically to decelerate imposed pronation. These include the tibialis anterior and posterior, extensor hallucis longus and digitorum, and the soleus/gastrocnemius group. This function indirectly acts as a shock-absorbing strategy by the body and when not optimum leads to anterior shin splints.[4] During midstance there is a dual function of many muscles based on the subphase of midstance. Early in midstance, the tibialis posterior and soleus act eccentrically and in the later phase they contract concentrically to supinate the subtalar and midtarsal joints. In the early midstance phase, the toe flexors also fire eccentrically, assisting the tibialis posterior and soleus in decelerating forward movement of the tibia. During push-off (propulsion) all of the intrinsic foot muscles act to stabilize the foot firing concentrically. The peroneus longus fires concentrically to plantarflex the first ray, as does the flexor digitorum longus. Other first toe muscles fire eccentrically to assist in stabilizing the first metatarsal joint.

Evaluation

History

Careful questioning of the patient during the history taking can point to the diagnosis (**Table 14–1**).

Clarify the type of complaint.

- Is the complaint one of pain, stiffness, looseness, crepitus, deformity, or a combination of complaints?

Table 14–1 History Questions for Foot/Ankle Complaints

Primary Question	What Are You Thinking?	Secondary Questions	What Are You Thinking?
Did you injure your foot?	Inversion or eversion sprain, strain, fracture	Sprain your ankle?	Inversion sprain likely with lateral pain; eversion with medial pain
		Twist ankle with foot planted?	Possible distal tibial or fibular fracture or diastasis
		Did your big toe get forced backward?	Turf toe (capsular sprain of first MTP joint)
		Sudden outside foot pain with pushing-off (e.g., jumping)?	Possible cuboid subluxation or metatarsal fracture (fifth)
		Stubbed toe and still painful?	Fracture of toe
		Heel pain landing from a jump?	Fat pad irritation, bone bruise, fracture
Acute onset of pain with no trauma?	Rheumatoid or crystalline arthritides, plantar fasciitis	Heel pain associated with hand pain?	Rheumatoid arthritis
		Heel pain associated with sacroiliac or low back pain?	Reiter's syndrome or ankylosing spondylitis

(continues)

Table 14–1 History Questions for Foot/Ankle Complaints (continued)

Primary Question	What Are You Thinking?	Secondary Questions	What Are You Thinking?
		Sudden pain in arch?	Plantar fasciitis
Gradual onset of first toe pain?	Hallux valgus, hallux rigidus, sesamoiditis	Hurt more when you pull your big toe back?	Hallux rigidus
		Is your big toe deviated out?	Hallux valgus (associated bunion)
		Pain on the bottom of your big toe?	Sesamoiditis
Gradual onset of pain in other parts of the foot?	Stress fracture, neuroma, tarsal subluxation, metatarsalgia	Stand for long periods of time on hard surfaces or run a lot of miles?	Stress fracture
		Pain on bottom of ball of foot?	Dropped metatarsal (subluxation) or neuroma
		Pain worse with tight shoes?	Metatarsalgia
Numbness and tingling in foot?	Nerve root, tarsal tunnel syndrome, interdigital neuritis	Associated with low back pain?	Nerve root
		On bottom of your foot?	Tarsal tunnel syndrome
		In between your toes?	Interdigital neuritis
			Diabetes
			B12 deficiency

Key: MTP, metatarsal phalangeal.

- Localize the complaint to the ankle, midfoot, or forefoot and then determine whether it is anterior, posterior, medial, or lateral.

Clarify the mechanism if traumatic.

- Plantarflexion/inversion injury to the ankle—Consider inversion ankle sprain with injury to the anterior talofibular, calcaneofibular, and (rarely) posterior talofibular ligaments.
- Dorsiflexion/eversion injury to the ankle—Eversion ankle sprains tear the deltoid ligament and are often associated with dislocation.
- Twisting injury at the ankle with foot fixed (ski boot type injury)—Consider distal tibial and fibular fracture or diastasis.
- Sudden dorsiflexion of the first toe—Turf toe is a sprain of the first MTP joint; the opposite mechanism occurs with sand toe.
- "Stubbing" the toe (especially the fifth toe)—Consider sprain or fracture.
- Lateral foot pain with push-off while jumping—Consider cuboid subluxation and metatarsal fracture.

- Heel pain when landing from a jump—Consider fat pad irritation and bone bruise to the calcaneus; when excessive force is applied, a calcaneal fracture is possible.

Determine whether the mechanism is one of overuse.

- In what position does the patient work? Does the patient stand or walk on hard surfaces?
- What type of footwear does the patient wear? Unsupportive footwear allows foot sprain/strain, high heels force the toes into the toe box and allow shortening of the Achilles tendon.
- If the patient is an athlete, determine the training program, running surface, and type of shoe.
- Are the demands of the sport or activity matched by the shoe design? Cleats may provide support in some settings and in others anchor the foot, causing injury; high-top shoes may provide some ankle stability in some sports while limiting needed motion in others.
- How often does the athlete replace his or her shoes? For high-level activity, every four to six months may be best; at the very least, every nine months.

Determine whether the patient has a current or past history/diagnosis of the foot/ankle complaint or other related disorders.

- Are there associated low back, pelvis, hip, or knee complaints or diagnoses?
- Does the patient have gout, diabetes, arterial insufficiency, varicose veins, or familial predisposition to hallux valgus?

Pain Localization

The following are possible causes of pain based on localization (**Figure 14–2**, A to C, and **Table 14–2**):

Forefoot

- First MTP joint
  1. Acute traumatic—turf toe, sesamoiditis
  2. Nontraumatic—hallux valgus, hallux rigidus, gout

- Fifth metatarsal
  1. Acute traumatic—transverse (Jones) fracture, avulsion fracture, spiral fracture
  2. Nontraumatic—peroneus brevis insertional tendinitis, Iselin's disease (traction apophysitis)
- Metatarsals
  1. Acute traumatic—stress fracture
  2. Nontraumatic—interdigital neuroma (between second and third interspaces), Freiberg's (second metatarsal), stress fracture

Midfoot

- Medial
  1. Acute traumatic—fracture, rupture of plantar fascia, navicular subluxation
  2. Nontraumatic—accessory navicular, Köhler's disease, navicular subluxation, stress fracture, plantar fasciitis

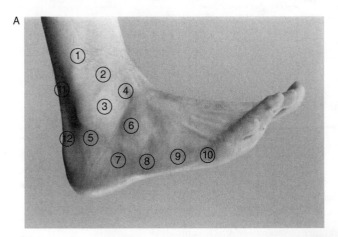
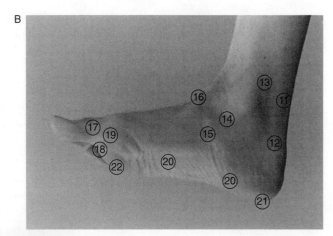
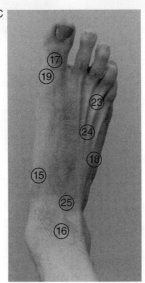

Figure 14–2 (A) Lateral aspect of ankle and foot; (B) medial aspect of ankle and foot; (C) dorsal aspect of ankle and foot.

Table 14–2 Foot and Ankle Pain Localization

#	Significant Structures	Overt Trauma	Insidious or Overuse
1	Peroneus longus and brevis tendons; sural nerve	Contusion of structures	Peroneal tendinitis
2	Anterior tibiofibular ligament	Diastasis with possible associated damage to interosseous membrane	Scar formation from previous ankle injury; talar subluxation
3	Anterior talofibular ligament	Inversion ankle sprain	Scar tissue from previous ankle sprains
4	Peroneus tertius, extensor tendons, superficial peroneal nerve	Contusion of structures	Peroneus tertius or extensor tendinitis
5	Calcaneofibular ligament, peroneal tendons and retinaculum	Inversion ankle sprain with possible torn ligament or retinaculum	Snapping peroneal tendons dislocating due to retinaculum looseness or rupture
6	Extensor digitorum brevis, distal calcaneus, bifurcate ligament	Bifurcate ligament rupture; avulsion fraction of distal calcaneus	Strain of extensor digitorum brevis
7	Cuboid	Cuboid subluxation	Cuboid subluxation
8	Base of fifth metatarsal; peroneus brevis insertion	Avulsion fracture (often secondary to inversion sprain); transverse (Jones) fracture	Iselin's disease (apophysitis), insertional tendinitis
9	Metatarsal shaft	Metatarsal fracture	Stress fracture
10	Fifth MTP joint	Fracture of phalange	Tailor's bunion
11	Achilles tendon	Achilles rupture	Achilles tendinitis
12	Subcutaneous and retrocalcaneal bursae, Haglund's process	Bursitis	Chronic bursitis, pump bump caused by irritation from Haglund's process
13	Tibialis posterior tendon; tibial nerve	Rupture of tibialis posterior tendon	Tibialis posterior tendinitis; tibial nerve compression
14	Deltoid ligament	Eversion ankle sprain	Ligament sprain from overpronation
15	Navicular tubercle	Secondary to eversion sprain; subluxation	Subluxation; accessory navicular, tarsal coalition
16	Tibialis anterior tendon	Strain from plantarflexion injury	Tendinitis
17	Dorsal first MTP joint	Turf toe (hyperextension) or sand toe (hyperflexion) injury to joint capsule	Hallux rigidus
18	Sesamoids	Sesamoid fracture or sesamoiditis	Sesamoiditis
19	Lateral aspect of first MTP joint	Capsular sprain	External bunion associated with hallux valgus; gout
20	Plantar fascia	Plantar fascia rupture	Plantar fasciitis
21	Calcaneus, fat pad	Calcaneal fracture	Fat pad syndrome or inflammation associated with rheumatoid arthritis and Reiter's syndrome
22	Metatarsal heads	Metatarsal subluxation	Morton's neuroma; subluxation
23	Interdigital space	Interdigital neuritis	Interdigital neuritis
24	Metatarsals; extensor tendons	Metatarsal fracture, subluxations	Stress fractures, tendinitis
25	Extensor retinaculum, joint capsule, talus	Capsular sprain, talar subluxation, retinaculum sprain	Capsular sprain, talar subluxation, retinaculum sprain

Note: See Figure 14–2 for localization of numbered areas.

- Lateral
    1. Acute traumatic—fracture, cuboid subluxation
    2. Nontraumatic—cuboid subluxation, peroneus brevis tendinitis
- Anterior
    1. Acute traumatic—fracture, subluxation
    2. Nontraumatic—talar exostosis, anterior tibial nerve compression, subluxation

Hindfoot

- Posterior
    1. Acute traumatic—Achilles rupture, Achilles tendinitis
    2. Nontraumatic—pump bump, Achilles tendinitis, retrocalcaneal bursitis, blisters
- Plantar
    1. Acute traumatic—calcaneal fracture, bone bruise
    2. Nontraumatic—fat pad syndrome, plantar fasciitis, subluxation, Sever's disease

Traumatic and Overuse Injuries

With direct trauma from a blow or dropping an object on the foot, it is always important to consider fracture of the impacted bone. When a sudden pain is felt following landing on the ball or heel, fracture should be suspected. A sudden propulsion (such as quick, forceful push-off for a sprint or jump) may on occasion cause a spiral fracture of the fifth metatarsal. When the pain is located at the first toe, it is important to determine whether there was a hyperextension or a hyperflexion of the toe, each of which is suggestive of capsular sprain.

With ankle injury it is always important to determine the position of the foot: plantarflexed/inverted (lateral stabilizing ligaments) or dorsiflexed/everted (medial stabilizing ligaments). It is extremely important to determine the ability of the patient to bear weight, and the degree and onset of swelling. All of these are important screening questions and observations in determining the need for radiographic screening for fracture. Generally, the inability to bear weight associated with significant swelling correlates with the degree of damage.

Overuse injuries are often subtle. It is important to determine the types of shoes worn by the patient and the types of ground surfaces encountered. It is important in athletes to review the specific requirements of the sport and the ability of the shoes to accommodate. How often does the athlete replace worn-out shoes? Many overuse injuries will be uncovered as a shoe problem (too flexible or loss or lack of shock absorption); too soft or too hard a ground surface; or, in the examination, an underlying varus/valgus deformity of the rearfoot or forefoot. If there is an underlying biomechanical problem, the repetitiveness and frequency of participation become important modifiers.

Weakness

Weakness may be less appreciable directly but indirectly evident because the toes catch on rugs or hit a curb or step when climbing stairs. This indicates neural compromise, especially when the condition is nonpainful. Inability to dorsiflex the ankle indicates primarily tibialis anterior (L4-L5) weakness or perhaps inability to dorsiflex the toes (extensor digitorum) or the big toe (extensor hallucis longus, L5). The physical examination should focus on differentiating between nerve root and peripheral nerve damage. Inability to rise up onto the toes is suggestive of S1 nerve root involvement, especially when nonpainful. Other rare possibilities are rupture of the tibialis posterior in an elderly patient or a patient with rheumatoid arthritis (RA), or Achilles tendon in an athlete.

Instability

Instability is primarily an ankle-related complaint. It is important to determine the number and severity of ankle sprains in the past. It is also important to determine whether footwear relieves this complaint.

Restricted Motion

Restricted motion is not a common foot complaint. The primary occurrence is at the first MTP joint. This is suggestive of hallux rigidus, especially when dorsiflexion is stiff and painful. When the patient complains of ankle stiffness, it is important to determine whether there is any associated pain or crepitus. Pain suggests mechanical blockage from a talar or calcaneal exostosis or scar tissue from a previous ankle injury. When dorsiflexion of the ankle is limited, contracture of the Achilles is likely; however, some equinus deformities due to congenital malformation of the tarsal bones are possible. This is differentiated in the exam through postisometric attempts at increasing movement. The patient may also claim that stretching makes no difference when there is an underlying congenital cause. When end-range positions feel blocked, the examiner should be directed to test for accessory motion restrictions.

Superficial Complaints

There are numerous dermatologic complaints of the feet. It is important first to determine whether the patient is diabetic or has signs/symptoms suggestive of diabetes. Next, it is important to ask about shoe wear. Black toenails and other compressive consequences are common when the shoe is too short and the patient is athletic. Fungal infection between the toes is common and is usually responsive to over-the-counter medications. The patient should be questioned regarding showering in public facilities, the environment of the shoes during activity (are the shoes made of a material that "breathes"?), and how hot/sweaty the feet become with activity. All may be predispositions for fungal growth.

When the patient complains of deformity, the location is often pathognomonic. A bunion at the first MTP indicates hallux valgus. Bony protrusion at the anterior ankle is often due to talar exostosis. Deformity at the posterior heel suggests Haglund's deformity (prominent postero-superior lateral border of the calcaneus) or a pump bump (associated retrocalcaneal bursa).

Numbness and tingling on the bottom of the foot should suggest nerve root or peripheral nerve compression. It is again important to determine whether the patient is diabetic. When the symptom is on the bottom of the foot, an S1 nerve root problem (especially when associated with low back pain complaints) is likely. When the numbness/tingling extends across the bottom of the foot, tarsal tunnel syndrome due to posterior tibial nerve compression is likely. This is often associated with an overpronated foot. When numbness occurs between the toes, interdigital neuritis due to transverse compression of the metatarsals is likely. This is often due to too narrow a shoe.

Examination

The Foot

Prior to examining the feet, it is often helpful to examine the patient's footwear. If the patient is an athlete, it is important for him or her to bring in training shoes. Looking at wear patterns on the shoe may be helpful. Generally, the normal wear pattern is at the ball of the foot and at the lateral heel. Excessive lateral wear at the heel coupled with a caved-in appearance of the inside

of the shoe would suggest pes planus, the opposite for pes cavus. The inside of the shoe should be examined to determine whether any irregularities may act as friction sources to the skin or underlying tendons. Check the shoe for flexibility and shock-absorption characteristics. Is there a firm heel counter? The fit of the shoe is also important to gauge while the patient is standing. Is there sufficient toe room? Is the shoe supportive of the medial longitudinal arch? Does the lacing fit too tightly over the talus or extensor tendons?

Much can be gained through observation of the foot. Look for indications of wear and tear on the foot. These are often clues to various foot deformities.

- Callus or corn formation at the dorsal aspect of the proximal interphalangeal (PIP) joint is seen with both hammer toes (flexion deformity of the PIP joint) and claw toes (dorsal subluxation of the MTP joint). A callus is also found at the plantar MTP joint with claw toes. Mallet toe (flexion contracture of the distal interphalangeal [DIP] joint) causes callus formation at the DIP joint and distal toe.
- Bunion development on the medial aspect of the first MTP joint is indicative of hallux valgus.
- Bunion development is also seen on the fifth MTP joint and is referred to as a tailor's bunion or a bunionette. It is often due to forefoot valgus.
- Callus formation under the second through third or fourth metatarsal heads is found with forefoot varus.
- Callus formation under the first, second, and sometimes third metatarsal heads is found with forefoot valgus.

If the patient is complaining of numbness and/or tingling of the foot, a search for neural irritation begins with a test of nerve root integrity with deep tendon reflex testing and sensory testing. The foot is primarily innervated by the L4-S2 nerve roots. If intact, a search for local nerve irritation focuses on the patient's localization. When there is numbness/tingling on the bottom of the foot, Tinel's test (tapping) of the posterior tibial nerve behind the medial malleolus may reveal tarsal tunnel syndrome. If the location of the symptom is more in the toes (possible associated motor loss), Tinel's test is performed at the anterior ankle at the anterior tibial branch of the deep peroneal nerve. If the patient's symptom extends from the medial knee down through the medial foot, testing with compression at the adductor tunnel or Tinel's test performed below the medial joint line of the knee may reveal saphenous nerve involvement. If sensation is decreased between the first two toes, the deep peroneal nerve is compromised. If there is numbness between the other toes, interdigital nerve compression is likely. When there is pain and numbness and tingling on the bottom of the ball of the foot, palpation for a neuroma between the second and third or third and fourth metatarsal spaces should be performed. Passive extension of the toes may increase the complaint, and some relief may be provided by passive flexion.

Determination of forefoot and rearfoot valgus and varus is usually performed with the patient prone. The opposite leg is brought into flexion on the table to neutralize rotation of the examined extremity. The initial positioning of the foot is an attempt at finding subtalar neutral (**Figure 14–3**). The approach is described generally in two ways:

1. The foot is grasped at the fourth and fifth metatarsal heads and passively dorsiflexed until resistance is felt. The foot is then supinated and pronated until a point is found where slightly more movement in either direction causes the talus to "fall off" to one side or the other. This is the neutral position.

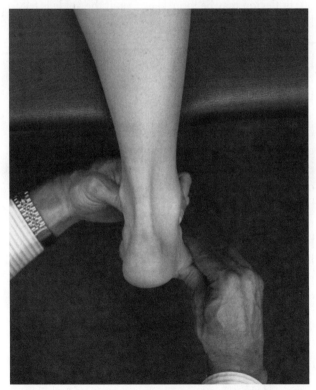

Figure 14–3 Neutral position of foot. Palpating the talus with the index finger and thumb, the examiner pronates and supinates the foot until the talus is felt equally by both contacts. The fourth and fifth metatarsal heads are then passively dorsiflexed.

2. The foot is grasped at the fourth and fifth metatarsal heads and distracted downward to remove dorsiflexion. The foot is then passively inverted and everted while the examiner palpates the talus with the thumb and middle finger. There will be a point at which the talus is felt by both thumb and finger or not at all by either. This is the neutral position.[5]

At this point a determination of the degree of hindfoot varus and valgus can be determined by connecting intersecting lines through the tibia (Achilles) and the calcaneus. If the calcaneus is within 2° to 8° of varus, the leg-to-heel alignment is normal. When the heel is inverted, hindfoot varus is present; if everted, hindfoot valgus is present. Through the use of a plastic goniometer placed against the metatarsal heads, the degree of forefoot valgus or varus should be measured.[6]

The patient can also be examined from behind in the standing position. The angle formed by the lower third of the Achilles and the calcaneus can be determined, indicating statically a tendency toward pronation (hindfoot valgus) or supination (hindfoot varus). When the patient is asked to raise onto his or her toes, a medial longitudinal arch should form. If there is no arch in this position, tarsal coalition (fibrous or bony connection between tarsal bones) or rupture of the tibialis posterior tendon is likely. Various forms of navicular positioning testing have been suggested. One is the Feiss line. This line represents a connection between the apex of the medial malleolus and the length of the first metatarsal. The navicular tuberosity is usually at a point along this line. When the patient stands with equal weight between the feet (about 6 in. apart), the navicular should remain in close proximity to this line. The farther it drops away, the more pronated the individual. A similar test is the navicular drop test (**Figure 14–4**, A and B). A paper card is placed alongside the foot with the patient not bearing weight. The navicular tuberosity position is marked on the card. The patient then bears his or her weight onto the foot and the distance between the original mark and the mark of the new navicular tubercle position is measured. Greater than about 0.5 in. implies a hyperpronated foot.

Radiographic assessment of the foot is dictated by whether the intention is a search for fracture or whether a biomechanical appreciation of the foot is desired. Fracture is usually evident on non-weight-bearing views. The standard series consists of an anteroposterior (AP [dorsiplantar]) view, an oblique (lateral aspect of foot elevated 30°) view, and a lateral view. On the AP view,

A

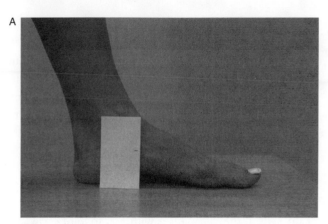

B

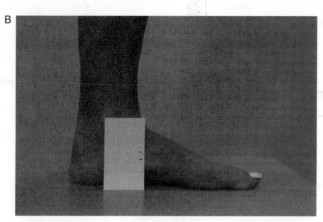

Figure 14–4 The navicular drop test for pronation. (A) The patient's navicular tubercle is marked while the patient is not bearing weight. (B) The position is then again marked when the patient bears weight onto the foot. If the difference between marks is greater than 5⁄8 in., the patient is probably functionally a pronator.

the forefoot and part of the midfoot are well visualized. The oblique view gives an excellent alternate perspective of the metatarsals. The talonavicular and calcaneocuboid joints and sinus tarsi are also demonstrated on this view. Calcaneonavicular coalition (bony bridging) is best seen on the medial oblique view. The lateral view is excellent for viewing the calcaneus, talus, navicular, cuboid, first cuneiform, and head of the fifth metatarsal. In addition to fractures, bony exostosis may be seen on the talus, calcaneus, or fifth metatarsal head. Additional views are designed to visualize the phalanges, sesamoids, calcaneus, and talus.

If the intention is to obtain a more functional perspective of the foot, weight-bearing films are often used. Numerous lines of mensuration are used to evaluate the biomechanical relationship of the foot on these views, a description of which is beyond the scope of this text. However, the most commonly used is the Cyma line.[7] On the lateral view, the articulation between the talonavicular and calcaneocuboid (Chopart's joint) forms a continuous S-shaped line. A break in the line anteriorly at the talus indicates pronation; a break posteriorly indicates supination.

The Ankle

The ability to bear weight is an important screening maneuver with ankle sprains. If the patient is able to bear weight, palpation of specific bony landmarks including the malleoli, navicular, and cuboid areas will help determine the need for radiographs.[8] The ankle is tested primarily for stability. Three tests are commonly used. The first is the anterior drawer test (**Figure 14–5A**). This test is performed with the patient supine and the ankle plantarflexed 15° to 20°.[9] This position places the anterior talofibular ligament perpendicular to the tibia. The

examiner pulls forward by stabilizing on the anterior distal tibia with one hand and the other hand pulls forward while cupping the calcaneus posteriorly. While analogous to the anterior drawer test of the knee, the more collateral ligamentous system is being tested in the ankle. With an inversion sprain the anterior talofibular ligament may be damaged. The anterior drawer test will reveal some laxity when compared with the opposite ankle. To eliminate stabilization from the Achilles, testing with the knee in 90° of flexion may be more sensitive. If the ankle is felt to be unstable in dorsiflexion, damage to the collateral and deep system of ligaments is likely. The talar tilt test is simply an inversion stress applied to the ankle. The best position is side-lying with the patient's knee flexed 90° with the hands cupped around the ankle, imparting an inversion force (**Figure 14–5B**). The talar tilt tests for integrity of the calcaneofibular ligament. The Kleiger test is an eversion test of the ankle.[10] With the patient seated on the examination table, the non-weight-bearing foot is everted out to test for the medial deltoid ligament complex.

The stabilizing function of muscles and the presence of tendinitis may be evaluated by basic resisted movement patterns coupled with stretch patterns. Also, resisting the movement pattern starting from the stretched position will reveal tendinitis not evident from neutral position testing.

- Dorsiflexion/eversion—mainly due to the peroneus tertius; stretching into plantarflexion/inversion may also increase pain.
- Dorsiflexion/inversion—mainly due to the tibialis anterior; stretching into dorsiflexion/eversion may also increase pain.
- Plantarflexion/eversion—mainly due to the peroneus longus and brevis; stretching into plantarflexion usually is more painful than dorsiflexion.

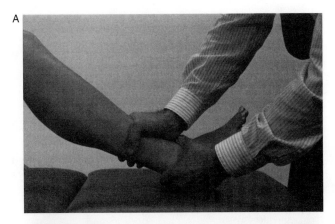

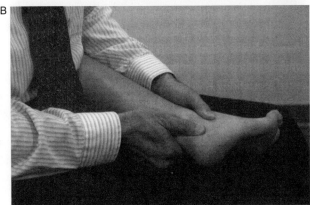

Figure 14–5 (A) The anterior drawer test. With the knee flexed and the ankle flexed to 15°, the examiner stabilizes the tibia while pulling forward on the calcaneus. (B) Inversion test for lateral ankle stability.

- Plantarflexion/inversion—mainly due to the tibialis posterior; stretching into dorsiflexion may also increase pain.

Radiographic assessment of the ankle is primarily used to rule out associated fracture. Ankle injury is extremely common, yet only 15% of patients will be found to have a fracture. The authors of the study have estimated that approximately $500 million is spent on ankle radiographs in the United States and Canada each year. According to this study, if the rules or guidelines were used, there could be an estimated savings of over $100 million without loss of quality of care.[11] Due to many factors—including the fear of malpractice, patient demands, and habit—radiographs are ordered on the majority of patients. The team of physicians who designed the Ottawa Ankle Rules found that the only consistent (sensitive and specific) history and examination findings that were relevant were pain in the malleolar region and either (1) tenderness at either malleolus or (2) the inability to bear weight immediately after the injury or in the emergency department.

For the mid-foot, the relevant findings were pain in the mid-foot area and either (1) tenderness at the base of the fifth metatarsal, (2) tenderness at the navicular, or (3) the inability to bear weight immediately after the injury or in the emergency department (**Exhibit 14–1**).

No significant fractures were missed when these rules were used at two major hospital emergency departments or outpatient clinics evaluating more than 2,300 adults. A significant fracture is defined as greater than 3 mm in breadth. Many small malleolar tip fractures do not require casting or pinning.

Researchers in a recent study used a modified version of the Ottawa Rules, called the "Buffalo" Rule, which switched the site of tenderness from the posterior borders of the malleoli to the midline away from ligament attachments to avoid false-positive responses.[12] Of 153 patients, there were six clinically significant fractures. Sensitivity for the ankle was 100%, with a specificity of 40%; specificity for foot fractures was 79%. There were no false-negative results. Potential reduction in ankle x-rays was 46%; for foot x-rays it was 79%. Standard views include an AP, a lateral, and a mortise view (AP with 20° of internal rotation of the foot). Stress views may be indicated when there is a need to distinguish between a single-ligament and a two-ligament injury. The talar tilt is the degree of opening between the tibia and talus when stressed into inversion as viewed on an AP view. More than 10° of tilt indicates injury to the anterior talofibular and calcaneofibular ligaments (positive predictive value between 85% and 99%).[13] The mortise view is helpful in revealing osteochondral fracture of the talus (seen less clearly on the straight AP view) and diastasis due to interosseous membrane rupture between the tibia and fibula.

The Heel

The primary differential of plantar heel pain is between plantar fasciitis and fat pad syndrome. In patients with a history of rheumatoid conditions, radiographs may prove helpful in detecting characteristic changes, yet these conditions would rarely present solely as heel pain. The primary distinction between fat pad syndrome and plantar fasciitis is the location of tenderness. Fat pad tenderness is directly in the middle of the heel. This tenderness is decreased by squeezing the bottom of the heel together and pressing over the same tender area. By squeezing the heel together, the remaining fat pad is approximated, providing more cushioning; tenderness should decrease substantially. Plantar fasciitis is painful at the medial heel because of the attachment to the medial tuberosity of the

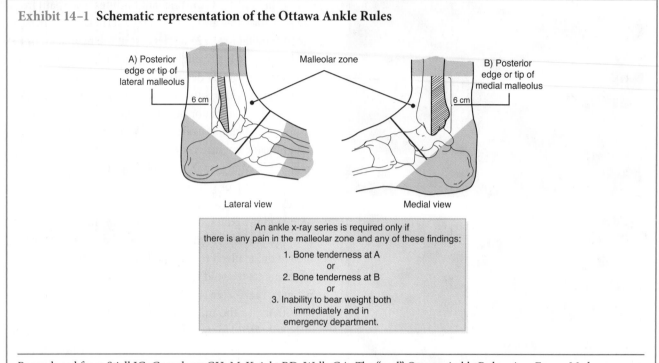

Exhibit 14–1 Schematic representation of the Ottawa Ankle Rules

A) Posterior edge or tip of lateral malleolus

Malleolar zone

B) Posterior edge or tip of medial malleolus

6 cm

6 cm

Lateral view

Medial view

An ankle x-ray series is required only if there is any pain in the malleolar zone and any of these findings:

1. Bone tenderness at A
or
2. Bone tenderness at B
or
3. Inability to bear weight both immediately and in emergency department.

Reproduced from Stiell IG, Greenberg GH, McKnight RD, Wells GA. The "real" Ottawa Ankle Rules. *Ann Emerg Med.* 1996;27:103–104, with permission from Elsevier.

calcaneus. Pain or tenderness may be increased through passive tension. This is accomplished by dorsiflexing the first toe and, if not positive, adding dorsiflexion of the ankle. The pain with plantar fasciitis is often across the bottom of the foot along the medial longitudinal arch.

Radiographic examination is warranted if there is trauma such as landing on the feet, if the patient is an adolescent (Sever's disease), or if there is a history of rheumatoid disease. Radiographs for plantar fasciitis are usually misleading because of the appearance of a heel spur. The heel spur is falsely accused of being the cause of the patient's pain. Resolution of pain without changes in the spur is the usual course of events. It is believed that the spur is a consequence of plantar fascial tension rather than a cause of plantar fasciitis.[14]

Management

Traumatic Injury

- Most fractures of the foot and ankle should be referred for reduction and casting; some exceptions include small, nondisplaced avulsion fractures at the fifth metatarsal or lateral malleolus (period of immobilization may be needed) and most toe fractures, which can be buddy-taped for two to three weeks.
- Sprains of the MTP capsules can be managed with appropriate taping, mild mobilization, and support.
- Ankle sprains are managed based on the degree of injury. Even full-ligament rupture (third-degree) can be managed conservatively with a cast and graduated return to weight-bearing and activity, although comanagement or previous experience is suggested prior to following this approach (**Table 14–3**).

Overuse and/or Biomechanical Injury

- Overuse injuries are often treated symptomatically with ice, myofascial stretching, and modification of activity; long-term management includes modification of footwear, terrain, maintenance of proper accessory motion, functional training of supportive muscles focusing on eccentric or concentric needs, and possible prescription of orthotic support.
- Stress fractures can be managed by immobilization with non-weight-bearing for two to six weeks, depending on activity level; aerobic conditioning

Table 14–3 Ankle Inversion Sprain Rehabilitation

Parameter	Acute Stage	Subacute Stage	Chronic Stage
Criteria	Lateral ankle swelling is dependent on degree of injury; pain and possible instability found with ankle inversion stress; radiograph to rule out fracture.	Swelling has decreased; some lateral ankle pain with inversion stress.	No swelling, mild lateral ankle pain on inversion stress.
Goals	Reduce swelling and pain; avoid full weight-bearing.	Progress to full weight-bearing through the use of crutches and ankle support (Air-Splint, taping, or brace).	Proprioceptively stabilize the ankle; correct any underlying predispositions; consider taping with aggressive sport activity.
Concerns	Possible fracture of tibia, fibula, talus, metatarsals; bifurcate ligament rupture; peroneal tendon dislocation.	Talar dome fracture not evident on radiograph.	Too early a return to sports activity; during restrengthening athlete needs external support.
Requirements for progression to next stage including approximate time needed	Partial weight-bearing possible; reduction in swelling and pain; 1–3 days.	Full weight-bearing without crutches; no swelling evident; full ROM 2–3 days.	Able to balance on one leg and hop on one leg without pain; 1–2 weeks.
Manipulation/mobilization	Based on the degree of injury; general talar or tibial adjustment (opposite position of injury-dorsiflexion/eversion) may assist.	General talar or tibial adjustment may assist.	Determine need for navicular, cuboid, calcaneal, and talar adjusting.
Modalities	Ice 3–5 times/day for 20 minutes (1 hour in between); rest, elevation, TENS or EMS (high-volt galvanic at 80–120 Hz with ice for 20 min/1–2 times/day).	Ice after activity; combination ultrasound/EMS at 1.0 watt/ cm^2,1–15 Hz for 6–8 minutes.	Ice after activity.
External brace, support, etc.	Air-Splint or open Gibney type of ankle taping, or Unna boot splint; crutch walking with toe touching only.	Air-Splints or lace-up brace; patient weaned off crutches after 1–2 days of gradual weight-bearing.	Figure-of-eight elastic bandage support with walking if necessary; taping for sports activities.
ROM/flexibility	Mild passive ROM.	BAPS board begun with the patient seated; postisometric relaxation approach to stretching.	Continue stretching with postisometric approach.
Open-chain exercise	Mild isometrics in neutral.	Isometrics at end-range into dorsiflexion and eversion; passive PNF diagonal patterns; side-lying straight leg raises for peroneals and hip abductors.	Elastic tubing exercises for dorsiflexors and evertors; resisted PNF diagonal patterns.
Closed-chain exercise	None.	Gradual two-legged toe raises and half squats	Toe raises against resistance.
Proprioceptive training	Toe touching with crutch use.	Consider weight-bearing with TENS application; taping or support acts as a proprioceptive stimulus.	Progression to weight-bearing exercises on BAPS (wobble) board; follow progressive training.

(continues)

Table 14–3 Ankle Inversion Sprain Rehabilitation (continued)

Parameter	Acute Stage	Subacute Stage	Chronic Stage
Associated biomechanical items	Check for weakness of hip abductors; evaluate for pronation or supination.	Shoes should contain a rigid heel counter; orthotic prescription should be performed if deemed necessary and swelling has decreased enough for casting.	Orthotic fitting.
Lifestyle/activity modifications	Crutch walking only for first 1–3 days with grade 2 injuries.	Crutch walking should involve partial weight-bearing, continuing to elimination of crutch use.	Stretch prior to activities such as running and jogging.

Key: ROM, range of motion; TENS, transcutaneous electrical nerve stimulation; EMS, electrical muscle stimulation; BAPS, biomechanical ankle platform system (Medipedic [Jackson, Michigan]); PNF, proprioceptive neuromuscular facilitation.

may be continued with non-weight-bearing activities (e.g., pool running).

Preventive Management

- Preventive management for ankle sprains includes isometric training of the peroneals, hip abductors, and tibialis anterior with stretching of the Achilles; proprioceptive training using taping, proprioceptive neuromuscular facilitation (PNF) techniques, or balance exercises with balance boards.
- Patient education regarding proper selection of shoes and foot hygiene is an important tool by which to avoid future problems.

An in-depth discussion of shoe design and prescription is beyond the scope of this text; however, some basics can be reviewed (**Figure 14–6**). The commonly

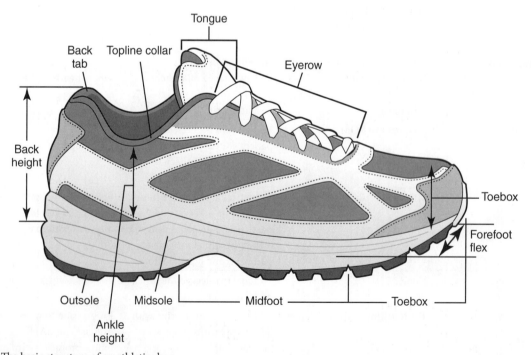

Figure 14–6 The basic structure of an athletic shoe.

used terminology and maxims for shoe construction are as follows:

- The heel counter should be deep and firm to provide stability and cushioning.
- The shank should be strong and should not deform with weight-bearing (the shank represents the portion on the bottom of the shoe that corresponds to the medial longitudinal arch).
- The toe box should be spacious enough to avoid compression of the metatarsals.
- The shoe should be long enough to avoid compression of the toes at the end of the toe box.
- If used in a sporting activity, the shoe should be specific to the sport.

The mold upon which the shoe is constructed is referred to as the *last*. There are essentially two types, straight last and curved last. The straight last is a better design for the pronated foot. The curved last design is for a forefoot angled medially. This shoe design is better for the supinated foot and/or those with hallux valgus. There are generally three types of last construction: (1) the board-lasted shoe, (2) the slip-lasted shoe, and (3) the combination-last shoe (**Figure 14–7**). When a patient's foot is severely pronated, the board-lasted shoe is usually best because of the support provided by a hard fibrous material placed on the inner surface of the shoe.

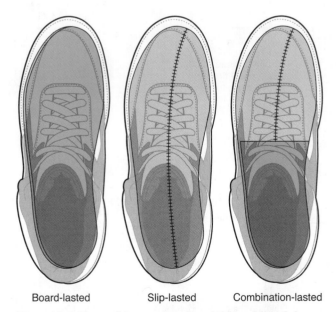

Board-lasted   Slip-lasted   Combination-lasted

Figure 14–7 Types of shoe construction: (A) board-lasted shoe, (B) slip-lasted shoe, (C) combination last shoe.

The slip-lasted shoe is constructed by stitching the upper into a one-piece moccasin and then gluing it to the sole. This provides a lighter, more flexible shoe; however, it has less stability. This shoe construction is probably better for the cavus foot. The combination-last shoe combines a board-lasted heel with a slip-lasted forefoot, the best of both worlds. This shoe construction is best for those with rearfoot varus or mild pronators.

A prescription for orthotics is often given to the patient with foot pain. An orthotic is a device that is usually placed in the shoe to accommodate for biomechanical abnormalities or to cushion painful areas. The biomechanical orthotic can be constructed according to individual need or purchased as an off-the-shelf product. The type of orthotic is often based on the seriousness or complexity of the problem and the patient's ability to purchase the product. The three common types of customized orthotics are the non-weight-bearing, casted orthotic; non-weight-bearing, vacuum-applied orthotic; and weight-bearing foam impression orthotic. There is much emotional debate as to the best way to cast the feet. The foam impression orthotic supporters claim that it is a "functional" orthotic giving an individual impression of the patient's foot in a closed-packed position. The argument against this approach is that the feet are casted in an imperfect position and allowed to splay and elongate with weight-bearing. The non-weight-bearing cast proponents claim that the foot is casted in the neutral "perfect" position and that the type of orthotic and the measurements used in the prescription allow for more individualized approaches through the use of forefoot and rearfoot posting. Also, if the individual has exostosis, bunions, or other abnormalities, the orthotic can be modified to accommodate.

There are generally two types of posting, rearfoot and forefoot. A rearfoot varus (medial) post is used to control or limit the calcaneal eversion and associated internal rotation of the tibia shortly after heel strike. Of course, the opposite principle is used for rearfoot valgus (lateral) posting; it is used to evert the calcaneus and therefore bring the subtalar joint closer to the optimal neutral position. Forefoot varus may be compensated for by a medial post, whereas forefoot valgus is best supported by a lateral post. This is particularly helpful when rearfoot compensation occurs to accommodate for forefoot abnormalities. Heel lifts are occasionally used for problems involving the Achilles tendon. When the Achilles tendon is tight, it may augment the effect of rearfoot problems. The use of a heel lift (3 to 6 mm) may decrease the tension of the Achilles and therefore its effect on rearfoot motion. A partial heel lift, referred to as a medial or lateral wedge, may also be used temporarily as an insert to test the feasibility of posting for patients who are reluctant to purchase the more expensive casted orthotic.

Algorithms

Algorithms for traumatic or sudden onset of foot pain, nontraumatic or insidious onset of foot pain, and initial ankle sprain evaluation are presented in **Figures 14–8** through **14–10**.

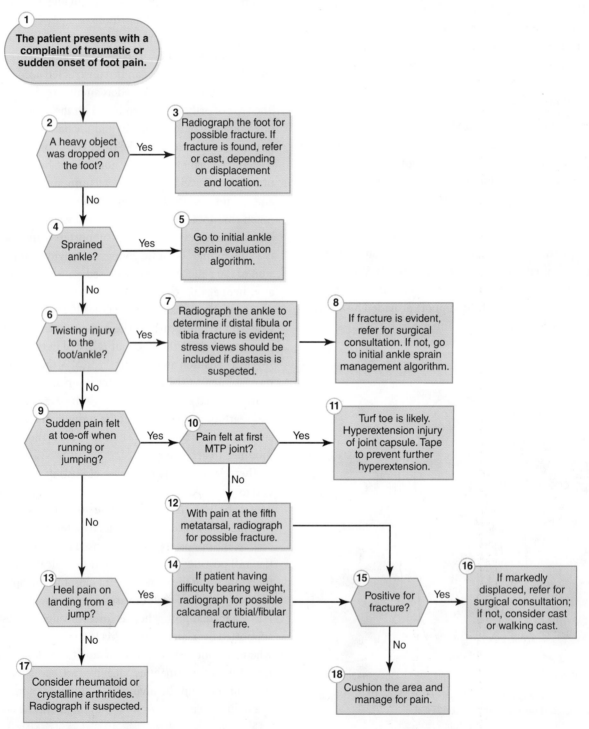

Figure 14–8 Traumatic or Sudden Onset of Foot Pain—Algorithm

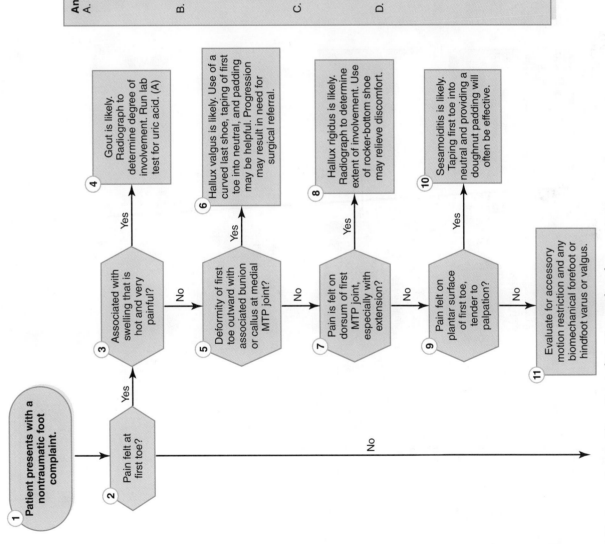

Annotations

A. Gout is a metabolic disease associated with excessive urates in the body. Deposition of urate crystals at the first toe (podagra) causes an acute inflammatory reaction. Late changes on radiograph include punched-out areas (radiolucent urate tophi).

B. Tarsal coalition is a congenital condition where fibrous, cartilaginous, or osseous bridging occurs between two or more tarsal bones. CT is often needed to visualize because many coalitions are not ossified. A flat-foot deformity due to coalition may be responsive to orthotics, but the success rate is not high; surgery is often needed in active individuals.

C. Iselin's disease is a traction apophysitis of the base of the fifth metatarsals. It is a rare disorder that, like Osgood-Schlatter disease of the knee, responds to taping or other support, and modification of the inciting activity.

D. A distinction must be made between Jones fractures and avulsion fractures. Avulsion fractures are usually due to inversion ankle sprains where the peroneus brevis may avulse part of the base of the fifth metatarsal. These are relatively stable and displacement is small. Transverse or Jones fractures are usually slightly distal to the base and are known for a higher potential of nonunion.

continues

1 Patient presents with a nontraumatic foot complaint.

2 Pain felt at first toe?

Yes

3 Associated with swelling that is hot and very painful?

Yes

4 Gout is likely. Radiograph to determine degree of involvement. Run lab test for uric acid. (A)

No

5 Deformity of first toe outward with associated bunion or callus at medial MTP joint?

Yes

6 Hallux valgus is likely. Use of a curved last shoe, taping of first toe into neutral, and padding may be helpful. Progression may result in need for surgical referral.

No

7 Pain is felt on dorsum of first MTP joint, especially with extension?

Yes

8 Hallux rigidus is likely. Radiograph to determine extent of involvement. Use of rocker-bottom shoe may relieve discomfort.

No

9 Pain felt on plantar surface of first toe, tender to palpation?

Yes

10 Sesamoiditis is likely. Taping first toe into neutral and providing a doughnut padding will often be effective.

No

11 Evaluate for accessory motion restriction and any biomechanical forefoot or hindfoot varus or valgus.

No

Figure 14–9 Nontraumatic or Insidious Onset of Foot Pain—Algorithm

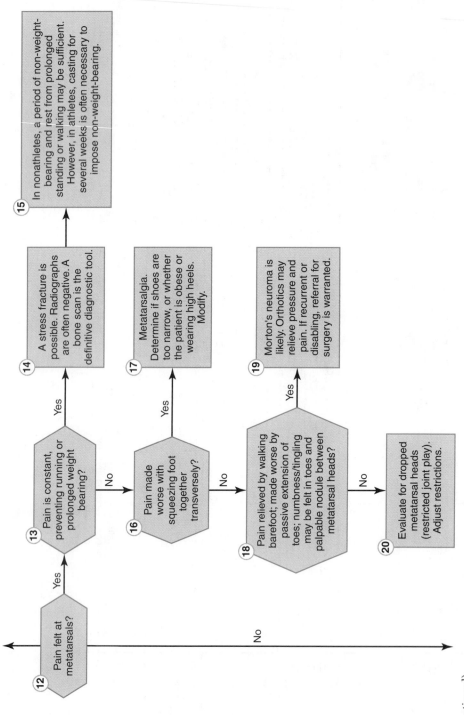

Figure 14-9 (Continued)

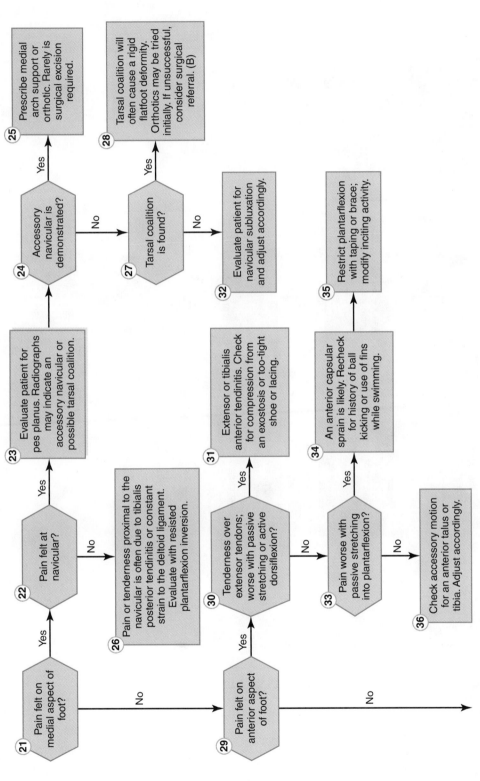

Figure 14-9 (Continued)

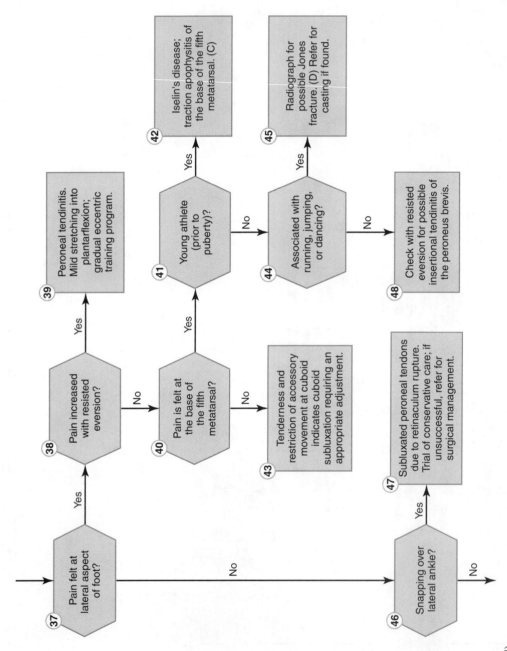

Figure 14–9 (Continued)

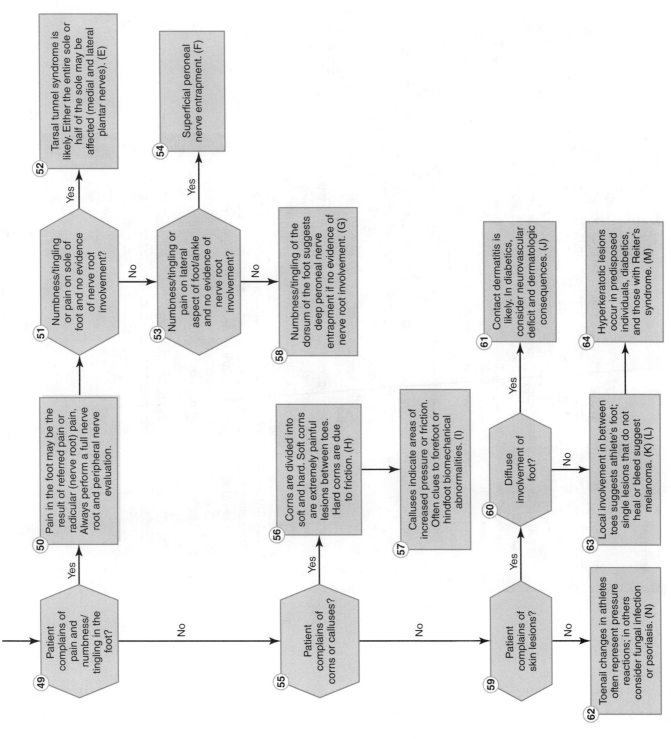

49 Patient complains of pain and numbness/tingling in the foot?

— Yes →

50 Pain in the foot may be the result of referred pain or radicular (nerve root) pain. Always perform a full nerve root and peripheral nerve evaluation.

↑

51 Numbness/tingling or pain on sole of foot and no evidence of nerve root involvement?

— Yes →

52 Tarsal tunnel syndrome is likely. Either the entire sole or half of the sole may be affected (medial and lateral plantar nerves). (E)

↓ No

53 Numbness/tingling or pain on lateral aspect of foot/ankle and no evidence of nerve root involvement?

— Yes →

54 Superficial peroneal nerve entrapment. (F)

↓ No

58 Numbness/tingling of the dorsum of the foot suggests deep peroneal nerve entrapment if no evidence of nerve root involvement. (G)

— No →

55 Patient complains of corns or calluses?

— Yes →

56 Corns are divided into soft and hard. Soft corns are extremely painful lesions between toes. Hard corns are due to friction. (H)

→

57 Calluses indicate areas of increased pressure or friction. Often clues to forefoot or hindfoot biomechanical abnormalities. (I)

— No →

59 Patient complains of skin lesions?

— Yes →

60 Diffuse involvement of foot?

— Yes →

61 Contact dermatitis is likely. In diabetics, consider neurovascular deficit and dermatologic consequences. (J)

↓ No

63 Local involvement in between toes suggests athlete's foot; single lesions that do not heal or bleed suggest melanoma. (K) (L)

↑

64 Hyperkeratotic lesions occur in predisposed individuals, diabetics, and those with Reiter's syndrome. (M)

— No →

62 Toenail changes in athletes often represent pressure reactions; in others consider fungal infection or psoriasis. (N)

Figure 14–9 (Continued)

Annotations (continued)

E. Tarsal tunnel syndrome may be due to trauma or hyperpronation. Orthotic management with appropriate foot manipulation is usually effective. However, surgical decompression may be necessary with causes other than pronation.

F. Involvement of the superficial peroneal nerve is usually due to ankle sprains. If orthotic support is ineffective, refer for lidocaine/cortisone injection.

G. The deep peroneal nerve may be compressed by tightly laced shoes or talar osteophytes. Shoe modification may be effective. Talar osteophytes may need surgical excision.

H. Hard corns are seen with hammer toes and claw toes; especially at the fifth toe. Treatment involves paring and padding the area, and shoe modification.

I. Calluses under the first metatarsal head is found with forefoot valgus; under the second, third, and fourth with forefoot varus.

J. The diabetic foot is prone to vascular insufficiency and infection. Neurologic compromise often eliminates the painful warning needed to alert the patient to a problem.

K. Athlete's foot is a fungal infection that occurs mainly in the lateral toewebs. Made worse by toe approximation from shoes, warm weather, and activity. Try OTC drugs first. Keep feet dry and use shoes that can aerate.

L. Malignant melanoma is rare; however, any bleeding lesion or nonhealing lesion requires dermatologic referral.

M. Hyperkeratosis may be hereditary or acquired. Fissures may develop and predispose the diabetic to infection. Fissures may be glued together (Krazy glue); general treatment is with topical keratolytics and buffing away thick layers.

N. When the shoe box is too tight, pressure on toenails may result in "black" toenails or other changes. Psoriatic involvement usually occurs on all the toes. Fungal infection usually occurs with "skipped" normal nails.

Figure 14–9 (Continued)

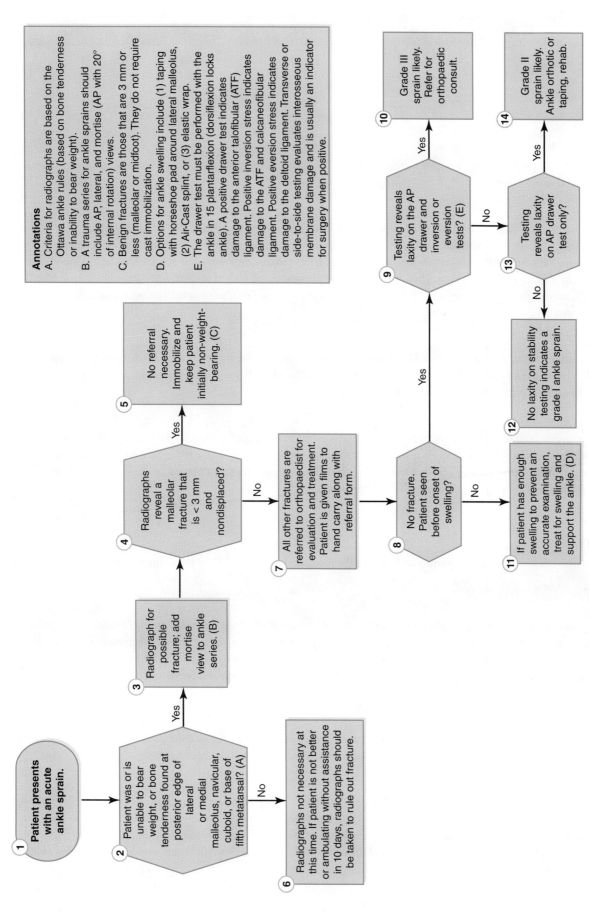

Figure 14–10 Initial Ankle Sprain Evaluation—Algorithm

Selected Foot Disorders*

FIRST TOE

Sesamoiditis

Classic Presentation

The patient presents with pain on the bottom of the great toe. He or she may remember the onset occurring while pushing-off with the toe or after forced dorsiflexion.

Cause

Either direct trauma or overpull from the flexor hallucis brevis may cause irritation of the sesamoids. The sesamoids serve as anchors and help to form the pulley for the flexor hallucis longus. They are the attachment points for the flexor hallucis brevis and adductor hallucis and abductor hallucis. Predisposition to sesamoiditis appears related to concomitant hallux valgus, too-flexible footwear, and repetitive running or walking on hard surfaces. These small bones may be associated with many processes, including a local bursitis, chondromalacia, fracture, stress fracture, bipartite development, OA, and secondary involvement with collagen/vascular, rheumatoid, or gouty processes.

Evaluation

Tenderness is felt at the plantar surface of the first MTP joint. Of the two sesamoids, the medial is often involved and more tender to palpation.[15] This is particularly evident when the first toe is passively dorsiflexed. Radiographs may reveal an underlying process such as a stress fracture, osteochondritis, bipartite sesamoids, or OA.

Management

The treatment for sesamoiditis is to tape the toe to prevent dorsiflexion and to use initially a doughnut-shaped padding to relieve direct pressure on the sesamoids. If there is an associated hallux valgus, it may be helpful to tape the great toe into adduction. Preventive measures are to determine the need for a less flexible shoe and recommend against playing or working on hard surfaces if this is a viable option. There are surgical procedures, but they are rarely needed.

Hallux Valgus

Classic Presentation

The patient presents with a complaint of deformity and pain on the medial side of the first MTP joint. The patient often is a middle-aged woman.

Cause

Hallux valgus involves lateral deviation (abduction) of the proximal phalanx of the first toe. There is a strong hereditary component with accelerating factors such as forefoot varus, Morton's deformity, inflammatory arthritis, and the frequent wearing of high heels. The deviation causes pressure to occur at the first MTP joint with subsequent development of a localized bursitis and bunion formation. Further deviation creates a sling effect whereby pull of the flexor hallucis longus and brevis and extensor hallucis longus tendons creates more deviation.[16]

Evaluation

The deformity is apparent, with the first toe deviating outward and the medial MTP joint visibly enlarged. If there is an apparent inflammatory process occurring or a history of a rheumatoid condition, a radiograph may be necessary.

Management

When deviation progresses, the patient must decide whether or not to have surgery. There are many different types of surgeries, and the recovery time with each varies. Conservative options are usually an attempt to slow the process of deviation. Taping to bring the first toe into neutral and padding over the bunion area are often tried first. Keeping the joint mobile with adjustments may be beneficial. Additional approaches include paring down the bunion, buying shoes with larger toe boxes, and avoiding the wearing of high heels. Some practitioners suggest a restraining device worn during sleep.

*See also Chapter 13, Lower Leg Complaints.

Hallux Rigidus

Classic Presentation

The patient presents with first toe pain felt on the dorsal surface. The patient is usually elderly or may be an athlete with repetitive capsular sprains.

Cause

Osteoarthritic and capsular changes occur at the first metatarsal joint as a result of aging or repeated capsular sprains.[17] Other causes may be an underlying inflammatory arthritic or systemic disease. When this process occurs at other metatarsal heads, it is referred to as Freiberg's infraction—aseptic subchondral cancellous bone necrosis. Hallux rigidus is analogous to or may be Freiberg's infraction of the first toe.

Evaluation

The patient has decreased flexion and extension at the first MTP joint. Pain is reproduced with motion, especially into dorsiflexion. A dorsal bunion also may be evident. Radiographically, there is often a dorsal ring of osteophytes at the metatarsal head.

Management

Mobilization may free up some motion at the joint. The mainstay of conservative management is the use of a stiff-soled shoe or a rocker-bottom shoe that artificially creates toe-off through a rounded metatarsal bar. Failure to resolve usually requires surgical excision of the osteophytes.

Turf Toe

Classic Presentation

The patient often is an athlete complaining of first toe pain especially when the toe is bent back. There may be a history of a trauma that forced the toe into dorsiflexion.

Cause

Turf toe is a sports term for a hyperextension (dorsiflexion) injury of the first toe. The plantar capsule of the MTP joint is sprained.[18] The cause is either sudden dorsiflexion or chronic dorsiflexion through wearing shoes that are too flexible. It may also occur as a result of trips or falls. A similar condition found with sports played on sand, such as beach volleyball, involves forced plantarflexion that causes a sprain of the dorsal capsule (sand toe). Here the toes are rolled under during the injury.

Evaluation

The evaluation is rather straightforward with a suggestive history and pain on dorsiflexion (or plantarflexion with sand toe).

Management

Treatment involves taping of the toe to prevent the aggravating movement pattern and the use of stiff-soled shoes. If these are not successful, immobilization in a cast for several days may be necessary.

Gout

Classic Presentation

The patient is usually middle-aged or older complaining of an acute attack of first toe pain. The toe appears swollen and red.

Cause

Gout is a metabolic disease characterized by retention of urates in the body. The urates accumulate in various body sites as crystalline depositions referred to as tophi. These serve as irritative foci, causing an inflammatory arthritis with eventual bone destruction after repeated attacks. Tophi are deposited in the first toe, the knee, the olecranon bursal area, and behind the ears. Gout can be secondary to other conditions that interfere with renal clearance, such as chronic renal disease, multiple myeloma, and diuretic use.[19]

Evaluation

The location of pain and the severity of this monoarticular attack usually make the diagnosis clear. When acute, the joint is red, swollen, and very tender. Laboratory evaluation often will demonstrate a high uric acid level, especially in the acute phases (> 7.5 mg/dL). Early radiographic changes may not be visible. Later changes include punched-out areas in bone (urate tophi are radiolucent). Identification of urate crystals in joint fluid or tophi gives the definitive diagnosis.

Management

During acute attacks, the use of nonsteroid anti-inflammatory drugs is the most effective treatment. Prophylactic management involves avoidance of specific foods or alcohol that appear to incite attacks; however, the general contribution of a diet high in meat is less important than once believed. One of the most important measures is consistent maintenance of a high fluid intake (not diuretic liquids such as coffee, tea, or sodas) and avoidance of diuretic medication. Medication strategy varies depending on the suspected cause. Allopurinol blocks xanthine oxidase, reducing uric acid formation, whereas colchicine inhibits the inflammatory reaction to urate crystals but does not lower uric acid levels.[20]

METATARSALS

Metatarsalgia

Classic Presentation

The patient complains of pain on the bottom of the foot, specifically at the sole.

Cause

Metatarsal pain may be due to a number of factors. It appears that chronic stretching of the transverse ligaments may be the underlying reason.[21] This may be the result of excessive weight, repetitive activity, hammer toes, or pes planus or cavus. Direct trauma from jumping or landing on the toes with running or jogging, or standing for long periods of time in high-heeled shoes may contribute to metatarsal pain. Shoes with too narrow a toe box will also cause compression and pain. Subluxated metatarsal heads may be the cause or part of the problem.

Evaluation

Increased stress at the metatarsals may be evident with calluses or corns (especially over the second metatarsal head). Evaluate the foot for pes planus/cavus, "dropped" metatarsal heads, and toe deformity.

Management

Remove or modify any underlying problems such as repetitive trauma or inappropriate footwear. During the acute phase, use of a metatarsal pad placed just proximal to the metatarsal heads, leaving room for the first and fifth metatarsal heads, is often successful. Local ultrasound may also be of some benefit. Adjustment of metatarsal heads is warranted when restricted movement is determined.

Morton's Neuroma

Classic Presentation

The patient complains of pain on the bottom of the sole. The onset was insidious. The patient notices less pain when barefoot.

Cause

The process often begins as an entrapment neuropathy with progressive degeneration and deposition of amorphous deposits on the nerve fibers.[22] Entrapment occurs most commonly on the plantar surface by the intermetatarsal ligament.

Evaluation

There is pain often in the second or third intermetatarsal space. Occasionally, a mass may be palpated in this space, representing the neuroma. Although transverse compression may increase the pain, it is nonspecific (other causes could include a stress fracture or subluxation). Passive extension of the MTP joints or interphalangeal joints may increase pain or create a sense of numbness/tingling or burning into the related toes. Plantarflexion of the joints often will relieve this response.

Management

Conservative management includes forefoot mobilization and a temporary metatarsal pad. If unsuccessful, casted orthotics may be of benefit. Acute management also may include the use of phonophoresis with cortisone (if allowed by individual state law). Preventive measures are to buy shoes that are long enough to prevent cramming of the toes and to ensure a proper-sized toe box and forefoot areas. Surgical excision is an option in recalcitrant cases.

Stress Fractures

Classic Presentation

The patient presents with a complaint of rather constant pain of the forefoot, especially with weight-bearing. There is almost always a history of prolonged walking or running.

Cause

Stress fractures occur over time when the bone resorptive process exceeds osteoblastic activity. This will occur when constant stressors are applied without sufficient unstressed periods to heal or when the stresses consistently exceed the structural integrity of the bone. The second metatarsal is most affected because of its length and position in serving as a biomechanical axis.

Evaluation

The bone may be tender to touch and pain may be increased with squeezing the foot together. Tuning fork evaluation probably will not significantly increase pain. The high level of suspicion based on the history and the location of the pain warrants radiography, but it is usually unrevealing. A bone scan is the definitive tool in detecting stress fractures, revealing an increased uptake at the fracture site.

Management

For a nonathlete, it may be sufficient to use a stiff shoe or rigid orthotics for several weeks. If pain persists, non-weight-bearing with crutches for a few weeks is necessary. For the athlete, it may be necessary to prescribe a walking cast or to cast the foot in order to impose a non-weight-bearing period for several weeks. Calcium intake should be increased during this period, and long-term bone status should be evaluated in serious female athletes.

Fifth Metatarsal Fractures

Classic Presentation

The patient often will complain of a sudden onset of lateral foot pain following an inversion ankle sprain. Other patients may report sudden lateral foot pain during running or jumping.

Cause

There are generally three types of fractures possible. The least common is a spiral fracture. An avulsion fracture of the styloid process of the base of the fifth metatarsal is usually the result of a sudden peroneus brevis pull during an inversion ankle sprain. A transverse fracture of the proximal diaphysis of the fifth metatarsal (Jones fracture) is usually due to repetitive stress.

Evaluation

There is point tenderness and pain at the proximal fifth metatarsal. The definitive diagnosis is radiographic.

Management

Avulsion fractures usually heal well with the symptomatic treatment of the associated ankle injury. There is a caution that if there is wide displacement of the fragment, a painful bump will form. Therefore, displacement necessitates an orthopaedic consultation. Transverse fractures have a reputation for nonunion.[23] If the patient is placed early enough in a short leg cast for six to eight weeks, healing usually will be acceptable; delayed healing, however, may require as much as three months of casting. Spiral fractures should be referred for orthopaedic consultation because of the variety of rotational patterns that affect the healing process; however, it has been demonstrated that nonsurgical management is often possible.[24]

OTHER CONDITIONS

Osteochondrosis of the Navicular

Classic Presentation

The patient is usually a child (average age of six years) who complains of inner foot pain. The parent reports that the child walks on the outer side of the foot.

Cause

The cause of this condition is still being debated. Some authors believe that it is a normal variant of ossification; others think that it is an avascular necrosis. There may be a history of trauma. It is also referred to as Köhler's disease.

Evaluation

There may be tenderness at the navicular. The definitive diagnosis is radiographic. The bone will appear more radiopaque and underdeveloped. These radiographic changes develop over two to four years.

Management

The symptomatic presentation often self-resolves in three to nine months.[25] During this period, use of arch supports will often relieve the discomfort. In rare cases, a below-knee walking cast is required. The natural history of the disorder is entirely benign with no apparent increase in degenerative joint disease.

Fat Pad Syndrome

Classic Presentation

An older individual presents with a complaint of heel pain. The pain is in the middle of the heel; it is much worse with weight-bearing.

Cause

As an individual ages, the fat pad on the bottom of the heel degenerates, leaving little shock absorption for the calcaneus. Shoes that do not have firm heel counters and/or are too wide allow the remaining fat pad to flatten out, decreasing the thickness and therefore shock absorption.[26]

Evaluation

Pain and tenderness are found in the middle of the heel. When the fat pad is supported on either side and pressure is reapplied, the pain is decreased. Plantar fasciitis is more often at the medial aspect of the calcaneus, not in the middle. Stretching of the plantar fascia or dorsiflexors of the first toe or ankle does not increase pain with fat pad syndrome. Radiographs are rarely needed unless the patient is not responsive to care.

Management

Both support of the remaining fat pad and substitution of the pad are the two approaches used. Use of various heel cups may be helpful. The heel cup is often made of shock-absorbent material and provides some medial/lateral support. Some patients do better with a more rigid support in the heel counter of the shoe to prevent splaying of the fat pad. Misdiagnosis of plantar fasciitis is common, so many patients are subjected to unnecessary cortisone injections and surgery.

Plantar Fasciitis

Classic Presentation

The patient complains of a sharp heel pain that radiates along the bottom of the inside of the foot. The pain is often worse when getting out of bed in the morning.

Cause

Either pronation or supination may be the cause. The flatfoot (hyperpronation) with associated forefoot abduction has a stretching effect on the plantar fascia, leading to repetitive tension overload. The high-arched foot (supinated) is relatively rigid. Forces usually absorbed through movement of the foot and ankle are transmitted to the plantar fascia and lower leg. In this way plantar fasciitis can be analogous to shin splints.

Evaluation

Pain or tenderness is increased with direct pressure over the medial tubercle of the calcaneus (the fascial insertion). This pain often will radiate along the bottom of the foot. It is also possible to reproduce the pain through stretching of the first toe into dorsiflexion alone or coupled with dorsiflexion of the ankle. Plantar fasciitis is estimated to be found in 10% of runners. A calcaneal spur is found in 50% of patients, but also found in 10% to 27% of asymptomatic patients; symptoms may be bilateral in 10%. More than 80% improve within 12 months regardless of type of care. Radiographs usually are not necessary. Although heel spurs often are seen, they are not the cause but the reaction to chronic fascial tension.[27] Laboratory testing is reserved for patients with known rheumatic disease or a situation where suspicion is raised by other joint complaints.

Management

Support of any underlying biomechanical predispositions includes orthotics for pronation or supination. This is based on the frequency of pain or the degree of incapacitation when pain does occur. Temporary solutions include taping the arch for support (low-dye taping) and gradual stretching. Myofascial release to the plantar fascia may be helpful. Underwater ultrasound coupled with stretching appears to be effective in many cases. Adjusting of any foot subluxations (especially navicular and first MTP joint) and strengthening of foot-support musculature should be a part of the treatment plan. Ninety-five percent of patients respond to conservative care.[28]

Several treatment approaches have gained popularity, including the use of magnetic insoles and the use of shockwave therapy (similar to lithotripsy for kidney stones). A recent randomized, controlled trial on the use of magnetic insoles found that there was no difference between patients wearing magnetic insoles and those wearing sham-magnetic insoles.[29]

A recent study involved researchers testing the use of shockwave therapy for plantar fasciitis.[30] A "placebo" group was treated with a less-than-therapeutic intensity. Five prior studies indicated good results; however, in this randomized, controlled trial, both groups improved at 6 and 12 months measured by pain, function, and an SF36. The researchers concluded that there was no difference between the sham treatment and "real" treatment over a one-year period. The question that still exists is whether short-term relief may be an advantage of shockwave therapy, returning patients to a more functional, pain-free level sooner than 12 months. A more recent study[31] indicated that there was a small difference in improvement over time with about 61% of patients treated with shockwave therapy versus 42% of patients with placebo who improved over a couple of months. Various injectables are utilized in an attempt to solve long-standing plantar fasciitis problems. There seems to be some emerging evidence for the use of platelet-rich plasma (PRP) for the management of chronic plantar fasciitis.[32,33] This injection of platelet concentrated autogenous fluid might provide the ingredients for better healing. More studies are needed.

Tarsal Tunnel Syndrome

Classic Presentation

The patient complains of numbness and tingling across the bottom of the foot, often at the sole or first toe. The onset is insidious and not associated with low back or leg pain.

Cause

The posterior tibial nerve may be stretched or compressed in the tarsal tunnel, a fibro-osseous tunnel formed by the flexor retinaculum, calcaneus, distal tibia, and malleolus. The contents of the tunnel include the tendons of the posterior tibialis, flexor digitorum longus, and flexor hallucis and the posterior tibial artery, vein, and nerve. Due to highly variable anatomy, the distal branches of the posterior tibial nerve (the medial calcaneal, medial plantar, and lateral plantar nerves) may be selectively affected.[34] Hyperpronation is often the cause of tarsal tunnel syndrome due to tightening of the flexor retinaculum or arch of the abductor hallucis. However, trauma, swelling, ganglions, and anatomic variation of blood vessels or the abductor hallucis may also cause compression.

Evaluation

Neurologic testing for nerve root involvement is negative. Numbness and tingling may be reproduced by percussion over the posterior tibial nerve just behind the medial malleolus (Tinel's sign) or along a line that continues to the navicular tuberosity, continuing down into the medial arch. In one study that evaluated patients with documented tarsal tunnel syndrome, 45% reported numbness, 39% reported pain, and 16% reported both.[35] Symptoms were produced in 82% of patients, usually within 10 seconds, by applying a passive dorsiflexion of the ankle and toes with eversion of the ankle. This testing approach may be a helpful addition to standard Tinel testing. Sensory deficit may occur in the medial (medial plantar nerve) or lateral (lateral plantar nerve) plantar surface of the foot. Usually two-point discrimination is decreased or hypoesthesia to pinprick are found. Motor weakness is less common. With difficult cases, nerve conduction studies may be needed.

Management

If trauma or swelling is involved, the initial course of care is to reduce the swelling with ice, compression, elevation, and physical therapy modalities. If pronation appears to be the cause, a trial use of orthotics will often solve the problem. Associated adjusting of restricted navicular, calcaneal, or talar movement may be beneficial. If a trial of several weeks is unsuccessful, referral for podiatric consultation is suggested for possible need of surgical release of the retinaculum or excision of a ganglion or other compressive structure.

Talar Osteophytes

Classic Presentation

Talar osteophytes may be anterior or posterior. Patients with anterior osteophytes complain of pain on dorsiflexion of the foot and occasionally numbness/tingling or weakness in the toes. Patients with posterior osteophytes complain of pain on forced plantarflexion of the foot.

Cause

Osteophytes on the neck of the talus or anterior tibia may cause an impingement of the local synovium leading to a hypertrophy and swelling.[36] With tight shoes, the anterior type of osteophyte may compress the deep peroneal nerve; however, this is more common with entrapment under the inferior extensor retinaculum.[37] Posterior compression may occur as a result of an os trigonum (small nonunited bone) or an elongated lateral process of the posterior tubercle of the talus (Stieda's process).[38] When there is pain on forced plantarflexion or dorsiflexion, lateral radiographs will usually reveal osteophytes or accessory bones that may represent the offending structure. If sufficient trauma is involved, it is important to consider a possible avulsion fracture.

Management

Surgical excision is usually necessary for the anterior talar osteophyte; however, the pain with posterior processes may resolve with activity modification; if not, lidocaine injection or surgery should be considered.

Ankle Sprains

Classic Presentation

A 20-year-old patient (could be any age) presents with a complaint of ankle pain and swelling following a twisting injury. He does not recall how it happened but now it is swollen, and he has difficulty placing weight on it.

Cause

The vast majority of ankle sprains are plantarflexion inversion sprains involving the lateral ligaments in a sequence of injury: the anterior talofibular ligament, calcaneofibular ligament, and then the posterior talofibular ligament. The more rare eversion sprain damages the medial ligament complex referred to as the deltoid ligament. Causes may include stepping on an uneven surface, landing on the outside heel, or running with too much cross-over or over-supination. Ligament laxity plays an important and ever-increasing role with subsequent sprains.

A number of complications and co-injuries may occur, which prolong recovery due to persistent pain or mechanical interference in the performance of rehabilitation exercises. Commonly seen complications are:

- Osteochondral fracture of the talar dome or loose body
- Subluxating or dislocating peroneal tendons
- Bifurcate ligament sprains
- Fracture of the base of the fifth metatarsal
- Achilles tendon injury

What is often not appreciated is the potential injury to the distal stabilizing elements of the tibia and fibula; the inferior tibiofibular ligament. This is also referred to as an ankle syndesmosis injury. Like all ligament damage, there are varying degrees of tearing and a variety of subsequent reactions in the tissue to attempt healing and stabilization. When full rupture occurs, fracture and/or dislocation is likely. This is referred to as diastasis and is easily viewed on radiographs. Lesser degrees of injury are notoriously difficult to assess both clinically and radiographically, yet may result in a prolonged recovery time. A sequelae to damage to the distal syndesmosis is synostosis. Although this is commonly secondary to fracture, it may occur as a result of damage to the inferior tibiofibular ligament. Pain is worse with the push-off. Persistent pain or swelling after activity is common. Dorsiflexion with the ankle in neutral is significantly restricted. Radiographically there is clear evidence of ossification between the distal tibia and fibula. Soft tissue impingement is possible. There is an extra distal fascicle of the anteroinferior tibiofibular ligament, which can cause impingement at the distal fibula and talus, causing damage to the talar surface. Pain is increased at the distal ankle with passive dorsiflexion and relieved by plantar flexion. Patients often report an anterior popping sensation.

Evaluation

The Ottawa Ankle Rules were founded on the basis that the only consistent (sensitive and specific) history and examination findings that were relevant were pain in the malleolar region and either (1) tenderness at either malleolus, or (2) the inability to bear weight immediately after the injury or in the emergency department.

For the midfoot the relevant findings were pain in the midfoot area and either (1) tenderness at the base of the fifth metatarsal, (2) tenderness at the navicular, or (3) the inability to bear weight immediately after the injury or in the emergency department. Depending on the timing in relationship to the injury, swelling may neutralize the value of stability testing. Stability testing includes the anterior drawer test followed by inversion testing if the drawer testing is positive (i.e., indicating a torn anterior talofibular ligament that allows strain to the lateral restraint of the calcaneofibular ligament). Caution must be used in ruling out any other injury that often complicates recovery, including tearing of the lateral retinaculum (which binds the tendons of the peroneals to the lateral malleolus), bifurcate ligament injury, interosseous ligament injury in the tarsal tunnel, and foot and ankle fractures. Radiographs, if taken, should include the standard series plus an ankle mortise view to search for an osteochondral fracture.

There are several tests used to evaluate the syndesmotic injury:

1. Syndesmosis ligament palpation—Palpation over the anterior talofibular ligament causes an increase in pain if the test is positive.
2. Squeeze test—Manually compressing the fibula to the tibia above the midpoint of the calf increases pain over the distal tibiofibular ligament area if the test is positive.
3. External rotation test—With the patient sitting with the knee at 90° flexion and the ankle held in neutral, pain is increased with passive external rotation of the foot and ankle if the test is positive.
4. Passive dorsiflexion test—This test was modified to indicate whether limited range of motion or increased pain on passive dorsiflexion could be affected by an examiner adding compression externally while the passive dorsiflexion was repeated. A positive result is an increase in ankle range of motion or a decrease in end-range pain with external examiner compression at the distal tibiofibular joint.

5. Moving the calcaneus and talus side-to-side in an effort to elicit a "thud" as the talus abuts against the fibula or tibia. This indicates excessive movement due to a torn tibiofibular ligament. The external rotation test had the highest degree of interrater reliability. Positive test results for the combination of the external rotation test and the dorsiflexion-compression test correlated with a prolonged recovery time.

A 2013 systematic review[39] of the literature on the value of these tests concluded that an inability to hop, syndesmosis ligament tenderness, and the dorsiflexion-external rotation stress test (sensitive findings) may be combined with pain out of proportion to the injury and the squeeze test (specific findings) to arrive at a high level of suspicion.

Management (see Table 14–3)

The standard approach is ice, elevation, and compression. Weight-bearing should be protected, with use of crutches for more serious injury. The main goal is to enable the patient to bear weight as soon as possible. Strengthening for plantarflexion inversion injury includes primarily the tibialis anterior and peroneals.

The focus in managing ankle sprains has switched to prevention. Following are some new concepts. Ankle sprains account for 25% of time lost in athletics. And money, too—some football teams spend as much as $50,000 annually on tape! One study evaluated the maximum resistance to inversion under weight-bearing conditions.[40] Although there was a 10% increase in resistance initially, it was lost after 40 minutes of vigorous activity. This is consistent with other studies. What is unique about this study is that the use of prewrap and tape together increased resistance to inversion by an additional 10%. This is counter to what is traditionally taught about the effect of prewrap.

In an interesting study testing the proposition that taping has a proprioceptive effect more than a structural one, 22 university students with functional instability of the ankle were randomized into two groups for training on an ankle disk.[41] Both groups trained for 10 minutes daily for 10 weeks. Group 1 trained with strips of tape over the lateral ankle while group 2 trained without tape. Group 1 achieved decreased sway patterns after four weeks of training, returning to normal at six weeks, while group 2 took two weeks longer for both aspects. The results suggest that taping may increase stability due to a proprioceptive training effect.

Boyce et al.[42] found in a prospective, randomized trial that patients improved faster with the use of an elastic bandage compared to those with no compressive support when measuring swelling and pain scores at 10 days postinjury. In a different randomized, controlled, clinical trial patients with Grade I and II ankle sprains were assigned to Air-Stirrup braces alone, elastic wraps alone, combined Air-Stirrups with elastic wraps, or walking casts.[43] Patients with the combined brace and wrap had an earlier return to preinjury function compared to the other groups.

In one small study of 12 athletes with a history of ankle sprains within the previous six months, both injured and uninjured ankles were evaluated for laxity, dorsiflexion range of motion, and joint play.[44] Posterior talar glide was significantly reduced in the injured ankles. Although dorsiflexion returned to normal, posterior talar glide remained restricted.

There is an increased number of literature reports of manipulation used for ankle sprains. One report[45] evaluated the effect of a Mulligan-type mobilization on subacute, Grade II lateral ankle sprains. This approach is referred to as mobilization with movement (MWM). A posterior talar glide is applied while the patient actively dorsiflexes the ankle. The intent is to provide a pain-free acquisition of previously unattainable movement. Although there was an increase in talocrural dorsiflexion, there was no effect on pain. This approach was again tested in individuals with recurrent ankle sprains and was found to improve weight-bearing dorsiflexion more than controls.[46]

A similar mechanical effect was demonstrated in a study by Lopez-Rodriguez et al.[47] Changes in posterior load, measured by a standing device, were found in subjects who had ankle manipulation (talocrural caudal manipulation or posterior glide manipulation). There was no mention of a measure of pain, swelling, or other symptoms. A literature review of mobilization and exercise for ankle sprains indicated that there was value in using exercise for prevention of recurrence.[48] The evidence for ankle mobilization was focused on increased talocrural motion or posterior glide but no improved clinical outcome was reported.

A small study involving osteopathic manipulation of the ankle in an emergency department setting indicates significant symptom improvement.[49] Patients managed with single osteopathic manipulation and standard ankle care were compared to those who simply received standard care. Those who received the manipulation had immediate results that were significant for improvement in edema, pain, and range of motion. In a follow-up, both groups improved. However, the manipulation group appeared to have better range of motion.

The results from a small case series by Jennings et al.[50] suggest that cuboid manipulation may have a role in patients with lateral ankle pain following an ankle sprain. The patients who responded had a history of ankle sprain from one to six weeks prior to presentation.

Another study attempted to determine the effect of using a standard talar adjustment on range of motion.[51] This randomized, controlled, blinded study evaluated 41 subjects (21 experimental, 20 for control); all were asymptomatic. Pretest and post-test measurement of dorsiflexion was performed. Ankles were adjusted with a standard prone gapping maneuver. Adjusting did not increase dorsiflexion ROM. Ankles that demonstrated the greatest pretest dorsiflexion were more likely to cavitate.

A single-blinded comparative study evaluated the outcome of treating Grade I and II ankle sprains with an ankle mortise separation adjustment or detuned ultrasound (placebo).[52] Both groups improved over a period of four weeks; however, there was significantly more improvement in the adjusted group for pain, range of motion, and function. A recent review summarizes the literature, which indicates a benefit for manipulation in the management of ankle sprains.[53]

In one recent study, researchers attempted to evaluate the cross-over effect of training either the dominant or nondominant ankle in 10 uninjured subjects.[54] Training involved isokinetic, concentric, and eccentric training in all four motions three times per week for eight weeks; a control group did no training. At the end of the eight weeks, the control group showed no improvement in torque strength. The trained group showed up to a 40% increase in peak torque and a cross-over benefit of 19% for eccentric inversion.

From a recent Cochrane review by Kirkhoffs et al.[55] it appears that there is insufficient evidence for either surgical or conservative management of acute lateral ligament complex injuries. Given the cost of surgery and potential complications, it would seem that, for the time being, conservative approaches would initially be preferred.

In one study,[56] there were several factors predictive of chronic ankle instability following ankle sprain. These include increased inversion laxity, anterior laxity, balance problems, and decreased plantarflexion and dorsiflexion peak torque. It was suggested by the authors that these could be avoided with proper initial rehabilitation.

The Evidence—Foot and Ankle

Translation into Practice Summary (TIPS)

There is little literature evidence for the history and examination of the foot and ankle with the exception of ruling-in the need for radiographs to determine if fracture is present. There is no literature on the evaluation of ankle instability although there are numerous tests.

The Literature-Based Clinical Core

- The Ottawa Knee Rule and Burnese are good for determining the need for x-ray for foot/ankle fractures. The addition of a tuning fork applied to the distal fibula may add to the specificity.
- The impingement sign is good for both ruling-in and ruling-out anterolateral ankle impingement.
- There is no evidence regarding the reliability or validity of testing for ankle instability.
- Assessment of static foot alignment, proprioception, sensation, swelling, and functional testing are all relatively reliable; however, they are of unknown clinical value.
- Dynamic measurement of hindfoot motion during gait is not of clinical utility due to the poor reliability and undetermined validity.

The Expert-Opinion-Based Clinical Core

- A history of recent plantarflexion/inversion injury with swelling is a strong indicator for lateral ankle sprain.
- A history of recent eversion injury with swelling is a strong indicator of medial ankle sprain.
- Stress testing positives of laxity for the anterior drawer and inversion stress indicate increasing severity of ligament damage including anterior talofibular to anterior talofibular to posterior talofibular damage. Eversion testing tests for the deltoid ligament complex.
- High-ankle sprains (syndesmotic injury) should be considered with all ankle sprains. Testing that may be of value includes passive external rotation, passive dorsiflexion test, and squeeze tests to demonstrate instability at the distal tibiofibular joint or recreate/exacerbate pain.
- Tarsal tunnel syndrome testing involves Tinel's and passive dorsiflexion of the ankle and toes with eversion. Tests seem sensitive but may not be specific.
- Midheel pressure for fat pad syndrome is a good test for distinguishing between planter fasciitis and fat pad syndrome.
- The Thompson test (calf squeeze) is a good first test for screening for Achilles rupture.
- Homan's test is not valuable in an ambulatory population in distinguishing between deep vein thrombosis and calf strain.
- In-office gait analysis may be good at picking up asymmetrical functional issues but is of unknown value in distinguishing between those in need of orthotics and not. Functional support testing with in-shoe orthoses or taping may be of more value.
- Compartment syndromes should be considered in patients with exercise-induced pain coupled with sensory or motor loss isolated to the calf to the foot without indications of low back involvement.

APPENDIX 14–1

References

1. McCrae JD. *Pediatric Orthopedics of the Lower Extremity*. New York: Futura Publishing; 1985.
2. McPoil TG, Knecht HG, Schuit D. A survey of foot types in normal females between the ages of 18 and 30 years. *J Orthop Sports Phys Ther*. 1989;(10)4:406–409.
3. Michaud TC. Ideal motions during the gait cycle. In: *Foot Orthoses and Other Forms of Conservative Foot Care*. Baltimore: Williams & Wilkins; 1993:27–56.
4. Reber L, Perry J, Pink M. Muscular control of the ankle in running. *Am J Sports Med*. 1993;21:805–810.
5. Elveru RA, Rothstein JM, Lamb RL. Goniometric reliability in a clinical setting: subtalar and ankle joint measurements. *Phys Ther*. 1988;68:672.
6. Root ML, Orien WP, Weed JN. *Clinical Biomechanics: Normal and Abnormal Function of the Foot*. Los Angeles: Clinical Biomechanics Corp; 1977;2:26–31.
7. Weismann S. *Radiology of the Foot*. Baltimore: Williams & Wilkins; 1984.
8. Steill IG, McKnight RD, Greensburg GH, et al. Implementation of the Ottawa ankle rules. *JAMA*. 1994;271:827–832.

9. Nyska M, Amir H, Dekel S. Radiologic assessment of a modified anterior drawer test of the ankle. *Foot Ankle*. 1992;13:400–403.

10. Kleiger B. Mechanisms of ankle injury. *Orthop Clin North Am*. 1974;5:127.

11. Stiell IG, McKnight D, Greenberg GH, et al. Implementation of the Ottawa Ankle Rules. *JAMA*. 1994;271:827–832.

12. Springer BA, Arciero RA, Tenuta JJ, Taylor DC. A prospective study of modified Ottawa ankle rules in a military population: interobserver agreement between physical therapists and orthopaedic surgeons. *Am J Sports Med*. 2000;29(6):864–868.

13. Cox JS, Hewes TF. Normal talar tilt angle. *Clin Orthop*. 1979;140:37–40.

14. Williams PL, Smibert JG, Cox R, et al. Imaging study of the painful heel syndrome. *Foot Ankle*. 1987;6:345.

15. Richardson G. Injuries to the hallucal sesamoids in the athlete. *Foot Ankle*. 1987;7:229.

16. Hattrup SJ, Johnson KA. Hallux valgus: a review. *Adv Orthop Surg*. 1985;8:404.

17. Hattrup SJ, Johnson KA. Hallux rigidus: a review. *Adv Orthop Surg*. 1986;9:259.

18. Clanton TO, Ford JJ. Turf toe injury. *Clin Sports Med*. 1994;13:731–741.

19. Roubenoff RR. Gout and hyperuricemia. *Rheumat Dis Clin North Am*. 1990;16:539.

20. Pratt PW, Ball GV. Gout treatment. In: Schumaker HR, ed. *Primer on the Rheumatic Diseases*. 10th ed. Atlanta: Arthritis Foundation; 1993.

21. Reid DC. Selected conditions of the foot. In: Reid DC. *Sports Injury Assessment and Rehabilitation*. New York: Churchill Livingstone; 1992:129–184.

22. Graham CE, Graham DM. Morton's neuroma: a microscopic evaluation. *Foot Ankle*. 1984;5:150.

23. Zogby RG, Baker BE. A review of non-operative treatment of Jones fracture. *Am J Sports Med*. 1987;15:304.

24. O'Malley MJ, Hamilton WG, Munyak J. Fractures of the distal shaft of the fifth metatarsal: dancer's fracture. *Am J Sports Med*. 1996;24:240–243.

25. Ippolito E, Pollini PTR, Falez F. Kohler's disease of the tarsal navicular: long term follow up of 12 cases. *J Pediatr Orthop*. 1984;4:416.

26. Miller WE. The heel pad. *Am J Sports Med*. 1982;10:9.

27. Furey JG. Plantar fasciitis: the painful heel syndrome. *J Bone Joint Surg Am*. 1975;75:672.

28. Baxter DE. The heel in sport. *Clin Sports Med*. 1994;13:685–693.

29. Winemiller MH, Billow RC, Laskoski ER, Harmsen WS. Effect of magnetic vs sham-magnetic insoles on plantar heel pain: a randomized controlled trial. *JAMA*. 2003;290:1471–1478.

30. Buchbinder B, Ptaszmik R, Gordon J, et al. Ultrasound-guided extrapcorporeal shock-wave therapy for planter fasciitis: a randomized controlled trial. *JAMA*. 2002;288(11):1364–1372.

31. Gerdesmeyer L, Frey C, Vester J, et al. Radial extracorporeal shock wave therapy is safe and effective in the treatment of chronic recalcitrant plantar fasciitis results of a confirmatory randomized placebo-controlled multicenter study. *Am J Sports Med*. 2008;36(1):2100–2109.

32. O'Malley MJ, Vosseller JT, Gu Y. Successful use of platelet-rich plasma for chronic plantar fasciitis. *HSS J*. 2013;9(2):129–133.

33. Kumar V, Millar T, Murphy PN, Clough T. The treatment of intractable plantar fasciitis with platelet-rich plasma injection. *Foot (Edinb)*. 2013;23(2-3):74–77.

34. Schon LC, Baxter DE. Neuropathies of the foot and ankle in athletes. *Clin Sports Med*. 1990;9:489–509.

35. Kinoshita M, Okuda R, Morikawa J, et al. The dorsiflexioneversion test for diagnosis of tarsal tunnel syndrome. *J Bone Joint Surg Am*. 2001;83A:183501838.

36. Parks JCH, Hamilton WG, Patterson AH, et al. The anterior impingement syndrome of the ankle. *J Trauma*. 1980;20:895.

37. Murphy PC, Baxter DE. Nerve entrapment of the foot and ankle in runners. *Clin Sports Med*. 1985;4:753.

38. Reid DC. Selected lesions around the talus. *Curr Theor Sports Med*. 1990;2:241.

39. Sman AD, Hiller CE, Rae K, et al. Diagnostic accuracy of clinical tests for ankle syndesmosis injury. *Br J Sports Med*. 2013. doi: 10.1136/bjsports-2013-092787. [Epub ahead of print]

40. Manfroy PP, Ashton-Miller JA, Wojtys EM. The effect of exercise, prewrap, and athletic tape on the maximal active and passive ankle resistance of ankle inversion. *Am J Sports Med*. 1997;25(2):156–163.

41. Matsususaka N, Yokoyama S, Tsurusaki T, et al. Effect of ankle disk training combined with tactile stimulation to the leg and foot on functional instability of the ankle. *Am J Sports Med*. 2001;29(1):25–30.

42. Boyce SH, Quigley MA, Campbell S. Management of ankle sprains: a randomised controlled trial of the treatment of inversion injuries using an elastic support bandage or an Aircast ankle brace. *Br J Sports Med*. 2005;39(2):91–96.

43. Beynnon BD, Renstrom PA, Haugh L, Uh BS, Barker H. A prospective, randomized clinical investigation of the treatment of first-time ankle sprains. *Am J Sports Med.* 2006;34(9):1401–1412.

44. Denegar CR. The effect of lateral ankle sprain on dorsiflexion range of motion, posterior talar glide, and joint laxity. *J Orthop Sports Phys Ther.* 2002;32(40):166–173.

45. Collins N, Teys P, Vicenzino B. The initial effects of a Mulligan's mobilization with movement technique on dorsiflexion and pain in subacute ankle sprains. *Man Ther.* 2004;9(2):77–82.

46. Vicenzino B, Branjerdporn M, Teys P, Jordan K. Initial changes in posterior talar glide and dorsiflexion of the ankle after mobilization with movement in individuals with recurrent ankle sprain. *J Orthop Sports Phys Ther.* 2006;36(7):464–471.

47. Lopez-Rodriguez S, Fernandez de-Las-Penas C, Alburquerque-Sendin F, Rodriguez-Blanco C, Palomeque-del-Cerro L. Immediate effects of manipulation of the talocrural joint on stabilometry and baropodometry in patients with ankle sprain. *J Manipulative Physiol Ther.* 2007;30(3):186–192.

48. van der Wees PJ, Lenssen AF, Hendriks EJ, Stomp DJ, Dekker J, de Bie RA. Effectiveness of exercise therapy and manual mobilisation in ankle sprain and functional instability: a systematic review. *Aust J Physiother.* 2006;52(1):27–37.

49. Eisenhart AW, Gaeta TJ, Yens DP. Osteopathic manipulative treatment in the emergency department for patients with acute ankle injuries. *J Am Osteopath Assoc.* 2003;103(9):417–421.

50. Jennings J, Davies GJ. Treatment of cuboid syndrome secondary to lateral ankle sprains: a case series. *J Orthop Sports Phys Ther.* 2005;35(7):409–415.

51. Fryer GA, Mudge JM, McLaughlin PA. The effect of talocrural joint manipulation on range of motion at the ankle. *J Manipulative Physiol Ther.* 2002;25(6):384–390.

52. Pellow JE, Bramingham JW. The efficacy of adjusting the ankle in the treatment of subacute and chronic grade I and grade II ankle inversion sprains. *J Manipulative Physiol Ther.* 2001;24(1):17–25.

53. Brantingham JW, Bonnefin D, Perle SM, et al. Manipulative therapy for lower extremity conditions: update of a literature review. *J Manipulative Physiol Ther.* 2012;35(2):127–166.

54. Uh BS, Beynnon BD, Helie BV, et al. The benefit of a single-leg strength training program for the muscles around the untrained ankle: a prospective, randomized, controlled study. *Am J Sports Med.* 2000;28(4):568–573.

55. Kerkhoffs GM, Handoll HH, de Bie R, Rowe BH, Struijs PA. Surgical versus conservative treatment for acute injuries of the lateral ligament complex of the ankle in adults. *Cochrane Database Syst Rev.* 2007(2):CD000380.

56. Hubbard TJ, Kramer LC, Denegar CR, Hertel J. Contributing factors to chronic ankle instability. *Foot Ankle Int.* 2007;28(3):343–354.

APPENDIX 14–2

Foot/Ankle/Lower Leg Diagnosis Table

Diagnosis	Comments	History Findings	Positive Examination Findings	Radiography/Special Studies	Treatment Options
Subluxation or Fixation of Talus Navicular Cuboid Cuneiforms Metatarsal-phalangeal Interphalangeal Joints	• Should be used when chiropractic manipulation is used as Tx for any foot/ankle/ lower leg problem/ Dx. • Can be primary Dx if patient is asymptomatic or mildly symptomatic (e.g., mild stiffness or pain level <2/10). • Must indicate chiropractic exam findings to support Dx.	*Nonspecific*	*Palpation*—Local tenderness or other signs of subluxation *Ortho*—None *Neuro*—None *Active ROM*—Variable restriction *Passive ROM*—End-range restriction *Motion palpation*—Specific articular restriction or symptoms produced on end-range	• Radiography not required for the diagnosis of subluxation. • Radiographic biomechanical analysis may assist in treatment decisions.	• Chiropractic adjustive technique. • Decisions regarding specifically which technique(s) is/ are applied and modifications to the given approach will be directed by the primary Dx and patient's ability to tolerate pre-adjustment stresses.
Eversion Sprain of Ankle (specify degree) Plantarflexion/ Inversion Sprain (specify degree)	• The vast majority of ankle sprains are plantarflexion/ inversion. • Sprains may be associated with other soft tissue damage, fracture, and subluxation.	*Mechanism*—Eversion strains the medial ankle with damage to the deltoid ligament and its components; plantarflexion/ inversion strains the lateral ankle ligaments, in particular, anterior talofibular and the calcaneofibular ligaments	*Ortho*—Stability testing may indicate degree of damage: *Anterior drawer*—Performed at 15°–20° plantarflexion (anterior talofibular) Talar tilt—Inversion test Kleiger test—Eversion test Swelling usually equal to degree of damage: • Pain with mild swelling, no instability = grade 1 • Moderate swelling, some instability = grade 2 • Gross swelling and instability = grade 3	• Radiography recommended to determine if fracture is present if patient is unable to bear weight or there is bony tenderness at either malleolus, cuboid, or navicular.	• Refer for surgery if gross instability, dislocation, or fracture is found. • For grades 1 and 2, P.T. to reduce swelling; consider mild manipulation. • Orthotic support (taping or brace) based on degree of injury. • Myofascial therapy. • Biomechanical advice with regard to sports; possible recommendation of protective brace or taping in early rehab. • Strengthening and preventive exercises.

Condition		Mechanism/Symptoms	Ortho	Radiography	Treatment
Hallux Valgus Bunion of First MTP Joint	The vast majority of patients are female, and wearing high heels may be an accelerating factor.	*Mechanism*—Abduction of the proximal phalanx of the first toe causes a sling effect from pull of local tendons; protrusion medially causes development of a painful bunion. *Symptoms/Signs*—Medial big toe pain often worse with tight-fitting shoes	*Ortho*—None; based on observation	• Radiography only necessary if there is an associated arthritide as the cause (e.g., RA) or to determine degree of deviation.	• Use of orthotics may be helpful to compensate for associated factors such as forefoot varus. • Avoidance of high heels and tight-fitting shoes. • Use of taping or night-sling to hold first toe in alignment may be helpful temporarily. • Surgery may eventually be needed.
Metatarsalgia	• General term to indicate pain at metatarsals; usually due to some underlying biomechanical stress. • Differentiate from stress fracture of metatarsals.	*Mechanism*—Chronic stretching of transverse ligaments due to various causes, including excessive weight, repetitive trauma, hammer toes, or direct trauma. *Symptoms/Signs*—Pain at bottom of foot increased by tight shoes	*Palpation*—Tenderness found at metatarsals, often at the sole. *Ortho*—Transverse compression of metatarsals increases pain; tuning-fork test negative	• Radiography not usually necessary initially except to rule out fracture with acute trauma or stress fracture with repetitive trauma (e.g., runners). • Bone scan may be needed if radiographs are not indicating stress fracture yet still suspected based on history.	• Use of metatarsal pads (proximal to metatarsal heads) may provide some symptom relief. • Correct or modify suspected biomechanical faults.
Hallux Rigidus	• Must be differentiated from capsular sprains and gout.	*Mechanism*—Due to either osteoarthritic changes of aging or repetitive capsular sprains in athletes; secondary to other arthritides	*Ortho*—Restricted flexion and extension of first MTP joint; worse with passive dorsiflexion. *Observation*—Dorsal bunion may be present	• Radiography may be necessary to rule out other arthritides or sesamoid involvement. • A dorsal ring of osteophytes may be evident with hallux rigidus.	• Use of a stiff-soled shoe or rocker-bottom shoe may help. • Failure of conservative regimen should result in podiatric or orthopaedic referral.

(continues)

Foot/Ankle/Lower Leg Diagnosis Table (continued)

Diagnosis	Comments	History Findings	Positive Examination Findings	Radiography/Special Studies	Treatment Options
Turf Toe or Other Digit Sprains	• Common injury in sports where athletes play on artificial surfaces, wear worn-out shoes, or play barefoot.	*Mechanism*—Hyper-extension of the toe(s) may result in capsular sprain on plantar surface; hyperflexion may result in similar problem on dorsal surface, often found with beach volleyball	*Ortho*—Pain increases with direction of injury force; passive dorsiflexion or plantarflexion; swelling is usually minimal	• Radiography not usually necessary.	• Taping to limit motion and correction of any underlying biomechanical causes, such as worn-out shoes, helps prevent further injury.
Plantar Fasciitis	• Plantar fasciitis is not due to heel spur; rather, the constant strain on fascia is cause of heel spur. • Patient may be treated successfully without elimination of heel spur.	*Mechanism*—Strain or stretching of plantar fascia may be due to pes planus or pes cavus foot. *History*—Sharp pain across bottom of foot; often worse when first walking in the morning	*Palpation*—Discrete tenderness at medial tubercle of the calcaneus *Ortho*—Pain increased by passive dorsiflexion of first toe or coupled with passive dorsiflexion of ankle	• Radiography may reveal an associated heel spur; however, resolution of heel spur should not be used as an outcome measure for treatment success.	• Temporary symptomatic relief may be accomplished through taping. • Ice and mild stretching. • Orthotic prescription for compensation of pronation or supination problems. • Correct any suspected biomechanical faults. • Myofascial therapy.
Achilles Tendinitis (Tendinosis) Tendinosis is a newer term used to indicate intratendinous degeneration due to atrophy (aging, microtrauma, vascular compromise, etc.). This is considered noninflammatory with hypocellularity, variable vascular ingrowth, local necrosis, and/or calcification, with accompanying fiber disorientation.	• Found mainly in athletes who run or jump as main component of sport.	*Mechanism*—Primarily due to eccentric strain of Achilles tendon with repetitive activities; area affected is 2 cm proximal to insertion *History*—With full tear, patient unable to plantarflex foot; with partial tears, complaints of burning along distal end of tendon	*Palpation*—Knotty swelling found just proximal to insertion with chronic tendinosis; with acute, discrete tenderness, with or without swelling *Ortho*—Thompson test indicates loss of passive plantarflexion effect of Achilles, indicating rupture; partial tears are not detectable *ROM*—Passive dorsiflexion coupled with resisted plantarflexion or toe raises may increase pain	• Radiography not generally useful; however, with full ruptures disruption of Kager's triangle may be evident. • Partial tears may be evident with diagnostic ultrasound. • Definitive Dx may require MRI.	• Full ruptures may be managed conservatively with plantarflexion immobilization or treated surgically (conservative treatment results in high re-tear rate). • Tendinitis in general may be initially managed with ice, stretching, and temporary taping support. • Long-term management includes orthotic prescription, if necessary, and stretching of Achilles.

Tibialis Anterior or Tibialis Posterior Tendinitis/Tendinosis	• Should be differentiated from shin splints if possible. • Tibialis tendinitis is differentiated by tenderness or pain along tendon rather than at the origin (shin splints represents a broader involvement and more periosteal involvement at origin).	*Mechanism*—Chronic strain to anterior tibialis is often due to running or walking on hard surfaces or shoes tied too tightly, whereas posterior tendinitis is usually secondary to hyperpronation *History*—Pain on anterior if across top of ankle; posterior pain on medial side of ankle and foot *Palpation*—Tenderness along tendon; often toward distal end *Ortho*—Worse with stretch of tendon or contraction corresponding muscle	• Radiography not necessary unless there is a suspicion of an underlying arthritide such as RA.	• Ice and taping may bring symptomatic relief initially. • Myofascial release may be effective for subacute or chronic problems. • Correction or compensation of associated biomechanical faults through orthotic prescription may be necessary.
Shin Splints	• Ill-defined disorder that may represent periosteal involvement of tibia. • Two types: anterior and posterior.	*Mechanism*—Anterior type found more in anterior/lateral muscle origin due to diminished shock-absorption capabilities of foot; posterior type *History*—Patient with anterior type may have Hx of running or standing on hard surfaces; patients with posterior type may have Hx of hyperpronation problems *Palpation*—Tenderness is just lateral to middle tibia with anterior type and posteromedial at the middle or lower tibia with posterior type *Ortho*—Pain may be increased by stretching involved tendons; tuning fork negative	• Radiographs should be ordered when chronic or when stress fracture is suspected (runners and/or females with menstrual irregularities). • Persistence of pain indicates need for bone scan to rule out stress fracture.	• Taping is often effective for symptom relief. • Buying new running shoes is often corrective for runners. • Correction or compensation of biomechanical faults is often necessary for prevention.
Morton's Neuroma	• Must differentiate from metatarsalgia; both may be reproduced by transverse compression. • The natural history of neuromas is to resolve and return regardless of Tx approach.	*Mechanism*—Entrapment of a digital nerve by intermetatarsal ligaments leads to amorphous deposits *Signs/symptoms*—Pain on bottom of forefoot, less when barefoot; insidious onset *Palpation*—A nodule may be palpable on plantar surface in intermetatrsal space (more common in 2nd or 3rd) *Ortho*—Passive dorsiflexion of MTP or interphalangeal joints may increase pain; decreases with passive plantar flexion	• Radiography not usually indicated.	• Forefoot mobilization and temporary metatarsal pad may be beneficial. • Orthotics may be needed. • Surgical excision may be needed eventually.

(continues)

Foot/Ankle/Lower Leg Diagnosis Table (continued)

Diagnosis	Comments	History Findings	Positive Examination Findings	Radiography/Special Studies	Treatment Options
Tarsal Tunnel Syndrome	• Must be distinguished from nerve root cause due to low back involvement.	*Mechanism*—Posterior tibial nerve is stretched or compressed in tarsal tunnel; often due to hyperpronation; may be due to trauma or swelling *History*—Numbness and tingling across bottom of foot	*Neuro*—Nerve root testing is negative; reproduced by passive dorsiflexion and eversion of the foot/ankle; Tinel's sign at medial ankle may reproduce complaints; sensory deficit on bottom of foot present; motor signs are rare	• Radiographs not usually indicated. • Nerve conduction studies may be needed to confirm.	• If swelling is cause, efforts directed at decreasing swelling. • If biomechanical in origin, correct or compensate through orthotic prescription or mobilization/manipulation.
Myofasciitis	• Used when specific trigger points are identified on physical examination. • Also may be used if a strain is not evident from the history but there are indicators of muscle tenderness, stiffness, or pain.	*Onset*—Nonspecific regarding onset *Symptoms*—Patient usually complains of pain, aching, and/or tenderness in specific muscle or tendon areas that may radiate pain in nonderamtomal pattern	Trigger points are evident as localized tenderness in a muscle that corresponds to traditional (Travell/Simons) trigger point charts; these points may be local or refer pain when compressed	• Not required or recommended.	• Myofascial approaches, such as myofascial stripping, trigger point massage, or spray and stretch, are the standard. • Home stretching and podification of activity suggestions.
Laxity Hypermobility	• This is an adjunctive code to identify causation or the result of a patient's primary diagnosis, such as a sprain or strain due to hypermobility. • Use Laxity code if laxity is confined to the involved joint only; use Hypermobility if multiple joints are lax.	A history of a single event, traumatic injury to the joint is not found; however, either overuse (microtrauma) or generalized inherent looseness is evident	Capsular or ligament testing reveals "looseness" that falls within the physiologic range of normal	• Not usually recommended unless when differentiating pathological laxity from congenital or overuse acquisition.	• Strengthening program. • Bracing or functional taping during rehabilitation or during strenuous activities.

Neurologic Complaints

Weakness

Context

As with many patient complaints, it is imperative to have the patient define his or her complaint: What does "weak" mean to the patient? Without a clear description, the doctor may be led to the assumption that a neurologic or muscular etiology is the cause when, in fact, weakness is actually fatigue associated with an infectious, metabolic, oncologic, pharmacologic, or psychologic (e.g., depression) disorder. Patients experiencing pain with movement will often express a sense of weakness. In addition, patients may interpret a sense of clumsiness, tightness, instability, or uncoordinated movement as "weakness." Determine first, then, whether the patient has general weakness or is substituting or misinterpreting another physical sign/symptom as weakness (**Exhibit 15–1**). If the complaint is more generalized, see Chapter 21, Fatigue, and Chapter 23, Sleep and Related Complaints.

In the context of chiropractic practice, it is most common to find a regional complaint of weakness with associated signs of pain and/or numbness and tingling. It would be unusual to find a patient with signs of central nervous system origin (unless previously diagnosed); the chiropractor must be vigilant, however, in searching for these findings. When weakness is associated with a concomitant complaint of region-specific pain, there must be a diligent search for an anatomic lesion. If there is an objectifiable strength deficit, a major concern is the permanency of this loss.

General Strategy

History

- Determine what the patient means by a complaint of "weakness." Is it a general sense of fatigue or tiredness or a specific regional or joint weakness?

- Is there a history of trauma that would lead one to suspect rupture of a muscle, ligament, or tendon? (Eventually this would be a painless weakness.)
- Is the onset sudden, with diffuse areas of neurologic weakness and/or associated signs of difficulty with speech, cognition, consciousness, or affect? (These deficits are suggestive of a cerebrovascular event.)
- Is the onset insidious with either persistence or progression of symptoms, or an addition effect of more neurologic signs? (The latter is typical of expansile lesions such as tumors.)
- Is there an improvement of neurologic signs, but recurrence? (This is suggestive of a vascular process or multiple sclerosis.)
- Has there been a period of disuse (immobilization with either a sling or cast) or support worn an extended period of time?
- With a specific regional weakness, are there associated sensory complaints such as pain, numbness/tingling, or unusual sensations? (Localize and attempt to match the complaint with a specific nerve root or peripheral nerve pattern.)

Examination

- First determine whether there are signs of an upper motor neuron lesion (UMNL) or a lower motor neuron lesion (LMNL).
- If there is a single regional weakness, attempt to localize it segmentally by associating any deficits in motor or sensory function.
- If a clear distinction is not found for differentiating the site of a lesion, further studies, including electrodiagnostic studies or magnetic resonance imaging (MRI), or both, must be considered.

Exhibit 15–1 Defining Patient's Complaints of Weakness

Patient complains of weakness

Differentiate between specific regional weakness and general weakness

Specific Weakness		General Weakness

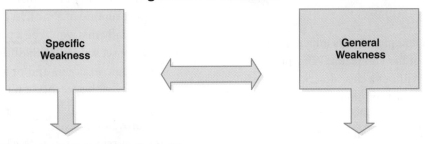

Differentiate objective from subjective if possible (e.g., restricted movement or joint laxity misinterpreted by patient as weakness due to perceived increased effort)

Neurologic	Muscular	Myoneural		Depression	Infection	Hormonal (thyroid or adrenal)

Neurologic causes usually affect the distal extremities.
    Ask the patient about writing or holding a cup for the upper limb; ask about tripping over rugs or curbs for lower.
Muscular disorders (e.g., muscular dystrophy) generally affect the larger, more proximal muscles.
    Ask the patient about gross proximal movements such as getting out of a seat for the lower extremity, combing the hair or reaching above the head for the upper.
Myoneural problems (e.g., myasthenia gravis) affect more the cranial nerves.
    Ask questions about jaw weakness while chewing food, or double vision.

Chronic fatigue syndrome

Metabolic (drugs, anemia, or other causes of poor oxygen delivery: congestive heart failure, chronic obstructive pulmonary disease, etc.)

    Tiredness or fatigue associated with a loss of enjoyment in life, difficulty sleeping, and a sense of worthlessness suggests a depression.
    Tiredness or fatigue that occurs only upon exertion implies metabolic causes such as anemia or poor oxygen delivery. Investigate with lab tests and auscultation.
    Both hypo- and hyperthyroidism may cause a sense of tiredness.
    Chronic fatigue syndrome requires certain criteria for the diagnosis:
  • incapacitating, decreasing ability to perform activities of daily living by 50% or more with fatigue not due to exertion only.
  • must have had for more than 6 months.
  • not relieved by sleeping.

Further differentiation with electromyographic or nerve conduction velocity testing may be necessary.

Management

- Weakness due to a UMNL should always be referred to a neurologist immediately.
- Weakness associated with myasthenia gravis should be referred for medical management.
- Most cases of nerve root or peripheral nerve weakness can be managed conservatively for one month, monitoring for worsening or progression (which would warrant referral for a second opinion).

Relevant Anatomy and Physiology

Although integration for smooth and coordinated muscle function is a complex process involving both ascending and descending pathways, for general strength the examiner's focus is on the corticospinal (and corticobulbar) tracts. Information that has been integrated at a higher level is sent to the anterior horn cells via the corticospinal tracts. From this point, information is sent out to the spinal nerves that divide into anterior and posterior primary rami. The posterior rami innervate the deep muscles of the back. The anterior rami form four plexuses that eventually, through a process of recombination (roots to trunks to division to cords), form peripheral nerves. All peripheral nerves interact with the target muscle(s) at the myoneural junction.

Corticospinal tract function includes inhibitory influences. Increased excitability due to cortical divorce from the alpha motoneuron results in increased muscle tone with passive movement. The hyperexcitable alpha motoneuron also causes an increase in deep tendon reflexes. A number of older reflexes that disappear with maturation of the nervous system are unmasked (e.g., Babinski's reflex). Although pathologic reflexes are hyperreflexic, the fact that the reflex is intact indicates a functioning alpha motoneuron and peripheral motor nerve.

An important anatomic design is the laminated arrangement of spinal tracts within the spinal cord. Fibers innervating the lower parts of the body are more superficial and lateral. Compressive lesions would present with a temporal presentation of sequential, ascending weakness. This lamination is also true of ascending sensory tracts. Therefore, an accompanying ascending sensory loss may be found.

For neurologic weakness to occur there must be a lesion somewhere along the corticospinal or corticobulbar paths (cortex, brainstem, spinal cord) or at the anterior horn cell, myoneural junction, or muscle. There are some generalizations that will guide the examiner in discriminating among the various neurologic and muscular causes. The first discrimination is whether there are any signs of a UMNL or an LMNL.

- A UMNL indicates pathology in the cerebral hemispheres, brainstem, or spinal cord. Interruption of inhibitory influences eventually leads to increased reflexes and an increase in muscle tone and spastic paralysis; pathologic reflexes such as Babinski's appear also.
- An LMNL indicates pathology in the anterior horn cell or motoneuron. Interruption of the reflex loop leads to absent or decreased deep tendon reflexes. Disconnection from the motoneuron leads to atrophy and fasciculations. Muscle tone may be normal or decreased (flaccid paralysis).

Stroke

Stroke is the third leading cause of death in the United States. Although it indicates a vascular cause of neurological deficit, the use of the term *stroke* is not always consistent with some vascular events such as subarachnoid hemorrhage, subdural hematomas, and epidural hematomas not included under the category of stroke due to more diffuse involvement of the central nervous system.

Stroke is an acute onset of neurological deficit that is vascular in origin and lasts at least 24 hours. It represents a focal area of damage in the brain that leads to diffuse clinical consequences based on the region affected. Therefore events that are shorter in duration or have more diffuse involvement have a different categorization. A transient ischemic accident (TIA) represents an event that resolves usually within 24 hours after onset, often in the first 30 minutes. Statistically, one-third of patients who suffer a TIA will have a full stroke within the next five years. Reversible, ischemic, neurological deficit (RIND), also called a minor stroke, is reserved for events that fully recover but take more than 24 hours; often several days. TIAs and RIND represent ischemic (i.e., blockage) events, not hemorrhage. Other cerebrovascular events that are more diffuse and do not classically fit under the definition of stroke are termed *global cerebral ischemia*. Global cerebral ischemia is more often the consequence of myocardial infarction or subarachnoid hemorrhage.

Chiropractors are not in a clinical position or level of expertise to diagnose where in the brain a stroke is occurring, but generally signs and symptoms will inevitably reveal the side of involvement and often the vascular area involved if clinically divided into an anterior versus a posterior circulation. Generally, weakness and sensory findings manifest on the opposite side of the lesion below the neck. Aphasia usually indicates the left cortex. The anterior circulation derived from the internal carotid artery supplies much of the cortex and subcortical white matter, the basal ganglia, and the internal capsule. When it is involved there is a combination of motor or sensory findings, language/speech deficits, and memory loss. The posterior circulation derived from the vertebral arteries, the branching basilar arteries, and their branches supply mainly the cerebellum, thalamus, brainstem, and parts of the occipital and temporal areas. Signs and symptoms are generally related to brainstem dysfunction including coma, drop attacks, vertigo, nausea, and ataxia.

Following are some examples of how more localization of the lesion site can be determined based on testing for specific neurological deficits:

- Because medial brainstem lesions involve the pyramidal tracts, lesions will usually cause contralateral spastic hemiplegia with no sensory loss. Further localization can be made through examination for deficit in the oculomotor nerve (i.e., midbrain), the abducens nerve (i.e., pons), and the hypoglossal nerve (i.e., medulla).
- Because lateral brainstem lesions will more often involve the spinothalamic tracts, with sensory loss as the main feature primarily involving pain and temperature. At the caudal pons and medulla where the spinothalamic and spinal trigeminal tracts travel closely together, there will be ipsilateral loss of pain and temperature in the face with contralateral loss in the trunk and limbs. Further distinction can be made by testing cranial nerves VII, VIII, IX, and X. At higher levels, localization involves testing the motor and principal trigeminal nuclei for the midbrain, the superior cerebellar peduncle, and the rostral pons and caudal midbrain, and for the rostral midbrain, the medial lemniscus and trigeminothalamic tracts.
- One of the most commonly involved areas with stroke is the internal capsule. This area includes the pyramidal tracts, the somatosensory tracts, and, closely located, the corticobulbar tracts. Involvement of the dorsal internal capsule would

then result in contralateral findings of spastic hemiplegia, contralateral lower face weakness, and contralateral anesthesia. If more ventral, the lesion may affect the optic radiation with an additional finding of contralateral homonymous hemianopsia.

There are generally two types of stroke: (1) thromboembolic (ischemic) stroke, representing occlusion or blockage of blood supply to the target area, and (2) hemorrhagic stroke, representing usually rupture and bleeding, often under high pressure due to arterial involvement. These are further divided and classified by the location of the lesion. Hemorrhagic is intracerebral, whereas ischemic stroke is either from a local thrombus or from a distantly originating embolus. There is also a combination of effects when an ischemic infarct leads to hemorrhagic conversion because the blood vessels become fragile and rupture.

Embolic infarct forms distally and travels to the brain, whereas thrombotic infarct is a blood clot that forms locally, usually due to atherosclerosis. Generally, embolic occur suddenly with rapid onset of symptoms, whereas thrombotic may be slow to develop. Other helpful discriminators are that stroke events that have the same clinical signs each time are generally from the cerebral circulation while those that differ each time are often cardiac in origin and are embolic. Some generalizations include that large-vessel infarcts generally occur from emboli (although proximal thrombus may occur). Small-vessel infarcts occlude small penetrating vessels to deep structures such as basal ganglia, thalamus, and internal capsule or the brainstem. Some small-vessel infarcts are sometimes referred to as lacunar because they form small cavities (lakes). Specific lacunar syndromes have been identified. So where do emboli develop prior to reaching the cerebral circulation? Following are some common examples:

- Cardioembolic—30% of those that have electrocardioversion for arrhythmias throw emboli
- Dissection—dependent on type of dissection, emboli can be thrown
- Patent foramen ovale—an atrial septal defect, this is associated with emboli and may have a relationship to migraine headache
- Deep vein thrombosis—more commonly travel to the lungs
- Other than thromboembolism, air, fat, and septic emboli are also possible

The most common nontraumatic cause of hemorrhagic stroke is chronic hypertension. Hemorrhagic stroke usually causes symptoms by compressing adjacent tissue (which then may produce ischemia). Hemorrhagic stroke tends to cause more severe headache and neurological depression than ischemic stroke. Neurologic deficits do not generally correspond to any single blood vessel.

A distinction must be established between general cardiovascular risk with associated complications of myocardial infarction, stroke, and peripheral vascular disease and stroke that is not atherosclerotic but instead is related to dissection (i.e., intimal tearing) or reflexogenic vasospasm. This latter type is more often the cause of vertebrobasilar (VB) stroke.

It is clear that many of the risk factors for atherosclerosis and subsequent stroke can be modified, whereas those related to vascular weakness other than hypertension are difficult to modify other than management of the underlying condition.

Evaluation

History

After having the patient clarify whether he or she feels weak, tired, or fatigued, the most revealing line of questioning is in relation to daily activities (**Table 15–1**).

Table 15–1 History Questions for Weakness: Determining the General Cause

Primary Question	What Are You Thinking?	Secondary Questions	What Are You Thinking?
Do you feel weakness of your arm or leg, hands or feet?	A yes would imply a neurologic or muscular disorder; a no requires further questioning.	**Do you feel generally weak (tired or fatigued)?**	Think more of metabolic and endocrine problems, infection, or depression.
		Are you taking any medications?	Antihypertensives, antihistamines, and barbiturates are common culprits.
		Is this feeling always there or only when you exert yourself?	If the feeling is only with exertion consider cardiopulmonary/vascular causes (including anemia).
Are specific daily activities difficult because of weakness?	Attempt to determine whether a specific body-area weakness is upper or lower, proximal or distal.	**Lower extremity** • proximal—getting up from chair, toilet, car • distal—tripping over rugs, curbs, cords	Proximal usually indicates an endocrine or myopathic problem (painless weakness).
		Upper extremity • proximal—combing hair, reaching overhead • distal—writing, typing, opening jars	Distal usually indicates a neurologic disorder.
		Head • whistling, blowing, chewing, speaking, swallowing, keeping soap out of eyes while showering	Cranial nerve dysfunction often implies a medullary or pontine disorder, especially if accompanied with extremity findings. Fatigue after repeated action points to myasthenia gravis.
Is there associated numbness and/or tingling?	A neurologic cause is likely. Look for a patch of skin that correlates with a dermatome or peripheral nerve pattern.	**Is the numbness constant or intermittent?**	Constant would imply a neurologic cause (possibly metabolic/endocrine); intermittent would imply transient or early neurologic compression.
Is there pain associated with the weakness?	Weakness is often the result of neurologic inhibition due to pain (example: knee gives out).	**If it is not painful now, was there ever trauma (injury) to the area?**	Rupture of muscles, tendons, or ligaments may result in loss of function that is eventually painless.

Ask the patient to describe the activity that causes the feeling of weakness in an attempt to determine whether he or she means a specific regional weakness, an unco-ordinated or clumsy sensation, or the exertion fatigue felt with some systemic and cardiopulmonary disorders. If it appears to be a regional complaint, further clarify by extracting a description that localizes upper or lower extremity and proximal or distal weakness. This line of questioning focuses on the generalization that neurologic diseases usually start distally, whereas myopathies usually become more evident proximally. For example, difficulty using the fingers or hands would be more suggestive of a neurologic cause, whereas difficulty with combing the hair or reaching behind the back would be more sug-gestive of a myopathy. In the lower extremities, tripping over rugs or curbs is more suggestive of a neural cause, whereas difficulty rising from a seated position is more often myopathic (especially if nonpainful).

Some characteristic patterns of "weakness" that suggest a global fatigue may help guide the examiner through questioning (see Chapter 21, Fatigue).

- Patients with an infectious cause are often tired after exertion. This may also occur with anemia or cardiopulmonary disorders.
- The weakness associated with endocrine and electrolyte disorders is often felt more proximally. Either hypo- or hyperthyroidism may cause weakness. It is more often (80% to 90%) found with hyperthyroidism. Also, hypo- or hyperadrenal disorders may present with a complaint of weakness. Electrolyte imbalances, high or low, may lead to weakness. Evaluation with a general screening lab workup may give direct or indirect indications of these causes.
- Fatigue or tiredness that seems worse after eating may indicate hypoglycemic reactions, reaction to alcohol consumption, or a delayed reaction from overingestion of caffeine.
- Medications often will have a sedative effect that may be augmented by the use of alcohol or other drugs such as antihypertensives, antihistamines, codeine, and barbiturates.
- Fatigue or tiredness throughout the day may be suggestive of a sleep disorder, including the possibility of depression. A characteristic insomnia pattern is often associated with reactive depression; with endogenous (neurochemical) depression, the patient often awakens early and finds it difficult to fall back to sleep (see Chapter 20, Depression).

A sense of weakness may be a misinterpretation by the patient. For example, if a patient has hip stiffness, it may feel as if lifting the knee toward the chest is weak; muscle testing in the midrange, however, might indicate normal strength. Instability may present similarly. If a patient has laxity of the shoulder, overhead movements may feel "weak" because of the inability of the shoulder muscu-lature to compensate for ligamentous/capsular laxity at higher levels of elevation.

Muscle cramps are most often related to sports or occupation. However, a multitude of diseases have pos-sible associated cramping, including Parkinson's disease, numerous central nervous system disorders/diseases, diabetes, peripheral nervous and peripheral vascular disease, and hemodialysis. Muscle cramps occur in almost half of pregnant women. Oral supplementation of calcium appears effective in most cases. If cramping is associated with walking, consider vascular insuf-ficiency and intermittent claudication and hyper- and hypothyroidism. Medications associated with cramping include, but are not limited to, cisplatin and vincristine. Cramping may be described for various drug-induced myalgias, from cimetidine and cholestyramine. Severe vomiting or hyperventilation may cause relative alka-losis with calcium, resulting in cramping and paresthe-sias. Rarer causes (often metabolic deficiency diseases) include the following:

- McArdle's disease—muscle phosphorylase deficiency
- Carnitine palmitoyltransferase II deficiency—genetic disorder of lipid metabolism
- Brody's disease—phosphoglycerate kinase deficiency (myoglobinuria)
- Tarui's disease—phosphofructokinase deficiency
- Isaac's syndrome—neuromyotonia
- Stiff man syndrome—back and abdominal cramping

For similar or overlapping complaints with weakness, such as tremors and ticks, and for the possibility of more serious inherited disorders, see **Tables 15–2** and **15–3**.

Examination

Following are some pattern generalizations that may help guide the examination:

- Cerebrum—Generally a combination of UMNL and associated problems with cognitive functions or mood suggests a cortical pathologic process.

Table 15–2 Muscular Disorders

Procedure	Comments
Muscular Dystrophies Duchenne's dystrophy	Both Duchenne's and Becker's are X-linked recessive disorders. Duchenne's involves a defect in dystrophin and has an onset within the first five years of life. Becker's usually has normal dystrophin. The pelvis area is affected first, then eventually limb involvement with both. With Becker's there is a slow progression with a normal longevity; however, with Duchenne's there is eventual respiratory muscles involvement, with death occurring within about 15 years of the onset. Duchenne's is detectable using DNA probes in late pregnancy. Diagnosis after birth is prompted by weakness which must be differentiated electromyographically and with serum creatine kinase levels.
Facioscapulohumeral	An autosomal dominant disorder that can occur at any age. It affects the face and shoulder girdle, although the pelvis and legs are eventually affected. There is minor disability with a normal longevity.
Limb-girdle (Erb's)	A variable genetic inheritance, usually autosomal recessive, with onset from ages 10 to 30 years. The pelvis and shoulder may be affected first. A wide variety of presentation and prognosis with the possibility of severe disability at middle age.
Myopathies Congenital	There are many, yet rare, disorders that may cause myopathy. These include glycogen storage diseases, such as Pompe disease, or errors in lipid metabolism, such as carnitine deficiency. There usually is multisystem involvement; however muscle-only may occur, such as nemaline myopathy or central core myopathy. Clinically the disease would be seen in an infant or child who cannot move, with flaccid limbs. Must be differentiated from cerebral palsy.
Steroid (acquired)	Patients on high-dose steroid therapy such as Prednisone are prone to developing steroid myopathy. Clues are that the CK and nerve conduction tests are normal but EMG demonstrates short-duration, low-amplitude motor unit potentials (MUPs) with early and rapid recruitment. Muscle biopsy demonstrates type 2 fiber atrophy.
Mitochondrial	A diverse group of disorders that affects skeletal muscle. This may be seen microscopically as "ragged red fibers" (accumulation of abnormal mitochondria) using the modified Gomori stain. Patients may have either ophthalmoplegia or limb weakness (especially after exercise).
Channelopathies Myotonic dystrophy (Steinert's disease)	Most common adult-onset muscular dystrophies occurring in 5 per 100,000 individuals. This is an abnormal trinucleotide repeat problem along chromosome 19 and possibly chromosome 3. Characterized by abnormal muscle relaxation, many individuals notice this after shaking hands with inability to relax. Other features include proximal and distal weakness, diabetes mellitus, early cataracts, premature balding, hypersomnia, and abnormalities of the heart and GI system. Serum creatine kinase Z(CK) levels are generally 10 times normal. Associate electrodiagnostic testing is found. Selective genetic analysis of blood and muscle confirm the diagnosis.
Myotonic congenita	An inherited trait involving the long arm of chromosome 7. Individuals have myotonia without weakness initially. Complaints are stiffness and weakness, worse with inactivity or cold and improved with exercise. Muscle hypertrophy may be present. Treatment is with a variety of drugs used with other myotonic conditions, including quinine, procainamide, or phenytoin, among others.
Inflammatory Dermatomyositis and polymyositis	This inclusion body myositis begins insidiously in middle age. Progression is usually proximal, first evident in the lower extremities. Serum creatine kinase levels may be normal and sometimes increased. Responsiveness to corticosteroids is not encouraging. Recent suggestions of intravenous immunoglobulin are still being investigated.
Familial Periodic Paralysis Hypokalemic	The most common familial periodic paralysis. This autosomal dominant disorder involves gene mutations of the dihydropyridine receptor that is involved with chloride channels. Other conditions that affect potassium levels must be evaluated, such as renal, endocrine, and GI causes. This rare condition (1.25 per 100,000) is characterized by attacks, which occur during adolescence, of paralysis that is precipitated by carbohydrate ingestion, alcohol, cold exposure, stress, and resting after exercise. Hypokalemia is a consequence, not a cause, of the disease.
Hyperkalemic	A possible defect in the sodium channel gene on the long arm of chromosome 17, attacks usually occur after exercise lasting less than an hour. They are relieved by several medications, including glucose, glucose and insulin, or calcium gluconate (intravenous). Prevention is sometimes attempted with daily acetazolamide or chlorothiazide.

Table 15–3 Movement Disorders

Type and Causes	Clinical Presentation/Management
Tremors Essential	Also called benign essential (familial) tremor, this autosomal dominant tremor is a fine-to-coarse tremor that is usually not present at rest but apparent with skilled acts. Tremor mainly involves the hands and head, usually not the lower extremity. It is enhanced by emotional stress and sometimes dramatically relieved (temporarily) with a small amount of alcohol.
Resting	A resting tremor is seen primarily with Parkinson's disease, disappearing with movement.
Cerebellar	Cerebellar tremors are often associated with multiple sclerosis and are intention tremors. The limb oscillates as it approaches an intended object. Other tremors include sustained tremor seen primarily with the proximal muscles when maintaining a fixed or weight-bearing posture. Titubation is a more gross tremor of the head and body that remits with lying down. Asterixis, or "liver-flap," is seen with some hepatic or metabolic encephalopathies.
Dyskinesias Myoclonus	Myoclonus is the brief, jerking movement felt by many individuals while falling asleep. Abnormal myoclonus, felt as brief involuntary contractions of a muscle or group of muscles, may occur secondary to other disorders such as uremia, Alzheimer's, epilepsy, slow viruses (Creutzfeldt-Jakob's disease), hypoxia, or head trauma. If there is an underlying metabolic disorder, it must be addressed. Anti-epileptic medication or 5-HTP with carbidopa may be used.
Tics • Simple tics	Repetitive, brief, rapid involuntary movements that may develop as mannerisms and resolve with time.
• Tourette syndrome	An autosomal dominant disorder with variable penetrance. Simple tics may progress to complex tics involving respiratory or vocal manifestations, including compulsive vocalizations with swearing. Some of the tics are under the individual's control for a few seconds. Treatment usually involves medication such as benzodiazepines or antipsychotics such as haloperidol.
Choreas and athetoses	Choreas are brief, purposeless movement of the distal extremities and face that are involuntary. The most common causes are Huntington's chorea, Sydenham's chorea related to rheumatic fever, SLE, and drug induced. Athetoses are writhing movements, flowing in nature, and often involve the proximal limb musculature. Both are due to dopaminergic overactivity in the basal ganglia.
Hemiballismus	Hemiballismus is a violent movement disorder where the arm (occurs on one side usually) or leg is flung about continuously. Usually the result of infarct or tumor of the contralateral subthalamic nucleus. Usually self-limiting over two months. Treatment is usually with antipsychotics.
Huntington's	An autosomal dominant disorder that involves degeneration of parts of the CNS, including the caudate nucleus and small cell bodies. GABA and substance P levels decrease. The individual experiences deterioration that is progressive, leading to choreiform movements, and intellectual and motor decline. The onset is usually middle age with both sexes affected equally. No treatment is available. Medication is used to manage choreiform movements and agitated behavior.
Dystonia	Dystonia is a sustained abnormal posturing or a disruption of a movement pattern due to altered muscle tone. There are several types, including generalized (a rare hereditary problem with fixed plantarversion and inversion of the foot), focal which is confined to a single region, and segmental which is a focal dystonia that spreads to an adjacent region. Several disorders are associated or named dystonias, including: • Meigs' syndrome (blepharo-oromandibular syndrome)—involuntary blinking, grimacing, or jaw grinding that begins in middle-aged individuals (should be differentiated by tardive dyskinesia usually associated with medication side effects). • Torticollis—deviation of the head and neck to one side, which can be voluntarily corrected initially. • Spastic dystonia—spasms of laryngeal muscles resulting in a voice change, sounding hoarse, cracking, or strained. • Occupational dystonia—associated with a specific, usually repetitive, activity such as writer's cramp. • Symptomatic dystonia—associated with specific diseases such as Wilson's, lipidosis, and cerebral palsy, among others. For local dystonias, botulism A toxin is injected into the area, which often results in relief of muscle spasm.

Table 15–3 Movement Disorders (continued)

Type and Causes	Clinical Presentation/Management
Drug-induced	Several classes of medications may cause blocking of dopamine receptors in the CNS resulting in extra-pyramidal signs, including Parkinson's, tardive dyskinesias, and acute dystonia. These medications include benzothiazine, antipsychotics, and antiemetics.
Parkinson's	Two types: Primary involves degeneration of the pigmented cells of the substantia nigra, locus coeruleus, and other areas involved in dopaminergic cells. Secondary Parkinson's is usually the result of medications that act as dopamine blockers (see above). Signs include a pill-rolling tremor (5–8 Hz), difficulty initiating and stopping movement, muscle rigidity, slowness of movement, and a mask-like facial appearance. Dementia affects approximately half of patients.
Progressive Supranuclear Palsy (Steele-Richardson-Olszewski syndrome)	Degeneration of the basal ganglia and brainstem leading to loss of voluntary eye movement control, pseudobulbar palsy, axial dystonia, and eventually dementia. Onset is during middle age. The first sign may be inability to look up with eye movement only; must use neck extension to look up, as when climbing stairs.
Cerebellar/ Spinocerebellar	Abnormalities related to the cerebellum may result in dystonias. The range of disorders includes infarcts, hemorrhages, infections, and tumors. Tumors include neuroblastoma cystic astrocytoma. Neurologic disease or disorders include multiple sclerosis, Chiari malformation (cerebellar tissue extends into cervical spinal canal), or basilar invagination with platybasia (flattening of the base of the skull as is sometimes seen in Paget's disease of bone). Degenerative disease results in ataxia and includes: • Friedreich's ataxia—an autosomal recessive disorder, with onset during childhood or early adolescence, resulting in upper extremity ataxia and dysarthria. Large-fiber sensory loss leads to loss of vibration and position sense. • Abetalipoproteinemia (vitamin E deficiency) and Refsum's disease—similar characteristics to Friedreich's ataxia. • Cerebellar ataxias—inherited disorder that affects middle-aged individuals with most of the pathologic aspects occurring in the cerebellum. • Multiple systems atrophy (olivopontocerebellar atrophy)—a group of variable disorders including Déjérine-Thomas disorder, Shy-Drager syndrome (autonomic involvement), and Machado-Joseph disease.

- Cerebellum—Combinations of ataxia, vertigo, and/or dysarthria suggest a cerebellar pathologic process. Cerebellar disorders usually result in problems with the rate, range, and force of movements. The cerebellum is often divided into three functional areas. The vestibulocerebellum (archicerebellum) includes the flocculonodular lobe and is involved in maintaining equilibrium, coordinating eye and neck movements, and is integrated with the vestibular nuclei. The middle vernis of cerebellum (paleocerebellum) is important for stance and gait. Finally, the lateral hemispheres (neocerebellum) control primarily ballistic types of movements and fine, coordinated movements of the limbs, particularly the arms.

- Brainstem—Cranial nerve problems are often predominant with a crossed pattern of involvement (i.e., the face on the lesion side and the body on the opposite side). The corticospinal tract crosses at the lower medulla.

- Spinal cord—A spinal cord lesion usually has a sensory level; sensory disturbance is found below the level of the lesion. At the level of the lesion an LMNL is often present; below are UMNL signs. In addition, if the lesion is expansive, loss of pain and temperature is often associated with an upper limb weakness that gradually descends to the trunk and lower extremity. Compressive lesions will produce the opposite (if anterior), an ascending pattern of motor weakness. If localized posteriorly, a loss of proprioception is evident.

- Nerve root—Weakness is often associated with low back or neck pain. In addition, there are accompanying sensory complaints such as numbness and/or tingling. More specifically, the pain should follow a related dermatome with weakness in a specific myotome. If there is a corresponding deep tendon reflex (DTR), it will be decreased or absent.

- Peripheral nerve—Like nerve root problems, a distinctive sensory pattern often accompanies peripheral nerve irritation or compression. This pattern should be distinct from the nerve root pattern, as should the distinctive muscle weakness grouping (assuming a motor component to the nerve). DTRs may be affected.

- Myoneural junction—Myoneural dysfunction is usually more evident with muscles supplied by cranial nerves. Characteristically, repeated contraction causes progressive weakness, with recovery with rest. This is typical of myasthenia gravis.
- Myopathy—Typically, myopathic weakness is evident first proximally. Examples include muscular dystrophy and inflammatory disorders of muscle. There are no sensory findings, and reflexes should be intact. Further investigation with laboratory or electromyographic (EMG) testing is necessary.

A high level of suspicion will have been gained by a thorough history. If there is a sense of a UMNL it is prudent to begin with a search for signs, including hyperreflexia, a pathologic reflex (Babinski's), and eventually changes in muscle tone (spastic weakness). If the lesion appears to be spinal, a search for a sensory level is extremely helpful. A sensory level is a combined finding where there is a sensory disturbance below the level of the lesion accompanied by signs of an LMNL at the level and signs of a UMNL below the level.

The standard grading scale for muscle strength is as follows:

- Grade 5—complete range of motion (ROM) against maximal resistance
- Grade 4—complete ROM against gravity and some resistance
- Grade 3—complete ROM against gravity
- Grade 2—complete ROM if gravity is eliminated
- Grade 1—palpable or visible evidence of muscle contraction, yet no movement
- Grade 0—no evidence of muscle contraction

This standard approach is based on ROM and resistance to gravity or examiner resistance. The distinction between grades 2 and 3, for example, is that with a grade 2 strength the patient is only able to slide his or her leg across the table (gravity is eliminated), while a patient with a grade 3 strength is able to lift the leg off the table (against gravity). The faults of this system lie in the evaluation being dependent on full ROM (isotonic contraction) and the limited choices for grading. Most

patients should be examined using isometric muscle testing in an effort first to determine whether pain is causing inhibition or whether true weakness is present. Also, it is important to determine whether normal strength is present within the ROM available.

Although orthopaedic muscle testing has been used to correlate muscle weakness with other localizing neurologic findings (dermatome and deep tendon reflex), other information may be gained. When a muscle is found to be weak it is important to determine why. If the muscle tests weakly and painfully, this response serves little function as a nerve root localizer, yet it is extremely valuable as a soft tissue localizer. In other words, pain often inhibits contraction. Therefore, it is difficult to determine true neurologic function when contraction is painful. If a muscle tests weakly but is painless, there is a high level of suspicion of neurologic weakness or a tendon rupture. Often a palpable bulge or deformity, combined with other findings, clearly differentiates between the two events.

When a muscle is weak and the test is painless, the neurologic differentiation is still incomplete. What becomes apparent when trying to narrow down the possibilities is the overlap among different levels of branching of the peripheral nervous system with regard to motor innervation. For example, if a patient was found to have weakness of the triceps, the extensor carpi radialis, and the extensor carpi ulnaris, the first suspicion may be radial nerve damage. If the brachioradialis is still strong, however, and the small muscles of the thumb (such as the abductor, opponens, and adductors) are also found to be weak, radial nerve damage is not likely. The two remaining peripheral nerves (median and ulnar) may account for the small muscle weakness, but they could not account for the triceps and extensor carpi weaknesses. This is also true of the divisions and trunks of the brachial plexus. However, the common root level of all weak muscles is C8 and T1. Neither has an associated deep tendon reflex. Neither alone could account for all the weak muscles; therefore, a search for where both could be affected reveals the suspected site at the lower trunk of the brachial plexus. This would be strongly reinforced with a finding of sensory abnormality over the dermatomes for C8 and T1; medial arm down to fifth and fourth fingers.

When performing manual muscle testing, it is important to realize some inherent weaknesses. As mentioned above, pain may cause a muscle to test weakly, and although not necessarily helpful in localizing a neurologic level, it does indicate a structure in need of attention. The other variables that influence a patient's ability to contract a muscle are numerous. These include time of day, gravity, velocity of the test maneuver, technique and instructions of the examiner, ambient noise, and inability to stabilize the muscle origin.[1] Some practical examples of this variation are as follows:

- If one tests the internal tibial rotators with the knee flexed to 90°, but the hip is placed in different positions, strength will vary with hip placement even though the tibia remains the same.
- If the patient feels unstable, she or he may not be able to contract the appropriate muscle(s) fully or may recruit other muscles to assist.
- If the examiner fails to instruct or prewarn the patient, a force may be applied too quickly for the patient to react, resulting in movement at the joint that could be interpreted as weakness by the examiner.

When a pattern is not clear and a lesion site is not obvious, electrodiagnostic studies may clarify the source (**Table 15–4**). Electrodiagnostic studies, mainly EMG and nerve conduction velocity (NCV) studies, are limited according to the experience and expertise of the examiner. When performed appropriately, however, these studies may help differentiate and in some cases identify the degree of damage when a neuronal pathology exists. EMG uses needle insertion into muscle to test muscle and nerve.[2] The spontaneous activity generated or the response generated with contraction helps distinguish between axon injury and demyelination disorders. NCV uses surface electrodes to measure velocity and the amplitude of an evoked response to an electrical stimulus. Both motor and sensory nerves can be tested.

When an anterior horn cell (or its fibers) is damaged, a specific group of muscle fibers is affected. Surviving neurons are able to sprout collateral fibers to reinnervate the denervated muscle fibers. These changes are reflected on the EMG.

- Because denervated muscle fibers are highly irritable, prolonged activity occurs with needle insertion (this may also occur with myopathy).
- At rest with the needle inserted, spontaneous activity consisting of fibrillations, positive sharp waves, and fasciculations indicate a neurogenic abnormality.
- During contraction of the muscle a reduction in the density pattern, interference pattern, and mean amplitude of motor unit potentials (MUPs) occurs with neurogenic disorders. With myopathies, the duration and amplitude of MUPs are decreased, but the interference pattern is unaffected.

NCV studies involve electrical stimulation at one or more sites along a peripheral nerve measured at a correlated muscle. For a motor NCV, the time it takes from each point of stimulation to the appearance of the muscle potential is referred to as the latency. The conduction velocity is calculated by dividing the distance between two points of stimulation and the time it takes to travel between the two points. Latencies are prolonged and velocities are decreased when there is an internodal demyelination or localized axonal narrowing as seen with specific neuropathies (e.g., carpal tunnel syndrome). More important, however, are the compound muscle action potential (CMAP) and the sensory nerve action potential (SNAP) amplitudes, which are more sensitive

Table 15–4 Electrodiagnostic Studies

Condition/Structure	NCV	SNAP/CMAP	EMC	SSEP
Nerve root/anterior horn (radiculopathy) (axonal degeneration)	Probably normal	Usually reduced in 2–3 weeks; SNAP normal if lesion is proximal to DRG	Fibrillation potentials, positive sharp waves, decreased recruitment; MUPs decreased	Interpeak latency between Erb's point and dorsal columns may localize to nerve root
Peripheral neuropathy	Slowed velocity, increased latency (within 1 week)	Unaffected unless conduction block	Not segmental or specific for nerve root	May help localize based on latency
Brachial plexus lesions	Not usually useful	SNAPs decreased or absent	No fibrillation in paraspinal muscles	Sometimes valuable in localizing

Key: NCV, nerve conduction velocity; SNAP, sensory nerve action potential; CMAP, compound muscle action potential; SSEP, somatosensory-evoked potentials; DRG, dorsal root ganglion; MUP, motor unit potential.

to traumatic peripheral nerve injury.[3] Following are some generalizations that may be helpful:

- Axonal degeneration will demonstrate normal velocities with NCV studies, but a reduced amplitude of evoked responses. EMG evidence takes about three weeks to surface, revealing spontaneous activity at rest, such as fibrillations and positive sharp waves; during contraction, there is a reduction in the density pattern, interference pattern, and mean amplitude of the MUPs.
- Demyelination disorders will demonstrate early changes in the nerve conduction velocity with relatively normal evoked amplitude responses.

When a proximal weakness pattern is found, further testing for a myopathic cause should include laboratory testing (e.g., lactate dehydrogenase) and muscle biopsy.

Management

Medical management is necessary for patients with UMNL, myasthenia gravis, Guillain-Barré syndrome, and drug- or toxin-induced neuropathy, or in the event that no known cause can be found. Most other causes of regional or specific weakness can be managed conservatively through a combination of spinal adjusting and muscular re-education. The reader is directed to chapters on specific disorders for a more detailed description of conservative management recommendations.

Algorithm

An algorithm for evaluation and management of weakness is presented in **Figure 15–1**.

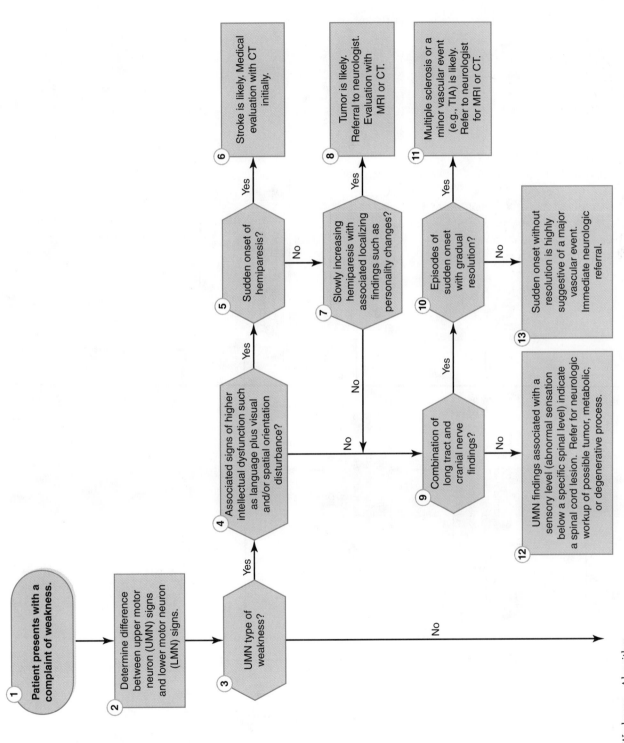

Figure 15–1 Weakness—Algorithm

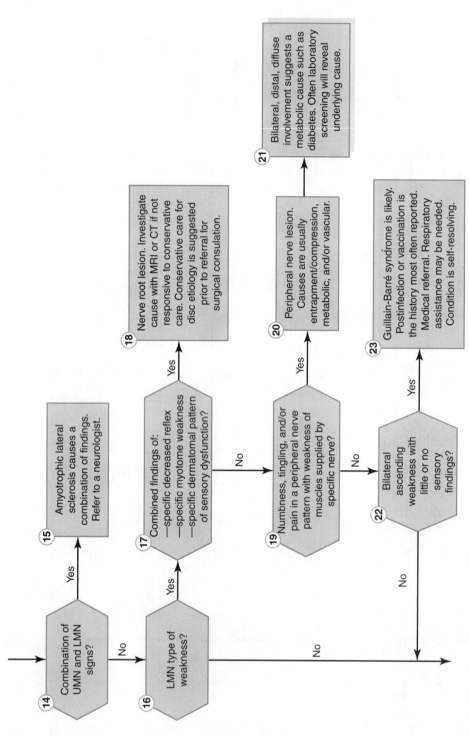

Figure 15–1 (Continued)

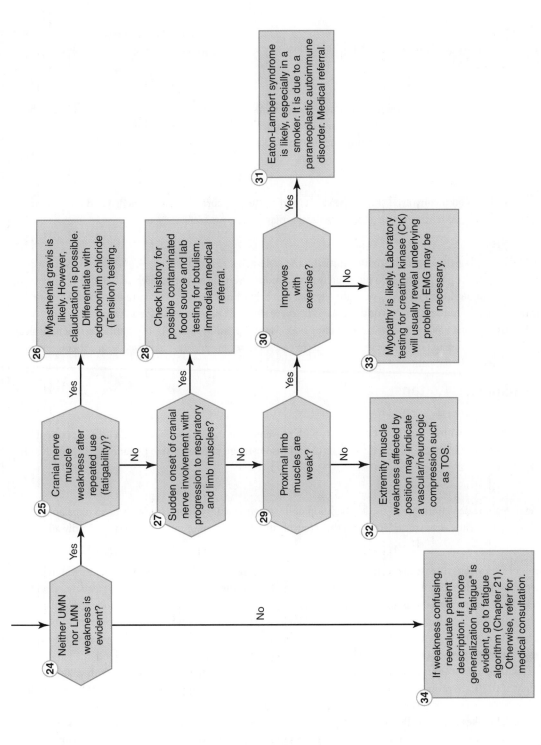

Figure 15–1 (Continued)

Selected Neurologic and Muscular Diseases*

Bell's Palsy

Classic Presentation

The patient complains of facial weakness and distortion and is unable to close one eye. There may be an associated ear pain. The patient does not recall any cause, just simply "woke up with it."

Cause

The cause is unknown; however, it is believed that a viral infection may cause an inflammatory reaction in the facial nerve near the stylomastoid foramen or in the facial nerve path through the temporal bone. Other causes of facial nerve involvement include stroke, cerebral tumor (mainly involves lower face), Ramsay Hunt syndrome (herpes vesicles visible in the ear), mastoid infection, fracture, or cerebellopontine angle tumors (associated hearing loss).

Evaluation

The patient's face appears expressionless on the involved side. If the case is severe, the palpebral fissure is widened and the patient cannot close the eye on the involved side. A deficit in taste and a hyperacusis may also be present.

Management

There is still a debate as to whether Bell's palsy should be treated initially. The general belief is that because 60% of patients recover completely without treatment and that the patients who do not usually have a more severe form, corticosteroids should be given only if the palsy is complete. It has not been demonstrated conclusively that this helps, but it does appear to reduce pain. The best approach is to monitor the degree of involvement for two or three days. If severe after this time, referral for a limited course of corticosteroids is warranted. Eye drops and a patch may be needed until eye closure is possible. Faradic stimulation or other physical therapy approaches may prevent contracture of facial muscles in long-term cases. Poorer prognosis is assumed with patients who are elderly, have hyperacusis, or have severe initial pain.

Parkinson's Disease (Paralysis Agitans)

Classic Presentation

The patient is older (aged 45 to 65 years) with a complaint of difficulty with movement and associated tremors. Often the patient has no specific complaint, yet on physical examination, the cardinal signs of parkinsonism are present. These include rigidity, bradykinesia, tremor, and walking difficulties.

Cause

Parkinson's disease is due to dopamine depletion caused by degeneration of the nigrostriatal system. This leads to an imbalance between dopamine and acetylcholine. The extrapyramidal system that controls the smoothness of movement is profoundly affected.

Evaluation

The cardinal clinical features of Parkinson's disease are resting tremor, bradykinesia, rigidity, and asymmetric onset.[4] Researchers performing a systematic review of the literature attempted to determine the value of common signs and symptoms associated with the diagnosis of Parkinson's.[5] Their recommendations are to pay particular attention to the following: patients who report difficulty turning in bed, opening jars, and rising from a chair. Important signs include rigidity, tremor, bradykinesia, micrographia, and a shuffling gait. The glabella tap and heel-to-toe tests may also be valuable. As the disease progresses, the patient appears to have a blank, emotionless facial expression. Seborrhea of the skin is also frequently seen. Although muscle strength is good, the patient is slow to react. There is often a visible tremor (four to six cycles per second) that is present at rest and is less severe with voluntary movement. Passive movement of the limbs reveals a characteristic rigidity (i.e., cogwheel or ratchet). Tapping over the bridge of the nose (two times per second) creates a sustained blink response (Myerson's sign). The patient's walk will often demonstrate a classic festinating gait in which the patient takes many small, shuffling steps and has difficulty stopping. The arms do not swing automatically with walking. Some of the early signs are difficult to differentiate from signs of old age. Even in later stages it is difficult to distinguish between autopsy-diagnosed multiple-system atrophy, supranuclear palsy, and cortical-basal ganglionic degeneration. On heavily weighted T2 magnetic resonance imaging (MRI), there is narrowing of the substantia nigra para compacta in patients with Parkinson's disease. Other MRI findings may help differentiate Parkinson's disease from other similar disorders.

---

*See also regional chapters for specific neuropathies or nerve root disorders.

Management

Treatment is aimed at either blocking the effects of acetylcholine with anticholinergic drugs or restoring dopamine levels with levodopa (precursor to dopamine). Early parkinsonism is not usually treated. Mild parkinsonism is treated with amantadine. With progression, levodopa is effective in treating many of the features of parkinsonism; however, it is associated with various dyskinesias and an "on–off" phenomenon characterized by abrupt fluctuations in symptoms. Sinemet is most often given.[6] It is a combination of levodopa and carbidopa. Carbidopa-levodopa (Sinemet) is sometimes given with other medications such as bromocriptine (ergot derivative). **Table 15–5** is a list of commonly used medications and their side effects. One study[7] indicated that estrogen replacement in early Parkinson's disease may lower symptom severity. Other approaches include posteroventral pallidotomy, bilateral fetal nigral transplantation, and electrical stimulation of the subthalamic nucleus.[8]

Multiple Sclerosis
Classic Presentation

The patient is younger (less than age 55 years) presenting with a history of dizziness, numbness, tingling, or weakness that resolved over a few days. Other similar neurologic events have occurred in the past.

Cause

Multiple sclerosis (MS) is a disease characterized by patchy demyelination with reactive gliosis in the spinal cord, optic nerve, and white matter of the brain.[9,10] The cause is unknown, but MS is suspected to be an immune disorder. MS occurs mainly in individuals who live in temperate zones and especially in individuals of western European ancestry. The combination of a genetic predisposition coupled with decreased sunlight exposure may trigger the process for susceptible individuals. The relapsing/remitting type (RRMS) accounts for 85% of presentations. For most patients the onset is predominantly between ages 20 to 40 years but for the progressive relapsing type of MS (least common) its onset more often is in patients older than age 40 years. There is an apparent genetic

Table 15–5 Parkinson's Medications

Drug Class	Examples	General Mechanism	Interactions/Side Effects
Carbidopa	Sinemet Lodosyn	Prevents peripheral metabolism of levodopa in effect making more available to the brain. Also prevents the inhibitory effects of pyridoxine (B6) on levodopa. Used in the management of Parkinson's.	May cause visual disturbances, GI symptoms, confusion, involuntary movements, hallucinations, dyskinesia, hypotension, and depression with suicidal tendencies.
Levodopa (L-Dopa)	Dopar Larodopa	L-dopa is the metabolic precursor to dopamine. Its advantage is it crosses the blood–brain barrier. Helps restore levels of dopamine in extra-pyramidal areas of the brain. Used in the treatment of Parkinson's.	May cause choreiform and other involuntary movements, increase tremor and cause bradykinetic episodes (on-and-off phenomenon). Many other side effects occur including hallucinations, paranoid delusions, severe depression and suicidal tendencies. There are a host of other system effects that include possible dark sweat or urine and all the other common side effects of many medications.
Selegiline	Eldepryl	Increases dopaminergic activity partial action due to MAO inhibition and inhibition of dopamine reuptake. Used as adjunctive treatment for Parkinson's.	May cause visual disturbances, GI symptoms, confusion, hallucinations, dyskinesia, and hypotension.
Bromocriptine	Parlodel	Reduces prolactin levels and through a series of events activates dopaminergic receptors in the hypothalamus which then releases prolactin inhibiting factor. Used for amenorrhea/galactorrhea or female infertility, but also used as adjunctive therapy to levodopa for Parkinson's.	May cause headaches, agitation, nervousness, mania, orthostatic hypotension, Raynaud's, depression, acute MI, or shock.

relationship due to the association of MS and HLA-DRB1. As part of a cascade of research on what appears to be an epidemic of vitamin D deficiency, a study[11] has found that high circulating levels of vitamin D are associated with a lower risk of multiple sclerosis. Another suspected associated risk is smoking.[12] The role of Epstein–Barr virus is still debated[13] but a 2007 study[14] does indicate that high titers of antibodies for Epstein–Barr virus B2LF1 are a strong predictor of MS.

Evaluation

MS is characterized by episodic attacks that initially resolve but eventually leave residual neurologic deficits. The initial episode often will resolve in days, and the patient may remain symptom-free for months or years. Eventually, however, symptoms recur. Symptoms usually will involve a region and consist of numbness, tingling, weakness, diplopia, dizziness, or urinary sphincter dysfunction (urgency or hesitancy). Optic nerve involvement is common and often the first source of signs/symptoms. The frequency of initial attacks is prognostic for future disability severity. The clinical diagnosis is based on two or more distinct episodes at least three months apart with two distinct neurological deficits with partial resolution eventually. On physical examination, in addition to finding scotomas or nystagmus on the eye exam, flexion of the neck may produce the Lhermitte sign of electric-shock sensations down one or both arms. MRI will demonstrate multifocal areas of patchy demyelination in the brain or cervical spinal cord. T2 images show these areas as hyperintense due to breach of the blood–brain barrier. T1 images demonstrate hypointense lesions (black or gray holes). On serial images lesions may disappear due to resolution of edema. Laboratory evaluation may reveal mild lymphocytosis or increased protein count in the cerebrospinal fluid (CSF; more often in acute attacks). Immunoglobulin G and oligoclonal bands are more often seen in the CSF. Other findings include an abnormal colloidal gold curve, mild mononuclear pleocytosis with lymphocytic predominance (< 40 cells/mL), and myelin debris.[15]

Management

There is no cure for MS. During acute exacerbations, corticosteroids are sometimes used to speed recovery. In addition to prednisone and methylprednisolone, immunosuppressive therapy with interferon-beta 1b (e.g., Betaseron) is used. Other drugs include Copaxone, Tysabri, and Gilenya. Monitoring of liver function is important. Nutritional approaches are unproven, yet some research[16] suggests that an increase in polyunsaturated fatty acids and metabolic enzyme supplements assist in providing an adequate lipid pool for oligodendrocytes. Also, antioxidants such as vitamins A, beta-carotene, E, C with bioflavonoids, and selenium may help with myelin membrane peroxidation.[17] Relapses commonly occur in women two to three months after childbirth. **Table 15–6** lists some medications and side effects for the management of multiple sclerosis. Seventy percent of patients live active lives, although within 10 years 50% are using a cane or wheelchair. Life expectancy is approximately the same as those without the disease.

Table 15–6 Multiple Sclerosis Medications

Drug Class	Examples	General Mechanism	Interactions/Side Effects
Interferon Beta 1a and 1b	Avonex, Rebif, Betaseron	A recombinant DNA medication that has effects that are antiviral, antitumor, antiproliferative, and immunomodulatory. Used in the management of relapsing multiple sclerosis.	**Common to have side effects including headache, fever, chills, anxiety, nervousness, GI disturbances, alopecia, abnormal mood, emotional lability, and confusion. Possible lab effects on thrombocytes and granulocytes.**
Isoniazid	INH, Isotamine, Laniazid, Nydrazid, Teebaconin	An anti-TB medication that interferes with the synthesis of bacterial proteins, lipids, and nucleic acids. Used also for high-risk individuals as a preventive. Additional use for tremors with multiple sclerosis.	**May cause paresthesias, peripheral neuropathies, tinnitus, dizziness, hallucinations, increased liver enzymes, decrease in B vitamin absorption, RA and SLE-like syndromes, or possible agranulocytosis and aplastic anemia (rare).**
Natalizumab	Antegren	A humanized monoclonal antibody used to treat multiple sclerosis and Crohn's disease. A receptor blocker that binds to alpha-4-beta-1 and alpha-4-beta-7 integrins, natalizumab prevents lymphocytes and eosinophils from moving from the bloodstream to outer tissue sites involved in inflammation. For multiple sclerosis it is used in combination with interferon beta 1-a).	**Most common side effects are abdominal pain and headache.**

Guillain-Barré Syndrome

Classic Presentation

The patient complains of bilateral leg weakness following either a viral infection or immunization. The patient may also complain of distal paresthesias.

Cause

The cause is unknown; however, it is believed to be a demyelinating, autoimmune disorder. Association to a postviral illness may be found; however, association to vaccines has not been proven.

Evaluation

The patient will have primarily motor signs, including loss of deep tendon reflexes. Because of autonomic involvement, there are fluctuations in blood pressure, abnormalities in sweating, and sphincter dysfunction. The weakness progresses variably, involving the arms and face in some patients. About 10% of patients have respiratory involvement. Examination of CSF demonstrates a high protein content; however, this may take two to three weeks to become evident.

Management

The condition is self-resolving in 80% to 90% of patients within months. During this period of time, a minority of patients will require respiratory assistance. About 10% of patients will have residual disability, and about 3% will have relapses. Prednisone should not be given because of the possibility of prolonging recovery time. Plasmapheresis and intravenous immunoglobulin may be of benefit.

Myasthenia Gravis

Classic Presentation

The patient is often a young woman complaining of double vision, difficulty swallowing, or weakness of the arm with repeated use or weakness of the jaw muscles when chewing.

Cause

Ocular myasthenia gravis (MG) occurs in 15% of cases but 50% of these progress to generalized MG (85% of MG patients). In 10% to 20% of infants born to MG mothers, transient MG symptoms occur, resolving in weeks to months. D-penicillamine may cause drug-induced MG. The peak age groups for myasthenia gravis (MG) are men older than 50 years, women aged 20 to 40 years, and then around age 70 years. Neuromuscular transmission is blocked by autoantibodies that bind to acetylcholine receptors, making them unavailable. The disease may be idiopathic or associated with a thymoma, thyrotoxicosis, rheumatoid arthritis, or lupus erythematosus. Thymomas are more common in older men. The initiation of MG may be related to prior viral infection including polio, measles EBV, or HIV.

Evaluation

A recent review by Scherer et al.[18] evaluated the ability to determine if a patient has MG based upon the history and examination. Sixty-five percent of patients will have double vision and a drooping eyelid. However, less than one-fourth will have bulbar weakness, report slurred or nasal speech, alteration of the voice, or difficulty chewing or swallowing. Unintelligible speech during prolonged speaking and the presence of the peek sign increased the likelihood of an MG diagnosis, although absence did not rule it out. The peek sign is elicited by having the patient gently close the eyes. Within 30 seconds (due to orbicularis oris weakness) the eyelid will start to elevate slightly revealing the sclera (peek sign). Using the eye with a higher degree of ptosis, three tests can be performed: the ice test, the rest test, and the sleep test. A latex glove finger filled with ice is placed over the ptotic eyelid for two minutes with the ice test. A latex glove finger filled with cotton is used as a placebo measure in the rest test, again held over the eyelid for two minutes. The sleep test involves having the patient close his or her eyes in a dark room for 30 minutes. A positive response is a complete response to one of the tests, or an improvement of 2 mm increase in the palpebral fissure. Other tests include the curtain test, which involves the examiner holding one lid open while the other gradually closes. If ptosis worsens when propping up the opposite eyelid or with sustained upward gaze a positive curtain sign is found. Strongly diagnostic is a response to an anticholinesterase medication, the Tensilon test (also called the edrophonium test). Lab testing includes an assay for anti-ACh receptor antibodies. Those without anti-AChR antibodies sometimes have antibodies to muscle-specific tyrosine-kinase (MuSK), which occurs more in females who have both bulbar and respiratory weakness. If thymoma is the cause, the lab test is for antistriated muscle (anti-SM) antibody (85% of patients over 40 years with thymoma).[19]

Repeated muscle contraction or eye movement leads to fatigue, although initial movement or contraction is strong. Reflexes and the sensory examination are normal. In older men, a chest radiograph and/or computed tomography may be considered in a search for a thymoma. Electrophysiologic testing will reveal a decreasing response to stimulation. Laboratory testing includes a new test to assay the circulating levels of acetylcholine receptor antibodies (sensitivity is 80% to 90%). Medical evaluation involves drug testing using a short-acting anticholinesterase, which causes a temporary increase in strength.

Management

Standard anticholinesterase medications include pyridostigmine (Mestinon) neostigmine (Prostigmin), and ambenonium (Mytelase). For immunosuppression, oral corticosteroids may be used. **Table 15–7** lists these medications and their potential side effects. Those who have antibodies to MuSK may have a bad reaction to cholinesterase inhibitors but do better with plasmapheresis selected immunotherapy like Rituximab (monoclonal antibody against antigen on B cells). Thymectomy often is dramatically effective, and it is often recommended to patients under age 60 years. However, this choice should be reserved for those with progression or those unresponsive to medical management.

Amyotrophic Lateral Sclerosis

Classic Presentation

The patient is an adult who complains of muscle weakness and cramping in the hand. Progressively, signs and symptoms multiply, including difficulty in swallowing, chewing, coughing, or breathing.

Cause

Amyotrophic lateral sclerosis (ALS) is part of a group of motor neuron diseases with degeneration of the anterior horn cells and motor nuclei of the lower cranial nerves, corticospinal and corticobulbar tracts. The disorder occurs between ages 30 and 60 years and is progressive. Although most cases are sporadic, there are some familial cases.

Evaluation

This disorder is characterized by a combination of upper motor neuron and lower motor neuron lesion signs. Therefore, in addition to muscle atrophy and fasciculations, there are often brisk deep tendon reflexes. Sensory examination is normal, and the sphincters are not affected. EMG will reveal abnormal spontaneous activity in a resting muscle and a decrease in recruitment ability.

Management

There is no treatment for ALS. The disease usually progresses to death over a period of about two to two-and-a-half years in most patients. The five-year survival rate is only 20%.

Syringomyelia

Classic Presentation

The patient is usually young. The parents are concerned about either the observation that the child injures his or her hands or arms and does not notice or the observation of a scoliosis.

Cause

A syrinx occurs in the central spinal cord either as a developmental problem or due to destruction or degeneration of gray and white matter secondary to trauma or an intramedullary tumor. Many cases are associated with herniation of the cerebellar tonsils, medulla, and fourth ventricle into the spinal canal. This developmental disorder is referred to as an Arnold-Chiari malformation. In this condition, the syrinx is actually a dilation of the central canal.

Evaluation

The patient will lose pain and temperature sense in a shawl-like distribution over the upper trunk and arms. Atrophy and areflexia also may be evident. Scoliosis is often present, and sometimes it represents a distinct opposite of the normal right-thoracic, left-lumbar curves, namely a left-thoracic, right-lumbar curve pattern. MRI evaluation will demonstrate both the Arnold-Chiari malformation with the cerebellar tonsils below the foramen magnum and also the level and extent of the syrinx.

Management

Treatment is surgical with decompression, including laminectomy in the upper cervical region and shunting of fluid into the peritoneum in some cases.

Neurofibromatosis

Classic Presentation

The patient is often a child brought by parents concerned about multiple skin lesions on the trunk area. Otherwise the patient is often asymptomatic. In other cases, parents are concerned about a child's hearing or eyesight problem.

Cause

Neurofibromatosis is a familial disorder that is either autosomal dominant or sporadic, occurring with no known cause. The characteristic lesions involve the Schwann cells and nerve fibroblasts. There are two distinct types, type 1 and type 2. The patient with type 1 will present with multiple hyperpigmented nodules. The patient with type 2 often presents with problems with hearing or eyesight.[20]

Evaluation

Finding the characteristic café-au-lait lesions over the trunk, pelvis, or flexor creases of the arms is virtually diagnostic if six or more large lesions are found. The neurofibromas are slowly progressive and in type 1 may lead to the rare but deforming Recklinghausen's disease. With type 1, plexiform neuromas (overgrowth of subcutaneous tissue) and bone distortion occur. With type 2, intracranial tumors affect cranial nerves controlling eyesight, balance, and hearing.

Management

There is no known treatment. Surgical removal of tumors of the skin and nerves is the only recourse for patients at this time.

Muscular Dystrophy (Duchenne Type)

Classic Presentation

Muscular dystrophy (MD) is a group of inherited myopathic disorders, each of which presents differently. The most common is the Duchenne type (pseudohypertrophic). The patient is between the ages of 1 and 5 years. The parents note that their child has difficulty in rising from a bent-over position, has a waddling gait, and falls often.

Cause

Duchenne's is an X-linked recessive gene disorder. The defective gene leads to a marked reduction or absence of an important protein, dystrophin.[21]

Evaluation

The characteristic difficulty in rising from a bent-over position may cause the patient to walk up the legs with his or her hands. Proximal muscle testing may indicate weakness. The disease affects the limbs first, then the shoulders. Pseudohypertrophy may occur as a result of fatty replacement of muscle. Mild mental retardation is also found. Laboratory studies will reveal markedly elevated creatine kinase (CK) levels. DNA analysis is the primary follow-up tool. If CK levels are elevated, deletion and duplication analysis is performed first; then, if negative, DMD testing for full sequencing for the DMMD gene for point mutations is performed. Other tests include dystrophin protein assay and muscle biopsy.[22]

Management

There is no treatment for the disease. However, for slowing the decline of muscle function prednisone may be helpful. Progression is rapid, leading to the need for a wheelchair. Patients progressively decline and finally die before age 20 years in most cases. Females on the maternal side of an affected child should be tested for elevations of CK or lactate dehydrogenase on several occasions. It is important to note that 50% of female carriers have twice the normal CK levels. These elevated markers may indicate the need for genetic counseling. Also, genetic studies in early pregnancy can determine whether the child will have Duchenne's. In late pregnancy DNA probes can be used on fetal tissue to diagnose Duchenne's in the fetus. There may be some potential hope for the use of gene therapy in the future.[23]

APPENDIX 15–1

References

1. Souza TA. Which orthopedic tests are really necessary? In: Lawrence DJ, Cassidy JD, McGregor M, et al. eds. *Advances in Chiropractic*. St. Louis, MO: Mosby Year Book; 1994;1:101–158.

2. Meyer JJ. Clinical electromyographic and related neuro-physiologic responses. In: Lawrence DJ, Cassidy JD, McGregor M, et al., eds. *Advances in Chiropractic*. St. Louis, MO: Mosby Year Book; 1994;1:29.

3. Long RR. Nerve anatomy and diagnostic principles. In: Pappas AM, ed. *Upper Extremity Injuries in the Athlete*. New York: Churchill Livingstone; 1995:43.

4. Gelb DJ, Oliver E, Gilman S. Diagnostic criteria for Parkinson disease. *Arch Neurol*. 1999;56:33–39.

5. Rao G, Fisch L, Srinivasan S, et al. Does this patient have Parkinson disease? *JAMA*, 2003;269(3):347–353.

6. Standaert DG, Stern MB. Update on the management of Parkinson's disease. *Med Clin North Am*. 1993;77:169.

7. Saunders-Pullman R, Gordon-Elliot J, Parides M. The effect of estrogen replacement on early Parkinson's disease. *Neurology*. 1999;52:1417–1422.

8. Jankovic J. New and emerging therapies for Parkinson disease. *Arch Neurol*. 1999;56:785–790.

9. Frohman EM, Eagar T, Monson N, Stuve O, Karandikar N. Immunologic mechanisms of multiple sclerosis. *Neuroimaging Clin N Am*. 2008;18(4):577–588.

10. Frohman EM, Racke MK, Raine CS. Multiple sclerosis—the plaque and its pathogenesis. *N Engl J Med*. 2006;354(9):942–955.

11. Munger KL, Levin LI, Hollis BW, Howard NS, Ascherio A. Serum 25-hydroxyvitamin D levels and risk of multiple sclerosis. *JAMA*. 2006;296(23):2832–2838.

12. Ascherio A, Munger KL. Environmental risk factors for multiple sclerosis. Part II: Noninfectious factors. *Ann Neurol*. 2007;61(6):504–513.

13. Ascherio A, Munger KL. Environmental risk factors for multiple sclerosis. Part I: the role of infection. *Ann Neurol*. 2007;61(4):288–299.

14. Massa J, Munger KL, O'Reilly EJ, Falk KI, Ascherio A. Plasma titers of antibodies against Epstein-Barr virus BZLF1 and risk of multiple sclerosis. *Neuroepidemiology*. 2007;28(4):214–215.

15. Polman CH, Reingold SC, Banwell B, et al. Diagnostic criteria for multiple sclerosis: 2010 revisions to the McDonald criteria. *Ann Neurol*. 2011;69(2):292–302.

16. Lyon JM. Multiple sclerosis; is there a better treatment? *Top Clin Chiro*. 1996;3(4):36–50.

17. Weinshenker BG, Issa M, Baskerville J. Meta-analysis of the placebo-treated groups in clinical trials of progressive MS. *Neurology*. 1996;46:1613–1619.

18. Scherer K, Bedlack RS, Simel DL. Does this patient have myasthenia gravis? *JAMA*. 2005;293(15):1906–1914.

19. Angelini C. Diagnosis and management of auto-immune myasthenia gravis. *Clin Drug Investig*. 2011;31(1):1–14.

20. Mulvihill JJ. Neurofibromatosis 1 (Recklinghausen's disease) and neurofibromatosis 2 (bilateral acoustic neurofibromatosis): an update. *Ann Intern Med*. 1990;113:39.

21. Mendell JR, Sahenk Z, Prior TW. The childhood muscular dystrophies: diseases sharing a common pathogenesis of membrane instability. *J Child Neurol*. 1995;10:150–159.

22. Bushby K, Finkel R, Birnkrant DJ, et al. Diagnosis and management of Duchenne muscular dystrophy, part 2: implementation of multidisciplinary care. *Lancet Neurol*. 2010;9(2):177–189.

23. Karpati G, Acsadi G. The potential for gene therapy in Duchenne muscular dystrophy and other genetic muscle diseases. *Muscle Nerve*. 1993;16:1141.

Numbness, Tingling, and Pain

# CHAPTER 16

Context

Patients complaining of pain do not necessarily have pathologic involvement of neural tissue but do have a response due to trauma or irritation of nociceptive nerve fibers. Patients complaining of numbness or tingling, however, are more likely to have disease, ischemia, or injury of neural tissue. The list of possible causes is enormous and can be narrowed down only by combining the findings of location, onset, and associated neural localizing findings (i.e., motor deficit or deep tendon reflex abnormality) (**Exhibit 16–1**). Although trauma or direct irritation often may be the source of these complaints, it is important to remember the sometimes transient response of neural tissue to ischemia (e.g., diabetes) or metabolic imbalance (e.g., uremia) that may occur with systemic processes.

Chiropractors are often faced with the presentation of a patient who claims numbness but when clinically evaluated has no objectifiable loss. Important discriminators are finding associated neurologic signs indicating nerve root or peripheral nerve pathology; however, these also are often absent. Possible explanations for this lack of evidence include the presence of a transient process, misinterpretation of the sensation by the patient, a "referred" sensory abnormality, and malingering.

Sensory perversions are often divided into two categories: paresthesia and dysesthesias. Paresthesias are spontaneous, abnormal sensations, described by patients as "pins and needles" or tingling. Dysesthesias are irritating sensations evoked by normally non-nociceptive stimuli such as light touch. Sometimes used synonymously with dysesthesias is hyperpathia—normal stimuli are pain producing. Hypesthesia implies that there is an elevated threshold to stimulus. For example,

pain is felt with a pinprick, but the applied pressure needed for pain perception is greater than would normally be required.

General Strategy

History

- Ask the patient to define what he or she means by a complaint of numbness, tingling, or other unusual sensations.
- Attempt to localize to a specific body region (distinguish between single and multiple areas, and whether the sensation is felt more distally in the hands or feet).
- Determine any associated symptoms such as pain or weakness.
- Determine whether the onset was abrupt or gradual and whether or not was related to trauma.
- Determine whether the patient has a known diagnosis of or indications of diabetes, alcoholism, liver or renal disease, or anxiety or depression; obtain a thorough drug history.

Attempt to differentiate chronic nociceptive pain from chronic central pain

Evaluation

- Perform a neurologic examination focusing on sensory testing; begin distally in an attempt to determine selective loss or alteration of pain, temperature, light touch, vibration, and position sense.
- Examine the motor system in an attempt to correlate findings suggestive of nerve root or peripheral nerve involvement.

Exhibit 16–1 Narrowing the Possible Causes of Numbness

Patient complains of numbness

Differentiate between objective and subjective numbness with a sensory examination

Subjective numbness is suggestive of referral or a transient process
(no demonstrable sensory or motor findings; often diffuse, following
no specific dermatomal pattern)

Distinguish among various neurologic possibilities

Nerve root	Peripheral nerve	Nerve plexus	Central nervous system, including spinal cord

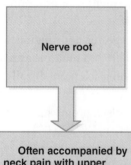

Often accompanied by neck pain with upper extremity numbness and low back pain with lower extremity numbness. —decrease in corresponding deep tendon reflex —weakness in corresponding myotome —hypoesthesia in corresponding dermatomal pattern	Usually a history of overuse or direct trauma. Examination reveals weakness of corresponding muscle if there is a motor component and hypoesthesia of the peripheral nerve patch of skin.	Classic example is thoracic outlet syndrome with pressure on the neurovascular elements of the brachial plexus. Traction trauma or tumor is also a possible cause. Although symptoms may be diffuse, most plexus lesions affect a specific section such as the lower plexus with involvement, for example, of the medial arm.	Involvement is often bilateral. Central cord processes may also affect temperature. Patchy involvement may indicate multiple sclerosis. Complete spinal cord involvement has associated motor findings.

- When a clear picture is not evident, it may be necessary to proceed to electrodiagnostic or other specialized testing based on the suspected cause.

Management

- Most cases of isolated peripheral nerve or nerve root problems can be managed initially by the chiropractor; monitor for progression or unresponsiveness to determine need for neurologic consultation.
- Some metabolic disorders, such as uremia, often require referral for management; others, such as diabetes, can be comanaged.

Relevant Anatomy

The following is a brief and generalized overview of the sensory nervous system. Participants in the sensory system include nerve cell bodies, nerve fibers, and sensory receptors. The types of sensations that are conveyed are generally divided into (1) pain and temperature, (2) touch, and (3) proprioception and vibration.

Free nerve endings are the primary receptors for pain and temperature. The signal is then carried to the first nerve cell body in the dorsal root ganglion (DRG). Fibers leaving the DRG enter the spinal cord by accessing Lissauer's tract (dorsolateral tract) and ascending or descending one or two segments before synapsing in the substantia gelatinosa. At this level interactions with interneurons influence transmission. From the second-order neuron. A delta (small myelinated) fibers cross the anterior commissure and ascend in the contralateral lateral spinothalamic tract, ascending to the thalamus to synapse primarily in the ventral posterolateral (VPL) nucleus of the thalamus. C fibers also cross in the spinal cord to ascend primarily in the anterior spinothalamic tract and terminate in the intralaminar and parafascicular nuclei of the thalamus. Both then continue to the somatic sensory area of the cortex. The lateral spinothalamic tract also carries touch and deep pressure sensations.[1]

For sensation of the head and related structures, the trigeminal nerve is the primary supply. Nerve cell bodies are found in the trigeminal ganglion. The spinal nucleus of the trigeminal nerve is devoted to pain and temperature. The main sensory nucleus serves the other sensory components such as discriminative touch. These signals travel in the trigeminal lemniscus in the brainstem to the ventral posteromedial (VPM) nucleus of the thalamus.

Other than conscious pain conveyed through the anterolateral system, several pathways convey signals through medial pain pathways that affect emotion, motivation, withdrawal, arousal, and autonomic reactions to nociceptive stimulation. These tracts may also trigger responses that contribute to the central or supraspinal inhibition of pain. Following is a brief summary of these pathways and functions.

- **Spinoreticular tract**—Terminating in the reticular formation, this tract and the reticular formation provide information that influences autonomic nervous system (ANS) reflexes and the emotional experience and response to pain.
- **Spinomesencephaloic tract**—Nociceptive signals terminate in the periaqueductal gray (PAG) of the midbrain and may also connect with the limbic system leading to a perception of diffuse, poorly localized pain, and also a fear response. Due to termination in the PAG, the spinomesencephalic tract may activate a descending inhibitory system that results in analgesia due to the release of serotonin.
- **Spinolimbic tract**—This pathway also provides for a non-localized perception of pain. Other manifestations are suggested through its synaptic connections to the midline thalamic nuclei, resulting in arousal and motivational effects via projections to both the frontal and cingulate cortex. It may also be involved in supraspinal inhibition of pain.

Nociceptive information projects through these tracts to at least four areas of the brain above the brainstem:

- To the parietal cortex for localization of pain only, but not the painful experience
- To the cingulate cortex of the limbic system for the emotional experience of pain
- To the temporal lobe for the imbedding of memory of the pain and what evokes pain
- To the hypothalamus for activation of the endocrine and autonomic nervous system

Descending systems, which are activated by the PAG of the midbrain and originate in the raphe nuclei and locus ceruleus, release serotonin (5-HT) and norepinephrine respectively. These neurotransmitters stimulate the endorphin-releasing interneurons and primary pain neurons, thereby "closing" the pain gate.

Larger, myelinated fibers participate in conveying information for proprioception and vibration. These include type Ia fibers for primary endings (annulospiral endings) in muscle spindles (intrafusal fibers) for stretch, and for Golgi tendon organs and ligament receptors for tension. Medium-size, myelinated nerves carry non-conscious proprioceptive information on type II fibers from muscle spindles (flower-spray endings) and joint mechanoreceptors (Pacinian corpuscles for movement and vibration and Ruffini for end-range stretch). Medium-size, myelinated type A-beta fibers carry fine touch and vibration through cutaneous and subcutaneous receptors. These include:

- Superficial (cutaneous): Meissner's corpuscles—light touch and vibration; Merkel's disks—pressure, and hair follicle receptors—displacement
- Subcutaneous: Pacinian corpuscles—touch and vibration; Ruffini's corpuscles—stretching of skin

For conscious proprioception, fibers carry information to the first-order neurons in the dorsal root ganglion and then to the posterior column of the spinal cord and ascend without crossing to synapse on second-order neurons in the nucleus gracilis and cuneatus in the medulla. They then cross to ascend in the medial lemniscus to the third-order neurons mainly in the VPL of the thalamus. After synapsing, the third-order neuron fibers ascend via the internal capsule to the corona radiata, accessing the neurons of the postcentral gyrus.

Other tracts convey non-conscious proprioceptive information to primarily the cerebellum. There are four tracts with the two devoted specifically to non-conscious proprioception. The other two are for the reporting of internuncial activity at the spinal cord level. These four tracts include the following:

- Posterior spinocerebellar—Conveys information primarily for the lower extremity and lower trunk. This information is muscle spindle information and some cutaneous information such as vibration. Fibers travel in the posterior columns (gracile fasiculus) to the posterior thoracic nucleus (dorsal nucleus; Clarke's nucleus or column) found only in T1-L1 (L2) segmentally. These remain ipsilateral (uncrossed) traveling to the cerebellum through the inferior cerebellar peduncle.
- Cuneocerebellar—Conveys information primarily from the upper extremity and upper trunk. Fibers

travel in the cuneate fasiculus synapsing in the accessory cuneate nucleus in the medulla just superior and outside of the cuneate nucleus

- Anterior spinocerebellar—This tract relays information regarding the activity of spinal reflex arcs. They double-cross; initially cross and then cross back after entering the cerebellum through the superior cerebellar peduncle.
- Rostral spinocerebellar—This tract also relays information regarding the activity of spinal reflex arcs. It enters the inferior cerebellar peduncle without crossing.

Two other tracts that may be involved in behavioral reaction and learning related to pain include:

- **Spinotectal tract**—Follows spinothalamic tract but ends in the superior colliculus; turning the eyes toward the painful stimulus.
- **Spinoolivary tract**—Sends tactile info to the inferior olivary nucleus (just lateral to the pyramids); involved in motor learning and modifying learned reflex activities.

The general architecture of the spinal cord may give clues to certain patterns of sensory loss or weakness. Therefore, a compressive myelopathy, for example, may produce an ascending pattern of sensory loss if progressive. A spinal lesion more centrally located (e.g., syringomyelia) would interrupt fibers that cross, such as those conveying pain and temperature, while sparing the dorsal column pathways, leaving vibration and proprioception unaffected.

It is believed that paresthesias and dysesthesias are the result of either damage to large fiber axons or demyelination. This is most common with structural damage that occurs with peripheral nerve or nerve root compression or toxic/metabolic disorders that cause neuropathy. Numbness is more often the result of loss or damage to smaller sensory fibers affecting both pain and temperature perception.

Through stimulation of nociceptor afferents pain causes a complex multisystem response which potentially involves the following:

- Reflex muscle spasm via synaptic activation of α motorneurons.
- Stimulation of the sympathetic nervous system resulting in vasoconstriction. Resulting ischemia may activate more nociceptors.
- Nociceptive stimulation of the hypothalamus causing the release of catecholamines,

adrenocorticotropic hormone (ACTH), cortisol, glucagon, anti-diuretic hormone (ADH), and other catabolic hormones, along with a concomitant decrease in the anabolic hormones insulin and testosterone

Chronic pain is a very common problem that is often divided into nociceptive chronic pain and neuropathic pain. With chronic pain of nociceptive origin, there is a pain generator present such as tissue damage from infection or pressure pain from a tumor. Neuropathic pain, though, is an example of pain becoming a disease rather than indicating tissue damage. In other words, the stimulus for pain no longer remains, but alterations in the peripheral or central nervous system continue to propagate pain. Peripherally there are several proposed mechanisms, including ectopic foci development, ephaptic transmission, and structural reorganization. When myelin damage is present, it is sometimes a reaction by the nervous system to produce excessive ion channels that are inserted into the demyelinated tissue which then becomes sensitive to stimulation. Another reaction that occurs with myelin damage is ephaptic transmission, also called cross-talk. This occurs when an action potential from a damaged neuron stimulates a neighboring neuron. Finally, structural reorganization can occur with changes in the dorsal horn where retraction of C fiber terminals is replaced with A-beta fiber axon terminals synapsing in areas that would normally receive only C fibers. This may result in normal sensation becoming painful.

Some specific proposed mechanisms for this induced chronic state and associated medical approaches are listed below.[2] Note that many of these medications are used for other disorders such as depression and seizures.

- In the DRG there is up-regulation of membrane channels in the nociceptive neurons:
  - sodium channel inhibitors—tricyclic antidepressants, carbamazepine, oxcarbazepine, phenytoin, lamotrigine, mexiletine, lidocaine
  - potassium channel inhibitors—gabapentin
  - calcium channel inhibitors—gabapentin and lamotrigine
- Sprouting sympathetic axons form "baskets" around nerve cell bodies. Inhibitors may include tricyclic antidepressants, bupropion, and venlafaxine.
- Sodium channels spread along axons at the site of peripheral nerve damage resulting in spontaneous discharges. Inhibitors are the same as listed above for sodium channels.
- Projections from the DRG to the interneurons in the spinal cord allow further transmission of pain signals through the release of substance P, calcitonin, gene-related peptide protein (CGRP), and glutamate.
- The second-order neurons in the spinal cord activated by glutamate through the α-amino-3-hyroxy-5-methyl-4-isoxazole propionic acid (AMPA) receptors are prompted to fire spontaneously (central sensitization) through activation of the N-methyl-α-aspartate (NMDA) receptors through an increase in intracellular calcium and activation of protein kinases (PK). Potential inhibitors are gabapentin, dextromethorphan, opiates, selective serotonin reuptake inhibitors, topiramate, lamotrigine, and others.
- Ectopic activation of second-order neurons can also be caused by dynorphin, which is found in patients with chronic pain, through activation of NMDA receptors.
- Down-regulation of γ-aminobutyric acid receptors decreases inhibition of second-order neurons.
- Sprouting of central terminals of non-nociceptive neurons in the DRG leads to hyperalgesia and tactile allodynia, which may be inhibited by levodopa.

Neuropathies, particularly peripheral neuropathies, are often divided into two general types based on the involved structure: axonal degeneration and paranodal or segmental demyelination. Although many disorders do not clearly fall into one category or the other, this distinction is important from the standpoint of physiologic testing. In evaluating nerve conduction, two responses are measured: the velocity (or latency) and the amplitude of the evoked response. Electrodiagnostic testing can evaluate either the sensory or motor component. In general, axonal degeneration results in relatively normal conduction; the evoked amplitude of the response, however, is decreased (with eventual electromyography [EMG] changes evident). Demyelination generally causes the reverse, with conduction velocity decreased yet normal evoked amplitudes (EMG is often normal).

Painful neuropathies may be divided into cause and type, primarily based upon specific underlying disease processes (see **Tables 16–1** and **16–2**). A broader classification includes two significant subtypes:

1. Small-fiber painful sensory neuropathy—Only the A-δ (small myelinated) and nociceptive C (unmyelinated) nerve fibers are involved. This

probably represents the most common cause for patients 50 years of age and older. An underlying cause is rarely determined.

2. Small-fiber/large-fiber painful sensory neuropathy—This is partially a result of damage to small nerve fibers. Additionally, A-β and A-α nerve fibers are

Table 16–1 Some Peripheral Neuropathies

Type	History, Exam, and Special Testing Indicators
Idiopathic, small-fiber neuropathy	Usually seen in patients over 50 years of age. Normal muscle strength, DTRs, and position and vibration sense. Reduction in pinprick in lower extremities. EMG and NCS are normal. Reduction in sudomotor function and, if performed, abnormal skin biopsy indicating small-fiber damage.
Diabetic peripheral neuropathy	Family and personal history. Adult onset with associated obesity, hypertension, hyperlipidemia. DTRs decreased with a reduction in distal sensation. Also may be associated with orthostatic hypotension. Abnormal EMG and NCS. Positives on laboratory for >126 mg/dl for blood glucose or HbA1c is 6.5% (47 mmol/mol) or higher.
Inherited neuropathy	Usually a family history. Examination reveals pes cavus/hammer toes presentation with decrease in DTRs and distal sensation loss. EMG and NCS are abnormal.
Connective tissue disease neuropathy	History of one of several diseases that may include rheumatoid arthritis, systemic lupus erythematosus, mixed connective tissue disease, Sjögren's, or sicca syndrome. Reduction of DTRs and distal sensation. Abnormal EMG and NCS. Usually positive for antinuclear antibodies, extractable nuclear antigens, or rheumatoid factor.
Peripheral nerve-vasculitis neuropathy	Usually diagnosed with a systemic vasculitis. Examples include polyarteritis nodosa temporal arteritis, Takayasu's arteritis, and that associated with connective tissue disorders. Multiple and symmetric involvement of sensory and motor findings. Abnormal EMG and NCS. One of the following may be positive: rheumatoid factor, antinuclear antibodies, hepatitis C, cryoglobulins, antineutrophilic cytoplasmic antibodies.
Monoclonal gammopathy of undetermined significance (MGUS) neuropathy	Found in older patients (age > 50 years). Variable findings on neurological exam including decreased DTRs and distal sensation perception. Usually abnormal EMG and NCS. On lab, monoclonal gammopathy.
Paraneoplastic neuropathy	History of smoking, family history, exposure to asbestos or dyes, paints, printing rubber, textiles, or leather. Reduction in DTRs and reduction in distal sensation. Abnormal EMG and NCS. Anti-Hμ antibodies.
Familial amyloid polyneuropathy	Family history. Sensory loss if primarily small-fiber with reduction in DTRs. Postural hypotension is commonly found. Abnormal EMG and NCS with possible NCS indicators of carpal tunnel syndrome.
Acquired amyloid polyneuropathy	History of plasma cell dyscrasia or monoclonal gammopathy. Sensory loss if primarily small-fiber with reduction in DTRs. Postural hypotension is commonly found. Abnormal EMG and NCS with possible NCS indicators of carpal tunnel syndrome. Monoclonal gammopathy if underlying cause.
Neuropathy of renal failure	Renal disease in history. Reduced DTRs with variable findings on sensory testing. Abnormal EMG and NCS. Laboratory indications of renal dysfunction.
Hereditary sensory autonomic neuropathy	Family history is positive. History of foot ulcers or painless injuries. Pes cavus with hammer toes and decrease in DTRs with variable sensory findings. Abnormal EMG and NCS.
Sarcoid neuropathy	Evidence of pulmonary sarcoidosis. Neurological exam indicates either multiple mononeuropathies or polyneuropathy. Abnormal EMG and NCS with elevated angiotensin-converting enzyme and abnormal chest findings, including perihilar lymphadenopathy and effusion.
Arsenic neuropathy	Exposure to pesticides, wood preservatives, or copper smelting. Reduction of DTRs, loss of all types of sensation with distal motor weakness, with Mees' lines. Abnormal EMG and NCS. Elevated arsenic levels in plasma, urine, nails, and hair.

Table 16-1 Some Peripheral Neuropathies (continued)

Type	History, Exam, and Special Testing Indicators
Fabry's disease	Early age onset (< 20 years old) with associated renal failure or stroke. Normal motor, reflex, and sensory exam. Normal EMG and NCS. Reduced levels of α-galactosidase A in serum, leukocytes, or tears.
Celiac disease	GI symptoms. Sensation exam variable with distal sensation common and reduced DTRs. EMG and NCS may be normal or abnormal. Positive serologic testing for celiac disease IgA antigliadin and IgA endomysial antibodies.
HIV-related neuropathy	One or more of the following may be positive: homosexual, drug abuse, blood transfusion, or treatment with antinucleosides. Sensation exam variable with distal sensation loss common and reduced DTRs. EMG and NCS abnormal. HIV antibody positive.

involved, changing the clinical picture due to the functional relationship to proprioception, vibration sensation, muscle strength, and muscle stretch reflexes such as deep tendon reflexes (DTRs).

The clinical presentation of each type is summarized below:

- Exclusive or dominant involvement of small fibers— There is a discrepancy between the severity of pain complaint and objective findings on examination. Patient is often over the age of 50 years. Although older patients may have some decrease in pinprick sensation, these patients have an abnormal degree, including involvement from the feet to the level of the knees (rarely above the knees). While touch sensation may be affected, other sensations are usually unaffected, such as proprioception and vibration. Muscle strength and DTRs are normal.

- Mixed neuropathies involving small and large fibers—These usually will decrease proprioception, vibration sense, and will include muscle weakness and decreased or absent DTRs. Although it is

Table 16-2 Some Named Sensory Mononeuropathies

Name	Nerve	Causes
Numb chin syndrome	Mental nerve	Often ominous, indicating possible metastatic process
Facial sensory neuropathy	Trigeminal nerve	Other than typical trigeminal neuralgia, consider sarcoidosis, Sjögren's syndrome, scleroderma, toxins, or neoplasm
Cheiralgia paresthetica	Superficial radial nerve	Direct trauma, handcuffs, intravenous lines, blood draws
Digitalgia paresthetica	Digital nerves of fingers or toes	Usually due to compression from direct trauma in hands (e.g., bowler's thumb) or pressure from transverse ligaments in toes
Notalgia paresthetica	Posterior rami of T2-T6	Subluxation of related vertebrae or due to pressure from multifidus muscle
Intercostal neuralgia	Intercostal nerves	Diabetes, herpes zoster (shingles), pregnancy, subluxations including rib subluxations
Maigne's syndrome	Posterior rami of T11-T12	Subluxation of related vertebrae
Meralgia paresthetica	Lateral femoral cutaneous nerve	Diabetes, obesity, prolonged sitting, pregnancy, holster, tool belt, surgical table
Gonyalgia paresthetica	Infrapatellar branch of saphenous nerve	Idiopathic, knee trauma, surgery, "influenza knee," viral, diabetes

common for vibration sensation in the elderly to be decreased, the vibration loss often extends into the ankles with mixed neuropathies.

- A recent animal study by Dilley and Bove[3] demonstrated that nerve inflammation disrupts axoplasmic transport and induces a mechanical sensitivity in C fiber nociceptor axons through the accumulation and insertion of mechanosensitive elements.

Complex Regional Pain Syndromes—Types I and II (formerly known as Reflex Sympathetic Dystrophy and Causalgia, respectively)

Reflex sympathetic dystrophy (RSD), now called complex regional pain syndrome (CRPS1), is often the result of severe trauma such as fractures, crush injuries, myocardial infarction, strokes, peripheral nerve injury, or certain medication use. The clinical result is a combination of pain and swelling that includes mainly the distal extremities (usually one) and involves vasomotor instability (including Raynaud's), trophic skin changes, and bone demineralization (Sudeck's atrophy). The accepted belief regarding the cause of RSD is aberrant sympathetic reactivity following injury or other precipitating event. The first phase may be pain and swelling with an increase in sweating and hair growth in the involved area. Classically, the next phase (occurring three to six months later) is characterized by the skin gradually changing to a shiny appearance that is cool to the touch. Eventually (three to six months after the second phase) this may progress to atrophic skin and the development of flexion contractures. When this occurs in the shoulder it is referred to as shoulder-hand syndrome. Causalgia, or CRPS II, is similar, but it is believed to be due to damage to a peripheral nerve. It too is a regional pain syndrome. Evaluation will likely include radiographs to detect osteopenia (Sudeck's atrophy) secondary to RSD. Evaluation of sympathetic dysfunction may include the use of thermography and sudomotor testing. Management is disappointing, with a host of approaches having been taken, from early mobilization and physical therapy in the earlier stages to the use of medical intervention. Drugs that have been incorporated include adrenergic blockers, calcium channel blockers, phenytoin, NSAIDs, opioids, and calcitonin. Stellate ganglion blocks are often used for upper-extremity CRPSs. More recently gabapentin (Neurontin) and pregabalin (Lyrica) are commonly prescribed.

Evaluation

History

The onset is often suggestive of an underlying cause.

- Sudden traumatic onset—When a related, localized area of the body is affected, a traumatic neuropathy is likely; when associated with neck or back trauma, an associated dermatome or myotome-related complaint of pain or weakness may help localize to a segmental level; bilateral complaints suggest spinal cord involvement.
- Sudden nontraumatic onset—This is more suggestive of a vascular cause. When relatively localized to a single area, vascular infarction as occurs occasionally with diabetes is likely; when more generalized or affecting a side of the body, a central vascular event is more likely (stroke or transient ischemic attack). Multiple sclerosis may also present with a rather sudden onset as either a localized or more diffuse pattern.
- Chronic onset—It is always important to ask about the patient's current medications (this may reveal a side effect of a medication or suggest a past diagnosis), and also any past diagnoses with a focus on diabetes, alcoholism, hepatic or renal disease, rheumatoid arthritis (RA), pregnancy, and depression or anxiety.

Complaints of numbness localized to the face or more generalized over the body with no apparent cause should raise the suspicion of anxiety with consequent hyperventilation. Distal numbness in a "stocking-and-glove" distribution is characteristic of metabolic and particularly diabetic neuropathy. This distribution is often bilateral.

If a complaint of numbness is related to a specific occupational or sports activity, it is important to identify any element of either direct compression of a specific nerve or possibly muscle or fascial entrapment. This requires the patient to demonstrate a working posture and any repetitive maneuvers employed.

Complaints associated with diabetes may have a metabolic cause (myelin affected) or be due to neural ischemia. Numbness that seems associated with pregnancy may be due to either fluid compression or vitamin deficiency. If numbness or tingling is present in a patient with RA, fluid compression is likely the primary cause.

Patients with coexisting spinal complaints often will be able to contribute localizing information with regard to pain and weakness. Coupling an outlined pain pathway or movement weakness with the area of numbness or tingling will usually discriminate between a peripheral nerve problem and a nerve root problem. This is further distinguished on the physical examination (**Figures 16–1** and **16–2**).

Examination

The examination must focus on finding which sensory component is affected.[4] Test the patient with his or her eyes closed and alternate the sensory stimulus, applying the stimulus in a random pattern. For example, using a pin and brush alternately touch the patient in a random fashion so that a pattern cannot be detected by the patient. Test the patient for the following:

- Alternate touching with the sharp and dull edge of a pin or broken tongue blade
- Light touch with a brush, wisp of cotton, or gentle touch from examiner's finger pads
- Temperature with small hot and cold test tubes

- Vibration with a struck tuning fork (128 vibrations per second)

Most neuropathies begin with distal sensory loss (the longer nerves affected most often). If no abnormalities are found distally, it is unusual to find proximal loss. If distal loss is found, progress upward to better define the involved area. With all sensory testing, it is important to compare sides. Specifically when testing with a pinwheel or touch, it is important to perform simultaneous testing because of the effect known as sensory extinction. Unilateral testing will be unrevealing, but when both bilateral areas are tested, a sensory deficit is exposed indicating a cortical sensory disorder. Other cortical sensory testing includes the following:

- Stereognosis—Have the patient identify an object placed in his or her hand while the patient's eyes are closed.
- Two-point discrimination—With either a two-point discriminator or a premeasured opened paper clip determine the patient's ability to feel both points of stimulation at the same time; in general, discrimination at the fingertip is 2 to 4 mm; dorsum of fingers, 4 to 6 mm; palms, 8 to 12 mm; and dorsum of hand, 20 to 30 mm.
- Graphesthesia—Write letters or numbers on the palm of the patient's hand with his or her

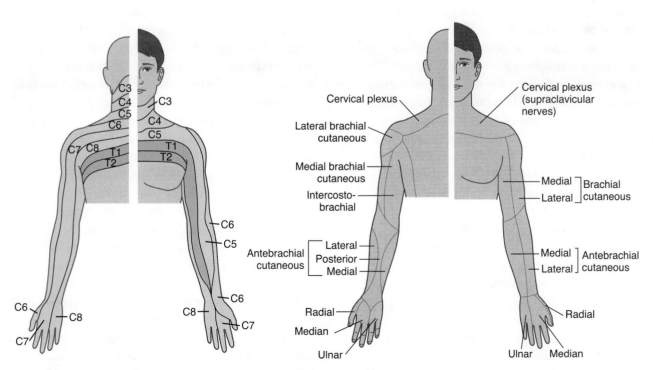

Figure 16–1 Dermatomes of the upper extremity and the cutaneous innervation of the arm by the peripheral sensory nerves.

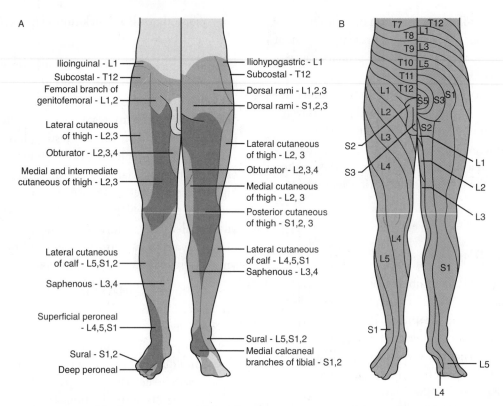

Figure 16–2 Sensory innervation of the lower extremity. (A) Peripheral nerve innervation. (B) Dermatomal (root) innervation.

eyes closed; ask the patient to identify what you are writing.

Proprioception is evaluated by testing joint position sense. The third and fourth digits of the upper and lower extremities have the most sparse innervation and therefore may reveal loss earlier than other digits.[5] The joint is grasped on the lateral surfaces and separated as much as possible from the other digits, being careful not to touch the other digits. The patient, with eyes closed, is asked whether the joint is being held up or down by the examiner. Another evaluation of position sense is the Romberg test. The ability of the patient to keep his or her standing balance with the eyes closed indicates an intact proprioceptive system. If the patient is able to balance (weight equally distributed between both legs) with the eyes open, yet loses balance with the eyes closed, he or she is relying on visual input for balance control. Abnormalities of vibration or position sense indicate problems with large fiber neurons and/or dorsal column disease.

In chiropractic practice, a common presentation is neck or low back pain with associated extremity complaints of pain, numbness, or tingling. Although it is

hoped that a pattern match will be made with these complaints and an objective demonstration of sensory loss, motor loss, or an associated deep tendon decrease, this is often not the case. For example, patients with neck pain may complain of a diffuse sense of numbness or paresthesias in the hand. They are unable to localize to a dermatome, and objective testing fails to clarify the diagnosis. It may be helpful first to attempt provocation maneuvers. For the nerve root, this includes standard orthopaedic testing of the related spinal area, such as cervical compression/distraction for the upper extremity or the straight leg raise or Kemp's test for the lower extremity. Additional provocation testing for peripheral nerves is accomplished by either tapping (if the nerve is superficial) or compression through direct pressure or muscle contraction. Patients who associate the complaint with an activity can be asked to repeat or hold the position (whichever is appropriate) in an attempt to reproduce the complaint.

When the area of involvement overlaps between a dermatome and a peripheral nerve skin patch, selected muscle testing, provocation tests, or an associated tendon reflex may help differentiate the source. For example, if the patient had a sensory area loss over the anterior thumb and two fingers, either median nerve involvement or a C6 nerve root lesion is possible. However, a median nerve disorder would not affect the brachioradialis reflex and a C6 nerve root disorder would not cause a positive Tinel's sign over the median nerve (unless there is a double-crush syndrome).

When the complaint is diffuse or nondermatomal, consideration of referral sources should be next. These may include facet irritation or trigger points. Reproduction may be possible with trigger point palpation, but facet involvement is difficult to demonstrate clinically except for the relief sometimes provided by an adjustment.

If the diagnosis is still in question, consideration of electrodiagnostic or special imaging studies is warranted. In most cases it would be appropriate to treat for a one-month period prior to utilizing these expensive procedures. The use of electrodiagnostic studies (EDS), such as electrical muscle stimulation (EMS) and nerve conduction studies (NCS), is focused on distinguishing among several possibilities:

- Mononeuropathy: an example is local/focal entrapment such as tarsal tunnel syndrome
- Differentiating multiple mononeuropathies: usually involves peripheral nerve vascular disease (vasculitis)
- Polyneuropathies: usually symmetric
- Axonal neuropathies: diabetes, for example
- Demyelinating neuropathies: multiple sclerosis, for example

A normal EDS evaluation indicates that the cause is non-neuropathic, possibly due to local inflammation, arthritis, referral pain, or central nervous system pain such as a myelopathy. A search for small-fiber involvement may include the following tests:

- Sudomotor reflex test: quantitates sweating and is approximately 80% sensitive for small-fiber damage[6]
- Skin biopsies: demonstrate loss of intraepidermal nerve fibers (not widely available)
- Quantitative sensory testing: assesses small-fiber damage through measurement of pain and temperature thresholds in the skin (not as sensitive or specific as sudomotor testing or skin biopsies)

EMG and nerve conduction velocity (NCV) studies are reserved for difficult cases. EMG uses needle insertion into muscle to test muscle and nerve.[6] The spontaneous activity generated upon insertion or the response generated with muscle contraction helps distinguish between axon injury and demyelination disorders. NCV studies use surface electrodes to measure velocity and the amplitude of an evoked response to an electrical stimulus. Both motor and sensory nerves can be tested. Important concepts are as follows:

- Axonal degeneration will demonstrate normal velocities with NCV studies, but a reduced amplitude of evoked responses. EMG evidence takes about three weeks to surface, revealing spontaneous activity at rest, such as fibrillations and positive sharp waves; during contraction, there is a reduction in the density pattern, interference pattern, and mean amplitude of the motor unit potentials (MUPs).
- Demyelination disorders will demonstrate early changes in the nerve conduction velocity with relatively normal evoked amplitude responses.

Management

Management is based on the suspected cause. Most peripheral nerve and nerve root disorders can be managed by a chiropractor for one month, being sure to monitor for any worsening or nonresponse to care that might require referral. Chronic pain requires different approaches. The potential central modulation that facilitates many cases of chronic pain requires a combination of behavioral and medical approaches if not responsive to conservative care. Predictors of chronicity should always be considered in baseline measures of incoming patients including regional functional outcome tools and global assessments of function such as the SF-36. Another strong predictor that can be measured and responded to in management is fear avoidance behaviors that tend to prolong recovery. Many musculoskeletal disorders such as low back pain, neck pain, and headache become chronic and may require a multimodal approach. Neuralgias secondary to diabetes and herpes are often in need of specific medications. Metabolic disorders often require medical evaluation and management; diabetes, however, often can be comanaged. See more thorough discussions of individual disorders in related chapters of this text.

Conservative management is based on the premise that "closing the pain gate" can be accomplished without the use of medication. Cutaneous stimulation through vibration, massage, myofascial stripping, taping, and bracing likely affect cutaneous and subcutaneous receptors that send their signals through large fiber afferents reaching the spinal cord prior to pain signals. Counter-irritation using transcutaneous electrical stimulation (TENS), acupuncture, or capsaicin are also used.

Proposed mechanisms for the chiropractic adjustment are that:

- Stimulation via mechanoreceptor activity in the posterior columns provides large-fiber dampening of pain transmission at the spinal cord level.
- Stimulation of nuclei in the brainstem through the spinomesencephalic tract and at the PAG activate descending fibers back down the spinal cord to inhibit pain.
- Reflex inhibition of tight muscles via group Ib inhibitory interneurons: Group Ib afferents from Golgi tendon organs, as well as cutaneous and joint mechanoreceptor afferents, can stimulate Ib inhibitory interneurons that are located in lamina VII of the spinal gray. These Ib interneurons inhibit α motoneurons, which leads to relaxation of spasmed muscle.
- A fast-stretch applied to a tight muscle stimulates Golgi tendon organs and activates lb afferents, which then produce reflex inhibition (inverse stretch reflex) of the same tight muscle that was stretched. The net result is relaxation of the tight muscle.

Current medical management of painful neuropathies has been estimated as achieving only a 30% to 50% reduction in pain.[7] There is a range of medications prescribed, including antidepressants and antiseizure medications. Some of the representative medication classes and examples follow:

- Antidepressants: includes tricyclic antidepressants and selective serotonin reuptake inhibitors
- Anticonvulsants: includes carbamazepine, phenytoin, gabapentin, and lamotrigine
- Antiarrhythmics: includes mexiletine
- N-methyl-D-aspartate glutamate
- Narcotic and non-narcotic analgesics
- Levodopa
- Topical agents: capsaicin and topical lidocaine

For a more complete list of medications see Tables 1-12 through 1-14 in Chapter 1: General Approaches.

Algorithm

An algorithm for evaluation and management of numbness is presented in **Figure 16–3**.

APPENDIX 16–1

Web Resources

Pain

American Pain Foundation
(888) 615-PAIN (7246)
http://www.painfoundation.org
American Society of Anesthesiologists
(800) 562-8666
http://www.asahq.org/patientEducation /managepain.htm
American Cancer Society
(800) 227-2345
http://www.cancer.org

APPENDIX 16–2

References

1. Brodal A. *Neurological Anatomy.* 2nd ed. New York: Oxford University Press; 1981.
2. Mendell JR, Sahenk Z. Painful sensory neuropathy. *N Engl J Med.* 2003;348:1243–1255.
3. Dilley A, Bove GM. Disruption of axoplasmic transport induces mechanical sensitivity in intact rat C-fibre nociceptor axons. *J Physiol.* 2008;586(2):593–604.
4. Walker HK, Hall WD, Hurst JW, eds. *Clinical Methods: The History, Physical, and Laboratory Examinations.* 2nd ed. Boston: Butterworth; 1980:942.
5. DeMeyer W. *Technique of the Neurological Examination: A Programmed Text.* 2nd ed. New York: McGraw-Hill; 1974:293–323.
6. Meyer JJ. Clinical electromyographic and related neuro-physiologic responses. In: Lawrence DJ, Cassidy JD, McGregor M, et al., eds. *Advances in Chiropractic.* St. Louis, MO: Mosby Year Book; 1994;1:29.
7. Sindrup SH, Jensen TS. Pharmacologic treatment of pain in polyneuropathy. *Neurology.* 2000;55:915–920.

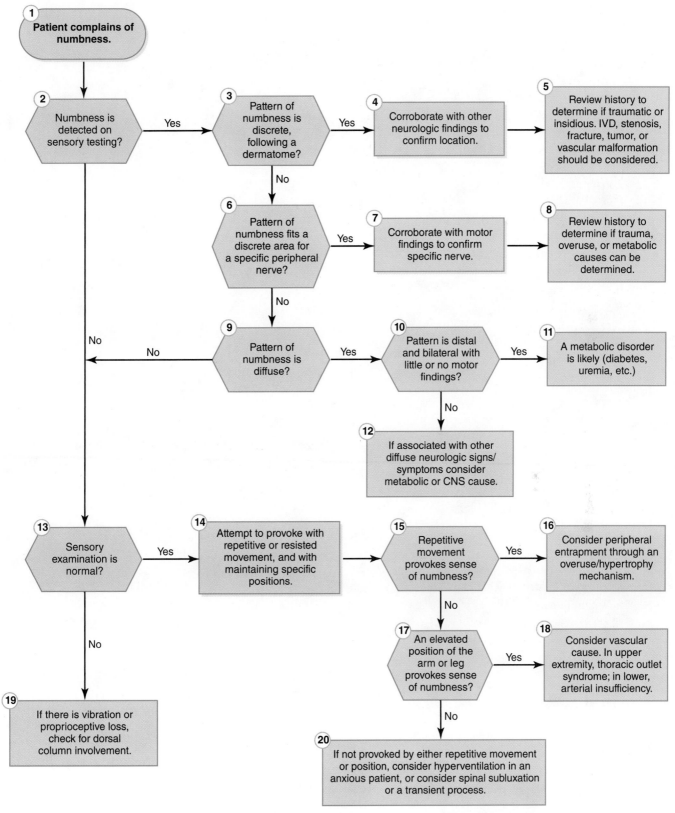

Figure 16–3 Numbness—Algorithm

Headache

Context

Severe headache causes significant financial impact on the individual, the employer, and the healthcare system. Considering only the cost of lost work and productivity, migraine headaches have a price tag of approximately $13 to $17 billion annually.[1, 2] This equals 112 million "bedridden days" per year. Direct costs for migraines are approximately $100 per patient annually for a total U.S. annual cost of $1 billion. More important to the individual is the finding of a recent study[3] indicating that migraine headache's negative impact on patients' quality of life is greater than that of other chronic conditions such as osteoarthritis, hypertension, or diabetes. One recent study found that children evaluated at a headache center had a quality of life comparable to children with rheumatoid diseases or cancer.[4] It has been estimated that up to 10% of children ages 5 to 15 years and 28% of adolescents experience migraine headaches.[5, 6] Fifty-seven percent of men and 76% of women report at least one significant headache per month.[4, 7] Approximately 27 million Americans have suffered from migraine headaches.[8]

Although they are a common human ailment, headaches, more often than not, do not warrant a visit to the doctor's office. Whether obviously associated with flu, excessive drinking, skipped breakfast, or other factors, the patient is quite aware of a connection to the headache. Many patients resort to over-the-counter (OTC) medications. In fact, headaches may be the most common reason for the use of OTC analgesic medications.[9] When a patient does seek an opinion or treatment, the headache has become either unbearable (affecting lifestyle) or worrisome (the patient thinks there may be a tumor), or there has been head trauma. Of patients reporting headaches, 27% have sought alternative management. Chiropractic care was the most common alternative therapy sought by these patients.[10]

In the chiropractic office one of the most common headache presentations is associated with whiplash. In fact, headache is one of the two most reported complaints after whiplash. Many studies indicate that a high percentage of whiplash patients (70% to 90%) develop a headache.[11-16]

Chronic headache that is unresponsive to treatment is a difficult scenario. First on the list of mechanical possibilities should be temporomandibular (TMJ) disorders.[17-19] Some differentials include tenderness of the pterygoids, tenderness of the TMJ, clicking in the TMJ, and abnormal mandibular movement patterns on opening and closing.[20] Overlap with clinical indicators of tension-like headache is common.

Migraine[21,22]

- Migraine is prevalent in 6.5% of males and 18.2% of females.
- Prevalence increases from age 12 years to 40 years and then declines.
- 51% of patients report at least a 50% reduction in work or school productivity.
- 27.9 million Americans suffer from migraine (increase over 10-year period likely related to growth in population).
- Less than half of patients who met the criteria for migraine were diagnosed correctly (possibly due to finding that only 49% of internal medicine residents and 62% of family practice residents felt prepared to treat headache patients).[21]
- In one study, in patients that met the IHS criteria for migraine, 42% were diagnosed with sinus headache and 32% were diagnosed with tension headache.[21]

Episodic Tension-Type

- Prevalence of 38% of U.S. adults

Cluster

- Prevalence of < 0.1% of U.S. adults

Cervicogenic

- Prevalence of 18% of U.S. adults

Only about 2% of patients in-office and 4% of patients in an emergency department setting will be diagnosed with a headache indicating serious pathology (e.g., tumor, AVM, aneurysm).[23] The categorization of headaches by the International Headache Society (IHS) distinguishes among the primary headache patterns and includes a category for cervicogenic headache.[24] The categories use specific criteria upon which to base the headache diagnosis. Unfortunately, the cervicogenic headache criteria are quite restrictive and exclusive of the other primary headache categories. In other words, there is a perception by the IHS that there could be no overlap or cervicogenic component to the other headache types. Yet research indicates that there is likely a pure category of cervicogenic headache, a category that has a significant contribution from a cervicogenic component, and yet another category that is unrelated. Using the criteria set forth by the IHS, one study[25] determined a cervicogenic headache prevalence of about 18% in a random population sample of adults.

Although the vast majority of headaches are benign (not life-threatening), the doctor initially must screen for secondary causes prior to assuming one of four common primary patterns: migraine, tension-type, cervicogenic, and cluster headaches. Screening the patient with headaches historically is the most fruitful, time-effective, and inexpensive approach (**Exhibit 17–1**). Expensive imaging approaches are rarely needed.

General Strategy

History and Examination

- Determine whether the patient has a secondary cause for the headache, such as trauma, metabolic disease, toxic (drug) effect, infection, or intracranial pathology (see **Table 17–1**).
- Determine whether the patient's headache fits one of three categories of primary headache: migraine, tension-type, and cluster, or whether cervicogenic is likely.
- Determine whether there are any obvious triggers or patterns to the headache.
- Evaluate the patient for musculoskeletal factors that may cause or influence headaches.

Management

The chiropractor should determine which cases are appropriate for referral. Referral is, in fact, rarely needed given the low incidence of serious causes. The red flags that warrant further investigation and possible referral include but are not limited to the following:

- Including sudden, severe headache (worst headache of their lives)
- A new headache in an older patient (possible tumor or temporal arteritis)
- Headache due to head trauma (possible subdural or epidural hematoma)
- Associated residual neurologic signs or symptoms (possible tumor or vascular event)
- Cognitive changes (e.g., confusion, drowsiness, giddiness)
- Vomiting without nausea (indicating increased intracranial pressure)
- Persistent or progressive headache
- Nuchal rigidity with or without fever (possible meningitis or subarachnoid hemorrhage, respectively)
- Suspicion of drug or alcohol dependence
- Headache associated with a diastolic blood pressure greater than 115 mm Hg (possible hypertensive headache)
- Persistent or severe headache in a child

For patients without these red flags, consider the following options for conservative care:

- Modify patient behavior (sleep, diet, and exercise) when determined by history as a significant factor.
- Manage with chiropractic manipulative therapy for an initial high-frequency period of one to three weeks, followed by a gradual tapering.
- Consider use of supplemental support or herbal alternatives including feverfew.

Exhibit 17–1   Historical Screening of the Patient with Headaches

Patient presents with a history of headaches

⬇

Differentiate Referral from Nonreferral Case

History Questions
History of head trauma? (Consider subdural or epidural hematoma.)
Slow or insidious onset of new headache? (Consider tumor or vascular event such as an aneurysm or arteriovenous malformation [AVM].)
Associated neurologic deficits? (Consider all the above.)
New temporal headache in a older patient, especially when associated with vision deficit or aching trunk area? (Consider temporal arteritis.)
Occurs only with exertion and is progressively worse? (Consider vascular cause such as aneurysm or AVM.)
Associated with nuchal rigidity with or without fever? (Consider subarachnoid hemorrhage without fever and meningitis with fever.)

⬇

Differentiate by Type

Vascular/Neurologic	Tension-Type/Cervicogenic	Metabolic/Toxic	Miscellaneous
Decreased blood to the brain (atherosclerosis) Increased pressure on vasculature (vasodilation or hypertension)	**Direct pull on periosteum, muscle spasm, referred pain, or nerve entrapment**	**Decreased glucose to the brain (diabetes, hypoglycemia), increased metabolism (hyperthyroidism), drug toxicity**	**Other causes such as sinus, eyestrain, cerebrospinal fluid (CSF) pressure changes, etc.**

Migraine
Is there a family history?
Are there visual changes before the headache? (aura)
Is the headache incapacitating?
Do they last for hours or days? (Differentiate between classic and common.)
Associated with sensitivity to light or sound?
Nausea and/or vomiting?

Cluster
Is the patient a middle-aged or a young man?
Is the pain orbital and associated with tearing or drooling?
Do they last a short time (45 minutes to 2 hours)?
Does alcohol or smoking make them worse or trigger them?
Does the headache wake the patient up at night?

Is there a history of a whiplash-type injury prior to headaches?
Are the headaches suboccipital or bandlike?
Are they worse in the afternoon?
Stress related?
Aspirin helpful to some degree?

Is there a history of hypo- or hyperthyroid disease, diabetes, anemia, or cardiopulmonary disease (e.g., COPD)?
Is the patient taking medications?
Is there a relationship to certain foods?
Is the patient occupationally exposed to toxic materials?

Is there a history of spinal tap? (Possible CSF pressure cause.)
Is the headache associated with upper respiratory infection signs/symptoms or made worse by bending forward? (Possible sinus infection.)
Associated with exercise? (related to hydration/diet, blood pressure, muscle strain, etc.)
Is the patient's eyesight normal or corrected? (Possible eyestrain or myogenic from forward head position.)

Table 17–1 Metabolic Causes of Headache

Common	Less Common
Hypo- and hyperthyroidism	Hypo-hyperadrenalism (Addison's/Cushing's)
Anemia and polycythemia	Pheochromocytoma
Hypoxemia	Carbon monoxide poisoning
Hypoglycemia	Vitamin A toxicity
Hypertension (especially malignant HTN)	Paget's disease (cranial bone involvement)
Uremia	Cranial tumors
Hypercarbia	Chronic leukemia
Hyponatremia	Hemoglobinopathies Parathyroid disease

- If chiropractic management is unsuccessful, refer for or use nonpharmacologic treatment such as acupuncture or biofeedback.
- If nonpharmacologic management is unsuccessful, refer for medical management.

Theories of Causation of Primary Headaches

Although the treatment of headaches chiropractically has anecdotally been supported for years, only recently have models of causal relationships between headaches and cervical dysfunction and studies to confirm effectiveness been advanced. Recent research suggests that the older theories of vascular dilation with migraines[26, 27] and muscle contraction with tension-type headaches[28] do not adequately explain how these headaches occur. From genetic research, migraine appears to be an ionopathy, a disorder based on abnormal ion channels—primarily calcium channels that allow hyperexcitability.[29] Structurally, it appears that one of the primary sites is the dorsolateral pons.[30] It appears that a neurologic event occurs associated with an imbalance of serotonin.[31–34] This serotonin imbalance appears to be site-specific. In other words, too little or too much serotonin may contribute to headache development, depending on where it occurs. In general, too little available serotonin centrally is the primary cause.

Dysfunction of brainstem modulation of sensory input is proposed as a major element of migraine and other headache pain. Large cranial blood vessels, proximal intracranial blood vessels, and the dura are innervated by the ophthalmic division of the trigeminal nerve. Posterior fossa structures are innervated by branches off the C2 nerve roots. Input from the trigeminal-innervated structures pass through the trigeminal ganglion synapsing in the trigeminocervical nucleus (complex). Information is then sent through the quintothalamic tract after decussating in the brainstem. Modulation of this nociceptive information is believed to come from the dorsal raphe nucleus, locus coeruleus, and nucleus raphe magnus.

Stimulation of cranial parasympathetic outflow occurs between neurons in the pons in the superior salivatory nucleus. This parasympathetic output is mediated through the pterygopalatine, otic, and carotid ganglia. This is referred to as the trigeminal-autonomic reflex and may be over-responsive in those with cluster and migraine headache.

For migraine headaches, increased local vascular concentrations of serotonin may act as part of an inflammatory cascade of chemical mediators including substance P.[35, 36] Neurogenic vascular inflammation results from antidromic stimulation of the trigeminal ganglion with release of tachykinins and calcitonin gene-related peptide causing plasma protein extravasation and vasodilation with degranulation of mast cells. In addition, it has been suggested that factors that may control this local neurogenic inflammation include a local C fiber nerve ending/mast cell feedback loop. The control of mast cells by histamine acting at H3 receptors may mitigate neurogenic inflammation.[37] Recent interest has focused on dopamine and its role in migraine with aura. Most migraine symptoms can be induced with dopaminergic stimulation or ameliorated with dopamine receptor antagonists.[38] Also the role of inheritance of the dopamine D2 receptor (DRD2) NcoI allele is currently being studied.

Convergence of afferent information from cervical spinal nerves and the trigeminal nerve in the trigeminocervical nucleus may serve to explain a referred pain mechanism for both migraine and tension-type headaches, and perhaps for cluster headaches.[39] The trigeminocervical nucleus (**Figure 17–1**) is a continuous column of neurons formed by the caudal end of the spinal nucleus of the trigeminal nerve and the dorsal horn of the upper cervical spinal nerves (C1-C3). Descending fibers from the nucleus raphe magnus and other midbrain and pontine nuclei normally have an inhibitory effect on the spinothalamic neurons (directly and through interneurons),

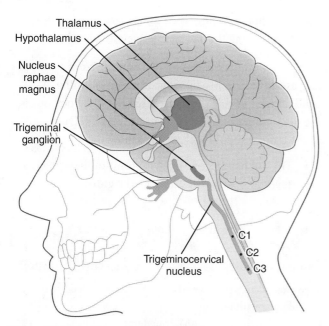

Figure 17–1 The Trigeminocervical Nucleus.

preventing transmission of pain signals. Deregulation may allow a lowering of the stimulus threshold necessary for pain perception, perhaps through a decrease in secreted serotonin. Therefore, afferent information that is not nociceptive in nature may become so due to lowering of the pain threshold and/or expansion of the receptor field. The result may be either referral to the head and face from irritation in the neck or referral of neck pain from irritation of intracranial pain-sensitive structures (e.g., intracerebral blood vessels causing posterior or suboccipital pain). Therefore structures innervated by C1-C3 including C2-C3 intervertebral disk annular fibers, deep muscles, joints, ligaments, and connections to the dura mater may be sources of referred pain to the head.

A more recent theory proposed by the inadvertent success of cosmetic surgery (i.e., brow lift surgery), is that there are peripheral triggers of trigeminal irritation or dysfunction. This theory is based on the possibility of local entrapment of superficial nerves in craniofacial muscles. This is further supported by the relief from migraine headaches through botulinum toxin injection of some of these muscles. A review of current evidence and approaches can be found in a review by Kung et al.[40]

A recent anatomic finding may further explain the relationship between response to chiropractic manipulation and headache. At the atlantooccipital junction, there appears to be a connective tissue attachment between the rectus capitis posterior minor muscle and the posterior

spinal dura.[41,42] A proposed mechanism of increased dural tension through upper cervical dysfunction has been suggested as a cause of headache; in particular, cervicogenic headache.

Another structure implicated in the production or control of migraine and cluster headaches is the sphenopalatine ganglion (SPG), a branch of the facial nerve. The SPG apparently contains a small percentage of trigeminal fibers and projects parasympathetic fibers to the cerebral vasculature.[43] Also, the SPG is a major source of nitric oxide synthase (NOS). It appears that the SPG may mediate vasodilation of cerebral blood flow when the trigeminal ganglion or the locus coeruleus is stimulated via NOS-containing nerve fibers that innervate the proximal anterior and middle cerebral arteries.

Hormonal influences on central serotoninergic and opioid neurons may play a role in migraine headache in women. Plasma levels of serotonin have been found to increase significantly in women with migraine with aura and those with tension-type headaches. This fluctuation was not evident in migraine sufferers without aura. It is unclear whether this is a reflection of central serotonin effects.[44] Menstrual migraine appears to be due to estrogen withdrawal.[45] Sixty percent of migraine attacks in women are associated with menses, but only 14% are exclusively related.[46] Sustained increased estrogen levels with pregnancy and decreased levels with menopause appear to be related to changes in headache patterns. Migraine sufferers usually improve during pregnancy, especially after the first trimester. This improvement is suspected to be related to sustained high levels of estrogen. However, 25% of women notice no change in their headache pattern.[47] The effect of contraceptives on migraine headache is less clear. Several studies report no difference between those who took oral contraceptives and a placebo group.[48] Other studies suggest an increased severity and incidence.[49] Migraine prevalence definitely decreases with age; menopause, however, may trigger the onset or return of migraine.[50] Again, some studies indicate that estrogen replacement therapy increases or exacerbates migraine while others indicate estrogen alone or in combination with testosterone helps relieve migraine.

There is evidence that some patients with migraine share genetic markers with patients who have epilepsy.[51] This may explain why antiepileptic medication is more effective in this subgroup. There is no evidence, though, that those with migraine have a higher incidence of epilepsy except for the familial hemiplegia subgroup.

History

Careful questioning of the patient during the history taking can point to the diagnosis (**Tables 17–2** and **17–3**).

- Determine any obvious triggers or causes of headaches from environmental, dietary, or medication sources.
- Determine any red flags suggestive of referral for medical management.

- Attempt to distinguish among three primary headaches, using the patient interview and headache diary.

Although the sequence of questioning is not as important as the comprehensiveness of the questioning, it is prudent next to rule out causes that might be obvious to the doctor but not necessarily to the patient. Questions to the patient should include the following:

- Do you have signs and symptoms of flu (especially fever or cough without nuchal rigidity)?

Table 17–2 History Questions for Headache

Primary Question	What Are You Thinking?	Secondary Questions	What Are You Thinking?
Did you hit your head?	Fracture, subdural or epidural hematoma, post-concussion syndrome.	**Did you lose consciousness and have difficulty with memory?**	Post-concussion syndrome.
		Are you having difficulty with memory, walking, or talking?	Subdural hematoma.
Are you taking any medications?	Side effect of drug, drug indicates past diagnosis, withdrawal from drug.	**Did you recently stop taking medication?**	Withdrawal phenomenon.
		Was the medication given for your headaches?	Rebound effect.
		Were you recently prescribed a medication?	Side effect of drug (vasodilators, etc.).
		Do you use recreational drugs? Drink (alcohol) heavily?	Side effect or withdrawal phenomenon (with possible alcohol abuse use CAGE questions).
Is this a "new" headache?	Especially in older persons: tumor, temporal arteritis, or CNS vascular event.	**(To an older patient) Is the headache throbbing at your temple?**	Temporal arteritis.
		Is there associated vision loss with this temple headache?	Temporal arteritis.
		Do you have an associated complaint of a deep, throbbing ache in the upper trunk (neck and shoulder) area?	Temporal arteritis.
		Have you had the headache for several weeks without improvement?	Possible tumor.
		Is it worse when bending forward?	Possible tumor (especially with no signs of sinus involvement).
Do you have any disorders or diseases that you know about?	Headache is often associated with disorders such as diabetes, thyroid, COPD, hypertension, AIDS, cancer, etc. Perhaps the underlying disorder is the main cause.	**Is the disorder being managed by a physician?**	Disorder not well-controlled.
		Do you follow the management recommendations (diet, medication, lifestyle changes)?	Disorder not well-controlled.

Key: CAGE, questions asked of an alcoholic: Do you need to Cut down? Does your drinking Annoy people? Do you feel Guilty about drinking? Do you use alcohol in the morning as an Eye opener?; NSAIDs, nonsteroid anti-inflammatory drugs; CNS, central nervous system; COPD, chronic obstructive pulmonary disease; AIDS, acquired immunodeficiency syndrome.

Table 17–3 History Questions for Suspicion of Migraine Headaches

Primary Question	Possible Causes for Positive Response	Differentiating Questions	Suspicion
Do you have any unusual vision changes prior to the headache?	Migraine, TIA, cluster headache, glaucoma, eyestrain.	Do you see flashing lights, zig-zag lines, and/or blind spots?	Migraine with aura.
		Do these go away in a short time (minutes to 1.5 hours)?	Migraine with aura (longer would suggest TIA).
		Is the pain mainly around your eye with increase in tearing?	Cluster headache (possible migraine).
		Do you see halos around lights or lose your vision on the periphery (outsides)?	Acute glaucoma.
Are they incapacitating?	Unless new in an older patient, it is likely to be migraine or cluster headache.	Do they last for hours or days?	Migraine is likely.
		Do they last less than 2 hours and cluster (several a day) over weeks?	Cluster headache.
Do certain foods, alcohol, or smoking bring on the headache or make it worse?	Migraine and cluster headaches.	Do you notice that wine, cheese, or cured meats cause headaches?	Migraine likely.
		Does alcohol or smoking either trigger or make your headache worse?	Cluster headache likely.
Is the headache related to sleep?	Migraine and cluster headaches.	Does either under- or oversleeping trigger a headache?	Migraine likely.
		Does it often wake you at night?	Cluster headache likely.
Is there a family history of similar headaches?	Migraine, tension, depression.	Has a parent, grandparent, or sibling been diagnosed with migraine headaches?	Migraine.
Have you been diagnosed with migraine and been given medication?	Migraine, rebound migraine.	Have you taken sumatriptin or other serotonin receptor agonist or NSAIDs more often than twice a week or suddenly stopped taking them?	Rebound migraine.

Key: TIA, transient ischemic attack; NSAIDs, nonsteroid anti-inflammatory drugs.

- Have you recently been given a new prescription?
- Have you recently discontinued use of a prescription drug?
- Have you recently stopped smoking, drinking coffee, drinking alcohol, or using recreational drugs?
- Do you use recreational drugs?
- Do you get headaches after reading or have you had a recent change in eyeglass prescription?
- Are you occupationally exposed to toxic chemicals?

A recent study has pointed out the need to consider caffeine as a source of headaches in children.[52] Children who suffered from chronic daily headache who had a relatively high intake of sodas (1.5 liters of cola per day) were gradually withdrawn from cola consumption over one to two weeks to avoid caffeine-withdrawal headaches.

Findings showed that 33 out of 36 children were headache-free, which was sustained at a 24-week follow-up.

Migraine prevalence has been found to increase before menopause and decrease after natural menopause.[53] This is particularly true of women most susceptible to hormonal shifts, such as those suffering from premenstrual syndrome. Low estrogen and high follicle-stimulating hormone seem to correlate with lower migraine prevalence. Additionally, one study indicated that migraine without aura was associated with an occurrence of headache during the two days preceding menses and on the first two days of menses.[54]

Exertion/Activity-Related Headaches

One of the major concerns with headache associated with exertion is the possibility of an underlying tumor or vascular weakness that may lead to sudden death.

It appears as though this concern is worth addressing; however, although 50% to 60% of patients with brain tumors have headaches, only 25% experience exertion-related headaches.[55] When aneurysms rupture, the usual progression is a quick onset of headache followed by loss of consciousness and death. In patients with a slow leak, however, a severe headache may appear over several days or weeks. This "sentinel" headache appears in 30% to 60% of patients with eventual rupture.[56] Associated symptoms may include nausea, vomiting, visual disturbances and photophobia, aphasia, nuchal rigidity (without fever), and weakness. Immediate referral is necessary. Evaluation will include computed tomography (CT) scan for structural brain lesions and a lumbar puncture to detect a subarachnoid bleed.

It is important to screen athletes regarding some common culprits of benign exertional headaches, including dehydration, hyperventilation, hypoglycemia and/or poor diet, alcohol use, caffeine withdrawal, and heat intolerance. They are more likely to be triggering mechanisms in the poorly conditioned athlete. When headache is associated with a specific activity, clues may be found with regard to the mechanism in some cases. For example, one common presentation is weightlifter's headache.[57] There are probably two possible explanations for this occurrence: (1) increased intracranial pressure is caused by the Valsalva-like maneuver with lifting, or (2) stretching or strain occurs in the cervical musculature/tendons.

Valsalva maneuvers increase intracranial venous sinus pressure. This in turn leads to a general increase in intracranial pressure, reducing cerebral blood flow. This effect is generally short-lived and benign. If the headache is persistent or severe, further evaluation with CT scan or magnetic resonance imaging (MRI) may be necessary. Overstrain due to maximum lift effort or abnormal posturing of the neck during activity may lead to a primarily subluxation/soft tissue–caused headache. Historical review of the mechanism of onset with regard to neck position and the onset of symptoms is valuable. Confirmation by physical examination, spinal palpation, and resolution with chiropractic care are likely with this etiology.

Migraine headaches occur in some athletes involved in short, strenuous activities, including weight lifting and short-distance running or swimming.[58] Although the mechanism is not clear, it has been proposed that hyperventilation leads to a decrease in partial pressure of carbon dioxide (PCO_2) with resulting vasoconstriction. This leads to a migraine aura followed by vasodilation leading to the headache.

Acute altitude change from 3,500 m to 5,000 m may lead to acute mountain sickness, which presents as a throbbing headache that may be associated with malaise, nausea, and vomiting in some cases.[59] The onset is generally within the first three days after ascent. After several days of acclimation, the headache resolves.

A distinct subcategory of sport-related headaches is found in divers.[60] There are a variety of mechanisms to consider.

- Skip breathing may lead to increased PCO_2, vasodilation, and subsequent headache.
- Cervical and facial muscles may be overstrained through stabilizing the mouthpiece.
- A tight mask may compress the supraorbital and supratrochlear nerves.
- Dental cavities may be sensitive to the barometric pressure changes with deep diving.

Posttraumatic Headaches

In automobile accidents and collision or contact sports, head and neck trauma are common. With direct trauma to the head, varying degrees of injury may occur, including cerebral contusion, sub- or epidural hemorrhage/hematoma, and intracranial artery dissection. Although it may seem logical that when damage is severe, headache would be immediate, this is not always the case. Slow leaks, as mentioned above, may take several hours, days, and rarely weeks to cause significant symptomatology. It would be prudent, though, to check all patients with head trauma for focal neurologic signs (in particular cranial nerves) and mental status.

Concussion

Concussion is considered a subset of mild traumatic brain injury (MTBI), which carries with it the possibility of complex pathophysiological processes that may not be immediately evident post-trauma. The definition of concussion does not include loss of consciousness. The biggest concern after concussion is post-concussion or post-concussive syndrome (PCS) where symptoms and neurological dysfunction may persist for weeks or months. Some of the most common signs/symptoms include headache, dizziness, difficulty concentrating, irritability, and other emotional and behavioral manifestations (e.g., mood changes, depression, restlessness, aggression, emotional lability, and apathy).

There are at least 3.8 million concussions in the United States annually, given that as many as 50% of concussions may go unreported.[61] Clearly the high-risk sports are those that are without protection and/or those that involve violent contact with the opposite team player; the highest incidence of concussion is in football, hockey, rugby, soccer, and basketball. It should be remembered that concussions occur in all sports, and in non-sports head trauma such as falls.

Headaches are the most common symptom; however, most athletes report the headache as similar to previous headaches but more frequent and longer lasting.

Although guidelines differ,[62,63] there is general agreement that:

- Concussion evaluation should be performed by healthcare professionals with specific training and experience in the assessment and management of concussion.
- Education of athletes as to the danger of concussion and what to look for in themselves and their teammates is of utmost importance. Educating parents, coaches, referees, and school administrators is important for recognition and proper management.
- Although various evaluation tools are available, a standardized assessment of function should be administered to athletes prior to sport participation to establish a baseline, with the caveat that issues such as balance need to be evaluated with sports equipment on.
- Using a baseline comparison, the same evaluation tool should be utilized immediately after any suspected concussion.

A commonly utilized tool is the Sport Concussion Assessment Tool 3 (SCAT3).[64] This comprehensive approach uses an initial assessment similar to the Glasgow Coma Scale, immediately followed by observation and documentation of any concussion signs. Next, symptoms and symptom severity, neurocognitive function, and balance function are assessed. It is important to note that there is no evidence to support the use of a composite/total score. In other words, each section should be assessed separately. In a study[65] evaluating high school athletes using a baseline SCAT2 (the older version) it was found that concentration testing in high school athletes is unreliable because of high baseline error. In other words, baseline concentration scores should not be used as a comparator after concussion.

A return-to-play (RTP) clearance involves a gradual, step-by-step increase in physical demands and sports-specific activities, as well as a consideration of the risk for contact. If symptoms occur with activity, no further progression should occur and the athlete should be restarted at the preceding symptom-free step. The primary concern with a premature RTP is decreased reaction time leading to an increased risk of a second concussion with a known risk for prolongation of symptoms. A very serious concern, especially in the pediatric and young adult population, is second-impact syndrome (SIS).[66] In SIS, a rapid hydrocephalus occurs, greatly increasing intracranial pressure, which may result in death.

Other testing for neuropsychological function may be performed to evaluate cognitive function. Tests include:

- The Stroop Color Test and the 2&7 Processing Speed Test (to detect problems with mental processing including speed).
- Rivermead Post-Concussion Symptoms Questionnaire, which measures the severity of post-concussion symptoms.
- The Hopkins Verbal Learning A (HVLA) test and the Digit Span Forward examination, which test verbal learning and recall including digit sequence recall.

A post-concussion migraine headache has been reported especially with soccer and English football.[67] This type of migraine resembles the classic migraine (migraine with aura) and usually resolves within 48 hours. A strikingly different type of headache is one in which there are associated signs of pupillary dilation and sweating. In between attacks there may be a partial Horner's syndrome. This type of headache is sometimes called traumatic dysautonomic cephalgia. It is thought to be caused by sympathetic fiber injury in the neck; it has been treated medically with β-blockers.

Finally, an insidious and potentially life-threatening condition associated with head trauma and headache is second-impact syndrome.[68] An athlete who suffers what appears to be minor head trauma develops cerebral edema that is not resolved at the time of a second head injury. Rapid swelling and subsequent death may occur. The recognition of this condition has led to recommendations that are far more conservative than in the past. Close observation of the athlete following head trauma and restriction from participation when there is LOC or persistent amnesia are common guideline recommendations.

Other Headaches

Patients with coexisting metabolic disease may experience headaches related to the disorder. See Table 17–1 for a list of these disorders.

Patients may report severe headache related to intercourse. This headache, called orgasmic or coital, is uncommon; however, when it occurs it is described as similar to migraine and can occur with sexual arousal or orgasm. Although almost always benign, given the exertional aspect of the occurrence, investigation for intracranial pathology, including neoplasm and aneurysm, should be pursued.

Paroxysmal headache refers to sudden jolts of head pain that occur for no apparent reason. These typically last for a few minutes to as much as an hour. Mostly benign, there is a possibility of involvement of the intracranial ventricular system, especially when associated with "drop attacks," vomiting, or loss of consciousness. Specifically, cystic masses of the third ventricle are possible and warrant special imaging investigation.

The insidious onset of short, stabbing headache pain has been divided into a group of disorders that includes cluster headache and a benign form that has no associated structural lesion. Chronic paroxysmal hemicrania (formerly called Sjaastad syndrome) is similar to cluster headache but the attacks are less severe. This type of headache is found primarily in women and seems responsive to indomethacin but not other NSAIDs. (Cluster headaches are not responsive to indomethacin and are found primarily in males.)

The New Headache

Most primary headaches have their initial onset at an early age and are recurrent. Therefore, a middle-aged or older individual complaining of a headache that feels "different" should warrant concern. A common scenario would be an older patient complaining of a temporal headache. If there are associated complaints of either an aching upper trunk area or vision difficulties, consider temporal arteritis. This systemic process becomes evident as a pulsating, hard, nodular temporal area associated with headache. Unfortunately, this process occludes other arteries and often leads to blindness. Biopsy and medical treatment (corticosteroids) are necessary to identify temporal arteritis and prevent blindness, respectively.

Headaches that are constant and/or severe without reprieve are likely to indicate an intracranial process and should necessitate a referral for further evaluation prior to an attempt at chiropractic treatment. Approximately 9% of cerebrovascular events are missed on the patient's first visit to the emergency department, with patients with a subarachnoid hemorrhage (SAH) missed about 20% of the time.[69] SAH is due to a ruptured berry-aneurysm 75% of the time, and 10% of the time is due to an arteriovenous malformation (AVM). The standard with unexplained severe headache in the emergency department is the "CT-LP" rule, which begins with a cranial CT and with negative findings moves to a lumbar puncture. Researchers were interested in seeing if there was a historical cluster that might identify the patient who is likely to have an SAH so that CT could be bypassed and move to the lumbar puncture, saving time, expense, and perhaps the patient's life. In a 2013 publication,[70] researchers presented a study that defined the Ottawa SAH Rule. In this cross-sectional study any one of six findings led to a sensitivity of 100% for SAH in patients with acute-onset headache (i.e., peaking within an hour). These include age ≥ 40 years, neck pain or stiffness, witnessed loss of consciousness, onset during exertion, thunder-clap headache (instantly peaking pain), and limited neck flexion on examination. The specificity, though, is quite low, at only around 15%. So although able to effectively rule out SAH, it may not be of much value in differentially diagnosing other causes of similar presentations.

Primary Headaches

Question the patient regarding the three primary headaches: migraine (with and without aura), tension-like, and cluster. There are often key clues to one of these differentials.

Using IHS criteria:[71]

Migraine with Aura

Patient must have at least two attacks with three of the following characteristics:

1. There are one or more resolved aura symptoms.
2. At least one aura symptom that develops gradually over 5 to 20 minutes and lasts for less than 60 minutes, or two or more aura symptoms occur in sequence.

3. Aura does not last more than one hour (if more than one aura symptom, proportionally rated).
4. The headache follows the aura (headache-free interval less than one hour) or headache begins before or simultaneously with aura.

Also, history, including both a physical and neurological examination, does not suggest another cause. The aura includes reversible disturbances, usually either visual (e.g., zig-zag lines, flickering lights, or vision loss), sensory (e.g., pins-and-needles sensation or numbness), or dysphasic speech disturbances.

Migraine without Aura

Patient must have had at least five attacks lasting 4 to 72 hours (untreated or unsuccessfully treated) (in children, 2 to 48 hours) with at least two of the following:

1. Unilateral location (59% of patients)
2. Pulsating quality (85% of patients)
3. Moderate to severe intensity that inhibits or prohibits daily activities
4. Aggravated by or causing avoidance of routine physical activities such as climbing stairs or comparable activity

Patient must also have with at least one of the following:

1. Associated nausea (73% of patients) and vomiting
2. Photophobia (80% of patients) and phonophobia (76% of patients)

Also, history—physical and neurological examination—does not suggest another cause. Premonitory symptoms for both types of migraine headaches occur hours to a day or two prior to the headache and include symptoms such as fatigue, neck stiffness, difficulty concentrating, sensitivity to light or sound, nausea, blurred vision, yawning, and pallor. These are not to be confused with the aura, which has a distinct preheadache occurrence.

It is important to note the following history findings from the research literature for migraineurs:

- 70% of migraine sufferers have a family history (1.9-fold increased risk of migraine without aura if found in first-degree relatives)[72]
- 75% report associated neck pain[73]
- 46% report tearing or nasal congestion[74]
- 50% report the following triggers:[75,76]
  o change of weather
  o stress
  o lack of sleep or fatigue
  o alcohol
  o food triggers (including but not limited to chocolate, fried foods, dairy products, and nitrates including those in cured meats and fish)
- Comorbid conditions include[77–79] psychiatric disorders (including major depression and bipolar disease),[80] generalized anxiety disorders and associated panic and phobia disorders, vestibular disorders such as Ménière's,[81] Raynaud's syndrome, multiple sclerosis, mitral valve prolapse syndrome, patent foramen ovale,[74] and malignant hypertension.

Women with migraine are at higher risk for ischemic stroke especially if they:

- use combined oral contraceptives (COCs) and hormone replacement therapy
- smoke

This risk is significant only for women who suffer from migraine with aura. Female patients having migraine with aura headaches who do take COCs or hormonal replacement therapy should be referred back to the prescribing doctor. Female patients with migraine who smoke should be counseled to the increased risk for stroke and placed in a smoking cessation program. Chronic migraine is a category reserved for those suffering 15 or more headaches per month for at least three months in the absence of medication overuse.

Cervicogenic

Cervicogenic headache is distinct in that it is caused by an abnormality of structures in the neck. The older HIS criteria were relatively specific and included the following. Headache is usually on one side of the head only. It tends to last between three hours to a week, recurring at intervals varying between as little as two days to as long as three months. Patients may have migraine-like associated symptoms of nausea, vomiting, and sensitivity to light.

- Pain is localized to the neck or suboccipital region and may project to other areas around the head, including the orbital area.
- Pain is provoked or aggravated by specific neck movements (such as flexing the neck or bending forward) or maintained neck positions.
- At least one of the following is found:
  1. restricted neck movements
  2. change in neck muscle contour, texture, tone, or response to active or passive stretching or contraction

3. abnormal tenderness of neck muscles
- Radiological evaluation reveals at least one of the following:
  1. movement abnormalities in flexion/extension
  2. abnormal posture
  3. fracture, congenital abnormalities, bone tumors, rheumatoid arthritis, or other pathology (not to include spondylosis or osteochondrosis)

The most recent classification by the HIS has eliminated the specificity of duration and of location. There is a criterion stating that headache resolves within three months due to successful treatment of the underlying cause. The newer classification also lists cervicogenic as either a primary or secondary headache diagnosis, primarily based on which headache appears first. A separate classification is given for headaches secondary to neck or head trauma (e.g., headache associated with whiplash).

Cluster

Cluster headaches are part of a large group of disorders now referred to as trigeminal autonomic cephalalgias (TAC) based on new understanding regarding their cause. They share the clinical features of headache with associated cranial parasympathetic autonomic features. This is believed to be due to activation of a trigeminal parasympathetic reflex with secondary clinical features that are sympathetic. For cluster headaches, patients must have experienced at least five episodes of headaches to qualify. There is severe unilateral, orbital, supraorbital, or temporal pain that peaks in 10 to 15 minutes, lasting 15 to 180 minutes with pain resolving rapidly. In addition, cluster headaches exhibit the following features:

- Cluster headaches tend to occur at night more than other headaches. Cycles are over a few weeks or months, with some lasting years, and the frequency of attacks is from one to eight per day. Headache macro cycles are usually months or years apart.
- Headaches are associated with at least one of the following: conjunctival injection, rhinorrhea, lacrimation, miosis, nasal congestion, ptosis, forehead and facial sweating, or eyelid edema.

A chronic version lasts for more than a year, and remission lasts less than one month. Also, 5% of patients have a partial Horner's syndrome. It is important to note that a similar, less severe presentation is called chronic paroxysmal hemicrania. This type of headache is more common in females and seems to be responsive to indomethacin but not other NSAIDs. Another TAC disorder is short-lasting, unilateral, neuralgiform headache attacks with conjunctival injection (SUNCT). These are distinct attacks that last for brief periods and are clinically dominated primarily with lacrimation and unilateral redness of the ipsilateral eye.

Episodic Tension-Type

Patient must have at least 10 previous headaches with a total of less than 180 days of headache in a given year, with each headache lasting 30 minutes to 7 days. There will be at least two of the following:

1. Pressing or tightening description (nonpulsatile)
2. Mild to moderate in intensity
3. Bilateral
4. Not aggravated by climbing stairs or similar activity

Also, there is no nausea or vomiting, and photophobia and phonophobia are absent (may have one or the other alone). Episodic, tension-type headaches are further classified as infrequent, frequent, and chronic.

It is important to determine past therapies and their effects on the patient's headaches. Most important is the determination of medication. When a patient with migraine takes either ergotamine or nonsteroid anti-inflammatory drugs (NSAIDs) continuously for more than three days or stops taking the drug suddenly, a rebound effect occurs in many patients, creating a headache often worse than the original—a common cause of emergency department visits. Ibuprofen and naproxen do not appear to be common culprits. The most commonly used medications that appear associated with rebound include but are not limited to:

- Ergotamines including Migranal
- The triptans including sumatriptan (Imitrex; others include Zomig and Amerge)
- Caffeine-containing OTC analgesics such as Excedrin
- Decongestants
- Butalbital medications including Fiorinal and phrenilin
- General vasoconstrictors such as Midrin
- Narcotics including Percocet or Tylenol #3

Examination

- Rule out secondary causes of headaches, searching for signs indicating tumor, infection, intracranial hemorrhage, glaucoma, etc.

- Determine whether any musculoskeletal abnormalities appear to be contributing or causing (cervicogenic) a patient's headaches.
- Determine the need for radiography or special imaging.

The primary role of the standard physical examination is to rule out secondary causes of headache such as tumor, infection, intracranial hemorrhage, and glaucoma. In patients with either a history of head trauma or associated neurologic signs or symptoms, a thorough neurologic examination must be performed. Emphasis on cranial nerve, vestibular, and pathologic reflex testing is necessary to rule out referable disorders. If the neurologic symptoms are transient, and therefore objective evidence on neurologic examination is lacking, refer for further evaluation (unless classic for the prodrome of migraine with aura). Although rarely confused with a "headache," glaucoma should be considered in patients complaining primarily of an orbital location to their pain. A quick evaluation is performed by shining a light tangentially across the eye, looking for a crescent-shaped shadow covering more than half the nasal side of the iris. This indicates a closed angle. In screening for intracranial pressure, ophthalmoscopic examination of the fundus for papilledema is necessary.

The examination process specific to those using manual therapy may provide the only clues to primary headache. The literature to date suggests that several musculoskeletal abnormalities are more prevalent in primary headache sufferers, including the following:

- Intersegmental hypomobility (primarily in the upper cervical area)[82–86]
- Specific tender points[87,88]
- Dysfunctional motion of the cervical spine[89–91]
- Postural imbalance (forward head position and round-shoulder appearance)[92,93]

Radiologic and Special Imaging for Headaches

Radiologic or advanced imaging for headaches is still controversial. Although research indicates possible radiographic findings such as hypomobility or a lordotic/hypolordotic cervical curve, the addition of this information clinically may be irrelevant to the diagnosis. For patient management, it may be arguable that this information allows one to pursue correction of these apparent biomechanical associations.

The literature suggests that the use of special imaging is rarely justified with headache sufferers. This is based on the following:

- Of all the patients with tumor or other conditions requiring cranial surgery only 5% had headache as a primary complaint (other neurologic findings were suggestive).[94]
- The yield for a positive scan was as low as 1/11,200 patients with headaches.

Similar findings have been demonstrated in the pediatric population.[95] However, common sense dictates that if the headache is severe, especially in a child, or unrelenting and not responsive to medication, imaging is an important tool for ruling out serious disorders.

Management

- Modify lifestyle factors that may be contributors.
- Treat with chiropractic manipulative therapy and adjunctive therapies.
- Refer for other nonpharmacologic treatment if chiropractic manipulative therapy (CMT) is ineffective.
- Refer for medical management if other nonpharmacologic treatment is ineffective.

Although it is important to narrow down the diagnostic impression for purposes of referral or correction of minor triggers, it must be remembered that many primary sufferers—in particular, patients with migraine and tension-like headache—may have other secondary contributing factors. In addition, the chiropractic manipulative treatment of these patients has not been demonstrated to be specific to headache type. It is therefore important to tailor the treatment to the patient with a focused approach to the primary headache and a holistic approach to contributing factors, including musculoskeletal, environmental, and psychologic. Management decisions and interpretations must also take into account the fact that the placebo effect in most studies of headache suggests an average positive response in the 30% range.[96]

General Approach

The literature for primary headache treatment is, like many conditions, muddled by lack of definition. There are also problems with well-controlled trials. However, taken as a whole, the literature reveals a relationship between cervical dysfunction and headaches.[97–105] More specifically, and most recently, randomized studies indicate improvement with manipulation and possibly advantages with the use of manipulation over the use of antidepressant medication in the treatment of chronic tension-like and migraine headaches.[106–108] Two recent reviews of the literature tend to support the role of manipulation in the management of tension-like and cervicogenic headache.[109,110] One is a Duke University study that completed a process begun by the Agency for Healthcare Research and Quality entitled *Evidence Report: Behavioral and Physical Treatments for Tension-type and Cervicogenic Headache.* Although the analysis of the literature supports chiropractic manipulation in the management of cervicogenic headaches, there was no evidence to support manipulation over various soft tissue procedures for episodic tension-type headache.

Consideration for other adjunctive or alternative therapies is based on suggestions listed below:

- Biofeedback. Biofeedback is a form of operant conditioning in which the patient uses electromyographic (EMG) or thermal cues to attempt control of either skeletal muscle (with EMG cues) or smooth/vascular muscle (with thermal cues). EMG uses surface electrodes with a video display for patient monitoring. Thermal biofeedback records peripheral temperature through the use of an index finger sensor with measurements displayed on a screen. Although the mechanism is not clear, it appears that biofeedback can be a useful tool in the treatment of headaches. One study[111] indicated good long-term success. Specifically, one study[112] indicated a better result with trapezius biofeedback than with frontal biofeedback or relaxation therapy. Biofeedback may also be helpful in decreasing chronic headache sufferers' dependency on medication.[113]
- Exercise. Although not used specifically for headache, it is anecdotally reported and supported in one study[114] that aerobic exercise may be of some benefit to patients with headache. Perhaps the mechanism is due more to psychologic well-being aspects than to direct measurable factors.
- Physiotherapy. When spinal pain or muscle tenderness is associated with a headache, physical therapy may be added to augment the effect of manipulation.
- Acupuncture. Although many anecdotal reports claim success with acupuncture, when compared

with physiotherapy, acupuncture consistently is less effective, although it does appear to help.[115–118] One small controlled study[119] indicated no significant difference over time between acupuncture and a placebo treatment.

Specific Recommendations for Specific Headaches

Some specific recommendations are made for specific headache types with the caution that there is often overlap among these headaches, and therapy that works for one may be beneficial with another.

Migraine

Patients with an aura to their headache can and should be managed with a treatment trial of manipulation (provided that high-risk indicators are absent). Specific recommendations would include the following:

- Keep sleep schedule as regular as possible, avoiding under- or oversleeping.
- Avoid skipping meals.
- Avoid food triggers.
- Manage stress through training and time-management techniques.

Nutritional support may be helpful (see **Table 17–4**).

Women suffering from migraine with aura who are taking contraceptives or hormonal replacement therapy (HRT) should be referred to the prescribing medical doctor due to a small increase in risk for stroke. Those on contraceptives or HRT who smoke should be counseled on the need to stop smoking due to a significant increased risk of stroke when combined with having migraine headaches.

Tension-type and Cervicogenic

Management is often more difficult given that some of the factors may be external and more under patient control and choice. Following are some recommendations:

- Correct any postural imbalances, in particular in the cervicothoracic regions.
- Pay particular attention to instruction of proper ergonomics in workstation environments.
- Consider the addition of myofascial and trigger point therapy.

Table 17–4 Nutritional Support for Migraine Headaches

Substance	How Might It Work?	Dosage	Special Instructions	Contraindications and Possible Side Effects
Feverfew (tanacetum parthenium)	May prevent constriction of blood vessels through inhibition of platelet serotonin release and maintain central levels of serotonin.	100-mg capsule (0.6% parthenolide) one time daily (up to 500 mg of parthenolide in one study).	Take with meals on a consistent basis. May take 4–6 weeks to work.	Contraindicated in pregnancy, when lactating, in children under 2 years of age. Side effects may include gastrointestinal upset or rash. Withdrawal symptoms include nervousness, tension, insomnia, and joint stiffness.
5-HTP (5-Hydroxytryptophan)	Increases serotonin levels, which may decrease symptoms of pain, insomnia, depression, headache, etc.	50–100 mg three times daily.	Best taken with meals. Should be taken with pyridoxal 5 phosphate (included in recommended supplement).	Do not combine with Imitrex or other SSRI or MAOI antidepressants. Taking more than recommended dose may lead to serotonin syndrome. Safety unknown for pregnant or lactating women.
Omega-3 (EPA & DHA)	Source of omega-3 fatty acids increases anti-inflammatory prostaglandins.	1,000 mg of EPA and 700 mg of DHA daily for at least 2 months.	None.	Long-term use of fish oils at more than 3–4 g/day may cause problems due to elevated blood sugar, cholesterol, or glucose levels. Side effects may include nose bleeds or gastrointestinal upset.
Calcium and vitamin D	May have effect on arterial smooth muscle tone.	800 mg of calcium per day and 400 IU of vitamin D per day.	None.	Individuals with chronic kidney disease, sarcoidosis, kidney stones, or hyperparathyroidism should not take extra calcium.
Riboflavin	May correct a mitochondrial energy metabolism dysfunction.	400 mg/day.	None.	May cause mild diarrhea or polyuria. Fluorescent yellow urine.
Multivitamin/mineral (containing magnesium, vitamins B2, B6)	B6 helps break down histamine. Magnesium helps maintain vessel tone and prevents neuronal overexcitability.	Should include 360 mg of magnesium per day.	None.	More than 350–500 mg of magnesium per day may cause diarrhea in some individuals.

Key: SSRI, selective serotonin reuptake inhibitor; MAOI, monoamine oxidase inhibitor; EPA, eicosapentaenoic acid; DHA, docosahexaenoic acid.

Note: The above have not been approved by the Food and Drug Administration for the treatment of this disorder.

- Educate the patient in self-stretching and exercise techniques.

Cluster

- Avoid alcohol and smoking.
- Use 100% oxygen (7–10 L/min for 10–12 minutes).

Sinus

- One chiropractic study[120] suggests a nasal-specific technique that is popular among a small group of chiropractors.
- The application of warm compresses or butterfly diathermy may be helpful.

- OTC decongestants may help temporarily.
- If specific to airplane travel, the use of a decongestant nasal spray may help.

When a conservative approach is taken, it is important to understand the difficulties associated with treatment of asymptomatic patients. In other words, although a patient may have a history of migraines, it is often the case that he or she does not have the headache at the time of the examination and initial care. How does one determine outcome without an outcome measure? Traditionally it has been an acceptable course to attempt reduction of the associated findings of muscle hypertonicity or spinal segmental fixation (which in themselves can be considered outcome measures) and suggest appropriate lifestyle changes. The course of care often extends for two to three weeks. If the patient has infrequent headaches, it is likely that this period will not extend into the next predicted headache occurrence. If the patient has not had a headache, it would seem appropriate to discontinue constant care until the patient is symptomatic, at which time an aggressive, high-frequency approach for two to three weeks followed by a return to more of a maintenance status is appropriate. To be considered effective, treatment should have aborted the attack, decreased the intensity, or reduced the duration of an attack. If not, perhaps one more trial during a symptomatic period is reasonable. If two or three predicted headache occurrences do not occur or are reduced in intensity, treatment may have been effective. It would not seem appropriate to continue this treatment course, however, without these positive indicators. Referral for other conservative approaches or medical treatment seems appropriate when a conservative trial is ineffective.

The medical treatment of migraine headaches is primarily abortive or prophylactic. Abortive medications include mainly ergot derivatives and sumatriptan succinate (serotonin receptor agonist). Prophylactic medications include those used for other conditions such as antihypertensives, antidepressants, and antiseizure drugs. If the patient suddenly withdraws any of these prescribed medications, he or she runs the risk of a rebound effect. This is particularly true with ergotamine and NSAIDs. Also, ergotamine, aspirin, or NSAIDs should not be taken more than a few days consecutively because of the same risk of rebound migraine.

Medical treatment for cluster headaches includes many of the same medications used for abortive treatment of migraine including sumatriptan and ergots. In addition, intranasal lidocaine and prescribed oxygen may be helpful in aborting an attack.

Algorithms

Algorithms for evaluation and management of headache and chiropractic management of primary headaches are presented in **Figures 17–2** and **17–3**.

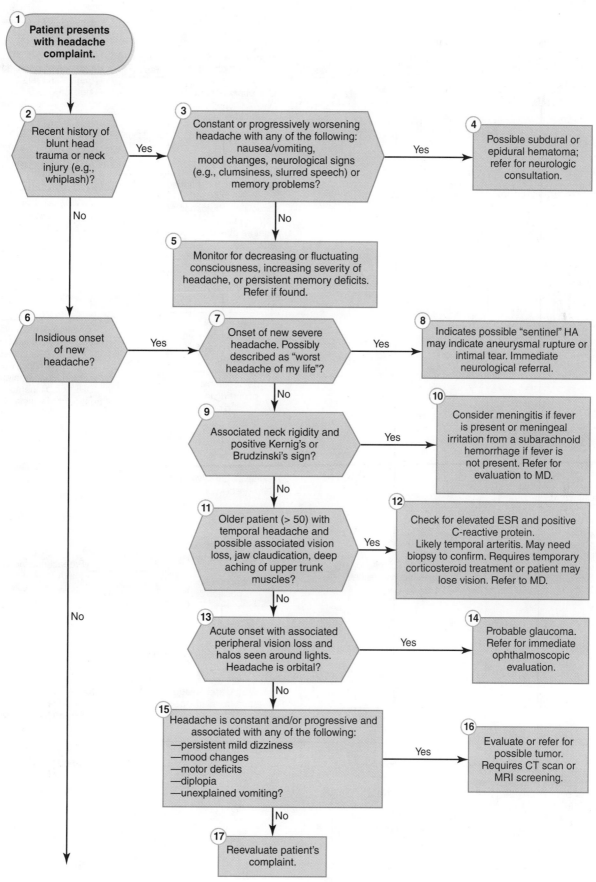

1 Patient presents with headache complaint.

2 Recent history of blunt head trauma or neck injury (e.g., whiplash)? — Yes →

3 Constant or progressively worsening headache with any of the following: nausea/vomiting, mood changes, neurological signs (e.g., clumsiness, slurred speech) or memory problems? — Yes →

4 Possible subdural or epidural hematoma; refer for neurologic consultation.

No ↓ (from 3)

5 Monitor for decreasing or fluctuating consciousness, increasing severity of headache, or persistent memory deficits. Refer if found.

6 Insidious onset of new headache? — Yes →

7 Onset of new severe headache. Possibly described as "worst headache of my life"? — Yes →

8 Indicates possible "sentinel" HA may indicate aneurysmal rupture or intimal tear. Immediate neurological referral.

No ↓ (from 7)

9 Associated neck rigidity and positive Kernig's or Brudzinski's sign? — Yes →

10 Consider meningitis if fever is present or meningeal irritation from a subarachnoid hemorrhage if fever is not present. Refer for evaluation to MD.

No ↓ (from 9)

11 Older patient (> 50) with temporal headache and possible associated vision loss, jaw claudication, deep aching of upper trunk muscles? — Yes →

12 Check for elevated ESR and positive C-reactive protein. Likely temporal arteritis. May need biopsy to confirm. Requires temporary corticosteroid treatment or patient may lose vision. Refer to MD.

No ↓ (from 11)

13 Acute onset with associated peripheral vision loss and halos seen around lights. Headache is orbital? — Yes →

14 Probable glaucoma. Refer for immediate ophthalmoscopic evaluation.

No ↓ (from 13)

15 Headache is constant and/or progressive and associated with any of the following:
—persistent mild dizziness
—mood changes
—motor deficits
—diplopia
—unexplained vomiting? — Yes →

16 Evaluate or refer for possible tumor. Requires CT scan or MRI screening.

No ↓ (from 15)

17 Reevaluate patient's complaint.

Figure 17-2 Headache—Algorithm

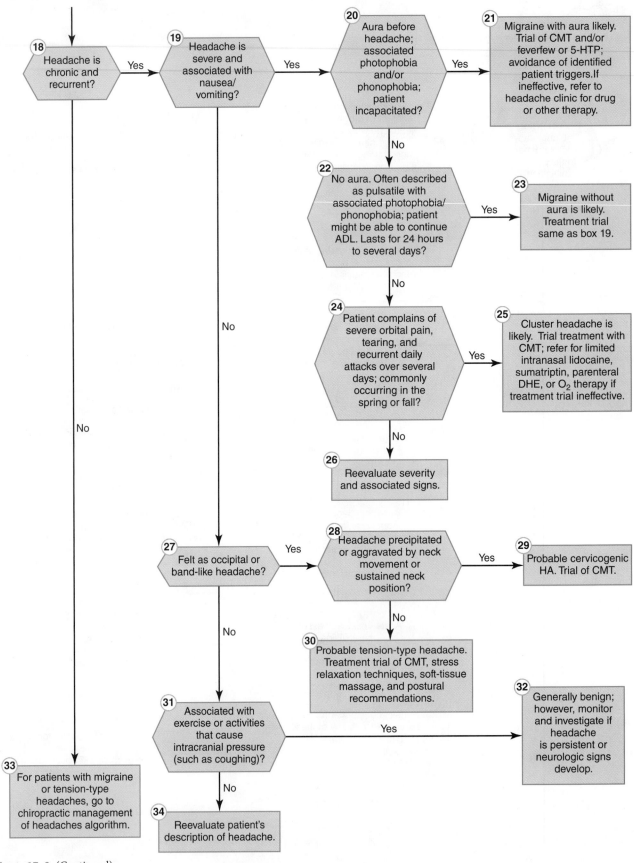

18 Headache is chronic and recurrent? — Yes →

19 Headache is severe and associated with nausea/vomiting? — Yes →

20 Aura before headache; associated photophobia and/or phonophobia; patient incapacitated? — Yes →

21 Migraine with aura likely. Trial of CMT and/or feverfew or 5-HTP; avoidance of identified patient triggers. If ineffective, refer to headache clinic for drug or other therapy.

No ↓

22 No aura. Often described as pulsatile with associated photophobia/phonophobia; patient might be able to continue ADL. Lasts for 24 hours to several days? — Yes →

23 Migraine without aura is likely. Treatment trial same as box 19.

No ↓

24 Patient complains of severe orbital pain, tearing, and recurrent daily attacks over several days; commonly occurring in the spring or fall? — Yes →

25 Cluster headache is likely. Trial treatment with CMT; refer for limited intranasal lidocaine, sumatriptin, parenteral DHE, or O₂ therapy if treatment trial ineffective.

No ↓

26 Reevaluate severity and associated signs.

27 Felt as occipital or band-like headache? — Yes →

28 Headache precipitated or aggravated by neck movement or sustained neck position? — Yes →

29 Probable cervicogenic HA. Trial of CMT.

No ↓

30 Probable tension-type headache. Treatment trial of CMT, stress relaxation techniques, soft-tissue massage, and postural recommendations.

31 Associated with exercise or activities that cause intracranial pressure (such as coughing)? — Yes →

32 Generally benign; however, monitor and investigate if headache is persistent or neurologic signs develop.

No ↓

33 For patients with migraine or tension-type headaches, go to chiropractic management of headaches algorithm.

34 Reevaluate patient's description of headache.

Figure 17–2 (Continued)

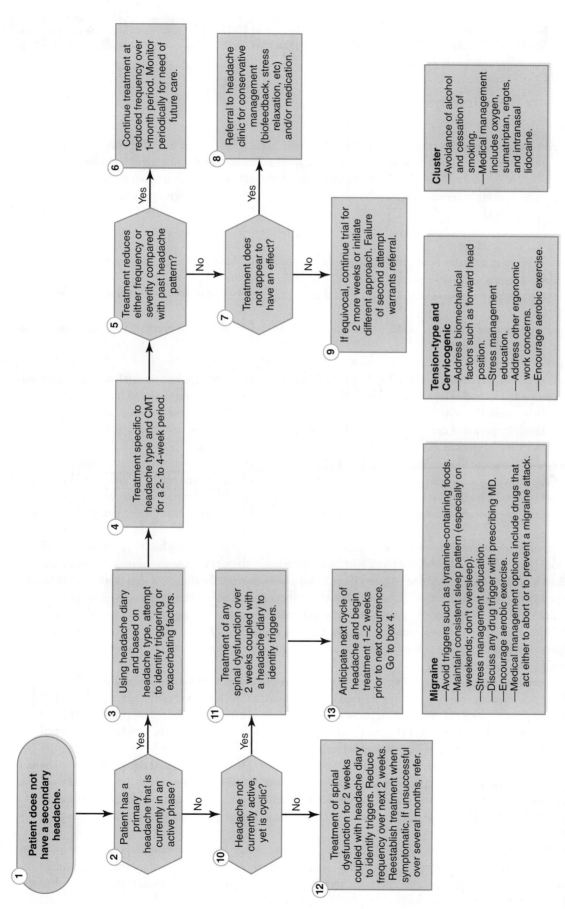

1 Patient does not have a secondary headache.

2 Patient has a primary headache that is currently in an active phase?

3 Using headache diary and based on headache type, attempt to identify triggering or exacerbating factors.

4 Treatment specific to headache type and CMT for a 2- to 4-week period.

5 Treatment reduces either frequency or severity compared with past headache pattern?

6 Continue treatment at reduced frequency over 1-month period. Monitor periodically for need of future care.

7 Treatment does not appear to have an effect?

8 Referral to headache clinic for conservative management (biofeedback, stress relaxation, etc) and/or medication.

9 If equivocal, continue trial for 2 more weeks or initiate different approach. Failure of second attempt warrants referral.

10 Headache not currently active, yet is cyclic?

11 Treatment of any spinal dysfunction over 2 weeks coupled with a headache diary to identify triggers.

12 Treatment of spinal dysfunction for 2 weeks coupled with headache diary to identify triggers. Reduce frequency over next 2 weeks. Reestablish treatment when symptomatic. If unsuccessful over several months, refer.

13 Anticipate next cycle of headache and begin treatment 1–2 weeks prior to next occurrence. Go to box 4.

Migraine
—Avoid triggers such as tyramine-containing foods.
—Maintain consistent sleep pattern (especially on weekends; don't oversleep).
—Stress management education.
—Discuss any drug trigger with prescribing MD.
—Encourage aerobic exercise.
—Medical management options include drugs that act either to abort or to prevent a migraine attack.

Tension-type and Cervicogenic
—Address biomechanical factors such as forward head position.
—Stress management education.
—Address other ergonomic work concerns.
—Encourage aerobic exercise.

Cluster
—Avoidance of alcohol and cessation of smoking.
—Medical management includes oxygen, sumatriptan, ergots, and intranasal lidocaine.

Figure 17–3 Chiropractic Management of Primary Headaches—Algorithm

Selected Headache Disorders

Migraine with Aura (Classic Migraine)

Classic Presentation

The patient is often female and presents with a complaint of unilateral throbbing headaches that are preceded by an aura. The prodrome consists of a progressively increasing (fortification) scotoma (blind spot) surrounded by flashing lights (scintillation). This lasts for about 30 minutes and is replaced by a disabling headache that lasts for several hours to as long as one to three days, causing the patient to seek a dark, quiet environment. There is often associated nausea and vomiting. There is a family history of similar headaches.

Cause

Once believed to be purely vascular, migraine headaches are believed to be neurogenic. Migraine with aura accounts for only 10% to 15% of all migraines. Current research findings[121] suggest one or a combination of the following:

- Trigeminal axons are prompted to release vasoactive peptides that cause vascular inflammation; this inflammation irritates meningeal nerve fibers.
- There is a dysfunction of the serotoninergic-based, central inhibitory pain system allowing a lowering of the pain threshold so that even normal stimuli may cause pain.
- There is an inherited problem with dopamine metabolism.
- A spreading wave of cortical depression occurs (changes proceeding from a wave of hyperpolarization followed by depolarization). This correlates with a spreading wave of decreased cerebral blood flow that lasts for one to several hours and then transitions into a phase of hyperemia. This reactive hyperemia does not necessarily correlate with the headache. Many times the headache occurs during the period of decreased cerebral blood flow. The aura is due to hyperexcitability of the occipital cortex in many patients with visual symptoms.[122]
- The trigeminal afferent input and the upper spinal nerve (C1-C3) input converge in the trigeminocervical nucleus in the spinal cord; because of this convergence, misinterpretation of the pain origin may lead to a referred headache phenomenon.
- Based on recent observations, it appears that branches of the trigeminal nerve may be entrapped in craniocervical musculature triggering chronic migraine attacks. Botox injection or cosmetic surgical release has resulted in migraine relief in some patients.

There appear to be a wide variety of triggers for migraine, including variation in sleeping or eating habits, environmental pollutants, certain medications (including vasodilators), and food. With food, the primary triggers include chocolate, caffeine, nitrates, cheese, nuts, wine, and a host of other individualized triggers. There is also a hormonal relationship, as is seen in women. Although in adults there is a clear female predominance, there is some evidence that under the age of 12 years, migraine is more common in boys.[123] There is a gradual shift to female predominance such that at age 20 years the female-to-male ratio is 2:1 and between 42 and 44 years it is about 3:1. The one-year prevalence for migraine was 11.7%: 5.6% in men and 17.1% in women.[124] Thirty-one percent of migraneurs have a headache attack occurrence of three or more times per month with 3.7% reporting severe impairment. At least 25.7% meet the criteria for preventive treatment.

When the aura is the prominent feature or if it outlasts the headache, it is referred to as a complicated migraine.[125] When the prodromal signs or symptoms predominate they are often referred to as migraine equivalents. There are three types of complicated migraines: ophthalmoplegic, where the third, fourth, and sixth cranial nerves are involved, often causing diplopia and eye pain; hemiplegic, where there is paresis on one half of the body, often lasting days; and basilar, where the vertebrobasilar system is involved, leading to accompanying vertigo, diplopia, tinnitus, and ataxia.

There are many subtypes of migraine. A particular concern is a basilar migraine where symptoms and signs of brainstem dysfunction predominate. In such cases, vertigo, dysarthria, tinnitus, hypoacusia, diplopia, visual symptoms in both temporal and nasal fields in both eyes, ataxia, decreased level of consciousness, and bilateral paresthesias may occur. It appears that in addition to the pons, the cerebellum may be involved due to dysfunctional calcium channels. These patients may respond better to the antiepileptic preventive medications available.[126]

The risk of stroke is higher in all patients with migraine, although the higher risk associated with contraceptives places more danger on women taking combined oral contraceptives (COCs).[127] Two studies by Kurth et al.[128,129] examined the cardiovascular risk for individuals with migraine. One study focused on men and found that they had a higher risk for myocardial infarction. The distinction between migraine with or without aura was not available. For females, there was no increased risk for migraine without aura.

However, for migraine with aura, cardiovascular disease, myocardial infarction, ischemic stroke, coronary revascularization, and angina were found to be higher in active migraine sufferers. This was supported by another study by Diener et al.[130]

Evaluation

The physical examination is rarely revealing and is usually used to rule out secondary causes that may resemble migraine with aura, such as a TIA or glaucoma. The aura is generally visual, with the most common descriptions as blind spots, flashing lights, and zig-zag lines. Occasionally it is described as having a "bubbling" appearance, movement like "an old-time movie" (strobe-like), and "morphing" of images (often circular into angular), among others. Aura may also be as simple as blurriness of vision. Any neurological manifestation is possible, including olfactory, paresthesias (common is digitolingual [tongue and down the arm to fingers]), temporary weakness of facial muscles or limbs, and other neurological manifestations. The combination of an aura that is often visual that occurs prior to a severe headache and an early age onset—often in early adulthood—is highly suggestive. Migraine with aura occurs less frequently than other headaches, often only once or twice a month or less. In making clinical decisions regarding imaging, a 2006 review by Detsky et al.[131] revealed that the best predictors of migraine could be applied using a mnemonic: POUNDing (Pulsating, duration of 4–72 hOurs, Unilateral, Nausea, Disabling). If four of the criteria are met, the accuracy for diagnosing migraine is high, and it decreases with fewer criteria being met. Additionally, they found that on pooled analysis the prediction for serious intracranial problems was increased for cluster headache, abnormal findings on neurologic exam, undefined headache (i.e., unable to categorize into one of the primary types), aggravated by exertion or a Valsalva-type maneuver, and headache with vomiting. When these features are present, patients should be referred for neuroimaging.

Migraine headache in children may be dissimilar to that seen in adults. For example, migraine with or without aura has its peak at an earlier age in males. For migraine with aura, it is age 5 years; migraine without aura, ages 10–11 years.[132] Another distinction is that headaches are more often bilateral in children, often frontotemporal. Occipital headache in children, whether unilateral or bilateral, should be further investigated due to the possibility of a structural lesion. Family history is important. If both parents have migraines, the risk is about 70% for the children, whereas if one parent has migraine, the risk is about 45%. About 20% of children with migraines report visual aura. The distinction may be that spots, colors, dots, or lights are often reported. The aura is generally short-lived, being 30 minutes or less. The description of pounding or pulsating is less common, as are reports of phonophobia and photophobia. Finally, headaches are generally shorter, lasting on average less than two hours. They may be more frequent in children.

Management

Migraine may respond to chiropractic manipulation.[107,108,133] A treatment trial is worth pursuing. Other conservative options include biofeedback and acupuncture. Linde et al.[134] evaluated, in a randomized controlled trial, the effects of acupuncture on migraine. Interestingly, the results indicated that 51% randomized to an acupuncture group and 53% randomized to a sham acupuncture group improved (i.e., reduction in headache days by at least 50%). Recommendations for nutritional and herbal support include the use of feverfew, 5-HTP (5-hydroxtryptophan), omega-3 fatty acids, magnesium, calcium and vitamin D, and riboflavin.[135–147] (See **Table 17–5**.) Supplementation with magnesium before menses may prevent some women's menstrual migraines.[148]

Medication options are primarily abortive and prophylactic.[149] The primary abortive drugs are ergotamine derivatives and sumatriptan, a serotonin receptor agonist (avoid both during pregnancy). Patients taking ergots, aspirin, or NSAIDs for longer than three days should be warned of a rebound migraine that can occur. This may also occur with sudden withdrawal from other medication. From a medical approach, first-line therapy is over-the-counter medications. One study showed that two tablets of a combination of acetaminophen, aspirin, and caffeine (Excedrin Extra-Strength) was effective for most cases of migraine.[150] This approach is recommended prior to the administration of prescription drugs. A 2013 Cochrane review supports the use of 1,000 mg of aspirin for abortive management of migraine.[151] The concern, of course, is that this level of medication carries with it gastrointestinal risk; primarily gastric ulcers and bleeding. Newer drugs include angiotensin II receptor blockers and topiramate for prophylaxis. Evidence-based guidelines for the protocol of prescription drug management have been published by the U.S. Headache Consortium (a collaborative of seven professional organizations).[152] Also, a review of effectiveness for the various triptans is available in a study by Goadsby et al.[153] With triptans there are concerns related to cardiovascular conditions and pregnancy. The effectiveness of triptans is approximately only 60%.

A series of Cochrane reviews[154–156] in 2012 evaluated the effectiveness of triptans based on the route of delivery. All three routes of intranasal, oral, or rectal demonstrated effectiveness but with a concern of increased adverse events compared with placebo.

Prophylactic treatments include antidepressants and antihypertensives. Additional therapies that have some literature support include subcutaneous histamine (prophylactic),[157] intranasal lidocaine (abortive),[158] and pulsed electromagnetic field therapy.[159,160]

For those patients refractory to conservative management, a medical alternative uses a sequenced approach. This begins with injection of either Botox or anesthetic such as lidocaine.[161] If this relief is sustained, than repeated injection may be necessary. If initially effective in the short term but not the long term, cosmetic surgery to decompress a branch of the trigeminal nerves in entrapped fascial or occipital musculature is now being performed. Long-term studies are still needed.

Migraine without Aura (Common Migraine)

Classic Presentation

The patient is often female complaining of a unilateral, pulsatile headache that is recurrent, which began to occur when she was a young adult. There are no associated visual or other neurologic signs or symptoms. The headache is severe; however, the patient is usually able to continue daily activities. Associated nausea and vomiting occur, with vomiting sometimes providing relief of the headache.

Cause

See migraine with aura above. Migraine without aura accounts for the vast majority of migraine headaches (80% to 85%). It appears that cerebral blood flow and cerebral blood volume may be reduced during the headache phase in patients with migraine without aura.[162] Interestingly, oxygen metabolism and extraction seem unaffected.

Evaluation

The physical examination is used primarily to screen for other secondary causes. The presentation is the primary diagnostic indicator. The main difference between migraine with aura and migraine without aura is the aura. Migraine without aura is usually somewhat less severe; however, it may last longer.

Management

The same principles are applied as outlined above for migraine with aura.

Tension-Type

Classic Presentation

The patient describes a headache with frequent occurrence that is often worse in the afternoon or early evening. The pain is usually bilateral, often suboccipital or supraorbital. The headaches last for days or weeks. Aspirin or over-the-counter NSAIDs seem to provide relief.

Cause

Although it was once believed that tension-type headaches were due to muscle tension, it is now recognized that although there are often tender trigger points in the neck and suboccipital area, there is no higher incidence of muscle hypertonicity when compared with other headache types. There is a growing group of researchers who believe that chronic tension-like headaches may represent part of a headache continuum.[163] These patients often begin with migraine attacks that gradually transform (transformed migraine) into more frequent, less severe, tension-type headaches. This may be related to chronic abuse of medication.

Evaluation

There are no diagnostic findings specific to tension-type headaches. It is not unusual to find tender trigger points and tight muscles in the neck, although these are not exclusive to tension-type headache sufferers. A history of frequent, often bilateral, attacks that are relieved by pain medication is a strong basis for a tension-type headache diagnosis.

Management

Studies are mixed regarding whether chiropractic manipulation is beneficial for tension-type headache sufferers.[106,164] A recent study that indicated no advantage with chiropractic manipulation utilized a small group of patients, which may reduce the strength of the findings. It is important for patients to avoid continual use of pain medications because of the gastrointestinal consequences.

Cervicogenic

Classic Presentation

The presentation is dependent on the criteria and definition of the term *cervicogenic*. The belief that other headaches have a cervicogenic component causes some overlap. Those with a pure cervicogenic headache without overlap may present with a complaint of daily headaches with no associated neurologic signs. There is often reduced movement in neck motion associated with neck pain.

Cause

Cervicogenic headache is due to referral from soft tissue and articular structures in the neck. Similar to the concept introduced above with migraine headaches, convergence in the trigeminocervical nucleus allows referral of pain from neck origins to the head.

Vernon[165] refers to several causes, including extrasegmental (myofascial structures), intersegmental (deep muscles and ligaments), infrasegmental (nerve roots and dorsal ganglions), and intrasegmental (referral via trigeminocervical nucleus).

Evaluation

It appears that patients with cervicogenic headache may have indications of restricted movement, in particular at the upper cervical/occiput region.[133] The headache may be made worse in some patients with head movement. Radiographically, there may be indications of arthrosis, but this is not specific for cervicogenic headaches.

Management

Manipulation is recommended as the primary treatment approach. One study[166] specifically focused on the outcome of patients who met the IHS criteria for cervicogenic headache and found a possible positive effect.

Cluster

Classic Presentation

The patient is often a middle-aged male complaining of incredibly painful headaches that are orbital in location. The headaches cluster over days or weeks and then end, to appear again several weeks or months later. The headaches last an average of 30 minutes and are the most painful feeling the patient has felt. The patient has a history of smoking and possibly alcohol abuse.[167]

Cause/Occurrence

Cluster headaches are believed to be primarily neurovascular and part of a group of trigeminal-autonomic cephalalgias that includes paroxysmal hemicrania and syndrome of short-lasting unilateral neuralgiform headaches with conjunctival (SUNCT syndrome).[168] Specifically, cluster headaches are characterized by cranial parasympathetic activation and sympathetic impairment.[169] Researchers now believe that cluster headache is due to activation of the ipsilateral inferior hypothalamic gray matter, the ventroposterior thalamus, the anterior cingulate cortex, and bilaterally in the insular based on position emission tomography (PET).[170,171] Triggers during the cluster period include alcohol and some foods.

The frequency of attacks is on average several times per day, often at night, lasting for one to several weeks. Recurrence may not occur for months or even years later. The natural history is for headaches to decrease in frequency and intensity as the patient ages. There are always exceptions to this statistical average.

Evaluation

The physical examination is unrevealing unless the patient is seen during an attack. During an attack there is often lacrimation associated with a runny nose on the same side as the headache. In a minority of cluster patients, there may be a Horner's syndrome (ptosis, miosis, anhidrosis). Unlike the patient with migraine, the patient with cluster headaches is often agitated and animated during attacks, sometimes beating the head against a wall in an attempt for relief. Some patients commit or attempt suicide because of the severity and recurrence of the headaches.

Management

The average clinic course is that headaches will gradually diminish over years. It is important to understand the natural history and convey this to the patient given that there is a high suicide rate among patients with cluster headache due to the psychological struggle of believing this is a lifelong sentence.

A new experimental approach for intractable cluster headaches has been electrical stimulation of the hypothalamus. A recent review suggests cautious optimism with this approach.[172]

Unlike migraine and tension-type headaches, there is no clear literature indication of chiropractic manipulation success with cluster headaches. However, given that it appears there may be a similar underlying mechanism, a trial of treatment during a cluster period seems warranted if the patient is amenable. Medical treatment is quite similar to that for migraine including the triptans. A 2010 Cochrane review[173] concluded that triptans were an effective management approach to cluster headache management. It appears that nonoral administration is likely more effective than oral. Additional treatments include 100% oxygen[174] (7 L/min for 15 minutes) and intranasal (5%–10% solution) lidocaine[175] (4% solution). Oxygen therapy is less effective in older patients and those with chronic cluster attacks. Lidocaine is thought to have an anesthetic effect on the sphenopalatine ganglion. Intravenous magnesium may also be a treatment strategy in some clinics.[176] In a small study[177] patients with medically intractable cluster headache had electrodes implanted in the suboccipital region for the purpose of occipital nerve stimulation. The device seemed to provide relief for the majority of patients.

For refractory cluster headache, gamma knife radiosurgery of the trigeminal nerve root entry zone has been advocated, as have radiofrequency lesions of the sphenopalatine ganglion.[178,179]

Temporal Arteritis

Classic Presentation

The patient is older (> 50 years) complaining of a unilateral headache in the temporal region. The headache is associated with a tender nodule at the superficial temporal artery at the side of the forehead. The patient may also complain of generalized aching and muscular fatigue in the upper trunk area. There may also be complaints of visual dysfunction or blindness of sudden onset.

Cause

Temporal arteritis (giant cell arteritis) is a generalized vasculitis affecting small- and medium-sized arteries. This inflammatory process affects more than just the temporal artery; however, it is largely asymptomatic with other areas of involvement. When the ophthalmic artery is involved, an ischemic optic neuropathy with blindness occurs. One study[180] suggests the possibility of an infectious cause due to cyclic incidence rates over time in a population-based investigation.

Evaluation

The onset of a new headache in an older patient brings temporal arteritis to the list of possibilities. Although it is called "temporal," only about half of patients feel it in the temples. However, 50% to 70% have scalp tenderness near the area of involvement.[181] Other indicators are jaw claudication, C-reactive protein above 2.45 mg/dL, neck pain, and an erythrocyte sedimentation rate (ESR) above 47 mm/hour. C-reactive protein is more sensitive (100%) than ESR (92%).[182] The combination of elevations gives the best specificity (97%). Visual changes may present as sudden loss of vision due to blockage of the retinal artery.[183] Some patients complain of diplopia. Dull, aching pain (polymyalgia rheumatica) in the upper trunk area is reported in about 40% of patients with temporal arteritis. Medical biopsy of the temporal artery will confirm the presence of multinucleated giant cells.

Management

The patient with temporal arteritis must be referred because of the high likelihood of blindness if left untreated. Temporal arteritis is treated with corticosteroids. The length of time varies based on the severity of the disease. Some authors recommend the use of color Doppler sonography to monitor progression.[184]

APPENDIX 17–1

Web Resources

International Headache Society and Links
http://ihs-classification.org/en/
American Headache Society
http://www.ahsnet.org/guidelines.php

APPENDIX 17–2

References

1. Osterhaus JT, Gutterman DL, Plachetka DR. Health care resource and lost labour costs of migraine headache in the United States. *Pharmacoeconomics.* 1992;2:67–76.

2. Hu XH, Markson LE, Lipton RB, et al. Burden of migraine in the United States: disability and economic costs. *Arch Intern Med.* 1999;159:813–818.

3. Eisenberg DM, Kessler RC, Foster C, et al. Unconventional medicine in the United States: prevalence, costs, and patterns of use. *N Engl J Med.* 1993;32:246–252.

4. Powers SW, Patton SR, Hommel KA, Hershey AD. Quality of life in childhood migraine: clinical impact and comparison to other chronic diseases. *Pediatrics.* 2003;112(1):e1–e5.

5. Abu-Arefeh I, Russel G. Prevalence of headache and migraine in school children. *BMJ.* 1994;309:765–769.

6. Split W, Neuman W. Epidemiology of migraine among students from randomly selected secondary schools in Lodz. *Headache.* 1999;39:494–501.

7. CDC. Prevalence of chronic migraine headaches: United States, 1980–1989. *Morbid Mortal Weekly Rep.* 1991;40:331–338.

8. Stewart WF, Lipton RB, Celentano DD, et al. Prevalence of migraine headaches in the United States: relation to age, income, race, and other sociodemographic factors. *JAMA.* 1992;267:64–69.

9. Kaufmann DW, Kelly JP, Rosenberg L, et al. Recent patterns of medication use in the ambulatory adult population of the United States: the Sloan Survey. *JAMA.* 2002;287:337–344.

10. Cypress B. Headache as the reason for the office visit. National Ambulatory Medical Care Society, United States 1977–78. *NCHC Adv Data.* 1981;67:1–6.

11. Balla J, Jansek R. Headaches arising from the cervical spine. In: Hopkins A, ed. *Headache Problems: Diagnosis and Management.* London: WB Saunders; 1988:243–247.

12. Schutt CH, Dohan FC. Neck injury to women in auto accidents. *JAMA.* 1968;206:2689–2692.

13. Norris SH, Watt J. The prognosis of neck injuries resulting from rear-end vehicle collisions. *J Bone Joint Surg Br.* 1983;65:608–611.

14. Hohl M. Soft tissue injuries of the neck in automobile accidents. *J Bone Joint Surg Am.* 1974;56:1665–1672.

15. Braff MM, Rosner S. Symptomatology and treatment of injuries of the neck. *NY State J Med.* 1955;55:237–242.

16. Dies S, Strapp JW. Chiropractic treatment of patients in motor vehicle accidents: a statistical analysis. *J Can Chiro Assoc.* 1992;36:139–142.

17. Graff-Radford SB. Temporomandibular disorders and headache. *Dent Clin North Am.* 2007;51(1):129–144, vi–vii.

18. Svensson P. Muscle pain in the head: overlap between temporomandibular disorders and tension-type headaches. *Curr Opin Neurol.* 2007;20(3):320–325.

19. Lupoli TA, Lockey RF. Temporomandibular dysfunction: an often overlooked cause of chronic headaches. *Ann Allergy Asthma Immunol.* 2007;99(4):314–318.

20. Bernhardt O, Gesch D, Schwahn C, et al. Risk factors for headache, including TMD signs and symptoms, and their impact on quality of life. Results of the Study of Health in Pomerania (SHIP). *Quintessence Int.* 2005;36(1):55–64.

21. Lipton RB, Stewart WF, Diamond S, et al. Prevalence and burden of migraine in the United States: data from the American Migraine Study II. *Headache.* 2001;41(7):646–657.

22. Edmeads J, Mackell JA. The economic impact of migraine: an analysis of direct and indirect costs. *Headache.* 2002;42(6):509–513.

23. Bigal ME, Bordini GA, Specialia JG. Etiology and distribution of headaches in two Brazilian primary care units. *Headache.* 2000;40:241–247.

24. Olesen J, et al. *Classification of Diagnostic Criteria for Headache Disorders, Cranial Neuralgias and Facial Pain.* Copenhagen: The International Headache Society; 1990.

25. Nilsson N. The prevalence of cervicogenic headache in a random population sample of 20–59 year olds. *Spine.* 1995;20:1884–1888.

26. Olesen J, et al. Timing and topography of cerebral blood flow, aura and headache during migraine attack. *Ann Neurol.* 1990;28:791.

27. Anderson A, et al. Delayed hyperemia following hypo-perfusion in classic migraine. *Arch Neurol.* 1988;45:154.

28. Boxtel A, Goudszaard P. Absolute and proportional resting EMG levels in chronic headache patients in relation to the state of headache. *Headache.* 1984;24:259.

29. Goadsby PJ. Recent advances in the diagnosis and management of migraine. *BMJ.* 2006;332(7532):25–29.

30. Afridi SK, Matharu MS, Lee L, et al. A PET study exploring the laterality of brainstem activation in migraine using glyceryl trinitrate. *Brain.* 2005;128 (Pt 4):932–939.

31. Takasha T, Shimomura T, Kazuro T. Platelet activation in muscle contraction headache and migraine. *Cephalalgia.* 1987;7:239.

32. Anthony M, Lance J. Plasma serotonin in patients with chronic tension-like headache. *J Neurol Neurosurg Psychiatry.* 1989;52:182.

33. Rajiv J, Welch K, D'Andrea G. Serotonergic hypofunction in migraine: a synthesis of evidence based on platelet dense body dysfunction. *Cephalalgia.* 1989;9:293.

34. Lance J, et al. 5-Hydroxytryptamine and its putative aetiological involvement in migraine. *Cephalalgia.* 1989;9 (suppl 9):7.

35. Moskowitz MA. Neurogenic inflammation in the pathophysiology and treatment of migraine. *Neurology.* 1993; 43(suppl 3):516–520.

36. Nakano T, Shimomura T, Takahashi K, Ikawa S. Platelet substance P and 5-hydroxytryptamine in migraine and tension-type headache. *Headache.* 1993;33:528–532.

37. Millan Guerrero RO, Isais Cardenas MA, Ocampo AA, Pacheco MF. Histamine as a therapeutic alternative in migraine prophylaxis: a randomized, placebo-controlled, double-blind study. *Headache.* 1999;39:576–580.

38. Peroutka SJ. Dopamine and migraine. *Neurology.* 1997;49:650–656.

39. Bogduk N. A neurological approach to neck pain. In: Glasgow EE, Twomey IV, Seall ER, Klehnhams AM, Edzack D, eds. *Aspects of Manipulative Therapy.* 2nd ed. New York: Churchill Livingstone; 1985:136–146.

40. Kung TA, Guyuron B, Cederna PS. Migraine surgery: a plastic surgery solution for refractory migraine headache. *Plast Reconstr Surg.* 2011;127(1):181–189.

41. Hack GO, Koritzer RT, Robinson WL, Hallgren RC, Greenman PE. Anatomic relation between the rectus capitis posterior minor muscle and the dura mater. *Spine.* 1995;20:2484–2486.

42. Rutten HP, Szpak K, van Mameren H, et al. Anatomic relation between the rectus capitis posterior minor muscle and the dura mater (comment). *Spine.* 1997;22:924–925.

43. Maizels M, Geiger A M. Intranasal lidocaine for migraine: a randomized trial and open-label followup. *Headache.* 1999;39:543–551.

44. D'Andrea G, Hasselmark L, Cananzi AR, et al. Metabolism and menstrual cycle rhythmicity of serotonin in primary headaches. *Headache.* 1995;35:216–221.

45. Silberstein SD, Merriam GR. Estrogens, progestins, and headache. *Neurology.* 1991;41:786–793.

46. Epstein MT, Hockaday JM, Hockaday TD. Migraine and reproductive hormones throughout the menstrual cycle. *Lancet.* 1975;1:543–548.

47. Ulknis A, Silberstein SD. Review article: migraine and pregnancy. *Headache.* 1991;31:372–374.

48. Raskin NH. *Headache.* 2nd ed. New York: Churchill Livingstone; 1988:35–98.

49. Philips BM. Oral contraceptive drugs and migraine. *Br Med J.* 1968;2:99.

50. Goldstein M, Chen TC. The epidemiology of disabling headache. *Adv Neurol.* 1982;33:377–390.

51. Haan J, Terwindt GM, van den Maagdenberg AM, Stam AH, Ferrari MD. A review of the genetic relation between migraine and epilepsy. *Cephalalgia.* 2008;28(2):105–113.

52. Hering-Hanat R, Gardoth N. Caffeine-induced headache in children and adolescents. *Cephalgia.* 2003;23:332–335.

53. Wang SJ, Fuh JL, Lu SR, et al. Migraine prevalence during menopausal transition. *Headache.* 2003;43(5):470–478.

54. Steward WF, Lipton RB, Chee E, et al. Menstrual cycle and headache in a population sample of migraineurs. *Neurology.* 2000;55:1517–1523.

55. Rooke ED. Benign exertional headache. *Med Clin North Am.* 1988;52:801–809.

56. Klara PM, George ED. Warning leaks and sentinel headaches associated with subarachnoid hemorrhage. *Milit Med.* 1982;147:660–662.

57. Paulson GW. Weightlifter's headache. *Headache.* 1983;23:193–194.

58. Kinsella FP. Exercise induced migraine. *Br Med J.* 1990;83:126.

59. Appenzeller O. Altitude headaches. *Headache.* 1972;12:121–129.

60. Diamond S, Solomon GD, Freitag FG. Headache in sports. In: Jordan BC, Tsairis P, Warren RF, eds. *Sports Neurology.* Gaithersburg, MD: Aspen Publishers, Inc; 1989:127–132.

61. Abrahams S, McFie S, Patricios J, Posthumus M, September AV. Risk factors for sports concussion: an evidence-based systematic review. *Br J Sports Med.* 2014;48(2):91–97.

62. West TA, Marion DW. Current recommendations for the diagnosis and treatment of concussion in sport: a comparison of three new guidelines. *J Neurotrauma.* 2013. Oct 16. [Epub ahead of print]

63. Harmon KG, Drezner JA, Gammons M, et al. American Medical Society for Sports Medicine position statement: concussion in sport. *Br J Sports Med.* 2013;47(1):15–26.

64. Guskiewicz KM, Register-Mihalik J, McCrory P, et al. Evidence-based approach to revising the SCAT2: introducing the SCAT3. *Br J Sports Med.* 2013;47(5):289–293.

65. Jinguji TM, Bompadre V, Harmon KG, et al. Sport Concussion Assessment Tool-2: baseline values for high school athletes. *Br J Sports Med.* 2012;46(5):365–370.

66. Simma B, Lutschg J, Callahan JM. Mild head injury in pediatrics: algorithms for management in the ED and in young athletes. *Am J Emerg Med.* 2013;31(7):1133–1138.

67. Mathews WB. Footballer's migraine. *BMJ.* 1972;2:326–327.

68. Saunders RL, Harbaugh RE. The second impact in catastrophic contact sports head trauma. *JAMA.* 1984;525:538–539.

69. Kowalski RG, Claassen J, Kreiter KT, et al. Initial misdiagnosis and outcome after subarachnoid hemorrhage. *JAMA.* 2004;291(7):866–869.

70. Perry JJ, Stiell IG, Sivilotti MLA, et al. Clinical decision rules to rule out subarachnoid hemorrhage for acute headache. *JAMA.* 2013;310(12).doi:10.1001/jama.2013.278018.

71. Headache Classification Subcommittee of the International Headache Society. *The International Classification of Headache Disorders,* 2nd ed. Blackwell Publishing, Oxford, UK. 2004; pages 1–150.

72. Russell MB, Olesen J. Increased familial risk and evidence of genetic factor in migraine. *BMJ.* 1995;311:541–544.

73. Kaniecki RG. Migraine and tension-type headache: an assessment of challenges in diagnosis. *Neurology.* 2002;58(suppl 6):515–520.

74. Bambatti P, Fabbrini G, Pesari M, et al. Unilateral cranial autonomic symptoms in migraine. *Cephalgia.* 2002;22:256–259.

75. Lipton RB. Editorial. Fair winds and foul headaches; risk factors and triggers of migraine. *Neurology.* 2000;54:280–281.

76. Martin VT, Behbehani NM. Toward a rational understanding of migraine trigger factors. *Med Clin North Am.* 2001;83:911–941.

77. Shecter AL, Lipton RB, Silberstein SD. Migraine comorbidity. In: Silberstein SD, Lipton RB, Dalessio DJ, eds. *Wolff's headache and other head pain.* New York: Oxford; 2001: 108–118.

78. Lanny C, Giannesini C, Zuber M, et al. Clinical and imaging findings in crytogenic stroke patients with and without patent foramen ovale: the PFO-ASA Study. Atrial-Septal Aneurysm. *Stroke.* 2002;33:706–711.

79. Merkingas KR, Rasmussen BK. Migraine comorbidity. In: Olesen J, Tfelt Hansen P, Welch KMA, eds. *The headaches.* 2nd edition. Philadelphia: Lippincott Williams & Wilkins; 2000: 235–240.

80. Fasmer OB. The prevalence of migraine in patients with bipolar and unipolar affective disorders. *Cephalgia.* 2001;21(9):894–899.

81. Neuhauser H, Leopold M, von Brevern M, et al. The interrelations of migraine, vertigo, and migrainous vertigo. *Neurology.* 2001;56:436–441.

82. Jull G. Manual diagnosis of C2-3 headache. *Cephalalgia.* 1985;5(suppl 5):308–309.

83. Jull GA. Headaches associated with the cervical spine: a clinical review. In: Grieve GP, ed. *Modern Manual Therapy of the Vertebral Column.* New York: Churchill Livingstone; 1986.

84. Jull G, Bogduk N, Marsland A. The accuracy of manual diagnosis for cervical zygapophyseal joint pain syndromes. *Med J Aust.* 1988;148:233–236.

85. Dwyer A, Aprill C, Bognuk N. Cervical zygapophyseal joint pain patterns, I: a study in normal volunteers. *Spine.* 1990;15:453–457.

86. Fligg B. Motion palpation of the upper cervical spine. In: Vernon HT, ed. *Upper Cervical Syndrome: Chiropractic Diagnosis and Management.* Baltimore: Williams & Wilkins; 1988.

87. Vernon HT, Steunab I, Hagino C. Cervicogenic dysfunction in muscle contraction headache and migraine: a descriptive study. *J Manipulative Physiol Ther.* 1992;15:418–429.

88. Bovim G. Cervicogenic headache, migraine and tension-like-type headache: pressure-pain threshold measurements. *Pain.* 1992;51:169–173.

89. Pfaffenrath V, Dandekar R, Mayer E, Hermann G, Pollman W. Cervicogenic headache: results of computer-based measurements of cervical spine mobility in fifteen patients. *Cephalalgia.* 1988;8:45–48.

90. Dvorak J, Froelich D, Penning L, Baumgartner TT, Panjabi MM. Functional radiographic diagnosis of the cervical spine: flexion/extension-like. *Spine.* 1988;13:745–755.

91. Kidd RF, Nelson R. Musculoskeletal dysfunction of the neck in migraine and tension-like headache. *Headache.* 1993;33:566–569.

92. Watson DH, Trott PH. Cervical headache: an investigation of natural head posture and upper cervical flexor muscle performance. *Cephalalgia.* 1993;13:272–282.

93. Nagaszwa A, Sakakihara T, Takahashi A. Roentgenographic findings of the cervical spine in tension-like-type headache. *Headache.* 1993;33:90–95.

94. Weingarten S, et al. The effectiveness of cerebral imaging in the diagnosis of chronic headaches. *Arch Intern Med.* 1992;152:2457.

95. McAbee G, et al. Value of MRI in pediatric migraine. *Headache.* 1993;33:143.

96. Couch J. Medical management of recurrent headache. In: Tollison C, Kunkel R, eds. *Headache: Diagnosis and Treatment.* Baltimore: Williams & Wilkins; 1993.

97. Parker GB, Pryor DS, Tupling H. Why does migraine improve during a clinical trial? Further results from a trial of cervical manipulation for migraine. *Aust N Z J Med.* 1980;10:192–198.

98. Hoyt H. Osteopathic manipulation in the treatment of muscle contraction headache. *J Am Osteopath Assoc.* 1979;78:322–324.

99. Wight JH. Migraine: a statistical analysis of chiropractic treatment. *J Am Chiro Assoc.* 1978;12:363–367.

100. Vernon H. Chiropractic manipulative therapy in the treatment of headaches: a retrospective and prospective study. *J Manipulative Physiol Ther.* 1982;5:109–122.

101. Vernon HT. Spinal manipulation and headaches of cervical origin: a review of literature and presentation of cases. *J Managed Med.* 1991;6:73–79.

102. Whittingham W, Ellis WB, Molyneux TP. The effect of manipulation (toggle recoil technique) for headaches with upper cervical joint dysfunction: a pilot study. *J Manipulative Physiol Ther.* 1994;17:369–375.

103. Mootz RD, Dhami MSI, Hess JA, Cook RD, Schorr DB. Chiropractic treatment of chronic episodic tension-like-type headache in male subjects: a case series analysis. *J Can Chiro Assoc.* 1994;38:152–159.

104. Bryans R, Descarreaux M, Duranleau M, et al. Evidence-based guidelines for the chiropractic treatment of adults with headache. *J Manipulative Physiol Ther.* 2011;34(5):274–289.

105. Bronfort G, Haas M, Evans R, Leininger B, Triano J. Effectiveness of manual therapies: the UK evidence report. *Chiropr Osteopat.* 2010;18:3.

106. Boline P, Kassak K, Bronfort G, Nelson C, Anderson AV. Spinal manipulation vs amitriptyline for the treatment of chronic tension-like-type headaches: a randomized clinical trial. *J Manipulative Physiol Ther.* 1995;18:148–154.

107. Nelson CF, Bronfort G, Evans R, et al. The efficacy of spinal manipulation, amitriptyline and the combination of both therapies for the prophylaxis of migraine headache. *J Manipulative Physiol Ther.* 1998;21:511–519.

108. Tuchin PJ, Pollard H, Bonello R. A randomized controlled trial of chiropractic spinal manipulative therapy for migraine. *J Manipulative Physiol Ther.* 2000;23:91–95.

109. Bronfort G, Assendelft WJ, Evans R, et al. Efficacy of spinal manipulation for chronic headache: a systematic review. *J Manipulative Physiol Ther.* 2001;24:457–466.

110. McCrory DC, Penzien DB, Hasselbad C, Gray RN. Evidence Report: Behavioral and Physical Treatments for Tension-type and Cervicogenic Headache. Duke University Evidence-based Practice Center. FCER; 2001.

111. Cott A, Parkinson W, Fabich M, Bedard M, Martin R. Long-term efficacy of combined relaxation biofeedback treatments for chronic headache. *Pain.* 1992;51:49–56.

112. Arena JG, Bruno GM, Hannah SL, Meader KJ. A comparison of frontal electromyographic biofeedback training, trapezius electromyographic biofeedback training, and progressive muscle relaxation therapy in the treatment of tension-like headache. *Headache.* 1995;35:411–419.

113. Blanchard EB, Taylor AE, Dentinger MP. Preliminary results from the self-regulatory treatment of high-medication-consumption headache. *Biofeedback Self Regul.* 1992;17:179–202.

114. Fitterling JM, Martin JE, Gamling S, Cole P. Behavioral management of exercise training in vascular headache patients: an investigation of exercise, adherence, and headache activity. *J Behav Analysis.* 1988;21:9–19.

115. Carlsson J, Fahlcrantz A, Augustinsson LE. Muscle tenderness in tension-like headache treated

with acupuncture or physiotherapy. *Cephalalgia.* 1990;10:131–141.

116. Carksiib HM, Augustinsson LE, Blomstrand C, Sullivan M. Health status in patients with tension-like headache treated with acupuncture or physiotherapy. *Headache.* 1990;30:593–599.

117. Carlsson J, Rosenthall U. Oculomotor disturbances in patients with tension-like headache treated with acupuncture or physiotherapy. *Cephalalgia.* 1990;10:123–129.

118. Vincent CA. The treatment of tension-like headache by acupuncture: a controlled single case design with time series analysis. *J Psychosom Res.* 1990;34:553–561.

119. Tavola T, Gala C, Conte G, Invermizzi G. Traditional Chinese acupuncture in tension-like-type headache: a controlled study. *Pain.* 1992;48:325–329.

120. Folweiler DS, Lynch OT. Nasal specific technique as part of a chiropractic approach to chronic sinusitis and sinus headache. *J Manipulative Physiol Ther.* 1995;18:38–41.

121. Nelson CF. Headache diagnosis. In: Lawrence DJ, Cassidy JD, McGregor M, et al., eds. *Advances in Chiropractic.* St. Louis, MO: Mosby-Year Book; 1994;1:77–99.

122. Aurova SK, Almad BK, Welch KMA, et al. Transcranial magnetic stimulation confirms hyperexcitability of occipital cortex in migraine. *Neurology.* 1998;50:1111–1114.

123. Bille B. Migraine in children: prevalence, clinical features, and a 30-year follow-up. In Ferrari MD, Ltaste X, eds. *Migraine and other headaches.* Carnforth, United Kingdom: Parthenon, 1989.

124. Lipton RB, Bigal ME, Diamond M, Freitag F, Reed ML, Stewart WF. Migraine prevalence, disease burden, and the need for preventive therapy. *Neurology.* 2007;68(5):343–349.

125. Bartleson JD. Treatment and persistent neurological manifestations of migraine. *Stroke.* 1984;15:383–386.

126. Lewis D, Paradiso E. A double-blind, dose comparison study of topiramate for prophylaxis of basilar-type migraine in children: a pilot study. *Headache.* 2007;47(10):1409–1417.

127. Etminan M, Takkouche B, Isorna FC, Samii A. Risk of ischaemic stroke in people with migraine: systematic review and meta-analysis of observational studies. *BMJ.* 2005;330(7482):63.

128. Kurth T, Gaziano JM, Cook NR, et al. Migraine and risk of cardiovascular disease in men. *Arch Intern Med.* 2007;167(8):795–801.

129. Kurth T, Gaziano JM, Cook NR, Logroscino G, Diener HC, Buring JE. Migraine and risk of cardiovascular disease in women. *JAMA.* 2006;296(3):283–291.

130. Diener HC, Kurth T, Dodick D. Patent foramen ovale, stroke, and cardiovascular disease in migraine. *Curr Opin Neurol.* 2007;20(3):310–319.

131. Detsky ME, McDonald DR, Baerlocher MO, Tomlinson GA, McCrory DC, Booth CM. Does this patient with headache have a migraine or need neuroimaging? *JAMA.* 2006;296(10):1274–1283.

132. Linet MS, Ziegler DK, Stewart WF. Headaches preceded by visual aura among adolescents and young adults. A population-based survey. *Arch Neurol.* 1992;49(5):512–516.

133. Vernon H. Spinal manipulation and headaches: an update. *Top Clin Chiro.* 1995;2(3):34–47.

134. Linde K, Streng A, Jurgens S, et al. Acupuncture for patients with migraine: a randomized controlled trial. *JAMA.* 2005;293(17):2118–2125.

135. Murphy JJ, Hepinstall S, Mitchell JRA. Randomized double-blind placebo controlled trial of feverfew in migraine prevention. *Lancet.* 1988;2:189–192.

136. Johnson ES, Kadam NP, Rosche W, et al. Efficacy of feverfew as prophylactic treatment of migraine. *Br Med J.* 1985;291:569–573.

137. Pittler MH, Vogler BK, Ernst E. Feverfew for preventing migraine. *Cochrane Database Syst Rev.* 2000; CD002286.

138. Mittra S, Datta A, Singh, SK, Singh A. 5-Hydroxytryptamine-inhibiting property of feverfew; role of parthenolide content. *Acta Pharmacol Sin.* 2000;21(12):1106–1114.

139. Ernst E, Pittner M. The efficacy and safety of feverfew (Tanacetum parthenium L): an update of a systematic review. *Public Health Nutrition.* 2003;3(4):509–514.

140. Shoemen J, et al. Effectiveness of high-dose riboflavin in migraine prophylaxis: a randomized controlled trial. *Neurology.* 1998;50(2):466–470.

141. Mauskop A, et al. Petasites Hybridus (Butterbar Root) extract is effective in the prophylaxis of migraine. Results of a randomized, double-blind trial. *Headache.* 2000;40(5):420–424.

142. Birdsall TC. 5-Hydroxytryptophan: a clinically effective serotonin precursor. *Altern Med Rev.* 1998;3(4):271–280.

143. McCarren T, Hitzemann R, Allen C, et al. Amelioration of severe migraine by fish oil (omega-3) fatty acids. *Am J Clin Nutr.* 1985;41(4):874–878.

144. Glueck CJ, McCarren T, Hitzemann R, et al. Amelioration of severe migraine with omega-3 fatty

acids: a double-blind placebo controlled clinical trial. *Am J Clin Nutr.* 1986;43(4):710–712.

145. Facchinetti F, Sances G, Borella P, et al. Magnesium prophylaxis of menstrual migraine: effects on intracellular magnesium. *Headache.* 1991;31:298–301.

146. Thys-Jacobs S. Vitamin D and calcium in menstrual migraine. *Headache.* 1994;34:544–546.

147. Thys-Jacobs S. Alleviation of migraines with therapeutic vitamin D and calcium. *Headache.* 1994;34:590–592.

148. Schoemen J, Jacquy J, Lemaerts M. Effectiveness of high-dose riboflavin in migraine prophylaxis: a randomized controlled trial. *Neurology.* 1998;50:466–470.

149. Kumar KL, Cooney TG. Headaches. *Med Clin North Am.* 1995;79:261–286.

150. Lipton RB, Stewart WF, Ryan RE Jr, et al. Efficacy and safety of acetaminophen, aspirin, and caffeine in alleviating migraine headache pain: three double-blind, randomized, placebo-controlled trials. *Arch Neurol.* 1998;55:210–217.

151. Kirthi V, Derry S, Moore RA. Aspirin with or without an antiemetic for acute migraine headaches in adults. *Cochrane Database Syst Rev.* 2013;4:CD008041.

152. Mather DB, Young WB, Rosenberg JH, et al. *Evidence-based guidelines for migraine headache: pharmacological management of acute attacks.* 2000. Available at http://www.aan.com/public/practiceguidelines/headache_gl.htm.

153. Goadsby PJ, Lipton RB, Ferrari MD. Migraine—current understanding and treatment. *NEJM.* 2002;346:257–270.

154. Derry CJ, Derry S, Moore RA. Sumatriptan (intranasal route of administration) for acute migraine attacks in adults. *Cochrane Database Syst Rev.* 2012;2:CD009663.

155. Derry CJ, Derry S, Moore RA. Sumatriptan (oral route of administration) for acute migraine attacks in adults. *Cochrane Database Syst Rev.* 2012;2:CD008615.

156. Derry CJ, Derry S, Moore RA. Sumatriptan (rectal route of administration) for acute migraine attacks in adults. *Cochrane Database Syst Rev.* 2012;2:CD009664.

157. Milian Guerrero RO, Isais Cardenas MA, Ocvampa AA, Pacheco ME. Histamine as a therapeutic alternative in migraine prophylaxis: a randomized, placebo-controlled, double-blind study. *Headache.* 1999;39:576–580.

158. Maizels M, Aeiger AM. Intranasal lidocaine for migraine: a randomized trial and open label follow-up. *Headache.* 1999;29:543–551.

159. Silberstein SD, Saper JR. Migraine diagnosis and treatment. In: Dalessio DJ, Silberstein SD, eds. *Wolff's Headache and Other Pain.* 6th ed. New York: Oxford University Press; 1993:96–170.

160. Sherman RA, Acosta NM, Robson L. Treatment of migraine with pulsing electromagnetic fields: a double-blind, placebo-controlled study. *Headache.* 1999;39:567–575.

161. Ilhan Alp S, Alp R. Supraorbital and infraorbital nerve blockade in migraine patients: results of 6-month clinical follow-up. *Eur Rev Med Pharmacol Sci.* 2013;17(13):1778–1781.

162. Bednarczyk EM, Remler B, Weikart C, Nielson AD, Reed RC. Global cerebral blood flow, blood volume, and oxygen metabolism in patients with migraine headache. *Neurology.* 1998;50:1736–1740.

163. Nelson CF. The tension-like headache, migraine headache continuum: a hypothesis. *J Manipulative Physiol Ther.* 1994;17:156–167.

164. Bove G, Nilsson N. Spinal manipulation in the treatment of episodic tension-type headache: a randomized controlled trial. *JAMA.* 1998;280:1576–1579.

165. Vernon HT. Vertebrogenic headache. In: *Upper Cervical Syndrome: Chiropractic Diagnosis and Management.* Baltimore: Williams & Wilkins; 1988.

166. Nilsson N. A randomized controlled trial of the effect of spinal manipulation in the treatment of cervicogenic headache. *J Manipulative Physiol Ther.* 1995;18:435–440.

167. Kudrow L. Cluster headache: clinical, mechanism, and treatment aspects. *Panminerva Med.* 1982;24:45–54.

168. Goadsby PJ, Lipton RB. A review of paroxysmal hemicranias, SUNCT syndrome, and other short-lasting headaches with autonomic feature, including new cases. *Brain.* 1997;120(1):193–209.

169. Goadsby PJ. Pathophysiology of cluster headache: a trigeminal autonomic cephalgia. *Lancet Neurol.* 2002;4:251–257.

170. May A, Bahra A, Buchel C, et al. Hypothalamic activation in cluster headache attacks. *Lancet.* 1998;352:275–278.

171. May A, Goadsby PJ. Hypothalamic involvement and activation in cluster headache. *Curr Pain Headache Rep.* 2001;5(11):60–66.

172. Leone M, Franzini A, Broggi G, Bussone G. Hypothalamic deep brain stimulation for intractable

chronic cluster headache: a 3-year follow-up. *Neurol Sci.* 2003;24(2);suppl 2:S143–145.

173. Law S, Derry S, Moore RA. Triptans for acute cluster headache. *Cochrane Database Syst Rev.* 2010(4):CD008042.

174. Fagan L. Treatment of cluster headache: a double-blind comparison of oxygen by air inhalation. *Arch Neurol.* 1985;42:362–363.

175. Kittrelle JP, Grouse DS, Seybold ME. Cluster headache; local anesthetic, abortive agents. *Arch Neurol.* 1985;42:496–498.

176. Mauskop A, Altura BT, Cracco RQ, Altura BM. Intravenous magnesium sulfate relieves cluster headaches in patients with low serum ionized magnesium levels. *Headache.* 1995;35:597–600.

177. Burns B, Watkins L, Goadsby PJ. Treatment of medically intractable cluster headache by occipital nerve stimulation: long-term follow-up of eight patients. *Lancet.* 2007;369(9567):1099–1106.

178. Ford RG, Ford KT, Swaid S, et al. Gamma knife treatment of refractory cluster headache. *Headache.* 1998;38:3–9.

179. Sanders M, Zuurmond WW. Efficacy of sphenopalatine ganglion blockade in 66 patients suffering from cluster headache: a 12- to 70-month follow-up evaluation. *J Neurosurg.* 1997;87:876–880.

180. Salvarani C, Gabriel SE, O'Fallon WM, Hunder GG. The incidence of giant cell arteritis in Olmsted County, Minnesota: apparent fluctuations in a cyclic pattern. *Ann Intern Med.* 1995;123:192–194.

181. Chmelewski WL, McKnight KM, Angudelo CA, et al. Presenting features and outcomes in patients undergoing temporal artery biopsy. *Arch Intern Med.* 1992;152:1690–1695.

182. Hayreh SS, Podhajsky PA, Raman R, Zimmerman B. Giant cell arteritis: validity and reliability of various diagnostic criteria. *Am J Ophthalmol.* 1997;123:285–296.

183. Couch JR. Headaches to worry about. *Med Clin North Am.* 1993;77:141–166.

184. Lauwerys BR, Puttemans T, Houssaiu FA, Devogelaer J P. Color Doppler sonography of the temporal arteries in giant cell arteritis and polymyalgia rheumatica. *J Rheumatol.* 1997;24:1570–1574.

APPENDIX 17–3

Headache Diagnosis Matrix

Diagnosis	Comments	History Findings	Positive Examination Findings	Radiography/Special Studies	Treatment Options
Tension-Type Headache	• Tension headache is the Dx used when there are no indications of neurologic involvement, symptoms are generally mild and responsive to OTCs. • Note that if it is suspected that headache is specifically due to subluxations of the cervical spine, should be called (cervicogenic headache).	*Age of Onset*—Any age *Onset Characteristics*—Generally insidious with onset often occurring in afternoon *Location*—Sub-occipital and band-like in temporal area most common *Severity*—Generally mild, however, wide variation *Duration*—Lasts for hours to days *Associated S & S*—Generally not associated with nausea or vomiting. Generally responsive to over-the-counter pain medication to some degree	*Nonspecific*—Localized tenderness in area of pain and/or in cervical region	• Radiography not recommended or required.	• Chiropractic adjustive technique (CAT). • Avoid repetitive use of OTCs. • Attempt to change occupational biomechanics if appropriate. • Suggest methods to reduce stress.
Migraine with Aura (Classic Migraine)	• The aura is a neurologic event lasting from one-half hour to a couple of hours, classically manifested as visual dysfunction such as flashing lights and scotomas. • In complex migraines, the aura is the predominant event and may be as severe as temporary hemiparesis.	*Age of Onset*—Any age is possible; most common onset is late teens/early twenties and then again postmenopausal; predominantly female *Onset Characteristics*—Preceded by aura by one-half hour or so *Location*—Unilateral, pulsatile, often temporal or orbital *Severity*—Quite severe *Duration*—Lasts for hours (occasionally days) *Associated S & S*—Generally associated with nausea or vomiting, photophobia	*Neurological findings*—Indications of temporary sensory or motor deficits may be found during aura, especially with cranial nerves *Nonspecific*—Localized tenderness in area of pain and/or in cervical region	• In cases where neurologic signs or symptoms are predominant, CAT scan or MRI may be needed to rule out other causes.	• Trial of CAT. • Feverfew or other supplementation. • Maintain regular sleeping and eating patterns. • Avoid known triggers. • Referral for biofeedback or acupuncture if ineffective. • Referral for medical management with sumatriptan. • Note that rebound migraine occurs when medication is stopped suddenly or taken for longer than 3 days.

Migraine without Aura (Common Migraine)	• Difficulty may exist in differentiating severe tension headaches from migraine without aura. • Temporal or orbital location with pulsatile characteristics and poor response to OTCs characterizes migraine without aura.	*Age of Onset*—Any age is possible; most common onset is late teens/early twenties and then again postmenopausal; predominantly female *Onset Characteristics*—No aura; insidious onset *Location*—Unilateral, pulsatile, often temporal or orbital *Severity*—Quite severe *Duration*—Generally last for days *Associated S & S*—Generally associated with nausea or vomiting	*Nonspecific*—Localized tenderness in area of pain and/or in cervical region	• In cases where neurologic signs or symptoms are predominant, CAT scan or MRI may be needed to rule out other causes.	• Trial of CAT. • Feverfew or other supplementation. • Maintain regular sleeping and eating patterns. • Avoid known triggers. • Referral for acupuncture if ineffective. • Referral for medical management with sumatriptan or similar serotonin update inhibitors.
Migraine Variant Includes Cluster Headache & Allergic Headaches	• Cluster headaches are particularly painful and psychologically difficult for the patient to handle; suicide is contemplated by many patients.	*Age of Onset*—Most common onset is 30s to late 40s; male predominant *Onset Characteristics*—Often same time each day; clusters over days or weeks. Smoking may initiate; alcohol exacerbates *Location*—Unilateral, orbital *Severity*—Very severe *Duration*—Lasts for 45 minutes to 2 hours *Associated S & S*—Unilateral lacrimation, rhinorrhea; generally associated with nausea or vomiting; generally not responsive to over-the-counter pain medication	*Neurological*—During attacks, a temporary Horner's syndrome may be present in a minority of patients *Nonspecific*—Localized tenderness in area of pain and/or in cervical region	• In cases where neurologic signs or symptoms are predominant, CAT scan or MRI may be needed to rule out other causes.	• Trial of CAT. • Feverfew or other supplementation. • Maintain regular sleeping and eating patterns. • Avoid known triggers. • Referral for acupuncture if ineffective. • Referral for medical management with O_2 therapy, intranasal lidocaine, or sumatriptan.

(continues)

Headache Diagnosis Matrix (continued)

Diagnosis	Comments	History Findings	Positive Examination Findings	Radiography/ Special Studies	Treatment Options
Cervicogenic Headache	• Used only when patient does not have clear indicators of one of the primary headache types, such as migraine or tension-type, and it is suspected that the headache is purely cervicogenic in origin.	*Onset*—May be posttraumatic or have an insidious onset *Symptoms*—Pain is localized to neck or occipital region; however, may radiate to various areas of the head and face	*Palpation*—Tenderness in neck musculature or changes in tone, contour *Ortho*—Headache may be exacerbated or reproduced by head/neck movements *ROM Findings*—Limitation or resistance to neck movements	• Radiographs indicate one or more of the following: movement abnormalities of flexion/extension, abnormal posture, or fractures/dislocations, congenital abnormalities, RA, tumors, or other distinct pathologies.	• Mobilization, manipulation (need corresponding subluxation code). • Stretching, postural exercises. • Myofascial therapy. • Physiotherapy.

Dizziness

# CHAPTER 18

Context

In most studies of primary care,[1] internal medicine,[2] and emergency departments,[3] dizziness ranks among the top three patient complaints. Statistics for chiropractic clinics are not as clear.[4] In the context of chiropractic practice, probably the most frequently seen cases are those associated with motor vehicle cervical spine/head injuries and in the elderly. Dizziness may be one of the top three symptoms reported after acceleration/deceleration injury to the neck.[5-8] It is unclear how many cases are due to insult to neck proprioceptors versus the vestibular apparatus or vascular supply to the head and neck.

Dizziness may occur in as many as 50% of the elderly.[9] In nearly 20% of all older persons, the dizziness is severe enough to consult a health professional. Although it appears that there are age-related declines in vestibular, visual, auditory, and somatosensory functions in normal older individuals, these changes correlate weakly to actual changes in gait and balance.[10]

At a dizziness and balance clinic for patients over age 65 years, the distribution of cause for dizziness was 32%, due to benign paroxysmal positioning vertigo;[11] 22% was due to either fear of falling or disuse equilibrium, and 13% was due to vestibular loss. All other causes accounted each for 5% or less of cases. Although dizziness is a frequent complaint,[12] only a little more than half of patients receive treatment.[13] The elderly population in particular is more prone to the vertiginous effects of medications and the lack of compensation that a younger population has for dysfunction of one of the components of balance. Vision, proprioception, and vestibular function are all integral to balance. When one is dysfunctional, the nervous system may accommodate through input and adaptation from the other systems. In the elderly, there may be a general deterioration of all neural systems, perhaps complicated by other diseases such as diabetes or atherosclerosis, making adaptation less effective and dizziness more disabling.

As with many patient complaints, the chiropractor must ask the patient to further describe a complaint of dizziness in order to gain a clearer understanding of which body systems are involved. Often this simple step in evaluation will narrow down the cause into a general category (**Exhibit 18-1**). Dizziness may be perceived as spinning of the room or self, motion imbalance or lack of coordination while walking, or simply lightheadedness or the sensation of almost fainting (i.e., presyncope). The sensation of spinning or motion is generally attributed to dysfunction of the vestibular and central processing systems, whereas a sensation of imbalance or lack of coordination is more likely due to cerebellar or proprioceptive dysfunction. In the senior, it is important to remember that myelopathy due to spinal stenosis is a common cause of a sense of imbalance. Lightheadedness or a sense of almost fainting suggests a vascular or psychologic cause. Some studies indicate a psychologic component in as many as 37% to 40% of patients with chronic dizziness, depending on the facility.[14, 15]

General Strategy

History

- Obtain a more detailed description of a patient's complaint of "dizziness."
- Differentiate vertigo from nonvertiginous causes of a dizziness complaint.
- Determine onset and length of attacks and whether they are recurrent to help differentiate further.

Exhibit 18–1 Narrowing the Cause of Dizziness

The Dizzy Patient

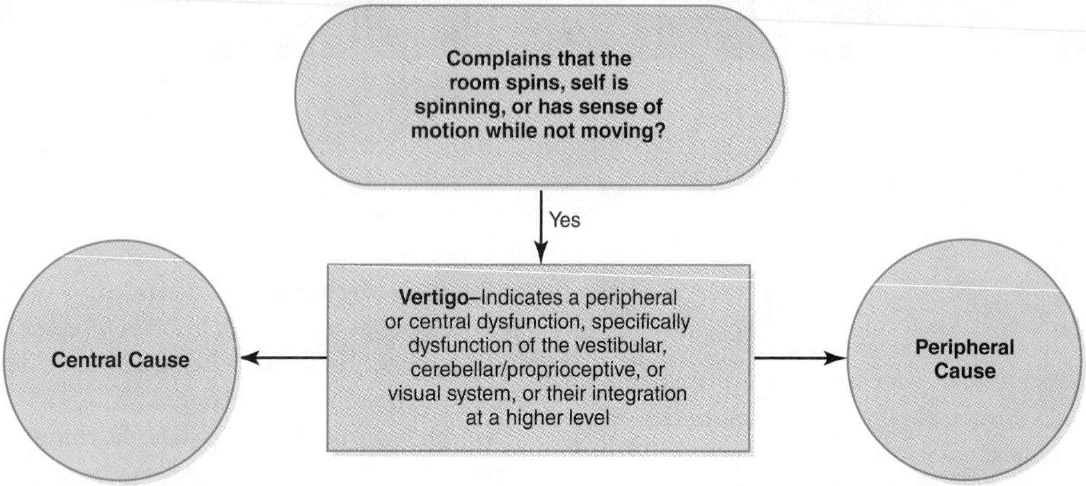

Complains that the room spins, self is spinning, or has sense of motion while not moving?

Yes

Vertigo–Indicates a peripheral or central dysfunction, specifically dysfunction of the vestibular, cerebellar/proprioceptive, or visual system, or their integration at a higher level

Central Cause

Peripheral Cause

History Cluster

Dizziness is
• often constant
• mild to moderate
• often associated with other neurologic signs

Key History Questions

Is the dizziness continuous?
This is suggestive of a central cause.

Is the dizziness severe?
Central causes usually result in less severe dizziness.

Is there associated hearing loss?
Peripheral causes such as Ménière's and labyrinthitis are suggested. Acoustic neuroma may be considered central or peripheral and is associated with hearing loss.

Is the dizziness recurrent?
This is found mainly with peripheral disorders, especially Ménière's disease.

Is there a specific position that causes the dizziness to occur?
This is found most commonly with benign positional vertigo, especially when it lasts for only seconds to as long as a few minutes.

History Cluster

Dizziness is
• moderate to severe
• self-resolving or recurrent
• often positionally related
• may have signs of an inner ear disorder

Examination Cluster

• Vertical nystagmus found; may change direction if rotational
Positional testing reveals:
• no latency with nystagmus/ vertigo
• does not fatigue or adapt
If an associated hearing loss is found, audiometry reveals:
• poor speech discrimination
• tone decay

Examination Cluster

• Nystagmus is horizontal or rotational
• Nystagmus/dizziness reduced with visual fixation on an object
Positional testing reveals:
• latency of seconds prior to onset of nystagmus/dizziness
• fatigues and adapts to provocative position
Hearing loss is most prominent with Ménière's, with a loss in the low-tone region

Classic Presentations Not to Be Missed

1. Patient presents with a sudden onset of dizziness due to a particular head position. Vertigo lasts for at most a minute or two. The patient has a history of trauma or is older. Physical examination reveals horizontal nystagmus that fatigues and adapts.
   Diagnosis: Benign Positional Vertigo

2. Patient presents with a history of recurrent attacks of vertigo. Sudden attacks come without warning and are associated with severe vertigo. They last hours to as long as a day or two. There is often a report of fullness in the ear and tinnitus. May be a history of diabetes or problems with fluid retention.
   Diagnosis: Meniere's Disease

3. Patient presents with a sudden onset of dizziness that is constant. It slowly improves over days or weeks, often with an associated hearing loss.
   Diagnosis: Labyrinthitis

4. Same presentation as above with no hearing loss.
   Diagnosis: Vestibular Neuronitis

5. Patient presents with a history of a whiplash injury and no obvious examination findings except that dizziness is reproduced by body rotation with the head held constant.
   Diagnosis: Vertebrogenic Vertigo

- Determine whether the patient senses any hearing loss.
- Ask about associated neurologic or systemic complaints.
- Ask about current medications.
- Differentiate between peripheral and central causes if vertigo is likely.

Narrowing the Cause of Dizziness

Evaluation

Screen with a battery of tests to:

- Determine whether there are any objective hearing deficits.
- Determine whether there are any associated systemic or neurologic problems.
- Determine the patient's vascular, endocrine, and psychologic status if nonvertiginous, particularly diabetes.
- Determine to what degree cervical spine dysfunction may be contributory.
- Evaluate seniors for signs of myelopathy.

Management

- Consider referral or comanagement in the following scenarios:
  - The patient has had head trauma and is demonstrating other associated neurologic signs, or a skull fracture is suspected.
  - Prescription medication is suspected as the underlying cause (refer to the prescribing physician if possible).
  - The dizziness is incapacitating, requiring medication during the symptomatic phase (comanagement may be possible).
  - The dizziness appears to have a strong psychologic component.
  - The patient appears to have a cardiopulmonary cause such as an arrhythmia, heart block, or congestive heart failure.
  - The patient is suspected of having a perilymphatic fistula.
  - The patient needs further audiologic or special imaging evaluation, especially in the consideration of brain tumors, cerebrovascular accidents,

demyelinating diseases (e.g., multiple sclerosis), or cerebellar or extrapyramidal disorders (e.g., Parkinson's disease).
  - The patient has hearing loss.
- Treat peripheral vertigo with chiropractic manipulative techniques, habituation exercises, and other conservative approaches.
- Refer if treatment is ineffective or the dizziness creates significant functional impairment.

Relevant Anatomy and Physiology

Balance and spatial orientation are maintained by an integrated, neuronal feedback loop. A slow adjustment can be made to compensate when input from any component is dysfunctional unless more than one component is involved. The components of this system are: (1) vestibular, (2) visual, and (3) proprioceptive. The vestibular labyrinth sends information to the vestibular nuclei in the medulla and lower pons via the vestibular branch of cranial nerve VIII. The cerebellum, receiving input from the spinocerebellar tracts (proprioception), also sends information to the vestibular nuclei. Conscious proprioception is conveyed through the posterior column/medial leminiscus (PCML) pathways. These may be adversely affected directly through myelopathy often due to the compressive effects of spinal stenosis or commonly at distal receptors affected by diabetes. The midline cerebellar structures have a strong inhibitory effect on the vestibular nuclei. In turn, the vestibular nuclei project to the cerebellum to all spinal levels through the vestibulospinal tracts, and to the medial longitudinal fasciculus (MLF) and the pontine reticular formation. Fibers in the MLF project to nuclei of the third, fourth, and sixth cranial nerves, stimulating reflex conjugate eye movement in reaction to head position change. The cerebral cortex, although not part of the vestibular system per se, modulates motor activity and coordination as a result of information supplied from various sensory inputs.

The vestibular receptor at each end of each semicircular canal is referred to as the ampullae (i.e., crista ampullaris). Within the ampulla is the cupula. Displacement of hair cells implanted in the neuroepithelium of the cupula occurs with angular movement (e.g., rotation) as a result of endolymphatic fluid movement. This component of equilibrium is often referred to as kinetic. In addition to the semicircular canals are the utricle and saccule. Together the utricle and saccule are referred to as otolith organs. They contain a small patch of sensory epithelium referred to as the maculae. Again, as with the ampullae, hair cells are sensitive to displacement through contact with a gelatinous material containing calcium carbonate crystals (i.e., otoliths). The utricle and saccule are sensitive to gravity and linear acceleration. This is often referred to as static equilibrium. Specifically, the utricle is more sensitive to forward and backward movement, whereas the saccule is more sensitive to vertical movement. A high rate of tonic firing from the vestibular sensory organs occurs, and when a unilateral disorder disrupts this tonic firing a sense of dizziness (and clinically manifested nystagmus) occurs. When there is bilateral damage to vestibular sensory organs, there is often no "imbalance" and the individual may not experience vertigo. A slow process such as an acoustic neuroma may not cause vertigo, because damage occurs gradually and compensation by the central nervous system is able to accommodate. Dislodging of otolith crystals may cause stimulation with certain head positions, causing vertigo that usually lasts for seconds to minutes. Any ipsilateral increase or decrease in labyrinth discharge will create a sense of movement.

Proprioception is conveyed through the integration of muscle spindles, joint receptors, and cutaneous mechnanoreceptors that transmit external and internal information about the body that results in both conscious and non-conscious perspectives about where the body is in space. Information specific to the cerebellum travels in the spinocerebellar tracts as non-conscious information that the cerebellum can use to compare with descending information sent from the cerebrum in the corticospinal tracts (collaterals sent through the pons to the cerebellum through the middle cerebellar peduncle) allowing fine adjustments to movement. This information and that from the posterior columns (i.e. conscious proprioception) may be interfered with through compression of the spinal cord; in particular, in elderly patients with spinal canal stenosis and subsequent myelopathy. Loss of proprioception in the feet often results in a perception of unsteadiness or being off-balance. This is common with diabetes. Proprioceptive information from the upper cervical musculature and joints may play a major role in a patient's perception of balance. The high density of receptors in the upper cervical region[16] participates in several reflexes. Although many assume that these are primarily capsular afferents, the scientific basis for this

assumption has been questioned. The original study[17] used the vertebral joints of quadrupeds for examination. It was found that in addition to nociceptors, the capsules contained proprioceptive type I afferents (tonic discharge; static position detection) and type II afferents (discharge only with movement). However, recent studies[18-20] indicate that human facet joints contain mainly nociceptors with only a few type I or type II proprioceptors. It appears that perhaps the majority of proprioceptors are located in other tissue, in particular the deep cervical muscles such as the interspinales, multifidus, rotator spinae, intertransversarii, and longus cervicis. The cervico-ocular reflex causes the eyes to rotate to the opposite side of head rotation. It becomes especially significant as a compensation for damage to the vestibular apparatus. The vestibulocollic reflex is more of an effector reflex, allowing vestibular information to modulate cervical muscle activity. To complete the interaction, input from the neck can also modulate vestibular reflexes.[21]

Theoretically, trauma or dysfunction in the cervical spine may have effects on these reflexes, or if there is damage to the vestibular apparatus, these reflexes may help compensate. Cervicogenic vertigo is believed to be a result of cervical joint dysfunction, muscle strain, or injury from trauma such as a whiplash-like accident. The basic science support for this possibility comes from numerous studies that have shown ataxia, nystagmus, and/or disequilibrium with local anesthetic injection[22] into the deep posterolateral neck, electrical stimulation[23] of strained muscles, and transection of suboccipital muscles or upper cervical root section in animals. Vibration of muscle tendons or the head can create a postural illusion leading to nystagmus and motion sickness.[24] Overstimulation from joint dysfunction or muscle spasm or damage to the upper cervical proprioceptors theoretically may result in an imbalance of proprioceptive information. Through vestibular reflexes the result may be a sense of disequilibrium.

The vascular supply to the ear and the vestibular apparatus and nuclei may be compromised, leading to the perception of dizziness. Although it was once believed that a sympathetically mediated vascular reflex could be the cause of vertigo in patients with cervical dysfunction, it appears that vertebral blood flow is minimally responsive to sympathetic stimulation.[25] The main vascular supply to the head is from branches off the vertebral or basilar arteries (the basilar artery is formed by the two vertebral arteries). The main artery is the anterior inferior cerebellar artery. The caudal portion of the vestibular nuclei is supplied more specifically by the posterior inferior cerebellar arteries via the lateral medullary or posterior spinal arteries. The vestibular and basilar arteries supply more than the vestibular nuclei; as a result, other symptoms accompany vertebrobasilar insufficiency, including diplopia, ataxia, "drop attacks," dysarthria, and various forms of body paralysis or weakness (although dizziness is often a prominent symptom).

Generally, dizziness is caused by decreased cerebral, cerebellar, or brainstem perfusion or dysfunction of one or all of the neural balance systems: (1) visual, (2) vestibular, and (3) proprioception/cerebellar. This dysfunction is usually due to trauma, vascular compromise, infection of the labyrinths, or neural inflammation or degeneration both centrally and peripherally (such as in multiple sclerosis). For less common causes of dizziness see **Table 18–1**.

Table 18–1 Differential List of Less Common Causes of Dizziness

Disorder	Clinical Clues	Management
Acute Ramsey-Hunt Syndrome—varicella virus infection of cranial nerves VII and VIII	In addition to facial paralysis (Bell's palsy) there is also possible hearing loss, tinnitus, and dizziness. Important to check otoscopically on all patients with signs of varicella infection.	Medical management includes acyclovir and possibly prednisone within first few days
Brainstem infarct—vertigo due to infarcts in posterior fossa structures that contain vestibular pathways		
• Anterior inferior cerebellar artery—branches including the cerebellar, pontine, and labyrinth	Infarct of anterior inferior cerebellar artery—vertigo, nausea/vomiting, and imbalance. Common cochlear or labyrinth artery presentation is same, plus hearing loss/tinnitus. Infarction of pontine branch—central signs including dysarthria, Horner's, peripheral facial paralysis, trigeminal sensory loss, and contralateral pain/temperature loss.	MR arteriography used to assess posterior circulation with transcranial Doppler for basilar artery flow. Warfarin often used. Management includes decrease in risk factors for cerebrovascular disease and vestibular exercises. Central compensation may not be complete if the infarct involves the vestibular portion of the cerebellum.
• Posterior inferior cerebellar artery—supply to posterior inferior cerebellum and dorsolateral medulla	Lateral medulla infarct results in Wallenberg's syndrome—crossed sensory findings, ipsilateral lateropulsion ataxia, Horner's sign. Nystagmus may be pure torsional or mixed.	Same as above for anterior, inferior cerebellar artery
Chronic vestibular hypofunction—chronic vestibular loss may be the residual of vestibular disease or when bilateral due to ototoxicity (e.g., gentamicin). The most common is idiopathic likely due to degeneration with age.	Patients may complain of unsteadiness while walking, oscillopsia with head movements (i.e., false sense of movement). There is no spontaneous nystagmus, positive on head thrust tests and negative Romberg.	Vestibular rehabilitation is key to treatment. A programmed sequence of vestibular training allowing for central compensation is often effective. A supervised program is more effective than handing the patient an instruction sheet.
Disuse disequilibrium and fear of falling—in the elderly, a combination of lack of exercise and mobility in general can lead to disuse disequilibrium. Fear of falling may result from disuse disequilibrium and exacerbate the problem by the patient's unwillingness to ambulate.	Patient expresses fear of falling especially with eyes closed and walking in areas where no support is evident. Past history of a fall is likely. The vestibular examination is normal. Tandem walking is often abnormal, as is Romberg's with eyes closed. The Tinetti risk assessment questionnaire may be helpful to determine risk and strategy for management.	Daily home program that includes exercise for endurance, balance, and lower extremity strength. Balance exercises are modeled after vestibular rehabilitation exercises.

(continues)

Table 18–1 Differential List of Less Common Causes of Dizziness (continued)

Disorder	Clinical Clues	Management
Leukoaraiosis—white matter disease of the brain due to significant small vessel disease seen most frequently in older patients with diabetes and hypertension	Gait and balance problems similar to Parkinson's and normal pressure hydrocephalus. Positive retropulsion test. Patient asked to take one step backward when examiner pulls back on patient's hip. Positive is either falling backward like a log or taking several steps backward.	Because features overlap with Parkinson's, including age, nonresponse to carbidopa/levodopa (Sinemet) indicates possibility. MRI reveals leukoaraiosis. Only available management is prevention of further progression and an attempt at vestibular training exercises, which have variable success.
Spells of dizziness Central positioning vertigo—caused by lesion near the fourth ventricle near the cerebellum, including tumors, multiple sclerosis, and strokes	Patient complains of onset with change of position. Hallpike maneuver response is usually an up- or downbeat nystagmus with no latency and no fatigue to repeated positioning.	Imaging, often using MR with or without gadolinium, reveals lesions. Surgical correction is likely.
Perilymphatic fistula—a hole connecting the inner and middle ear due to barotrauma (e.g., scuba diving), head trauma, tumor (cholesteatoma), or movement of a prosthetic middle ear bone into the inner ear	A history of barotrauma such as scuba diving or heavy weight lifting may be found. Also, lifting weights may cause oscillopsia and vertigo. Pressure changes provoke dizziness due to flow of fluid between the two compartments. Valsalva maneuver may also provoke oscillopsia, as will blowing out through pinched nostrils. Using the insufflation device of the otoscope may also provoke. Hallpike maneuver may or may not provoke a peripheral type of response.	Surgical exploration with patching of round or oval window with autogenous tissue is usually effective. Patient usually ambulating after one week postsurgery.
Superior canal dehiscence—less than 1% of the population is born with a thin bony top of the superior semicircular canal. Mild head trauma or pressure change may cause an opening with contact between the membranous canal and overlying dura.	Patients may complain of a "rumbling" sensation in the head with talking or coughing. Dizziness occurs with changes of position, Valsalva maneuver, or with loud noises (Tullio's phenomenon). An ocular tilt response may occur with blowing out through a pinched nose, resulting in one eye moving up and in and the other down and out.	Petrous bone CT will usually reveal the loss of bone. Treatment usually involves surgically placing a bone plate over the superior SCC or, if not surgically possible, having patient avoid pressure changes and using earplugs to avoid the Tullio phenomenon.
Transient ischemic attacks (TIA)—TIAs of the vertebrobasilar vascular area will often cause transient symptoms.	TIAs of the vertebrobasilar area may be due to dissection or thrombus. The attacks generally last only a few minutes and, in addition to sudden dizziness, may also include "drop attacks," visual disturbances, and/or weakness. Risk factors for cerebrovascular disease are evident in those with repeated spells of dizziness.	MR arteriography is the diagnostic tool of choice. Transcranial Doppler may reveal decreased blood flow in the basilar artery. Warfarin is often used when there is vertebral or basilar artery stenosis.
Migraine—a variant of migraine; may be the "aura" prior to headache	Some patients with migraine experience vertigo. Dizzy spells generally last 45 minutes to 60 minutes and do not always result in a subsequent headache. The dizziness may appear vestibular because it is provoked by head movement.	Management is similar for migraine headaches in general. Avoidance of triggers, regular lifestyle maintenance (e.g., regular sleeping and eating habits). Chiropractic manipulation should be considered when serious causes of dizziness have been ruled out.
Psychogenic/anxiety—commonly associated with anxiety, bouts of attacks that include dizziness as one of a complex of symptoms	When the patient uses multiple terms to describe the dizziness (vague), depression or anxiety is likely. Common descriptions include floating and rocking. There is often a history of stress. Associated complaints including shortness of breath or chest tightness, paresthesias, and sweating are not uncommon. They often occur together, escalating over about 10 minutes when in a stressful or uncomfortable situation.	Behavioral modification may be very effective. If not, selective serotonin reuptake inhibitors (SSRIs) are often prescribed. Alprazolam (Xanax) is an anti-anxiety medication that may also be prescribed.

Evaluation

History

The most important step in the evaluation of a complaint of dizziness is to ask the patient to qualify or more clearly describe his or her complaint. The patient may be reluctant or unable to describe the complaint further, and it may be necessary to prompt him or her with some common descriptions (**Tables 18–2** and **18–3**). Patient descriptions correlate well with four general categories of dizziness: (1) vertigo, (2) syncope or presyncope, (3) disequilibrium, and (4) psychogenic (hyperventilation, depression).

If the patient feels as though the room or he or she is spinning, one would be more likely to think of classic vertigo. Vertigo includes any abnormal sensation of motion when there is no motion or an exaggerated sense

of motion in response to a body movement. The next step in evaluation would be to determine causes that are central and those that are peripheral. *Peripheral vertigo* refers to dysfunction of the labyrinths or vestibular nerve. *Central vertigo* refers to disorders affecting the central connections to the cerebellum and brainstem.

A distinction among the various types of peripheral vertigo may be evident through a comparison of common history elements with regard to onset, duration, recurrence, and associated hearing loss (90% accurate for the most common disorders).[26]

- Benign paroxysmal positional vertigo (BPPV) is suggested when there are brief episodes of moderate to severe vertigo associated with specific provocative head positioning; it gradually diminishes over a month or two without associated hearing loss.

Table 18–2 History Questions for Dizziness

Primary Question	What Are You Thinking?	Secondary Questions	What Are You Thinking?
Do you or the room spin?	Vertigo. Peripheral or central causes.	**Is it continuous or intermittent, coming and going?**	Continuous indicates central; recurrent indicates peripheral.
Does it feel like you are about to faint or are lightheaded?	Vascular or endocrine cause.	**Does this occur when you stand?**	Orthostatic hypotension. Ask about medications.
		Does this occur when you haven't eaten?	Hypoglycemic reaction.
		Does this occur when you cough?	Cough syncope (glossopharyngeal).
		Does this occur when you are "stressed out"?	Anxiety. Adrenal disorder.
		Does this occur when you turn your head?	Subclavian steal, atherosclerotic cause.
		Does it occur when you wear a tight collar?	Sick sinus syndrome.
		Are you diabetic?	Patient may not know. Need to evaluate with lab.
Are you "dizzy" only when you walk?	Cerebellar or proprioception problem.	**Is it worse with your eyes closed or in a dark room?**	Proprioceptive problem, probably dorsal columns.
		Do you fall always to the same side?	Cerebellar cause should be investigated.
Are you taking medication?	Side effect or indication of underlying disorder that could cause dizziness.	**Are you taking muscle relaxants, medication with codeine, or barbiturates?**	Central nervous system depression.
		Are you taking cimetidine (Tagamet), pain medications, or high blood pressure medications?	Common drugs that may cause dizziness.

Table 18–3 Specific History Questions for Vertigo

Primary Question	What Are You Thinking?	Secondary Questions	What Are You Thinking?
Is the dizziness continuous or progressive?	If yes, a central cause is likely. If no, suspect a peripheral cause.	Is the dizziness relatively mild and not affected much by position?	Central cause such as acoustic neuroma, multiple sclerosis.
Is the dizziness recurrent?	Most commonly benign positional vertigo and Ménière's disease.	Is the onset abrupt and related to a specific position change?	Benign paroxysmal positional vertigo (BPPV).
		Does it last for seconds to a couple of minutes?	BPPV.
		Is it abrupt but lasts for hours to a day or so?	Ménière's disease is likely.
		Is there associated fullness and a ringing in the ear during attacks?	Ménière's disease is likely.
Is there associated hearing loss?	Peripheral causes include labyrinthitis and Ménière's disease. Central causes include acoustic neuroma and other pontine tumors.	Have you had this for weeks with a gradual decrease in dizziness?	Labyrinthitis.
		Are these recurrent attacks with associated hearing loss?	Ménière's disease.
Was there a somewhat fast onset with a slow decrease in dizziness?	Labyrinthitis and vestibular neuronitis.	Is there hearing loss?	Labyrinthitis more likely (no hearing loss with vestibular neuronitis).

- Ménière's disease is suggested if there is an abrupt onset of severe vertigo lasting for several hours to one day that is recurrent and associated with attack-related tinnitus (cause of most severe tinnitus; roaring sound), hearing loss, and a sensation of fullness in the ear.
- Vestibular neuronitis or labyrinthitis is suggested if there is a rather abrupt onset of severe vertigo (cause of most severe vertigo and nausea) associated with a prior respiratory infection lasting for several days and gradually diminishing over weeks; the distinguishing factor is whether hearing loss is evident, suggesting labyrinthitis.
- Chronic bilateral vestibulopathy results in nonspecific dizziness or disequilibrium. Often it creates the illusion that the environment is moving when the head is moved (i.e., oscillopsia). The most common cause is ototoxicity due to aminoglycoside use (i.e., certain antibiotics).
- Migraine-associated vertigo is suggested if vertigo precedes a headache. However, isolated vertigo attacks may also occur (i.e., migraine equivalent). Benign recurrent attacks of vertigo suggest migraine-associated vertigo.[27] Basilar migraine is clinically evident via posterior-fossa symptoms (e.g., vertigo, ataxia, dysarthria, and tinnitus) associated with abnormal visual phenomena. Basilar migraine is more common in adolescent girls.
- Transient vertebrobasilar insufficiency is more common in older patients as a cause of vertigo. It is unclear whether the cause is ischemia of the labyrinth, brainstem, or both; however, the source of blood supply to these structures and the vestibular nuclei and eighth cranial nerve is the vertebrobasilar circulation. Transient ischemic attacks (TIAs) are typically abrupt in onset; last for several minutes; and may be accompanied by nausea, vomiting, and vertigo. If the posterior circulation is involved, visual blurring, blackouts, diplopia, drop attacks, headache, and weakness and numbness of the extremities may accompany the vertigo. Risk factors are those for atherosclerosis including hypertension, coronary artery disease, diabetes, and hyperlipidemia.

The International Headache Society classification of migraine has a subcategory referred to as benign paroxysmal vertigo of childhood. This refers to multiple episodic attacks of disequilibrium, anxiety, or vomiting in otherwise healthy children. There is no suggestion of cause or management.

Vertigo that is mild and/or constant is always suggestive of a central problem, especially if associated with other neurologic signs or symptoms.

A more rare description of rocking, swaying, or bobbing sometime occurs after prolonged travel on a cruise ship or airplane. This is mal de debarquement syndrome. It is sometimes associated with migraine headaches.

Another description may be that the patient feels as though he or she is about to faint. This feeling also may be described as lightheadedness. This description is clearly one of decreased cerebral perfusion. It would be important then to determine whether this occurs while sitting, which would be more classically a common faint position, or whether it occurs on rising, which would be more suggestive of orthostatic hypotension. With orthostatic hypotension as a suspicion, a drug history would be the first avenue of concern. This inquiry would be followed by questioning regarding signs suggestive of diabetes, anemia, or cardiopulmonary causes such as congestive heart failure.

One of the most important context questions is, when does it occur? Lightheadedness on rising is suggestive of orthostatic hypotension, whereas difficulty with ambulation is suggestive of a proprioceptive problem. If the patient has more difficulty with dimly lit areas (especially an elderly patient), when not wearing corrective lenses, or with eyes closed a proprioceptive problem is likely. If the dizziness is apparent with certain head positions such as rotation, vertigo is more likely—more specifically benign positional vertigo.

When the patient complains of associated neurologic symptoms such as slurred speech or electric shock sensations down the arms, multiple sclerosis must be considered, especially in a middle-aged patient. Additional considerations are the use of drugs/alcohol and cervical trauma. It is important to obtain a thorough drug history to determine whether illicit use of drugs may be the cause or the side effect of a prescription medication. Medication interactions may cause dizziness, especially in the elderly. Some drugs that may cause dizziness are:

- Anticonvulsants, alcohol, and tranquilizers—through central nervous system (CNS) depression or cerebellar dysfunction
- Antihypertensives—postural hypotension
- Aminoglycosides—vertigo due to asymmetric hair cell loss, disequilibrium due to vestibulospinal reflex loss, and oscillopsia due to vestibular-ocular reflex loss

Examination

The examination process is dictated by suspicions generated from the history. If the patient's history is suggestive of a vascular cause, evaluation of cardiopulmonary status and perhaps laboratory evaluation are warranted. If the patient's history is more suggestive of vertigo, an evaluation for nystagmus is essential, as is some form of provocative testing. If the dizziness appears to be more disequilibrium, a search for cerebellar and proprioceptive dysfunction is the focus of the examination. Given that there is some variation and ambiguity in patient descriptions, a standard battery of screening tests should be performed on most patients in an attempt to clarify or confirm historical suspicions.

Nystagmus is a jerking eye movement that represents an external observation of a disproportional stimulus from the labyrinths. There are usually fast and slow components to this jerking eye movement. Generally, when there is a normal amount of vestibular neural output in one ear, the pathologic ear with decreased output will be the side of slow beating. It is important to recognize that some degree of end-range nystagmus is possible, especially in individuals with poor vision. Observation of nystagmus is possible visually and electrically. Electronystagmography (ENG) is a helpful adjunct to the more gross visual observation used in most offices. ENG may also detect peripheral and cerebellar nystagmus that has been hidden by gross observation because of the patient's ability to incorporate optic fixation reflexes. This is accomplished with special lenses or with the eyes closed. Gross observation can be passive, looking for spontaneous nystagmus without head movement, or active, using provocative maneuvers to elicit nystagmus. Assisting gross observation is the use of Frenzel lenses. These lenses are used to abolish the patient's ability to fixate visually on an object and have the added benefit of magnifying the patient's eyes. Generally, nystagmus accompanies a sensation of spinning. When there is no vertigo but nystagmus is present, a central neurologic cause should be suspected and a neurologic consultation should be sought.

The type of nystagmus may be helpful in distinguishing between peripheral and central causes. In general, the following statements can be made:

- A peripheral cause is suggested if the nystagmus is horizontal or horizontal-rotational, decreased by visual fixation, increased with gaze toward the fast phase of nystagmus, occurring in one direction yet bilateral, associated with position change, and associated with moderate to severe vertigo.

- A central cause is suggested if the nystagmus is variable, being often vertical, unaffected by visual fixation, present with the eyes open or closed, and associated with constant, mild vertigo.

Provocative testing can be positional or with the introduction of water into the ear—caloric testing. Caloric testing is cumbersome and is considered relatively insensitive for detecting inner ear causes.[28] Most chiropractors do not perform caloric testing, so the focus will be on positional, provocative maneuvers. The classic positional test is to begin with the patient in a seated or supine position and quickly place the patient in the opposite position. The Nylen-Bárány (also called the Bárány, Hallpike, or Dix-Hallpike maneuver) test starts with the patient seated, head turned 45° to the involved side, and quickly brings the patient into a supine position with the head tilted to the side of involvement and slightly extended (**Figure 18–1**). The responses that are monitored are as follows:

- Latency—a few seconds of latency are indicative of benign positional vertigo due to delay in crystalline movement and causing stimulation.
- Severity of dizziness—peripheral causes generally produce more severe dizziness.

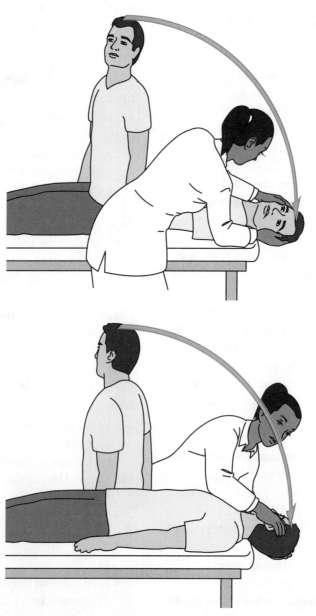

Figure 18-1 Nylen-Bárány maneuver.

- Direction of nystagmus—most peripheral nystagmus is rotational or horizontal; central causes often produce a vertical nystagmus.
- Adaptation and fatigue—if the nystagmus decreases after holding the position for 10 to 20 seconds or if the response to positioning decreases in severity with repeated attempts (dispersion of crystal particles), benign positional vertigo is suggested.

A simple in-office test of the horizontal vestibulo-ocular reflex is referred to as the head thrust test.[29] By prepositioning the patient's head 30° downward from neutral, the sensitivity of the head thrust test is increased. The patient's head is quickly turned from a neutral (forward facing) position observing whether the eyes are facing neutral. To perform the test, have the patient look straight ahead (i.e., at the examiner), head tilted 30° downward, then quickly rotate the head 10° to the left. The patient visually focuses on the examiner's nose. The examiner observes for corrective rapid eye movements (saccades), which indicate a decreased vestibular response. In other words, the eyes move with the head rather than remaining fixed to the visual target. If these "catch-up" saccades occur after a head thrust into one position but not the other, a vestibular lesion on the same is likely (e.g., eighth cranial nerve or root's entry into brainstem). Repeat on the right. Sensitivity and specificity are in the 80% range.

Testing for cervicogenic vertigo is performed with the rotating chair test. The examiner has the patient sit on a rotating chair. The first part of the test is to have the patient rotate his or her head from side to side several times to determine whether he or she becomes vertiginous. The examiner then stabilizes the patient's head while the patient rotates his or her body. Theoretically, the second maneuver eliminates direct semicircular canal participation yet allows stimulation of proprioceptors and the vestibular nuclei. It is suggested that vertigo reproduced with the head stationary and the body rotating indicates cervicogenic vertigo.

An attempt to differentiate vascular and other causes of dizziness may be made with a battery of tests. These tests are designed to detect vascular compromise via decreases in blood pressure or auscultation of bruits. If absent, a position of rotation and extension to each side is performed in an attempt to provoke signs of vertebrobasilar insufficiency such as dizziness, nystagmus, or visual signs such as diplopia. Unfortunately, there is

no clear evidence to support the use of these "screening" procedures.[30] They are considered insensitive and nonspecific.[31] Traditionally, chiropractors have used the maneuvers to protect the patient and also themselves (in the event of a post-manipulative vascular event). Yet there is disagreement as to whether this practice should be continued. It appears as though patients with dizziness provoked by extension or extension and rotation may in fact have other causes such as cervicogenic, benign positional vertigo, or a normal variant response. Brandt and Daroff[32] demonstrated that even healthy individuals may experience a to-and-fro vertigo and postural imbalance with head extension. Closing the eyes or standing on foam rubber augments this effect.

Patients who complain of imbalance or unsteadiness while standing or walking should be screened with proprioceptive testing. The main test is Romberg's. If the patient sways or loses balance only when standing with the eyes closed, a proprioceptive problem is the cause (i.e., a positive Romberg test). With the eyes open, visual input compensates. The Fukuda test is an extension of the Romberg test. The patient closes his or her eyes and walks in place. A positive response occurs when the patient rotates, usually to the side of the lesion.

Given spinal stenosis is so common in the senior patient, it is important to understand and test for signs of myelopathy. If the anterior cord is involved pain, pathological reflexes and/or hyperactive deep tendon reflexes or motor weakness may be evident whereas, if the posterior cord is involved, loss of dexterity, gait abnormalities, poor coordination, clumsiness, or sensory loss may the dominant signs and symptoms. Overlap may occur so that headache, neck stiffness, shoulder pain, paresthesia in one or both arms or hands, or other radiculopathic signs may also be present.

For patients with myelopathy, the following tests have been found to be specific but not sensitive:

- Gait or Balance—Both abnormal gait (ataxia, wide-based gait, or spastic gait) and a positive static or dynamic Romberg sign
- Pathological Signs—Hoffmann's sign, Babinski's, and clonus
- Deep tendon reflex changes—Hyperreflexia

The inverted supinator sign is probably the most sensitive test. It is similar to the brachioradialis reflex test with the patient's forearm placed in slight pronation on the examiner's knee. The examiner delivers a few quick strikes with a percussion hammer near the radial styloid process. A pathological response is slight finger flexion or elbow extension.

Specialized testing options to clarify a diagnostic suspicion further include ENG, brainstem auditory-evoked response (BAER), duplex Doppler scanning, dynamic posturography, and magnetic resonance imaging (MRI). In general, ENG is used to objectify a suspicion of vestibular pathology; BAER is used to identify a central lesion. Using surface electrodes and the delivery of a series of clicks through headphones, the neural signal can be divided into five potentials. Latency between potentials identifies the side of potential lesion. For example, latencies between I and II indicate an acoustic nerve lesion; between I and V or III and V indicates a brainstem lesion. Duplex Doppler scanning is used to determine blood flow in extracranial (and intracranial with transcranial three-dimensional Doppler) vessels, dynamic posturography is used mainly as a research tool, and MRI is used to identify a brain tumor or multiple sclerosis.

Management

- Refer to a medical doctor if systemic disease, drugs, or psychologic dysfunction is suspected as the cause.
- Refer for further evaluation if hearing or other neurologic deficits are found, a tumor or bacterial infection is suggested, or a perilymphatic fistula is suspected.
- Treat peripheral vertigo with chiropractic manipulative techniques, habituation exercises, and other appropriate conservative approaches.
- Refer if treatment is ineffective or dizziness creates significant functional impairment.

Given that the vast majority of dizziness complaints are benign, initial referral often is not necessary. Obviously, if a tumor, infection, hearing deficit, or drug interaction is suspected, referral is requisite. In the rare but serious event of vertebrobasilar ischemia, the most common symptom following the event is dizziness. Other symptoms/signs to consider include the five "Ds"—dizziness, diplopia, drop attacks, dysarthria, and dysphagia, and the three "Ns"— nystagmus, numbness, and nausea. Never readjust the patient if the patient complains of any of the above following an adjustment. See **Table 18–4** for a capsule summary of vertebrobasilar accidents. If the patient is vomiting and disabled by the dizziness, referral for medication seems appropriate,

although comanagement is often possible. Most causes of vertigo are usually due to abnormality of the vestibular nerve or labyrinth. Of these, the most common cause of vertigo is benign positional vertigo.[33, 34] In patient populations of both post-whiplash and the elderly, benign positional vertigo is common. Acceleration/deceleration injuries, in addition to causing a cervicogenic form of vertigo, may simulate Ménière's disease, or in some instances cause it.

Cervicogenic Vertigo

A history of neck trauma, muscle spasm, and restricted cervical range of motion (ROM); negative tests for peripheral or central causes of vertigo; or positive findings on the chair rotation test suggest a cervicogenic cause of vertigo. Theoretically, joint dysfunction may produce reflex muscle spasm or alter input to the vestibular nuclei.[35] The chiropractic approach is to reduce muscle spasm and free restricted movement through manipulation, with possible adjunctive therapy such as electrical stimulation, deep heat, myofascial therapy, or traction. Some practitioners[36, 37] claim a high degree of success. Generally, the research[38–40] supports a possible positive effect with cervical adjusting alone or in combination with other approaches such as vertigo exercises or biofeedback.

There are several difficulties with the designation of cervicogenic vertigo. It appears that there is often an overlap between cervicogenic vertigo and other peripheral vestibular vertigos such as benign positional vertigo and Ménière's disease. Second, although it is called *vertigo* it appears that many patients feel more of a disequilibrium, where they are pulled to one side, although rotary vertigo is also reported.

Benign Paroxysmal Positional Vertigo

There are several conservative approaches to BPPV. One approach is habituation exercises (**Exhibit 18–2**). These exercises are designed to fatigue the response to the positional stimulation of vertigo. In one study[41] in which patients acquired the provoking position several times every three hours, the success rate was quite high and was achieved in 3 to 14 days. A more sophisticated approach, the Vestibular Habituation Therapy test battery, attempts to identify various body and head position changes to develop an individualized series of training exercises. One study[42] indicated a 70% to 80% success rate in six to eight weeks of treatment with this approach.

Table 18–4 Vertebrobasilar Ischemia (VBI)/Accident Fact Sheet

Type	Summary Information
What is known about the ability to detect risk?	• There is no age or gender predilection. • Risk factors such as smoking, hypertension, alcohol consumption, or others have not been firmly established. • Testing is insensitive to the patient most at risk and may result in false positives for those not at risk.
How does VBI occur?	Trauma to arterial wall causing damage and/or vasospasm with the following possibilities: • Subintimal hematoma • Intimal tear with or without emboli • Dissection with subintimal hematoma (stenosis) • Dissection with pseudo aneurysm development • Perivascular bleeding
What are the most common presenting signs/symptoms of impending/existing VBI?	• Severe neck or head pain was the most common presenting complaint (often described as different than any previously experienced). • Dizziness is the most common symptom of VBI.
What are the possible risk factors for VBI?	• Precursor lesions • Fibromuscular dysplasia • Medial cystic necrosis • Behçet's disease • Rheumatoid arthritis • Giant cell arteritis • Osteogenesis imperfecta • Ligamentous hypermobility (e.g., Ehlers-Danlos syndrome, Marfan syndrome, osteogenesis imperfecta)
Is VBI testing, such as George's, sensitive or specific for VBI?	• Standard in-office testing cannot detect arterial anomalies, or pathology that predisposes to VBI. • Cannot detect arterial structural damage that exists prior to treatment. • Tests cannot be used to predict whether damage or reflexogenic spasm will occur. • Cannot distinguish between proprioceptive "dizziness" versus vascular "dizziness."
When do the signs of VBI appear with regard to occurrence?	• Symptoms of VBI appear in the practitioner's office 69% of the time. • Another 9% within 1 hour. • Another 14% within 24 hours (92% within first 24 hours).
What are the most common symptom/sign indicators of VBI?	Dizziness, drop attacks, diplopia, dysarthria dysphagia, nausea, numbness, nystagmus (the 5 Ds and 3 Ns)
What is the damage associated with VBI?	• Wallenberg syndrome—occlusion of PICA • Locked-in syndrome—basilar artery occlusion • Other brainstem injuries • Occipital, cerebellar, or thalamic injury
What is the prognosis for those patients who suffer VBI?	• The reported rate of death from dissections of the carotid and vertebral arteries is less than 5%. • 90% of stenosis resolves eventually. • 66% of occlusions are recanalized. • 33% of aneurysms decrease in size. • Improvement occurs primarily in the first 2–3 months after the dissection.
Are there specific adjustment techniques associated more with the occurrence?	Mechanisms are reported in the literature and have varied descriptions that may be overlapping or misleading. • 60%—Rotation • 10%—Rotation with extension • 4%—Rotation with flexion and hyperextension

Exhibit 18–2 General Habituation Exercises

The patient is taken through a structured, progressive program in an attempt to increase balance, increase independent eye-from-head movement, fatigue the peripheral response of specific head positions, and increase confidence in moving in a poorly lighted area.

The exercises are performed first seated and progress to standing. The exercises are first performed slowly and progressively increased to rapid performance. Following is a general outline of some exercises:

1. After determining the provocative head positions, have the patient either acquire the position and hold it for 30 seconds or repeatedly acquire the position several times until the sense of vertigo diminishes.
2. The patient practices moving the eyes up and down and side to side with the head remaining stationary.
3. Repeat the exercises while focusing on a finger held in front of the face.
4. Bend over to pick up objects 20 to 30 times.
5. Throw a ball from hand to hand while watching the ball (20 to 30 times).
6. Walk across a room 10 times with eyes open.
7. Walk across a room while turning the head slowly from side to side, attempting to focus on pictures or cards placed on the wall.
8. Walk across a room 10 times with eyes closed.

Based on a theory of cupulolithiasis and canalolithiasis, therapeutic maneuvers have been designed to "reposition" debris in the canals in an attempt to decrease inadvertent stimulation. One theory is that debris gets stuck to the cupula, making it heavier and more responsive to head movement. This is referred to as cupulolithiasis. The canalolithiasis theory is similar; however, the debris supposedly is floating in the long arm of the posterior semicircular canal, influencing the flow of endolymph and causing a secondary movement effect on the cupula. When a patient is sitting, a congealing of crystals occurs at the most dependent section of the posterior semicircular canal. Moving the head back and to the side (in the plane of the posterior canal) allows the crystalline clot to have a plunger effect. Standard maneuvers have been developed with numerous variations employed. Several reports indicate a relatively high rate of success, often with a single treatment. The average rate of success is between 66% and 92%, depending on the type of maneuver used and the time frame in which it is measured.[43, 44] Some argue that, because BPPV will resolve spontaneously in about one month in many cases, results measured after this time would not appear to be different from results with no treatment at all.[45] For the vertiginous patient, however, an earlier relief of symptoms is welcome. Two maneuvers are discussed below.

The modified Epley maneuver (**Figure 18–2**) attempts to move debris from the long arm of the posterior semicircular canal to the common crus.[43] The patient sits on the examination table with the head turned 45° toward the involved side. The examiner quickly lays the patient on his or her back, maintaining the head in 45° rotation. The patient is maintained in this position for 20 seconds, at which time the doctor rotates the patient's head to the opposite side over a 20-second period. Then the entire patient is rolled onto a side-lying position with the head turned 45° down (toward the floor) and left in the position for 20 seconds. With the head deviated toward the side that is not affected, the patient slowly sits up. Instructions are given following the maneuver to prevent otoconia movement. The use of a soft collar is a reminder not to quickly move the head, especially into neck extension.

The second approach is called the Semont maneuver (**Figure 18–3**). The attempt is to remove debris from the cupula (i.e., cupulolithiasis). The patient begins seated. The patient turns the head 45° away from the affected side. The patient is quickly brought down on his or her side, maintaining the previous head position. Vertigo is often experienced. The patient is maintained in this position for about four minutes, at which time he or she is quickly brought onto the opposite side, maintaining the same head position. If vertigo does not occur, move the patient's head through a few quick, short-arc ROM oscillations. After four minutes, the patient is brought back to the seated position slowly.

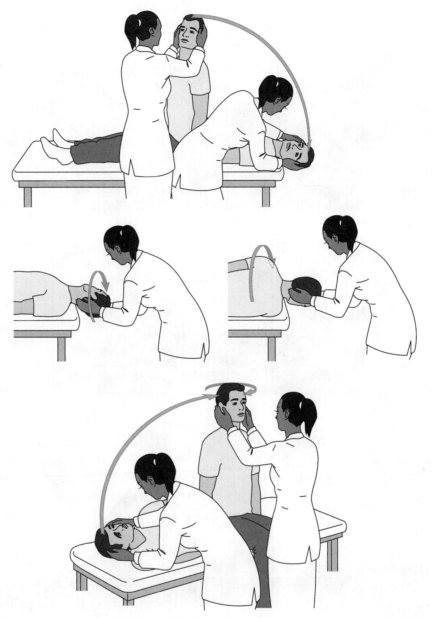

Figure 18–2 Modified Epley manuever.

Following either maneuver the patient should be given the following instructions:

- Wait 10 minutes before leaving the doctor's office; avoid sudden head movement; have another person drive you home.
- Sleep in a half-reclined (recumbent) position either in a recliner or propped up on pillows on the couch for the following two to three days; avoid sudden movements; avoid sleeping on the "bad" side.
- Avoid movements that will reproduce the vertigo; especially avoid head extension maneuvers such as looking to the ceiling, looking up to shave your chin (men), extension positions at the hairdresser or dentist, sporting activities (especially aerobics, sit-ups, swimming).
- Try to move slowly into the provoking position after one week; if still dizzy see the doctor for habituation exercises.

Ménière's Disease

The basic premise for management of Ménière's disease is that there is an imbalance in the production of endolymph. A recent study[46] suggests a dysfunction

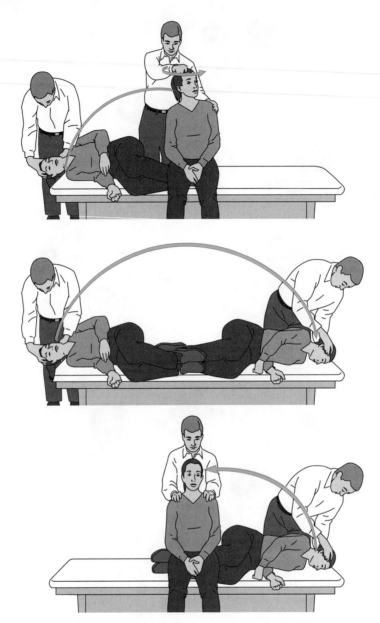

Figure 18–3 Semont's maneuver.

of antidiuretic hormone (ADH)-dependent control at the inner ear. Medical treatment has focused on the reduction of excess endolymph with the prescription of diuretics and salt-reduction diets. With this approach, approximately two-thirds of patients improve.

The natural course of Ménière's disease is gradually to "burn out" over months to years; however, the patient is often left with permanent hearing loss. Chiropractically, a course of nonmedical (herb) diuretic therapy coupled with a low-sodium diet may be helpful, combined with chiropractic manipulative therapy (CMT) for a short course to determine effectiveness. Some studies indicate the possibility of improvement with CMT.[47]

Medications used in the treatment of vertigo are usually one of several types, including antihistamines (meclizine, cyclizine), anticholinergics (scopolamine), and sedative/hypnotics (diazepam). These drugs are rarely needed except with severe attacks. It is worth mentioning that there is evidence that using these drugs in cases where there is vestibular disease decreases the ability of the CNS to compensate.

Algorithm

An algorithm for evaluation and management of dizziness is presented in **Figure 18–4**.

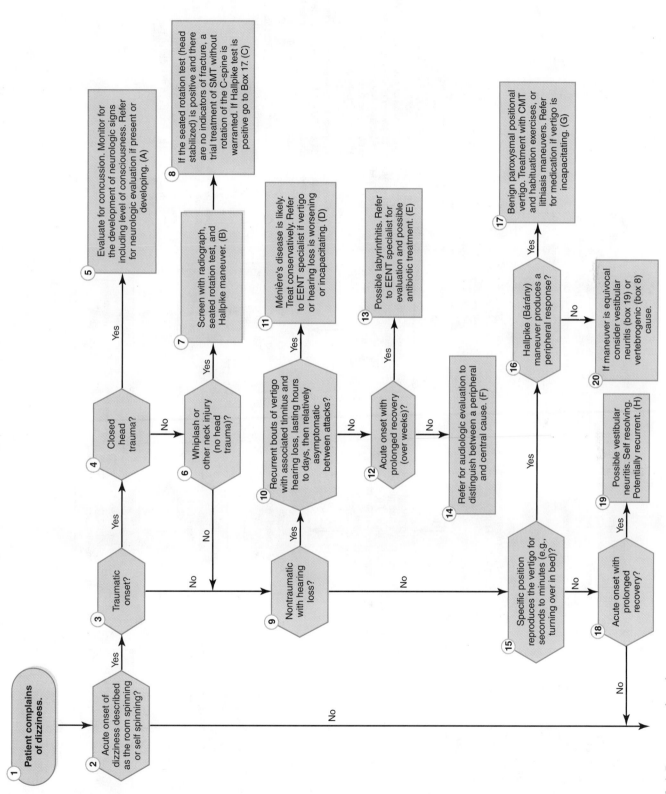

Figure 18–4 Dizziness—Algorithm

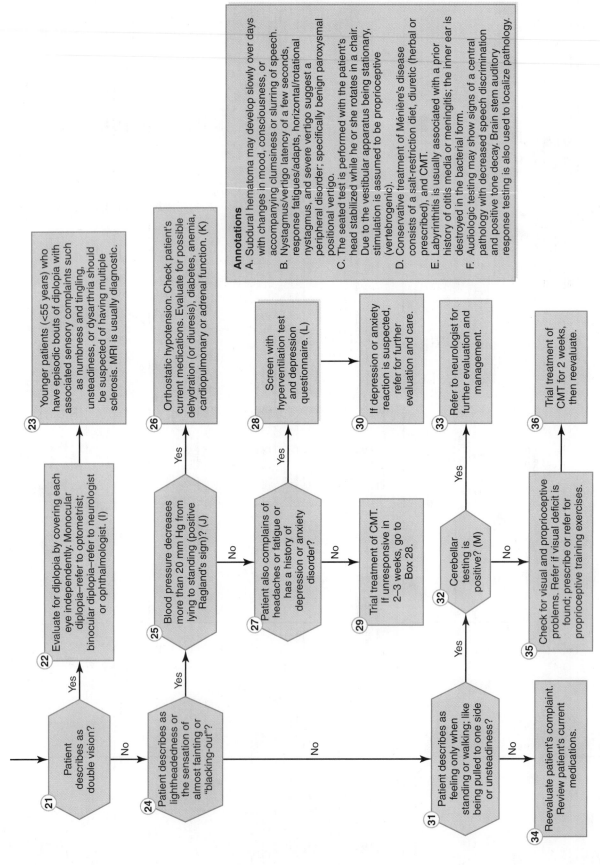

Annotations

A. Subdural hematoma may develop slowly over days with changes in mood, consciousness, or accompanying clumsiness or slurring of speech.

B. Nystagmus/vertigo latency of a few seconds, response fatigues/adapts, horizontal/rotational nystagmus, and severe vertigo suggest a peripheral disorder; specifically benign paroxysmal positional vertigo.

C. The seated test is performed with the patient's head stabilized while he or she rotates in a chair. Due to the vestibular apparatus being stationary, stimulation is assumed to be proprioceptive (vertebrogenic).

D. Conservative treatment of Ménière's disease consists of a salt-restriction diet, diuretic (herbal or prescribed), and CMT.

E. Labyrinthitis is usually associated with a prior history of otitis media or meningitis; the inner ear is destroyed in the bacterial form.

F. Audiologic testing may show signs of a central pathology with decreased speech discrimination and positive tone decay. Brain stem auditory response testing is also used to localize pathology.

23. Younger patients (<55 years) who have episodic bouts of diplopia with associated sensory complaints such as numbness and tingling, unsteadiness, or dysarthria should be suspected of having multiple sclerosis. MRI is usually diagnostic.

22. Evaluate for diplopia by covering each eye independently. Monocular diplopia–refer to optometrist; binocular diplopia–refer to neurologist or ophthalmologist. (I)

21. Patient describes as double vision? — Yes →

No ↓

24. Patient describes as lightheadedness or the sensation of almost fainting or "blacking-out"? — Yes →

25. Blood pressure decreases more than 20 mm Hg from lying to standing (positive Ragland's sign)? (J) — Yes → 26. Orthostatic hypotension. Check patient's current medications. Evaluate for possible dehydration (or diuresis), diabetes, anemia, cardiopulmonary or adrenal function. (K)

No ↓

27. Patient also complains of headaches or fatigue or has a history of depression or anxiety disorder? — Yes → 28. Screen with hyperventilation test and depression questionnaire. (L) → 30. If depression or anxiety reaction is suspected, refer for further evaluation and care.

No ↓

29. Trial treatment of CMT. If unresponsive in 2–3 weeks, go to Box 28.

No ↓ (from 24)

31. Patient describes as feeling only when standing or walking; like being pulled to one side or unsteadiness? — Yes → 32. Cerebellar testing is positive? (M) — Yes → 33. Refer to neurologist for further evaluation and management.

No ↓ (from 32)

35. Check for visual and proprioceptive problems. Refer if visual deficit is found; prescribe or refer for proprioceptive training exercises. → 36. Trial treatment of CMT for 2 weeks, then reevaluate.

No ↓ (from 31)

34. Reevaluate patient's complaint. Review patient's current medications.

Figure 18–4 (Continued)

Annotations (continued)

G. Habituation exercises require the patient to maintain the head in the provocative position or repeatedly acquire the position to fatigue the response. Lithiasis maneuvers attempt to reposition degenerative debris in the posterior semicircular canal.

H. Vestibular neuritis is thought to be due to a viral infection. There is no associated hearing loss. Recovery may be assisted with proprioceptive or habituation types of exercise.

I. Monocular diplopia suggests a refractive error or cataract (diplopia disappears when involved eye is covered; persists when uninvolved eye is covered). Binocular diplopia represents more often a neurologic cause such as extraocular muscle weakness due to tumor, diabetes, or myasthenia gravis (double vision disappears when either eye is covered; is present only when both eyes are open).

J. The normal sympathetic response to standing is vasoconstriction of splanchnic vessels (in particular veins) to maintain cerebral blood pressure. A drop in blood pressure after standing for 2 minutes suggest orthostatic hypotension.

K. Common drugs that may cause orthostatic hypotension include antihypertensives and antidepressants.

L. Short depression questionnaires include the Beck Depression Inventory and the Zung Self-Rating Depression Scale. The hyperventilation test is performed with the patient supine. The patient is instructed to breathe deeply for 2 minutes as the examiner feigns auscultation. If the patient reports the same sense of dizziness, anxiety-related hyperventilation may be the cause.

M. Cerebellar testing includes past-pointing, heel-to-shin, and quick repetitive pronation/supination of the hands. Direction of sway with Romberg's test may indicate the site of lesion in both labyrinth and cerebellar disorders. If swaying or loss of balance occurs only with the eyes closed, a proprioceptive problem peripherally or in the spinal cord (dorsal columns) should be investigated.

Figure 18–4 (Continued)

Selected Causes of Vertigo

Benign Paroxysmal Positional Vertigo

Classic Presentation

The patient reports episodes of vertigo that occur with certain head positions. The vertigo lasts for seconds to a couple of minutes. Common head positioning changes that precipitate attacks are head extension ("top shelf vertigo") or rotation, bending over and straightening back up, or rolling over in bed.

Cause

It is believed that BPPV is due to degenerative debris (otoconia) floating in the posterior semicircular canal. Either the debris sticks to the cupula, making it heavier and more responsive (cupulolithiasis), or the debris floats in the long arm of the canal, inappropriately causing endolymph to move the cupula (canalolithiasis).[48] Trauma and age appear to be important factors.[49] BPPV is the most common cause of vertigo.[34]

Evaluation

In addition to the patient's complaining of head positioning-specific onsets lasting for a few seconds, BPPV is also provoked by positioning maneuvers. The Hallpike (Nylen-Bárány) maneuver quickly positions the sitting patient into a supine posture with the head turned 45° to the same side.[50] A positive response is a small latency of a few seconds before vertigo and nystagmus begin. The vertigo is severe, and the nystagmus is usually horizontal-rotational to the same side. If the patient is left in the position or returned to the position several times, the vertigo fatigues.

Management

There are two main approaches: habituation exercises and otoconia repositioning maneuvers. Single-treatment responses appear to be effective (55% to 70%) when using a repositioning maneuver.[43] The intention of the maneuvers is to move the debris so that it no longer causes inappropriate stimulation. The two most commonly used methods are the modified Epley maneuver for canalithiasis and Semont maneuver for cupulolithiasis (see Figures 18–2 and 18–3). Habituation exercises take advantage of the fatigue and adaptation response of holding the head in the provocative position or repeatedly acquiring the provocative head position. In addition, exercises can be used to train independent eye movement and balance control. Rarely is medication or surgery considered a viable option.

Ménière's Disease

Classic Presentation

The patient complains of paroxysmal (sudden and recurrent) attacks of severe vertigo accompanied by low-tone hearing loss, low-tone tinnitus, and a sense of fullness in the ear. The episodes last for several hours to a day, with vertigo-free periods lasting for weeks or months. Hearing loss is progressive, while vertigo attacks appear to "burn out" over time. Some patients have sudden "drop" attacks without loss of consciousness.

Cause

Distention from either overproduction or retention of endolymph appears to be the cause in most cases. Specifically, there appears to be a problem with the endolymphatic sac's (immune processing area) and/or duct's filtration and excretion function with a possible autoimmune etiology. An association between high levels of ADH and stress has been found in Ménière's patients.[51] Head trauma or previous infection may be factors. Pregnant females may be more prone to attacks. Ménière's disease is considered the fourth most common cause of vertigo.[52]

Evaluation

Recurrent, sudden onset of vertigo with associated hearing loss or tinnitus is fairly diagnostic of Ménière's disease. Hearing loss is usually low tone, and the patient may also be found to have a positive recruitment phenomenon with sensitivity to loud sounds; a small increase in sound intensity is perceived as large. Both ears are affected in 30% to 50% of patients over time.[53] Patients who fit the vertigo pattern but do not have auditory dysfunction may have recurrent vestibulopathy. Some of these patients have basilar migraine while others progress to typical Ménière's disease.

Management

The primary conservative approach is based on the theory that increased fluid causes distention and symptoms. Therefore, diuretic therapy (herbal or prescribed) in combination with a salt-restriction diet may be effective in managing the vertiginous component of Ménière's disease; however, there is some debate as to whether this is a natural history overlap of effect.[54–56] For a few patients, surgical intervention using decompression of the endolymphatic sac has been performed; however, a Cochrane review found little scientific support for its use.[57] Other approaches include transtympanic gentamicin, intratympanic steroid therapy, and, for intractable cases, vestibular nerve section,[58] although, in one study,[59] half of patients had residual subjective complaints but 85% were satisfied with their decision. The possibility of an overlap between Ménière's disease and cervicogenic vertigo warrants a treatment trial of cervical manipulation in patients with Ménière's disease.

Vestibular Neuronitis (Neuritis)

Classic Presentation

The patient complains of severe vertigo that occurred rather suddenly and lasted for days to weeks. There is often associated nausea and vomiting. The patient says that lying still may help. There is no associated hearing loss.

Cause

The cause is unknown. However, it is postulated that there is a viral infection of the vestibular nerve because of the report of an antecedent respiratory infection in some patients.[60] Of patients with vestibular neuritis, 50% report having had a common cold.[61] There is an age-range peak at around 40 to 50 years of age. It is postulated that this disorder is a reactivation of a dormant herpes infection in the Scarpa's ganglion within the vestibular nerve. Involvement appears to be with the superior division of the vestibular nerve. The initial attack of severe vertigo, nausea, and disequilibrium generally lasts a few days. Although constant dizziness improves over days, rapid head movements will provoke vertigo and disequilibrium often for several weeks. Although often used interchangeably, labyrinthitis is usually reserved for involvement of both the vestibular and cochlear nerves. The primary differentials for vestibular neuritis are:

- Labyrinthitis, which is differentiated by also having hearing loss and often signs of bacterial infection (e.g., fever, chills, ear pain)
- Infarction or hemorrhage of the inferior cerebellum (25% of patients with risk factors for stroke who appear to the emergency department with complaints of severe vertigo, nystagmus, and disequilibrium have an infarction of the cerebellum)[62]

Evaluation

It is important to differentiate vestibular neuritis (peripheral) from cerebellar stroke (central). Nystagmus is made worse by looking in the direction of the unaffected side (Alexander's law) and is reduced by visual fixation with vestibular neuritis. Central nystagmus is not reduced by visual fixation and may change direction. There are often other neurologic signs and symptoms with cerebellar involvement such as dysarthria, ataxia, and difficulty with repeated supination/pronation or finger-to-nose testing and the patient's complaint is usually one of disequilibrium; not vertigo. Caloric testing demonstrates hyporesponsiveness or nonresponsiveness with vestibular neuritis.[63]

Management

Central compensation occurs, and the condition resolves over time. Even when nystagmus is present, it is important to begin vestibular training with having the patient focus on a target with head movement in all directions, and eye–head coordination exercises. Helpful exercises are to have the patient focus on a target while moving the head up and down and side to side. Balance exercises are incorporated as soon as possible. Medication may be needed during the acute phase. Antihistamines such as meclizine or cyclizine or anticholinergics such as scopolamine are often prescribed. The most effective medications for suppression of vestibular symptoms are the benzodiazepines such as lorazepam (Ativan) or diazepam (Valium). However, their use should be restricted to those who are able to stay home. Sublingual benzodiazepines are a good first-line approach. The caveat for the use of any vestibular suppressants is that it delays central compensation so symptoms may last longer.

Labyrinthitis

Classic Presentation

The patient complains of an acute onset of vertigo with (bacterial) or without (viral) hearing loss. Although the vertigo may improve over a week, sudden head movements may provoke the vertigo for weeks.

Cause

The distinction between labyrinthitis and vestibular neuritis is often not clear in the literature. One distinction is to call labyrinthitis that is bacterial, suppurative labyrinthitis. Another distinction is to call viral labyrinthitis serous. It is believed that either a viral or bacterial infection causes damage to the inner ear. Common viral causes include cytomegalovirus, mumps, varicella, or rubella. Common bacterial causes include Streptococcus pneumoniae, Haemophilus influenza, and Neisseria meningitidis. Bacterial infection may follow otitis media or meningitis, leading to complete destruction of the inner ear. Viral infection is less fulminant and may be reversible.[64]

Evaluation

The findings are the same as for vestibular neuritis plus there is some hearing deficit. Otoscopic evaluation may reveal an otitis media.

Management

Antibiotic therapy is beneficial with bacterial labyrinthitis. With viral causes, a tapered course of oral prednisone may be helpful, but results are varied. Physical therapy training for balance control may be utilized during the recovery period.

Perilymphatic Fistula

Classic Presentation

There is no classic presentation because the onset, intensity, and frequency vary. However, many patients have a history of barometric pressure changes, as with diving or air flight, or internal pressure development through intense weight lifting.[65]

Cause

An opening develops between the middle and inner ear (oval or round window rupture), allowing leakage of perilymph. Perilymphatic fistulas are a rare cause of vertigo.

Evaluation

Findings are variable; however, there is often a response to bearing down and provocation with pressure created by a pneumatic otoscope, which causes increased pressure in the ear.[66]

Management

Surgical management is often corrective.

Cervicogenic Vertigo

Classic Presentation

The patient complains of vertigo that is associated with maintaining certain head positions (not acquiring the position). There may be associated complaints of neck or suboccipital pain. There appears to be a history of trauma (such as a whiplash injury) in about one-third of patients.

Cause

It is believed that either overstimulation of upper cervical proprioceptors or degeneration of these proprioceptors or their pathways may cause an imbalance of information leading to a perception of vertigo or dysequilibrium.[37]

Evaluation

Findings of upper cervical soft tissue involvement and restricted movements are possible. The Fitz-Ritson rotation test may help differentiate.[33] The examiner stabilizes the patient's head while the patient rotates his or her body in a chair. If the patient becomes dizzy, a vertebrogenic source is suggested because it is believed that vestibular stimulation is eliminated with this maneuver.

Management

Chiropractic manipulation may be beneficial and should be applied as a treatment trial.[67] It is important to consider that because of the proprioceptive input of the upper cervical area, chiropractic manipulation may serve to benefit other causes of vertigo or that there may be an overlap between cervicogenic vertigo and other types.

Acoustic Neuroma

Classic Presentation

A patient in his or her 50s or 60s presents with a complaint of mild but constant hearing loss and dizziness sometimes with associated tinnitus. The onset is gradual and may be ignored initially. There are rarely acute attacks. Dizziness may be described as spinning but more often as off-balance.

Cause

A benign schwannoma of the vestibular nerve is called an acoustic neuroma. It is located in the cerebellopontine angle, where other cranial nerves are susceptible to compression. Most commonly this involves the facial nerve. As the tumor grows it may cause brainstem compression. Ninety-five percent of the time these are unilateral (bilateral may occur with neurofibromatosis). Associated risk factors may be smoking, pregnancy, and epilepsy.

Evaluation

Unless the tumor is large and pressing on other cranial nerves, there are likely to be no additional clinical findings. Auditory testing may reveal poor speech discrimination. Hearing loss is sensorineural. Stacked auditory brainstem response (ABR) is 95% sensitive and 88% specific for lesions < 1 cm (standard ABR only for lesions > 1 cm). When the suspicion is high, an MRI should be ordered. It is the definitive diagnostic tool.

Management

Age and growth rate need to be considered prior to a decision for surgical excision. Growth is about 5 mm in the first year of detection but less than 1 mm in the fourth year following detection.[68] Fifty-seven percent of neuromas shrink and 70% of extracanalicular lesions grow less than 2 cm per year.[69,70] Preservation of hearing is better with conservative management than with radiotherapy or surgery. A distinguishing factor is speech discrimination. Sixty-nine percent of patients with 100% speech discrimination on initial detection maintain their hearing 10 years after detection.[71] Options that are nonconservative include gamma-knife single-dose stereotactic surgery and three standard surgical approaches including retromastoid/retrosigmoid, middle cranial fossa, and translabyrinthine that use microscopic approaches.

APPENDIX 18–1

References

1. Kroenke K, Lucas CA, Rosenberg ML, et al. Causes of persistent dizziness: a prospective study of 100 patients in ambulatory care. *Ann Intern Med.* 1992;17:898–904.

2. Kroenke K, Mangelsdorff AD. Common symptoms in ambulatory care: incidence, evaluation, therapy, and outcome. *Am J Med.* 1989;86:262–266.

3. Herr RD, Zun L, Mathews JJ. A directed approach to the dizzy patient. *Ann Emerg Med.* 1989;18:664–672.

4. National Board of Chiropractic Examiners. *Job Analysis of Chiropractic.* Greeley, CO: NBCE; 1993:64.

5. Hinoki M. Neurootological studies on vertigo due to whiplash injury. *Equilibrium Res Suppl.* 1971;1:5–29.

6. Hinoki M. Vertigo due to whiplash injury: a neurological approach. *Acta Otolaryngol (Stockh).* 1985;419:9–29.

7. Chester JB, Jr. Whiplash, postural control, and the inner ear. *Spine.* 1991;16:716–720.

8. Hildingson C, Wenngren B, Bring G, Toolamen G. Oculomotor problems after cervical spine injury. *Acta Orthop Scand.* 1989;60:513–516.

9. Colledge NR, Wilson JA, MacIntyre CC, MacLennan WJ. The prevalence and characteristics of dizziness in an elderly community. *Age Ageing.* 1994;23:117–120.

10. Baloh RW, Ying SH, Jacobson KM. A longitudinal study of gait and balance dysfunction in normal older people. *Arch Neuro.* 2003;60:835–839.

11. Tusa RJ. Dizziness. *Med Clin N Am.* 2003;87:609–641.

12. Sullivan M, Clark M, Katon J, et al. Psychiatric and otologic diagnoses in patients complaining of dizziness. *Arch Intern Med.* 1993;153:1479–1484.

13. Jonson P, Lipsitz L. Dizziness and syncope. In: Hazzard W, Bierman J, Blass J, Ettinger W, Halter J, eds. *Principles of Geriatric Medicine and Gerontology.* 3rd ed. New York: McGraw-Hill; 1994.

14. Sloane PD, Harman M, Mitchell CM. Psychological factors associated with chronic dizziness in patients aged 60 and older. *J Am Geriatr Soc.* 1994;42:847–852.

15. Kroenke K, et al. Psychiatric disorders and functional impairment in patients with persistent dizziness. *JAMA.* 1993;810:530–535.

16. Fitz-Ritson D. Neuroanatomy and neurophysiology of the upper cervical spine. In: Vernon H, ed. *Upper Cervical Syndrome.* Baltimore: Williams & Wilkins; 1988:48–85.

17. Wyke B. Neurology of cervical spinal joints. *Physiotherapy.* 1979;65:72–76.

18. Suzuki I, Park BR, Wilson VJ. Directional sensitivity of, and neck afferent input to, cervical and lumbar interneurons modulated by neck rotation. *Brain Res.* 1986;367:356–359.

19. Sanes JN, Jennings VA. Centrally programmed patterns of muscle activity in voluntary motor behavior in humans. *Exp Brain Res.* 1984;54:23–32.

20. Rose PK, Keirstand SA. Segmental projection from muscle spindles: a perspective from the upper cervical spinal cord. *Can J Physiol Pharmacol.* 1986;64:505–507.

21. Brink EE, Jannai K, Hirai N, Wilson VJ. Cervical input to vestibulocolic neurons. *Brain Rev.* 1981;217:13–21.

22. DeJong PTVM, DeJong JMBV, Cohen B, Johngkees LBW. Ataxia and nystagmus induced by injection of local anesthetics in the neck. *Ann Neurol.* 1977;1:240–246.

23. Suzuki M. The effect of electricity of flowing electrode. *J Physiol Soc Jpn.* 1955;17:223–234.

24. Goodwin GM, McCloskey DI, Mathews PBC. The contribution of muscle afferents to kinesthesia shown by vibration-induced illusions of movement and by the effects of paralyzing joint afferents. *Brain.* 1972;95:705–748.

25. Bogduk N, Lambert G, Duckworth JW. The anatomy and physiology of the vertebral nerve in relation to cervical migraine. *Cephalalgia.* 1981;1:1–14.

26. Kentala E. Characteristics of six otologic diseases involving vertigo. *Am J Otol.* 1996;17:883–892.

27. Savundra PA, Carroll JD, Davies RA, Laxon LM. Migraine-associated vertigo. *Cephalalgia.* 1997;17:501–510.

28. Moller MR, Moller AR. Vascular compression syndrome of the eighth nerve. *Neurol Clin.* 1990;8:421–439.

29. Schubert MC, Tusa RJ, Grime LE, Herdman SJ. Optimizing the sensitivity of the head thrust test for identifying vestibular hypofunction. *Phy Ther.* 2004;84:151–158.

30. Ferezy JS. Neurovascular assessment for risk management in chiropractic practice. In: Lawrence DJ, Cassidy DJ, McGregor M, et al., eds. *Advances in Chiropractic.* St. Louis, MO: Mosby-Year Book; 1994;1:455–475.

31. Bolton PS, Stick PE, Lord RSA. Failure of clinical tests to predict cerebral ischemia before neck manipulation. *J Manipulative Physiol Ther.* 1989;12:304–307.

32. Brandt TH, Daroff RB. The multisensory physiological and pathological vertigo syndromes. *Ann Neurol.* 1980;7:195–203.

33. Drachman DA, Hart CW. An approach to the dizzy patient. *Neurology.* 1972;22:323–334.

34. Nedzelski JM, Barber HO, Milmoyl L. Diagnosis in a dizziness unit. *J Otolaryngol.* 1986;15:101–104.

35. Brant T. Cervical vertigo—reality or fiction? *Audiol Neurotol.* 1996;1:187–196.

36. Fitz-Ritson D. Assessment of cervicogenic vertigo. *J Manipulative Physiol Ther.* 1991;14:193–198.

37. Cote PC, Mior SA, Fitz-Ritson D. Cervicogenic vertigo: a report of three cases. *J Can Chiro Assoc.* 1991;35:89–94.

38. Galin R, Rittmeister M, Schmitt E. Vertigo in patients with cervical spine dysfunction. *Euro Spine J.* 1998;7:55–58.

39. Wing L, Hargrave W. Cervical vertigo. *Aust N Z J Surg.* 1974;44(3):275–276.

40. Bracher ESB, Ameida CIR, Almeida RR, et al. A combined approach for the treatment of cervical vertigo. *J Manipulative Physiol Ther.* 2000;23:96–100.

41. Brandt T, Daroff RB. Physical therapy for benign paroxysmal positional vertigo. *Arch Otolaryngol.* 1980;106:484–485.

42. Norre ME. Rationale for rehabilitation treatment for vertigo. *Am J Otolaryngol.* 1987;8:31–35.

43. Herdman SJ, Tusa RJ, Zee DS, et al. Single treatment approaches to benign paroxysmal positional vertigo. *Arch Otolaryngol Head Neck Surg.* 1993;119:450–454.

44. Harvey SA, Hain TC, Adamiec LC. Modified liberatory maneuver: effective treatment for benign paroxysmal positional vertigo. *Laryngoscope.* 1994;104:1206–1212.

45. Li JC. Mastoid oscillation: a critical factor for success in canalith repositioning procedure. *Otolaryngol Head Neck Surg.* 1995;112:670–675.

46. Takeda T, Kakigi A, Saito H. Antidiuretic hormone (ADH) and endolymphatic hydrops. *Acta Otolaryngol Suppl (Stockh).* 1995;519:219–222.

47. Lewit K. Ménière's disease and the cervical spine. *Rev Czech Med.* 1961;2:129–139.

48. Brandt T. Benign paroxysmal positional vertigo. In: Brandt T, ed. *Vertigo: Its Multisensory Syndromes.* New York: Springer-Verlag; 1991:139–151.

49. Davies RA, Luxon LM. Dizziness following head injury: a neurootological study. *J Neurol.* 1995;242:222–230.

50. Dix MR, Hallpike CS. The pathology, symptomatology, and diagnosis of certain common disorders of the vestibular system. *Proc R Soc Med.* 1952;45:341–354.

51. Sawada S, Takeda T, Saito H. Antidiuretic hormone and psychosomatic aspects in Ménière's disease. *Acta Otolaryngeol Suppl (Stockh).* 1997;528:109–112.

52. Brandt T. Vertigo—a systematic approach. In: Kennard C, ed. *Recent Advances in Clinical Neurology.* Edinburgh: Churchill Livingstone; 1990:59–84.

53. Paparella MM, Alleva M, Bequer MG. Dizziness. *Primary Care.* 1990;17:299–308.

54. Ruckenstein MJ, Rutka JA, Hawke M. The treatment of Ménière's disease: Torok revisited. *Laryngoscope.* 1991;101:211–218.

55. Sajjadi H, Paparella MM. Ménière's disease. *Lancet.* 2008;372(9636):406–414.

56. Thirlwall AS, Kundu S. Diuretics for Ménière's disease or syndrome. *Cochrane Database Syst Rev.* 2006(3):CD003599.

57. Pullens B, Verschuur HP, van Benthem PP. Surgery for Ménière's disease. *Cochrane Database Syst Rev.* 2010;2:CD005395.

58. Brookes GB. The role of vestibular nerve section in Ménière's disease. *Ear Nose Throat J.* 1997;76:652–656.

59. Reid CB, Eisenberg R, Halmagyi GM, Fagan PA. The outcome of vestibular nerve section for intractable vertigo: the patient's point of view. *Laryngoscope.* 1996;106:1553–1556.

60. Schuknecht HF, Kitamura K. Vestibular neuritis: second Louis H Clerf lecture. *Ann Otol Rhinol Laryngol Suppl.* 1981;31(6):901–919.

61. Furuta Y, Takusa T, Fukuda S, et al. Latent herpes simplex virus type I in human vestibular ganglia. *Acta Otolarygol Suppl (Stockh).* 1993;503:85–89.

62. Norving B, Magnisson M, Holtas S. Isolated acute vertigo in the elderly: vestibular or vascular disease. *Acta Neurol Scand.* 1995;91:43–48.

63. Brandt T. Vestibular neuritis. In: Brandt T, ed. *Vertigo: Its Multisensory Syndromes.* New York: Springer-Verlag; 1991:29–40.

64. Paparella MM, Sugiura S. The pathology of suppurative labyrinthitis. *Ann Otol Rhinol Laryngol.* 1967;76:554–586.

65. Lehrer JF, Rubin RC, Poole DR, et al. Perilymphatic fistula—a definitive and curable cause of vertigo following head trauma. *West J Med.* 1984;141:57–60.

66. Rizer FM, House JW. Perilymph fistulas: the House Ear Clinic experience. *Otolaryngol Head Neck Surg.* 1991;104: 239–243.

67. Huise M. Disequilibrium caused by a functional disturbance of the upper cervical spine. *Manual Medicine.* 1983;1:18–23.

68. Battaglia A, Mastrodimos B, Cueva R. Comparison of growth patterns of acoustic neuromas with and without radiosurgery. *Otol Neurotol.* 2006;27(5):705–712.

69. Smouha EE, Yoo M, Mohr K, Davis RP. Conservative management of acoustic neuroma: a meta-analysis and proposed treatment algorithm. *Laryngoscope.* 2005;115(3):450–454.

70. Stangerup SE, Caye-Thomasen P, Tos M, Thomsen J. The natural history of vestibular schwannoma. *Otol Neurotol.* 2006;27(4):547–552.

71. Stangerup SE, Thomsen J, Tos M, Caye-Thomasen P. Long-term hearing preservation in vestibular schwannoma. *Otol Neurotol.* 2010;31(2):271–275.

Seizures

Context

It is important to remember that not all seizures are epileptic[1] and not all epilepsy results in convulsive activity. Patients diagnosed as epileptic often are subject to restrictions (sports, driver's license, etc.) and biases. Therefore, it is incumbent on the evaluating doctor to make an effort to distinguish epilepsy from other causes of "seizures." Epileptic seizure activity may be benign or cause death through status epilepticus (an uninterrupted seizure) or cause the deaths of others if the patient is operating a car or other potentially lethal machinery. Those with true epilepsy often can be helped through medication or surgery.

Epilepsy and unprovoked seizures affect approximately 2.3 million Americans.[2, 3] Approximately 3% of individuals will have epilepsy during their lives. Although approximately 6% of adults will experience at least one afebrile seizure in their lifetime, only half of these adults will have recurring seizures (epilepsy).[4, 5] This must be considered prior to initiating medical management decisions. About 60% of childhood-onset epilepsy is due to birth and neonatal injuries, 15% to central nervous system (CNS) infections, and 12% to head trauma. With adult-onset epilepsy, 60% is due to CNS infarcts or hemorrhage, 10% to tumors, and 9% to CNS infections. Approximately 60% of seizures do not recur after one year, with 15% resolving some time later. Unfortunately, 25% are intractable. There appears to be a higher incidence in black men and in the elderly. Most of the black male occurrence is in middle-aged groups, possibly reflecting consequences of trauma or cerebrovascular disease.[6] Tumor accounts for the majority of seizures in patients between ages 25 and 64 years.[7] Other causes include cysts and vascular malformations. In the over-65-years age group, stroke, cardiovascular disease, tumor, and Alzheimer's disease are the main causes of seizures. Twenty-four percent of epileptic

patients are elderly, with 38% of new cases occurring in the elderly (with stroke accounting for one-third of cases).[8] If an adult has a seizure following moderate to severe head trauma, he or she is likely to develop epilepsy. Most will develop seizures within two years of the incident. Fortunately, about one-half will experience only a single seizure, 25% will have two to three future seizures, and the remaining 25% will have multiple seizures.

The incidence of a single, nonepileptic (nonrecurrent), unprovoked convulsive episode in children appears to be between 0.5% and 1%.[9] Most occur within the first year of life. Twenty percent of epileptic cases develop before age 5 years; 50% develop before age 25 years. Absence epilepsy (petit mal) accounts for 10% to 15% of childhood epilepsy, myoclonic epilepsy for 5%, and idiopathic localization-related epilepsy for 10%.

If a patient has a family history, the chance of a second seizure within the next two years is 35%. Even without a family history, the chance of a second seizure within the following 24 hours of a first seizure is about 15%.[10] These important facts must be kept in mind by the chiropractor, who with the best of intentions is trying to save the patient from the potential side effects of medication.

The direct and indirect costs for epilepsy in the United States were estimated at $3.6 billion in 1975.[11] The total cost to the nation in 1995 was estimated at $12.5 billion.[3] The impact on individuals with regard to educational achievement, employment, and psychological stresses is significant and sometimes insurmountable.

Patients do not often present to chiropractic offices with a complaint of seizures. However, there is the occasional patient who has anecdotally heard of or spoken to someone with seizures who felt that he or she had been helped by chiropractic care. Such patients usually are unhappy with the side effects of medication or are not completely controlled by their medication. They present as "last hope" patients. Although the author has heard from colleagues of resolution of seizures with chiropractic care, there are unfortunately few case studies and no large studies to help support the anecdotal "miracle" cures. One of the difficulties with interpretation of therapeutic effect is that the outcome measure has been eliminated. In other words, if the outcome measure is a reduction or elimination of seizure activity, the patient on medication is often well-controlled, eliminating the outcome to be measured. It is to be hoped that, within the next few years, those chiropractors who feel that they have had an effect will join together in publication to help generate interest in larger studies.

The context of a seizure patient's entering a chiropractic setting is fraught with difficulty. Often the patient is being controlled by medication and is dissatisfied with the drug's effect on his or her general sense of well-being.

The chiropractor is in the position of not being able to withdraw medication gradually to determine a therapeutic effect with manipulation. If a sudden withdrawal does occur, there is a strong risk of a rebound effect with an increased severity or frequency of attacks, including status epilepticus. It is imperative that the patient understand that any changes in medication are dictated only through consultation with the prescribing physician. Neither the patient nor the chiropractor should attempt withdrawal or reduction of seizure medication.

Realistically, the chiropractor may be especially helpful if he or she is at the scene of an epileptic occurrence. With his or her knowledge of different seizure types, the chiropractor may assist in management of an acute seizure. A list of "do's and don'ts," as recommended by the Epilepsy Foundation of America, is given in **Table 19–1**.

Table 19–1 Seizure Recognition and First Aid

Type of Seizure	Symptoms	First Aid	Don'ts
Tonic/clonic (grand mal)	Sudden cry, fall, rigidity (grand mal) Followed by muscle jerks, shallow breathing, bluish skin, possible loss of bladder or bowel control Usually lasts a couple of minutes Person may be confused and/or fatigued, followed by return to full consciousness	Look for medical identification Protect from nearby hazards Loosen tie or shirt collar Protect head from injury Turn on side to keep airway clear Reassure when consciousness returns If brief, single seizure, ask if hospital evaluation desired If multiple seizures or if one seizure lasts longer than 5 minutes, call an ambulance If person is pregnant, injured, or diabetic, call for aid at once	Don't put any hard implement in the mouth. Don't try to hold tongue; it can't be swallowed. Don't try to give liquids during or just after a seizure. Don't use artificial respiration unless breathing is absent after muscle jerks subside, or unless water has been inhaled. Don't restrain.
Single partial	Jerking may begin in one area of body, arm, leg, or face Patient stays awake and is aware Jerking may proceed from one area of the body to another, sometimes becoming a convulsive seizure May not be obvious to an onlooker Patient experiences a disturbed environment	No first aid necessary unless seizure becomes convulsive, then first aid as above No immediate action needed other than reassurance and emotional support Medical evaluation recommended	
Complex partial	Often starts with blank stare Followed by chewing, then random activity Person appears unaware of surroundings, dazed, mumbling Actions clumsy, not directed May run, appear afraid, and struggle or flail at restraint Lasts a few minutes, but postseizure confusion can last substantially longer	Speak calmly and reassuringly to patient and others Guide gently away from obvious hazards Stay with person until completely aware of environment Offer to help getting home	Don't grab unless sudden danger (such as cliff edge or approaching car) threatens. Don't try to restrain. Don't shout. Don't expect verbal instructions to be obeyed.

Courtesy of Epilepsy Foundation of America, © 1989, 1996.

General Strategy

Look for causes other than epilepsy (**Exhibit 19–1**):

- Determine whether the patient lost consciousness or whether there was convulsive activity of a body

part without loss of consciousness—nonepileptic causes often result in loss of consciousness due to hypoxia with associated convulsive activity.

- Determine whether the patient was given information from any witnesses detailing the

---

Exhibit 19–1 Differentiating between Epilepsy and Other Causes of Symptoms

Patient presents with a history of a "seizure."

Differentiate between epilepsy and other causes of convulsive activity.

Hypoxia or hypoglycemia	**Fever**	**Drugs**
Is there a relationship to eating (hypoglycemia)? Is there a history of hyperventilation (anxiety) or fainting? Is there a history of a heart problem (arrhythmia or murmur)? Is there a history of breath-holding?	*Do seizures only occur with a high fever? If they occur also at other times, is there a relationship to other factors?*	*Has the patient abruptly discontinued taking a prescription drug? Is there a history of "recreational" drug usage? Has the patient acquired prescription drugs from more than one physician?*

Differentiate among known causes of epilepsy.

1. **Vascular** (includes arteriovenous malformation, aneurysm, hemorrhage)
2. **Tumor**
3. **Head trauma**
4. **Metabolic**

If the patient has associated neurlogic symptoms such as headache, dizziness, change in personality, changes in level of consciousness, or obvious neurologic deficits such as paralysis, weakness, or persistent numbness and tingling, an organic brain lesion is likely. Are there triggers that the patient can identify, such as use of a computer, watching a fan, specific sounds or smells, etc.?

Differentiation requires a thorough neurologic examination. Referral to a neurologist should result in an EEG, CT, or MRI evaluation, and possibly an angiogram.

length of time that he or she was unconscious or length of any convulsive activity.

- Determine whether the patient had any pre- or postictal signs or symptoms.
- Determine the position and environment that the patient was in and whether these are consistent with any previous episodes.
- In an infant or child, determine whether there was an associated fever.
- Always determine the patient's use of medications and alcohol, and any sudden stopping of the medication regimen.
- Is there any history of toxic exposure (specifically, lead intoxication in children)?
- Is the patient diabetic?

If epilepsy is suspected, attempt to determine the cause and any triggers.

- Is there a family history? There may be a genetic predisposition (especially with generalized absence seizures or febrile seizures).
- Did the seizures begin before age 2 years? Ask about birth trauma and metabolic causes. Specifically determine whether there is a history of cerebral palsy, mental retardation, tumors/cysts, or hydrocephalus (all are often associated with epileptic seizure activity).
- Did the seizure activity begin between ages 2 and 20 years? Idiopathic epilepsy is likely.
- Did the seizures begin later than age 30 years? If yes, consider tumor; if over age 60, consider a vascular event or Alzheimer's.
- Is there a recent or past history of head trauma?
- What accompanies the seizure? Any auras? Any automatisms (i.e., purposeless repetitive movements such as scratching)? Any postictal findings such as extreme tiredness, headaches, or incontinence during the attacks?

Determine whether further testing is necessary.

- If a nonepileptic cause is suggested, lab testing may be necessary.
- For a firm diagnosis of epilepsy, an electroencephalogram (EEG) is necessary; often several 24-hour EEGs are needed using provocation such as strobe light stimulation or hyperventilation.
- If a tumor is suspected, refer for neurologic consultation, which is likely to include magnetic resonance imaging (MRI).

Definitions and Classifications

Specifically, an epileptic seizure is an event characterized by excessive electrical discharge due to a hyperexcitable group of neurons. The diagnosis of epilepsy is reserved for a recurrent history of such attacks. A seizure, however, is any attack of cerebral origin regardless of the cause. It becomes clear, then, how difficult it is to use these terms discriminately. Convulsions are involuntary contractions of muscles. They may be the result of epilepsy or a host of other causes. Convulsions do not always occur with epilepsy. Unfortunately, a patient could easily be mislabeled without a search for other causes.

Epilepsy that is inherited, without a known cause, is termed idiopathic. When associated with a suspected disorder or lesion, epilepsy is labeled symptomatic. Cryptogenic epilepsy refers to seizures that are secondary to a disorder or lesion, but whose cause is unknown. The most common classification system used is that proposed by the International League Against Epilepsy (ILAE).[12] This revised classification system is complex; however, there are some general points that would be useful to the nonspecialist. There are generally two classifications of epileptic seizures (see **Table 19–2**):

1. Generalized—simultaneous involvement of all or large parts of both cerebral hemispheres. Generalized seizures are often metabolic in origin.
2. Localization-related, also known as partial seizures—initiated in a discrete cortical site accompanied by related focal EEG and clinical manifestations. Partial seizures are the most common seizure disorder in adults, usually due to small, focal lesions such as scars or pressure effects from head trauma, strokes, and tumors. These seizures are further divided into simple partial seizures, in which consciousness is unimpaired, and complex partial seizures, in which consciousness is impaired. Complex partial seizures (psychomotor or temporal lobe epilepsy) account for 40% of all epilepsies.

Epilepsy is often classified based on clinical features such as complex partial seizures and generalized tonic-clonic seizures. Given that these are more syndromes than specific types of seizures, another classification scheme is based on type of seizure, the association or lack thereof of neurological or developmental abnormalities, and electroencephalogram (EEG) findings.

Table 19–2 Specific Aspects of Some Selected Types of Epilepsy

Classification	Clinical Features	Possible Mechanism/Cause
Generalized Absence epilepsy (petit mal)	Begins between age 4–8 years, but may occur as late as age 20 years. Rapid onset. Often after relaxing following physical or mental activity individuals stare, stopping other activity for up to about 10 to 30 seconds, then return to normal without memory of the event. This may occur tens or hundreds of times/day. May be confused with daydreaming or attention deficit disorder. The classic EEG pattern is three/second, generalized spike-waves. Seizures are provoked by hyperventilation in most individuals.	It is now believed that the mechanism is an abnormal circuit that causes rhythmic activation of the cortex (same as non-REM sleep), a thalamocortical circuit dysfunction. The reason for this dysfunction is not known. Theories include problems with T-type calcium channels, GABA receptor dysfunction, or brainstem modulation problems. Each may be targeted by specific medications, such as ethosuximide and valproic acid for T-type calcium channel blockade, or benzodiazepines inhibiting GABA receptors.
Generalized epilepsy with febrile seizures plus	A genetic (autosomal dominant with incomplete penetrance) disorder that results in febrile seizures plus one other type, such as absence, myoclonic, atonic, or tonic-clonic.	A mutation in the gene for voltage-gated sodium channel β1 subunit (SCN1B) associated with chromosome 19q. Leads to hyperexcitability of cortical neurons.
Benign familial neonatal convulsions	Autosomal dominant, single-gene mutation syndrome. Seizures begin within a few days of birth and resolve in a few weeks with or without treatment. There are no associated neurological or metabolic abnormalities.	Mutations in genes for potassium channels on chromosomes 20q and 8q, resulting in prolonged depolarizations that increase neuronal hyperexcitability.
Primary generalized tonic-clonic seizures (grand mal)	Loss of consciousness either without warning or preceded by myoclonic jerks. There is first stiffening (tonic stage) for about one minute followed by clonic jerks (i.e., convulsions involving all four limbs) that may last on average 1–3 minutes. Individual is slow to recover with possible tongue biting or incontinence during the seizure. Individuals are disoriented and recover slowly. Sometimes individuals are combative. Routine EEG (no seizure) reveals spike-wave patterns at 3–5 Hz.	Complex inheritance patterns.
Partial Simple partial seizures (focal)	Consciousness is not impaired. Signs and symptoms are motor, sensory, autonomic, or psychic, indicating seizure generation area. When motor-dominant and spreading down a limb, referred to as a Jacksonian seizure. When this persists as weakness or paralysis that lasts hours to days, it is referred to as Todd's paralysis. Routine EEG (no seizure) reveals focal slowing and/or sharp-wave activity.	Lesions or pressure cause altered neuronal function. This may include scarring from infection, vascular malformations, tumor, and trauma.
Complex partial seizures such as medial temporal-lobe epilepsy or psychomotor	Seizures usually begin with olfactory or gustatory hallucinations and epigastric rising sensations, or psychic symptoms such as déjà vu. If the seizures progress to a disconnection with the environment, the individual may stare blankly, speak incoherently, or exhibit automatisms such as lip smacking, or picking at clothing. Routine EEG (no seizure) reveals focal slowing and/or sharp-wave activity.	The most common lesion found is hippocampal sclerosis. There is some debate as to whether this is the cause or an effect of seizures.
Secondary generalized partial seizures (tonic-clonic or grand mal)	Same as primary except preceded by motor, sensory, autonomic, or psychic signs and symptoms, indicating seizure generation area. Then there is a loss of consciousness either without warning or preceded by myoclonic jerks. Tonic increase in muscle tone followed by clonic jerks that may last on average 1–3 minutes. Individual is slow to recover with possible tongue biting or incontinence during the seizure. Individuals are disoriented and recover slowly. Sometimes individuals are combative. Routine EEG (no seizure) reveals focal slowing and/or sharp-wave activity.	

When epilepsy results in loss of consciousness, there are two defined phases. The seizure itself is termed the *ictal phase*. The time following the seizure is referred to as the *postictal phase*.

Hallucinatory visual, auditory, olfactory, or other sensory aberrations are common. When they occur preceding loss of consciousness and last a few seconds, they are referred to as an aura. When they last longer than a few seconds, they are classified as a complex partial seizure. Additional signs of a complex partial seizure are referred to as automatisms. These include repetitive activity such as scratching an area of skin, lip smacking, or any repetitive movement.

Status epilepticus is a prolonged seizure that lasts longer than 30 minutes and may lead to death if not interrupted by medical intervention. The risk for permanent injury increases when the seizure lasts longer than five minutes. In children, about one-third who suffer from an episode of status epilepticus will have permanent neurologic damage (i.e., hemiparesis, microcephaly, mental retardation).[13]

Relevant Anatomy and Physiology

A seizure involves a sudden, abnormal electrical discharge in the brain. The normal asynchronous interaction of the cortical neurons suddenly becomes synchronous. Although the etiology of seizure activity is often unclear with epilepsy, generally it can be said that a decrease in either oxygen or glucose, an imbalance in electrolytes, or generalized toxic events may lead to a seizure episode. Other causes are direct damage through pressure or scarring of an area of the brain. Pressure is often due to either a tumor or vascular event, whereas scarring is often due to infection. The result is a dysfunctional cortical area that is, in many instances, hyperexcitable. With infection or trauma, it is not uncommon for the seizure to occur six months to as much as several years later, after scar tissue has formed. During a seizure, electrical impulses increase. For example, impulses of 80 per second are suddenly increased to 500 per second. In addition, this increased activity is uncoordinated. The resulting seizure activity is dependent on the specific area affected. Therefore, an epileptic "seizure" runs the gamut of emotional, motor, and sensory manifestations with and without loss of consciousness.

New Models of Epilepsy

Some new theories of partial epilepsy are:[14]

- *Neurogenesis:* Based on animal models, it appears that seizures can trigger increased mitotic activity in the dentate gyrus (specific to temporal lobe epilepsy), increasing differentiation and creation of new dentate granule cells.
- *Mossy-fiber sprouting:* Found with temporal lobe epilepsy, these extend to pyramidal neurons as part of the hippocampal output pathway.
- *Cortical malformations:* These may be involved with partial or generalized epilepsy. Theory is based on a disruption of development in the cerebral cortex classified as disorders of neuronal proliferation, neuronal migration, or disruption or reorganization of the cortex. These may be involved more with refractory epilepsy and specifically in cases once believed to be cryptogenic. Neurons within dysplastic areas may lack potassium channels or GABA-mediated inhibitory mechanisms.
- *Glial cell:* Glial cells, although primarily supportive, also serve functions of buffering that help maintain uptake of potassium and glutamate (among other metabolic balances). The result may be increased levels of extracellular potassium, decreasing the threshold for neuronal firing (hyperexcitability).

Evaluation

History

There appears to be an age-related association to epilepsy. The following list is based on age:

- Infancy–childhood: developmental, infection, trauma, cerebrovascular disease (CVD)
- Adult: brain tumor, trauma, developmental disorder, infection, CVD
- Late adulthood–elderly: CVD, brain tumor, degenerative disease, trauma

Important aspects of the history that might suggest a nonepileptic form of seizure include the following (**Table 19–3**):

- Loss of consciousness that was brief, with no postictal complaints
- No aura prior to loss of consciousness

Table 19–3 History Questions for Seizures

Primary Question	What Are You Thinking?	Secondary Questions	What Are You Thinking?
Did you lose consciousness?	Epilepsy, hypoxia, head trauma, syncope	Were you out for less than a minute? Did you hit your head? Did you feel any unusual feelings before passing out? How did you feel after regaining consciousness? Were you out longer than a couple of minutes? Were there any witnesses? Any history of irregular heart rhythm or do you feel any chest symptoms? (For a child) Did the child hold breath before passing out?	Syncope. Seizure due to hypoxia. Posttraumatic seizure or subdural/epidural hematoma. Warrants neurologic referral. An epigastric sensation or confusion would suggest epilepsy; lightheadedness suggests syncope. Extreme fatigue, soreness, headache, incontinence, tongue bleeding suggest grand mal seizure. Epileptic attack usually lasts 3–5 minutes. Describe sequence; especially how the person fell; any automatisms. Arrhythmia may cause LOC with convulsions due to hypoxia. Breath-holding is possible with children when they are angry.
Are you taking medications?	Side effect, withdrawal symptom.	Have you had a recent change in your prescription? Have you recently stopped taking the medication? Do you use recreational drugs or alcohol? How much?	Check Physicians' Desk Reference for side effect of medication. Antiseizure medication will often cause seizures when abruptly stopped. If abuse is suggested, refer to a counseling or specialized center.
(For infants or children) Did this occur with a high fever?	Febrile seizures.	Do they occur only with fever or at other times?	Febrile seizures usually do not indicate progression to epilepsy.
Is there a family history?	Epilepsy, inherited metabolic problems.	Any known metabolic disorders?	These usually occur in infancy. If epilepsy, chance of more seizures is increased.
Did this occur while you were conscious?	Partial epileptic seizures.	Did the seizure happen in your arm/leg?	Especially if it moves slowly up the arm it is suggestive of partial seizure.

Key: LOC: loss of consciousness.

- History of arrhythmias, diabetes, use of antidepressants and other medications, use of recreational drugs, psychologic problems, or possible electrolyte imbalance

There are generally two history findings that confuse the distinction between epileptic and nonepileptic seizures: (1) loss of consciousness (LOC), and/or (2) convulsions. Obtaining an eyewitness account and the patient's recollection of presyncope and postsyncope events goes a long way in differentiating between epilepsy and other causes. If LOC occurred upon standing, after prolonged standing (especially in a hot environment), or after feeling lightheaded and nauseated, the cause is less likely to be epilepsy. If the patient collapsed as opposed to falling stiffly when passing out, the cause again is less likely to be epileptic. Finally, if the patient did not experience significant ictal or postsyncopal signs or symptoms such as tongue biting, urinary or fecal incontinence, extreme fatigue, headache, or persistent achiness, the cause probably is not epileptic. Movement disorders such as shuddering attacks, nonepileptic myoclonus, tics and spasms, and paroxysmal choreoathetosis may be mistaken for epilepsy. Betts[1] feels that as many as 20% of patients referred to specialist centers for intractable epilepsy have nonepileptic seizures.

Febrile seizures are alarming to parents. However, only about 1% of cases proceed to tonic-clonic seizures, and only 5% of children will have status epilepticus.[15] Although the cause may be direct, such as with meningitis, most seizures are benign and do not indicate a propensity for future epilepsy or other neurologic dysfunction.[16] A family history is often found. With generalized absence seizures a family history is also found, often suggesting an inherited tendency toward a low-seizure threshold reaction to physiologic stresses such as sleep deprivation, fever, psychic stress, and repetitive stimulation (e.g., light flashes/photosensitivity).[17] One study[18] of inducing factors found that in adolescents common triggers were fatigue after exercise (15.2%), sleep disturbance (9.1%), and psychic stress and emotional change (15.1%).

The following are important facts about seizures and related causes or triggers:

- One rare but significant cause of seizure activity is an arrhythmia such as ventricular tachycardia of the torsades de pointes type. It is identified on an electrocardiogram as a P/long or prolonged QT interval (idiopathic QT syndrome).[19]
- Although antidepressants (and other drugs) have been targeted as causes of seizures, the rate is only 0.3% to 0.6%.[20] Predictive risk factors include a previous history of seizures, alcohol or sedative withdrawal, or multiple drug usages.
- One of the causes of nonepileptic seizures is a response to sexual abuse in childhood.[21] Two reactions have been studied. One is referred to as a "swoon," considered a cutoff reaction. The other is referred to as an abreactive type that may represent an acting out of the memory of abuse.
- Although video games have been accused of increasing the occurrence of epileptic seizures, one study[22] indicates that the risk is no greater than that for the general population.
- Seizures that are likely to be epileptic are those that are recurrent and often stereotypic for that patient.
- Recent evidence[23] suggests a relationship between migraine headache and epilepsy. Migraine is particularly prevalent in patients with centrotemporal epilepsy (63%; rolandic epilepsy). In patients with absence seizures, 33% had migraine, 7% had partial epilepsy, and 9% had a history of cranial trauma.[24]

Examination

The examination of a seizure patient should focus on nonepileptic causes first. This would include a cardiovascular examination, including blood pressure after lying down for three minutes and then standing (check for orthostatic hypotension), auscultation for any obvious chronic lung or heart abnormalities, and a thorough neurologic evaluation to determine any underlying neurologic disease. Further evaluation would include laboratory testing to determine the possibility of a metabolic association. Electrolyte, glucose, and blood cell evaluation should be used as an initial screen. Further evaluation is warranted when a specific metabolic disorder is suggested; this evaluation is best performed by the medical specialist. More and more, a reaction to use of or discontinuation of illicit drugs and alcohol is found, especially in the adolescent, young, and middle-aged adult in whom no other obvious cause has been found. Laboratory evaluation is often helpful. When pseudoseizures are suspected (due often to psychologic factors), a postictal prolactin estimation may help clarify whether a "true" seizure has occurred. After a major tonic-clonic seizure, there is usually a significant rise in serum prolactin levels.[25] This is not as noteworthy with partial seizures. If a baseline can be established and a subsequent level taken postseizure, an elevated level would be more suggestive of a true seizure.

The primary diagnostic tool in evaluating seizures is EEG. EEG coupled with clinical findings is likely to distinguish between generalized and localization-related (partial) seizures. Epileptiform EEG patterns (spikes and sharp waves) are characteristic of epileptic seizures. Although only 29% to 50% of patients with epilepsy show abnormalities on the first EEG, multiple testing yields abnormal findings in 59% to 92% of patients. This is increased with the use of provocative techniques such as hyperventilation or strobe light stimulation. Also sleep EEG and sleep deprivation–induced procedures are sometimes employed. Indications for the site of a source of initial seizure activity are sometimes represented by focal slowing in the form of delta waves indicating the presence of a mass or lesion. Another indicator is what is referred to as phase reversal between two adjacent electrodes, which helps localize specifically where the initiating ictal focus is originating from, again suggesting a mass or lesion.

When structural brain disorders are suspected (often based on the finding of localization-related seizures), MRI and other specialized imaging procedures may be helpful. MRI is usually more sensitive than computed tomography (CT) scan in uncovering cerebral lesions as causes of epilepsy.[26] Positron emission tomography (PET) may demonstrate abnormalities in about 70% of patients with temporal lobe epilepsy.[27] However, its use is probably more valuable for research purposes because it is generally unavailable and does not provide information beyond that gained from other imaging techniques.

Management

If the patient is having a seizure, based on a knowledge of the most common seizure types, quickly determine intervention needs based on recommendations from the Epilepsy Foundation of America (see Table 19–1).

If the patient is not having a seizure but has had a past diagnosis of epilepsy, review the history to determine whether the patient has had a full evaluation to differentiate between nonepileptic and epileptic seizures. If the patient has had a recent episode that has not been evaluated prior to presentation in your office, obtain a thorough history to determine any indicators of seizure type and refer the patient with your recommendations. If the patient wants chiropractic care, it is important to comanage the case with the prescribing physician to avoid patient misinterpretation and resultant changes in medication schedule.

The majority of epileptic cases are managed with medication. Those that are unresponsive and fit other criteria may be successfully treated with a variety of surgical procedures. The only predictors of seizure intractability are short-term unresponsiveness to medication, history of status epilepticus, and an initially high seizure frequency.[28] Many cases will resolve over time; however, 66% of patients remain on lifetime medication, in particular those who have seizures later in life. Some studies[29, 30] indicate that when epilepsy was untreated or minimally treated in some societies, the remission or inactivity rate was quite high (44%). With medical care, about 50% of children on medication for two years will remain seizure-free with gradual withdrawal of the drug(s) over a period of six weeks to one year. In four years, this rate increases to 70%.[31] Those who do not have remission over time are usually patients for whom the following factors apply:[32]

- There is a high frequency of seizures.
- There was a long period of time before medical therapy was initiated or before the seizures could be controlled through medication.

- There are associated neurologic problems such as mental retardation.

The primary drugs used in the treatment of epilepsy include carbamazepine, phenytoin, phenobarbital, and valproic acid. With the understanding that seizure activity represents, in part, hyperexcitability, the mechanism of action for many of the medications prescribed for epilepsy becomes more evident. The development of effective medications is premised on the basis that neurotransmitters that are primarily excitatory need to be diminished or blocked and those that are inhibitory need to be enhanced. Following are some common examples:

- Phenytoin (e.g., Dilantin) and carbamazepine (e.g., Tegretol) are part of a medication category termed glutamate antagonists. They block glutamate ionotropic receptors rendering ion channels less permeable to sodium and/or calcium.
- Benzodiazepines and barbiturates used in the management of many disorders are used as therapy for seizures due to their glutamate inhibition by GABA through hyperpolarization.
- Sodium valproate is able to effectively block the conversion of GABA to glutamate by blocking the transaminase enzyme responsible for this conversion.
- Ethosuximide is a specific T-channel blocker affecting the excitability of thalamic relay neurons. This then blocks these neurons from entering a burst-firing mode.

Note that anti-epileptic medications are used for other disorders based on these neuronal inhibitory effects, including prophylactic management of chronic headache and neuralgias such as trigeminal neuralgia and postherpetic neuralgias.

The major concern with medical management of epilepsy is the chronic effect on psychomotor and cognitive function.[33] Phenytoin and phenobarbital are of particular concern with long-term usage. A possible problem with AEDs is CNS toxicity, including sedation, dizziness, imbalance, diplopia, and nausea. Usually these are transient. Morbilliform rashes occur in 5% to 7% of patients. Common side effects for the three primary drugs include:

- Valproic acid (Depacon): tremor and weight gain
- Phenytoin (Dilantin): in young patients, gingival hyperplasia and hirsutism

- Carbamazepine (Carbatrol, Tegretol, Tegretol-XR) and oxcarbazepine (Trileptal): hyponatremia in patients who drink large amounts of fluids or are on diuretics

The specific prescription must account for several other variables, however, including seizure type, age of patient, ability to control with one medication, and other concomitant systemic or neurologic disorders (other medications, diabetes, other diseases). Partial seizures are managed with carbamazepine, phenytoin, phenobarbital, primidone, or valproic acid. Valproic acid is effective for most patients with generalized seizures. Valproic acid and ethosuximide are used for absence attacks.

Another concern with anti-epileptic medication is the risk to pregnant patients of having malformed infants. Although 90% of all pregnancy outcomes are unremarkable, the remaining 10% are abnormal and may be attributed to the possible teratogenic effect of seizure medication.[34] Unfortunately, none of the four major medications has been identified as the single culprit. There has been a suspicion that the birth defects were, in part, due to the seizures themselves or inherited tendencies from the mother. A recent study indicates that the cause is the AED when comparing mothers with epilepsy taking AEDs and those who did not.[35] The defects include major malformations, microcephaly, growth retardation, and some minor abnormalities of the face and fingers. It appears that supplementation with folic acid did not have an effect on decreasing these malformations. Suggestions for pregnant epileptics are to seek monotherapy drug treatment at the lowest effective dosage and to adhere to a diet with adequate amounts of folate (or supplement).

In addition to the standard primary medications, other medications are also being used. These include:

- Ethosuximide (Zarontin) and valproic acid (Depacon) as first-line treatment of childhood absence seizures
- Lamotrigine (Lamictal) and oxcarbazepine as initial treatment of partial-onset epilepsy
- Lamotrigine as an alternative treatment for absence seizures
- For patients who do not respond well to first-line therapy, topiramate (Topamax), levetiracetam (Keppra), gabapentin (Neurontin), tiagabine (Gabitril), and zonisamide (Zonegran)

Only about 50% of newly diagnosed epilepsy patients become seizure-free with first-line medical treatment.[36] About two-thirds will achieve good seizure control.

A generally held concept is that if the patient is seizure-free for two years, the patient can be gradually withdrawn from epileptic medication. More recently, with increasing data regarding risk of recurrence, it has been suggested that perhaps for some children, withdrawal could begin as early as six months or one year if the patient is seizure-free.[37] This is a complex decision; however, it is known that patients with partial seizures, neurologic abnormalities, epileptiform activity on EEG, or patients who have siblings with seizures have a much higher risk of recurrence. The parent and patient must be reminded that the prescribing physician must direct any decrease in medication use and that sudden withdrawal, in particular, could result in an increase in seizure occurrence or even status epilepticus.

For intractable childhood seizures, a diet developed in the 1920s, referred to as the ketogenic diet, may be of benefit. This radical diet is almost the antithesis of the "healthy" diet. The positive effects appear to be due to ketone body accumulation in the brain. A ketogenic approach consists of a diet high in fat and low in protein and carbohydrate.[38] A standard ratio is 4:1, which represents the ratio of grams of fat to grams of protein and carbohydrates. There is a very strict protocol, which includes a gradual introduction to the diet in a supervised, hospital environment and continued use at home after extensive training of parents coupled with a strong supporting staff of experts. Two recent large studies[39,40] reported the success rate in intractable patients to be about 55% if success is based on a 50% or more reduction in seizure occurrence. Both studies showed similar dropout rates after one year: about half of the starting number. They were due to ineffectiveness or the difficulties that arise from this extremely precise, restrictive diet. About one-fourth of the patients had a 90% reduction, and 10% actually became seizure-free. The subjects were patients for whom drug therapy was not effective. Apparently the diet must be strictly followed for long periods of time for the effect to be significant.

Experimentation with a new Food and Drug Administration–approved therapy shows some promise. The therapy, called vagal nerve stimulation (VNS), uses a small programmable pulse generated to deliver short bursts of electrical energy to the vagus nerve.[41] The device is implanted under the skin of the left upper chest, and the patient or partner can use a magnet to activate the generator if a seizure onset is perceived. The only known side effects at this time are hoarseness or change in voice quality.

Surgery is reserved for a special subgroup of epileptic patients. If it appears that the cortical area that is the cause of the seizure is identifiable and that surgical excision can safely remove this epileptogenic region without significant neurologic impairment, surgery may be an option. Most often these patients will be those with complex partial seizures and unilateral temporal lobe seizures.

For refractive epilepsy several options are available depending on the age, location, and type of lesion. Following is a list of current surgical options with related types that may be treated:[42]

- Resective surgery: The epileptogenic area must be delineated using several approaches to a convergent localization that allows accuracy in resection. Temporal lobe epilepsy is one example of epilepsy that may be responsive to resection.
- Multiple subpial transections: This is based on the knowledge that functional cortical organization is primarily vertical. Intracortical fibers that are generally responsible for seizures are horizontally oriented. Small parallel cortical slices are made perpendicular to the long axis of the gyrus in an effort to spare function. This procedure is used alone or in combination with resective surgery for seizures arising in or around motor, sensory, or language cortical areas.
- Gamma-knife surgery: This is a stereotactic delivery of radiation to a very specific point in the brain that has been identified using MRI. A delay

effect in results may occur as much as one to three years post-procedure. Currently, three types of epilepsy are being evaluated for success using this treatment: hypothalamic hamartomas, vascular malformations, and mesial temporal lobe sclerosis. In selected cases, success rates for cessation of seizures are around 75%.

- Vagal nerve stimulation: This is an adjunctive therapy with an effect of desynchronizing the EEG of the left vagal nerve stimulation through a subcutaneous lead. The device may decrease frequency of seizures by about 25%, but is not used as a cure-all.
- Deep brain stimulation: Experiments have been done to stimulate areas including the anterior thalamus, the centromedian thalamic nucleus, the caudate nucleus, the posterior hypothalamus, and hippocampus. Multicenter studies are now under way to determine effectiveness.

With correct patient selection, about half of patients remain seizure-free while another quarter or more have a significant reduction in seizure activity.[43]

Debate over the recommendations for driving privileges will continue. In 1994, the Joint Commission on Drivers' Licensing of the International Bureau for Epilepsy and the ILAE made joint recommendations.[44] They recommended against physicians being required to report all cases of epilepsy. They suggested an individual case-by-case assessment with the general recommendation

Table 19–4 Anti-seizure Medications			
Drug Class	**Examples**	**General Mechanism**	**Interactions/Side Effects**
GABA Agonists Benzodiazepines and barbiturates	Clonazepam Klonopin Rivotril	A benzodiazepine derivative that potentiates GABA and acts to inhibit seizure activity. Used alone or in combination with other medications for absence seizures, myoclonic seizures, Lennox-Gastaut, akinetic seizures, restless legs syndrome.	**Palpitations, dry mouth, anorexia, drowsiness, ataxia, sedation, respiratory distress, GI symptoms, diplopia, facial edema, hallucinations and other psychogenic problems.**
	Diazepam Apo-diazepam Valium Diastat Diazemuls Novo-Dipam Vivol	Drug of choice for status epilepticus; however, used as an anti-anxiety, sedative, muscle relaxant also. A long-acting benzodiazepine acting at the limbic, hypothalamic areas producing sedation.	**Vertigo, dizziness, fatigue, laryngospasm, thorax or chest pain, incontinence or urinary retention, hiccups, hypotension, cardiovascular collapse.**

(continues)

Table 19–4 Anti-seizure Medications (continued)

Drug Class	Examples	General Mechanism	Interactions/Side Effects
	Phenobarbital Barbital Luminal Solfoton	A long-acting barbiturate used primarily for the management of epilepsy (grand mal). Inhibits the reticular activating system, causes CNS depression, and raises the threshold for stimulation of the cerebral cortex. Also used for pre- and postoperative sedation in pediatrics and pylorospasm in infants.	**Causes CNS depression with possible extreme of coma and death. May cause usual GI symptoms, hyperkinesia, insomnia, nightmares, headaches, bradycardia, syncope, megaloblastic (macrocytic) anemia, agranulocytosis, thrombocytopenia, folic acid or vitamin D deficiency, if taken during pregnancy, birth defects (10%).**
	Gabapentin Neurontin	Related to gamma aminobutyric acid (GABA). Used as an adjunctive treatment of seizures; also used for herpes zoster.	**May cause tiredness, ataxia, dizziness or other CNS effects.**
	Topiramate Topamax	May affect GABA or kainite/AMPA receptors. Used in the treatment of partial seizures.	**May cause ataxia, dizziness, speech and psychomotor impairment.**
	Valproic acid Depacon	Possible augmentation of GABA neurotransmission by blocking conversion to glutamate; blocks transaminase. Used in the treatment of all seizure types.	**Severe hepatotoxicity possible, thrombocytopenia, and hyperammonemia.**
Glutamate Antagonists	**Carbamazepine** Carbatrol Tegretol Tegretol-XR	Sodium, potassium, and calcium currents are reduced across neuronal membranes decreasing neuronal transmission. Has an antidiuretic effect. Used in the treatment of seizures and facial neuralgias, also sometimes schizophrenia.	**CNS toxicity including sedation, dizziness, imbalance, and nausea/vomiting. Agranulocytosis or aplastic anemia. Also possible cause of birth defects.**
	Phenytoin Dilantin	Sodium, potassium, and calcium currents are reduced across neuronal membranes decreasing neuronal transmission. Used in the treatment of epilepsy (except absence seizures).	**CNS toxicity including sedation, dizziness, imbalance (ataxia), nausea, diplopia (nystagmus); also birth defects, hepatotoxicity, bone marrow suppression, and GI disturbances. Usually these are transient. Morbilliform rashes occur in 5% to 7% of patients; in young patients gingival hyperplasia and hirsutism**
	Lamotrigine Lamictal	May have an effect on glutamate/aspartate release and help in stabilizing neurons. Used in the treatment of seizures; in particular, partial seizures.	May cause dizziness, headache, nausea, diplopia, blurred vision, ataxia, tiredness.
T Channel blocker	**Ethosuximide** Zarontin	A succinimide anticonvulsant used in the treatment of seizures. Specifically, absence seizure, myoclonic and akinetic epilepsy. Acts to depress the motor cortex and elevate CNS threshold for stimulation.	May cause drowsiness, hiccups, ataxia, dizziness, headaches, lethargy, sleep disturbances, myopia, nausea, vomiting, epigastric discomfort, eosinophilia, thrombocytopenia, positive direct Coombs test, hirsutism, pruritic skin rash, gingival hyperplasia, and weight loss.

that there be a seizure-free period of one to two years. However, they felt that physicians should report those patients whom they believe pose a danger to themselves and to public safety. Risk factors for seizure-related motor vehicle crashes have recently been studied.[45] Only 54% of patients who crashed were driving legally. These individuals were not seizure-free. Twenty-five percent of patients had more than one seizure-related crash. Having a 12-month or longer seizure-free period reduced the odds of having a crash by 93%. Staying on or modifying medication and having reliable auras (fair warning to pull off the road) also aid in decreasing the odds of an accident.

With regard to sports participation, it is known that the following are risk factors and should either be avoided or the activity modified:

- Sleep deprivation or excessive fatigue

- Hypoglycemia associated with a poor diet (especially before activity)
- Hyponatremia (electrolyte loss) and hypernatremia (dehydration)
- Hypothermia (i.e., physical exhaustion and heat)
- Hypoxia associated with high altitudes

Sports participation should be avoided with high-contact sports. Solo participation or unsupervised participation in sports that involve speed or potential drowning should be performed in tandem or with supervision.[46]

Algorithm

An algorithm for evaluation and management of seizure is presented in **Figure 19–1**.

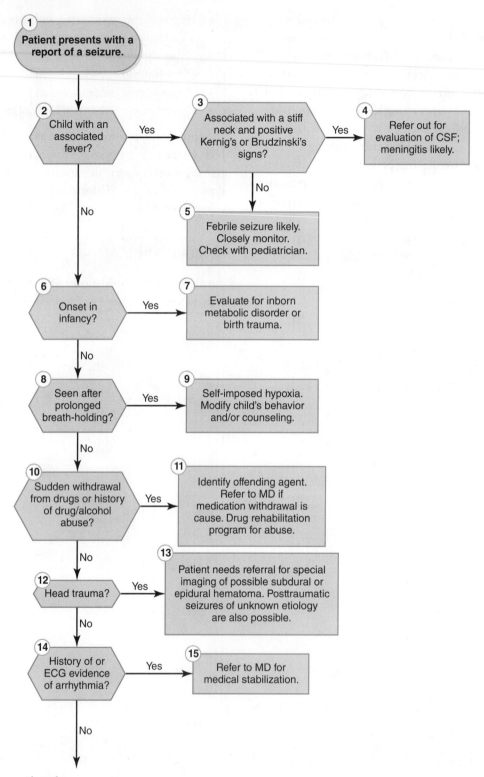

Figure 19–1 Seizure—Algorithm

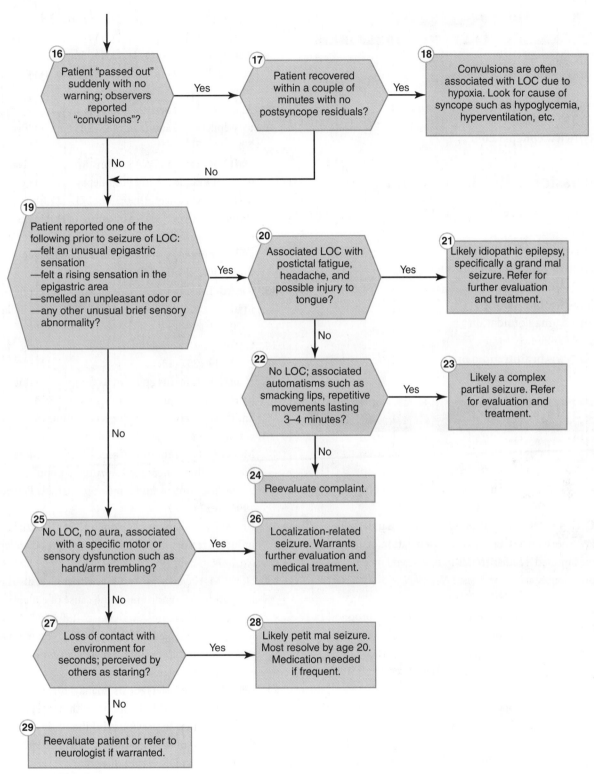

Figure 19–1 (Continued)

APPENDIX 19-1

Web Resources

Epilepsy Foundation
(800) 332-1000
http://www.epilepsy.com

Concussion with Brain Injury

National Institute of Neurological Disorders and Stroke
(800) 352-9424
http://www.ninds.nih.gov
Brain Injury Association of America
(800) 444-6443
http://www.biausa.org
Brain Trauma Foundation
(212) 772-0608
http://www.braintrauma.org

APPENDIX 19-2

References

1. Betts T. Pseudoseizures: seizures that are not epilepsy. *Lancet.* 1990;336:163–164.
2. Cockerell OC, Eckle I, Goodridge DM, Sander JW, Shorwon SD. Epilepsy in a population of 6,000 reexamined: secular trends in first attendance rates, prevalence, and prognosis. *J Neurol Neurosurg Psychiatry.* 1995;58:570–576.
3. Begley CE, Amegers JF. Epilepsy incidence, prognosis, and use of medical care in Houston, Texas, and Rochester, Minnesota. Presented at the American Epilepsy Society Annual Meeting; December 9, 1998; San Diego, CA.
4. So NK. Recurrence, remission, and relapse of seizures. *Cleve Clin J Med.* 1993;60:439–443.
5. Hauser WAS, Rich SS, Annegers JF, Anderson VE. Seizure recurrence after a 1st unprovoked seizure: an extended follow-up. *Neurology.* 1990;40:1163–1167.
6. Hauser WA, Headorffer DC. *Epilepsy: Frequency, Causes and Consequences.* New York: Epilepsy Foundation of America; 1990.
7. Ettinger AB. Structural causes of epilepsy: tumors, cysts, stroke, and vascular malformations. *Neurol Clin.* 1994;12:41–56.
8. Stephen LJ. Epilepsy in elderly people. *Lancet.* 2000;355:4–8.
9. Hauser WA. The prevalence and incidence of convulsive disorders in children. *Epilepsia.* 1994;35(2P, suppl):S1–S6.
10. Murray IM, Halpern MT, Leppik IE. Cost of refractory epilepsy in adults in the USA. *Epilepsy Res.* 1996;23:139–148.
11. Hart YM, Sanders JWAS, Johnson AL, et al. National General Practice Study of Epilepsy: recurrence after a first seizure. *Lancet.* 1990;336:1271–1274.
12. Proposal for revised classification of epilepsies and epileptic syndromes: Commission on Classification and Terminology of the International League Against Epilepsy. *Epilepsia.* 1989;30:389–399.
13. Aicardi JM, Chevrie JJ. Convulsant status epilepticus in infants and children: a study of 239 cases. *Epilepsia.* 1970;111:187–197.
14. Chang BS, Lowenstein DH. Epilepsy. *N Engl J Med.* 2003;349:1257–1266.
15. Hauser WA. Status epilepticus frequency: etiology and neurological sequelae. *Adv Neurol.* 1983;34:3–13.
16. Smith MC. Febrile seizures: recognition and management. *Drugs.* 1994;47:933–944.
17. Monetti VC, Granieri E, Casetta I, et al. Risk factors for idiopathic generalized seizures: a population-based case control study in Copparo, Italy. *Epilepsia.* 1995;36:224–229.
18. Konishi T, Naganuma Y, Hongo K, et al. Seizure inducing factors in patients with childhood epilepsy. *No To Hattatsu.* 1992;24:238–243.
19. Hordt M, Haverkamp W, Oberwittler C, et al. The idiopathic QT syndrome as the cause of epilepsy and nonepileptic seizures. *Nervenarzt.* 1995;66:282–287.
20. Rosenstein DL, Nelson JC, Jacobs SC. Seizures associated with antidepressants: a review. *J Clin Psychiatry.* 1993;54:289–299.
21. Betts T, Boden S. Diagnosis, management, and prognosis of a group of 128 patients with non-epileptic attack disorder, II: previous childhood sexual abuse in the aetiology of these disorders. *Seizure.* 1992;1:27–32.
22. Quirk JA, Fish DR, Smith SJ, et al. First seizures associated with playing electronic screen games: a community-based study in Great Britain. *Ann Neurol.* 1995;37:733–773.
23. Lipton RB, Ottman R, Ehrenberg BL, Hauser WA. Comorbidity of migraine: the connection between migraine and epilepsy. *Neurology.* 1994;44(suppl 7):S28–S32.

24. Septien L, Pelletier JL, Brunote F, Giroud M, Dumas R. Migraine in patients with history of centrotemporal epilepsy in childhood: a Hm-PAO SPECT study. *Cephalalgia.* 1991;11:281–284.

25. Rao ML, Stefan H, Bauer J. Epileptic but not psychogenic seizures are accompanied by simultaneous elevation of serum pituitary hormones and cortisol levels. *Neuro-endocrinology.* 1989;49:33–39.

26. Theodore WH, Dorwan R, Holmes M, et al. Neuroimaging in refractory partial seizures: comparison of PET, CT, and MRI. *Neurology.* 1986;36:750–759.

27. Henry TR, Engel JM, Marziotta JC. PET studies of functional cerebral anatomy in human epilepsy. In: Meldrum BS, Ferrendelli JA, Wieser HG, eds. *Anatomy of Epileptogenesis.* London: John Libbey; 1988:155–178.

28. Sillampaa M. Remission of seizures and predictors of intractability in long-term follow-up. *Epilepsia.* 1993;34:930–936.

29. Placencia M, Sander JW, Roman M, et al. The characteristics of epilepsy in a largely untreated population in rural Ecuador. *J Neurol Neurosurg Psychiatry.* 1994;57:320–325.

30. Watts AE. The natural history of untreated epilepsy in a rural community in Africa. *Epilepsia.* 1992;33(3):464–468.

31. Thurston JH, Thurston DL, Hixon BB, Keller AJ. Prognosis in childhood with epilepsy: additional follow up of 148 children 15 to 23 years after withdrawal of anti-convulsant therapy. *N Engl J Med.* 1982;306:831–836.

32. Emerson R, D'Souza BJ, Vining EP, et al. Stopping medication in children with epilepsy: predictors of outcome. *N Engl J Med.* 1983;304:1125–1129.

33. American Academy of Pediatrics Committee on Drugs. *Behavioral and cognitive effects of anticonvulsant therapy.* Elk Grove Village, IL: American Academy of Pediatrics; 1985;76:644–647.

34. Delgado-Escueta AV, Janz D. Consensus guidelines: preconception counseling, management, and care of the pregnant woman with epilepsy. *Neurology.* 1992;42(suppl 5):149–160.

35. Holmes LB, Harvey EA, Coull BA, et al. The teratogenicity of anticonvulsant drugs. *N Engl J Med.* 2001;344:1132–1138.

36. Kwan P, Brode MJ. Effectiveness of first antiepileptic drug. *Epilepsia.* 2001;42:1255–1261.

37. Greenwood RS, Tennison M. When to start and stop anticonvulsant therapy in children. *Arch Neurol.* 1999;5:1073–1077.

38. Kinsman SL, Vining EP, Quaskey SA, et al. Efficacy of the ketogenic diet for intractable seizure disorders: a review of 58 cases. *Epilepsia.* 1992;33:1132–1136.

39. Freeman JM, Vinig EP, Pillas DJ, et al. The efficacy of the ketogenic diet—1998: a prospective evaluation of intervention in 150 children. *Pediatrics.* 1998;102:1358–1363.

40. Vining EP, Freeman JM, Ballaban-Gil K, et al. A multicenter study of the efficacy of the ketogenic diet. *Arch Neurol.* 1998;55:1433–1437.

41. Camfield PR, Camfield CS. Vagal nerve stimulation for treatment of children with epilepsy. *J Pediatr.* 1999;134:532–533.

42. Nguyen DK, Spencer SS. Recent advances in the treatment of epilepsy. *Arch Neurol.* 2003;60:929–935.

43. Engel J, Jr, ed. *Surgical Treatment of the Epilepsies.* New York: Raven Press; 1987:553–571.

44. Fisher RS, Parsonage M, Beaussart M, et al. Epilepsy and driving: an international perspective. Joint Commission on Drivers' Licensing of the International Bureau for Epilepsy and the International League Against Epilepsy. *Epilepsia.* 1994;35:675–684.

45. Krauss GL, Krumholz A, Carter RC, et al. Risk factors for seizure-related motor vehicle crashes in patients with epilepsy. *Neurology.* 1999;52:1324–1328.

46. Sirven JI, Varrato J. Physical activity and epilepsy: what are the rules? *Phys Sports Med.* 1999;27(3):86–94.

General Concerns

Depression

Context

Most individuals think of depression as a reaction to an unfortunate and emotionally painful occurrence in their life. However, this is not the clinical entity referred to as major depression. The physician expecting his or her patients to complain of depression or to account for a "sad" feeling with a cause-and-effect narrative will miss the diagnosis in many cases.[1] Following hypertension, depression is the next most common chronic condition seen in an average primary care medical office.[1] Of these patients, approximately 10% suffer from major depression. Approximately 10% of men and 20% of women are affected by depression at some point in their life.[2] A recent large-scale study rated the lifetime prevalence for a major depressive disorder at 16.2% in the United States.[3] Major depressive episodes last an average of eight months. If onset of major depression occurs during childhood or adolescence, the risk of recurrence after a single episode is 40% in the next two years and 72% in five years.[4] Prevalence of depression in children is 1% and in adolescents it is 5%. Twenty percent of these cases are at risk for bipolar disease. In people with medical illness, depression is as high as 36% with conditions such as chronic fatigue syndrome, fibromyalgia, stroke, diabetes, rheumatic diseases, heart disease, certain forms of cancer, and renal impairment at the top of the list. Depression also appears to be a risk factor for coronary heart disease.[5] Another study indicated that depression is a possible risk factor for Alzheimer's disease.[6] With depression the chance of being affected by other medical illnesses and the use of medical services increases. The prognosis for these diseases is often less optimistic for depressed individuals. Almost half of adult patients with a major depression are not diagnosed by their primary care physician. It is obvious

that it is difficult to diagnose a disorder for which one does not understand the criteria. Patients with a major depressive disorder will account for between 5% and 13% of patients seen in a primary care setting.[7] (Zung[8] reports this estimate to be as high as 30% of patients.) There are a number of questionnaires available to evaluate patients with possible depression. A recent review of these questionnaires was performed by researchers. Their conclusion was that a clinical interview by a mental health professional or a semi-structured interview made by a primary care physician is able to diagnose major depression with high reliability.[9] A list of websites for many of these questionnaires is given at the end of this chapter.

Chiropractors may feel that depression is outside their scope of practice. The chiropractor, however, can play an important role in developing a diagnostic impression of depression and perform an appropriate referral. Although it would seem logical that patients would complain of depression to their caregiver, most patients with depression actually complain of physical symptoms. This transference from mental to physical is an unconscious process referred to as somatization. The chiropractor is key in identifying a somatizing complaint given musculoskeletal complaint, in particular spinal pain, is commonly reported by patients with depression. It may be that the treatment of major depression is the domain of the medical specialist, but comanagement may be appropriate when associated with musculoskeletal complaints. More important, when treating a depressed patient for a musculoskeletal complaint, the outcome of treatment may be seriously affected by underlying depression.

Depression has a major impact on the quality of life and the productiveness of the individual. Suicide is more common in depressed patients, with a suicide rate eight times that of the general public.[10] The societal impact of depression can be enormous. The annual indirect and direct costs of depression have been estimated at $44 billion.[11, 12]

General Strategy

History and Evaluation

- Ask the patient about mood disturbance: feeling "blue," "sad," "low," "not right."
- Determine whether the patient can associate a life event with this feeling, such as loss of a loved one, moving, divorce, leaving home, getting married, lack of social support, or occupational or school stress.
- Screen with questions regarding sleep disturbances, appetite changes, energy level, and loss of interest in previously enjoyed activities if depression is suspected.
- Look for a cluster of complaints that appear unrelated and reported as mild but persistent such as headache, dizziness, increased effort to breathe, and multiple joint complaints in patients who are somatizing.
- Observe all patients for suggestive signs in appearance, behavior, and thought content.
- Determine any past history or family history of mental illness and any past suicide attempts.
- Determine whether there are any current medical conditions that have been diagnosed. Some disorders associated with depression include chronic fatigue syndrome, fibromyalgia, rheumatoid arthritis, multiple sclerosis, chronic heart conditions, acquired immunodeficiency syndrome (AIDS), stroke, diabetes, renal failure, and Parkinson's disease.
- Determine whether the patient has given birth within the last year.
- Obtain a thorough drug history. Some drugs that may cause affective changes are glucocorticoids, anabolic corticosteroids, oral contraceptives, antihypertensives (especially methyldopa, guanethidine, and clonidine), H_2 antagonists such as cimetidine, anticonvulsants, antiparkinsonian drugs, and digitalis. Always investigate the possibility of alcohol abuse (CAGE questions, discussed later). Always check for use of any

stimulants; they may cause depression upon withdrawal.
- Consider using a questionnaire for patients suspected of having depression. Choose from the Beck Depression Inventory (BDI), Center for Epidemiologic Studies Depression Scale (CES-D), or the Zung Self-Rating Depression Scale (SDS).

Management

- Patients who appear to have a reactive depression should be referred for counseling if the depression appears to be disabling or causing a major disruption in job performance.
- Patients who appear to have a major depressive disorder, bipolar disorder, or mood disorder or those who have possible depression secondary to another illness or drug or alcohol abuse should be referred for medical evaluation and management of the depression.

Terminology and Classification

Relevant Anatomy and Physiology

With the advent of more sophisticated neuroimaging tools, some of the neurochemical/endocrine and structural relationships to depression are becoming evident. Some of these new advances in understanding relate to the nervous system's response to stress. Although the effects of depression and stress are better understood, the underlying cause of depression is only recently addressed through a genomic approach matched with a theory of genes and environment.

There is a vicious cycle initiated with stress:

- The cortex sends signal to the amygdala (a preconscious signal may arrive first).
- The amygdala is prompted to release corticotrophin-releasing hormone (CRH).
- CRH stimulates the brainstem to activate the sympathetic nervous system.
- Sympathetic activation causes the adrenals to release epinephrine, and a separate pathway causes the release of glucocorticoids.
- If the stress is chronic, glucocorticoids prompt the locus coeruleus to release norepinephrine.

- Norepinephrine stimulates the amygdala to release even more CRH.

The effects of chronic stress on the brain include:

- Release of glucocorticoids, epinephrine, and norepinephrine, which increases the risk of depression through dopamine depletion.
- Decreased stimulation of the raphe nucleus, which then decreases the release of norepinephrine from the locus coeruleus; this decreases attentiveness and possibly memory.
- Decreased secretion of serotonin from the raphe nucleus and possibly decreased number of receptors in the frontal cortex; this effects sleep and mood.
- Possible cell death and shrinkage of the hippocampus; those with serious depression have been shown to have a 10% to 20% decreased hippocampal volume.

There is mounting evidence that an individual's susceptibility to depression following stress is genetically related. One study recently found that individuals with one or two copies of the short allele of the 5-HTT promoter polymorphism exhibit more depressive symptoms than individuals homozygous for the long allele when exposed to stressful situations.[13] It appears that an individual's response to environmental factors coupled with genetic predisposition plays an important role in whether depression results from exposure to stressful life situations.

The terminology and criteria used to describe mental illness may be confusing. Terminology is often updated with new terminology; however, the older terminology is still used. Many psychologic disorders are overlapping, making distinct diagnosis difficult. An attempt at standardization has been made by the American Psychiatric Association (APA) through a task force that has provided updated classification and criteria for mental disorders in a manual called *Diagnostic and Statistical Manual of Mental Disorders* (DSM). The fifth (latest) edition (DSM-V) was published in 2012.[14]

Depression fits under a broad category of mood disorders characterized by disturbances in emotional, behavioral, cognitive, and somatic function. Depression is further divided into the following main types:

- Adjustment disorders with depressed mood
- Depressive disorders
- Bipolar disorders
- Organic mood disorders

Adjustment Disorders

Adjustment disorder is the new terminology for what was called exogenous, reactive, or situational depression. This is a common occurrence when a stressful life situation such as moving, divorce, job stress, or physical illness is "reacted to" with depression. This is considered a maladaptive reaction when the degree of response and type of response are out of proportion to the stressor. Depression is usually mild and lacks some of the diagnostic criteria for major depression.

Another similar type of depression is bereavement or grief reaction. Although it is a normal reaction to be depressed at the loss of a loved one, there appears to be a natural course of incapacitation that does not usually exceed six months. A prolonged grief reaction is disabling for more than six months. The patient demonstrates signs of a major depression disorder (loss of sleep, loss of weight, overwhelming sadness with crying, and isolation from friends/relatives) indicating the need for medication and psychotherapy.

Depressive Disorders

Depressive disorders are divided into major depression disorder (MDD) and persistent depressive disorder (which includes chronic MDD and the previously termed *dysthymia* for milder signs/symptoms). Major depression may occur as a single episode or recurrently. The hallmark of MDDs is a major depressive episode (MDE). Major depression is believed to be due to an imbalance in neurotransmitters, possibly genetically determined. The diagnostic criteria for MDE require that an individual experience a minimum of five out of nine symptoms almost continuously for two weeks; the nine symptoms are as follows:

1. Depressed mood that lasts most of the day, often worse in the morning; felt by the individual or observed by others
2. Loss of interest in previously enjoyable activities; unable to have fun, disinterest in sex or previously enjoyed hobbies
3. Disturbed appetite or change in weight; involuntary loss of more than 5% of weight in a one-month period
4. Fatigue or loss of energy felt every day
5. Disturbed sleep indicated by insomnia or hypersomnia; the classic pattern is terminal

insomnia—the person wakes up several hours early and cannot get back to sleep

6. Psychomotor retardation or agitation
7. Feelings of guilt, worthlessness, or self-reproach
8. Suicidal thoughts or focus on death
9. Inability to concentrate or make decisions

The major required criteria are depressed mood and loss of interest or pleasure in life. The criteria are also exclusive in that the patient must also not have an underlying secondary cause such as hypothyroidism, drug effect, stress at work, another mental illness, or bereavement. An MDE is also seen with bipolar disorders.

A more chronic condition in which many of the same symptoms for MDE are present in a milder form for at least two years in adults or one year in children and adolescents is called persistent depressive disorder (previously termed *dysthymia*). Other types of major depression are seasonal affective disorder (SAD) and postpartum depression.[15] SAD appears to be a dysfunction of circadian rhythms occurring more frequently in the winter. These patients respond to full-spectrum light. Postpartum depression must be differentiated from postpartum blues. Postpartum blues ("baby-blues") occur in the majority of new mothers, peaking around the fourth day post-delivery and resolving after 10 days. Although of concern, this common problem does not usually affect the mother's functional ability. Within the first month post-delivery there are large fluctuations of hormones in the mother. These fluctuations may lead to periods of sadness and emotional lability; however, the condition is self-resolving within weeks. Postpartum depression, however, is more likely to occur weeks or months after delivery and is characterized by thoughts about harming the baby or feelings of incompetence with regard to taking care of the infant. This disorder may occur in varying degrees of severity in approximately 13% of pregnancies. Postpartum depression is possibly more related to neurotransmitter imbalance than hormonal imbalance and requires medical management. Postpartum depression occurs in susceptible women as a result of withdrawal of gonadal steroids. However, other factors, such as a family history of mood disorders, a stressful life event, and past history of depression, are all risk factors and predictive of those at risk.[16]

Bipolar Disorders

Bipolar disorders are often alternating episodes of depression and mania. Manic depression is further divided into bipolar I and bipolar II disorders. Bipolar I is dominated by manic episodes that may alternate with depressive episodes. Bipolar II is dominated by depressive episodes that alternate with less severe manic periods that cause less impairment. Manic episodes are characterized by feelings of elation or euphoria, overactivity, constant offerings of plans or new ideas, and easy distractibility. Although these are not inherently bad traits, the individual is prone toward lability with regard to mood and can become easily agitated. Quick decisions and commitments are often regretted and abandoned, leaving a trail of alienated friends and relatives. The onset of bipolar disorders is generally at an earlier age than unipolar depression. Spring and summer appear to be periods when manic episodes surface. When the cycle of mania and depression occurs four or more times per year, the patient is referred to as a "rapid cycler." Substance abuse is often found in manic depressives in an attempt to keep the "highs" of the disorder.

For children who present with persistent irritability and frequent episodes of extreme behavioral dyscontrol, a new diagnosis called disruptive mood disintegration disorder is used in an attempt to caution medical doctors on over-diagnosing manic depression in children with the associated prescription of related medications and their effects. Like major depression, bipolar disorders may manifest as a milder, yet more chronic, dysfunction. For manic depression this has been called a cyclothymic disorder or, more currently, hypomania. Like persistent depressive disorders, the symptoms are milder, yet are constant for a period of at least two years.

Organic Mood Disorders

Organic mood disorders have an identifiable cause. The major categories are concurrent illness and medication induced. Many illnesses, especially chronic illnesses, can cause depression. Disorders such as rheumatoid arthritis, multiple sclerosis, cancer, AIDS, Parkinson's disease, and chronic heart disorders are commonly associated with depression. Depression may also occur in response to hormonal changes.

Drugs are an important cause of depression. Drugs may cause depression as part of normal usage or as part of a substance abuse pattern. Common medications that have been noted as potential causes of depression are corticosteroids, oral contraceptives, antihypertensives, antiparkinsonian drugs, and digitalis. All stimulant drugs potentially can cause a limited cycle of depression associated with withdrawal, including caffeine.

Evaluation

The Agency for Healthcare Research and Quality (AHRQ), through the Depressive Guideline Panel, has developed *Clinical Practice Guidelines: Depression in Primary Care*.[2] It contains a suggested approach to diagnosis and management. The focus of the AHRQ approach is detection of depression via a systematic evaluation that begins with a patient's appearance, behavior, and thought process and content. Therefore, both examination and history are occurring simultaneously in the evaluation of depression.

History

Patients with the following conditions may present with depression as a chief complaint.

- Hypothyroidism
- Hyperthyroidism
- Neurosyphilis
- Premenstrual disorder
- Postpartum blues/depression
- Dementia

Also take a thorough medication history cognizant that the following (among others) affect mood:

- Glucocorticoids
- Anabolic corticosteroids
- Oral contraceptives
- Antihypertensives
- H_2 antagonists such as cimetidine
- Anticonvulsants
- Antiparkinsonian drugs
- Digitalis

Noting current comorbidities is important because depression is more prevalent for patients who have Parkinson's, myocardial infarction (MI), stroke, end-stage renal disease, cardiac disease, and cancer.

It is important for primary care or first-contact physicians to be cognizant of the symptoms of depression. Although patients reporting to mental health specialists will likely report feeling depressed, those reporting to primary care physicians usually report other symptoms

due to somatization. Somatization is an *unconscious* psychological process that expresses psychological distress as physical symptoms. Suspicion should be raised when a patient presents with multiple complaints, especially if these include complaints of coexisting fatigue, sleep disturbances, mild headaches, dizziness, chest pains, and multiple joint pains. Depression is more common in women and in those who are single, divorced, or separated or who have a serious disease or a personal or family history of depression.[17] It is equally important to realize that patients may not voluntarily report the symptoms of depression, and a subtle fishing expedition is often needed. One opening approach is the HATAH question: **H**ow **A**re **T**hings **A**t **H**ome? This often reveals issues related to the fatigue and agitation often associated with depression.

The assumption by physicians is that patients who are depressed will say so, yet asking that one question is estimated to rule in depression with a yes answer to only around a 20% to 37% post-test probability and a negative answer (no answer) leaving the post-test probability still at 6% to 12%. The characteristic indicators are mood depression and a loss of enjoyment of activities that used to be enjoyable (anhedonia). Asking two history questions regarding depressed mood and anhedonia (loss of life's pleasures) has a sensitivity of 96% but a specificity of 57%, which means that additional questions are needed if the patient indicates a depressed mood or anhedonia.[18] Absence of these positives virtually rules out depression (assuming the patient is being honest). The application of a questionnaire based on the DSM-V criteria for depression is called the PRIME-MD.[19] A simplified, two-question approach is the basis for the PRIME-MD2 used for the purpose of screening for depression. The focus is on sadness and anhedonia. The questions are prefaced with "over the last two weeks . . . ." The next sequence in the evaluation is the Patient Health Questionnaire 9 (PHQ-9),[20] which utilizes the DSM-V criteria (nine elements) as questions with one additional question regarding the effect of these symptoms on work, home environment, or getting along with people. The patient is asked "over the last two weeks . . .?" The patient rates each element by choosing:

- Not at all = 0 points
- A few days = 1 point
- Half of days = 2 points
- Nearly every day = 3 points

An example of how this could be applied in practice would be, if there were a prevalence of depression of around 7% in a given practice, the following would be how probability would be estimated. If there is a positive response to the PRIME-MD questions and a score >10 on the PHQ-9 increases the post-test probability of depression to 49% to 59% whereas a PHQ-9 score of <10 decreases the likelihood to 1% to 4%.[21]

Factors that increase the likelihood for depression by 1.5 to 3.5 times are being female, having a chronic medical illness or chronic pain syndrome, recent life changes or stressors, rating personal health as fair or poor, or unexplained symptoms. **Figure 20–1** is a basic approach to utilizing the PRIME-MD and PHQ-9 in the screening and referral points for patients with suspected depression.

Attempts to determine if the patient meets the criteria for an MDE are set forth by the DSM-V (see Depressive Disorders above) including effects on sleep, appetite (weight loss), fatigue, memory/concentration, psychomotor retardation, and suicidal thoughts. While interviewing the patient, statements indicating a sense of guilt or worthlessness may surface. The patient may also be slow to respond and have difficulty concentrating or even remembering information. This finding has led to the term *pseudodementia*, which should be considered as an alternative to Alzheimer's disease as a cause of "forgetfulness" in the elderly.

When depression is suspected, a distinction among the various types should be made when possible. Questions regarding life stressors such as relationships and occupation are good beginning points. Common causes include loss of a loved one, postpartum periods, moving, leaving home, performance expectations at work, loss of money/property, and being a victim of abuse or violence. Reactions to these adverse situations may become over-reactive or prolonged, requiring psychologic counseling, or evolve into major depression requiring medical care.

In looking for secondary causes, it is important to ask about coexisting disease and to perform a review of systems to determine the possibility of an undiagnosed condition. Questioning regarding substance or alcohol abuse is important. The CAGE questionnaire[22] should be considered if alcohol abuse is suspected. It includes the following questions:

- Have you ever felt you ought to **C**ut down on your drinking?
- Have people **A**nnoyed you by criticizing your drinking?
- Have you ever felt bad or **G**uilty about your drinking?
- Have you ever had a drink first thing in the morning to steady your nerves or get rid of a hangover (**E**yeopener)?

A medication history is important in determining a side effect of medication or a reaction from withdrawal of stimulants. An endogenous source is suggested when there are indicators for depression but no identifiable cause. A familial tendency may be evident.

A caution is warranted for detecting depression in specific groups:

- Men may mask their depression through the use of alcohol, drugs, or even working excessively long hours. Unlike women who may admit feelings of hopelessness, men tend to be more irritable, angry, and discouraged.
- Depression in the elderly is often manifested as physical symptoms and complaints.
- Children who are depressed may pretend to be sick or worry about a parent leaving them or dying.

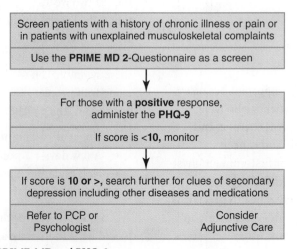

Figure 20–1 Algorithm for applying PRIME-MD and PHQ-9.

In older children, depression is more difficult to detect due to childhood/adolescent stages; however, getting into trouble at school, constant negativity, sulking, and antisocial behavior may be indicators.[23]

In addition to the above approaches for screening for depression, those patients with bipolar disorder require additional screening. Bipolar I (BP-1) is characterized by at least one manic or mixed episode that often alternates with episodes of major depression, whereas, bipolar II (BP-2) is a mood disorder that results in at least one episode of major depression and one episode of hypomania (milder form of mania). Three or more findings on a screening approach list called "DIG FAST" is helpful. These include:

- Distractibility—distracted often to irrelevant or trivial stimuli
- Insomnia—requires little sleep; often as little as three hours per night
- Grandiosity—inflated self-esteem and sense of infallibility
- Flight of ideas—the individual reports that their mind is "speeded-up" and racing and that the individual cannot slow down their thoughts
- Agitation or an increase in goal-directed activity
- Speech—individuals are overly talkative not leaving any opportunity for interruption
- Taking risks—individuals are excessively involved in seeking pleasurable activities that often carry a high potential for catastrophic consequences

Also, for self-assessment, individuals can take the Mood Disorder Questionnaire, which is easily accessible on-line.

Suicide

Given that depressed individuals have a higher incidence of suicide attempts, it is important to know the following about suicide attempts during a depressive episode:

- Risk factors include coexisting substance abuse, impulsivity and aggression, a history of abuse (physical and/or sexual), same-sex attraction and sexual activity, a personal or family history of suicide attempt, and access and/or plan for suicide.
- For children and adolescents, girls are more likely to attempt suicide; however, boys are more likely to succeed.
- 25% to 50% of BP-1 individuals attempt suicide, and 15% are successful

Even with treatment, it appears the risk for suicide may differ based on the type of medication used. For example, a recent study indicated that patients treated for bipolar disorder had a lower risk for suicide while being treated with lithium versus those treated with the most commonly prescribed mood-stabilizing medication in the United States, divalproex.[24]

Examination

The initial part of the examination begins while interviewing the patient. If the patient appears to be unkempt, and if his or her movements demonstrate either a slowness or conversely a restlessness or agitation, depression should be suspected.

The examination of a patient suspected of having depression is largely a search for underlying secondary causes. Thyroid screening may be appropriate when physical signs and history are supportive. Also, anemia, vitamin deficiency, cancer, or endocrine disorders may be unmasked by appropriate laboratory examination.

Management

For untreated major depression, 40% of patients will improve in six months to one year.[2] However, in 40%, symptoms last longer than one year, and in 20%, the improvement is not complete. Unfortunately, half of all patients with one depressive episode are likely to have at least one other. Also, with each recurrence, the chance of another recurrence dramatically increases (70% for those with two episodes, and 90% for three). Seventy-five percent of these recurrences were related to a provoking life event that caused major distress.[14] Many patients report a prodromal phase of both anxiety and mild depression prior to the recurrence.

The following are suggestions with regard to suspected depression.

- When the depression appears to be a reaction to an outside stressor and the symptoms are prolonged or acute, psychological counseling is warranted.
- If the depression appears to be the result of a medication, referral to the prescribing physician is imperative with a letter of explanation.
- When the cause is a secondary disorder, referral to the primary physician, if already diagnosed, is needed. If undiagnosed but suspected, referral to the appropriate specialist is necessary for proper management.

- If the suspected problem is major depression or manic depression, referral to a psychologist first may facilitate the referral to a psychiatrist. Many patients are reluctant to see a psychiatrist immediately.

The type of depression dictates the form of medical management. The types of management include psychotherapy, pharmacologic therapy, electroconvulsive shock therapy, and light therapy. Drug therapy alone is not a complete treatment for depression. Some form of psychotherapy should be combined with drug therapy or used as an initial approach with dysthymia. Psychotherapy approaches vary; however, the intention is to provide a supportive environment for management of the emotional component of dealing with depression. Cognitive and behavioral therapists use a directed approach, guiding the patient through assignments that target negative behavior and help direct appropriate responses. Psychoanalytic approaches attempt to focus the patient's attention on the past in order to interpret his or her current feelings in the context of his or her whole life experience. **Table 20-1** is a list of medications based on these categories.[25]

The basis upon which medical management has evolved follows the hypothesis development over several decades that is related primarily to the function of mainly three neurotransmitters: serotonin, norepinephrine, and dopamine. Also called the monoamines, these neurotransmitters are crucial to proper function related to, among others, emotion, sleep, appetite, sexuality, and reactions to stress. Medications either increase one or more of these monoamines, decrease their breakdown (e.g., monoamine oxidase inhibitors), or normalize receptor sensitivity. Although the neurotransmitters are often increased within hours of ingestion, it may take weeks for the effects to be felt by the patient. This delay may be due to a hypothesized receptor sensitivity reaction. Up-regulation may occur when decreased neurotransmitters are available leading to increased receptor sensitivity or an increased number of receptors. Medications may decrease this hypersensitivity or decrease the number of receptors through down-regulation. This may take several weeks, partially explaining the delayed effects of antihypertensive medications. The permissive hypothesis restates the cause of depression through a proposed *imbalance* of neurotransmitters versus their actual levels. For example, low levels of serotonin may allow proportionately high levels of norepinephrine to cause mania.

Following are examples of drug categories and mechanisms of action.

- Tricyclic (e.g., amitriptyline [Elavil, Endep] and doxepin HCl [Adapin, Sinequan]) and heterocyclic antidepressants (e.g., trazodone HCl [Desyrel])
- Selective serotonin reuptake inhibitor (SSRI; e.g., fluoxetine HCl [Prozac], paroxetine HCl [Paxil], and sertraline HCl [Zoloft])
- Monoamine oxidase (MAO) inhibitors

When stress reaction is managed medically, drugs such as Valium and Librium are used. These benzodiazepines inhibit the stimulation from the locus coeruleus to the amygdala, thereby decreasing subsequent sympathetic stimulation. These drugs are effective; however, due to their sedative and addictive properties they should be used with caution.

Lithium is still the standard for manic depression; however, patients with thyroid, kidney, or heart disorders should not take lithium. Other medications include two anticonvulsants, carbamazepine (Tegretol) and valproate (Depakote), and lamotrigine (Lamictal) and gabapentin (Neurontin). However, the role of gabapentin was apparently misrepresented, and although effective for other disorders it has not been shown to be effective for depression.

Newer drug approaches being tested include:

- Substance P: Mixed results have been found in clinical trials regarding substance P blockade as an indirect approach to managing anxiety and depression.
- Corticotropin-releasing hormone (CRH): Because CRH is released from the amygdala in response to stress, attempts are being made to block CRH receptors in the brainstem, breaking the cycle that is initiated by CRH.
- Brain-derived neurotrophic factor (BDNF): Injection of BDNF is being tested as a way of decreasing the neurological damaging effects of glucocorticoids.
- Gene therapy: For depression, genes placed in the hippocampus could create proteins that break down glucocorticoids.

For major depression without mania, most physicians will begin with a single tricyclic medication. It takes a minimum of three to four weeks and as much as six to eight weeks for the medication to be effective. If not effective, a second tricyclic or SSRI is used. Failing a response or for those patients with atypical depression (i.e., excessive sleep and weight gain), MAO inhibitors are prescribed. Antidepressants do work in approximately 80% of cases. The argument against drug therapy is that major depression may resolve without therapy in 6 to 12 months. Therefore, in those cases, drug therapy is simply assisting the person through a very difficult emotional period. Given that major depression may be self-resolving, it is recommended that the prescribing physician gradually reduce medication starting 6 to 12 months after symptoms have resolved. It should be noted that sexual dysfunction may be a side effect with many antidepressant medications. Some other possible side effects of these medications include:

- Drowsiness and sedation—tricyclics
- Insomnia and anxiety—SSRIs
- Orthostatic hypotension and cardiac arrhythmia—tricyclic and heterocyclic agents

- Weight gain—tricyclics, heterocyclics, and MAO inhibitors
- Delirium—interactions between tricyclic and heterocyclic compounds and SSRIs may cause what has been coined "serotonin syndrome," which results in excess cerebral serotonin stimulation

It is not unusual for a patient with a depressive disorder to have accompanying anxiety or a panic disorder. Up to 20% of patients with an MDD have a panic disorder. The panic disorder precedes MDD in about half of cases. It appears that these individuals are less responsive to therapy and are more prone to suicide attempts. Antianxiety drugs are often used as an adjunct to antidepressant medication. For patients with manic depression, the standard medication is lithium. Table 20–1 lists commonly prescribed medications for depression and manic-depression.

Electroconvulsive shock therapy (ECT), although sounding barbaric, is often an effective, painless approach to recalcitrant, disabling depression. ECT is

Table 20–1 Anti-Depressive Medications

Drug Class	Examples	General Mechanism	Interactions/Side Effects
Duloxetine	Cymbalta	Used in the management of depression, acts as a selective serotonin and norepinephrine reuptake inhibitor (SSNRI). Caution with narrow-angle glaucoma or patients taking MAOIs.	Fatigue, hot flashes, rashes, nausea, dry mouth, constipation, decreased appetite, decreased libido, insomnia, tremor
Aripiprazole	Abilify	A psychotropic drug used in the management of schizophrenia, bipolar disorder, and adjunctive therapy for major depressive disorder.	Not for elderly with dementia-related psychosis, also warnings for tardive dyskinesias, orthostatic hypotension, seizures, worsening of suicidal risk, neuroleptic malignant syndrome, hyperglycemia, and diabetes, cognitive impairment and body temperature regulation, nausea, vomiting, constipation, headache, dizziness, anxiety, insomnia
Imipramine	Impril Tofranil	Used for major depression and sometimes adjustment disorders, works by blocking reuptake of norepinephrine and serotonin by presynaptic neurons (classified as a tricyclic antidepressant). Reduces REM sleep and increases stage 3 NREM sleep.	Hypersensitivity reactions (anaphylaxis), drowsiness, extra-pyramidal symptoms, orthostatic hypotension, heart block, blurred vision, dry mouth, urinary retention
Alprazolam	Xanax	A benzodiazepine sedative causing CNS depression. Suggested sites of action are the limbic, thalamus, and hypothalamus. Used in the treatment of anxiety, panic attacks, insomnia, and muscle spasms. Also used as adjunctive therapy with depression (associated anxiety).	May cause lethargy; some concern over dependency/abuse and withdrawal problems

(continues)

Table 20–1 Anti-Depressive Medications (continued)

Drug Class	Examples	General Mechanism	Interactions/Side Effects
Amitriptyline	Elavil Endep	Increases levels of serotonin and to a lesser degree norepinephrine through inhibition of reuptake at the presynaptic neuron in the brain. It is used for depression and associated insomnia, restlessness, and nervousness. Also used for fibromyalgia and chronic pain.	May cause drowsiness, sedation, dizziness, orthostatic hypotension, tachycardia, increased appetite, weight gain, urinary retention, or constipation
Bupropion	Wellbutrin Zyban Wellbutrin SR	Inhibits the reuptake of dopamine, serotonin, and norepinephrine with the major effect on dopamine. Wellbutrin is used in the treatment of depression, while Zyban has been approved as an aid for smoking cessation.	Possible problems with seizures, hepatotoxicity, nausea, vomiting, headache, agitation, tremor, and anticholinergic effects
Citalopram	Celexa	A selective serotonin reuptake inhibitor (SSRI) (prevents reuptake at presynaptic neuron) making more serotonin available in the CNS. Used in the treatment of depression.	May cause fatigue, fever, arthralgia, myalgia, postural hypotension, anorexia, paresthesia, tremor, agitation, anxiety, migraine
Manic Depression			
Chlordiazepoxide	Libritabs Librium Medilium Novo-Poxide Sereen	A benzodiazepine that affects sleep by suppression of REM and increasing stage 4 NREM with an increase in total sleep time. Has a mild anxiolytic effect. Used primarily for anxiety and tension and assisting sleep in these individuals.	May cause drowsiness, lethargy, depression, orthostatic hypotension, dry mouth, vertigo, syncope, photosensitivity or urinary frequency
Chlorpromazine	Chlorpromanine Largactil Ormazine Promapar Promaz Somazina Thorazine Thor-Prom	A phenothiazine derivative that has alpha-adrenergic blocking effects, an anti-emetic effect through depression on chemoreceptor trigger zone, and antipsychotic effects through actions (blocks postsynaptic dopamine receptors) in the hypothalamus and reticular formation. Used in the management of manic phase of manic depression, for psychotic disorders such as schizophrenia, and for severe nausea and vomiting. Also, sometimes used for behavioral disorders in attention deficit disorder in children.	Many side effects; may cause neuroleptic malignant syndrome, sudden death, extrapyramidal symptoms, dizziness, tremors, drowsiness, EEG changes, pancytopenia, hypothermia, enlargement of parotid glands, infertility, reduced REM sleep dyskinesias, or seizures
Diazepam	Valium	A benzodiazepine. Binds to benzodiazepine site on GABA receptor complex. May cause dyskinesia inhibition through enhancement of GABA mediated chloride influx. Used for anxiety, nervous tension, and psychosomatic illness. May be used as an anticonvulsant or muscle relaxant.	May cause drowsiness, decreased consciousness, and other CNS effects
Doxepin	Adapin Sinequan Triadapin Zonalon	A tricyclic antidepressant that acts as a serotonin reuptake inhibitor and to a lesser degree norepinephrine also. Used in the management of depression and anxiety.	May cause drowsiness, orthostatic hypotension, dry mouth, metallic taste, photophobia, urinary retention, or weight gain
Lithium	Cibalith-S Lithonate Lithane Lithobid Eskalith	Competes with other ions and as a result accelerates catecholamine breakdown, inhibits the release of neurotransmitters, and decreases the sensitivity of postsynaptic receptors. Used in the treatment of acute mania and manic phase of mixed bipolar disorder.	May cause headache, lethargy, fatigue, recent memory loss, nausea, vomiting, abdominal pain, nephrogenic diabetes insipidus, fine hand tremors, muscle weakness, and reversible leukocytosis; rare peripheral vascular collapse

Table 20–1 Anti-Depressive Medications (continued)

Drug Class	Examples	General Mechanism	Interactions/Side Effects
Lorazepam	Ativan	A benzodiazepine used for anti-anxiety. Acts to enhance the effects of GABA particularly in the thalamus, hypothalamus, and limbic areas. It is the most potent of the benzodiazepines but has fewer interactions and less toxic than most other benzodiazepines. Also used for insomnia and panic attacks.	Many side effects disappear with continued use including anterograde amnesia, weakness, dizziness, sedation, restlessness, hallucinations, hyper- or hypotension, blurred vision, or depressed hearing
Nortriptyline	Aventyl Pamelor	Tricyclic antidepressants that act as a serotonin reuptake inhibitor and to a lesser degree norepinephrine also. Used in the management of depression and anxiety.	May cause drowsiness, orthostatic hypotension, dry mouth, metallic taste, photophobia, urinary retention, or weight gain
Paroxetine	Paxil	A selective serotonin reuptake inhibitor (SSRI) making more serotonin available in the CNS. Used in the treatment of depression and obsessive-compulsive disorders.	May cause nausea, vomiting, weakness, dizziness, agitation, insomnia, headaches, or abnormal ejaculation
Phenelzine	Nardil	A monoamine oxidase (MAO) inhibitor in the management of depression. Increases available levels of serotonin and norepinephrine. Also may affect the hepatic microsomal enzymes that metabolize drugs, prolonging the effects of these drugs.	May cause orthostatic hypotension, dry mouth, dizziness, constipation, anorexia, blurred vision, tremors, or muscle twitching; caution for hypertensive crisis when ingesting foods containing tyramine
Prochlorperazine	Compazine Stemetil	A phenothiazine derivative that has alpha-adrenergic blocking effects, an anti-emetic effect through depression on chemoreceptor trigger zone, and antipsychotic effects through actions (blocks postsynaptic dopamine receptors) in the hypothalamus and reticular formation. Used in the management of manic phase of manic depression, for psychotic disorders such as schizophrenia, and for severe nausea and vomiting. Also, sometimes used for behavioral disorders in attention deficit disorder in children.	Many side effects; may cause neuroleptic malignant syndrome, sudden death, extrapyramidal symptoms, dizziness, tremors, drowsiness, EEG changes, pancytopenia, hypothermia, enlargement of parotid glands, infertility, reduced REM sleep, dyskinesias, or seizures
Sertraline	Zoloft	A selective serotonin reuptake inhibitor (SSRI) making more serotonin available in the CNS. Used in the treatment of depression and obsessive-compulsive disorders.	May cause nausea, diarrhea, dry mouth, dizziness, insomnia, fatigue, or impotence
Tranylcypromine	Parnate	A monoamine oxidase (MAO) inhibitor used as a last-choice treatment for those unresponsive to other MAOs in the management of depression.	May cause orthostatic hypotension, dry mouth, dizziness, anorexia, blurred vision, tremors, or muscle twitching; caution for hypertensive crisis when ingesting foods containing tyramine
Trazodone	Desyrel	Inhibits the reuptake of dopamine, serotonin, and norepinephrine with the major effect on serotonin. Used in the treatment of depression and also for aggressive disorders.	May cause a decrease in appetite, rash, hypertension, or shortness of breath

delivered after the patient is given a muscle relaxant and placed under short-term anesthesia. Surface electrodes deliver electrical impulses to the patient's head with the patient anesthetized. Although the electrical stimulation usually results in seizure activity for about 30 seconds, there appears to be no damage. ECT is typically given three times per week for several weeks to be effective. The effects are often not permanent, and relapse is likely; therefore, antidepressant drugs are still used. The most common side effects are some transient memory loss,

posttreatment malaise, and interactions between the
ECT and current drug therapy.

Lifestyle modification may be important in the management or comanagement of depressed patients. Studies indicate that routine exercise, in particular aerobic exercise for three hours per week, may have a positive effect for depressed individuals.[26,27]

Two Cochrane reviews[28,29] conclude that there is effectiveness for the use of exercise in the management of major depression. Some studies[30,31] indicate that aerobic exercise is as effective as sertraline, an SSRI. It would seem the benefits are a combination of effects including endorphin release and perhaps a placebo effect. The placebo effect, though, is considered quite strong for patients taking antidepressant medications also.

Fairly recently, new studies are indicating a potential protective feature for coffee, green tea, caffeine, and moderate amounts of wine. In one study[32] of Japanese participants, there was a 51% lower prevalence in depression for those drinking four or more cups of green tea per day compared to one or fewer. For coffee, the effect was less robust but was still moderate for those drinking two or more cups per day. The results from two studies[33,34] indicated that there is a moderate benefit to drinking two to seven drinks per week and that this effect seems stronger in women.

Some studies[35,36] indicate that food allergies may trigger depression; therefore, an elimination-diet approach may be suggested in an attempt to determine any particular culprit. For patients with mild to moderate depression, various herbal and nutritional supplementation recommendations have been made. It is important to remember that patients who are severely depressed or suicidal should never be managed with these approaches. Also, with the use of any management strategy, it must be remembered that for some patients, self-resolution occurs in 6 to 12 months no matter what the intervention. The primary recommendations have been for St. John's wort and 5-hydroxytrytophan (5-HTP), both proposed to assist in normalizing serotonin levels.[37–39] St. John's wort (Hypericum perforatum) is often recommended for depression. A 2008 Cochrane review[40] concluded that St. John's wort was more effective than placebo and as effective as standard medication (with fewer side effects) for the treatment of major depression. Although in the past it was believed that hypericin was the major active ingredient, it appears that hypericin does not cross the blood–brain barrier. Hyperforin appears to be the major constituent, yet although it appeared to have similar effects on serotonin, dopamine, and other neurotransmitters, it does not seem to act like a standard SSRI. It may have an anxiolytic action. The Food and Drug Administration, concerned about the interaction between St. John's wort and medications for heart disease, depression, AIDS, and seizures among others, issued a Public Health Advisory in 2000 warning about these possible interactions. This interaction seems to be related to the affect of St. John's wort on drug metabolism through an interaction with the cytochrome P450 3A4 enzyme.[41]

Other recommendations include vitamin B6 for depression associated with premenstrual syndrome, vitamin B12 and/or folic acid for those with deficiency, tyrosine (amino acid) for women taking oral contraceptives, L-phenylalanine, phosphatidylserine (derived from the amino acid serine), dehydroepiandrosterone (DHEA) and other sources of omega-3 fatty acids (especially when associated with heart disease), and S-adenosylmethionine (SAM).[42–52] Because many depressed patients have anxiety as an associated problem, specific recommendations including kava-kava and valerian have been made. For mild bipolar disorders, short-term improvement may be seen with use of omega-3 fatty acids.[53] However, a Cochrane review[54] published in 2008 concludes that the effect is stronger for unipolar depression and less for the manic phase of a bipolar disorder. See **Table 20–2** for a more detailed recommendation list.

Table 20–2 Nutritional Support for Depression*

Substance	How Might It Work?	Dosage	Special Instructions	Contraindications and Possible Side Effects
5-HTP (5-Hydroxytryptophan)	Increases serotonin levels, which may decrease symptoms of pain, insomnia, depression, headache, etc.	50–100 mg, 3 times/day	Best with meals. Should be taken with pyridoxal 5 phosphate (included in recommended supplement).	Do not combine with Imitrex or other SSRI or MAOI antidepressants. Taking more than recommended dose may lead to serotonin syndrome. Safety unknown for pregnant or lactating women.

Table 20–2 Nutritional Support for Depression* (continued)

Substance	How Might It Work?	Dosage	Special Instructions	Contraindications and Possible Side Effects
St. John's wort (Hypericum perforatum)	Works synergistically with 5-HTP; also anti-inflammatory and analgesic properties.	(0.3% hypericin content) 300 mg, 3 times/day (as high as 600 mg, 3 times/day for some patients).	If taken with 5-HTP, reduce 5-HTP dose to 100 mg daily. Best taken at mealtime.	Possible mild stomach irritation; may cause photosensitivity of skin in fair-skinned individuals; rarely allergy, tiredness, weight gain, headache, or restlessness.
Omega-3s (EPA and DHA)	Omega-3 fatty acids may have a general dampening of signal transduction pathways associated with phosphatidylinositol, arachidonic acid, and other related systems.	1,000 mg of EPA and 700 mg of DHA daily for at least 2 months.	None.	Long-term use of fish oils at more than 3–4 g/day may cause problems due to elevated blood sugar, cholesterol, or glucose levels. Side effects may then include nose bleeds or gastrointestinal upset.
L-Phenylalanine	An amino acid that converts to mood-affecting substances including phenylethylamine.	3–4 g/day of phenylalanine for 1-month trial (some research indicated amounts as low as 75–200 mg/day may help).	None.	Large amounts of individual amino acids can cause nerve damage. Safe at 1,500 mg/day. Mild side effects may include nausea, heartburn, and transient headaches.
SAM (S-Adenosylmethionine)	Possibly raises levels of dopamine.	1,600 mg/day	None.	Occasional gastrointestinal upset. Some caution about patients with manic depression switching from depression to a manic episode. Apparently safe in pregnancy.
Kava-kava (Piper methysticum)	Possibly effective as an anxiolytic and muscle relaxer.	60 to 120 mg/day of kava pyrones (70%) for anxiety, stress, and restlessness; for sleep,180 to 210 mg of the extract taken 1 hour before going to bed.	Should not be taken with central nervous system depressants or ethanol.	Not habit-forming; however, may cause dizziness or a scaly skin condition if taken in excess.
Valerian (Valeriana officinalis)	Unknown; however, used for anxiety and as a sleep aid.	2 to 3 g taken 1–3 times/day.	Valerian smells bad even when encapsulated. The active ingredients are unstable; therefore, use only fresh valerian.	Should not be taken during pregnancy or with drugs used to treat anxiety or as sleep enhancers.
Magnesium and malic acid (calcium/magnesium CitraMate)	Increases products of cellular energy and serotonin function, alleviating fatigue.	1 capsule 1–3 times /day (80 mg magnesium and 240 mg malic acid).	Best taken with meals.	None at recommended dosage: however, increase in magnesium dose may cause diarrhea.

*See tables in Chapter 55 for recommendations for depression related to menstrual dysfunction.

Note: These substances have not been approved by the Food and Drug Administration for the treatment of this disorder.

Key: SSRI, selective serotonin reuptake inhibitor; MAOI, monoamine oxidase inhibitor; EPA, eicosapentaenoic acid; DHA, docosahexaenoic acid

APPENDIX 20–1

Web Resources

Depression/Psychiatry

American Psychiatric Association
(888) 357-7924
http://www.psych.org
National Mental Health Association
(800) 969-6642
http://www.depression-screening.org
Depression and Bipolar Support Alliance
(800) 826-3632
http://www.dbsalliance.org
National Institute of Mental Health
http://www.nimh.nih.gov
National Mental Health Association
(703) 684-7722
http://www.nmha.org
American Foundation for Suicide Prevention
(888) 333-2377
http://www.afsp.org

Postpartum Depression

Postpartum Support International
(800) 944-4773
http://www.postpartum.net

APPENDIX 20–2

References

1. Wells KB, Sturm R, Sherbourne CD, Meredith LS. *Caring for Depression*. Cambridge, MA: Harvard University Press, 1996.
2. Agency for Health Care Policy and Research. *Clinical Practice Guidelines: Depression in Primary Care*. Bethesda, MD: National Institutes of Health; 1993.
3. Kessler RC, Berglund P, Demler O, et al. The epidemiology of major depressive disorder: results from the National Comorbidity Survey Replication (NCS-R). *JAMA*. 2003;289:3095–3105.
4. Nirmaher B, Ryan ND, Williamson DE, et al. Child and adolescent depression: a review of the past 10 years. *J Am Acad Child Adolesc Psychiatry*. 1996;35:1427–1439.
5. Ferketick AK, Schwartzbaum JA, Frid DJ, Moeschberger ML. Depression as an antecedent to heart disease among women and men in the NHANES I study. National Health and Nutrition Examination Survey. *Archives of Internal Medicine*. 2000;160(9):1251–1258.
6. Green RC, Cupples LA, Kurz A, et al. Depression as a risk factor for Alzheimer's disease: The MIRAGE Study. *Arch Neurology*. 2003;60;753–759.
7. Coulehan JL, Schulber HC, Block MR, et al. Medical comorbidity of major depressive disorders in a primary medical practice. *Arch Intern Med*. 1990;150:2363–2367.
8. Zung WWK. Prevalence of depressive symptoms in primary care. *J Fam Pract*. 1993;37:337.
9. Williams Jr. JW, Noel PH, Gordes JA, Ramirez G, Pignone M. Is this patient clinically depressed? *JAMA*. 2002;287:1160–1170.
10. Monk M. Epidemiology of suicide. *Epidemiol Rev*. 1987;9:51–68.
11. Greenberg PE, Stiglin LE, Finkelstein SN, Berndt ER. The economic burden of depression in 1990. *J Clin Psychiatry*. 1993;54:405–418.
12. Stewart WF, Ricci JA, Chee E, et al. Cost of lost productive work time among U.S. workers with depression. *JAMA*. 2003;289:3135–3144.
13. Caspi A, Sugden K, Moffitt TE, et al. Influence of life stress on depression: moderation by a polymorphism in the 5-HTT gene. *Science*. 2003;301:386–389.
14. American Psychiatric Association. *Diagnostic and Statistical Manual of Mental Disorders*. 4th ed. Washington, DC: APA; 1994:339–345.
15. Rosenthal NE. Diagnosis and treatment of seasonal affective disorder. *JAMA*. 1993;270:2717.
16. Wisner KL, Parry BL, Piontek CM. Postpartum Depression. *N Engl J Med*. 2002;347(3):194–199.
17. Weissman MM. Advances in psychiatric epidemiology: rates and risk for depression. *Am J Public Health*. 1987;77:445–451.
18. Whooley MA, Avins AL, Miranda J, Browner WC. Case-finding instruments for depression: two questions are as good as many. *J Gen Intern Med*. 1997;12(4):439–445.
19. Hahn SR, Kroenke K, Williams JBW, Spitzer RL. Evaluation of mental disorders with the PRIME-MD. In: Maruish M, ed. *Handbook of Psychological Assessment in Primary Care Settings*. Mahwah, NJ: Lawrence Erlbaum; 2000:191–253.
20. Spitzer RL, Kroenke K, Williams JBW. The Patient Health Questionnaire Primary Care Study Group.

Validation and utility of a self-report version of PRIME-MD: the PHQ primary care study. *JAMA.* 1999;282:1737–1744.

21. Simel DL, Rennie D, eds. *The Rational Clinical Examination: Evidence-Based Clinical Diagnosis. The American Medical Association*: McGraw-Hill Education, LLC; 2009:247–263.

22. Ewing JA. Detecting alcoholism. The CAGE questionnaire. *JAMA.* 1984;252:1905–1907.

23. Brent DA, Birmaher B. Adolescent depression. *N Engl J Med.* 2002;347(9):667–671.

24. Goodwin FK, Fireman B, Simon GE, et al. Suicide risk in bipolar disorder during treatment with lithium and divalproex. *JAMA.* 2003;290:1467–1473.

25. El-Mallakh RS, Wright JC, Breen KJ, Lippman SB. Clues to depression in primary care practice. *Postgrad Med.* 1996; 100(1):396–404.

26. Martinsen EW. Benefits of exercise for the treatment of depression. *Sports Med.* 1990;9:380–390.

27. Martinsen EW, Medhus A, Sandivik L. Effects of aerobic exercise on depression: a controlled study. *Br Med J.* 1985;291:109–111.

28. Mead GE, Morley W, Campbell P, Greig CA, McMurdo M, Lawlor DA. Exercise for depression. *Cochrane Database Syst Rev.* 2009(3):CD004366.

29. Cooney GM, Dwan K, Greig CA, et al. Exercise for depression. *Cochrane Database Syst Rev.* 2013(9):CD004366.

30. Blumenthal JA, Babyak MA, Doraiswamy PM, et al. Exercise and pharmacotherapy in the treatment of major depressive disorder. *Psychosom Med.* 2007;69(7):587–596.

31. Hoffman BM, Babyak MA, Craighead WE, et al. Exercise and pharmacotherapy in patients with major depression: one-year follow-up of the SMILE study. *Psychosom Med.* 2011;73(2):127–133.

32. Pham NM, Nanri A, Kurotani K, et al. Green tea and coffee consumption is inversely associated with depressive symptoms in a Japanese working population. *Public Health Nutr.* 2013:1–9.

33. Gea A, Martinez-Gonzalez MA, Toledo E, et al. A longitudinal assessment of alcohol intake and incident depression: the SUN project. *BMC Public Health.* 2012;12:954.

34. Gea A, Beunza JJ, Estruch R, et al. Alcohol intake, wine consumption and the development of depression: the PREDIMED study. *BMC Med.* 2013;11(1):192.

35. King DS. Can allergic exposure provide psychological symptoms? A double-blind test. *Biol Psychiatry.* 1981;16:3–19.

36. Brown M, Gibney M, Husband PR, Radcliffe M. Food allergy in polysymptomatic patients. *Practitioner.* 1981;225:1651–1654.

37. Linde K, Ramirez G, Mulrow CD, et al. St. John's wort for depression—an overview and meta-analysis of randomised clinical trials. *Br Med J.* 1996;313:253–258.

38. Von Prang HM, Lemus C. Monoamine precursors in the treatment of psychiatric disorders. In: Wurtman RJ, Wurtman JJ, eds. *Nutrition and the Brain.* New York: Raven Press; 1986;7.

39. Shaw KA, Turner J, Del Mar C. Tryptophan and 5-Hydroxytryptophan for depression. *Cochrane Database of Systematic Reviews* 2002(1): CD003198. DOI: 10.1002/14651858.

40. Linde K, Berner MM, Kriston L. St John's wort for major depression. *Cochrane Database of Systematic Reviews* 2008(4): CD000448. DOI: 10.1002/14651858. CD000448.pub3

41. Markowitz JS, Donnovan JL, De-Vane CL, et al. Effect of St. John's Wort on drug metabolism by induction of cytochrome P450 3A4 enzyme. *JAMA.* 2003;290:1500–1504.

42. Kleijien J, Riet GT, Knipschild P. Vitamin B6 in the treatment of the premenstrual syndrome—a review. *Br J Obstet Gynecol.* 1990;97:847–852.

43. Holmes JM. Cerebral manifestations of vitamin B12 deficiency. *J Nutr Med.* 1991;2:89–90.

44. Reynolds E. Folate deficiency in depressive illness. *Br J Psychiatry.* 1970;117:287–292.

45. Beckman H, Strauss MA, Ludolph E. DL-Phenylalanine in depressed patients: an open study. *J Neural Transm.* 1977;41:123–134.

46. Sabvelli HC, Fawcett J, Gustovsky F, et al. Clinical studies on the phenylethylamine hypothesis of affective disorder: urine and blood phenylacetic acid and phenylalanine dietary supplements. *J Clin Psychiatry.* 1986;47:66–70.

47. Wolkowitz OM. Dehydroepiandrosterone (DHEA) treatment of depression. *Biol Psychiatry.* 1997;41:311–318.

48. Bell KM, Potkin SG, Carreon D, Plon L. S-Adenosylmethionine blood levels in major depression: changes with drug treatment. *Acta Neurol Scand.* 1994;154 (suppl):15–18.

49. Bressa GM. S-Adenosyl-1-methionine (SAMe) as antidepressant: meta-analysis of clinical studies. *Acta Neurol Scand.* 1994;154(suppl):7–14.

50. Edwards R, Peet M, Shay J, Horrobin D. Omega-3 polyunsaturated fatty acid levels in the diet and in red blood cell membranes of depressed patients. *J Affect Disord.* 1998;48:149–155.

51. Taylor MJ, Carney S, Geddes J, Goodwin G. Folate for depressive disorders. *Cochrane Database Syst Rev.* 2003(2):CD003390.

52. Taylor MJ, Carney SM, Goodwin GM, Geddes JR. Folate for depressive disorders: systematic review and meta-analysis of randomized controlled trials. *J Psychopharmacol.* Jun 2004;18(2): 251–256.

53. Stoll AL, Sevenus E, Freeman M, et al. Omega-3 fatty acids in bipolar disorder: a preliminary double-blind, placebo-controlled trial. *Arch Gen Psychiatry.* 1999;56:407–412.

54. Montgomery P, Richardson AJ. Omega-3 fatty acids for bipolar disorder. *Cochrane Database of Systematic Reviews* 2008(2): CD005169. DOI: 10.1002/14651858.CD005169.pub2

Fatigue

Context

How often do patients complain of feeling tired? It may seem to many practitioners that most do, most of the time. Some studies indicate as many as one out of four or five patients have a complaint of constant tiredness.[1] As a primary complaint, fatigue ranks seventh among all patient complaints in primary care. Statistically, this represents approximately 5% of patients in a primary care setting in the United States; studies[2, 3] in Canada indicate 7% of patients. Although patients often arrive self-diagnosed with chronic fatigue syndrome, it is extremely important to realize that this diagnosis is a difficult one, even for the physician; however, there are defined criteria. It is also important to note that some studies indicate that 50% to 80% of patients with chronic fatigue have a psychiatric problem, most often depression.[4]

The causes of fatigue are generally divided into organic and psychogenic. Each accounts for up to half of all cases (20% to 45% have an organic cause; 40% to 45% have a psychogenic cause).[5, 6] In approximately 10% to 30% of cases, however, no cause is identified. The good news is that approximately 75% of patients improve within a one- to three-year period.[7, 8] These are not necessarily the patients for whom a diagnosis was made. One study[9] provided interesting insight into the psychology of the doctor–patient relationship with regard to diagnosis of chronic fatigue syndrome (CFS). Seventy-five percent of doctors were reluctant to give their patients a diagnosis of CFS because of the uncertainty of the scientific understanding of the etiology and treatment. They also feared that the diagnosis might be a self-fulfilling prophecy if patients believed they had the disorder. Patients, however, felt that the negative effects of not having a diagnosis outweighed the negative effects of the diagnosis of CFS.

General Strategy

History

Determine what the patient means by a complaint of fatigue. Determine the following:

- Is the complaint more of tiredness (relieved by rest) as opposed to fatigue?
- Is the fatigue or tiredness disabling? Does it interfere with more than 50% of daily activities? If so, consider CFS.
- What is the timing of the fatigue or tiredness? If felt more in the morning it is suggestive of a functional cause; if it is worse as the day progresses it is more suggestive of a physiologic cause.
- Is the sense of fatigue only with exertion? A physiologic cause is suggested.
- What is the patient's typical daily schedule, including eating habits, work habits, and sleep habits (not enough or interrupted sleep, skipping breakfast, drinking large amounts of coffee in the morning, a large lunch, alcohol consumption during the day, athletic training schedule is excessive, etc.)?
- Are there any signs of infection such as fever or upper respiratory symptoms (e.g., sore throat or cough)?
- Is the patient taking medication(s)?
- Have there been any past diagnoses for the fatigue by any other physicians?

- Are there signs or symptoms suggestive of endocrine disorders such as thyroid problems, diabetes, cancer, anemia, or depression?
- Is depression a possibility? Consider the use of a depression questionnaire if suspected.

Evaluation

- Perform a focused examination based on the history.
- Order laboratory studies based on history and examination findings; Epstein-Barr testing is not recommended.

Management

- Management is based on the underlying cause.
- Half of all cases of CFS will self-resolve in two years; supportive advice and recommendations involve diet, rest, and exercise.
- Patients suspected of endocrine or oncologic causes should be referred to the appropriate specialist.
- For anemia, see Chapter 52.

General Discussion

The more common causes of tiredness and fatigue are usually easily recognized by patients. These include strenuous activity, lack of sleep, flu, pregnancy, and overwork. Often, though, patients do not associate fatigue with stress. Although the first list illustrates situations of increased demand or lack of rest (physiologic), stress borders the categories of physiologic and functional causes. Physiologic stress is often more acute and therefore more easy to associate with a specific cause. Functional or psychologic causes are often without an identifiable match (**Exhibit 21–1**).

CFS is a popular label for patients who feel fatigued or who have no other identifiable cause for their complaint. There are, however, specific criteria that may help separate CFS as a cause.[10, 11] The case definition requires that the patient have a "new" onset of fatigue (not lifelong). This does not result from exertion only nor is it substantially relieved by rest. The sense of fatigue causes a significant reduction in previous levels of occupational, educational, social, and personal activities. To fit the criteria, other symptoms such as short-term memory loss, postexertion fatigue lasting more than 24 hours, sore throat, or headache must persist for six months or more. These criteria alone will eliminate the majority of patients with a complaint of fatigue in an ambulatory setting. It is important to explain to patients that there is no single laboratory or physical examination finding by which to diagnose CFS.

CFS has had many names, including Epstein-Barr virus (EBV) disease, yuppie flu, neuromyasthenia, postviral fatigue syndrome, royal free disease, Iceland disease, and encephalomyelitis; it is often confused with fibromyalgia.[12] There is little support for most theories for CFS. There is no clear evidence that EBV or chronic yeast infection is the cause. Evidence[13] does suggest a chronic immunologically mediated inflammatory process involving the central nervous system. The immune response is believed to be secondary to a number of infectious and psychiatric illnesses. Interest in human herpes virus 6 (hHV 6) is based on lymphocyte cell cultures. This finding, however, probably is not an indication of primary infection but reactivation of a latent infection.[14, 15]

An association between neurally mediated hypotension (NMH) and chronic fatigue is recognized. Initially, NMH was identified as a cause of unexplained syncope in some individuals. In one study the patients had postexertional fatigue, while another study tested a sample of patients who met the criteria for CFS. Both groups had an abnormal response to the upright tilt test and good response to therapy using antihypertensive medication.[16, 17] The upright tilt test is designed to detect an abnormal cardiovascular reflex.

CFS and depression are related. Studies suggest that in many cases, depression precedes CFS; however, depression is found with all CFS patients. For this reason, the original criteria for CFS, which excluded patients with psychiatric disorders, have been modified to include those with nonpsychotic depression, somatoform disorders, and generalized anxiety or panic disorders.[18] In one study,[19] suicidal thoughts were found in 55% of CFS patients.

Two other interesting studies should be mentioned. The first study[20] illustrates a possible relationship between hypofunctioning of the corticotropin-releasing hormone neurons and CFS. The authors suggest a central deficiency of a potent arousal-producing neuropeptide. In the second study,[21] the authors suggest that the immunosupportive role of sleep is key to the understanding of the sleepiness associated with chronic fatigue. They point

---

Exhibit 21–1 Etiology of Fatigue

Acute infection: influenza, hepatitis

Chronic infection: tuberculosis, infectious mononucleosis, brucellosis, subacute infectious hepatitis, subacute bacterial endocarditis, asymptomatic urinary tract infection, hookworm, parasitic infection

Autoimmune condition: systemic lupus erythematosus, rheumatoid arthritis

Neurologic disorder: Parkinson's disease, multiple sclerosis, posttraumatic syndrome

Primary muscle disorder: polymyositis, muscular dystrophy, myasthenia gravis

Endocrine and metabolic disease: adrenal or aldosterone insufficiency, panhypopituitarism, Cushing's disease, hypothyroidism, hyperthyroidism, hypogonadism, hyperparathyroidism, hypercalcemic and hypocalcemic states, hyperaldosteronism, potassium depletion, uncontrolled diabetes mellitus, hypoglycemic states, renal insufficiency

Anemia or blood dyscrasia

Nutritional deficiency

Circulatory disorder: silent myocardial infarction, congestive heart failure, cardiomyopathy

Pulmonary insufficiency: emphysema, chronic bronchitis

Neoplastic disorder: lymphomas, carcinomas, occult tumors

Psychologic disorder: depression, anxiety

Chronic drug intoxication

Lack of sleep

Reproduced from L. J. Bowers, *Topics in Clinical Chiropractic*, Vol. 1, No. 1, p. 27, © 1994, Aspen Publishers, Inc.

---

out that some viruses cause excessive sleepiness and postulate that some infections may cause a dysfunction in the sleep/wakefulness cycle.

Evaluation

History

The initial focus of the history is to determine exactly what the patient means by a complaint of fatigue. Patients may describe their complaint as weakness, weariness, boredom, lack of energy, exhaustion, unwillingness or aversion to work, sleepiness, and difficulty breathing with exertion, among others. It is important for the chiropractor to listen patiently to this explanation. Although obtaining the history is time consuming, there are often valuable clues that will lead to a more expedient diagnosis with more judicious use of laboratory testing (**Table 21–1**).

The key initial distinction is between organic/physiologic causes and functional/psychologic causes. In general, the history clues that would point toward a functional cause include the following:

- Fatigue or tiredness is felt more in the morning and improves as the day progresses.

- Although the patient may feel like sleeping, sleeping does not improve his or her fatigue.
- The sense of fatigue is associated with work or situations that are perceived as stressful; improvement occurs with avoidance.
- There is a past or current history of depression, anxiety, or somatization disorder.

Clues that would point toward a physiologic cause include the following:

- Complaints of insomnia or disrupted sleep improve with napping.
- The patient feels best in the morning and feels worse with activity or as the day progresses; complaints improve with sleep.
- The patient has dyspnea or weakness on exertion.
- The patient attributes fatigue to a work or sports activity that is strenuous.
- The patient describes the fatigue as worse in the afternoon and has a history of large caffeine ingestion in the morning, a large lunch, skipped breakfast, or daytime alcohol ingestion.
- The patient is taking a medication such as antihypertensives, antipsychotics, chemotherapy for cancer, anticonvulsants (for seizure),

Table 21–1 History Questions for Fatigue

Primary Question	What Are You Thinking?	Secondary Questions	What Are You Thinking?
How long have you had a sense of fatigue?	Fatigue of recent onset is more likely physiologic and/or transient.	**Have you had the fatigue for longer than 6 months and does it significantly affect your performance of daily activities?**	More likely CFS unless other condition has been diagnosed.
(For more recent onset) Are you taking any medications?	Medications may be the cause or may be prescribed for an underlying disorder that can cause fatigue.	**Are you taking antidepressants, antiseizure medicine, or antihistamines? Do you use illicit drugs such as cocaine?**	Side effect of medications.
Does your fatigue occur only after exertion?	Physiologic cause, likely postinfectious or cardiopulmonary.	**Have you had a recent infection that included a sore throat, fever, and/or lymph node swelling?**	Postinfectious; consider mononucleosis.
		Is it difficult for you to breathe while lying on your back at night?	Congestive heart failure or obesity.
		Are you a high-level athlete training multiple hours a week?	Overtraining.
Is the fatigue more a sense of tiredness in the afternoon?	Consider dietary cause or sleep disturbance.	**Do you eat a large meal at lunch or have alcohol with lunch?**	Postprandial hypoglycemia.
		Do you drink multiple cups of coffee in the morning but not in the afternoon?	Rebound effect of caffeine.
		Do you or your sleep partner notice any problems with sleep?	Sleep disorder.
Do you feel "blue" or depressed?	Depression.	**Do you relate this feeling to a specific life event (e.g., loss of a loved one)?**	Reactive depression.
		Do you feel that activities that used to bring you enjoyment no longer do?	Depression.
		Have you noticed a change in eating or sleeping habits (increase or decrease in either)?	Depression.
Do you have a diagnosed condition?	Hyperthyroidism, cancer, depression, etc., cause fatigue.	**Have you had a significant loss of weight over the last 6 months?**	Possible cancer, especially in an older patient.
		Have you noticed a change in heat/cold tolerance, tremor, fast heart rate, or change in skin or hair?	Possible thyroid disorder.

tricyclic antidepressants, benzodiazepines, and antihistamines (antihistamines are the main ingredients in most over-the-counter sleep-inducing medications).
- The patient has a history of drug or alcohol abuse.

Examination

The examination focuses on a search for systemic, metabolic, or neurologic conditions that may cause fatigue. Often the symptoms elicited with the history will be suggestive of a particular system. Following are some of the more common causes with associated examination clues:

- Infection—fever, lymphadenopathy, associated upper respiratory complaints such as cough, urinary tract complaints such as burning on urination, and abdominal complaints such as nausea/vomiting, abdominal pain, or diarrhea; upper right quadrant tenderness or hepatomegaly suggests hepatitis; splenomegaly suggests mononucleosis

- Hypothyroidism—thyroid nodules or enlargement, coarse hair, dry skin, loss of outer third of eyebrows
- Hyperthyroidism—thyroid nodules or enlargement, moist skin, fine tremor, fine hair, occasionally pretibial myxedema
- Chronic renal failure—hypertension, cardiomegaly, edema, or pericardial friction rub
- Congestive heart failure—lower leg edema, ascites, adventitial lung sounds, hepatojugular reflux, cardiomegaly
- Chronic obstructive pulmonary disease—cyanosis, barrel chest, prolonged respiration, FEV_1 reduction, rhonchi, wheezes
- Cancer—weight loss, blood in stool, persistent or localized lymphadenopathy
- Anemia—tachycardia, conjunctival pallor, fatigue on exertion (step test), glossitis
- Acquired immunodeficiency syndrome (AIDS)—persistent lymphadenopathy, muscle wasting, leukoplakia

Laboratory evaluation of a fatigued patient is often unrevealing because of the high percentage of psychologically related complaints. However, a general screen often will reveal direct or indirect signs of a physiologic cause if present. The National Institutes of Health[22] recommended in 1991 that the following be included on an initial laboratory examination of the fatigued patient:

- complete blood cell count with differential
- serum chemistries (including electrolytes, blood urea nitrogen, glucose, and creatinine)
- liver function tests
- thyroid function tests
- antinuclear antibody (ANA) test
- urinalysis
- tuberculin (TB) skin test

The majority of the above tests are done in a standard screening laboratory; however, the ANA test, thyroid function tests, and the TB skin test are not. The expense of adding these tests should be considered, and the decision to order should be based on relevant historical or examination clues.

Tests that should be run if clinically indicated include the following:

- serum cortisol (Addison's disease)
- immunoglobulin levels (chronic fatigue syndrome and connective tissue disorders)
- rheumatoid factor (rheumatoid arthritis)
- Lyme serology (Lyme disease in endemic areas)
- human immunodeficiency virus (HIV) antibody (AIDS)

The study did not recommend testing for EBV in evaluating a patient suspected of having chronic fatigue syndrome because 95% of adults over age 30 years have serologic evidence of a past EBV infection.[23, 24] The study, however, did recommend the use of screening questionnaires for depression or other psychiatric problems (see Chapter 20).

When an underlying sleep disorder is suggested, referral to a sleep laboratory for confirmation is needed to determine the degree of involvement. Many patients feel they sleep poorly; however, they are demonstrated to sleep adequately with a sleep laboratory investigation.

Management

Management of fatigue is based on an identifiable cause. When there is an obvious lifestyle factor, such as diet, work, or stress, modification is often all that is needed. The chiropractor can play a clear role in advice regarding proper diet and exercise, stress management, and avoidance of excess in alcohol and drugs. When the underlying cause is suspected to be a medication, referral to the prescribing physician with a letter of explanation is necessary. All other patients with identifiable or suspected diseases should be referred to a primary care or specialist physician for comanagement.

It appears that a moderate exercise plan may be important in preventing worsening of fatigue.[25, 26] A number of different approaches have been used in the treatment of CFS, but there has been no consistent, reproducible benefit with any. Notably, a study[27] comparing immunologic therapy, psychiatric counseling, and placebo demonstrated no difference in effect among groups. The literature is full of therapeutic trials using essential fatty acids,[28] magnesium,[29] liver extract-folic acid/vitamin B12,[30] gamma globulin,[31] and acyclovir.[32] One gram of carnitine three times a day resulted in some improvement in a small group of patients.[33] Licorice that contains glycyrrhizin (not the DGL-type licorice) may cause an elevation in blood pressure and has been recommended as a possible alternative for patients with hypotension-associated CFS. One case study[34] used 2.5 g of licorice per day. It is important to note that these hypertensive aspects of licorice should be taken quite seriously prior to recommending licorice as a nutritional aid to CFS. One study[35] indicated a role for essential fatty acid prescription. None has demonstrated a consistent effect superior to the natural course of CFS or placebo.

Algorithm

Algorithms for evaluation and management of initial fatigue screening and organic fatigue screening are presented in **Figures 21–1** and **21–2**.

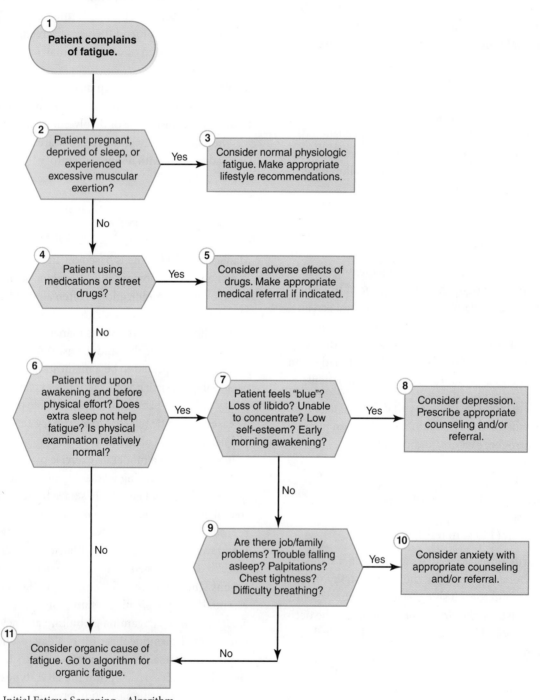

Figure 21–1 Initial Fatigue Screening—Algorithm

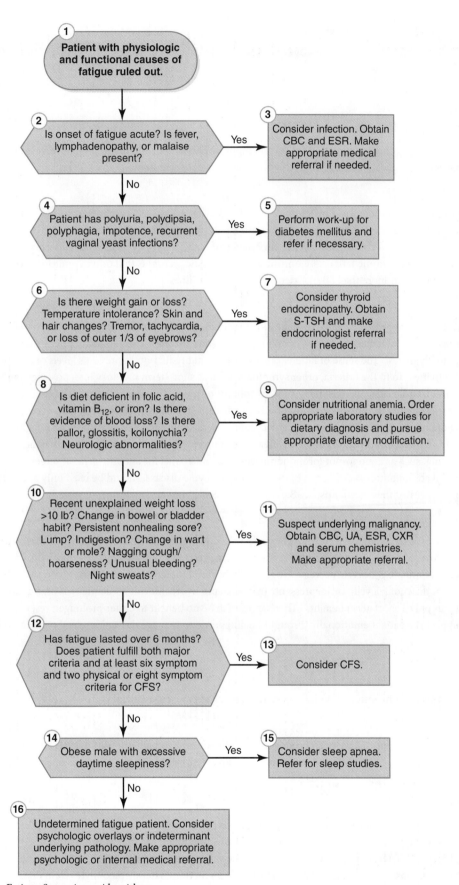

Figure 21–2 Organic Fatigue Screening—Algorithm

Selected Disorders Presenting as Fatigue*

Chronic Fatigue Syndrome

Classic Presentation

The patient complains of fatigue that has persisted for several months. This is not something felt before. It is disabling enough to interfere with normal activities of daily living. Rest feels good, but does not seem to make any difference.

Cause

The cause is unknown. In the past there was a belief that a specific viral agent such as Epstein-Barr was the cause. However, there is no evidence that there is a single cause. It appears that the cause is a dysfunction in immune function, often in reaction to an acute illness. One finding that helps support this theory is the persistence of high levels of cytokines (i.e., interferons and interleukins) after a viral infection in patients with chronic fatigue.[36] Confusing the diagnostic picture is that other conditions coexist, in particular fibromyalgia (overlap with CFS is more than 50%),[37] depression, or other illness.

Evaluation

The diagnostic criteria have changed. The 1988 case definition was revised in 1994 to a much more abbreviated list of criteria.[11] The case definition requires that the patient have a "new" onset of fatigue (not lifelong). This fatigue neither results from ongoing exertion nor is relieved substantially by rest. The sense of fatigue causes a significant reduction in previous levels of occupational, educational, social, and personal activities. To fit the criteria, other symptoms, such as short-term memory loss, postexertion fatigue lasting more than 24 hours, sore throat, and headache, must persist for six months or more. The clinical search for other causes of fatigue involves a thorough history and evaluation for possible thyroid or adrenal disease, psychologic cause or overlay (i.e., depression), somatization, Lyme disease, mononucleosis, anemia, cancer, or any chronic disease. The choice of laboratory or imaging testing is based on the suspected cause. The clinical examination can help differentiate fibromyalgia, and questionnaires may help reveal depression. Specific laboratory testing, such as a monospot for mononucleosis, anemia panel for anemia, general screen for cancer or chronic disease, and enzyme-linked immunosorbent assay (ELISA) testing for Lyme disease, should be used only after a thorough history and examination have suggested their need. Epstein-Barr or other specific viral testing is not suggested.

Management

It has been reported that 50% of patients will recover in two years.[38] However, a recent study[39] indicated that of those patients with severe CFS, only 4% recovered over the four years of the study. During recovery several strategies may help, including a proper diet, adequate rest periods, and mild to moderate exercise. Cognitive behavioral therapy is also important. To treat the sleep dysfunction associated with CFS, low doses of tricyclic antidepressants (e.g., doxepin hydrochloride [Sinequan] 10 mg/d) are prescribed. Low-dose hydrocortisone has only a short-term benefit.[40] There appears to be no benefit to either prolonged rest or immunotherapy.[41] It is important to help support the patient emotionally through the illness and to manage musculoskeletal complaints when necessary.

Fibromyalgia

Classic Presentation

The patient is often a woman complaining of both fatigue and generalized musculoskeletal pain.

Cause

The cause is unknown. Several theories have been proposed focusing on lowered pain-threshold levels and decreased serotonin levels. It is believed that an interruption of stage 4 (nonrapid eye movement) sleep due to intrusions of alpha rhythms is also contributory.[42]

Evaluation

The American College of Rheumatology set criteria for the diagnosis of fibromyalgia in 1990.[43] These include persistence of generalized musculoskeletal pain (both sides of the body, above and below the waist) for at least three months. There must also be tenderness at 11 of 18 sites (9 bilateral sites). These sites include the suboccipital area, the lower cervical spine (transverse processes of C5-C7), upper trapezius, supraspinatus, second rib (costochondral junction), lateral epicondyle (2 cm distal), gluteals, greater trochanter of the femur, and the medial fat pad at the knee (proximal to the joint line). The sensitivity of this approach is 88%;

*See also Chapter 20, Depression, Chapter 50, Thyroid Dysfunction, and Chapter 52, Anemia.

specificity is 81%.[44] Other symptoms include fatigue, sleep disturbance, persistent early morning stiffness, paresthesia, and headache. Approximately 2% of the general population has fibromyalgia (3.4% women; 0.5% men) and this incidence increases with age (7% of women aged 60–79).[45] Fibromyalgia is found in 10% to 40% of patients with rheumatoid arthritis and systemic lupus erythematosus (SLE). Of patients referred to Lyme disease clinics, 25% to 50% had fibromyalgia instead of Lyme disease.

Management

Unfortunately, there is no consistent effect with any therapy. However, approximately three quarters of all patients with fibromyalgia will recover over a one-year period.[46] It appears that the use of low-dose tricyclic antidepressants will help approximately half of these patients. Pregabalin (Lyrica) is a new medication that may help. Although many other conservative approaches have been suggested, including the use of oral malate and magnesium, vitamin E (see **Table 21–2**), exercise, physical modalities, homeopathy, and manipulation, none has been demonstrated in large studies to indicate a significant difference compared with control groups.[47] In one study, fibromyalgia patients were randomized to either an exercise group (exercise bicycle and treadmill) or a relaxation group (stretches and relaxation exercises) for one hour, twice a week, for 12 weeks.[48] At the end of the trial treatment, 35% of patients in the exercise group rated feeling "much better" or "very much better" versus 18% for patients in the relaxation group. The effect seemed to be maintained at a nine-month follow-up for the exercise group (38%), with a small increase in the relaxation group to 22%. A systematic review[49] published in 2009 concluded that there was strong evidence for the use of aerobic exercise and cognitive behavioral therapy. They concluded there was moderate evidence for muscle strengthening, massage, acupuncture, and balneotherapy (spa therapy). There was only limited evidence for spinal manipulation, vitamins, minerals, and herbs. It appears that vitamin D deficiency is common in patients with fibromyalgia and occurs more frequently in those who also have anxiety and depression.[50] Although the deficiency is not

Table 21–2 Nutritional Support for Fibromyalgia

Substance	How Might It Work?	Dosage	Special Instructions	Contraindications Possible Side Effects
5-HTP (5-hydroxytryptophan)	Increases serotonin levels, which may decrease symptoms of pain, insomnia, depression, headache, etc.	50-100 mg, 3 times/day	Best taken with meals. Should be taken with pyridoxal 5 phosphate (included in recommended supplement).	Do not combine with Imitrex or other SSRI or MAOI antidepressants. Taking more than recommended dose may lead to serotonin syndrome. Safety unknown for pregnant or lactating women.
St. John's wort (Hypericum perforatum)	Works synergistically with 5-HTP; also anti-inflammatory and analgesic properties.	(0.3% hypericin content) 300 mg, 3 times/day (as high as 600 mg, 3 times/day for some patients).	If taken with 5-HTP, reduce 5-HTP dose to 100 mg daily.	Possible mild stomach irritation; may cause photosensitivity of skin in fair-skinned individuals; rarely, allergy, tiredness, weight gain, headache, or restlessness.
SAM (5-densylmethionine)	Possibly raises levels of dopamine.	1,600 mg/day.	None.	Occasional gastrointestinal upset. Some caution about patients with manic-depression switching from depression to a manic episode. Apparently safe in pregnancy.
Vitamin E	Unknown.	100–300 IU/day.	None.	None as recommended.
Magnesium and malic acid (calcium/magnesium CitraMate)	Increases products of cellular energy and serotonin function, alleviating fatigue.	1 capsule 1–3 times/day (80 mg magnesium and 240 mg malic acid).	Best taken with meals.	None at recommended dosage; however, increase in magnesium dose may cause diarrhea.

Key: SSRI, selective serotonin reuptake inhibitor; MAOI, monoamine oxidase inhibitor.
Note: These substances have not been approved by the Food and Drug Administration for the treatment of this disorder.

necessarily causal, there appears to be a relationship that theoretically indicates the possibility of improvement with correction of the deficiency. One pilot study[51] using intravenous nutrient therapy found significant improvements in pain and energy. No participants had complete or lasting resolution, but the results are an indication for further research. The patients in this study were treated once per week for eight weeks. Patients had longstanding fibromyalgia (eight years or longer) and had not responded to other therapies. Finally, acetyl L-carnitine may be of benefit. A study[52] combining 500 mg/day capsules and weekly injections compared to placebo demonstrated some significant difference with more improvement in the L-carnitine group after the tenth week post-treatment.

Mononucleosis

Classic Presentation

The patient is usually young (age range 10 to 35 years) and complains of fever, fatigue, and sore throat.

Cause

Infection by Epstein-Barr virus (human herpes virus 4) is the cause of mononucleosis. It appears to be most often transmitted via saliva, with an incubation period of 5 to 15 days.

Evaluation

The patient usually has a fever, enlargement of the posterior cervical chain lymph nodes, and, in about half of cases, splenomegaly. Inspection of the throat will usually reveal an exudative pharyngitis or tonsillitis. All of the above findings may be nonspecific, yet suggest a laboratory evaluation. This evaluation may include a screen, which will reveal atypical lymphocytes, or suggest the need for specific testing including the heterophile antibody test (or the related monospot test), which will be positive for mononucleosis. It may take several weeks after acquiring the infection for these tests to become positive, however.

Management

Management is largely palliative for most patients. The sore throat may last several weeks while the fatigue may last for one to three months. Rare complications occur in older or immunosuppressed patients and include enlargement of lymphoid tissue compromising breathing (refer for corticosteroids), hepatitis, myocarditis, or encephalitis. These select patients should be managed medically.

Lyme Disease

Classic Presentation

Presentation is dependent on the course of the disease. With early disease, the patient presents with a skin rash and flu-like symptoms following a camping or hiking trip (or simply occupational exposure for those who work in high-risk areas). Later course presentations include multiple joint pains and fatigue.

Cause

Transmission of the spirochete *Borrelia burgdorferi* occurs from an *Ixodes* tick bite. High-risk areas include Massachusetts to Maryland, Wisconsin, Minnesota, California, and Oregon. Onset is most often in the summer or early fall. Most patients are children and young adults; however, anyone living or working in heavily wooded areas is at risk.

Evaluation

Early manifestations are a small red macule or papule (erythema [chronicum] migrans), often at the site of a tick bite, that expands and spreads into a rash. This is often followed by mild flu-like symptoms such as malaise or low-grade fever. An inflammatory arthritis appears in about 60% of people usually over weeks or months, with the larger joints such as the knee commonly affected. Multisystem involvement may also occur including the heart, central nervous system, or peripheral nervous system. Common serologic testing is not useful in early Lyme disease due to low sensitivity.[53] Later in the course of disease, positive or equivocal results on an ELISA, immunofluorescence antibody (IFA), or immuno-dot assay require supplemental testing using a Western blot assay. Negative results on a Western blot or ELISA indicate no serologic evidence of *B. burgdorferi* infection at the time of testing. Some laboratories can provide culturing of skin lesions and polymerase chain reaction of skin biopsy and blood, which may be helpful in the diagnosis.

Management

For early Lyme disease doxycycline or amoxicillin is used for 21 days or longer. With later involvement of joints, probenecid is added and the treatment is extended to 30 days. If neurologic involvement occurs, parenteral antibiotics are given. Generally, the long-term outcome is favorable for patients with Lyme disease.[54] A Lyme disease vaccine is available and recommended for those at high risk due to geographic location, occupation, or significant recreational exposure in high-risk areas.[55]

Hepatitis A

Classic Presentation

Although many patients are asymptomatic, some patients may present with anorexia and malaise. At some point in the illness, the patient may develop a fever just prior to becoming jaundiced.

Cause

Infection with the hepatitis A virus (HAV) is usually related to exposure by the fecal–oral route. This highly contagious viral infection is most common in daycare centers, homosexual men, and institutionalized individuals. Other means of transmission include eating undercooked shellfish, drinking contaminated water, and handling of imported chimpanzees or apes. Anywhere from 20% to 80% of the adult population has immunity (higher in lower socioeconomic group individuals). The incubation period is 15 to 45 days.

Evaluation

The patient may have hepatomegaly with upper right quadrant tenderness. Another characteristic sign is dark urine. At some point the patient may develop a fever that precedes the appearance of jaundice. Interestingly, the onset of jaundice occurs when the patient begins to feel better and the fever rapidly decreases. White blood cell count and erythrocyte sedimentation rate (ESR) are generally normal. Liver enzyme levels, such as alanine aminotransferase (ALT) and aspartate aminotransferase (AST), are quite high (more than eight times the normal level when jaundice appears); bilirubin also is elevated as is alkaline phosphatase. Diagnosis is by immunoglobulin M (IgM) anti-HAV in the early stage. IgM is found during the onset of jaundice.

Management

The disease is generally self-resolving; it lasts approximately six weeks with the possibility of two to three relapses. Increased calorie intake (especially in morning) and avoidance of hepatically metabolized drugs is all that is necessary. The patient is not a carrier. HAV vaccine is recommended for those at high risk.

Hepatitis B

Classic Presentation

Many patients are asymptomatic. If symptomatic, the patient presents with a complaint of chronic malaise or fatigue. If presenting during the prodrome, the patient may have signs of serum sickness such as urticaria, rash, and arthralgias.

Cause

Infection with the hepatitis B virus (HBV) is usually related to exposure by the parenteral route (needle use including infected transfused blood, contaminated needles in drug abusers, and tattoos). The most common individuals are homosexual men, drug abusers, visitors and immigrants from endemic areas, Alaska natives, neonates born to infected mothers, prisoners and the institutionalized, and medical workers exposed to accidental needle pricks. Infection at an early age in developing countries usually is unremarkable with only mild disease and no jaundice. The incubation period for HBV is 50 to 180 days. HBV is an infectious disease notifiable on the national level.

Evaluation

The patient may have hepatomegaly with upper right quadrant tenderness. Another characteristic sign is dark urine. At some point the patient may develop a fever that precedes the appearance of jaundice. Interestingly, the onset of jaundice occurs when the patient begins to feel better and the fever rapidly decreases. White blood cell count and ESR are generally normal. Levels of liver enzymes such as ALT and AST are quite high (more than eight times normal when jaundice appears); bilirubin also is elevated as is alkaline phosphatase. Diagnosis is by IgM anti-hepatitis B core antibody (HbcAb) in the acute or early convalescent serum. IgM is found during the onset of jaundice. Hepatitis B surface antibody indicates an immunization response. Eventually, over months, anti-hepatitis B surface antigen (HbsAG) is replaced by HbcAb.

Management

The disease is generally self-resolving; it lasts approximately six weeks with the possibility of two to three relapses. Increased calorie intake (especially in morning) and avoidance of hepatically metabolized drugs is all that is necessary. Patient is a carrier. All pregnant women should be screened for HbsAG on their first prenatal visit and later in pregnancy if at high risk. For prevention, after needle stick, within 14 days of sexual exposure, or at birth HBV, hyperimmune globulin should be administered followed by HBV vaccination. Standard immune globulin is also as effective. Due to the higher risk of liver cancer in chronic HBV individuals, immunization is recommended for all high-risk individuals. (*Note:* For chronic liver diseases, see **Table 21–3**.)

Table 21–3 Differential Diagnosis in Patients with Chronic Elevation of Liver Enzymes

Disease/Disorder	Definition	Clinical Features	Laboratory Findings	Treatment
Chronic hepatitis B	Either persistent carrier state with hepatitis or chronic active hepatitis.	Symptoms are nonspecific including malaise, anorexia, and fatigue. Past history of acute hepatitis B or past transfusion or IV drug abuser.	Moderate AST levels; positive for hepatitis B surface antigen and anti-hepatitis B core antibody.	Recombinant interferon-alpha; steroids are variably helpful for chronic active hepatitis B.
Hepatitis C	An acute progressive liver parenchymal infection by hepatitis C virus (HCV).	Symptoms are nonspecific including malaise, anorexia, and fatigue. Past history of acute hepatitis B or past transfusion or IV drug abuser.	ALT and AST elevation (six to eight times), bilirubin increased by five to ten times; positive for anti-HCV antibody detected by ELISA	Recombinant interferon-alpha for 6 months to reduce ALT and HCV viremia; relapse occurs 50% of time; 3- to 6-year remissions do occur.
Hemochromatosis	An autosomal recessive disorder with increased iron absorption and an accumulation of iron as hemosiderin in multiple organs including adrenals, liver, pancreas, heart, testes, kidneys, pituitary, and joints.	Family history, increased skin pigmentation, hepatomegaly and tenderness, systemic illness (e.g., heart, pancreas), arthritis (in particular hip).	Elevated serum transferrin saturation values; increased plasma iron, ferritin, liver enzymes; measurement of hepatic iron index in liver biopsy.	Weekly phlebotomy of 500 ml of blood for several months; subsequent phlebotomies are performed every 3 to 6 months; deferoxamine (iron chelating agent) is used in severe cases.
Alcoholic liver disease	Due to chronic alcohol damage fatty changes with diffuse inflammatory response and necrosis are found.	History of alcohol abuse.	High GGT, high MCV, AST:ALT ratio is greater than 2:1.	No alcohol; prednisone is used in severe cases.
Fatty liver steatonecrosis	Fat accumulation in the liver due to alcohol abuse, diabetes, and obesity.	Found with diabetes and obesity; more common in women.	Mild GGT, AST, and ALT elevation; glucose intolerance.	Control of underlying alcoholism, diabetes, or obesity.
Primary biliary cirrhosis	A disease of unknown origin with chronic cholestasis and progressive destruction of bile ducts.	Pruritus, fatigue, and jaundice; found with other disorders such as thyroiditis, arthritis, Sjögren's syndrome, scleroderma, and renal tubular acidosis.	High alkaline phosphatase and GGT; positive ANA; IgM increase.	Methotrexate and other major medications; prednisone not beneficial; supplementation of vitamins A, D, and K and calcium, pruritus treated with cholestyramine; liver transplant needed in severe cases.
Wilson's disease	A progressive and fatal disorder (unless treated) of copper metabolism inherited as a mutant gene on chromosome 13. Deposition of copper in the brain and liver is life-threatening.	Younger patient with Kayser-Fleischer rings (gold or greenish gold crescents on the cornea) confirmed by an ophthalmologist with a slit-lamp, associated with neuropsychiatric symptoms.	Deficiency of serum ceruloplasmin, excessive hepatic copper, Coombs negative hemolytic anemia, hypercupriuria.	Penicillamine, trientine, and zinc acetate are approved for treatment. Treatment must be lifelong whether symptomatic or not or death from CNS or liver pathology will occur.

Table 21–3 Differential Diagnosis in Patients with Chronic Elevation of Liver Enzymes (continued)

Disease/Disorder	Definition	Clinical Features	Laboratory Findings	Treatment
Alpha-1-antitrypsin deficiency	Alpha-1-antitrypsin is produced by the liver and it inhibits proteolytic enzymes throughout the body with the most significant effects in the lungs.	Positive for family history of liver and emphysematous lung disease.	Serum protein electrophoresis (low serum globulin); measure alpha-1-antitrypsin levels.	Genetic counseling Liver transplant necessary in severe cases Counseling regarding smoking to prevent severe emphysema

Key: ANA, antinuclear antibody; ALT, alanine aminotransferase (also called SGP); AST, aspartate aminotransferase (also called SGOT); ELISA, enzyme linked immunosorbent assay; IgM, gamma M immunoglobulin; GGT, gamma glutamyl transferase; MCV, mean corpuscular volume.

Hepatitis C

Classic Presentation

Many patients are asymptomatic. If symptomatic, the patient presents with a complaint of chronic malaise or fatigue. If presenting during the prodrome, the patient may have signs of serum sickness such as urticaria, rash, and arthralgias. There may be upper right quadrant abdominal pain during an acute attack.

Cause

Infection with the hepatitis C virus (HCV) is usually related to exposure by the parenteral route (needle use including infected transfused blood, contaminated needles in drug abusers, and tattoos). The most common individuals are homosexual men, drug abusers, visitors and immigrants from endemic areas, neonates born to infected mothers, prisoners and the institutionalized, and medical workers exposed to accidental needle pricks. Infection at an early age in developing countries usually is unremarkable with only mild disease and no jaundice. HCV is an infectious disease notifiable on the national level. There are 40,000 new cases of chronic hepatitis in the United States each year. Two-thirds of individuals with chronic HCV are undiagnosed. The CDC recently recommended screening for HCV for all individuals born between 1945 and 1965. It is the most common cause of chronic liver disease and need for liver transplants in the United States. There has been a reduction in new cases since all donor blood has been screened since 1992.

Evaluation

The patient may have hepatomegaly with upper right quadrant tenderness. Another characteristic sign is dark urine. At some point the patient may develop a fever that precedes the appearance of jaundice. Interestingly, the onset of jaundice occurs when the patient begins to feel better and the fever rapidly decreases. If patients do become symptomatic it is usually two weeks post-exposure, persisting for 2–12 weeks. White blood cell count and ESR are generally normal. Levels of liver enzymes such as ALT and AST are high with acute HCV; however, most liver enzymes are not greatly elevated in chronic HCV. HCV RNA is positive one to two weeks post-exposure. Anti-HCV is negative until at least two months post-exposure. For chronic HCV, ultrasound and liver biopsy may be necessary to determine the degree of liver damage.

Management

Initially therapy was with interferon monotherapy. Recent advances have enlisted the addition of drugs that have specific effects on viral replication. With the older therapy the viral clearance rate was less than 10%. Now the rate with the addition of these new medications is around 70%. The combination of peginterferon and ribavirin leads to a 70% to 80% response against HCV for genotype 2 or 3 but only a 45% to 70% response for other genotypes. This has led to a triple therapy approach using one of two new protease inhibitors added to the standard care. There is still controversy about the effect and risk of this new approach.[56] New studies are necessary. Treatment within 12 weeks of exposure is highly effective. Treatment is less effective for those >60 years old. (*Note:* For chronic liver diseases, see Table 21–3.)

Chronic Myelogenous Leukemia

Classic Presentation

The patient is usually middle-aged or older and complains of fatigue, night sweats, and a low-grade fever.

Cause

Overproduction of myeloid cells that are capable of differentiation is due to an abnormality of the Philadelphia chromosome (reciprocal translocation of long arms of chromosomes 9 and 22). The BCR-ABL oncogene on the Philadelphia chromosome facilitates the production of the BCR-ABL protein, which inhibits cell apoptosis and DNA repair. Sixty percent are symptomatic. Forty percent are asymptomatic and are identified only by a blood test. If allowed to progress, CML in the chronic phase progresses to an accelerated phase and then a final blast phase (becomes acute leukemia) within about three to five years. In the accelerated phase there may be upper left quadrant pain and referred left shoulder pain due to splenic rupture.

Evaluation

The patient will have splenomegaly at some point. The diagnosis is based on laboratory findings of a markedly elevated white blood cell count (> 150,000/mm³) with granulocytes in various stages of development. Blasts are less than 5%, and basophilia may be present. Uric acid levels may be elevated. Cytogenic testing can include detection of the Philadelphia chromosome t(9,22) using FISH or reverse-transcription-polymerase chain reaction.

Management

The disease is eventually fatal unless the patient is treated with medication or has a bone marrow transplant. Tyrosine kinase inhibitors (TKI) are the mainstay of treatment. As of 2014 there were five approved TKIs including the first-generation imatinib, and more potent second-generation products dasatinib, nilotinib, bosutinib, and ponatinib. For patients in the chronic phase of CML, dasatinib and nilotinib are more effective. A decision regarding which is appropriate for each individual patient is obviously an informed decision with the managing oncologist. Of patients on TKI therapy, 71% maintain results for at least seven years. The success rate is 70% to 80% for bone marrow transplant in patients under age 40 years who have the transplant within one year of the diagnosis.[57] (*Note:* For other leukemias, see Chapter 52.)

APPENDIX 21–1

References

1. Buchwald D, Gantz NM, Katon WJ, Manu P. Tips on chronic fatigue syndrome. *Patient Care.* 1991;25:45–58.

2. Kroenke K, Wood DR, Mangelsdorff D, et al. Chronic fatigue in primary care. *JAMA.* 1988;260;929–934.

3. Kroenke K. Chronic fatigue: frequency, causes, evaluation, and management. *Compr Ther.* 1989;15(7):3–7.

4. Cathebras PJ, et al. Fatigue in primary care: prevention, psychiatric comorbidity, illness, behavior, and outcome. *J Gen Intern Med.* 1992;7:276.

5. Morrison JD. Fatigue as a presenting complaint in family practice. *J Fam Pract.* 1980;10:776–781.

6. Kirk J, Douglass R, Nelson E, et al. Chief complaint of fatigue: a prospective study. *J Fam Pract.* 1990;30:33–41.

7. Levine PH, et al. Clinical, epidemiologic, and virologic studies in four clusters of the chronic fatigue syndrome. *Arch Intern Med.* 1992;152:1611.

8. Elnicki DM, Schockcor WT, Brick JE, et al. Evaluating the complaint of fatigue in primary care: diagnoses and outcomes. *Am J Med.* 1992;93:303–306.

9. Woodward RV, Broom DH, Legge DG. Diagnosis of chronic illness: disabling or enabling—the case of chronic fatigue syndrome. *J R Soc Med.* 1995;88:325–329.

10. Holmes GP, Kaplan JE, Ganz NM, et al. Chronic fatigue syndrome: a working case definition. *Ann Intern Med.* 1988;108:387–389.

11. Fukuda K, Straus SE, Hickie I, et al. The chronic fatigue syndrome: a comprehensive approach to its definition and study. *Ann Intern Med.* 1994;121:953–959.

12. Shafran SD. The chronic fatigue syndrome. *Am J Med.* 1991;90:730–739.

13. Holmes GP, Kaplan JE, Stewart JA, et al. A cluster of patients with a chronic mononucleosis-like syndrome. *JAMA.* 1987;257:2297–2302.

14. Krupp LB, Mendelson WB, Freidman R. An overview of chronic fatigue syndrome. *J Clin Psychol.* 1991;52:403.

15. Centers for Disease Control. Inability of retroviral tests to identify persons with chronic fatigue syndrome. *Morbid Mortal Weekly Rep.* 1993;42:183.

16. Bou-Holaigah J, Rowe PC, Kan J, Calkins H. The relationship between neurally mediated hypotension and the chronic fatigue syndrome. *JAMA.* 1995;274:961–967.

17. Rowe PC, Bou-Holaigah J, Kan J, Calkins H. Is neurally mediated hypotension an unrecognized cause of chronic fatigue? *Lancet.* 1995;345:623–624.

18. Schleudelberg A, et al. Chronic fatigue syndrome research: definition and medical outcome assessment. *Ann Intern Med.* 1992;117:325–331.

19. Lane TJ, Mann P, Mathew DA. Depression and somatization in the chronic fatigue syndrome. *Ann Intern Med.* 1991;91:335.

20. Gold PW, Licino J, Wong ML, Chrousos GP. Corticotropin releasing hormone in the pathophysiology of melancholic and atypical depression and in the mechanism of action of antidepressant drugs. *Ann N Y Acad Sci.* 1995;771:716–729.

21. Pollmacher T, Mullington J, Korth C, Hinze-Selche D. Influence of host defense activation in sleep in humans. *Adv Neuroimmunol.* 1995;5:155–169.

22. Gunn WJ, et al. Epidemiology of chronic fatigue syndrome: the Centers for Disease Control study. *Ciba Found Symp.* 1993;173:406–414.

23. Sumaya SV, et al. Seroprevalence study of Epstein-Barr virus infection in a rural community. *J Infect Dis.* 1975;131:403–408.

24. Buchwald D, Sullivan JL, Kormaroff AL. Frequency of "chronic" active Epstein-Barr virus infections in general medical practice. *JAMA.* 1987;257:2303–2307.

25. Futcher KY, White PD. Randomised controlled trial of graded exercise in patients with chronic fatigue syndrome. *Br Med J.* 1997;314:1647–1652.

26. McCully KK, Sisto SA, Natelson BH. Use of exercise for treatment of chronic fatigue syndrome. *Sports Med.* 1996;21:35–48.

27. Lloyd AR, Hickie I, Brockman A, et al. Immunologic and psychogenic therapy for patients with chronic fatigue syndrome: a double-blind, placebo controlled trial. *Am J Med.* 1993;94:187–203.

28. Behan PO, Behan WMH, Horrobin D. Effect of high doses of essential fatty acids on the postviral fatigue syndrome. *Acta Neurol Scand.* 1990;82:209–216.

29. Cox IM, Campbell MJ, Dowson D. Red blood cell magnesium and chronic fatigue syndrome. *Lancet.* 1991;337:757–760.

30. Kaslow JF, Rucker L, Onishi R. Liver extract-folic acid-cyanocobalamin versus placebo for chronic fatigue syndrome. *Arch Intern Med.* 1989;149:2501–2503.

31. Lloyd AR, Hickie I, Wakefield D, et al. A double-blind, placebo controlled trial of intravenous

immunoglobulin therapy in patients with chronic fatigue syndrome. *Am J Med.* 1990;89:561–568.

32. Strauss SF, et al. Acyclovir treatment of the chronic fatigue syndrome. *N Engl J Med.* 1988;319:1692–1698.

33. Plioplys AV, Plioplys S. Amantadine and L-carnitine treatment of chronic fatigue syndrome. *Neuropsychobiol.* 1997;35:16–23.

34. Beschetti R. Chronic fatigue syndrome and liquorice. *N Z Med J.* 1995;108:156–157.

35. Warren G, McKendrick M, Peet M. The role of essential fatty acids in chronic fatigue syndrome. *Acta Neurol Scand.* 1999;99:112–116.

36. Bates DW, Buchwald D, Lee J, et al. Clinical laboratory test findings in patients with chronic fatigue syndrome. *Arch Intern Med.* 1995;155:97–103.

37. White KP, Speechley M, Harth M, Ostbye T. Coexistence of chronic fatigue syndrome with fibromyalgia syndrome in the general population. A controlled study. *Scand J Rheumatol.* 2000;29(1):44–51.

38. Hicks JE, Jones JF, Renner JH, Schmaling K. Chronic fatigue syndrome: strategies that work. *Patient Care.* 1995;5:55–73.

39. Hill NF, Tiersky LA, Scavalla VR, et al. Natural history of severe chronic fatigue syndrome. *Arch Phys Med Rehabil.* 1999;80(9):1090–1094.

40. McKenzie R, O'Fallon A, Dale J, et al. Low-dose hydrocortisone for treatment of chronic fatigue syndrome. A randomized controlled trial. *JAMA.* 1998;280:1061–1066.

41. Reid S, Chalder T, Cleare A, et al. Chronic fatigue syndrome. *Br Med J.* 2000;320:292–296.

42. Smythe H. Fibrositis syndrome: a historical perspective. *J Rheumatol.* 1989;16(suppl 9):2–6.

43. Wolfe F, Smythe HA, Yunus MB, et al. The American College of Rheumatology 1990 criteria for classification of fibromyalgia: report of the Multicenter Criteria Committee. *Arthritis Rheum.* 1990;33:160–172.

44. Bennett RM. Nonarticular rheumatism and spondyloarthropathies—similarities and differences. *Postgrad Med.* 1990;87:97–104.

45. Goldenberg DL. Fibromyalgia syndrome a decade later: what have we learned? *Arch Intern Med.* 1999;159:777–785.

46. Mitchell RI, Carmen GM. The functional restoration approach to the treatment of chronic pain in patients with soft tissue and back injuries. *Spine.* 1994;19:633–642.

47. St. Claire SM. Diagnosis and management of fibromyalgia syndrome. *J Neuromusculoskeletal Syst.* 1994;2(3):101–111.

48. Richards SCM, Scott DL. Prescribed exercise in people with fibromyalgia: Parallel group randomized controlled trial. *Br Med J.* 2002;325:185–188.

49. Schneider M, Vernon H, Ko G, Lawson G, Perera J. Chiropractic management of fibromyalgia syndrome: a systematic review of the literature. *J Manipulative Physiol Ther.* 2009;32(1):25–40.

50. Armstrong DJ, Meenagh GK, Bickle I, Lee AS, Curran ES, Finch MB. Vitamin D deficiency is associated with anxiety and depression in fibromyalgia. *Clin Rheumatol.* 2007;26(4):551–554.

51. Massey PB. Reduction of fibromyalgia symptoms through intravenous nutrient therapy: results of a pilot clinical trial. *Altern Ther Health Med.* 2007;13(3):32–34.

52. Rossini M, Di Munno O, Valentini G, et al. Double-blind, multicenter trial comparing acetyl l-carnitine with placebo in the treatment of fibromyalgia patients. *Clin Exp Rheumatol.* 2007;25(2):182–188.

53. Brown SL, Hansen S L, Langone JL. Role of serology in the diagnosis of Lyme disease. *JAMA.* 1999;282:62–66.

54. Seltzer EG, Gerger MA, Cartter ML, et al. Long-term outcomes of persons with Lyme disease. *JAMA.* 2000;283:609–616.

55. Recommendations for the use of Lyme disease vaccine. *Morbid Mortal Weekly Rep.* 1999;48:11–13.

56. Liang TJ, Ghany MG. Current and future therapies for hepatitis C virus infection. *N Engl J Med.* 2013;368(20):1907–1917.

57. Clift RA. Treatment of chronic myeloid leukemia by marrow transplantation. *Blood.* 1993;34:1954.

Fever

Context

Although fever may not be a common presenting complaint to a chiropractic office, its presence among other signs or symptoms, or lack thereof, provides an important clue in differential diagnosis. Temperature should be measured in:

- Children on an initial visit who appear to have low energy, loss of appetite, or decreased playfulness
- All patients with signs of infection or generalized inflammation
- All seniors on initial presentation

Fever of unknown origin (FUO) is a temperature greater than 38.3°C (101°F) that is present several times over a three-week period (undiagnosed after one week) or a persistent fever for 10 to 14 days that remains undiagnosed.[1] It is unlikely but possible that this scenario may present to a chiropractor's office. If so, it is important to recognize the potential seriousness of this presentation. One study estimated that approximately 41% of children with true FUO had a chronic or fatal disease.[2] The primary focus of the following discussion is on proper assessment of temperature and a generalized approach to narrow possibilities.

There are many misconceptions with regard to fever. It is important to bear in mind the following:

- Fever is a protective response, and is not in and of itself bad.
- Fever does not always indicate infection.
- Although there is a reference normal temperature of 98.6°F, this does not represent a "fixed" normal.
- Fever is often regarded as a symptom; however, it is possible to feel "feverish" and not have a fever, or to feel normal and have a fever. It is also possible for someone with a fever to appear normal, sometimes even hyperactive; therefore, fever must be objectified.

The standard normal temperature of 98.6°F was established over 130 years ago by Wunderlich.[3] Recently, this has been called into question and reexamined. Mackowiak determined that the mean body temperature was not 98.6°F, but 98.2°F (close enough!).[4] More important is the recognition that there is a normal range of temperature that varies. Temperature is usually the lowest in the morning, highest in the late afternoon and early evening. This diurnal variation is as much as 1°F to 1.5°F. According to Mackowiak's study, fever in young and middle-aged adults is classified as a reading at or above 37.2°C (99.0°F) in the early morning; in the evening, at or above 37.8°C (100°F). There are other normal variations that must be acknowledged, as follows:

- Women have a rise in temperature at ovulation of 0.5°F to 0.75°F due to production of progesterone. The temperature returns to the normal basal reading at the beginning of menstruation.
- Children often have an exaggerated response to infection, generating a much higher temperature than adults with the same infection or cause.
- Senior patients generally have a lower mean temperature (average of 36.2°C [97.2°F]); their response to a pyrogenic stimulator is often less remarkable than that of a younger adult; seniors often do not feel that they have a fever when, in fact, they have one.
- Exercise can raise the body temperature.

FUO is a worrisome phenomenon. The medical criteria are fever higher than 38.3°C on several occasions for three weeks or longer in patients without neutropenia or immunosuppression. Of these patients, the statistical breakdown of cause is as follows:

- 25% have chronic, indolent infection.
- 25% have autoimmune disease.
- 10% have a malignancy.
- The remainder have miscellaneous or no known cause.

In cases of FUO, 5% to 35% go undiagnosed, with approximately 75% of these resolving without incident (the majority having an infectious etiology).[5] However, there are still concerns. As with a standard self-remitting fever, the most common cause of FUO is infection. The most common causes are tuberculosis and endocarditis. Other common infections that may not have obvious associated signs are sinus infections and urinary tract infections. The second most common cause of FUO is neoplasms, especially leukemias, lymphomas, and solid tumors of the abdomen. Obviously, a patient with FUO must be referred for a medical evaluation to uncover these potentially life-threatening and often curable disorders.

General Strategy

History

Screen for patients at risk, including those with a history that might suggest an infectious, inflammatory, hemorrhagic, or cancerous process.

Evaluation

- Determine the temperature using a mercury, electronic, or infrared device (rectal temperature readings are reserved for infants, or athletes suffering from hypo- or hyperthermia).
- Attempt to match other physical signs that localize to a specific organ system or process.

Management

- Refer the patient if an underlying serious process is discovered, if the fever is persistent for more than 10 days, if the fever is greater than 104°F, or if the fever is present off and on over a period of three weeks (FUO).
- Minor fevers (101°F or less) associated with signs of gastroenteritis, flu, or other common infections can be managed with time and monitoring; if necessary, aspirin (not for children) or acetaminophen every four hours is effective.
- Fevers of 102°F to 104°F do not usually require treatment; however, cold sponges, ice packs, or cold baths may help in reducing body temperature.

Relevant Physiology

Phagocytic leukocytes release endogenous pyrogens (proteins) into the bloodstream in response to a host of pyrogenic triggers. The endogenous proteins reach the thermoregulatory center in the anterior hypothalamus, causing the production and release of prostaglandins. The result is a new set-point for the body requiring measures to raise body temperature, including shivering and vasoconstriction. Following is a general list of conditions that may cause fever:

- Infections
- Connective tissue disorders
- Thromboembolic hemorrhage
- Various metabolic conditions
- Neoplasms
- Vascular events

Table 22–1 gives a more extensive list under each category. Generally, infection is the most common cause, resulting in a fever that is gone within one week. When fever persists beyond this time frame, the other categories of disorders should be considered. **Table 22–2** is a list of named fever disorders.

Hyperthermia

Heatstroke (Sunstroke)

With heatstroke, hyperthermia is due to a failure of the body's normal heat loss mechanisms. Usually sweating is markedly decreased, allowing for sustained body temperatures in the 40°C to 41°C (104°F–106°F) range for several hours, with associated circulatory collapse and death if untreated. The individual will often experience disorientation, headache, vertigo, and fatigue, leading to unconsciousness and convulsions. Pulse increases without a concomitant change in blood pressure. The skin is flushed, dry, and hot. If the patient survives, permanent brain damage and renal failure are possible. Emergency management (until hospital management) includes removing all clothes and wrapping the individual in wet blankets while fanning to increase loss of heat through evaporation. If the patient can be immersed in water, especially cold water, this should be done, watching for shivering. Shivering should be avoided because it increases core temperature. Temperature is monitored rectally every 10 minutes and not allowed to drop below 39.3°C (101°F).

Heat Exhaustion

Unlike heatstroke, the body's ability to dissipate heat is functional. Heat exhaustion is a loss of fluid and electrolytes through excessive sweating. Initially presenting as a fatigued, weak, and anxious individual, heat exhaustion will progress to circulatory collapse with the individual losing consciousness. With progressing circulatory collapse, the patient will have cold, clammy skin and a slow, difficult-to-palpate pulse. The core temperature is usually in the "fever" range of 38.3°C to 40.6°C (101°F–105°F). The primary concern is conserving fluid loss and assuring blood supply to the heart and brain. Placing the patient flat or with the head slightly down and replacing fluids slowly with an electrolyte solution such as a sports drink or slightly salted water should be initiated until the patient can be assessed medically.

Heat Cramps

Heat cramps may occur when excessive sweating results in significant fluid and electrolyte loss. This is most common with individuals involved in outdoor occupations and with athletes. It is more common in dry environments where sweating is not as obvious. Cramping is usually in the extremities; however, it may start in the abdominal muscles and simulate an abdominal (visceral) presentation. Replacement of water and electrolytes is preventive and palliative.

Table 22–1 Causes of Fever

Infection	Autoimmune disease	Neoplasms
Bacterial	Systemic lupus erythematosus	Primary neoplasms
Viral	Polyarteritis nodosa	• Colon
Rickettsial	Rheumatic fever	• Rectum
Fungal	Polymyalgia rheumatica	• Liver
Parasitic	Giant-cell arteritis	• Kidney
Mycobacterial	Still's disease	Neuroblastoma
Hematologic	Relapsing polychondritis	Liver metastasis
	Dermatomyositis	
Lymphomas	Adult rheumatoid arthritis	
Leukemias		
Hemolytic anemias		
Endocrine disease	**Cardiovascular disease**	**Abdominal disease**
Hyperthyroidism	Myocardial infarction	Inflammatory bowel disease
Pheochromocytoma	Pulmonary embolism	Liver abscess
		Alcoholic hepatitis
		Granulomatous hepatitis
Miscellaneous	**Central nervous system disease**	**Chemical**
Sarcoidosis	Cerebral hemorrhage	Drug reactions
Familial Mediterranean fever	Head injuries	
Factitious fever	Brain and spinal cord tumors	
	Degenerative CNS disease	
	Spinal cord injury	

Reproduced from Evans, R., *Topics in Clinical Chiropractic*, Vol. 2, No. 1, pp. 30–36, ©1995, Aspen Publishers, Inc.

Table 22–2 Some Named Fever Conditions

Type	Summary of Information
Colorado tick	An infection transmitted by tick bites in the western United States and Canada, most often in the "tick season" of March through November. Acute onset of a high fever, often with chills, other flu-like symptoms, and a light rash. There are often two to three bouts of fever lasting 1–3 days. There is leucopenia with a shift to the left. A reverse transcriptase PCR assay is diagnostic.
Dengue	Spread by mosquitoes, this viral infection previously was limited to Thailand, the Philippines, India, the Caribbean, Central America, and the northern half of South America, but has now reached the southern United States. Infection may be asymptomatic or present as a wide range of severity, including severe hemorrhage and fatal shock. There is a biphasic fever, with the first phase lasting a few days longer. There is also a biphasic rash appearance during remission from the first fever or beginning of second phase. This may be the only distinguishing clinical sign differentiating it from malaria or yellow fever. Leukopenia and thrombocytopenia will be present in the hemorrhagic form. There are rapid serologic assays available to help diagnose the condition. There is no specific treatment other than to maintain volume and use acetaminophen.
Hemorrhagic	A very diverse group of infections may cause hemorrhagic diastasis. Transmission is also variable, including transmission from ticks, rodents, and mosquitoes. Examples include the following fevers: yellow, dengue, Chikungunya, Ebola, Omsk, and Forrest fever among many others. A high fever with leucopenia, hemorrhagic diastasis, and altered mental status are common in the presentation. There is no specific treatment for most.
Mediterranean (familial)	An autosomal recessive disorder affecting people of the Mediterranean with a specific appearance in Sephardic Jews, Armenians, Arabs, and Turks. The (familial) disease is due to a lack of a specific protease. Patients develop severe abdominal pain, peritonitis, and fever that resolves within one to two days. There is a genetic test to confirm the diagnosis. Colchicine is used if amyloidosis develops.
Rheumatic	A sequelae to a beta-hemolytic infection of the pharynx, this immune response is quite rare in the United States. Antibodies are developed against primarily the heart (heart valves), joints, and nervous tissue. The Jones criteria are used, which include two major and two minor criteria. In essence, mitral valve or other cardiac involvement, erythema marginatum (skin lesions), Sydenham's chorea, and arthritis are the areas evaluated. The laboratory diagnosis is with the finding of antistreptococcal antibodies, which includes antistreptolysin O and antiDNase B. A nonspecific finding is an increase in ESR. Treatment is with penicillin or, in those who are allergic, sulfonamides or erythromycin. Salicylates are used for the fever and joint pain. Prophylaxis for recurrent attacks may be necessary.
Scarlet	An uncommon disorder caused by group A streptococcal infection that produces an erythrogenic toxin causing an abdominal rash and lateral chest, a "strawberry" tongue, and symptoms similar to other streptococcal pharyngitis diseases. Group A beta-hemolytic streptococci are found in culture from the throat, and the antistreptolysin O titers rise. Treatment is with penicillin or, in those who are allergic, sulfonamides or erythromycin. Salicylates are used for the fever and joint pain. Prophylaxis for recurrent attacks may be necessary.
Typhoid (enteric)	A salmonella typhi infection that produces malaise, headache, cough, sore throat, abdominal pain and, initially, constipation. The patient may develop a rash (rose spots), abdominal distention, splenomegaly, and bradycardia. Diagnosis is preferentially from blood culture of the organism. The fever gradually increases over 10–14 days, at which time the patient is feeling the worst. If there are no complications, the patient will gradually improve over the following 7–10 days. Transmission is through consumption of contaminated food or drink. Incubation is 5–14 days. There is growing resistance to the traditional antibiotics. Most recently, ceftriaxone and fluoroquinolones are used.
Yellow	Yellow fever is a viral infection spread by mosquitoes primarily in Africa and South America. There is a mild and a severe form. The mild form presents simply as "flu" symptoms. The severe form (15%) first appears as the mild form, and after a few days progresses to fever, bradycardia, GI bleeding, nasal bleeding, jaundice, hypotension, and delirium. Diagnostically, there is proteinuria and is usually confirmed by a specific rapid test IgM capture enzyme immunoassay (EIA). There is no specific treatment. Those who do not survive often have signs of intractable hiccups, black vomitus, anuria, and melena.
Malaria	Malaria is a parasitic infection transmitted by mosquitoes in many parts of the world, including the tropics and subtropics, accounting for 300 million infected individuals per year and 1.5–2.7 million deaths. There are four species of plasmodium; some are more endemic to certain regions. Malaria is still evident in Mexico, Haiti, the Dominican Republic, Central and South America, Africa, Southeast Asia, China, the Middle East, and Indonesia. Cases have been "imported" to the United States. Malarial attacks occur over hours, with shaking chills and fever. Associated flu-like symptoms are present. Symptoms seem to alter on an every-other-day or every-three-days cycle. The organism is demonstrated on thick or thin blood film. Approximately 2% of the RBCs are affected. A large armamentarium of antimalarial drugs is available. Some strains have become resistant to some of the standard approaches. Chemoprophylaxis is available for those traveling to high-risk areas.

Evaluation

Examination

Although generally the history is the starting point in evaluation, the order has been switched to emphasize the need for an accurate, consistent measurement of body temperature. The armamentarium for body temperature evaluation has expanded beyond the simple mercury thermometer.[6] Now available are mercury-in-glass, electronic, infrared, and strip thermometers. Mercury thermometers can be used orally, rectally, and in the axillary region. (The least reliable and most susceptible to variation is the axillary reading; it has largely been avoided when possible.) Oral mercury thermometers are accurate when properly used; however, readings take between four and eight minutes depending on whether or not the patient is febrile. Electronic thermometers take only about 30 seconds in comparison. They also use disposable, unbreakable probe covers. The new infrared thermometers have recently become less expensive and provide an accurate measurement in a few seconds. Paper strip thermometers are convenient, but they are not considered very reliable.

The standard for medical recording is in degrees Celsius (centigrade) (C). The conversion formulas are:

- degrees C = 5/9 (°F –32)
- degrees F = (9/5°C) + 32

Following is a suggested technique for taking an oral temperature with a mercury thermometer:

- If the patient has just had hot or cold liquids, wait 15 minutes prior to evaluation.
- If the patient has just smoked, wait two minutes.
- Shake the thermometer down to a temperature of 35.5°C (96°F).
- Make sure the thermometer has been sterilized and/or has a disposable probe slip in place.
- Place the thermometer at the base of the tongue on either side of the posterior sublingual pockets (not in the middle of the tongue).
- Instruct the patient to keep his or her lips closed.
- Leave the thermometer in place for three to four minutes if the patient is afebrile.
- Leave the thermometer in place for up to eight minutes if the patient is febrile.

For an infrared thermometer:

- Gently place the covered probe tip in the patient's ear.

- Do not force the thermometer into the ear or fully block the canal.
- Activate and read the temperature in approximately two to three seconds.

Rectal temperature is considered to be a more accurate measure; however, it is less convenient in most cases. When other devices are not available or when measuring for hypo- or hyperthermia, rectal temperature is preferred.

- Wear gloves.
- Lubricate the probe end of the rectal thermometer (it has a more short, blunt probe compared with the oral thermometer).
- Insert the thermometer about 1 inch toward the umbilicus.
- Leave the thermometer in for two and a half minutes.
- Rectal readings are generally 0.5°C (1°F) higher than oral readings.

A factitious fever should be suspected in patients who are emotionally disturbed. These patients are often women working in healthcare positions. Clues to a factitious fever include the following:

- The fever is out of proportion to patient's general appearance—no loss of weight, no prostration, no sweating.
- The pulse rate does not increase proportionately with the degree of fever.
- The urine temperature does not match the rectal temperature (rectal temperature is significantly higher).

The remainder of the examination is a generalized approach looking first for clues such as the following:

- Examination of the skin for patterns of lesions (and in the history a sequence of appearance) (found with common childhood diseases, venereal disease, and rheumatoid and connective tissue disorders)
- Auscultation of the heart for murmurs
- Auscultation of the lungs for rales
- Palpation of the calves for localized swelling (thrombophlebitis)
- Examination for tophi at the big toe, knees, elbows, and ears
- Examination of the abdomen with a complaint of associated abdominal pain

This generalized approach should provide clues that narrow the possibilities. Further testing with laboratory, radiographs, or special studies should be justified by the history and physical exam findings. Researchers performing a literature review evaluated the value of signs, symptoms, and tests for adult patients with meningitis.[7] The researchers concluded that given the seriousness of meningitis, most physicians proceed to lumbar puncture based on a few positives. In adult patients, the absence of the classic triad of fever, neck stiffness, and altered mental status virtually eliminates a diagnosis of meningitis (i.e., rules out meningitis). Kernig's and Brudzinski's signs have low sensitivity but possibly high specificity (rule-out) value. Jolt accentuation of a patient's headache may be useful. Seventy-three percent of patients with meningitis have a petechial rash according to this study.

History

Given the enormous numbers of pyrogenic stimulators, the diagnostic approach is a search for the above-listed categories. The approach is a broad-based evaluation looking for any clue that may suggest the underlying cause. It is highly unusual to have fever as the only indicator of a disease or disorder. Localizing findings by organ or system is usually revealing. See the applicable chapters of this text based on these accompanying signs or symptoms.

General indicators of a viral infection in an adult are a low-grade fever and associated general aches and pains, a headache, malaise, or fatigue. An adult with a bacterial infection presents with a fever above 103°F and the general symptoms of a viral infection plus some localizing findings in the throat, abdomen, or chest. Children, on the other hand, may run high temperatures with almost any illness, including viral infections, otitis media, measles, and roseola. Very high readings (>105°F) are medical emergencies suggesting intracranial hemorrhage or tumor, pancreatitis, or a bad urinary tract infection. If the temperature remains at this elevation, significant brain damage or malignant cardiac arrhythmias may occur.

When the fever is not obviously tied to a flu or upper respiratory infection, a potential valuable avenue of questioning is recent travel within or outside the United States.[8] Certain fungal infections are endemic to specific regions of the United States. Following the same line of questioning, contact with certain animals such as birds, dogs, cats, rats or other rodents, or livestock suggests a specific infectious organism.

In the past, it was recommended to determine a time curve for fever presentation in an attempt to attach a specific diagnosis to a specific pattern of fever activity. This approach is now not considered useful as a match-type approach. The temporal sequence, however, may provide valuable clues to the underlying cause.

Management

There are two overlapping goals of management: (1) control for excessive fever and ensure adequate hydration, and (2) treat the underlying cause if it poses a health risk to the patient. Control of fever is rarely necessary unless it reaches the range of 103° to 104°F. At this level of fever it may be necessary to use cold packs, alcohol or cold sponges, or cold baths. Generally, this level of fever is well tolerated. If medication is used it is important to give aspirin or acetaminophen every four hours without a break in routine. Giving it only at night may cause a reactionary occurrence of chills or sweats. It is important not to give aspirin to children, especially those with flu or chicken pox, because of the risk of Reye's syndrome (leads to brain and liver damage or death).

APPENDIX 22–1

References

1. Everett MT. Definition of FUO in general practice. *Practitioner.* 1977;218:388–393.
2. Kimmel SR, Gemmill DW. The young child with fever. *Am Fam Physician.* 1988;37:196–206.
3. Kluger MJ. *Fever: Its Biology, Evolution, and Function.* Princeton, NJ: Princeton University Press; 1979.
4. Mackowiak PA, Wasserman SS, Levine MM. A critical appraisal of 98.6 degrees F: the upper limit of the normal body temperature, and other legacies of Carl Reinhold August Wunderlich. *JAMA.* 1992;268:1578–1580.
5. Greenberg SB, Taber L. Fever of unknown origin. In: Mackowiak PA, ed. *Fever: Basic Mechanisms and Management.* New York: Raven Press; 1991.
6. Jarvis C. *Physical Examination and Health Assessment.* Philadelphia: WB Saunders Co; 1992:200.
7. Attia J, Hatala R, Cook DJ, Wong JC. Does this adult patient have acute meningitis? *JAMA.* 1999;282(2):175–181.
8. Strickland GT. Fever in the returned traveler. *Med Clin North Am.* 1992;76:1375–1392.

Sleep and Related Complaints

Context

If asked, most patients would have a complaint of disrupted sleep at some times in their lives. Often they can relate this to a specific event such as a stressful incident, alcohol ingestion, or pain. When it is a prolonged or chronic problem, the patient becomes concerned. The conscious effort to initiate sleep often may worsen the condition. It is interesting to note that underreporting is the standard for one of the most common sleep disorders: insomnia. A Gallup survey found that only 5% of insomniacs consulted a physician. Approximately 30% had mentioned it when presenting to a doctor for other complaints.

It is not always obvious what a person does or does not do during sleep. This is important when considering that the result of sleep dysfunction is excessive sleepiness often without a complaint of disrupted sleep. Instead, the primary complaint is tiredness or fatigue. With excessive tiredness or fatigue, there is the obvious disruption of functional ability with daily activities; however, the larger concern is the potential danger when driving a car or operating other potentially dangerous machinery.

Although many sleep problems are transient and/or benign, when a primary sleep disorder is detected, further evaluation at a sleep laboratory is necessary to identify clearly the cause and plan for subsequent management.

General Strategy

History and Evaluation

- Determine whether the patient is able to describe the complaint, attempting to clarify whether the problem is in falling asleep, constant interruption of sleep, inability to fall back to sleep after early morning awakening, "light" sleep, or other difficulty.
- Determine associated problems such as excessive daytime sleepiness.
- Determine possible causes or contributing factors, including the following:
    1. Diet related—alcohol, caffeine, food allergy
    2. Smoking (more than one pack per day)
    3. Drugs—cocaine, over-the-counter (OTC) stimulants such as nasal sprays, abuse of OTC sleep medications, prescription drugs
    4. Underlying disorders such as asthma, hypo- or hyperthyroidism, chronic obstructive pulmonary disease, congestive heart failure
    5. Painful conditions (headaches; hip, knee, shoulder, low back, and/or neck pain)
    6. Restless legs or muscle cramps
    7. Amount of sleep, jet lag, work habits
    8. Stress and possible depression
    9. Moderate exercise prior to sleep
    10. Past diagnosis or treatment of a psychologic /psychiatric disorder
- If the patient is presenting with a complaint of fatigue or tiredness, it may be necessary to obtain an eyewitness account of his or her sleep pattern.

Management

- If a primary sleep disorder is suspected, referral to a sleep laboratory is warranted.
- Make recommendations regarding sleep hygiene (**Exhibit 23–1**).
- Conservative management may be appropriate when sleep hygiene is the primary cause; however, specific sleep disorders should be referred to a specialist for management.

Exhibit 23–1 Sleep Hygiene

- Go to bed at a consistent time.
- Sleep in a comfortable room that is cool and free of stimulation (noise, light, restless sleep partner).
- Sleep on a comfortable bed (more firm is suggested).
- Do not eat large amounts of food prior to sleeping.
- Avoid alcohol, smoking, and caffeine prior to sleeping.
- Do not exercise heavily before sleeping.
- Avoid daytime napping.
- If focused on a bothersome mental concern, write it down and deal with it in the morning if possible.
- If unable to sleep after 30 minutes, get up and have a light snack or listen to soothing music; then return to bed.
- Avoid the use of OTC sleep medications.
- Weight reduction may be helpful to those with central sleep apnea.

- For obstructive sleep apnea, use of a dental appliance and loss of weight may be effective. If not, referral for Continuous Positive Airway Pressure (CPAP) will likely be beneficial.

Relevant Anatomy and Physiology

Sleep is a complex interactive function coordinated by many parts of the brain. The structures that facilitate sleep include the basal forebrain, the dorsal raphe nuclei, the midline thalamus, and the area around the solitary tract in the medulla. Waking is facilitated by the reticular activating system (pons and midbrain) and the posterior hypothalamus. This interaction is dependent on changing levels of serotonin, catecholamines, acetylcholine, and a host of other neurotransmitters. During sleep there are also fluctuations of hormonal levels that may play a role in the quality of sleep and wakefulness. One example is the decrease in epinephrine and cortisol coupled with elevated histamine and other mediator levels between midnight and 4 a.m. These changes correlate with worsening of asthma at night.[1]

Sleep is generally divided into two phases in relationship to changing eye movement and other electrophysiologic events: rapid eye movement (REM) sleep and nonrapid eye movement (NREM) sleep. These two distinct states cycle throughout the night at about 90- to 120-minute intervals. Most individuals pass through three to five cycles per night. They are not equal, however. NREM accounts for approximately 80% of total sleep.

Sleep is further divided based on EEG changes.[2] Normally, individuals pass through the following sequence based on these changes, waves, and rhythms:

- Alpha rhythm is evident in primarily occipital leads with the eyes closed and the individual relaxed.
- NREM
  1. Stage 1 characterized by theta waves.
  2. Stage 2 characterized by theta waves interrupted by sleep spindles and K-complex spikes.
  3. Stage 3 characterized by delta (slow) waves. (Patients awakened during delta sleep recall more thought fragments than actual dreams. Only 5% of patients recall vivid dreams.[3])
  4. After about one hour, stage 2 patterns are repeated followed by a longer time spent in slow-wave sleep.
  5. Approximately a one-minute delay is followed by REM sleep, although generally this does not occur on the first pass-through cycle of sleep.
- REM
  1. Characterized by beta waves (paradoxical sleep because more characteristic of wakefulness). Heart rate, respiration, blood pressure, and penile erections vary widely throughout REM sleep.
  2. Characterized by vivid dreaming, rapid eye movements but paralysis of trunk and limb musculature. This accounts for the occasional phenomenon of sleep paralysis wherein, upon wakening, an individual is temporarily not

able to move. Vivid dreaming during REM is purported to be due to visual cortex activation through a pathway connecting the pontine reticular formation and the lateral geniculate body to the occipital cortex (PGO pathway).

3. REM becomes more dominant throughout the last two sleep cycles prior to waking.

There is a maturation phenomenon associated with time spent in REM or NREM. Newborns spend 50% of their time in REM and enter REM soon after sleep initiation.[4] The time spent in REM decreases as the newborn matures to as little as 20% by six months of age. The corresponding switch to an adult pattern of NREM/REM cycling begins at around four months of age and is associated with a concomitant increase in the production of melatonin. This connection between melatonin and sleep has led to the recent use of melatonin in the elderly to help "normalize" sleep. In the elderly the amount of REM remains the same; however, there is a marked decrease in deep sleep.

Classification System

The International Classification of Sleep Disorders is the standard used for categorizations of sleep-related problems.[5] (See **Table 23–1**.) The primary divisions are:

1. Dyssomnias
2. Parasomnias
3. Sleep disorders associated with mental, neurologic, or other medical disorders
4. Proposed sleep disorders

Dyssomnias usually result in excessive daytime sleepiness or are involved with difficulty starting or maintaining sleep, and are further divided into (selected examples given):

- Intrinsic sleep disorders—most insomnias, narcolepsy, and sleep apnea
- Extrinsic sleep disorders—categories of external factors such as eating, drinking, toxins, altitude, and any environmental disruption

Table 23–1 Categorization of Sleep-Related Disorders: An Abbreviated List

Dyssomnias

Intrinsic	Extrinsic	Circadian Rhythm
Insomnia	Inadequate sleep hygiene	Time zone change (jet lag)
Hypersomnia	Environmental	Shift work
Narcolepsy	Altitude insomnia	Irregular sleep–wake pattern
Sleep apnea (central)	Adjustment sleep disorder	Delayed sleep-phase syndrome
Sleep apnea (obstructive)	Insufficient sleep syndrome	Advanced sleep-phase syndrome
Central alveolar hypoventilation syndrome	Sleep onset association disorder	Non-24-sleep–wake disorder
Periodic limb movement	Food allergy insomnia	
Restless legs syndrome	Nocturnal eating/drinking syndrome	
	Hypnotic-dependent sleep disorder	
	Alcohol/stimulant/toxin-dependent sleep disorder	

Parasomnias

Arousal Disorders	Sleep–Wake Transition	REM-Related	Other
Confusional	Rhythmic movement	Nightmares	Sleep bruxism
Sleep walking	Sleep starts	Sleep paralysis	Sleep enuresis
Sleep terrors	Sleep talking	Penile erection dysfunction	Abnormal swallowing
	Leg cramps	Painful erection	Paroxysmal dystonia
		REM sinus arrest	Sudden infant death
		REM sleep behavior disorder	Benign sleep myoclonus

(continues)

Table 23–1 Categorization of Sleep-Related Disorders: An Abbreviated List (continued)

Sleep Disorders Associated with Other Medical Conditions

Mental	Neurologic	Other
Psychosis	Cerebral degenerative disorders	Sleeping sickness
Mood disorders	Dementia	Nocturnal cardiac ischemia
Anxiety disorders	Parkinsonism	Chronic obstructive pulmonary disease
Panic disorders	Fatal familial insomnia	Sleep-related asthma
Alcoholism	Sleep-related epilepsy	Sleep-related gastroesophageal reflux
	Sleep-related headaches	Peptic ulcer disease
		Fibromyalgia

- Sleep–wake transition disorders—jet lag, shift work, and circadian rhythm sleep disorders

Parasomnias are not necessarily abnormalities of sleep but deal primarily with external or internal elements that tend to disrupt sleep and include disorders such as sleep-walking, sleep-talking, movement disorders, nocturnal leg cramps, nightmares, and sleep apnea. See **Table 23–2** for a further breakdown.

Evaluation

History

- Obtain a detailed history of the patient's complaint with regard to length of the problem and any recognizable contributing lifestyle events.
- Obtain a detailed history from the sleep partner if available (personal videotaping may be feasible).

Difficulty Falling Asleep

At some time in everyone's life, difficulty falling asleep has occurred. When this is chronic, it is important to ask questions regarding lifestyle and environment. The most productive avenue of investigation is to ask what occurs prior to going to bed, such as stimulation from exercise, caffeine, smoking, alcohol, stimulating reading, nasal sprays (active ingredient is often ephedrine), argument with family member, or paying bills. If this line of questioning is unproductive, a search for daily activities may yield a possibility. Does the patient take naps; smoke more than a pack of cigarettes during the day; or take steroids, dopaminergic agents, xanthine derivatives other than caffeine (e.g., theophylline for asthma), β-agonists, appetite suppressants, or decongestants?

Table 23–2 Characteristic EEG Findings with Various Causes and Disorders of Sleep

Disorder or Substance	Characteristic EEG Findings
Depression	Decreased total sleep time Fragmented sleep Early onset of REM sleep Shift of REM sleep to first half of night Decreased slow-wave sleep
Bipolar disorder	Total sleep time decreased Shortened REM latency Increased REM activity
Sleep panic attacks	Occurs in transition from stage 2 to stage 3 (NREM) in patients with a longer REM latency
Acute alcohol intake	Decreased sleep latency Reduced REM sleep in first half of night Increased REM in second half of night (REM rebound) Increase in stage 3 sleep Vivid dreaming and frequent awakenings
Chronic alcohol intake	Increase in stage 1 Decreased REM sleep
Alcohol or sedative withdrawal	Delayed onset of sleep REM rebound
Smoking (other stimulants)	Decreased total sleep time (mainly NREM) Increased sleep latency
Sedatives/hypnotics	Increased total sleep time Decreased sleep latency Decreased awakenings Variable effects on NREM sleep Antidepressants decrease REM

A curious but distressing disorder is restless legs syndrome. The patient complains of a dysesthesia that is relieved only by moving the legs. In fact, the urge to move the legs is irresistible. The dysesthesia can occur as often as every 20 to 30 seconds and delay sleep well into the early morning. Because of the associated hereditary tendency, it is important to ask whether relatives experience the disorder or have been diagnosed with a similar condition.

Early Morning Awakening with Difficulty Falling Back to Sleep

Questioning directed at possible depression should be initiated with any patient who reports waking up early and not being able to get back to sleep. A quick screening question is, "Are there activities/hobbies/relationships that used to give you pleasure, events that you would look forward to, but no longer hold any interest?" If it seems that the patient has lost interest in past hobbies or activities and feels a lack of drive or energy, endogenous depression is a possible cause when associated with this pattern of sleep disturbance.

Other possibilities include drug-induced early-morning waking. This is more likely to occur with the use of some short-acting benzodiazepines. Alcohol may cause a rebound REM effect, which also will result in early-morning waking. Another condition that may manifest similarly is advanced sleep phase syndrome. This is frequently seen in the elderly.

Frequent Awakenings (Interrupted Sleep)

Secondary effects of drugs, pain, an uncomfortable environment, alcohol, abuse, or stress could all result in frequent awakenings. If a screening for the causes of these complaints is unrewarding, however, it is likely that the patient has a primary sleep disorder. Those that cause frequent awakenings are divided into those that result in excessive daytime sleepiness and those that may not.

Does the patient notice repetitive, uncontrolled muscle jerks throughout the night? Some patients with sleep-related (nocturnal) myoclonus are aware of the jerks and partial awakenings throughout the night. Others are aware of waking often but do not recall the muscle jerks. In these cases, it is extremely helpful to have the report of a sleep partner to corroborate your suspicion. Another possibility is restless legs syndrome. This is characterized by an irresistible urge to move the legs because of a "creeping" sensation inside the calves. Many of these patients also have nocturnal myoclonus. Patients with restless legs syndrome may have an underlying cause. Therefore, it is important to determine whether a deficiency of iron or folate exists or whether the patient is pregnant or has uremia or a peripheral neuropathy. A common misinterpretation is the presence of hypnic jerks, which occur in many people sporadically. This phenomenon is the sudden jerking that occurs as one is falling asleep and does not represent a sign of myoclonus. Persistent leg cramps may also be a cause of frequent awakenings and may be due to excessive exercise, inadequate hydration, or deficiencies in potassium or calcium.

Excessive Daytime Sleepiness

Excessive daytime sleepiness (EDS) is caused by sleep apnea syndrome (43%), narcolepsy (25%), and insufficient sleep.[6] Sleep apnea that is central is not as likely as obstructive sleep apnea to result in EDS. Obstructive sleep apnea causes the patient to increase abdominal pressure as he or she recovers from an apneic episode. As a result the patient may have an apparently unrelated list of associated problems, including the following:

- Early-morning headache
- Urge to void early in the morning or often throughout the night
- Esophageal reflux
- Early-morning hypertension

Examination

The primary evaluation tool for sleep disorders is an overnight polysomnogram.[7,8] This consists of a series of measurements that are superimposed to present a composite picture of various sleep activities. These measurements include the following:

- An EEG
- An electrooculogram (EOG)
- An electromyogram (EMG)
- Arterial oxygen saturation (SaO_2)
- Oral airflow (N/OT)
- Thoracic movement (TSG)
- Heart rate (by a cardiotachometer)
- An electrocardiogram (ECG)

REM and NREM sleep are distinguished by characteristic patterns, especially with the EEG and EOG. These are summarized in Table 23–1.

The most common disorder discovered on polysomnography is obstructive sleep apnea (OSA) syndrome. It is characterized by excessive daytime sleepiness and breathing cessation (apnea) or a reduction of airflow (hypopnea) during sleep. The diagnosis is a combination of these. Following are the terms and criteria:[9]

- **Apnea:** breathing cessation for >10 seconds
- **Hypopnea:** reduced respiratory airflow by 30% with a 4% decrease in oxygen saturation
- **Apnea-hypopnea index (AHI):** number of apnea and hypopnea events recorded per hour of sleep
  1. Mild OSA: AHI ≥5–15/h
  2. Moderate OSA: AHI ≥15–30/h
  3. Severe OSA: AHI ≥30/h
- **OSA syndrome:** AHI ≥5 with evidence of daytime sleepiness

The quality of sleep and the degree of excessive daytime sleepiness can be determined by a number of questionnaires or by using laboratory measures such as the multiple sleep latency test (MSLT), which measures how quickly an individual falls asleep. However, the best combination of evaluation tools is still the Sleep Apnea Clinical Score (SACS). The items are easily determined by history and physical examination:

- Neck circumference
- Hypertension
- Habitual snoring
- Nocturnal gasping or choking

As a single indicator, neck circumference of 50 cm or higher is associated with a modestly increased risk. As neck circumference increases, fewer of the other three variables are required to increase the likelihood of OSA. Matching the value of this approach to a diagnostic threshold of AHI 10/h or higher (determined by polysomnography in a study population):

- SACS >15: increases the likelihood of OSA (LR, 5.2; 95% CI, 2.5–10).
- SACS ≤5: OSA is less likely (LR, 0.25; 95% CI, 0.15–0.42).

Although factors such as snoring and hypertension are important, the literature appears to indicate that although the absence of snoring makes a diagnosis of OSA less likely, neither snoring alone nor self-reported sleepiness and morning headaches discriminate between those with and without OSA.

Management

- Alter aspects of the patient's lifestyle that might assist sleep, such as reducing smoking, alcohol, caffeine, or OTC stimulants; keeping regular sleeping hours; or decreasing stress (see Exhibit 23–1).
- Refer to a sleep disorder clinic for evaluation and management of primary disorders.
- Refer for psychologic evaluation when sleep disturbance is typical of depression, such as early-morning waking with difficulty falling back to sleep.
- Treat any coexisting musculoskeletal complaints.

Some general measures apply to most patients with sleep difficulties. These include keeping a regular sleep cycle, avoiding stimulation such as exercise, reducing stimulants (nasal sprays, caffeine, smoking, etc.), and decreasing stress. If the patient has a more severe problem or a clear-cut primary or secondary sleep disorder, referral for sleep analysis and treatment is needed. Most sleep medications cause dependence. Zolpidem tartrate (Ambien) is used for the short-term treatment of insomnia. It is a nonbenzodiazepine hypnotic. Eszopiclone (Lunesta) affects GABA receptor complexes, which may be coupled to benzodiazepine receptors. It shortens sleep latency and improves sleep maintenance and does not cause dependence. Below are some selected conditions and the options for management.

Sleep Apnea

Sleep apnea may be central or obstructive. Central sleep apnea is associated with morbid obesity and appears to be associated with a central nervous system, primarily brainstem-related dysfunction that decreases sensitivity to CO_2 levels and the reflex triggering of breathing to expel excess CO_2. Obstructive sleep apnea is far more common and is characterized by periods of apnea due to mechanical or functional blockage to airflow.

Several conservative measures are recommended specifically for those patients with obstructive sleep apnea disorders. It is realistic to state that many of these alterable factors are effective only in mild cases and when the patient is or can be compliant. Given that two-thirds of patients with sleep apnea have moderate to severe obesity,[10] a loss of weight often will subjectively and objectively improve breathing.[11,12] This is due to increased lung volumes and decreased pharyngeal collapse.

Maintaining the weight reduction, however, is notoriously elusive.

Sleep position change may help, with the caveat that it is difficult to avoid certain positions while asleep. It has been demonstrated that apnea occurs less often in the lateral decubitus (side-lying) position than the supine position.[13] Avoidance of alcohol may eliminate a compounded effect on sleep apnea. Alcohol has been shown to depress hypoglossal nerve activity with genioglossal and other support muscle decreases in tone, leading to increases in upper airway resistance even in nonapneic sleepers.[14,15] If sedatives (or narcotics) are used to assist sleep, they should be discontinued if the patient has obstructive problems.

The mainstays for management of OSA are either mandibular advancement devices (MAD), also known as oral appliances, and nasal continuous positive airway pressure (CPAP).[16] Although many oral appliances have been utilized, little information on criteria for the devices or the specific patient group that would benefit has been provided. A fairly comprehensive study suggests, however, that an oral appliance may be beneficial with some patients.[17] Both snoring severity and apnea are improved. In a 2013 study[18] evaluating both the categorization of patients and the results of mandibular advancement using oral appliances, there was again confirmation of the effectiveness; however, there was no real distinction among the types of obstruction. Oral appliance therapy was modestly effective for all types of obstruction including primary retropalatal, retroglossal, and retroepiglottic. The researchers concluded that the success or failure of the device is not based on an anatomical identification of the region of maximal upper airway collapse.

It has been found that although oral appliances can be effective, as many as 35% of patients still needed additional therapy. The compliance rate for patients using oral appliances is approximately 75%. Although side effects are minimal, long-term effects on the temporomandibular joint might occur. Devices generally caused the mandible to advance and rotate downward, thereby enlarging the posterior airway. This may have a secondary effect on the soft palate.

Nasal CPAP was introduced in 1981 as a potential treatment option for obstructive sleep apnea. The general principle is simple: maintain air pressure through a mask that delivers a continuous stream of room air under high pressure, thereby creating a "pneumatic splint." Although the device appears to be extremely effective, there are several compliance issues that render it far less effective than had been hoped. The mere presence of the machine, the loudness of the blower, and the irritation to the mucosa

from constant air have led to a poor compliance rate after several months. Patients complain of nasal problems, throat soreness, and headaches, among other side effects. Patients who remain on CPAP for a minimum of several weeks have improvement in NREM and REM sleep and particularly in daytime function, with much less daytime tiredness. CPAP also improves hypertension and quality of life and even reduces depression and motor vehicle crashes. Improvements in technology may allow adjustment of pressure and oxygen concentration, decreasing some side effects and increasing compliance.

For those patients who do not improve, various forms of surgery are an option. Removing nasal polyps; correcting a deviated nasal septum; or removing tonsils, adenoids, or the uvula is often a first attempt. More radical approaches involve mandibular restructuring. A new technique using a laser to remove or shrink the uvula has a dramatic effect on snoring; however, the effect on apnea is variable.

Narcolepsy and Narcolepsy/Cataplexy Syndrome

Narcolepsy is characterized by sudden sleeping episodes during the day. This is a condition whereby the patient drops into REM sleep without warning. Usually this is for periods of about one hour, several times a day. In addition, the individual will experience sleep paralysis for a minute or two prior to or just after falling asleep. Also associated are hypnogogic hallucinations where the individual combines dreaming from his or her REM state with his or her waking environment. The narcoleptic syndrome involves brief attacks of cataplexy that involves muscle paralysis ranging from simply dropping the head or jaw, or dropping a held object, to full paralysis of the trunk and limbs without loss of consciousness.

It appears that narcolepsy has an autoimmune basis due to the strong association with human leukocyte antigens (HLA) DQw6 and DRw15.[19] There appears to be a decrease in cells in the walls of the hypothalamus and decreased production of an excitatory peptide orexin (hypocretin).[20] Symptoms tend to develop rather early, between ages 15 to 25 years, but it has been recorded as early as at age 2 years and as late as age 45 years. The ASDA criteria for narcolepsy state that no other known disorder is responsible. Symptoms and signs include:

1. For at least three months, daily or almost daily, lapses into sleep or naps. Indications of cataplexy, including sudden loss of all postural muscle tone related to intense emotion.

2. Excessive daytime sleepiness or sudden muscle weakness. Associated complaints would include sleep paralysis, hypnogogic hallucinations, and automatic behaviors.

3. Polysomnography findings include one of the following: sleep latency of less than 10 minutes and REM latency less than 20 minutes, multiple sleep latency test with latency of less than five minutes, and two or more sleep-onset REM periods.

Treatment includes central nervous system stimulants for the hypersomnolence (e.g., amphetamine or methylphenidate) and anticholinergics for the cataplexy (e.g., imipramine or protriptyline). Drugs such as modafinil may function by decreasing GABA-mediated neurotransmission while amphetamines (low-dose) and monoamine oxidase inhibitors (MAOIs) may maintain levels of norepinephrine released from the locus coeruleus.

Restless Legs Syndrome

Although many cases are benign, some patients have severe dysesthesia and irresistible leg movements in an attempt at temporary relief. These abnormalities can lead to serious sleep deprivation in some patients because of a prolonged sleep latency until after 3 a.m.

Iron supplementation may be beneficial with 65 mg of elemental iron given one to three times a day as needed. Other conservative options include magnesium, passion flower, and valerian root. Caution for those taking quinine. Many individuals are sensitive to quinine and there is no evidence for its use with RLS.

Medical approaches are similar to Parkinson's management. The newest is the use of Requip (ropinirole). The mechanism appears to be stimulation of postsynaptic dopamine D2-type receptors. Another treatment is a tablet containing 25 mg of carbidopa and 100 mg of levodopa (Sinemet) taken before bedtime, and occasionally a second dose during the night or during the day. Other drugs include Neurontin (gabapentin), Lyrica (pregabalin), and gabapentin enacarbil (Horizant). These are referred to as alpha-2 delta drugs, which affect calcium channels.

It is important to caution the doctor that these are not muscle cramps and will not respond to the usual recommendations. The disorder is quite distressing and requires medication in most serious cases.

Algorithm

An algorithm for insomnia or other complaints of sleep is presented in **Figure 23–1**.

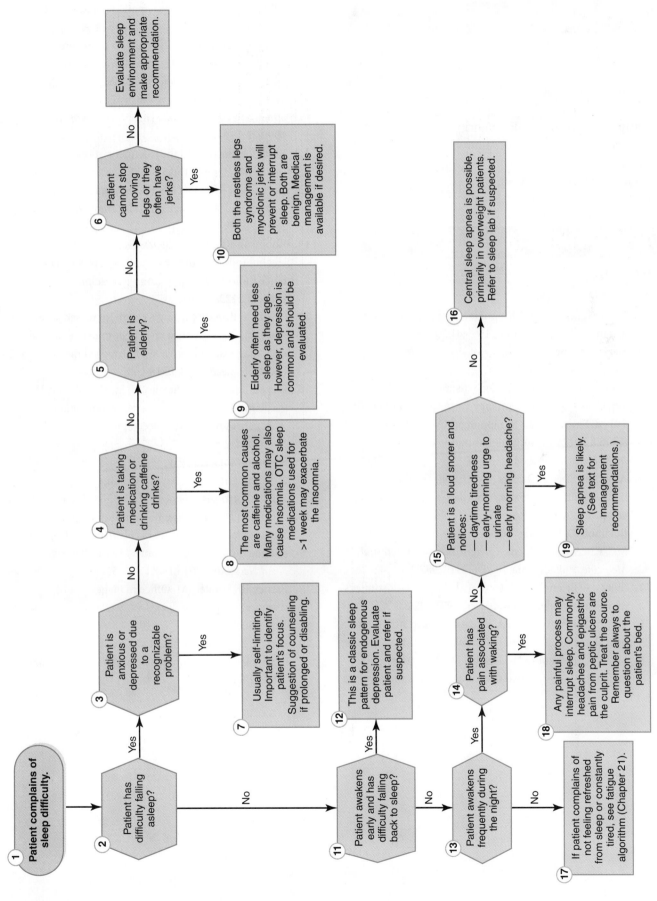

Figure 23–1 Insomnia or Other Complaints of Sleep—Algorithm

APPENDIX 23–1

Web Resources

National Sleep Foundation
(202) 347-3471
http://www.sleepfoundation.org
American Insomnia Association
(708) 492-0930
www.sleepassociation.org

APPENDIX 23–2

References

1. Kraft M, Martin RJ. Chronobiology and chronotherapy in medicine. *Dis Mon.* 1995;41:501–575.
2. Siegel JM. The neurobiology of sleep. *Semin Neurol.* 2009;29(4):277–296.
3. Kovasevic-Ristanovic R. Sleep disorders. In: Weiner WJ, Goetz CG, eds. *Neurology for the Non-Neurologist.* 3rd ed. Philadelphia: JB Lippincott Co.; 1989:281.
4. Sandyk R. Melatonin and maturation of REM sleep. *Int J Neurosci.* 1992;63:105–114.
5. American Sleep Disorders Association. The international classification of sleep disorders, revised: diagnostic and coding manual. Rochester, MN. *ASDA.* 1997.
6. Buchholz D. Sleep disorders. In: Bayless TM, Brain MC, Chermick RM, eds. *Current Therapy in Internal Medicine.* Philadelphia: BC Decker; 1987:2.
7. Iber C, O'Brien C, Schluter J, et al. Single night studies in obstructive sleep apnea. *Sleep.* 1991;14:383–385.
8. Thorpy MJ, McGregor PA. The use of sleep studies in neurologic practice. *Semin Neurol.* 1990;10:11.
9. Myers KA, Mrkobrada M, Simel DL. Does this patient have obstructive sleep apnea? The Rational Clinical Examination systematic review. *JAMA.* 2013;310(7):731–741.
10. Kales A, Cadieux RJ, Bixler EO, et al. Severe obstructive sleep apnea: onset, clinical course, and characteristics. *J Chronic Dis.* 1985;38:419–425.
11. Wittels EH, Thompson S. Obstructive sleep apnea and obesity. *Otolaryngol Clin North Am.* 1990;23:751–760.
12. Bray GA. Barriers to the treatment of obesity. *Arch Intern Med.* 1991;115:152–157.
13. Cartwright RD, Diaz F, Lloyd S. The effects of sleep posture and sleep stage on apnea frequency. *Sleep.* 1991;14:351–353.
14. Robinson RW, White DP, Zwillich CW. Moderate alcohol ingestion increases upper airway resistance in normal subjects. *Ann Rev Respir Dis.* 1985;132:1238–1241.
15. Scrima I, Broudy M, Nay K, et al. Increased severity of obstructive sleep apnea after bedtime alcohol ingestion: diagnostic potential and proposed mechanisms of action. *Sleep.* 1982;5:318–328.
16. Epstein LJ, Kristo D, Strollo PJ, Jr., et al. Clinical guideline for the evaluation, management and long-term care of obstructive sleep apnea in adults. *J Clin Sleep Med.* 2009;5(3):263–276.
17. Schmidt-Norwara WW, Meade TE, Hays MB. Treatment of snoring and obstructive sleep apnea with a dental orthosis. *Chest.* 1991;99:1378–1385.
18. Friedman M, Shnowske K, Hamilton C, et al. Mandibular advancement for obstructive sleep apnea: relating outcomes to anatomy. *JAMA Otolaryngol Head Neck Surg.* 2013;140(1):46–51.
19. Farney RJ, Walker JM. Office management of common sleep-wake disorders. *Med Clin North Am.* 1995;79:391.
20. Kim SJ, Lyoo IK, Lee YS, et al. Gray matter deficits in young adults with narcolepsy. *Acta Neurol Scand.* 2009;119(1):61–67.

Hypertension

# CHAPTER 24

Context

The most common primary diagnosis in the United States is hypertension.[1] Because it is essentially a silent disorder, 30% of individuals are unaware of their hypertension. Cardiovascular disease has been estimated to total more than $320 billion in healthcare costs in the United States alone.[2] Hypertension is a significant modifiable risk factor for cardiovascular disease.

As primary contact doctors, chiropractors are well positioned for detecting patients with high blood pressure/hypertension (HTN). Given that the majority of these patients will be asymptomatic for HTN, it is important to include screening on all new patients. Jamison et al.[3] have demonstrated that the chiropractor may serve an important role in screening for, and recommending, important lifestyle changes. HTN is found in as many as 50 million Americans; 18% of the adult white population, and 35% of the adult black population.[4] Sixty percent of these individuals have a blood pressure (BP) in the high-normal range. Patients with BP in the high-normal or mildly elevated range can be managed initially with diet and exercise prior to referral for drug management. These patients have been demonstrated to have a 40% increase in risk for cardiovascular disease; thus their management is not to be taken lightly.[5] A 2007 study by Hansen et al.[6] indicates that there is underdiagnosis of hypertension in children and adolescents. In a group of 507 children and adolescents, 3.6% had hypertension. Only 26% of those with HTN had an entry in their medical records and only 11% with prehypertension had an entry. Factors related to an increased associated risk were older age, increase in 1% height-for-age percentile, obesity, and frequency of prior abnormal blood pressure readings.

The risk of HTN increases with age and is greater in African-Americans than in whites.[4] Although some cases of HTN are due to secondary causes (5%), primary (essential) hypertension accounts for 95% of cases, with no identifiable cause. Secondary causes include the following:

- Estrogen use (5% of women taking oral contraceptives chronically are hypertensive)
- Renal disease and renal vascular HTN (1% to 2% of hypertensive patients)
- Primary aldosteronism and Cushing's disease (or chronic corticosteroid use; 0.5% of hypertensive patients)
- Coarctation of the aorta (prevalence is 0.1 to 0.5 per 1,000 children)[7]
- Pheochromocytoma
- Pregnancy (preeclampsia/eclampsia)
- Disorders associated with hypercalcemia such as thyroid conditions
- Sleep apnea

Uncontrolled HTN puts an individual at risk for coronary heart disease (CHD), congestive heart failure, cerebrovascular events, aortic aneurysms, renal disease, and retinopathy. Many of these disorders are life-threatening. Fortunately, the death rate from CHD and stroke has been reduced 50% or more over the last two decades.[8] This decline has been attributed to public awareness leading to improvements in diet, exercise, and medical intervention.

Relevant Physiology

Blood pressure is the result of cardiac output and peripheral vascular resistance (PVR). There are numerous factors that can influence either. Basically, the PVR can be increased by smooth muscle contraction or intrinsically elevated through blockages as seen with athero- and arteriosclerosis. Cardiac output increases as a result of sympathetic discharge from stress or increased metabolic demand. Output also increases with an increased vascular volume; there is more fluid to pump.

PVR is predominantly determined by an interplay among the autonomic nervous system, renal system, and neuroendocrine/hormonal actions. Sympathetic activity increases BP through increases in both PVR and cardiac output. The renin-angiotensin system also plays a key feedback role. Decreases in renal perfusion, increased sympathetic activity, hypokalemia, and arteriolar stretch all may act as initiators of this sequence. Renin secreted by the juxtaglomerular cells causes angiotensinogen to form angiotensin I that is then converted to angiotensin II. Angiotensin II is a potent vasoconstrictor and also causes the release of aldosterone, another vasoconstrictor.

The underlying cause of essential hypertension is unknown; however, it appears to be multifactorial. There may be a genetic predisposition that is most evident when both parents are hypertensive. Other factors that influence HTN are those that influence the development of atherosclerosis, such as diet and exercise, diabetes mellitus, and smoking. Salt intake is a factor in some patients; however, it is usually only one component of an individual's BP increase.[9] Obesity influences HTN through several mechanisms, the most obvious being an increase in intravascular volume with a consequent higher cardiac output.[10] Alcohol consumption also influences BP. The increase in BP is thought to be due to increased levels of catecholamines.[11] Patients with HTN who drink excessively have HTN that is more difficult to control. Smoking has a similar effect, possibly due to increased levels of norepinephrine.[12]

Theories regarding underlying pathology with essential HTN patients include the following:[13]

- Sympathetic nervous system hyperactivity or decrease in sensitivity of baroreflexes
- Renin-angiotensin-aldosterone system (RAAS) dysfunction
- Intracellular increases in sodium

Obesity has been tied to HTN. There is the obvious contribution from increased sympathetic activity and RAAS activity but additionally there have been some proposed mechanisms through an imbalance of bioactive molecules such as increases in leptin and resistin and decreases in adiponectin. Additionally, obese patients often have obstructive sleep apnea. The contributions of intermittent hypoxia coupled with increased endothelin-1 may also be factors.

One study found that the number of nephrons is reduced in patients with primary HTN and that this appears to be a cause versus a result of HTN.[14]

General Strategy

- Screen all patients for HTN.
- Check for possible signs and symptoms suggestive of a secondary cause of hypertension: in young patients, renal insufficiency, renal artery stenosis, or coarctation of the aorta are possible causes; in adults, renal artery stenosis, Cushing's disease, hyperthyroidism, and pheochromocytoma should be considered.
- Screen for major risk factors for HTN including smoking, dyslipidemia, diabetes mellitus, age older than 60 years, being male or a postmenopausal female, or a family history of cardiovascular disease (affected relatives are women under age 65 years or men under age 55 years).
- Screen for target organ disease such as left ventricular hypertrophy, angina or prior myocardial infarction (MI), prior coronary revascularization or heart failure, past history of stroke or transient ischemic attack (TIA), nephropathy, peripheral vascular disease, or retinopathy.
- Be vigilant for signs of HTN in the pregnant patient. Its development in later trimesters may be the first sign of preeclampsia/eclampsia.
- Use proper cuff size and procedure; make sure the patient has avoided alcohol for 12 hours and smoking and caffeine at least 30 to 60 minutes prior to examination.
- Recheck high findings at least two other times over the next week to confirm original reading (**Exhibit 24-1**); if severely high on the initial reading, refer for medical evaluation.
- Categorize patients based on level of HTN and associated risk factors.
- Refer patients with mild HTN and existing CHD and patients with moderate to severe HTN.
- Manage or comanage patients with mild HTN with diet, exercise, and possibly stress relaxation approaches.

Exhibit 24–1 **Screening for Hypertension**

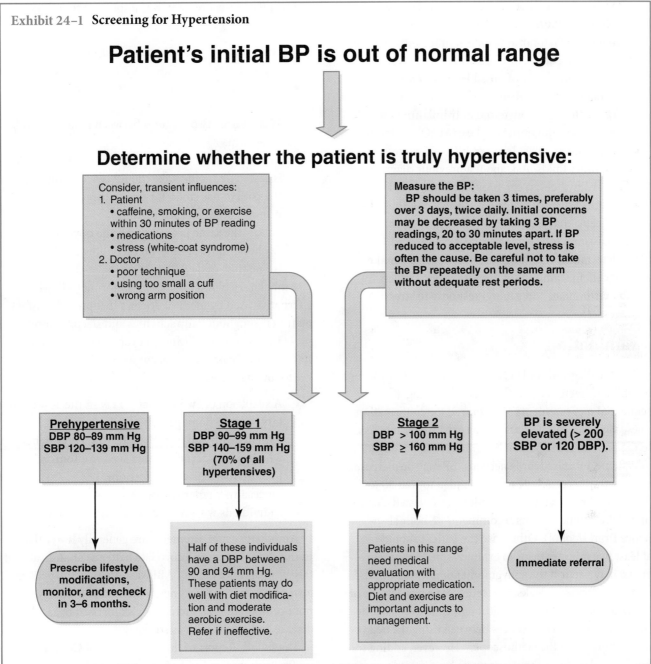

Patient's initial BP is out of normal range

Determine whether the patient is truly hypertensive:

Consider, transient influences:
1. Patient
   - caffeine, smoking, or exercise within 30 minutes of BP reading
   - medications
   - stress (white-coat syndrome)
2. Doctor
   - poor technique
   - using too small a cuff
   - wrong arm position

Measure the BP:
   BP should be taken 3 times, preferably over 3 days, twice daily. Initial concerns may be decreased by taking 3 BP readings, 20 to 30 minutes apart. If BP reduced to acceptable level, stress is often the cause. Be careful not to take the BP repeatedly on the same arm without adequate rest periods.

Prehypertensive
DBP 80–89 mm Hg
SBP 120–139 mm Hg

Stage 1
DBP 90–99 mm Hg
SBP 140–159 mm Hg
(70% of all hypertensives)

Stage 2
DBP > 100 mm Hg
SBP ≥ 160 mm Hg

BP is severely elevated (> 200 SBP or 120 DBP).

Prescribe lifestyle modifications, monitor, and recheck in 3–6 months.

Half of these individuals have a DBP between 90 and 94 mm Hg. These patients may do well with diet modification and moderate aerobic exercise. Refer if ineffective.

Patients in this range need medical evaluation with appropriate medication. Diet and exercise are important adjuncts to management.

Immediate referral

Always consider a secondary cause in individuals who are younger than age 20 or older than age 55, and/or when the onset is abrupt. Look for endocrine imbalances such as hyperthyroidism or adrenal disease, and in the older individual look for renal artery stenosis.

Evaluation

History

Historical clues are important in determining underlying causes of HTN and any end-organ dysfunction as a result of HTN. A significant finding in younger patients is a family history, especially if both parents have HTN. Other familial findings that are significant include stroke, diabetes, cardiovascular disease, and hyperlipidemia. Important personal history information to be elicited include the following:

- Note any symptoms suggestive of end-organ problems (congestive heart failure, stroke, kidney dysfunction, peripheral vascular problems).

- Determine whether there are indicators of a secondary cause (mainly renal, cardiac, or endocrine factors); a history of oral contraceptive use; alcohol abuse; use of antihypertensive medication; or use of possible hypertension-inducing herbs or drugs such as licorice root, corticosteroids, nonsteroid anti-inflammatory drugs, or monoamine oxidase (MAO) inhibitors.
- Ask about any past levels of high BP, cholesterol, and other lipids. Ask about a previous diagnosis of cardiovascular, cerebrovascular, or renal disease.
- Obtain a dietary history; if feasible, ask the patient to keep a diary indicating intake of sodium, potassium, folic acid, fat, and alcohol.
- Determine other lifestyle factors such as intake of caffeine, amount of exercise, work and family environment, and general response to stress.

Examination

Key to the diagnosis of HTN is an accurate BP measurement. Many factors can influence this reading, thus sequential measurements are required for confirmation. These variables can be classified as extrinsic or intrinsic to the patient. If the patient has smoked, taken alcohol or caffeine, exercised, or is nervous, BP may be increased transiently. It is generally recommended to wait 30 to 60 minutes after the patient has smoked or ingested alcohol or caffeine (some authors recommend 12-hour abstinence from alcohol). Otherwise the patient should rest at least five minutes prior to examination. Equipment errors may occur if the sphygmomanometer is not calibrated, the pressure leaks, the stethoscope has defects, or the wrong size cuff is used. Although controversial, one study indicated no differences between using the bell or the diaphragm of the stethoscope.[15] However, adding too much pressure from the stethoscope head may decrease the diastolic reading by as much as 10 mm Hg.[16] To accommodate different arm sizes, pediatric, adult, and oversized cuffs should be available. The bladder portion should cover four-fifths (80%) of the patient's arm circumference. Using too small a cuff will increase the BP reading, often substantially. Preferably, measurements should be taken with a mercury sphygmomanometer. Second choices include a recently calibrated aneroid manometer or a validated electronic device. Ambulatory readings performed by patients may be appropriate if there is a high level of suspicion regarding the "white coat" elevation seen in the office with some patients.

For in-office measurement, it is important to do the following:

- Seat patient in a chair with his or her back supported.
- Make sure the patient's arm is bare and at heart level.
- Wait at least two minutes between readings on the same arm.
- Measure the BP twice on one arm when the patient is seated or supine; take the BP twice again after the patient has stood for two to three minutes (two minutes between each reading).
- Follow the same procedure on the opposite arm.
- Recheck high readings on the following three days (same time of day).

Ambulatory blood pressure monitoring (ABPM) is an alternative used by medical doctors that provides information throughout daily activities and sleep.[17] Blood pressure is automatically taken every 15 to 30 minutes. It is used to obtain a more accurate profile for patients in the following scenarios:

- A suspicion of "white-coat" HTN in the absence of target organ damage
- Patients with apparent drug resistance; patients who have apparent hypotensive symptoms related to antihypertensive medications
- Fluctuating hypertension
- Individuals with suspected autonomic dysfunction

Ambulatory measurements are generally lower than in the clinic setting and correlate better as an indicator of target organ injury. Sleep ABPM is usually 10% to 20% lower than daytime readings. When these reductions do not occur, there is an increased risk for cardiovascular disease and events such as stroke.[17, 18]

The Eighth Report of the Joint National Committee on Prevention, Detection, Evaluation, and Treatment of High Blood Pressure has again redefined the classifications and recommendations for high blood pressure based on new evidence.[19-21] The previous committee felt the need to establish a new prehypertension category based on data that suggest those with a blood pressure between 120–139 mm Hg systolic and 80–89 mm Hg diastolic are at twice the risk of developing HTN compared to those below these levels.[22] Additionally, data from the Framingham Heart Study indicate that even those individuals who are normotensive at age 55 still have a 90% lifetime risk for developing HTN.[23] However, this was not compared to a control group of individuals who lived a healthy lifestyle or changed to a healthy lifestyle. For patients older than age 50 years, systolic blood pressure is a more important CVD risk factor than diastolic blood pressure and is more difficult to control.[24] Two-thirds of individuals over age 65 years have hypertension, and they also have the poorest success rates for blood pressure control.[25]

The JNC guidelines are based on recommendations from the National High Blood Pressure Education Program (NHBPEP), a coalition of 39 professional, public, and voluntary organizations coordinated by the National Heart, Lung, and Blood Institute (NHLBI). The JNC 7 guidelines categorize blood pressure into the following classifications with recommendations for those without compelling indications (comorbid conditions or risks):

- Normal: <120 mm Hg systolic and <80 mm Hg diastolic: medication not needed, lifestyle recommendations are encouraged
- Prehypertensive: 120–139 mm Hg systolic or 80–89 mm Hg diastolic: medication not needed, lifestyle modification given
- Stage 1 hypertension: 140–159 mm Hg systolic or 90–99 mm Hg diastolic: lifestyle modifications given, medications recommended starting with thiazide-type diuretics (consider others if ineffective)
- Stage 2 hypertension: >160 mm Hg systolic or >100 mm Hg diastolic; lifestyle modifications given; two-drug combination therapy recommended

To be consistent with the literature and recommendations of the JNC, systolic blood pressure is considered the point at which the first of two or more sounds is heard (phase 1) and diastolic blood pressure at the point before the disappearance of sounds (phase 5). Using the visual gauge is not accurate. The JNC also recommends giving patients their specific blood pressure readings and recommendations both verbally and in writing.

In addition to BP measurement, a search should be made for physical signs due to secondary causes or contributors to HTN. Measurement of height and weight is important to determine any level of obesity. Atherosclerosis may diminish pulses. Atherosclerosis and/or high volume or turbulent flow may cause bruits. Auscultation for thyroid, subclavian, aortic, and renal bruits should be performed. Auscultation of the heart may indicate murmurs, S3 or S4 sounds, and arrhythmias. Indication of congestive heart involvement is found

with distended neck veins, bilateral lower leg edema, and ascites. Fundoscopic evaluation includes a search for arteriovenous nicking, cotton-wool patches, or papilledema. The thyroid should be palpated and the patient examined for possible hyperthyroidism if indicated.

Laboratory evaluation may be helpful if an underlying cardiac or renal problem is suspected. Indications of kidney dysfunction include creatinine or the corresponding glomerular filtration rate (GFR) (<60 mL/min. is a cardiovascular risk factor). Diabetes is an important cause of HTN and high-risk individuals should be screened for this disease. In addition, a serum cholesterol and lipid panel are helpful in determining hyperlipidemia.

Management

The 2014 JNC guidelines have made some substantial changes in their recommendations. These changes are really simply establishing thresholds for drug management and seem to ignore lifestyle recommendations. They largely focus on two things; the level of HTN in need of management for those 60 years old and older, and the types of drugs utilized. Following is a summary of those recommendations that reflect the changes:

- For persons aged 60 years or older use a BP goal of less than 150 mm Hg and a diastolic goal of less than 90 mm Hg.
- Keep the threshold of 140/90 mm Hg for all other groups including adults with diabetes or nondiabetic chronic kidney disease (CKD).
- For HTN, initiate drug treatment with either an angiotensin-converting enzyme inhibitor, angiotensin receptor blocker, calcium channel blocker, or thiazide-type diuretic in the nonblack hypertensive population, including those with diabetes.
- As initial therapy in the black hypertensive population, including those with diabetes, a calcium channel blocker or thiazide-type diuretic is recommended.
- There is evidence to support initial or add-on antihypertensive therapy with an angiotensin-converting enzyme inhibitor or angiotensin receptor blocker in persons with CKD to improve kidney outcomes.

Although there are many contributing factors to the development of coronary heart disease (CHD), a recent study emphasized that 80% to 90% of individuals with CHD have the four "conventional" risk factors.[26] These are cigarette smoking, hypertension, diabetes, and hyperlipidemia. The focus must be on lifestyle changes, including smoking cessation and control of the other three factors that are interrelated.

The conservative management options for the chiropractor hinge mainly on lifestyle modification, including diet and exercise. This approach may be successful if these patients do not have cardiovascular disease or signs of organ damage; however, failure to reduce BP after a reasonable trial of perhaps 6 to 12 months should warrant referral for comanagement. Although there have been several isolated studies reporting reduction in HTN following adjustments of the spine, the current evidence[27] suggests that these effects do not appear to be consistent or permanent. There are only about six publications related to manipulation and its effect on blood pressure (see **Table 24–1**).[28-33] Three utilize a single treatment. Two of these utilized a pre- and posttreatment measurement of blood pressure without any further follow-up. The other four studies had a follow-up of between four to eight weeks. Only two studies demonstrated any significance in blood pressure reduction; however, one was posttreatment only. In the Goertz et al. study,[31] groups were divided into a dietary intervention group only and a combined dietary intervention group plus manipulation. The manipulation was administered three times per week for four weeks for a total of 12 treatments. There was no difference between the dietary intervention only and dietary intervention plus manipulation groups. The other study by Bakis[32] demonstrated a decrease, on average, of 17 points in the systolic blood pressure and 10 points in the diastolic blood pressure after eight weeks. This specific upper-cervical technique approach is currently being expanded to a larger study to determine the effect on a larger patient population with different doctors applying treatment rather than one doctor. In the

Plaugher et al. study,[33] the control group actually had a slightly lower average blood pressure than the manipulated group. Clearly more research is needed.

There is an increasing body of literature that supports the use of lifestyle modification for blood pressure control. A recent study reporting the results of the PREMIER Clinical Trial indicated that even recommending lifestyle changes can have an effect of lowering systolic blood pressure.[34] A supervised program can have even more effect.

Although lifestyle modifications have been undersold with regard to degree of effect, it has been shown that the effects of a 1,600-mg sodium DASH diet is equal or similar to single-medication treatment.[35] Making two or more modifications can result in even greater effects. **Table 24–2** is a summary of the effects of various lifestyle modifications, showing that even small changes can have a dramatic effect.

Physical inactivity is a major risk factor for CVD. Those individuals who are less active have a 30% to 50% higher risk for high blood pressure.[34] Specifically, aerobic exercise has been shown in a recent meta-analysis to decrease blood pressure in both normotensive and hypertensive individuals.[36] Interestingly, a decrease in blood pressure was not always associated with a decrease in weight, indicating that the effects of aerobic exercise on blood pressure may be independent of weight loss. For young adults, it is important to consider psychosocial factors for the risk of HTN. Researchers in one study demonstrated a dose–response increase in the long-term risk for HTN in those young adults with indications of time-urgency/impatience and hostility.[37] The relationship did not exist for achievement/striving/competitiveness, hostility, or depression in this study.

Specific lifestyle modifications include the following:

- Recommend a weight reduction program if the patient is overweight.

Table 24–1 Manipulation and Hypertension

Study	Technique	# Points	Follow-Up	# Treatments	Results
(2007) Bakris	NUCCA	50	8 weeks	1 (85%)	−17/−10
(2002) Goertz	Diversified	140	4 weeks	12	Not significant
(2002) Plaugher	Gonstead	23	8 weeks	20	Not significant
(2001) Knutson	Upper cervical	110	Post Tx	1	Not significant
(1998) Yates	Activator	21	Post Tx	1	−14/−13
(1985) Morgan	Osteopathic	29	6 weeks	6	Not significant

Table 24–2 Lifestyle Modifications to Manage Hypertension*†

Modification	Recommendation	Approximate SBP Reduction (Range)
Weight reduction	Maintain normal body weight (body mass index 18.5–24.9 kg/m²).	5–20 mm Hg/10 kg weight loss
Adopt DASH eating plan	Consume a diet rich in fruits, vegetables, and low-fat dairy products with a reduced content of saturated and total fat.	8–14 mm Hg
Dietary sodium reduction	Reduce dietary sodium intake to no more than 100 mmol per day (2.4 g sodium or 6 g sodium chloride).	2–8 mm Hg
Physical activity	Engage in regular aerobic physical activity such as brisk walking (at least 30 min per day, most days of the week).	4–9 mm Hg
Moderation of alcohol consumption	Limit consumption to no more than 2 drinks (1 oz or 30 mL ethanol; e.g., 24 oz beer, 10 oz wine, or 3 oz 80-proof whiskey) per day in most men and to no more than 1 drink per day in women and lighter-weight persons.	2–4 mm Hg

DASH, Dietary Approaches to Stop Hypertension.

*For overall cardiovascular risk reduction, stop smoking.

† The effects of implementing these modifications are dose- and time-dependent, and could be greater for some individuals.

- Emphasize a diet of vegetables, fruits, low-fat dairy products, and foods low in saturated and total fat.
- Reduce daily sodium intake to no more than 1 teaspoon of salt/day (2.4 g of sodium or 6 g of sodium chloride); one suggested approach is to cut down on processed foods (details provided in the National Institutes of Health DASH (Dietary Approaches to Stop Hypertension) Diet (see **Appendix 24–1**).
- Use food sources to increase potassium intake to at least 3.5 g/day by eating foods such as bananas, orange juice, yogurt, potatoes, prunes, or winter squash.
- Perform aerobic physical activity for 30 to 45 minutes per day most days of the week.
- Limit alcohol use to no more than 1 oz of ethanol alcohol per day for men (24 oz of beer, 10 oz of wine, or 2 oz of hard liquor) and half that amount for women or lighter-weight individuals.

The interrelationship among hypertension, atherosclerosis, obesity, diabetes, diet, and exercise should be considered when making recommendations for nutritional support. Specific recommendations for each disorder should be considered if found in an individual patient's profile of risk. Refer to the appropriate chapter for recommendations. Specific recommendations for HTN have included increases in calcium, potassium, magnesium, vitamin E, and folic acid.[38]

The role of potassium in the management of HTN has been underappreciated. It is clear from many population studies that societies with a high intake of dietary potassium have a dramatically low prevalence of HTN. For example, less than 1% of individuals in an isolated society have HTN versus one-third of adults in more industrialized countries.[39] One factor is the amount of naturally acquired dietary potassium. It is known that potassium restriction is the trigger for cells to take in sodium in order to maintain their volume and tone. The difficulty in detecting low levels is that serum potassium may be normal, however, skeletal/muscle potassium is low. Low potassium inhibits insulin secretion and is associated with glucose intolerance. The Institute of Medicine recommends 4.7 grams of potassium per day, which is twice the U.S. average. The forms of potassium that have the greatest antihypertensive effect are fruits, vegetables, and other foods rather than supplementation. However, it has been shown that potassium supplements can dramatically reduce the need for antihypertension medication. In one study, 82% of individuals needed less than half of their medication dosage and 38% required no medication after a one-year follow-up.[40]

There has been a concern regarding sodium restriction, suggesting that it may activate the renin-angiotensin system and adversely affect both the lipid profile and insulin sensitivity. The literature indicates that these concerns have no support. The role of dietary magnesium and calcium is still debated. Generally, recommendations are that supplementation of magnesium or calcium is not preventive or effective in treating HTN; however, there is still some debate with some subgroups of patients who might benefit.[41,42] Recent evidence suggests that folic acid may be helpful in reducing HTN. The foods highest in folic acid are broccoli, asparagus, and spinach. It has also been suggested that calcium supplementation may lead to a small reduction in systolic BP.[43] A study by Siani et al.[44] indicates that a diet with foods containing L-arginine versus L-arginine supplements had a more beneficial effect on hyperlipidemia and HTN. Arginine is a precursor to nitric oxide, which is a vasodilator. It is found in brown rice, chocolate, caffeine, nuts (e.g., walnuts, filberts, pecans, Brazil nuts), oatmeal, raisins, seeds, and whole wheat bread. The one concern is the balance between L-lysine and L-arginine, especially with patients who have a viral infection (e.g., herpes).

Pregnant women appear to be at increased risk of pre-eclampsia/eclampsia with calcium deficiency. Either supplementation at 2 g of calcium per day or drinking one or two glasses of milk per day has been shown to decrease the risk of HTN during pregnancy.[45] Interestingly, one study[46] demonstrated an increased risk when women drank three or more glasses of milk per day.

In 2007, the American College of Sports Medicine and the American Heart Association published their updated recommendations for physical activity and public health.[47] All healthy adults age 18–65 years need at least:

- Moderate-intensity aerobic physical activity (e.g., jogging) for a minimum of 30 minutes five days each week.
- Vigorous, intense aerobic exercise for a minimum of 20 minutes three days each week.
- Combinations of moderate and vigorous activity can be used to meet the minimum such as walking briskly for 30 minutes twice per week and jogging for 20 minutes two times during the same week, or moderate-intensity exercise in bouts of 10 minutes or more.
- To perform exercise to maintain strength and endurance two days a week.

They also recommend exceeding the minimum requirement for those individuals wishing to further improve their physical fitness, avoid gaining weight, or decrease their risk for chronic disease and associated disability. Moderate exercise in the range of 50% to 65% of MHR may decrease DBP 15 to 20 mm Hg in patients with mild HTN. Exercise at levels of 70% or above demonstrated an abrupt increase in DBP. One study[48] indicated that patients with mild HTN (DBP, 90 to 105 mm Hg; SBP, 140 to 180 mm Hg) showed no difference between those on an aerobic program and those on a waiting list with regard to blood pressure reduction. However, these patients were exercising at 70% or above the maximum oxygen consumption (VO2 max). Recent studies[49-51] indicate a benefit to using a routine of aerobic exercise, independent of other factors, in lowering blood pressure. This effect may diminish in magnitude with age.[52] With regard to mortality rates, a study[53] published in 2013 indicated that there was no advantage for running over walking as a choice of exercise for hypertensives.

The use of breathing exercises has been demonstrated in a number of small studies to lower blood pressure.[54-57] From these studies, it appears that reducing the respiratory rate to less than 10 per minute with prolonged expiration has cardiovascular benefits. Reduction rates vary among the studies but seem to be around 10 to 15 mm Hg for systolic blood pressure. There also appears to be an advantage to using a device designed to give feedback for the patient to guide their breathing. The studies indicate that performing breathing exercises at least 15 minutes daily for two months is most beneficial. The effect seems to be more dramatic in seniors and in those with higher baseline blood pressure measurements.

There is still some debate as to the benefit of stress reduction; however, the recommendations of the Canadian Medical Association suggest a role in individualized cognitive behavioral interventions.[58] One recent study[59] suggests that patients who spent time with a personal pet had half the increase in blood pressure compared to those who did not own a pet.

Medication Summary

Medications reduce the pressure in the cardiovascular system by reducing the force of contraction of the heart, reducing the amount of fluid in the system, or reducing the tension in the arteries/veins. **Table 24–3** is a list of medications commonly used for the control of

Table 24–3 Antihypertensives

Drug Class	Examples	General Mechanism	Interactions/Side Effects
Angiotensin converting enzyme (ACE) inhibitors	**Captopril** Capoten	ACE inhibitor used in the management of hypertension, congestive heart failure, diabetic nephropathy, left ventricular dysfunction, and post MI	Hypersensitivity reactions, angioedema, persistent cough, orthostatic hypotension, altered taste sensation, positive ANA titers
	Enalapril Vasotec	An ACE inhibitor. Blocks the conversion of rennin to angiotensin II, thereby decreasing the release of aldosterone. This blocks the potent vasoconstriction effects of these substances, resulting in a decrease in blood pressure without a compensation of increased heart rate or cardiac output.	May cause headache, dizziness, fatigue, postural hypotension, chronic cough, hoarseness, and rash. May increase potassium levels, BUN, or creatinine.
	Lisinopril Zestril	An ACE inhibitor. Blocks the conversion of rennin to angiotensin II thereby decreasing the release of aldosterone. This blocks the potent vasoconstriction effects of these substances resulting in a decrease in blood pressure without a compensation of increased heart rate or cardiac output.	May cause headache, dizziness, fatigue, postural hypotension, chronic cough, hoarseness, and rash. May increase potassium levels, BUN, or creatinine.
Alpha and beta blockers	**Atenolol** Tenormin	Beta blocker: A β-adrenergic antagonist blocking primarily β1 receptors (less bronchoconstriction effect than β2 blockers); decreases heart rate and rennin release used in the treatment of hypertension.	CNS depressive effects with concerns for those with diabetes, heart block and heart failure, asthma, and emphysema.
	Labetalol Trandate Normodyne	An antihypertensive that acts as an alpha-adrenergic blocker and nonselective beta blocker. Results are decreased peripheral resistance, decreased conduction at sinus node, AV node, and ventricular muscle. Often used with thiazide diuretics.	May cause postural hypotension, bronchospasm, dizziness, fatigue, malaise, tremors, and GI disturbance. May cause positive results on ANA or testing and SLE-like syndrome.
	Metoprolol Lopressor Toprol XL	Beta blocker: A β-adrenergic antagonist blocking primarily β1 receptors (less bronchoconstriction effect than β2 blockers) decreases heart rate and rennin release used in the treatment of hypertension.	CNS depressive effects with concerns for those with diabetes, heart block and heart failure, asthma, and emphysema.
	Nadolol Corgard	Beta blocker: Blocks both β1 and β2 adrenergic receptors, decreases heart rate and rennin release used in the treatment of hypertension. Also has bronchoconstriction effect due to β2 blockade.	May cause CNS depressive effects with concerns for those with diabetes, heart block and heart failure, asthma, and emphysema. Transient hypertension due to blockage of β2 receptors (which normally dilate large arteries).
	Prazosin Minipress	Alpha blocker: α-adrenergic antagonist causing dilation of arteries and veins used for the treatment of hypertension.	Postural hypotension, dry mouth, edema, congestion, headache, sexual dysfunction, and lethargy.
	Propranolol Inderal	Beta blocker: Blocks both β1 and β2 adrenergic receptors, decreases heart rate and rennin release used in the treatment of hypertension. Also has bronchoconstriction effect due to β2 blockade.	CNS depressive effects with concerns for those with diabetes, heart block and heart failure, asthma, and emphysema. Transient hypertension due to blockage of β2 receptors (which normally dilate large arteries).

(continues)

Table 24–3 Antihypertensives (continued)

Drug Class	Examples	General Mechanism	Interactions/Side Effects
	Terazosin Hydrin	An α1-adrenergic blocker used in the management of hypertension in combination with a β-adrenergic blocker and thiazide diuretic. Also used in the management of benign prostatic hypertrophy.	May cause weakness, dizziness, headache, weight gain, or syncope.
	Timolol Blocadren	Beta blocker: Blocks both β1 and β2 adrenergic receptors, decreases heart rate and rennin release used in the treatment of hypertension. Also has bronchoconstriction effect due to β2 blockade.	CNS depressive effects with concerns for those with diabetes, heart block and heart failure, asthma, and emphysema. Transient hypertension due to blockage of β2 receptors (which normally dilate large arteries).
α2 adrenergic agonists	**Clonidine**	An α2 adrenergic agonist used as an antihypertensive. It decreases cardiac output, heart rate, and blood pressure.	Rash, drowsiness, headache, impaired ejaculation, dry mouth, and if stopped suddenly, rebound hypertension.
	Methyldopa Aldomet	An α2-adrenergic agonist used as an antihypertensive. It decreases cardiac output, heart rate, and blood pressure.	May cause dry mouth, possible postural hypotension, and sedation. May experience nightmares or psychic disturbances.
Diuretics	**Furosemide** Lasix Fumide Lauramide Furomide	A sulfonamide "loop" diuretic that inhibits resorption of sodium and chloride at the loop of Henle and proximal and distal renal tubules. Used in the management of hypertension, fluid reduction for CHF, hepatic cirrhosis, and renal dysfunction.	May cause hypokalemia (supplement with potassium), GI complaints, circulatory collapse, or aplastic types of anemia.
	Vasopressin Pitressin	An extracted animal hormone from the posterior pituitary that has primarily an antidiuretic effect (no oxytocin effect). Effect is primarily due to increasing tubular resorption of water creating a concentrated urine. Used in the management of diabetes insipidus, for dissipation of gas shadows on abdominal films, or for reducing abdominal distention postsurgically. Has also been used as intranasal spray for maintenance treatment of diabetes insipidus and sometimes for enuresis.	Small doses may cause angina or MI and aggravate other pre-existing heart conditions. May cause headache, water intoxication, and anaphylaxis among other common drug side effects.
Calcium channel blocker	**Nifedipine** Adalat Procardia	A calcium channel blocker that causes smooth muscle relaxation of coronary and peripheral blood vessels, decreasing peripheral resistance without affecting serum calcium levels. Used in the management of hypertension usually in combination with a diuretic and also vasospastic (Prinzmetal or variant) angina.	May cause dizziness, lightheadedness, postural hypotension, facial flushing, palpitations, peripheral edema, hepatotoxicity, sore throat, and various GH symptoms.

hypertension. The following general classes of medications accomplish these actions:

- Diuretics (decrease fluid in system)
- Drugs that affect the sympathetic nervous system such as β-blockers and α-adrenergic blockers (reduce force of contraction of the heart and/or tension in the vascular system)
- General vasodilators

- Calcium channel blockers (similar effect on heart and vasculature as sympathetic drugs)
- Angiotensin-converting enzyme (ACE) inhibitors (inhibit the renin-angiotensin-aldosterone cycle)
- Angiotensin receptor blockers

Common and popular examples are: Lisinopril (ACE inhibitor), hydrochlorothiazide and furosemide (diuretics), and Norvasc (calcium channel blocker). Each drug has its potential side effects. The most characteristic side effects are as follows:

- Diuretics—Some diuretics will cause loss of potassium or magnesium and lead to some increase in low-density lipoprotein cholesterol.
- β-Blockers—β-blockers often have an effect of causing a decrease in energy or inducing general malaise.
- Calcium channel blockers—Some of the older types of calcium channel blockers have been associated with an increased risk for certain cancers.
- ACE inhibitors—Facial edema and a nonproductive cough may occur. The dry cough associated with ACE inhibitors may be alleviated with iron supplementation but not at the same time due to potential interference with the drug's absorption.

It is important that the patient consult his or her physician prior to decreasing or increasing the dose of medication. Older patients may forget to take their medication (or with diuretics, potassium supplementation) or decide to stop taking medication because of the cost. It is important to ask questions regarding any change in medication, in particular with those patients who appeared to be under control, yet now have a high BP.

Algorithms

Algorithms for evaluation and management of HTN are presented in **Figures 24–1** and **24–2**.

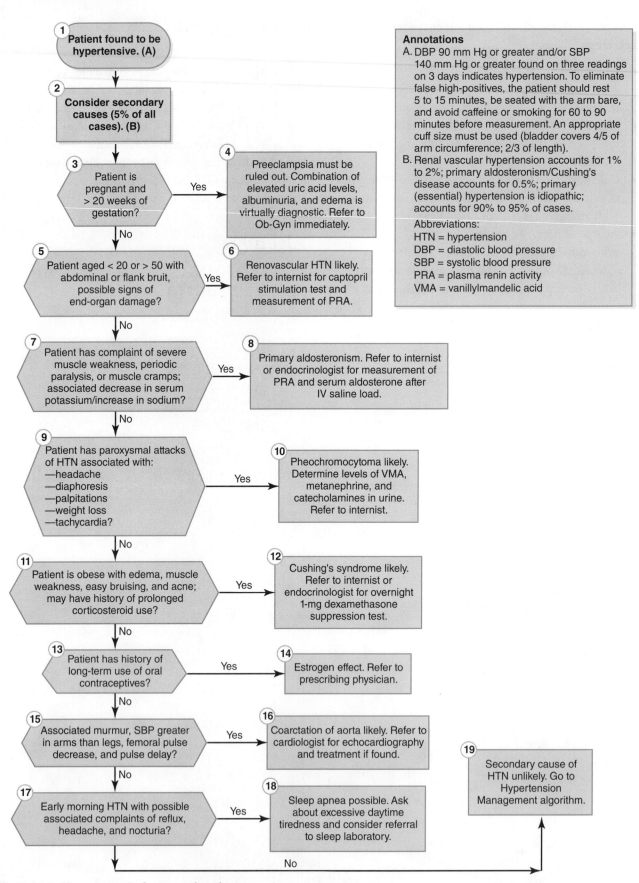

Figure 24-1 Hypertension Evaluation—Algorithm

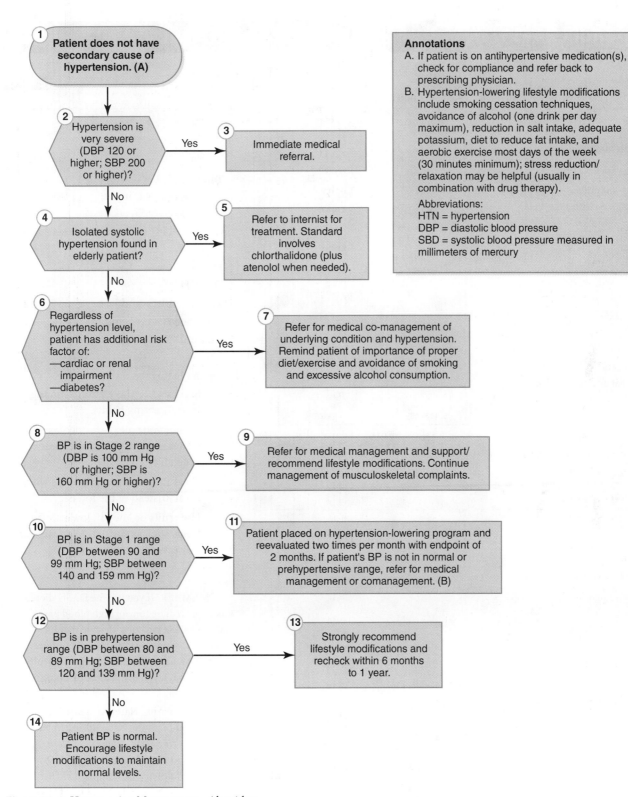

1 Patient does not have secondary cause of hypertension. (A)

2 Hypertension is very severe (DBP 120 or higher; SBP 200 or higher)? — Yes → **3** Immediate medical referral.

No ↓

4 Isolated systolic hypertension found in elderly patient? — Yes → **5** Refer to internist for treatment. Standard involves chlorthalidone (plus atenolol when needed).

No ↓

6 Regardless of hypertension level, patient has additional risk factor of:
—cardiac or renal impairment
—diabetes? — Yes → **7** Refer for medical co-management of underlying condition and hypertension. Remind patient of importance of proper diet/exercise and avoidance of smoking and excessive alcohol consumption.

No ↓

8 BP is in Stage 2 range (DBP is 100 mm Hg or higher; SBP is 160 mm Hg or higher)? — Yes → **9** Refer for medical management and support/ recommend lifestyle modifications. Continue management of musculoskeletal complaints.

No ↓

10 BP is in Stage 1 range (DBP between 90 and 99 mm Hg; SBP between 140 and 159 mm Hg)? — Yes → **11** Patient placed on hypertension-lowering program and reevaluated two times per month with endpoint of 2 months. If patient's BP is not in normal or prehypertensive range, refer for medical management or comanagement. (B)

No ↓

12 BP is in prehypertension range (DBP between 80 and 89 mm Hg; SBP between 120 and 139 mm Hg)? — Yes → **13** Strongly recommend lifestyle modifications and recheck within 6 months to 1 year.

No ↓

14 Patient BP is normal. Encourage lifestyle modifications to maintain normal levels.

Annotations
A. If patient is on antihypertensive medication(s), check for compliance and refer back to prescribing physician.
B. Hypertension-lowering lifestyle modifications include smoking cessation techniques, avoidance of alcohol (one drink per day maximum), reduction in salt intake, adequate potassium, diet to reduce fat intake, and aerobic exercise most days of the week (30 minutes minimum); stress reduction/ relaxation may be helpful (usually in combination with drug therapy).

Abbreviations:
HTN = hypertension
DBP = diastolic blood pressure
SBD = systolic blood pressure measured in millimeters of mercury

Figure 24–2 Hypertension Management—Algorithm

Appendix 24–1

National Institutes of Health

The DASH Diet ■ Sample Menu ■ Based on 2,000 Calories/Day

Food	Amount	Servings Provided
Breakfast		
orange juice	6 oz	1 fruit
1% low-fat milk	8 oz (1 C)	1 dairy
corn flakes (with 1 tsp sugar)	1 C	2 grains
banana	1 medium	1 fruit
whole wheat bread (with 1 tbsp jelly)	1 slice	1 grain
soft margarine	1 tsp	1 fat
Lunch		
chicken salad	3/4 C	1 poultry
pita bread	1/2, large	1 grain
raw vegetable medley:		
carrot and celery sticks	3–4 sticks each	
radishes	2	
loose-leaf lettuce	2 leaves	1 vegetable
part-skim mozzarella cheese	1.5 slice (1.5 oz)	1 dairy
1% low-fat milk	8 oz (1 C)	1 dairy
fruit cocktail in light syrup	1/2 C	1 fruit
Dinner		
herbed baked cod	3 oz	1 fish
scallion rice	1 C	2 grains
steamed broccoli	1/2 C	1 vegetable
stewed tomatoes	1/2 C	1 vegetable
spinach salad:		
raw spinach	1/2 C	
cherry tomatoes	2	
cucumber	2 slices	1 vegetable
light Italian salad dressing	1 tbsp	1/2 fat
whole wheat dinner roll	1 small	1 grain
soft margarine	1 tsp	1 fat
melon balls	1/2 C	1 fruit
Snacks		
dried apricots	1 oz (1/4 C)	1 fruit
mini-pretzels	1 oz (3/4 C)	1 grain
mixed nuts	1.5 oz (1/3 C)	1 nuts
diet ginger ale	12 oz	0

Total number of servings in 2,000 calories/day menu:

Food Group	Serving
Grains	= 8
Vegetables	= 4
Fruits	= 5
Dairy Foods	= 3
Meats, Poultry, and Fish	= 2
Nuts, Seeds, and Legumes	= 1
Fats and Oils	= 2.5

Tips on Eating the DASH Way

- Start small. Make gradual changes in your eating habits.
- Center your meal around carbohydrates, such as pasta, rice, beans, or vegetables.
- Treat meat as one part of the whole meal, instead of the focus.
- Use fruits or low-fat, low-calorie foods such as sugar-free gelatin for desserts and snacks.

REMEMBER! If you use the DASH diet to help prevent or control high blood pressure, make it part of a lifestyle that includes choosing foods lower in salt and sodium, keeping a healthy weight, being physically active, and, if you drink alcohol, doing so in moderation.

Reproduced from National Heart, Lung, and Blood Institute, National Institutes of Health, *The Sixth Report of the Joint National Committee on Prevention, Detection, Evaluation, and Treatment of High Blood Pressure*, NIH Publication 98-1080, November 1997.

APPENDIX 24–2

References

1. Cherry DK, Woodwell DA. National Ambulatory Medical Care Survey: 2000 Summary. *Advance Data.* 2002;328.

2. *2000 Heart and Stroke Statistical Update.* American Heart Association. Dallas, TX: American Heart Association, 1999.

3. Jamison JR. Reducing the personal risk of perceived disease: the chiropractic patients' self-care endeavor. *J Manipulative Physiol Ther.* 2001;24(6):378–384.

4. Burt VL, Whelton P, Rocella EJ, et al. Prevalence of hypertension in the U.S. adult population: results from the Third National Health and Nutrition Examination Survey, 1988–1991. *Hypertension.* 1995;25:305–313.

5. Joint National Committee on Detection, Evaluation, and Treatment of High Blood Pressure. *The Sixth Report of the Joint National Committee on Detection, Evaluation, and Treatment of High Blood Pressure.* Bethesda, MD: National Institutes of Health, National Heart, Lung, and Blood Institute; 1997. NIH publication 98-4080.

6. Hansen ML, Gunn PW, Kaelber DC. Underdiagnosis of hypertension in children and adolescents. *JAMA.* 2007;298(8):874–879.

7. Buyse M, ed. *Birth Defects Encyclopedia.* St. Louis, MO: Blackwell Scientific Publications; 1990:156.

8. Garraway WM, Whisnant JP. The changing pattern of hypertension and the declining incidence of stroke. *JAMA.* 1987;258:214–217.

9. Cutler J, Follman D, Eliot P, Suh I. An overview of randomized trials of sodium reduction and blood pressure. *Hypertension.* 1991;17(suppl 1): 127–133.

10. Pan W, Nanas S, Dyer A, et al. The role of weight in the positive association between age and blood pressure. *Am J Epidemiol.* 1986;124:612–623.

11. Smith W, Crombie I, Tavendale R, et al. Urinary electrolyte excretion, alcohol consumption, and blood pressure in the Scottish Heart Health Study. *Br Med J.* 1988;297:329–330.

12. Mann S, James G, Wang R, Pickering T. Elevation of ambulatory systolic blood pressure in hypertensive smokers: a case control study. *JAMA.* 1991;265:2226–2228.

13. Massie BM. Systemic hypertension. In: Tierney LM, Jr, McPhee SJ, Papadakis MA, eds. *Current Medical Diagnosis and Treatment.* 34th ed. Norwalk, CT: Appleton & Lange; 1995:373.

14. Keller G, Zimmer G, Mall G, et al. Nephron number in patients with primary hypertension. *N Engl J Med.* 2003; 348:101–108.

15. Cushman WC. Effect of back support and stethoscope head on seated blood pressure determination. *Am J Hypertension.* 1990;3:240–241.

16. Londe S, Klitzner TS. Auscultatory blood pressure measurement. Effect of pressure on head of the stethoscope. *West J Med.* 1984;141:193–195.

17. Pickering T. Recommendations for the use of home (self) and ambulatory blood pressure monitoring. American Society of Hypertension Ad Hoc Panel. *Am J Hypertension.* 1996;9:1–11.

18. Clement DL, De Bacquer DA, Duprez DA, et al. Prognostic value of ambulatory blood-pressure recordings in patients with treated hypertension. *N Engl J Med.* 2003; 348:2407–2415.

19. Chobanian AV, Bakris GL, Black HR, et al. The seventh report of the joint national committee on prevention, detection, evaluation, and treatment of high blood pressure: the JNC 7 report. *JAMA.* 2003;289(19):2560–2572.

20. The Seventh Report of the Joint National Committee on Prevention, Detection, Evaluation, and Treatment of High Blood Pressure. NIH Publication 03-5233, May 2003. National Institutes of Health.

21. James PA, Oparil S, Carter BL, et al. 2014 Evidence-based guideline for the management of high blood pressure in adults: report from the panel members appointed to the eighth joint national committee (JNC 8). *JAMA.* 2014;311(5):507–520.

22. Vasan RS, Larson MG, Leip EP, et al. Assessment of frequency of progression to hypertension in non-hypertensive participants in the Framingham Heart Study: a current study. *Lancet.* 2001;358:1682–1686.

23. Vassan RS, Beiser A, Seshadri S, et al. Residual lifetime risk for developing hypertension in middle-aged women and men. The Framingham Heart Study. *JAMA.* 2002;287:1003–1010.

24. Izzo JL, Levy D, Back HR. Clinical Advisory Statement: Importance of systolic blood pressure in older Americans. *Hypertension.* 2000;35:1021–1024.

25. Hyman DJ, Pavlik VN. Characteristics of patients with uncontrolled hypertension in the United States. *N Engl J Med.* 2001;345:479–486.

26. Khot UN, Khot MB, Bajzer CT. Prevalence of conventional risk factors in patients with coronary heart disease. *JAMA*. 2003;290:898–904.

27. Goertz C, Mootz RD. A review of conservative management strategies in the care of patients with essential hypertension. *J Neuromusculoskel Syst*. 1993;1:91–108.

28. Yates RG, Lamping DL, Abram NL, Wright C. Effects of chiropractic treatment on blood pressure and anxiety: a randomized, controlled trial. *J Manipulative Physiol Ther*. 1988;11(6):484–488.

29. Morgan JP, Dickey JL, Hunt HH, Hudgins PM. A controlled trial of spinal manipulation in the management of hypertension. *J Am Osteopath Assoc*. 1985;85(5):308–313.

30. Knutson GA. Significant changes in systolic blood pressure post vectored upper cervical adjustment vs resting control groups: a possible effect of the cervicosympathetic and/or pressor reflex. *J Manipulative Physiol Ther*. 2001;24(2):101–109.

31. Goertz CH, Grimm RH, Svendsen K, Grandits G. Treatment of Hypertension with Alternative Therapies (THAT) Study: a randomized clinical trial. *J Hypertens*. 2002;20(10):2063–2068.

32. Bakris G, Dickholtz M, Sr., Meyer PM, et al. Atlas vertebra realignment and achievement of arterial pressure goal in hypertensive patients: a pilot study. *J Hum Hypertens*. 2007;21(5):347–352.

33. Plaugher G, Long CR, Alcantara J, et al. Practice-based randomized controlled-comparison clinical trial of chiropractic adjustments and brief massage treatment at sites of subluxation in subjects with essential hypertension: pilot study. *J Manipulative Physiol Ther*. 2002;25(4):221–239.

34. Writing Group of the PREMIER Collaborative Research Group. Effects of comprehensive lifestyle modification on blood pressure control: main results of the PREMIER Clinical Trial. *JAMA*. 2003;289(16):2083–2093.

35. Sacks FM, Svetkey LP, Vollmer WM, et al. Effects on blood pressure of reduced dietary sodium and the dietary approaches to stop hypertension (DASH) diet: DASH-sodium collaborative research group. *N Engl J Med*. 2001;344:3–10.

36. Whelton SP, Chin A, Xue K, Jiang H. Effect of aerobic exercise on blood pressure: a meta-analysis of randomized, controlled trials. *Ann Intern Med*. 2002;136:493–503.

37. Yao LL, Liu K, Mathews KA, et al. Psychosocial factors and risk of hypertension: the coronary artery risk development in young adults (CARDIA) study. *JAMA*. 2003;90:2138–2148.

38. Burgess E, Lewcanczuk R, Bolli P, et al. Recommendations on potassium, magnesium, and calcium. *Can Med Assoc J*. 1999;160(9, suppl.):535–545.

39. He FJ, MacGregor GA. Fortnightly review: beneficial effects of potassium. *BMJ*. 2001;323(7311):497–501.

40. Siani A, Strazzullo P, Giacco A, Pacioni D, Celentano E, Mancini M. Increasing the dietary potassium intake reduces the need for antihypertensive medication. *Ann Intern Med*. 1991;115(10):753–759.

41. Yang CY, Chiu HF. Calcium and magnesium in drinking water and the risk of death from hypertension. *Am J Hypertens*. 1999;12:894–899.

42. Touyz RM, Milne FJ. Magnesium supplementation attenuates, but does not prevent, development of hypertension in spontaneously hypertensive rats. *Am J Hypertens*. 1999;12:757–765.

43. Bucher HC, Cook RJ, Guyatt GH, et al. Effects of dietary calcium supplementation on blood pressure. A meta-analysis of randomized controlled trials. *JAMA*. 1996;275:1016–1022.

44. Siani A, Pagano E, Iacone R, Iacoviello L, Scopacasa F, Strazzullo P. Blood pressure and metabolic changes during dietary L-arginine supplementation in humans. *Am J Hypertens*. 2000;13(5 Pt 1):547–551.

45. Cong K, Chi S, Liu G. Calcium supplementation during pregnancy for reducing pregnancy-induced hypertension. *Chin Med J*. 1995;108:57–59.

46. Richardson BE, Baird DO. A study of milk and calcium supplement intake and subsequent preeclampsia in a cohort of pregnant women. *Am J Epidemiol*. 1995;141:667–673.

47. Haskell WL, Lee IM, Pate RR, et al. Physical activity and public health: updated recommendation for adults from the American College of Sports Medicine and the American Heart Association. *Circulation*. 2007;116(9):1081–1093.

48. Blumenthal JA, Siegel WC, Appelbaum M. Failure of exercise to reduce blood pressure in patients with mild hypertension. *JAMA*. 1991;266:2098–2104.

49. Jessup JV, Lowenthal DT, Pollock ML, Turner T. The effects of endurance exercise training on ambulatory blood pressure in normotensive older adults. *Geriatr Nephrol Urol*. 1998;8:103–109.

50. Martel GF, Hurlbut DE, Lott ME, et al. Strength training normalizes resting blood pressure in 65- to 73-year-old men and women with high normal blood pressure. *J Am Geriatr Soc*. 1999;47:1215–1221.

51. Seals DR, Silverman HG, Reilling MJ, Davy KP. Effect of regular aerobic exercise on elevated blood pressure in postmenopausal women. *Am J Cardiol.* 1997;80:49–55.

52. Ishikawa K, Ohta T, Zhang J, et al. Influence of age and gender on exercise training-induced blood pressure reduction in systemic hypertension. *Am J Cardiol.* 1999;15:192–196.

53. Williams PT. Walking and running produce similar reductions in cause-specific disease mortality in hypertensives. *Hypertension.* 2013;62(3):485–491.

54. Elliot WJ, Izzo JL, Jr., White WB, et al. Graded blood pressure reduction in hypertensive outpatients associated with use of a device to assist with slow breathing. *J Clin Hypertens (Greenwich).* 2004;6(10):553–559; quiz 560–551.

55. Meles E, Giannattasio C, Failla M, Gentile G, Capra A, Mancia G. Nonpharmacologic treatment of hypertension by respiratory exercise in the home setting. *Am J Hypertens.* 2004;17(4):370–374.

56. Rosenthal T, Alter A, Peleg E, Gavish B. Device-guided breathing exercises reduce blood pressure: ambulatory and home measurements. *Am J Hypertens.* 2001;14(1):74–76.

57. Viskoper R, Shapira I, Priluck R, et al. Nonpharmacologic treatment of resistant hypertensives by device-guided slow breathing exercises. *Am J Hypertens.* 2003;16(6):484–487.

58. David Spence J, Barnett PA, Linden W, et al. Recommendations on stress management. *J Canadian Med Assoc.* 1999;160(9, suppl.):546–550.

59. Allen KM. Increased social support (pet ownership), but not ACE inhibitor therapy, attenuates cardiovascular reactivity to mental stress among hypertensive stockbrokers. Presented at American Heart Association 72nd Scientific Sessions; Nov. 7–10, 1999; Atlanta, GA.

Lower Leg Swelling

Context

Lower leg swelling may be the result of a variety of causes via a variety of mechanisms. In general, swelling is usually vascular, muscular, fatty, myxedematous, or tumorous. Bilateral leg swelling is suggestive of a systemic process and is often the result of fluid retention and stagnation due to congestive heart failure, salt-retaining drugs, liver or kidney disorders (hypoproteinemia), primary lymphedema, and dependency. Unilateral leg swelling is usually secondary to trauma, requiring a differentiation between thrombosis and a muscular tear, a task not always as simple as it may seem.

General Strategy

Unilateral Acute Leg Swelling

- Determine whether trauma was involved.
- Determine whether there is a history of contraceptive use or immobilization.
- Determine whether there was a sudden or gradual onset of pain with exercise.

Bilateral Chronic Leg Swelling

- Determine whether the onset was at an early age.
- Determine the patient's cardiopulmonary status.
- Determine whether the patient is taking drugs that cause salt retention or has a high-salt diet.
- Determine whether the patient stands for many hours at a time.
- Determine whether the patient has varicosities and, if so, test to determine which part of the venous system is involved.

Relevant Physiology and Anatomy

Review of simple physiologic principles reveals most of the common causes of edema (**Exhibit 25–1**). Fluid within the vascular system remains in the system unless drawn or forced outward by two processes. One process is simply pressure within the system. Hypertension, gravity, venous valvular incompetence, and venous or lymph blockage will increase hydrostatic pressure, forcing fluid into the interstitium. The second mechanism involves oncotic pressure. Key to the retention of fluid is the osmotic influence of protein, specifically albumin. Low albumin states are usually due to loss or decreased production. Production of albumin occurs in the liver. Albumin is usually retained by the kidney, yet in some pathologic states, such as long-term diabetes or chronic renal failure, albumin is lost in the urine.

Veins allow unidirectional (toward the heart) movement of blood. This is dependent on one-way valves. When these valves are incompetent or pressure and dilation exceed their restraining ability, blood flows retrograde and can be forced into the interstitium. The venous system has two levels of veins that connect via communicating veins. Blood in the deep system is pumped toward the heart through muscular contraction. Lack of muscular contraction or blockage in the deep system forces blood to flow retrograde through the communicating system to the superficial veins. The superficial system does not have the advantage of muscular contraction to aid in transport and as a result is more likely to demonstrate superficial signs of incompetence—varicosities.

Salt either in the diet or due to drugs or hormones such as estrogen, which cause the retention of salt, can increase vascular fluid and cause lower leg edema.

Exhibit 25–1 Common Causes of Edema

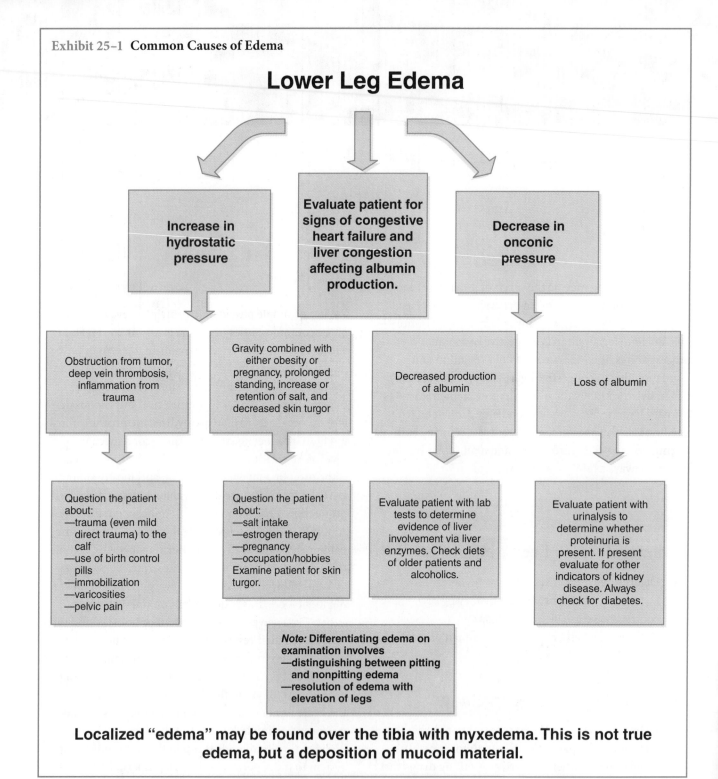

Lower Leg Edema

Increase in hydrostatic pressure

Evaluate patient for signs of congestive heart failure and liver congestion affecting albumin production.

Decrease in onconic pressure

Obstruction from tumor, deep vein thrombosis, inflammation from trauma

Gravity combined with either obesity or pregnancy, prolonged standing, increase or retention of salt, and decreased skin turgor

Decreased production of albumin

Loss of albumin

Question the patient about:
—trauma (even mild direct trauma) to the calf
—use of birth control pills
—immobilization
—varicosities
—pelvic pain

Question the patient about:
—salt intake
—estrogen therapy
—pregnancy
—occupation/hobbies
Examine patient for skin turgor.

Evaluate patient with lab tests to determine evidence of liver involvement via liver enzymes. Check diets of older patients and alcoholics.

Evaluate patient with urinalysis to determine whether proteinuria is present. If present evaluate for other indicators of kidney disease. Always check for diabetes.

Note: Differentiating edema on examination involves
—distinguishing between pitting and nonpitting edema
—resolution of edema with elevation of legs

Localized "edema" may be found over the tibia with myxedema. This is not true edema, but a deposition of mucoid material.

Localized "edema" may be found over the tibia with myxedema. This is not true edema, but a deposition of mucoid material.

Evaluation

History

Timing and position are helpful discriminators. Acute, unilateral swelling of the calf is most often due to deep vein thrombosis (DVT) or muscle tear. Associated indicators of DVT are a history of immobilization, use of birth control pills, or minor trauma to the area (especially in an older patient). It is more likely that a muscle strain occurred when the patient can identify a sudden onset with activity, especially with plantarflexion of the ankle. Slow onset of swelling that is relieved by elevation of the legs is suggestive of venous insufficiency or congestive heart failure. Diffuse swelling that is unrelieved by elevation suggests lymph blockage. Calf pain and swelling that appear with exercise are more likely due to a compartment syndrome in a younger person and DVT in an older person. Cancer such as pancreatic cancer should be considered in the differential for lower leg swelling when multiple swellings represent a superficial thrombophlebitis process.

A review of medications and diet may indicate a salt-retaining mechanism for swelling. Substances such as estrogen promote salt retention (this occurs as a natural consequence of estrogen production during a regular menstrual cycle).

Examination

Observation for the degree of swelling and whether it is localized may be extremely helpful, for example, in the following cases:

- In obese women, swelling that spares the ankles is often due to fat deposition (lipedema), especially if bilateral.
- Localized swelling that appears rather hard and sometimes tender may indicate an underlying bone or soft tissue tumor.
- Swelling localized behind the knee may indicate bursal swelling, a Baker's cyst, or a medial gastrocnemius rupture.
- Swelling localized to the tibial crest probably represents myxedema, which is found in some patients with hyperthyroidism.

- A unilateral swelling in the calf may represent thrombophlebitis.

Skin texture and appearance may be characteristic for some causes of leg swelling.

- Lymphedema—The skin becomes dry and scaly with progressive thickening.
- Chronic venous insufficiency—The skin may become golden brown (hemosiderin deposition) at the medial ankle or more diffusely.
- Cellulitis—Diffuse redness and warm skin or red streaks appear on the leg.
- Erythema nodosum—Discrete, nummular areas that are warm appear on the anterior leg.
- Reflex sympathetic dystrophy—In the early stage, the skin is hypersensitive and cool; later, the skin is taut, shiny, and thin.
- Gastrocnemius tear—Bluish purple discoloration appears at the medial malleolus.
- Congenital venous malformations—Flat, purplish red angiomata or dark purple verrucous lesions appear.
- Lymphatic obstruction—Eventually the skin is indurated with a texture like an orange peel (peau d'orange).

Another distinguishing factor is whether the swelling is pitting or nonpitting. Pitting edema is often found in conditions that produce a less viscous fluid; for example, the edema found with congestive heart failure. Swelling that is nonpitting is more often associated with lymph blockage as may occur with tumors. The excess proteinaceous fluid that is normally cleared from the interstitium by the lymphatics is allowed to accumulate.

Improvement of swelling with leg elevation may also help distinguish between lymphedema and edema due to venous involvement. There is a marked improvement with elevation when venous engorgement is the main problem. There is little improvement when the lymphatics are involved. Additionally, venous insufficiency is evaluated with several tests. Trendelenburg's test is used to determine whether varicosities are due to incompetence of the superficial, communicating, or deep veins. The patient's leg is elevated to drain the venous system. A tourniquet is tied tightly enough to occlude the superficial veins at the proximal thigh. The patient stands. If the varicosities fill, the deep and communicating systems are responsible (usually deep vein obstruction). If the varicosities do not appear, but do develop with removal of the tourniquet, the incompetency is in the superficial system.

A running debate as to how long to maintain anti-coagulant medication has led to a search for predictors of future risk while not on anticoagulants. Recently, one study noted that D-dimer is a global indicator of coagulation activation and fibrinolysis.[1] A high D-dimer level has been associated with increased risk for a first venous thrombosis. This study found that patients with a D-dimer level less than 250 ng/mL after withdrawal from oral anticoagulants has a low risk for recurrence of venous thrombosis.

If the patient has history and examination results suggestive of DVT, referral for noninvasive Doppler ultrasound is needed to confirm the suspicion. Doppler ultrasound is replacing the gold standard of venography in most cases. A positive finding is identification of an area of noncompressibility along the suspected vein.

Management

- Acute unilateral swelling that is suggestive of DVT should be referred immediately for evaluation with Doppler ultrasound or a venogram; if positive, medical management would include immobilization with elevation for approximately one week and anticoagulant therapy for three months or longer.
- Congestive heart failure should be referred for comanagement. Long-term management should include the use of natural diuretics when possible, reduction of salt, and a graduated, supervised diet and exercise program.
- Varicose veins may be treated conservatively through advice, including advice on the use of elastic stockings, use of frequent breaks with leg elevation, weight loss, and avoidance of prolonged standing. If these measures are unsuccessful or unacceptable by the patient, referral for a discussion of surgical options should be made.

Algorithm

An algorithm for evaluation and management of lower extremity edema is presented in **Figure 25–1**.

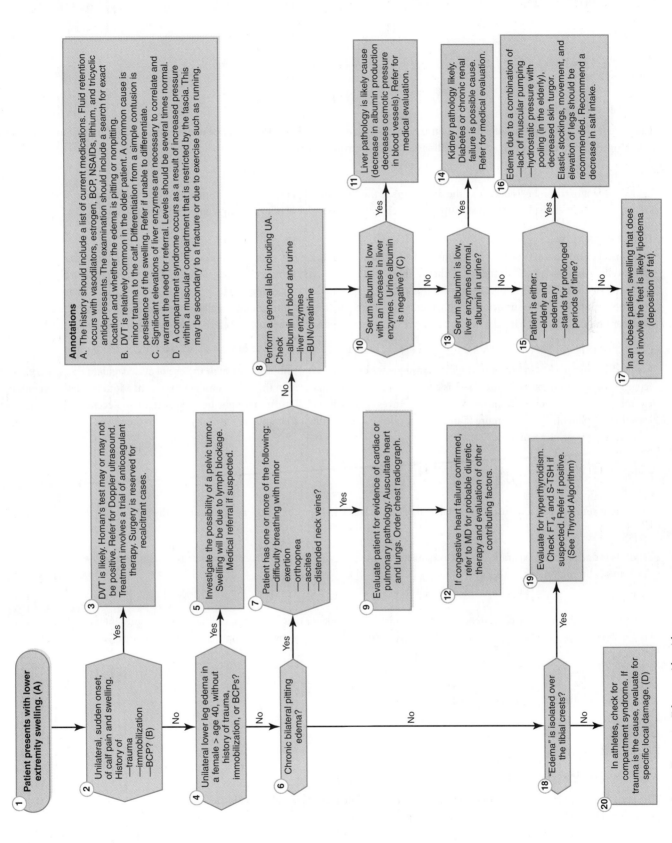

Annotations

A. The history should include a list of current medications. Fluid retention occurs with vasodilators, estrogen, BCP, NSAIDs, lithium, and tricyclic antidepressants. The examination should include a search for exact location and whether the edema is pitting or nonpitting.

B. DVT is relatively common in the older patient. A common cause is minor trauma to the calf. Differentiation from a simple contusion is persistence of the swelling. Refer if unable to differentiate.

C. Significant elevations of liver enzymes are necessary to correlate and warrant the need for referral. Levels should be several times normal.

D. A compartment syndrome occurs as a result of increased pressure within a muscular compartment that is restricted by the fascia. This may be secondary to a fracture or due to exercise such as running.

1. Patient presents with lower extremity swelling. (A)

2. Unilateral, sudden onset, of calf pain and swelling. History of
—trauma
—immobilization
—BCP? (B)

3. DVT is likely. Homan's test may or may not be positive. Refer for Doppler ultrasound. Treatment involves a trial of anticoagulant therapy. Surgery is reserved for recalcitrant cases.

4. Unilateral lower leg edema in a female > age 40, without history of trauma, immobilization, or BCPs?

5. Investigate the possibility of a pelvic tumor. Swelling will be due to lymph blockage. Medical referral if suspected.

6. Chronic bilateral pitting edema?

7. Patient has one or more of the following:
—difficulty breathing with minor exertion
—orthopnea
—ascites
—distended neck veins?

8. Perform a general lab including UA. Check
—albumin in blood and urine
—liver enzymes
—BUN/creatinine

9. Evaluate patient for evidence of cardiac or pulmonary pathology. Auscultate heart and lungs. Order chest radiograph.

10. Serum albumin is low with an increase in liver enzymes. Urine albumin is negative? (C)

11. Liver pathology is likely cause (decrease in albumin production decreases osmotic pressure in blood vessels). Refer for medical evaluation.

12. If congestive heart failure confirmed, refer to MD for probable diuretic therapy and evaluation of other contributing factors.

13. Serum albumin is low, liver enzymes normal, albumin in urine?

14. Kidney pathology likely. Diabetes or chronic renal failure is possible cause. Refer for medical evaluation.

15. Patient is either:
—elderly and sedentary
—stands for prolonged periods of time?

16. Edema due to a combination of
—lack of muscular pumping
—hydrostatic pressure with pooling (in the elderly),
—decreased skin turgor.
Elastic stockings, movement, and elevation of legs should be recommended. Recommend a decrease in salt intake.

17. In an obese patient, swelling that does not involve the feet is likely lipedema (deposition of fat).

18. "Edema" is isolated over the tibial crests?

19. Evaluate for hyperthyroidism. Check FT₄ and S-TSH if suspected. Refer if positive. (See Thyroid Algorithm)

20. In athletes, check for compartment syndrome. If trauma is the cause, evaluate for specific local damage. (D)

Figure 25–1 Lower Extremity Edema—Algorithm

Selected Causes of Lower Leg Swelling

ACUTE UNILATERAL

Deep Vein Thrombosis

Classic Presentation

The patient may complain of calf pain or tightness that is worse with walking. There may be a history of a minor trauma to the calf or a prolonged period of rest due to a chronic illness (or a long airline flight).

Cause

Eighty percent of thrombosis occurs in the deep veins of the calf, although other sites may include the femoral and iliac veins. Predispositions include prolonged rest, surgery (especially hip surgery), use of oral contraceptives in women, and cancer.

Evaluation

The clinical examination is often unrevealing. In fact, 50% of patients are not even symptomatic. When symptomatic, there may be mild swelling and tenderness in the calf. Other findings that are relatively nonspecific include a slight fever and tachycardia. The standard Homan's test, which involves passive dorsiflexion of the ankle in an attempt to increase pain, is nonspecific in an ambulatory population. When the suspicion is high, plethysmography or Doppler ultrasound is an acceptable noninvasive screening tool.[2] A D-dimer test should also be included. The definitive diagnosis may require the gold standard of ascending contrast venography.

Management

The medical approach is to prevent the lethal consequence of pulmonary embolism through the use of anticoagulant therapy (i.e., heparin) for several months. **Table 25–1** is a list of some medications used in the management of DVT. In addition, elevation of the legs for approximately one week is needed with the knees slightly flexed. Return to weight-bearing is gradual. Recent evidence suggests that for patients requiring more than three months of anticoagulant therapy, low-intensity warfarin therapy is warranted and is effective in preventing recurrence.[3]

Cellulitis

Classic Presentation

The patient complains of a diffuse, hot, swollen area on the leg. There may be a history of a break in the skin.

Cause

Cellulitis is due primarily to gram-positive organisms; however, *Escherichia coli* may also be a cause. Cellulitis may be seen as a complication of chronic venous stasis.

Evaluation

Finding an area that is red and swollen, with either a history or evidence of a break in the skin, is a classic presentation. If the patient has a history of venous stasis, finding a new area of tenderness is also suggestive. Attempts at isolating the organism are usually unsuccessful.

Management

Refer for antibiotic treatment in suspected cases.

SUBACUTE OR CHRONIC

Venous Insufficiency

Classic Presentation

The patient complains of chronic lower leg swelling. There are itching and a dull ache in the area that is worse with prolonged standing. There may be a history of phlebitis or leg trauma.

Cause

Damage to the deep vein valves is usually secondary to DVT or trauma.

Table 25–1 Medications Used for DVT

Drug Class	Examples	General Mechanism	Interactions/Side Effects
Heparin Dalteparin	Hepalean Heparin Hep-Lock Lipo-Hepin Liquaemin	Prepared from bovine lung tissue and porcine intestinal mucosa, this potent mucopolysaccharide anticoagulant enhances the inhibitory actions of antithrombin III. Used for the treatment of venous thrombosis and pulmonary embolism, prevention of thrombi/emboli following surgeries, and also used for the treatment of disseminated intravascular coagulation (DIC).	May cause spontaneous bleeding, transient thrombocytopenia, bronchospasm, anaphylaxis, osteoporosis, and hypoaldosteronism.
Warfarin	Coumadin Panwarfin Warfilone	An anticoagulant that decreases the synthesis of vitamin K–dependent coagulation factors. Similar to heparin but actions are accumulative and prolonged. Used prophylactically for embolic and thromboembolic conditions such as deep vein thrombosis, transient ischemic attacks, prosthetic valves, pulmonary embolism, and atrial fibrillation with embolization.	May cause bleeding at any site. Caution when adjusting patients on warfarin due to subarachnoid bleeds, bruising of skin, and other potential bleeding sites. May also cause anorexia, abdominal cramps, diarrhea, and may increase liver enzymes.
Clopidogrel	Plavix	An inhibitor of platelet aggregation acting by inhibition of ADP binding to its receptor. Used to prevent atherothrombotic events after recent MI (especially ST-segment elevation-related), stroke, or with peripheral artery disease, acute coronary syndrome.	Bleeding major and minor, abnormal liver function tests, hepatitis, confusion, hallucinations, taste disorders, angioedema, bronchospasm, hypotension and other autonomic nervous system events.
Streptokinase (tissue plasminogen activator: TPA is similar)	Kabikinase Streptase	Produced from beta-hemolytic streptococcus, this potent thrombolytic enzyme promotes conversion of plasminogen to plasmin. This process breaks apart clotting materials into a soluble form clearing blocked areas in acute thrombotic or embolic situations. Used for acute treatment of deep vein thrombosis, pulmonary embolism, coronary artery thrombosis, etc.	Given this is an antithrombotic agent, hypocoagulation exists which may lead to bleeding at any body site. May also cause an allergic reaction, anaphylaxis, unstable blood pression, ventricular arrhythmias, musculoskeletal pain, and flushing.

Evaluation

The patient will have edema that is reduced by elevation of the leg. Associated findings include varicosities and leg lesions. When the valves are incompetent, resulting venous stasis will eventually lead to the development of skin lesions around the medial ankle and anterior lower leg. These may include nonhealing ulcers.

Management

Like primary varicosities, the long-term management involves avoiding prolonged standing, elevating the legs as often as possible, wearing supportive elastic stockings, and reducing weight and salt intake. When acute stasis dermatitis is present, compresses using isotonic saline, Burow's solution (buffered aluminum), or boric acid may be applied for one hour four times daily. Over-the-counter corticosteroid creams may be helpful. Ulcerations require a medical consultation to determine the need for grafting.

Primary Varicosities

Classic Presentation

The patient may complain of cosmetic and/or painful discrete swellings on the inside of the leg. The pain is a dull, aching heaviness in the lower extremity that is worse with prolonged standing. Cramping may also occur; it is relieved by leg elevation.

Cause

Varicosities are abnormally dilated, tortuous superficial veins. Primary varicosities occur due to incompetence of the valves in superficial veins, and communicating veins (veins that connect the deep and superficial venous system), occurring most often in the long saphenous vein (inside of leg) and its tributaries. Patients who are overweight or pregnant or who stand for prolonged periods of time are more often affected. There does appear to be a genetic predisposition.

Evaluation

The diagnosis is primarily through visual inspection. The Trendelenburg test is an attempt to differentiate between deep vein occlusion and superficial vein valve incompetence. The patient's leg is elevated for 20 to 30 seconds. A tourniquet is tied around the upper thigh (enough to occlude the superficial venous system). The patient is then asked to stand. If the varicosities become apparent with the tourniquet still applied, deep vein occlusion or communicating vein incompetence is the cause. If varicosities appear only after removal of the tourniquet, superficial vein valve incompetence is the cause. Doppler ultrasound or duplex scanning may identify the sites of valve incompetence and help in planning surgery (if performed).

Management

Conservative management includes taking frequent breaks to elevate the legs, the use of elastic stockings, losing weight, and avoidance of prolonged standing. If conservative management is ineffective or cosmetically unacceptable by the patient, surgery involves ligation or removal of involved segments, preserving uninvolved segments for the potential need of vein grafting with cardiac bypass surgery. Sclerotherapy is reserved for small varicosities. The vein is injected with a sclerosing agent and compressed, obliterating the vein.

Congestive Heart Failure

Classic Presentation

The patient complains of bilateral leg edema. He or she has associated complaints of difficulty breathing with exertion or lying fully supine at night (orthopnea).

Cause

Right-sided heart failure is often secondary to left-sided failure. Pressure increases into the venous system, delaying return to the heart from the lower extremities.

Evaluation

The edema is reduced by elevation of the legs. Rales are often apparent on auscultation. The chest radiograph provides important confirmation of cardiac failure with a demonstration of cardiomegaly, dilation of the upper-lobe veins, haziness of vessel outlines, and interstitial edema. Electrocardiography may reveal associated arrhythmias or hypertrophy.

Management

Comanagement is recommended. The standard approach is the use of diuretics for early-stage failure. However, long-term management should include a change to a strict, low-fat diet, with gradual supervised exercise.

Reflex Sympathetic Dystrophy (Complex Regional Pain Syndrome: Type 1)

Classic Presentation

The patient will report having persistent pain and swelling following an episode of trauma.

Cause

There are many theories regarding reflex sympathetic dystrophy (RSD). Some investigators question the existence of this disorder. It is believed that sympathetic nervous system (SNS) dysfunction is at the core of this syndrome. Theories include hyperactivity of the SNS, abnormal connection between the sympathetic and sensory neurons, an autoimmune reaction, nerve sprouting following injury, or abnormal activation of receptors.[4]

Evaluation

RSD may progress through stages. In the early stage, the patient may complain more of a burning, sharp pain in the area. In the "moderate" stage, sympathetic signs may appear, including atrophic skin changes with cold, moist, or mottled skin. The generalized area becomes hypersensitive to stimuli and the pain becomes continuous. In more severe stages, the pain becomes throbbing and aching. Dystrophic changes become visible in the skin and nails. Muscular atrophy and contracture may become evident. Radiographically, localized osteoporosis (i.e., Sudeck's atrophy) occurs in the later stages of RSD. Bone scans will demonstrate an increased uptake on the involved side. Thermography will usually demonstrate a temperature differential between the two sides, but it is nonspecific.

Management

Conservative management would include manipulation of spine-related segments, physical therapy, and elevation to decrease swelling. Two reports suggest that chiropractic manipulation may increase distal blood flow; however, the reports are not specific to RSD.[5,6] Stress reduction may be helpful for some patients. Medically, sympathetic blockades through injectable blocks (e.g., bretylium and lidocaine),[7] ganglion blocks, implanted neuro-stimulators, and α- and β-adrenergic blocker drugs are all approaches that are employed.[8]

APPENDIX 25–1

References

1. Eiehinger S, Minar E, Bialonczyk, et al. D-dimer levels and risk of recurrent venous thromboembolism. *JAMA*. 2003;290:1071–1074.

2. Ritchlie DL. Noninvasive imaging of the lower extremity for deep venous thrombosis. *J Gen Intern Med*. 1993;8:271.

3. Ridker PM, Goldhaber SZ, Danielson E, et al. Long term, low-intensity warfarin therapy for the prevention of recurrent venous thromboembolism. *N Engl J Med*. 2003;348:1425–1434.

4. Vernon HT. Reflex sympathetic dystrophy and chiropractic. In: Lawrence DJ, Cassidy JD, McGregor M, et al., eds. *Advances in Chiropractic*. St. Louis, MO: Mosby-Year Book; 1995;2:183–194.

5. Figar S, Stary O, Hladka V. Changes in vasomotor reflexes in painful vertebrogenic syndromes. *Rev Czech Med*. 1964;10:238–246.

6. Stary O, Figar S, Andelova E, et al. The analysis of disorders of vasomotor reactions to lumbrosacral syndromes. *Acta Univ Carol Med Monogr (Praha)*. 1965;21:70–72.

7. Hord AH, Rooks MD, Stephens BO, et al. Intravenous regional bretylium and lidocaine for treatment of reflex sympathetic dystrophy: a randomized, double-blind study. *Anesth Analg*. 1992;74:818–821.

8. Charlton JE. Management of sympathetic pain. *Br Med Bull*. 1991;47:601–618.

Lymphadenopathy

Context

Patients present with a concern of either an enlarged or a tender lymph node, or upon examination the examiner discovers a suspicious enlargement. The patients' common concern is whether this is an indication of cancer. Statistically, their concern may be justified if they are over age 50 years, when approximately 60% of lymphadenopathy represents a malignancy. However, if they are under age 30 years, there is an approximately 80% chance that the cause is benign.[1]

The chiropractor's role is to determine whether an enlarged lymph node is simply an inadvertent discovery. For the patient this represents a "new" or enlarged nodule; however, in reality it represents a chronic, benign node or group of nodes unnoticed by the patient in the past. Additionally, it is important to attempt to differentiate among other causes of "nodules" (especially in the head and neck area in thin individuals), including the following:

- Sebaceous or dermoid cysts
- A cervical transverse process or cervical rib
- The carotid body (high cervical area)
- Nodularity in the brachial plexus

The next two important steps in the process of evaluation are, first, to distinguish among generalized, regional, and localized involvement. Second, it is important to determine whether there are associated signs of infection or indicators of malignancy. In general, follow-up with specific laboratory procedures should be reserved for specific suspicions or when there is little evidence to indicate a specific cause.

General Strategy

History

Determine whether the following apply:

- The patient's onset was acute? or chronic?
- The patient has associated signs of infection
- The complaint is generalized? more regional? localized?
- The patient has been exposed to others with similar signs
- The patient has been exposed to birds, cats, or dogs or their excrement
- The patient is taking medications that may cause a hypersensitivity reaction
- The degree of exercise is associated with the degree of inguinal enlargement

Evaluation

- Palpate the lymph nodes in an effort to distinguish the texture and whether or not the nodes are fixed.
- Determine the degree of involvement: a single node, all regional nodes, or generalized.
- Consider laboratory investigation when a specific disorder is suspected such as mononucleosis, hyperthyroidism, tuberculosis (TB), human immunodeficiency virus (HIV), connective tissue disorder, or fungal infection.
- Consider radiographs when TB, sarcoidosis, lung disease, or fungal infection is suspected.

- Refer for biopsy if the patient has indicators of high risk (e.g., solitary supraclavicular node).

Management

- Many causes are benign and self-resolve.
- When lymphadenopathy is an indicator of an underlying serious or medically responsive condition, referral for consultation is suggested.
- When lymphadenopathy is persistent beyond three weeks with no identifiable cause, refer for medical evaluation.

Relevant Anatomy and Physiology

The lymphatic system includes the lymph nodes, the lymphatic channels, and the spleen. The function of the lymphatic system is to remove excess protein-rich fluid and return it to the vascular system. The lymph nodes are sites of immune response. There are more than 500 lymph nodes in the body. Certainly, not all are peripherally located and therefore are not accessible. Hilar lymph nodes, for example, require radiographic or invasive investigation to determine involvement. Children have as much as twice the amount of lymphoid tissue as adults and are more likely to respond to an infectious, inflammatory, or other inciting reaction than adults, and in a more dramatic way.

Node involvement is found with a variety of processes including infectious, inflammatory, and neoplastic diseases; metastatic carcinomas; connective tissue disorders; endocrine/metabolic disorders; hypersensitivity reactions; and infiltrative disorders. It would seem impossible to narrow down this large list; however, there are some anatomic predispositions and some classic presentations that may help. Generalized lymphadenopathy usually represents a systemic process involving infection, connective tissue disease, or hematologic neoplastic disease. Lymphomas and leukemias are two general categories to consider. Lymphocytic leukemia is more likely to produce a generalized response. Carcinomas are more likely to cause a regional lymphadenopathy; however, carcinomas are more likely than sarcomas to produce general involvement. Sarcomas are much more likely to disseminate hematogenously and are therefore less likely to cause lymph node involvement.

When investigating enlargement of lymph nodes, it is important to understand the watershed area of the node(s). Draining for common involved areas is listed below:

- Occipital, postauricular, and posterior cervical nodes—the scalp
- Preauricular—the face and eye
- High superficial and deep cervical nodes, submaxillary, and submental—the pharynx and mouth
- Supraclavicular and scalene—the head and neck, arms, mediastinum, and abdomen
- Axillary nodes—arm and breast
- Epitrochlear—arm and hand
- Inguinal-femoral nodes—most of the lower extremity and buttocks, lower anus, genitalia, perineum, and the lower anterior abdominal wall (ovarian and testicular cancer do not usually enlarge the inguinal nodes)

Additionally, certain regional presentations represent systemic processes:

- Posterior cervical and postauricular— viral infections, intra-articular pathology, mononucleosis
- Preauricular—eyelids and conjunctivae
- High cervical nodes—carcinoma of the oral cavity (often submaxillary)
- Supraclavicular and scalene—often represents a neoplastic process (i.e., Virchow's node)
- Axillary—metastatic breast carcinoma, cat-scratch disease, streptococcal and staphylococcal infections of the arm, brucellosis, tularemia
- Epitrochlear—infections of the hand and forearm; occasionally mononucleosis and non–Hodgkin's lymphoma
- Inguinal—lymphogranuloma venereum, venereal disease, excessive exercise (i.e., marathon running or heavy lower extremity workouts)

Evaluation

History

Timing may be an important discriminator. Nodes that appear abruptly and are tender more often will represent an infectious or inflammatory process. Chronic or recurrent node enlargement often represents a neoplastic or connective tissue disorder. Associated signs of infection such as cough, sore throat, and fever are common in children with cervical lymph node enlargement.

Associated signs and symptoms often will help narrow down the possibilities:

- night sweats, fever, and weight loss suggest either lymphoma or tuberculosis
- joint pains, skin rash, and muscle weakness suggest a connective tissue disorder (e.g., lupus erythematosus)
- fever, sore throat, and cervical lymphadenopathy suggest mononucleosis

Determining the patient's exposure to particular environments or with others having similar signs and symptoms may be helpful in the following cases:

- HIV—homosexual contact among gay or bisexual men (although heterosexual contact is also a possibility), sharing needles (use of contaminated needles) with drug abuse (also consider syphilis)
- mononucleosis—saliva transmission
- cat-scratch fever or toxoplasmosis—contact with cats or cat litter, respectively
- fungal infection—travel to specific areas or contact with soil or bird excrement (e.g., coccidioidomycosis in the San Joaquin Valley of California)

Examination

It is recommended that the chiropractor palpate as many "normal" individuals as possible to gain a sense of the variations in lymph node presentation. Palpation of the area of enlargement is performed with a focus on the area of drainage and the most common causes of regional involvement. These are listed above. Additionally, it may be important to determine whether the lymph nodes are tender. This is more indicative of an inflammatory or infectious cause. Hard and matted lymphadenopathy that is fixed to underlying muscle is suggestive of cancer. If the nodes are more rubbery in consistency, lymphoma is more likely. The distinction between the two is not always easily made.

A prediction rule has been devised, called the "lymph node score." Its scoring involves adding certain risk factors with assigned risk points such as age >40 years old, the size of the lymph node, nontenderness, and supraclavicular location and subtracting items such as

lymph node tenderness and a correction factor to arrive at a final lymph node score. Scores less than 3 virtually rule out serious disorders while scores of greater than 5 or 6 warrant further evaluation for a serious cause (**Table 26–1**). The value of the physical exam expressed as likelihood ratios is graphically represented in **Exhibit 26–1**.

Evaluation of the throat, skin, and joints is essential in differentiating common upper respiratory infection from generalized connective tissue disease or fungal infections. The spleen and liver must be palpated for enlargement. These may be enlarged in several conditions, such as mononucleosis (cervical lymph node enlargement), lymphomas, and leukemias. Axillary lymph node involvement in a woman warrants a breast examination and follow-up mammography or biopsy if suspicious.

Some lymph node involvement is not palpable but is visible radiographically. Sarcoidosis is more often characterized by hilar lymphadenopathy visible on a chest radiograph. This is also true of bronchogenic carcinoma of the lungs. A chest radiograph may add evidence to a suspicion of fungal infection such as coccidioidomycosis or histoplasmosis if it demonstrates diffuse granulomatous involvement.

Table 26–1 Lymph Node Score

Finding	Points
Age > 40 years	+5
Lymph node tenderness	−5
Lymph node size	
< 1 cm^2	0
1–3.99 cm^2	+4
4–8.99 cm^2	+8
≥ 9 cm^2	+12
Generalized pruritus	+4
Supraclavicular nodes present	+3
Lymph node is hard	+2
Correction factor	−6*

*Included in every patient's score. For example, a 55-year-old asymptomatic patient with nontender but hard supraclavicular adenopathy measuring 6 cm^2 has a score of 12 (i.e., 5 + 8 + 3 + 2 − 6).

Reproduced from Vassilakopoulos TP, Pangalis GA. Application of a prediction rule to select which patients presenting with lymphadenopathy should undergo a lymph node biopsy. *Medicine* (Baltimore). 2000;79(5):338–347.

Exhibit 26-1   Likelihood Patient Has a Serious Cause of Lymphadenopathy

Approximating Probability: The likelihood ratios (LRs) in this graphical representation represent estimates of probability based on the aggregate of multiple reviews of each test finding. They are only approximations and only reliable indicators of a change in the context of a patient having an intermediate pre-test probability of between 20% to 80%. If the pre-test probability is very high or very low, the LR has little effect on changing the probability.

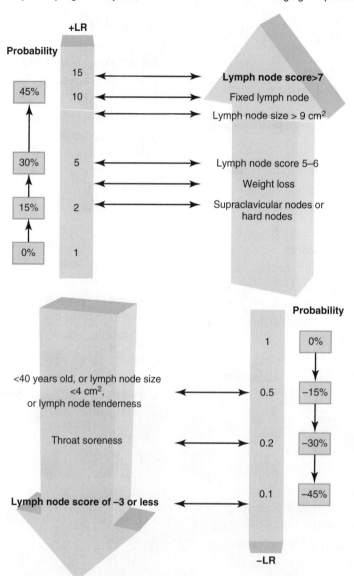

Determining which laboratory evaluations to perform is important given the large number of disease processes possible and the separate laboratory evaluation for each. Following are some examples:[3]

- mononucleosis—heterophile antibody or monospot test
- HIV—enzyme-linked immunosorbent assay (ELISA) test confirmed by Western blot test (testing may be performed by the patient through a mail service if desired)

- lupus erythematosus and mixed connective tissue disease—antinuclear antibody (ANA)
- TB—purified protein derivative (PPD) skin test and if positive, culture and smear
- coccidioidomycosis, histoplasmosis, lymphogranuloma venereum—complement fixation test

Biopsy of lymph nodes is often needed to determine the cause in persistent lymphadenopathy. Therefore, patients without an identifiable cause after two to four weeks or with a suspicious single node involvement in the supraclavicular area or axilla should be referred for biopsy. Lymph node biopsy is not entirely sensitive; however, a second attempt will often raise the positive yield. Biopsy is important in diagnosing neoplastic and fungal causes. Reactive hyperplasia is a nonspecific finding with viral and connective tissue disease causes. It must be remembered that lymph node biopsy of the neck in an elderly patient has been shown to increase the incidence of distant metastasis.

Sometimes it is necessary to biopsy other areas of the body when a specific disease is suspected, including the following:

- transbronchial lung biopsy for sarcoidosis
- renal biopsy for systemic lupus erythematosus
- bone aspiration and biopsy for leukemia

Management

Because of the large list of lymphadenopathy causes, there is no common management approach. Treatment is specific to the underlying cause. Chiropractically, it is important to act as a watchdog for lymphadenopathy, pursue a rational diagnostic approach, and consider referral when evidence suggests a serious disorder requiring further evaluation or amenable to medical management. Persistence of lymphadenopathy beyond three weeks with no identifiable cause is reason for medical consultation.

Algorithm

An algorithm for evaluation and management of lymphadenopathy is presented in **Figure 26–1**.

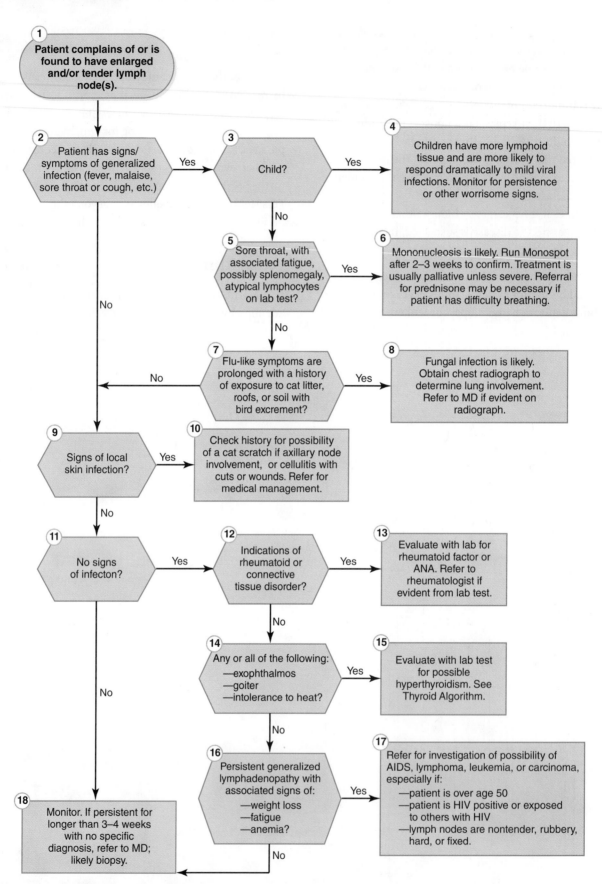

1 Patient complains of or is found to have enlarged and/or tender lymph node(s).

2 Patient has signs/symptoms of generalized infection (fever, malaise, sore throat or cough, etc.) — Yes →

3 Child? — Yes →

4 Children have more lymphoid tissue and are more likely to respond dramatically to mild viral infections. Monitor for persistence or other worrisome signs.

3 No ↓

5 Sore throat, with associated fatigue, possibly splenomegaly, atypical lymphocytes on lab test? — Yes →

6 Mononucleosis is likely. Run Monospot after 2–3 weeks to confirm. Treatment is usually palliative unless severe. Referral for prednisone may be necessary if patient has difficulty breathing.

5 No ↓

7 Flu-like symptoms are prolonged with a history of exposure to cat litter, roofs, or soil with bird excrement? — Yes →

8 Fungal infection is likely. Obtain chest radiograph to determine lung involvement. Refer to MD if evident on radiograph.

7 No →

2 No ↓

9 Signs of local skin infection? — Yes →

10 Check history for possibility of a cat scratch if axillary node involvement, or cellulitis with cuts or wounds. Refer for medical management.

9 No ↓

11 No signs of infecton? — Yes →

12 Indications of rheumatoid or connective tissue disorder? — Yes →

13 Evaluate with lab for rheumatoid factor or ANA. Refer to rheumatologist if evident from lab test.

12 No ↓

14 Any or all of the following:
—exophthalmos
—goiter
—intolerance to heat? — Yes →

15 Evaluate with lab test for possible hyperthyroidism. See Thyroid Algorithm.

14 No ↓

16 Persistent generalized lymphadenopathy with associated signs of:
—weight loss
—fatigue
—anemia? — Yes →

17 Refer for investigation of possibility of AIDS, lymphoma, leukemia, or carcinoma, especially if:
—patient is over age 50
—patient is HIV positive or exposed to others with HIV
—lymph nodes are nontender, rubbery, hard, or fixed.

16 No ↓

11 No ↓

18 Monitor. If persistent for longer than 3–4 weeks with no specific diagnosis, refer to MD; likely biopsy.

Figure 26–1 Lymphadenopathy—Algorithm

Selected Causes of Lymphadenopathy

Acquired Immunodeficiency Syndrome

Classic Presentation

The presentation of acquired immunodeficiency syndrome (AIDS) varies, dependent on the staging of the disease. Following is the earliest presentation. The patient is often a homosexual male (this is not always true; see below) who complains of generalized symptoms such as fever, sore throat, lymphadenopathy, and headache. The symptoms are resolved, but there is persistent lymph node swelling.

Cause

The HIV is a retrovirus that infects mainly T cells and cells related to monocytes. The major factor for immune dysfunction is the progressive depletion of T lymphocytes (primarily CD4+ lymphocytes), leading to decreased ability to fight disease. Lymphocyte functions such as cytotoxic and natural killer cell function are impaired. The antibody response to antigens is reduced.[4] There are several groups at risk, including sexually active, unprotected individuals, particularly homosexual males; drug users who share needles; hemophiliacs and others who received blood transfusions from 1978 through 1985; sexual partners of high-risk individuals; and children born to HIV-infected mothers.

Evaluation

Physical examination may reveal few signs in the early stages. Persistent generalized lymphadenopathy (PGL) is one of the few indicators. Later in the course of disease progression, acquisition of minor opportunistic infection is common, followed by progressive susceptibility to more life-threatening infections. Oral manifestations include thrush and leukoplakia. HIV may be tested by a screening for antibodies to viral protein using an ELISA. A positive test is then confirmed with a Western blot test. Home kits are now available, allowing the person to send a sample to a lab. An indicator of progression is the CD4+ cell numbers. These numbers correlate well with the acquisition of common opportunistic infections. The correlations are TB in patients with a count of 300; *Pneumocystis carinii* pneumonia with counts less than 200; cytomegalovirus and mycobacterium avium complex (MAC) when counts are less than 50.[5] HIV-related malignancies are common causes of death, including Kaposi's sarcoma and non-Hodgkin's lymphoma.

Management

AIDS is managed medically with zidovudine (AZT) (antiviral drug).[6] Alternative drugs include didanosine, zalcitabine, protease inhibitors, stavudine, or a combination of these drugs. Treatment of an acquired disease is specific to the disease, but is more difficult in these immunosuppressed individuals. Prevention is crucial to eliminate further spread. This includes condom protection and the use of sterilized needles.

Non-Hodgkin's Lymphoma

Classic Presentation

The patient may present with lymphadenopathy alone or complain of constitutional symptoms such as night sweats, fever, or weight loss.

Cause

Non-Hodgkin's lymphoma represents a broad array of lymphocytic cancers. The classification is based on the degree of aggressiveness, including low-grade, intermediate-grade, and high-grade classifications. Patients with HIV disease are particularly prone to non-Hodgkin's lymphoma.

Evaluation

Finding regional or disseminated lymph node involvement warrants referral for biopsy if persistent. Laboratory results vary and may include increased levels of serum lactate dehydrogenase and occasionally a leukemic response.

Management

Indolent lymphomas are not usually curable, but high-grade lymphomas may respond to chemotherapy. The survival period for indolent lymphoma is between six and eight years. The disseminated large-cell lymphomas can be cured in about half of patients.[7]

Hodgkin's Disease

Classic Presentation

Because of the bimodal age distribution, the patient may be in the 20s or over age 50 years. The patient complains of constitutional symptoms such as fever, weight loss, night sweats, or generalized pruritus. He or she may have noticed a painless mass in the neck and is concerned.

Cause

Hodgkin's disease is characterized by lymphoreticular proliferation of unknown cause. One study indicated a possible relationship between infectious mononucleosis and Hodgkin's lymphoma. The relationship was based on the finding that 55% of biopsied tumors from patients who had Hodgkin's lymphoma and infectious mononucleosis in the past were positive for Epstein-Barr virus.[8]

Evaluation

The patient presentation is nonspecific. Suspicion requires referral to a hematopathologist who can determine whether there is the presence of Reed-Sternberg cells on lymph node biopsy. Additionally, it is important to stage the disease. This is done with two approaches: (1) degree of involvement, and (2) whether or not symptomatic (A = asymptomatic; B = symptomatic). Stage I indicates one lymph node region involved, stage II indicates involvement of two lymph node regions, stage III indicates lymph nodes involved on both sides of the diaphragm, and stage IV is disseminated involvement of bone and liver.

Management

Treatment is often based on staging. Stage IA and stage IIA diseases are treated with radiotherapy, with a 10-year survival rate of 80%. Chemotherapy is used in patients with stages IIIB and IV (five-year survival rate of 50% to 60%).[9]

Chronic Lymphocytic Leukemia

Classic Presentation

The patient is older than age 50 years and complains of fatigue and lymph node swelling.

Cause

The cause is mainly a malignancy of B lymphocytes. The cells are immunoincompetent, leading to a predisposition to infection. Additionally, there is bone marrow failure and organ infiltration. Ninety percent of cases occur over the age of 50 years. The disease is slowly progressive.

Evaluation

About half of patients have splenomegaly or hepatomegaly. Patients with fatigue and lymphadenopathy should be screened with a laboratory evaluation. The white blood cell count is usually more than 20,000 with the majority of cells being lymphocytes.

Management

No treatment is used initially. Advanced stages are treated with chemotherapy and prednisone. The five-year survival rate is about 50%; the 10-year survival rate is 25%. Patients discovered with advanced disease usually survive less than two years.[10]

APPENDIX 26–1

References

1. Strauss GM. Lymphadenopathy. In: Greene HL, Fincher RME, Johnson WP, et al., eds. *Clinical Medicine.* 2nd ed. St. Louis, MO: Mosby-Year Book; 1996:383–387.

2. Vassilakopoulos TP, Pangalis GA. Application of a prediction rule to select which patients presenting with lymphadenopathy should undergo a lymph node biopsy. *Medicine (Baltimore).* 2000;79(5):338–347.

3. Hayes BF. Enlargement of lymph nodes and spleen. In: Branswald E, ed. *Harrison's Principles of Internal Medicine.* 12th ed. New York: McGraw-Hill; 1991.

4. Pantaleo G. The immunopathogenesis of human immunodeficiency viral infection. *N Engl J Med.* 1993;328:327.

5. Stein DS. CD4+ lymphocyte enumeration for prediction of clinical course of human immunodeficiency virus disease. *J Infect Dis.* 1992;165:352.

6. Cooper DA. Zidovudine in persons with asymptomatic HIV infection and CD4+ cell counts greater than 400 per cubic millimeter. *N Engl J Med.* 1993;329:297.

7. Armitage JO. Treatment of non-Hodgkin's lymphoma. *N Engl J Med.* 1993;328:1023.

8. Hjalgrim H, Askling J, Rostgaard K, et al. Characteristics of Hodgkin's lymphoma and infectious mononucleosis. *N Engl J Med.* 2003;349:1324–1332.

9. Urba WJ, Longo DL. Hodgkin's disease. *N Engl J Med.* 1992;326:678.

10. Foon KA, Rai KR, Gale RP. Chronic lymphocytic leukemia: new insights into biology and therapy. *Ann Intern Med.* 1990;113:525.

Skin Problems

Context

Dermatologic problems can be very difficult to diagnose because of the enormous number of causes and the variety of presentations. Chiropractors may serve a role as either a referral source or source of assurance to patients with many of the common, benign skin conditions. A discussion of skin problems is hampered without an atlas of color plate examples. The reader is encouraged to compare the following verbal descriptions with an atlas to compare better with specific patient presentations. The intention of the following discussion is to focus on several common scenarios in a chiropractic setting without a comprehensive discussion of all dermatologic possibilities.

It is important for the chiropractor to recognize the following skin presentations:

- Generalized skin changes such as pallor, cyanosis, jaundice, brown-tannish discoloration
- Danger signs with pigmented lesions
- The rashes associated with "childhood" diseases such as measles, chickenpox, and rubella
- Common causes of pruritus (itching)
- Lesions associated with venereal disease
- Lesions associated with rheumatoid/arthritic disorders

It is also important for the chiropractor to have a working knowledge of the vocabulary used to describe skin lesions to facilitate an intelligent discussion with a dermatologist in the course of consultation or referral. Following is a list of these terms (see **Figures 27–1** and **27–2** for illustrations).

Primary Lesions

Primary lesions develop on previously normal skin due to a specific causative factor. *Note:* Primary lesions often evolve from flat, nonpalpable lesions to fluid-filled palpable lesions or may coexist, leading to combined descriptions such as maculopapular or vesiculopustular.

Flat and Nonpalpable

- Macule—small (up to 1 cm) and circumscribed. Examples: freckles, flat nevi, petechiae, hypopigmentation
- Patch—larger than 1 cm. Examples: Mongolian spot, café au lait spot, vitiligo, chloasma

Palpable (Raised) and Solid

- Papule—small (up to 0.5 cm). Examples: mole, wart, lichen planus
- Nodule—large (0.5 to 2 cm) and deeper than a papule. Examples: fibroma, xanthoma
- Tumor—larger (>2 cm) benign or malignant, hard or soft. Examples: lipoma, hemangioma
- Plaque—papules coalesce, forming a flat, elevated lesion larger than 0.5 cm. Examples: lichen planus, psoriasis
- Wheal—local, transient, skin erythema due to an allergic reaction, mosquito bite, dermatographism
- Urticaria (hives)—wheals coalesce to form a large reaction that is pruritic

Palpable, Fluid-Filled Lesions (Rupture Releases Pus or a Clear Fluid)

- Vesicle—small, elevated lesion full of clear serum. Examples: chickenpox, shingles (herpes zoster)
- Bulla—larger lesions that are usually single-chambered. Examples: burns, friction blisters, pemphigus, a contact dermatitis

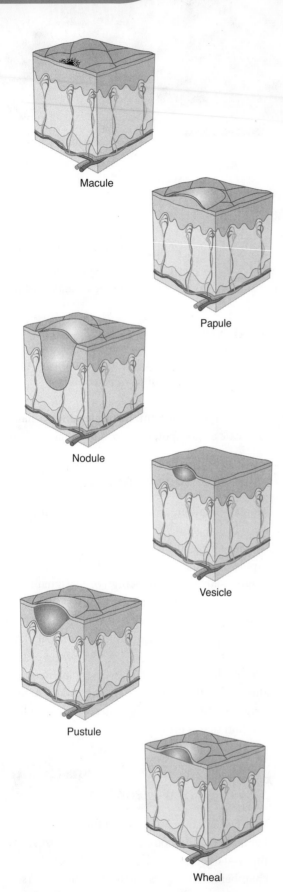

Macule

Papule

Nodule

Vesicle

Pustule

Wheal

Figure 27–1 Primary skin lesions.

- Pustule—circumscribed lesion filled with pus. Examples: acne, impetigo
- Cyst—encapsulated, fluid-filled lesion that may be in the dermis or subcutaneous. Example: sebaceous cyst

Other

Lesions involving hair include furuncle and carbuncle or comedo (blackhead).

Secondary Lesions

Secondary lesions are due to evolutionary changes in primary lesions.

Below-the-Skin Lesions

- Erosion—a superficial lesion involving only the epidermis, therefore no bleeding; heals without a scar; a scooped-out depression. Example: the appearance of skin after a vesicle has ruptured
- Ulcer—a deeper depression involving the dermis, therefore may bleed and heals with a scar; lesion is irregular. Examples: pressure sore, stasis ulcer, chancre
- Fissure—a linear crack extending into dermis; may be dry or moist. Examples: cheilosis (corners of mouth) or athlete's foot
- Excoriation—an abrasion that is self-inflicted, usually due to scratching from intense itching. Examples: insect bites, scabies, varicella, dermatitis
- Atrophic scar—thinning of epidermis with associated depression. Examples: striae or injection site for insulin
- Scar—when normal tissue is replaced with connective tissue (collagen) the area is fibrotic. Examples: healed wound from surgery, injury, or acne; a hypertrophic scar (common in African Americans) is called a keloid

Above-the-Skin Lesions

- Scaling—flakes of skin from dead epidermis that may be dry or greasy, silvery or white. Examples: psoriasis (silver), seborrheic dermatitis (yellow, greasy), eczema, or simply dry skin
- Crusting—when pustules or vesicles erupt they leave a thickened, dried-up exudate. Examples:

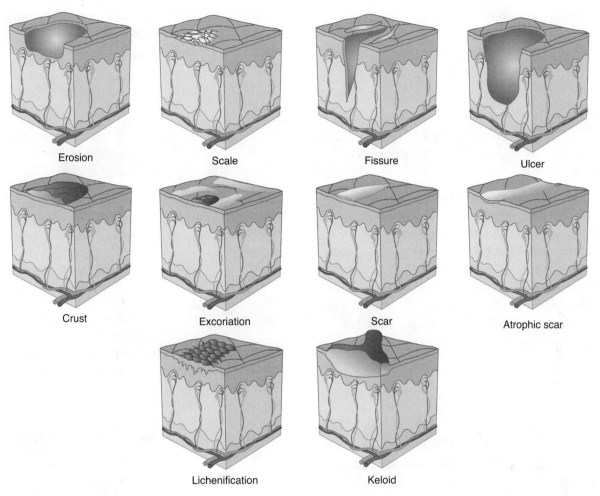

Figure 27–2 Secondary skin lesions.

impetigo, scab formation following abrasion, weeping eczematous dermatitis
- Lichenification (lichen = moss-like appearance)— an intermediate skin lesion due to prolonged, intense scratching leading to a thickened area of skin characterized by tightly packed papules

General Strategy

If the patient has a skin complaint, determine whether it is a lesion, pruritus, or skin color change. For skin lesions, do the following:

- Determine whether there is a single lesion or multiple lesions (always check for sites that may not be visible to the patient).
- Determine whether the onset was associated with other signs such as fever, malaise, or joint pains.
- Determine whether the initial lesions appeared in one area and spread or moved to another.

- Determine whether there is associated pruritus.
- Determine whether there are other contact individuals with similar presentations.
- Elicit a medication history, including topical skin applications.
- Determine whether a rash occurred after sun exposure (miliaria [heat rash]).
- Determine whether the patient was exposed to dyes or color film developers (lichen planus).
- With single pigmented lesions, determine any "danger signs," such as enlargement, change in color, ulceration, or change in sensation (melanoma).

With pruritus as the chief complaint (no obvious skin lesions):

- Determine whether the patient lives or works in an environment that is dry or whether central heating is used.
- Determine whether the patient may have been exposed to fiberglass.

- Determine whether the patient has signs or past diagnosis of renal failure.
- Determine whether the patient has signs of hypo- or hyperthyroidism.
- If the patient complains of specific itching of face, scalp, and genitalia without skin lesions, consider depression.

With skin color changes (not a color change of a lesion; see above):

- Determine whether the patient has had signs of flu and the skin color is yellow (jaundice).
- Determine whether the patient has associated signs of fatigue and has a brown-tan appearance without exposure to the sun (Addison's disease).
- Determine whether the color change is localized to an area of skin and whether this occurred at birth or was acquired (Mongolian spots, café au lait spots, vitiligo, some vascular nevi).

Evaluation

Contact and Allergic Dermatitis

One should first attempt to identify a contact allergen, especially when skin lesions appear to be regional (**Table 27–1**). Any environmental contact is a potential source. The most common are soaps, lotions, clothing, and poison oak or poison ivy. The onset and relationship to the potential contact allergen are usually clear.

Drug reactions are rare; however, they do occur in 2% to 3% of hospitalized patients. The onset is usually abrupt, resulting in a maculopapular rash involving the entire body or symmetrically the extremities. This may be accompanied by severe itching. The most common drugs are amoxicillin, trimethoprim-sulfamethoxazole, penicillin, or ampicillin. Fixed, single, or multiple lesions that become hyperpigmented are seen with reactions to barbiturates and tetracycline.

Childhood Diseases

With children, maculopapular rashes are caused by common childhood diseases, including chickenpox (varicella), measles (rubeola), German measles (rubella), and roseola. One helpful clue is a history of exposure to a patient with known disease (incubation period for most is two to three weeks). Second, the initial location of the

Table 27–1 Contact Dermatitis

Body Area	Cause
Face and neck	Hairsprays, shampoos, conditioners, hair dyes
Scalp	Perfumes, hair sprays, insect sprays
Sides of neck	Hatband
Forehead	Lipstick, mouthwashes, toothpaste
Around the mouth	Metal earrings
Earlobes	Soaps or cosmetics
Face	
Hands and forearms	
Fingers/hands	Soaps, soap under rings, rings, fingernail polish
Forearms	Soaps, insect spray, wrist bands or tennis elbow brace, tape
Axillae	Deodorants, dress shields, dry cleaning solutions
Trunk	Any new clothing (especially wool or clothing with a dye) or clothing with attached metal or rubber
Anogenital	Douches, contraceptive creams, dusting powder, colored toilet paper, medications used to treat pruritus ani or fungal infections in infants
Feet	Shoe or foot powders, treatment for athlete's foot
Generalized	Bath soaps, clothing, drug allergy

rash and its evolution will usually make the diagnosis clear. A brief description of each follows:

- Varicella—Mild, generalized symptoms of malaise, fever, or headache are followed by lesions that first appear on the trunk and then spread to the face and extremities; the sequence of evolution is important, starting as maculopapules, changing in hours to vesicles, pustules, and crusting (new lesions may appear over three to five days).
- Rubeola—The rash is preceded usually by a high fever 40–40.5 °C (104° F to 105°F); two days before the rash, Koplik spots (resembling table-salt crystals) appear on the mucous membranes of the mouth (these are pathognomonic for measles); the rash appears on the face and behind the ears about four days after the onset of symptoms and spreads to the trunk and extremities (including soles of feet and palms).

- Rubella—Preceded by mild symptoms, the rash first appears on the face as a fine, pink rash that spreads to the trunk and extremities quickly over two to three days; the rash disappears over one day in each area (some patients do not have a rash).
- Roseola—Roseola is most common in infants between ages 6 and 18 months; it is heralded by a high fever 39.4 °C to 40.5 °C (103°F to 105°F) for four to five days followed by a faint macular rash on the trunk that lasts a few days.

When erythematous lesions follow an upper respiratory infection or flu (especially in children), two possibilities should be investigated: (1) erythema multiforme, and (2) erythema nodosum. Erythema multiforme lesions are symmetric and may be bullous lesions involving the distal extremities or mucous membranes. They are referred to as target or iris lesions forming a concentric ring with a central purpura (grayish discoloration). Erythema nodosum commonly involves the pretibial area or arms. Red, tender nodules are found. There are numerous other causes in adults. Treatment of the above is mainly for the underlying disease; antibiotics are often used.

Scaling

When scaling is prominent there are a few common disorders to consider. Their distribution and characteristic presentation are often helpful. Following is a list with a brief description of each:

- Eczema (atopic dermatitis)—There is often a personal or family history of allergies or asthma; itching may be a prominent symptom with dermal inflammation occurring on the face, neck, upper trunk, hands and wrists, popliteal area of the knees, and antecubital area of the elbows. Constant itching may lead to lichenification. Eczema is chronic and recurrent.
- Psoriasis—Silvery scaling or red plaquing that is usually not itchy appears on the scalp and extensor surfaces of the extremities, particularly the knees and elbows (although some patients may have inverse psoriasis in body folds that is itchy); associated findings include pitting of fingernails or onycholysis (nail separation); some patients may have an associated arthritis of the fingers or sacroiliac joint. Psoriasis is chronic and recurrent.
- Seborrheic dermatitis—This disorder presents as either a dry or oily scaling with a predilection for the scalp, eyebrows, body folds, and presternal or interscapular areas; it is possibly yeast-related. Factors such as stress, nutrition, and seasonal effects (drier humidity in winter due to heated homes) play a role. Patients who are more prone include those with Parkinson's disease, those who are chronically hospitalized, and those with human immunodeficiency virus (HIV). Seborrheic dermatitis is chronic and recurrent.
- Pityriasis rosea—This disorder appears as oval-shaped, fawn-colored, scaly eruptions. A single patch, called a herald patch, appears one to two weeks prior to more extensive involvement of the cleavage lines of the trunk; the center of the lesions has a cigarette-paper appearance. Pityriasis rosea is more common in women and in the spring or fall (may be due to a virus); it is self-resolving over one to two months.
- Tinea capitis—A presentation similar to that of seborrheic dermatitis occurring in children is tinea capitis due to head lice. There are often small areas of hair loss (alopecia), with broken off or short stubs of hair visible. Accompanying cervical lymphadenopathy is often present. Tinea capitis is more common in African Americans.

Pruritus

Many skin disorders have itching as an accompanying complaint; however, when the main complaint is itching, a search may be narrowed by location or associated findings. Following are some common presentations:

- Dry skin—Dry skin from environmental causes is more common in the winter, with low-humidity environments in heated homes. Skin may also become dry from frequent bathing or use of soaps with some individuals. Dry skin is also part of the presentation of hypothyroidism.
- Metabolic disease—Uremia occurring with kidney failure (or with hemodialysis), obstructive liver disease, or malignant disorders (leukemia, lymphoma, or other cancers) may cause itching.
- Psychiatric disorder—Patients who complain of burning and itching that involve primarily the face, scalp, and genitalia with no obvious skin lesions may have an underlying depression.
- Genital/anal itching—In addition to the above-mentioned depression, anal itching may be due

to irritation from toilet paper, contact dermatitis, extension of psoriasis or seborrheic dermatitis, irritation from fecal content or diarrhea, or pinworm in children. Localized vaginal itching suggests yeast infection in women (frequent occurrence in diabetics); in athletes and in the obese, "jock itch" (tinea cruris) is a common cause of groin pruritus (sparing the scrotum in men).

- Scabies—When the itching is primarily at night, scabies should be considered. Scabies is caused by mite infestation acquired through bedding or an infested individual. The most common location of lesions is on the sides of fingers and on the palms, appearing as vesicles and pustules occurring as "runs" or "burrows."
- Urticaria—A hypersensitivity reaction mediated by immunoglobulin E, with quickly changing wheals or hives. The common causes are drugs, insect bites, heat (including hot showers) or cold, exercise or excitement, or reactions to vaccines or food (shellfish or strawberries). The response may be mild or lead to difficulty breathing; severe responses require epinephrine.
- Ringworm (tinea corporis or circinata)—Ring-shaped lesions appear on the face or arms after exposure to an infected cat. (Some patients have only scaly patches.)
- Lichen planus—Violet lesions along scratch marks with a symmetric distribution in a patient exposed to color dyes or in color film developers is suggestive.

Acne Vulgaris

Acne vulgaris is probably the most common skin condition; it is caused by sebaceous overactivity with subsequent plugging of follicles, leading to infection with the acne bacillus (*Propionibacterium acnes, Staphylococcus albus,* or *Pityrosporum ovale*). Overspill of sebum and fatty acids causes local irritation. Acne vulgaris often begins at puberty and is much more common and severe in males. A similar problem, rosacea, may occur in middle-aged patients and is associated with a higher incidence of migraine headaches. These patients may complain of burning or stinging of the face associated with flushing. It should be kept in mind that large, muscular, young men with acne may be abusing steroids.

The lesions with acne vulgaris are commonly found on the face and upper trunk area. The most common lesion is a comedone (blackhead). Papules, pustules, and cysts may also be seen. The general approach to treatment involves avoidance of touching the lesions, using an over-the-counter benzoyl peroxide cleanser, and avoidance of foods that seem to increase the occurrence. With moderate acne, antibiotic creams or oral antibiotics may be used. With severe acne, isotretinoin (Accutane) is often used.

Warts

Warts are a common complaint representing single or multiple papules often on the hands or feet. Anogenital warts are not uncommon in homosexual men. Warts are due to a viral infection and often heal spontaneously. Large, chronic warts in older individuals may represent squamous cell carcinoma and should be biopsied. Treatment for warts is usually with over-the-counter salicylic acid products or liquid nitrogen, or surgical or laser removal.

Venereal Disease

Venereal disease does not always present with skin lesions; however, those that do should be recognized and referred. Chancroid is caused by *Haemophilus ducreyi,* beginning with a vesicopustule that breaks down and forms a soft, painful ulcer with a necrotic base. The chancre of syphilis, in contrast, is clean, painless, and characterized by a hard base. Granuloma inguinale produces painless nodules with a bright-red friable base. Lesions tend to spread out and can become infected secondarily. Lymphogranuloma venereum is caused by *Chlamydia trachomatis,* producing a quickly vanishing ulcerative lesion on the external genitalia. The characteristic associated finding is inguinal lymphadenopathy producing soft, matted nodes. A patient with herpes simplex virus type 2 will usually present with burning and stinging in a patch of skin in the genital or buttocks area that evolves into a lesion made up of small, grouped vesicles that eventually crust and fall off. Inguinal lymph nodes are often enlarged. Although only a brief introduction, any of the above descriptions or any genital lesions in a sexually active person should be considered suspicious, and referral for laboratory confirmation should be achieved through medical referral. Antibiotics are used for the bacterial causes, and acyclovir is used for herpes simplex virus type 2.

Skin Lesions Associated with Polyarthritis/Rheumatic Conditions

Skin lesions are sometimes associated with conditions that cause joint pain, and therefore may present to a chiropractic office. The most common conditions are rheumatoid arthritis, seronegative arthritides, and connective tissue disorders. Most conditions have characteristic regional joint involvement and radiographic findings that support the diagnosis. However, skin involvement may assist in the diagnosis, or in a patient already diagnosed may represent an indicator of disease activity. Following is a brief list of these lesions:

- Reiter's syndrome—keratogenous lesions on the feet, oral ulcers (also uveitis and conjunctivitis)
- ankylosis spondylitis (although not specifically skin)—uveitis and conjunctivitis
- psoriatic arthritis—psoriatic lesions (usually extensor surfaces), pitting of nails
- rheumatoid arthritis—subcutaneous nodules (often extensor surfaces)
- systemic lupus erythematosus (SLE)—malar erythema, rash, hair loss, oral ulcers
- scleroderma—atrophic, edematous thickening of the skin
- sarcoidosis—erythema nodosum (tender nodules over pretibial area)
- dermatomyositis—discoloration of upper eyelids

Skin Cancer

Patients and chiropractors should be aware of the relative risks of developing skin cancer. They are:[1]

- a history of childhood sunburns
- excessive exposure to sunlight as a child
- excessive exposure through occupational and recreational activities
- fair skin, light hair, and light-colored eyes, especially Irish or Scottish descent
- the presence of more than 50 moles
- a poor ability to tan or tendency toward sunburn
- a family history of skin cancers
- exposure to therapeutic radiography (acne, cancer) or ultraviolet light (psoriasis)
- immunosuppression such as in acquired immunodeficiency syndrome or organ transplantation

Probably the single most important role the chiropractor may play in the evaluation of a patient's skin is the detection of suspicious lesions in need of dermatologic referral. The most important is malignant melanoma. The distinction between a benign lesion and a malignant lesion is summarized by the American Cancer Society mnemonic ABCD (Asymmetry, Border irregularity, Color variation, and Diameter > 6 mm). Therefore, a mole that is burning, stinging, itching, changing shape or color, or growing or bleeding requires a dermatologic evaluation. The original ABCD checklist has been revised to a United Kingdom seven-point checklist. This revised checklist has a very high sensitivity but low specificity.[2] The checklist is a stratified list of seven items divided into three major and four minor criteria. The major criteria are historical and the minor are primarily physical examination findings. The major criteria are changes in size, shape, and color; the minor criteria are inflammation, crusting or bleeding, sensory change, and a diameter greater than or equal to 7 mm. In the elderly and the diabetic, these lesions are often ignored by physicians who assume that they are the consequence of poor healing. Basal cell carcinoma is more common in fair-skinned, young adults with chronic sun exposure. The lesions are found on areas of skin exposed to sun and appear as papules or nodules with a characteristic "pearly" or translucent appearance. Squamous cell carcinoma, although occurring in a similar group of patients, is not as easily detected. The lesions are usually small, red, hard nodules that ulcerate.

The incidence rate for malignant melanoma has risen 4% per year since 1975, so that the rate of melanoma has gone from 1/1,500 persons in 1935 to a predicted risk of 1/75 in the year 2000 for those living in the United States.[3] However, the five-year survival rate has gone from 40% in the 1940s to a current rate of 87%. The smaller the lesion the higher the predicted rate of survival. If the lesion is less than 1 mm thick, the survival rate approaches 95%; however, if the lesion is greater than 4 mm thick, the survival rate drops to 50% over five years.[4]

The ability of nondermatologists to detect skin cancer is not impressive. By testing with color pictures, one study indicated that malignant melanoma was correctly identified by only 12% of nondermatologists; an atypical mole by 42% (98% of dermatologists correctly identified).[5] Another limiting factor is that malignant melanoma occurs in exposed areas only 20% of the time, requiring a full body examination. Many patients are embarrassed by full body examination. Even if the examination is performed (with a patient same-sex "chaperone"), a lesion may still be missed. More education in detection of skin cancer is needed in the education of nondermatologist healthcare providers.

Self-examination may be helpful in detecting some of the "danger" signs. One study indicated that patients instructed on self-examination for palpable arm nevi and larger (> 5 mm) nevi scored specificities of 63% and 68%, respectively.[6] The recommendation for self-examination, coupled with an annual examination in patients over age 40 years and every three years in younger patients, is important in detecting skin cancer.

Management

- If the underlying cause is obviously a contact dermatitis—unless complicated by infection—time and the use of over-the-counter medications such as corticosteroid creams, diphenhydramine hydrochloride (Benadryl), or calamine lotion for poison ivy are usually sufficient.
- For drug-reaction dermatitis, refer back to the prescribing physician or, if over-the-counter, have the patient discontinue use.
- Common childhood diseases (measles, rubella, chickenpox) usually resolve with minimal palliative care; all common childhood diseases should be monitored, and exposed individuals or institutions such as schools should be contacted. Each state has a list of reportable diseases; check individual state for reporting criteria. Monitor for complications.

- Seborrheic dermatitis and acne, if mild, may be helped minimally with over-the-counter medication; however, dermatologic referral is necessary in more involved cases.
- Refer all cases of venereal-related skin disease.
- Comanagement of collagen-vascular cases or referral is suggested.
- Refer all cases of suspected skin cancer to a dermatologist.
- Refer all cases that are not identifiable and worrisome to the patient to a dermatologist.

APPENDIX 27–1

References

1. Daniel CR III, Dolan NC, Wheeland RG. Don't overlook skin surveillance. *Patient Care.* 1996;30:90–107.
2. Whited JD, Grichnik JM. Does this patient have a mole or a melanoma? *JAMA.* 1998;270:696–701.
3. American Cancer Society. *Cancer Facts and Figures—1996.* Atlanta; 1996.
4. Drake A, Ceilley RI, Cornelisen RL, et al. Guidelines of care in malignant melanoma. *J Am Acad Dermatol.* 1993;28:638–641.
5. Wagner RF, Wagner D, Tomich JM, et al. Diagnosis of skin cancer: dermatologists vs nondermatologists. *J Dermatol Surg Oncol.* 1985;11:476–479.
6. Gruber SB, Roush GC, Barnhill RL. Sensitivity and specificity of self-examination for cutaneous malignant melanoma risk factors. *Am J Prev Med.* 1993;9:50–54.

Weight Loss

Context

Rapid or excessive weight loss is often viewed as an ominous sign indicating life-threatening cancer. It is true that 25% of patients die within the first year of significant weight-loss detection. However, studies indicate that although a significant percentage of patients (7% to 36%) have cancer, very few are occult malignancies.[1–4] Another significant percentage of patients (9% to 18%) are diagnosed as depressed. Fourteen percent to 17% of patients have a gastrointestinal disorder such as inflammatory bowel disease, malabsorption, or peptic ulcer. Twenty-three percent to 35% of patients have no identifiable cause for their weight loss.

Weight loss is a comparative measurement. Past documentation as a base reference is necessary to establish true weight loss. When this information is not available, the next reliable source is family members. The severity of weight loss with regard to significance is not clearly defined. An accepted standard is loss of more than 5% of total body weight within six months or 10% within one year. It is interesting to note that as many as 50% of patients who complain of significant weight loss are unsupported by past medical records or family members.[2] Only about one-third of patients with significant weight loss report it as the chief complaint. The remainder have systemic complaints that are elevated to a higher level of concern because of an associated weight loss.

The significance of weight loss increases with age. Either low body weight or unintentional loss of weight factors into increased morbidity and mortality.[5] Obviously, this is a multifactorial occurrence given that the elderly have a naturally higher morbidity and mortality rate. Compared with risk to seniors who are at ideal or high body weight, the risk of death is significantly higher with very low body weight. In a sense, those with higher body mass are protected because of an available "reserve" that buffers them from reaching the critical threshold beneath which skeletal and cardiac muscle wasting occur.

General Strategy

History

- Attempt to document a significant loss of weight from past medical records or corroborate the patient's report with family member support or at the very least a change in clothing or belt size.
- Determine whether weight loss is intentional. If it is, determine whether the patient is educated in proper dieting.
- If weight loss is intentional, determine whether the patient feels that although he or she appears thin, the patient's perception is that he or she is overweight.
- If weight loss is unintentional, determine whether the patient's food intake is normal or decreased.
- If food intake is normal, determine whether there is associated diarrhea.
- If food intake is decreased, determine whether the patient has pain or discomfort associated with eating.
- Obtain a full medication, drug, and alcohol history.
- Screen the patient for depression or other psychologic problems.
- Determine if there are any symptoms that might suggest cancer, hyperthyroidism, diabetes, or gastrointestinal pathology, including peptic ulcer disease or inflammatory bowel disease.
- Determine the patient's ability to feed himself or herself (financially, functionally, environmentally).

Evaluation

- Attempt to document true weight loss greater than 5% over six months or 10% over one year, comparing with any available past medical records.
- Look for indications of "occult" disease through examination of the mouth, skin, and lymph nodes.
- Look for any indications of hyperthyroidism, including a fine tremor, exophthalmos or lid lag, increased pulse, and respiratory rate.
- Evaluate the patient for chronic obstructive pulmonary disease (COPD) if suggested from history (chronic cough in a smoker for three consecutive months for two years).
- Evaluate the patient with laboratory testing for any suspected underlying metabolic problems such as anemia, diabetes, hyperthyroidism, cancer, liver, and kidney disease.
- Evaluate the patient with a chest radiograph (especially in smokers) and stool Hemoccult tests.
- Radiography of painful joints may reveal a metastatic or primary process. If negative yet the suspicion is high, a bone scan is warranted (especially in a patient with a past history of cancer).
- Refer for upper gastrointestinal studies, endoscopy, or colonoscopy in patients with suspected upper and lower gastrointestinal disease.

Management

- If occult processes are discovered or still suspected after evaluation, refer to an internist.
- Refer to a psychiatrist for depression and other psychologic problems.
- Refer to an eating disorders clinic if anorexia nervosa is suspected.
- Refer to a medical physician for evaluation of medication-induced weight loss or possible medical control of anorexia or cachexia if needed.

Relevant Physiology

Weight loss occurs because of a decrease in caloric intake, increase in utilization, or loss in the stool or urine. A number of factors may contribute to weight loss when caloric intake is the cause, including anorexia, nausea, altered sense of taste or smell, and altered perception of satiety. High on the list of causes are cancer, depression, and medications. Following are some proposed mechanisms in these patients:

- Humoral substances (bombesin and somatostatin) may cause early satiety or anorexia in patients with cancer, possibly due to a distention effect.[6]
- Cytokines (tumor necrosis factor, methyl N-methylnipecotate [adipsin], and interleukin 1) are causes of anorexia in patients with cancer, acquired immunodeficiency syndrome (AIDS), and infection.[7]
- Decreased norepinephrine and increased corticotropin-releasing factor levels may play a role in an early satiety effect or food aversion with depression.[8]
- In the elderly, the satiety effect of cholecystokinin is increased; zinc deficiency may cause anorexia.

Of course, a decrease in caloric intake may be voluntary, as is the case with anorexia nervosa, or involuntary because of isolation or economic hardship. Increased utilization may be due to demands of increased physical exertion as is seen in marathon runners and triathletes. Internal metabolic demands may come from hypermetabolic states such as hyperthyroidism (more rarely pheochromocytoma) or cancer. Weight loss may be the most common presenting complaint of the elderly with hyperthyroidism. Patients with either congestive heart failure or chronic pulmonary disease may lose weight due to an increased workload of breathing.

Medications may lead to significant weight loss through a variety of mechanisms. Following are some common examples:

- Nonsteroid anti-inflammatory drugs (NSAIDs), theophylline, quinidine, procainamide, and other drugs may cause nausea.
- Digoxin toxicity causes stimulation of the "vomit" center in the medulla, leading to anorexia, nausea, and vomiting.
- Angiotensin-converting enzyme (ACE) inhibitors may alter taste or smell.
- Tricyclic antidepressants, diuretics, and clonidine may cause dry mouth, which adversely affects swallowing.
- Amphetamines and other stimulants inhibit the appetite center in the hypothalamus, as does smoking.
- Alcohol may be used as a substitute for food.

- Loss of calories may occur through several processes, as follows:
  - maldigestion and malabsorption
  - diarrhea
  - renal excretion of glucose and protein

Significant loss of weight may carry with it the following consequences:

- increased rate of infection
- cardiac and muscle wasting
- decreased sensitivity to chemotherapy in patients with cancer

Evaluation

History

Careful questioning of the patient during the history taking can point to the diagnosis (**Table 28–1**).

Intentional weight loss is due to a limited number of causes. Questioning first determines the patient's knowledge of proper dieting. Second, if the patient is thin, it is important to determine whether he or she has a distorted image of self. If patients feel that they are overweight and yet their weight is 15% below normal, anorexia nervosa is likely. Another subgroup of patients may be wrestlers. To meet certain weight classifications, wrestlers often resort to short-term approaches to weight loss through water loss.

Unintentional weight loss is often accompanied by other signs or symptoms that help lead to the diagnosis. The most logical line of questioning begins with a discrimination between those patients who have a normal or increased appetite and those who do not. Patients who have a normal or increased appetite may be further subdivided into those with chronic diarrhea and those without. Patients with diarrhea are likely to have inflammatory bowel disease, malabsorption, parasitic infection, or pancreatic disease. These patients often will have other abdominal symptoms that help differentiate further (see Chapter 33). Patients with or without

Table 28–1 History Questions for Weight Loss

Primary Question	What Are You Thinking?	Secondary Questions	What Are You Thinking?
Are you intending to lose weight?	Dieting, anorexia nervosa	**(With a thin patient) Do you feel you are overweight and need to restrict your diet?**	Possible anorexia nervosa, especially with a young female
		(With an overweight patient) What kind of diet are you on?	Determine whether the patient understands the nutritional requirements and the yo-yo effect of many diet fads
Is your appetite normal or increased?	Conscious decision not to eat due to pain, poverty, or endocrine or hypermetabolic states if increased food intake	**Is it painful to eat?**	Temporomandibular joint (TMJ) or dental problems are most common; ask about ill-fitting dentures and painful oral lesions
		Do you have diarrhea?	Increased loss; determine underlying cause (inflammatory bowel disease likely)
		Do you have any back pain unrelieved by rest, or past history of cancer?	Cancer
Is your appetite decreased?	Side effect of medications, depression, cancer	**What medications are you currently taking?**	Check drug handbook to determine effect on appetite
		Do you feel sad or depressed, not enjoying life's activities as you used to?	Depression
		Do you have a chronic history of smoking?	Possible lung cancer
		Blood in stools?	Possible colorectal cancer

diarrhea should be screened for common symptoms related to the following:

- diabetes—polyphagia, polydipsia, polyuria, numbness and tingling in the hands or feet, or visual changes
- hyperthyroidism—nervousness, weakness, tremor, menstrual dysfunction, heat intolerance, etc.
- excessive exercise
- decreased eating—check for painful conditions associated with eating, including peptic ulcer, oral or anal conditions, and dysphagia; also check for limited diet and alcoholism

Patients who do not have a normal appetite should be questioned regarding medications, COPD, congestive heart failure, depression, liver disease, and kidney disease. Certainly, the combination of weight loss and spinal pain that has been unresponsive to conservative care for one month in a patient over age 50 years with a history of prior cancer is highly suggestive of metastasis.

Examination

The physical examination is less revealing than the history. Documentation of weight loss is the initial task. If convinced that there is significant weight loss, examination for signs of hyperthyroidism, congestive heart failure, COPD, and other lung pathology is warranted. Patients suspected of having anorexia nervosa may have coexisting signs of bulimia. These are usually the result of the erosive action of gastric juices or the loss of protein. Swollen parotid glands, hoarseness unrelated to respiratory symptoms, calluses on the backs of fingers, tooth erosions, or swollen hands or feet may be clues.

Given the broad list of possibilities, a general screening lab testing, including urinalysis, may indicate the underlying problem if anemia, kidney, liver, or diabetic disorders are the cause. Chest radiographs are often very revealing. One study indicated that 41% of weight loss cases had a significant abnormality on chest films, including a lung mass or infiltrate, congestive heart failure, or adenopathy.[2]

Management

The chiropractor may serve in a primary care role by referring cases to appropriate specialists, and comanaging other cases. Comanagement involves a supportive and an educational role. Instruction on proper diet, assistance with access to financial assistance programs, and food programs such as Meals on Wheels are among the many adjunctive tools that can be used. Patients who are depressed or suffering from prolonged bereavement due to the loss of a loved one will benefit from referral to a psychologist or psychiatrist. Patients with dental problems should be referred to a dentist. Those with motor skill or memory deficits should be referred to a therapist who specializes in these areas. Patients suspected of having anorexia nervosa must be referred to an eating disorders clinic. It is far beyond the scope of most healthcare professionals to manage this disorder. Simple advice or counseling is useless.

Neuropsychological disorders need a minimum of comanagement. Conditions such as Parkinson's disease, various causes of dementia, stroke, depression, and alcoholism require specialized care.

One option for some patients is referral to a medical physician for prescription of medication that increases appetite. There are several drugs available, as follows:

- Cyproheptadine (antiserotonergic drug), although generally effective, has not been shown to affect weight gain in patients with advanced cancer.
- Corticosteroids are used in patients with advanced cancer; however, it has yet to be demonstrated that the weight gain is not primarily fluid; in addition, side effects, including oral candidiasis and Cushing's-like effects, occur often.
- Megestrol acetate (progestational agent) is an expensive but effective medication with few side effects for patients with cancer.

Algorithm

An algorithm for evaluation and management of weight loss is presented in **Figure 28–1**.

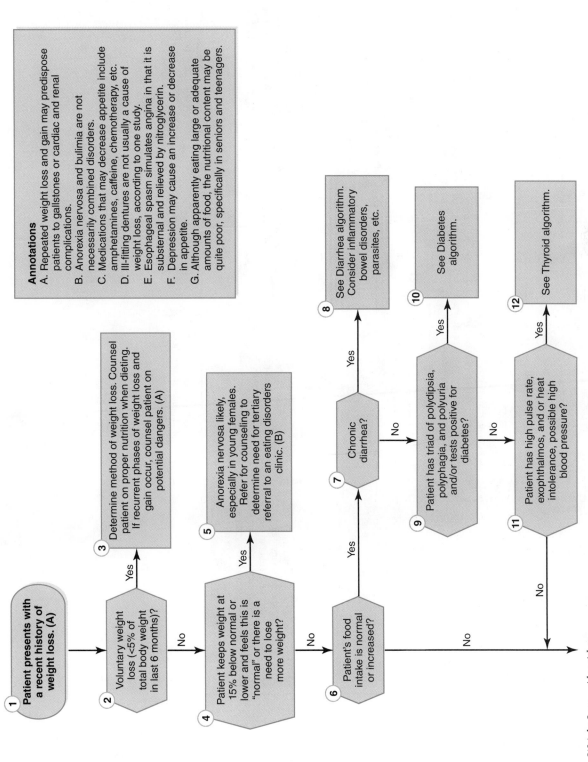

Annotations

A. Repeated weight loss and gain may predispose patients to gallstones or cardiac and renal complications.

B. Anorexia nervosa and bulimia are not necessarily combined disorders.

C. Medications that may decrease appetite include amphetamines, caffeine, chemotherapy, etc.

D. Ill-fitting dentures are not usually a cause of weight loss, according to one study.

E. Esophageal spasm simulates angina in that it is substernal and relieved by nitroglycerin.

F. Depression may cause an increase or decrease in appetite.

G. Although apparently eating large or adequate amounts of food, the nutritional content may be quite poor, specifically in seniors and teenagers.

1. Patient presents with a recent history of weight loss. (A)

2. Voluntary weight loss (<5% of total body weight in last 6 months)?

Yes →

3. Determine method of weight loss. Counsel patient on proper nutrition when dieting. If recurrent phases of weight loss and gain occur, counsel patient on potential dangers. (A)

No ↓

4. Patient keeps weight at 15% below normal or lower and feels this is "normal" or there is a need to lose more weight?

Yes →

5. Anorexia nervosa likely, especially in young females. Refer for counseling to determine need for tertiary referral to an eating disorders clinic. (B)

No ↓

6. Patient's food intake is normal or increased?

Yes →

7. Chronic diarrhea?

Yes →

8. See Diarrhea algorithm. Consider inflammatory bowel disorders, parasites, etc.

No →

9. Patient has triad of polydipsia, polyphagia, and polyuria and/or tests positive for diabetes?

Yes →

10. See Diabetes algorithm.

No →

11. Patient has high pulse rate, exophthalmos, and or heat intolerance, possible high blood pressure?

Yes →

12. See Thyroid algorithm.

No ↓

Figure 28–1 Weight Loss—Algorithm

(continues)

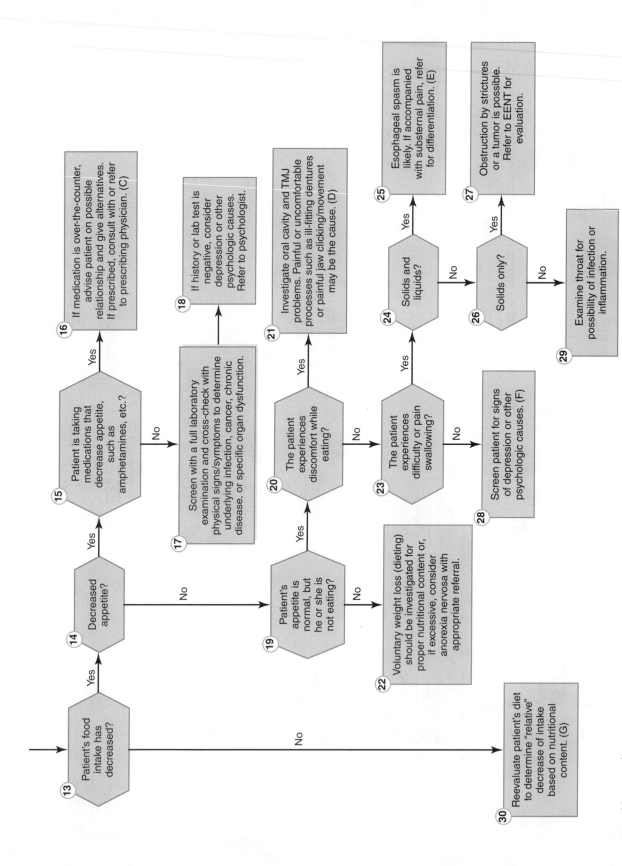

Figure 28–1 (Continued)

APPENDIX 28–1

References

1. Rabinovitz M, Pitlik SD, Leifer M, et al. Unintentional weight loss: a retrospective analysis of 154 cases. *Arch Intern Med.* 1986;146:186–187.

2. Marton KI, Sox HC, Krupp JR. Involuntary weight loss: diagnostic and prognostic significance. *Ann Intern Med.* 1981;95:568–574.

3. Wiley MK, Zahn PE. Evaluation of weight loss in the elderly. *Clin Res.* 1987;35:93.

4. Thompson MP, Morris LK. Unexplained weight loss in the ambulatory elderly. *J Am Geriatr Soc.* 1991;39:497–500.

5. Hardy C, Wallace C, Khansur T, et al. Nutrition, cancer, and aging: an annotated review. *J Am Geriatr Soc.* 1986;34:219.

6. Morley JE. Neuropeptide regulation of appetite and weight. *Endocr Rev.* 1987;8:256–278.

7. Lowry SF, Moldawer LL. Tissue necrosis factor and other cytokines in the pathogenesis of cancer cachexia. *Cancer Prin Pract Oncol Updates.* 1990;4:1–12.

8. Morley JE, Silver AJ. Anorexia in the elderly. *Neurobiol Aging.* 1988;9:9–16.

Weight Gain/Obesity

Context

Simply put, the most common cause of weight gain is an increase in caloric intake or a decrease in energy expenditure. Fluctuations in weight are common within a few pounds and generally reflect fluid retention and loss. Cyclic fluctuations are common in women in relation to menstruation. Substances that cause salt retention such as estrogen and steroids and appetite-stimulating drugs such as some antidepressants are less common causes. Familial obesity and low resting metabolic rates are uncommon. Only about 10% of obese patients have an underlying neurologic, endocrine, or genetic cause. Hypothyroidism may account for small increases in weight due to a slowed metabolic rate; however, significant weight gain is found in only 60% of patients and usually when the disease is advanced. Eighty percent of patients with adult-onset diabetes are obese.[1]

Obesity, to some extent, is a relative term. In the past a patient's weight was compared with actuarial tables that reflected averages based on height, weight, and gender. This simple approach was found to be misleading, not accounting for body build and the amount of muscle mass and body fat. A newer approach is to combine two methods. A determination of the body mass index (BMI) coupled with a body fat measurement accounts for some of these variables. Some studies use a BMI greater than or equal to 25 kg/m^2 whereas others use greater than or equal to 30 kg/m^2 to indicate overweight or obesity. Obviously, the percentage of overweight individuals increases when using the lower threshold.

Obesity has been categorized into the following classes:

Class 1: BMI of 30–34.9

Class 2: BMI 35–39.9

Class 3: BMI ≥ 40 (morbid or extremely obese)

When using 25 kg/m^2 as the threshold BMI indicator of overweight or obesity, the prevalence of overweight or obesity in the United States increased more than 25% over the last three decades.[2] Sixty-three percent of men and 55% of women fall into the category of a BMI of 25 kg/m^2 or greater, meaning being either overweight or obese. Averaged, this equals more than half of the adult population over the age of 17 years. Using 30 kg/m^2 as the threshold, the prevalence of overweight or obesity in the United States increased from 12% in 1991 to 17.9% in 1998.[3] These increases were independent of smoking status. It is alarming that the greatest magnitude of change was seen in younger individuals (18- to 29-year-olds) and those with higher education levels. Regionally, the greatest increases were seen in the mid- and south Atlantic states. Obesity prevalence increases were seen in all sociodemographic groups; however, the prevalence of obesity increased dramatically in the Hispanic population. More than one-third of U.S. adults (35.7%) are obese.[4]

More recent literature over the last several years appears to support earlier findings and emphasizes the growing concern regarding obesity, especially in the United States. Below is a summary of the findings from some of these studies:

- The prevalence of overweight has increased from release of the 1988–1994 NHAMES III report to release of the 1999–2000 report and then again in the 2009–2010 report. For obesity, there was an increase of 8% between these two time points in men with no significant change in women, holding at around 35.8%. The prevalence of obesity increased from 14.0% in 1999–2000 to 18.6% in 2009–2010 among boys; among girls the prevalence was 13.8% in 1999–2000 and 15.0% in 2009–2010. There seems to be leveling off currently with no significant change in obesity prevalence from 2007–2008 to 2009–2010. Yet there are more than 5 million girls and approximately 7 million boys who were obese during this same time period.[5,6]

- The prevalence of class 3 obesity is increased rapidly in the years 1990–2000 from 0.78% in 1990 to 2.2% in 2000, with the highest increase among African American women, individuals who have not completed high school, and short persons.[7] However, between 1988–1994 and 2007–2008 the prevalence of obesity increased in adults regardless of income or education levels.
- The age-adjusted prevalence of obesity was 30.5% in 1999–2000 compared to 22.9% in 1994.[8] The prevalence of overweight increased from 55.9% to 64.5%. Extreme obesity increased from 2.9% to 4.7%.
- Sadly, in 2009–2010, over 78 million U.S. adults and about 12.5 million U.S. children and adolescents were obese.[6]

These statistics become important in the context of one study that found that white men aged 20 years with BMIs greater than 45 are predicted to have 13 years of life lost (YLL), with eight years of life lost for women in the same age and range.[9]

Another issue regarding obesity is cultural perception. It may be acceptable, and sometimes desirable, to be overweight as one ages. This is often perceived as a sign of prosperity. It is important to recognize this cultural variation and be sensitive to different perspectives. However, morbid obesity carries with it enough risk that some degree of weight loss would need to be suggested.

Being obese carries some increased risk in several areas.[10] Individuals with the greatest weight had an increased prevalence of having two or more health disorders.

- Mortality rates are higher for patients with a BMI of 25 or higher compared with normal-weight individuals. The risk of death was from all causes including cardiovascular disease, cancer, and other diseases. African Americans were at lower risk than Caucasians when comparing rates of death with high-BMI individuals.[11] Rates for a condition known as non-alcoholic fatty liver disease has risen dramatically due to obesity. It is becoming a major reason for the need of a liver transplant.
- The obese are 3 to 10 times more likely to develop adult-onset diabetes (insulin resistance increases with weight gain).
- The obese have a higher incidence of cardiovascular disease, hypertension, dyslipidemia, and stroke.

- The obese are more likely to have sleep apnea or hypersomnolence syndrome, which carries with it the risk of arrhythmias, hypoxemia, cor pulmonale, and pulmonary hypertension. Specifically, there is a rising trend of atrial fibrillation found in the U.S. population with the highest risk factor being obese.
- The obese are more likely to have degenerative joint disease, especially in the hips and knees; it is also probably a risk factor for low back pain.
- The obese have an increased risk for cholelithiasis, thromboembolism, varicose veins, and blunted growth hormone response.
- A recent study[12] estimates that obesity-related morbidity accounts for approximately 6.8% of U.S. healthcare expenses. The estimated annual medical cost of obesity in the U.S. was $147 billion in 2008 U.S. dollars.
- Medical expenses for people who are obese were $1,429 higher than those individuals of normal weight.

A new observation may be important to understanding fat accumulation. Findings from several studies suggest that parasympathetic activity increases insulin sensitivity and fat synthesis.[13] Supporting this theory is the observation that there appears to be an association between reduced parasympathetic nervous system function and increased plasma-free fatty acid levels, and also an association between insulin resistance in patients with a combination of obesity and type-2 diabetes mellitus. An increase in parasympathetic tone occurs at night, promoting nocturnal deposition of fat and possibly explaining why fat deposits in some areas and not others. For example, visceral white adipose tissue (intra-abdominal fat) is more heavily innervated than subcutaneous fat. Systemic effects may be that elevated plasma levels of free fatty acids may lead to a pro-inflammatory and pro-atherogenic state. A low-grade systemic inflammation may factor into some of the morbidity associated with obesity. A laboratory test, C-reactive protein (CRP), is an indicator of systemic inflammation and is more commonly used with rheumatoid and other overtly inflammatory-based conditions. CRP has been shown to estimate future risk of coronary artery disease. There appears to be a correlation between a high BMI and acute-phase CRP in middle-aged and elderly individuals. However, these studies did not account for confounding causes such as other disorders. A recent study[14] demonstrated that a higher BMI is associated with higher CRP in adults aged 17 to 39 years. This association was independent of any coexisting disorders that might also influence CRP. This study also indicated that the distribution of fat was correlated with an increased CRP independent of BMI. A high waist-to-hip ratio was associated with an increase in CRP. This distribution indicates larger amounts of visceral fat. Elevated levels of CRP at 0.22 mg/dL were found in 27.6% of individuals.

General Strategy

History

- Determine the amount of weight gain and specify over what period of time.
- Determine what constitutes the patient's diet; follow with a diet diary.
- Determine whether the patient is taking any medications that may increase fluid retention or appetite.
- Determine the patient's family history with regard to obesity and diabetes.
- Determine whether the patient has recently stopped smoking.
- Determine any changes in exercise levels.
- Determine whether the patient is under stress and uses food for relaxation or reward.
- Determine whether the patient has any symptoms of hypoglycemia (insulinoma; rare).

Examination

- Weigh and measure height of the patient.
- Determine the BMI.
- Determine the patient's percentage of body fat with skin calipers or an impedance device (referral for water immersion method is less practical, but most accurate).
- Examine the patient for signs of fluid retention in abdomen and legs.
- Examine the patient for congestive heart failure if suspected from history (difficulty breathing while lying recumbent) and obtain a chest radiograph.
- Perform laboratory evaluation if the patient has historical and/or physical signs of diabetes, Cushing's disease, or hypothyroidism.

Management

- The majority of obese patients can be managed with a healthful diet and a graduated exercise program.

- It may be necessary to work with a team including a specialist in weight loss to better guarantee compliance with suggestions and provide a support network for those making substantial lifestyle changes.

Evaluation

History

It is extremely important to approach the obese patient from a health risk perspective and not be perceived as being judgmental or addressing the more cosmetic aspects of excess weight. As mentioned above, weight gain over a day or two is most often due to fluid retention. Therefore minor gain in weight over a number of days or during a woman's menstrual period is of little concern. The patient who is dieting, however, may feel discouraged. Also, when patients are exercising they must keep in mind that muscle weighs more than fat.

Examination

Estimation of a patient's relative body weight is best accomplished with a formula to determine the BMI. In addition, an estimate or measurement of body fat content is crucial to determining the degree to which weight is due to fat and muscle. The BMI is calculated by dividing kilograms of weight by meters of height. The conversion for pounds and inches is $750 \times$ lb/sq in. A BMI over 27 is equal to being about 20% overweight and warrants further investigation and management.

Management

Given that the most common cause of weight gain is overeating or eating an unbalanced diet, the chiropractor must decide how much time, investment, and interest can be donated to patient management. There are many centers that specialize in weight loss. **Table 30–1** is a summary of many popular diet plans with a general description of the plan's focus and the pros and cons of each. These centers do not focus on diet alone but address issues of mental attitude, motivation, and exercise. Quick fixes with diet drinks or fad diets are to be avoided. Statistically, most patients who diet eventually gain back weight over a period of a year or two. According to one study,[15] approximately one-third of adults who attempt to lose weight or maintain weight loss focus more on less fat than fewer calories.

Table 29–1 Summary of Some Popular Diets

Diet	Summary of Focus, Advantages, and Disadvantages
Atkins	Focuses on restricting carbohydrate calories and emphasizes fat and protein. Examples of foods allowed include red meat, chicken, turkey, seafood, eggs, high-fat dairy, oil, nuts, and vegetables that do not contain high amounts of starch (i.e., potatoes). Three phases of diet include induction, weight loss, and maintenance. High degree of initial satisfaction due to "desirable" foods allowed plus initial rapid weight loss (water). Concerns include risk of cardiovascular disease and kidney stones. Any diet that restricts calories will, in the initial phases, likely decrease blood pressure and reduce blood sugar, cholesterol, and triglycerides.
Eat Right for Your Type	Not really a weight loss diet, but a diet that is based on blood type, founded on the belief that a patient's blood type determines digestion and immune response. Diet has a list of foods to avoid and foods to emphasize based on blood type and can range from modified vegetarian to large portions of animal fat. Concerns are the lack of scientific evidence and the potential deficiencies in needed nutrients with some recommended plans.
Beverly Hills	A rapid weight loss plan with no long-term goals. The premise is that an individual can lose 10–15 pounds in 35 days. There is a heavy initial emphasis on fruits that will result in fluid loss but possible diarrhea. The claim is that eating one type of food in combination with another type, such as a protein with a carbohydrate, destroys specific digestive enzymes, leading to weight gain and poor digestion. Therefore, the contention is that eating food types separately encourages weight loss. Concerns are the same for all diets that emphasize rapid weight loss with severe food restrictions and no long-term approach.
Fit For Life	Main focus is specific food combinations eaten at specific times of the day; emphasis is on fruits and vegetables. There is no restriction specifically on calories or grams of fat due to the types of foods recommended (i.e., fruits/vegetables). A vegetarian-based diet with restrictions of protein, including lean protein meats and low-fat dairy products, may have an effect of imbalance or deficiency in certain needed nutrients. This is less of a weight loss diet than an approach to healthy eating with weight loss as a side benefit.
Jenny Craig	This is a highly structured program focused initially on prepackaged foods, weekly counseling that promotes lifestyle changes and teaches meal planning, exercise, and managing stress as important elements in maintaining weight loss. The advantages are the convenience of prepackaged foods and personal support. The disadvantages are the initial cost and the difficulty of following the initial plan while dining with others. More convenient for single individuals. Due to prepackaging and nutritional considerations, there are no concerns from a nutritional perspective. Slow, consistent weight loss with a focus on healthy lifestyle are important pluses.
Mayo Clinic	The diet is not endorsed by the Mayo Clinic. The focus is on eating large amounts of grapefruit, meat, and high fat until satiated. The contention is that grapefruit aids in the digestion of fat. Cautions are from the imbalance and restriction of complex carbohydrates. Also, some studies indicate that high amounts of grapefruit intake may promote kidney stones.
Nutrisystem	Another plan focused on prepackaged food. Some store-bought items are allowed. Advantage is the prepackaging and the online support. Disadvantages are cost and concern about the addition of appetite suppressants sold along with the food.
Optifast	This is a medically supervised weight loss approach with a focus on low-calorie liquid shakes and supplements. The diet is intended for the markedly obese (i.e., BMI over 30). Advantages are the medical supervision, which includes regular blood work, counseling with registered dieticians, and maintaining nutritional balance. Optifast quotes a study that indicated weight loss in 600 patients who lost 5%–10% of body weight and maintained this loss for up to five years. However, much of the weight was gained back during this time frame. In other words, initial weight loss was greater, but then weight was gained back to a plateau.
Pritikin	A low-fat diet, the Pritikin diet focuses on unprocessed fruits and vegetables, lean animal foods, and nonfat dairy products. Calorie intake is based on "calorie density," which is the amount of calories per pound, with a restriction to foods that contain 400 calories or less per pound. A generally healthy diet, the primary concern is long-term compliance (as with many diets).
Scarsdale	Another rapid weight loss approach to be used for only two weeks, this diet emphasizes lean animal foods, fruits, vegetables, and the use of herbal appetite suppressants. There is an extreme carbohydrate restriction with no snacks allowed. This provides rapid weight loss through fluid loss. As with all rapid weight loss approaches, the vast majority of individuals gain weight back. There is also some increased risk of the development of kidney stones and gallstones.

Table 29–1 Summary of Some Popular Diets (continued)

Diet	Summary of Focus, Advantages, and Disadvantages
South Beach	An MD-developed program that has three phases. The first phase is two weeks long and focuses on normal-sized helpings of lean meats (e.g., chicken, turkey, fish, and shellfish) and vegetables. Carbohydrates are restricted based on their glycemic index, so that the first two weeks eliminates alcohol, fruit, bread, rice, potatoes, pasta, baked goods, sugar, and pastries. Wine, fruits, and whole grains are phased in during the later two phases. Although considered a low-carb, low-fat diet, it is more about "good carbs" versus no carbs based on their glycemic index.
Weight Watchers	Weight loss is based on a point system for calorie restriction. Foods can be chosen within the point system restrictions. Prepackaged foods are available. There is also an emphasis on weekly support meetings that encourage healthy lifestyle choices and make use of weekly weigh-ins and associated peer pressure/support. Generally, a healthy diet approach.
Zone	This diet is a very low caloric diet (800–1200 calories) based on low carbohydrate, high protein, and moderate fat intake, emphasizing a balance of foods at each meal to stay within "the zone." Focus is on foods with a low glycemic index. Restricts refined carbohydrates low in nutrition and emphasizes fruit and low-starch vegetables. Low in whole grains and calcium.

Less than one-fifth of individuals combine a regimen of decreased caloric intake with a couple of hours of physical activity each week. Regular exercise such as brisk walking reduces body weight and body fat in overweight and obese postmenopausal women.[16] In a study of over 73,000 women ages 50 to 79 years, subjects who walked or were engaged in vigorous exercise 2.5 hours a week reduced the risk for cardiovascular events by about 30%.[17] Researchers in the Health Professionals Follow-Up Study assessed 44,000 men over 12 years for exercise and levels of daily activity. Men with the greatest activity had a 30% decreased risk over sedentary males for cardiovascular risk. Specific activities and risk reduction included weight training—33% reduction, rowing—18% reduction, and running—42% reduction.[18] Weight gain in women has been associated with a decrease in physical activity and increased levels of pain.[19] Pain may act as a deterrent to exercise, yet weight loss has been shown to decrease body pain.

The solution to permanent weight loss is total management by a specific individual or team with inclusion of a sensible exercise routine coupled with a sensible diet (see **Exhibit 29–1**). The time demand for education, exercise and diet prescription, and counseling/support may be well beyond the time availability and expertise of the chiropractor. Comanagement with a medical doctor or a clinic specializing in weight loss is often more appropriate. The newest medical approach is with a new class of drugs called lipase inhibitors. Orlistat (Xenical) prevents the breakdown of some fat (up to 30%) so that it can be excreted in the feces without being absorbed. Some degree of weight loss was achieved and maintained after 18 months in a study comparing treatment with orlistat compared to placebo.[20] Approximately 33% of patients on orlistat versus 25% of patients on placebo lost weight initially. Long-term maintenance of weight loss (≥10% of initial weight) was 28% for those on orlistat versus 14% on placebo.

Referral for medical consultation is warranted when drugs are suspected as the underlying cause or when metabolic problems such as Cushing's disease or hypothyroidism are suspected.

Exhibit 29–1 Low-Fat Foods

Here Are Some Low-Fat Foods To Choose More Often:

	Serving	Calories	Grams of Fat
Dairy Products			
Cheese:			
Low-fat cottage (2%)	1/2 cup	100	2
Mozzarella, part skim	1 oz	80	5
Parmesan	1 tbsp	25	2
			(continues)

Exhibit 29–1 **Low-Fat Foods** (continued)

	Serving	Calories	Grams of Fat
Milk:			
Low-fat (2%)	1 cup	125	5
Nonfat, skim	1 cup	85	trace
Ice milk	1 cup	185	6
Yogurt, low-fat, fruit flavored	1 cup	230	2
Meats			
Beef:			
Lean cuts, such as trimmed bottom round, braised or pot-roasted	3 oz	190	8
Lean ground beef, broiled	3 oz	230	16
Lean cuts, such as eye of round, roasted	3 oz	155	6
Lean and trimmed sirloin steak, broiled	3oz	185	8
Lamb:			
Loin chops, lean and trimmed, broiled	3 oz	185	8
Leg, lean and trimmed, roasted	3 oz	160	7
Pork:			
Cured, cooked ham, lean and trimmed, baked	3 oz	135	5
Center loin chop, lean and trimmed, broiled	3 oz	195	9
Rib, lean and trimmed, roasted	3 oz	210	12
Shoulder, lean and trimmed, braised	3 oz	210	10
Veal:			
Cutlet, braised or broiled	3 oz	185	9
Poultry Products			
Chicken, roasted:			
Dark meat without skin	3 oz	175	8
Light meat without skin	3 oz	145	4
Turkey, roasted:			
Dark meat without skin	3 oz	160	6
Light meat without skin	3 oz	135	3
Egg, hard cooked	1 large	80	6
Seafood			
Flounder, baked, no butter or margarine	3 oz	85	1
Oysters, raw	3 oz	55	2
Shrimp, boiled or steamed	3 oz	100	1
Tuna, packed in water, drained	3 oz	135	1
Other Foods			
Salad dressing, low calorie	1 tbsp	20	1

Reproduced from *Diet, Nutrition & Cancer Prevention: The Good News*, Publication No. 87-2878, 1986, National Institutes of Health.

APPENDIX 29–1

Web Resources

Obesity

Academy of Nutrition and Dietetics
http://www.eatright.org
Obesity Society
http://www.obesity.org
Centers for Disease Control and Prevention Body
Mass Index Web Calculator
**http://www.cdc.gov/nccdphp/dnpa/bmi
/calc-bmi.htm**

Dietary Supplements

U.S. Food and Drug Administration (includes a link to
MEDWATCH to report adverse events)
http://www.fda.gov
National Center for Complementary and Alternative
Medicine
http://www.nccam.nih.gov
National Institutes of Health Office of Dietary
Supplements
http://dietary-supplements.info.nih.gov

Nutrition Government Site

http://www.nutrition.gov

APPENDIX 29–2

References

1. Report of the U.S. Preventive Services Task Force. Screening for obesity. In: *Guide to Clinical Preventive Services.* 2nd ed. Baltimore: Williams & Wilkins; 1996:219.
2. Flegal MD, Carroll J, Kuczmarski RK, Johnson CL. Overweight and obesity in the United States: relevance and trends, 1960–1994. *Int J Obes Relat Metab Disord.* 1998;22:39–47.
3. Mokdad AH, Serdula MK, Dietz WH, et al. The spread of the obesity epidemic in the United States, 1991–1998. *JAMA.* 1999;282:1519–1522.
4. Flegal KM, Carroll MD, Ogden CL, Curtin LR. Prevalence and trends in obesity among US adults, 1999–2008. *JAMA.* 2010;303(3):235–241.
5. Ogden CL, Flegal KM, Carroll MD, Johnson CL. Prevalence and trends in overweight among U.S. children and adolescents, 1999–2000. *JAMA.* 2002;288:1728–1732.
6. Ogden CL, Carroll MD, Curtin LR, Lamb MM, Flegal KM. Prevalence of high body mass index in U.S. children and adolescents, 2007–2008. *JAMA.* 2010;303(3):242–249.
7. Freedman DS, Kettel-Khan L, Serdula MK, et al. Trends and correlates of class 3 obesity in the United States from 1990–2000. *JAMA.* 2002;288:1758–1770.
8. Flegal KM, Carroll MD, Ogeden CL, Johnson CL. Prevalence and trends in obesity among U.S. adults, 1999–2000. *JAMA.* 2002;288:1723–1727.
9. Fontaine KR, Redden DT, Wang C, et al. Years of life lost due to obesity. *JAMA.* 2003;289(2):187–193.
10. Must A, Spadano J, Coakley EH, et al. The disease burden associated with overweight and obesity. *JAMA.* 1999;282:1523–1529.
11. Calle EE, Thun MJ, Petrelli JM, Rodriguez C, Heath CW. Body mass index and mortality in a prospective cohort of U.S. adults. *N Engl J Med.* 1999;341:1097–1105.
12. Wolf AM, Colditz GA. Social and economic effects of weight loss in the United States. *Am J Clin Nutr.* 1996;63(suppl 3):466S–469S.
13. Boden G, Hoeldtke RD. Nerves, fat, and insulin resistance. *N Engl J Med.* 2003;349:1966–1967.
14. Visser M, Bouter LM, McQuillan G, et al. Elevated C-reactive protein levels in overweight and obese adults. *JAMA.* 1999;282:2131–2135.
15. Serdula MK, Mokdad AH, Williamson DF, et al. Prevalence of attempting weight loss and strategies for controlling weight. *JAMA.* 1999;282:1353–1358.
16. Jakicic JM, Marcus BH, Gallagher KI, et al. Effect of exercise duration and intensity on weight loss in overweight, sedentary women. *JAMA.* 2003;290(3):1323–1330.
17. Manson JE, Greenland P, LaCroix AZ, et al. Walking compared with vigorous exercise for the prevention of cardiovascular events in women. *N Engl J Med.* 2002;347,716–725.

18. Tanasescu M, Leitzmann MF, Rimm EB, et al. Exercise type and intensity in relation to coronary heart disease in men. *JAMA*. 288(16):1994–2000, 2002.

19. Fine JT, Golditz GA, Coakley EH, et al. A prospective study of weight change and health-related quality of life in women. *JAMA*. 1999;282:2136–2142.

20. Krempf M, Louvet JP, Allanic H, et al. Weight reduction and long-term maintenance after 18 months treatment with orlistat for obesity. *Intern J Obesity*. 2003:27;591–597.

Osteoporosis

# CHAPTER 30

Context

The signs of osteoporosis often appear suddenly with the development of a painful kyphosis or hip fracture. Over half of women over age 50 years will have a fracture due to osteoporosis.[1] There are approximately 700,000 vertebral fractures and 300,000 hip fractures per year in the United States with an annual cost of $18 billion. Less than 50% of patients with hip fracture recover pre-fracture function. There is a wide variation in reported mortality rates for individuals who suffer a hip fracture. This variation is due in part to differences between men and women and differences based on the time included in the measure. Most studies indicate an approximate range of 13% to 21.5%.[2, 3] Risk may be as high as 24% in women and 26% in men when measured at five years postfracture. It appears that if hip fractures are treated within 48 hours, this risk decreases.[4] Surprisingly, less than one-quarter of women who have sustained an osteoporotic fracture currently receive appropriate therapy.[5] The chiropractor's role with osteoporosis is both diagnostic and preventive. It is estimated that 50% of osteoporotic hip fractures and 90% of vertebral compression fractures are preventable.[6] Prevention should not be thought of as crisis intervention but a lifelong attempt at development and preservation of bone mass.

Osteoporosis is a loss of bone mass associated with deterioration of the microarchitecture of bone tissue. Osteoporosis is generally divided into bone loss associated with age, called senile or senescent osteoporosis (type II) and postmenopausal osteoporosis (type I). Women are susceptible to both types. Radiographically, osteoporosis is classified based on the area or region of involvement. Generalized osteoporosis is the most common form, found with both senile and postmenopausal causes. A regional osteoporosis may occur that is restricted to a bone or a portion of a limb. This is most often found with immobilization and Sudeck's atrophy (associated bone changes found with reflex sympathetic dystrophy). Localized osteoporosis may occur in specific areas of bone as a result of infection, neoplasm, or an inflammatory arthritis.

Osteoporosis is often classified as primary or secondary. Primary causes include senile and postmenopausal types. Secondary causes include hormonal dysfunction such as hyperthyroidism and hyperparathyroidism as well as the effect of reduced bone mass associated with the use of thyroid medication, corticosteroids, smoking, and alcohol.

The World Health Organization (WHO) distinguishes the degree of loss of bone mass by two terms:[7]

- osteopenia—bone density greater than 1 standard deviation (SD) below the normal mean but less than or equal to 2.5 SD below the normal mean
- osteoporosis—bone density greater than 2.5 SD below the normal mean

Women with a hip bone mineral density (BMD) T-score of −2.5 or less and an existing vertebral fracture had a 56% chance of additional vertebral fracture whereas those with normal BMD and no prevalent vertebral fracture had only a 9% risk.[8]

The difficulty with diagnosing and managing osteoporosis is that it is radiographically hidden until 30% to 50% of bone mass is lost. It is therefore important to be aware of more sensitive imaging options that allow for screening of high-risk patients. When osteoporosis is inadvertently discovered on radiographs, it is necessary to include a list of less common but possible differentials. The main differentials include osteomalacia, renal osteodystrophy, hyperparathyroidism, Paget's disease, and multiple myeloma. When an underlying pathologic process is discovered, referral for medical management or comanagement is warranted.

General Strategy

History

- Determine whether the patient has any known risk factors.
- Determine whether the patient has any indications of hormonal dysfunction.
- Determine whether the patient is taking corticosteroids, thyroid supplementation, estrogen, or calcium and Vitamin D supplementation or has adequate calcium content in his/her diet.
- Determine the patient's exercise routine, if any.
- Determine whether there is any history of cancer.

Evaluation

- Evaluate radiographs for vertebral compression fractures.
- Differentiate osteopenia caused by osteoporosis from other diffuse processes such as hyperparathyroidism or osteomalacia, and more regional processes such as reflex sympathetic dystrophy or bone cancer.
- Determine the degree of bone mass loss via dual energy x-ray absorptiometry (DEXA) for those patients at high risk or with known osteoporosis to establish a baseline for future determinations.

Management

- Establish a health-style habit of adequate calcium and exercise for all females beginning in adolescence.
- Refer patients with a suspicion of cancer, hyperthyroidism, adverse effects of corticosteroids, alcohol abuse, or hyperparathyroidism.
- Educate the patient with primary osteoporosis regarding management options such as estrogen replacement, calcitonin, or alendronate.
- Comanage patients with primary osteoporosis with an emphasis on exercise, diet, and precautions for falling.

Relevant Anatomy and Physiology

Osteoporosis is a consequence of bone quantity loss without an associated decrease of bone quality (mineralization is normal). Generally it is the result of increased resorption in the face of normal bone formation. The process of bone formation and resorption is a delicate balance governed by the interplay of a number of environmental, nutritional, and hormonal factors. Eighty percent of bone mass variation is due to genetics, whereas lifestyle factors account for only 20%.[9]

A productive imbalance occurs in early life when bone formation exceeds resorption. This peaks during and soon after puberty, gradually declining in the mid-20s to early 30s. A relatively small period of balance occurs when production equals resorption. Particularly in women, an imbalance in favor of resorption begins in the late 30s and early 40s. The rate of bone loss in women exceeds that of men, so that women lose about 50% of their total bone mass in a lifetime; men lose only about 25%.

Bone is composed of two-thirds mineral (mainly hydroxyapatite); the remaining one-third is a combination of collagen, water, proteoglycans, and other noncollagenous proteins. Type I collagen acts as a framework for deposition of minerals. The process of bone formation and repair is determined by an interaction of three cell types: osteoblasts, osteocytes, and osteoclasts. The role and cross-talk of these cells are not completely understood. Osteoblasts secrete the precursors that help form type I collagen. Osteocytes appear to be osteoblasts that serve more of a coordinating function, perhaps helping to mobilize bone minerals. Osteoclasts are multinucleated giant cells that use collagenases and proteolytic enzymes to break down bone. Osteoclasts are stimulated by a number of factors, including parathyroid hormone (PTH), cytokines (interleukin 1 and tumor necrosis factors), growth factors, and prostaglandin E_2.

Although it is known that a decrease in estrogen at menopause causes cortical bone loss and therefore increases the risk of fracture, evidence seems to suggest that some of the increased risk of fracture is mitigated by periosteal apposition. Periosteal apposition occurs with age-related bone loss and, to some extent, with menopause. The effect is an increase in bone size. A recent study indicates that this effect increases the ability of the distal radius to accommodate bending forces by up to 30%.[10] The explanation is that through periosteal apposition, the cortical shell is placed farther away from the long axis of bone, improving resistance to both bending and rotational forces.

Calcium metabolism is an important link in the chain of bone formation. Calcium intake must meet the demands of peak bone formation and exceed the daily loss of 100 mg to 250 mg. Calcium absorption is dependent on a normally functioning gastrointestinal environment. Key to absorption is adequate amounts of vitamin D (more closely resembles a hormone). Vitamin D is produced by the body through several conversion reactions beginning with ultraviolet stimulation of epidermal 7-dehydrocholesterol, which forms an unstable form of vitamin D. Further conversions in the liver and subsequently the kidney produce a potent form of vitamin D. Without sufficient sunlight, vitamin D production is halted, requiring supplementation. Almost half of healthy women who have none of the standard risk factors may still be at risk for osteoporosis. This risk is primarily due to low levels of vitamin D.[11]

Evaluation

History

Known risk factors for osteoporosis include the following:

- female gender
- white or Asian background
- early menopause
- family history
- lean body habitus
- lack of exercise or excessive exercise in the young
- glucocorticoids, phenytoin, aluminum antacids, lithium, loop diuretics, tetracycline, warfarin
- heavy alcohol consumption; smoking; low calcium intake or vitamin D deficiency; high phosphate, fiber, or sodium intake; more than four cups of coffee per day; carbonated drinks (several a day); and possibly a high animal-protein diet (although a low-protein diet may also place the female at risk)

Ethnicity percentages of osteoporosis as defined by WHO criteria are:[12]

- African American women = 12%
- Mexican Americans = 18.8%
- Other ethnic groups = 28.3%

For white females aged:

- 50–59 years = 14.8%
- 60–69 years = 21.6%
- 70–79 years = 38.5%
- 80 years and older = 70%

Interestingly, in skilled nursing homes, regardless of race and sex, those older than 75 years had a prevalence of 50% or more.[13]

Patients on any of the following medications may be at increased risk either due to the drug or the disease being managed:

- Steroids
- Aromatase inhibitors (e.g., Arimidex, Aromasin, Femara)
- Proton pump inhibitors
- GNRH inhibitors (e.g., Lupron)
- SSRIs
- Lithium
- Anticonvulsants

Given the popularity of proton-pump inhibitors for acid-reflux and duodenal ulcers, there is an increasing concern about their effect on decreasing acid secretion and the related effect of decreasing calcium absorption (among other minerals). A meta-analysis[14] published in 2011 found an increased risk of fracture related to the use of proton-pump inhibitors but not with the use of H2 antagonists. Increased gastrin levels may cause histamine production through hypertrophy of gastric enterochromaffin-like cells, which could lead to bone loss. In younger females, osteoporosis may be part of the "female athlete triad" (disordered eating, menstrual irregularity, and osteoporosis/osteopenia; see **Table 30–1**). Disordered eating has been estimated to occur in as many as two-thirds of young female athletes. Disordered eating is classified as restricted eating behaviors that do not necessarily become a clinical eating disorder such as anorexia nervosa.[15] In young competitive female runners, for example, disordered eating has a strong correlation to menstrual irregularity that is associated with a low BMD.[16] However, disordered eating is associated with a low BMD regardless of whether there is an associated menstrual irregularity.

In many patients, osteoporosis is a silent disorder until fracture occurs. Physical examination findings are usually the result of these fractures. An increased, acute-angle kyphosis is suggestive, especially if associated with an acute onset of spine pain following sneezing,

Table 30–1 Terminology Used with Bone Densitometry

Term	Definition
Bone density or bone mineral density (BMD)	The average concentration of mineral in a 2- or 3-dimensional image or defined section of bone. Also used to refer to the results of bone densitometry.
Bone mass	The amount of bone in the entire skeleton or in one specific location. There is no technology that measures bone mass.
Bone mineral content	The average concentration of mineral per unit area; also referred to as areal BMD.
Broadband ultrasound attenuation	The slope of the line of attenuation of sound energy across a spectrum of sound frequencies.
Speed of sound	The faster transmission of a specific frequency of sound through a given section of bone.
Trabecular bone density	Mineral density of bone that is trabecular only.
T-score	The difference in number of SDs below the mean BMD between a given individual patient value compared to a group of young adults of the same sex. The mean value and size of an SD vary with different techniques and sites that are measured.
Z-score	The difference in number of SDs above or below the mean BMD between that of a given patient and group of people of the same sex and age.
Osteopenia	WHO defines as a T-score between –1.0 and –2.5.
Osteoporosis	WHO defines as a bone density T-score at or below 2.5 standard deviation of normal. Also used is the finding of a vertebral fracture on radiographs.
Volumetric bone density	The bone mineral content divided by the volume of the bone section measured; measured with QCT.

WHO = World Health Organization

coughing, or a sudden jolt to the body such as stepping heavily off a curb. However, even vertebral fractures can be clinically silent. As many as two-thirds of vertebral fractures are asymptomatic; however, these fractures represent a two- to three-fold increased risk of future fracture. Green et al.[17] found that the following were helpful, in a review of clinical examination procedures that may assist in detecting occult fracture, or screen for those who may need further evaluation:

- A wall–occiput distance greater than 0 cm (in other words, with the patient standing with their heels and back to the wall, they are unable to touch the occiput to the wall).
- A rib–pelvis distance of less than two finger breadths (the examiner places his or her fingers between the lower rib and pelvis in the midaxillary line).
- Low teeth count.
- Self-reported humped back.

Additional examination findings will be found if the underlying cause of the osteoporosis is, for example, endocrine. Hyperthyroidism may be associated with osteoporosis, and either a history of previous diagnosis or physical examination findings may be suggestive. If the patient complains of intolerance to heat, fatigue, palpitations, and/or a change in the appearance of the eyes (exophthalmos), hyperthyroidism should be investigated. Hyperparathyroidism may also be associated with osteoporosis. Physical signs are generally absent; however, joint pains, especially of the knee, hip, wrist, or shoulder, may be reported. Radiologic confirmation is necessary.

Examination

The primary tools for evaluation of osteoporosis are radiographic. Physical examination focuses on indirect indicators of compression fractures such as an increased kyphosis. Signs of secondary causes of osteoporosis focus on hyperthyroidism and Cushing's disease or Cushingoid appearance due to long-term corticosteroid use. From a preventive perspective, it is important to screen the elderly for proprioceptive deficits. This would include an evaluation of balance, vision, and sensory function.

BMD is an excellent predictor of fracture risk; however, there is no known threshold that indicates fracture risk. Therefore, BMD is considered a "continuous" risk factor, meaning that the lower the BMD, the higher the risk of fracture, with no specific point that reflects a dramatic increase in risk. Although there are numerous methods of measuring BMD, and the BMD can be used to predict fracture, its use is still controversial as to who should be screened. A recent scientific review found evidence for measuring BMD in white women older than 65 years.[18] It may also be valuable to measure BMD in younger postmenopausal women with risk factors. Other guidelines from the National Osteoporosis Foundation and U.S. Preventive Services Task Force (USPSTF) recommend screening of women 65 years or older regardless of ethnicity.[19] Both groups suggest that women aged 60 to 65 years with risk factors should also be screened. Risk factors include personal history of hip fracture, current cigarette smoking, use or planning on use of oral corticosteroids for longer than three months, body weight less than 57.2 kg, and any metabolic condition such as hyperthyroidism or malabsorption that places the patient at risk.

There are classic radiographic findings with osteoporosis; however, their appearance indicates advanced involvement. Loss of between 30% and 50% is necessary before osteopenia becomes radiographically evident as an increase in radiolucency. Additional findings are cortical thinning (pencil-thin cortex) and trabecular changes. Trabecular resorption may leave the remaining stress-surviving trabeculae more visible, in contrast to a background of radiolucency. The remaining trabeculae of the spine are the vertical, stress-bearing ones. The horizontal trabeculae are preferentially lost. Changes in the vertebral shape with osteoporosis include vertebra plana (pancake vertebra), wedged vertebra, and biconcave (fish, hourglass) vertebra.

More sensitive techniques include single- and dual photon absorptiometry (SPA and DPA), quantitative computed tomography (QCT), DEXA, and possibly ultrasonography (US).[20]

- SPA and DPA use a radionuclide source measuring photon attenuation at the examination site. The SPA beam can be used only where soft tissue thickness is constant. It measures only the appendicular skeleton primarily at the distal radius and calcaneus. DPA is similar but emits photons at two different energy levels and has a better record in predicting future fractures. DPA is also able to evaluate axial and appendicular loss. Although both cortical and trabecular bone can be evaluated, DPA cannot distinguish between the two. Other limitations include the scan time (20 to 40 minutes), which may introduce distortion of image quality if the patient moves.

- DEXA—Although DPA, QCT, and DEXA measure both types of bone, DEXA is now the measurement tool of choice because it replaces the nuclide source with an x-ray source with a reduction in scan time and improvement in image quality. Although having some of the same disadvantages of DPA, DEXA can compensate by including both lateral and posterior images of the spine. DEXA is known to have a low level of error and high degree of accuracy. DEXA is used to assess the bone mineral density and estimate the degree of standard deviation compared to a normal mean. Vertebrae L1 through L3 or L4 are used to measure spine BMD. Spine BMD may increase after age 65 years due to degenerative arthritis.

- QCT requires a long scan time, resulting in more irradiation than with DEXA and DPA. It is also more expensive. The advantage is in measuring and distinguishing between cortical and trabecular bone in the spine. Use of dual-energy or bipolar QCT may improve some limitations with regard to fat and water content variations. Peripheral scanners are also available; however, their value has not yet been established.

- Ultrasonography—The newest approach to bone assessment is US. The U.S. Food and Drug Administration (FDA) has approved US as a screening tool to determine which patients might need further evaluation with DEXA. US provides broadband ultrasound attenuation, which is a value indicative of bone integrity. Due to the use of sound waves instead of radiation, US is safer. US may provide valuable information about future fracture risk, and it has been shown to provide a strong correlation with DEXA measures of bone density.

- Peripheral densitometry—These are smaller devices that use DXA or SXA to measure bone density at the forearm or heel. Although they take less time and cost much less than DEXA, they are less predictive for vertebral fractures, and the T-scores vary from one type of device to another.

- Quantitative ultrasound—The patterns of absorption of different sound frequencies (broadband ultrasound attenuation) are derived from sampling at the calcaneus and femoral neck. The combination of these BMD assessments is a good predictor of hip fracture risk.

Most major medical groups do not recommend screening all women with these techniques.[21]

Recommendations for the use of one of these specialized tools include the following:

- as an aid in decision-making regarding the need for estrogen replacement therapy (high-risk individuals)
- for monitoring patients on long-term glucocorticoids
- for monitoring patients with hyperparathyroidism who are at risk for skeletal disease (i.e., those who may need parathyroid surgery)

Laboratory evaluation is valuable only in the differential evaluation. Most bone-related lab levels, such as calcium, phosphorus, and alkaline phosphatase, are usually normal unless there has been a recent fracture. Urinary hydroxyproline levels may be elevated. Newer approaches include measures of specific biochemical markers. Bone density is estimated based on these indicators of bone turnover. Serum and urinary markers include enzymes associated with either osteoblastic or osteoclastic activity, elements released during resorption, or proteins that are produced by osteoblasts. These include:

- bone formation markers—bone-specific alkaline phosphatase, osteocalcin (protein found in bone and dentin measured by enzyme-linked immunosorbent assay [ELISA] technique), and pro-collagen I extension peptides
- bone resorption markers—urinary pyridinoline and deoxypyridinoline (collagen phosphate cross-links), total and dialyzable hydroxyproline

Management

- For all women, establish a lifestyle habit of maintaining an adequate amount of calcium and vitamin D combined with an appropriate level of exercise; also recommendations for avoidance of known contributors to osteoporosis acceleration including smoking, alcohol, caffeine, carbonated drinks, etc.
- When a secondary cause of osteoporosis or a compression fracture is found or suspected (i.e., cancer, Paget's disease, hyperparathyroidism, or osteomalacia) medical consultation is necessary.
- If a compression fracture appears radiographically unstable, refer for medical consultation (see Chapter 6 for details).

- For all older women, establish a prevention program for falls including an environmental evaluation, exercise program, and nutritionally supportive regimen.
- For all osteoporotic patients, provide a comprehensive program including patient education, appropriate exercise, and appropriate nutrition (see **Table 30–2**) coupled with psychosocial support.

Management decisions are based primarily on several factors including age, BMD, previous fracture, and 10-year fracture risk. Smoking and rheumatoid arthritis are also important considerations in management.

Medical management strives to maintain the T-score, as opposed to improving it, in all cases. An improvement of one on the T-score value is equal to a 10% improvement in bone strength. In judging the effect of medical management, comparisons can be made only if the follow-up DEXA is performed on the same machines due to variations in equipment. Also there is a 2% to 3% standard deviation factor that must be accounted for. Therefore, there must be at least a 3% change in the vertebral measurement and a 3% to 4% change in the hip to be considered significant (either plus or minus). If the BMD is normal, most guidelines recommend rechecking in three to five years. If a patient is under medical management, checking every two years is required. Drug therapy is highly effective at reducing vertebral and sometimes hip fractures, yet that reduction is still in the 50% range.

Education of the osteoporotic patient is a key component to management. In addition to the educational advice of the doctor, several organizations such as the National Osteoporosis Foundation (NOF), the Older Women's League (OWL), and the National Dairy Council provide educational pamphlets and materials to patients and doctors.

Although there is some debate as to the degree of effect, a combination of calcium supplementation and exercise can, at the very least, reduce bone loss in the majority of postmenopausal females. Supplemental calcium not only decreases bone loss in postmenopausal females but also reduces the risk of vertebral fracture by up to 45% (nonvertebral fracture and hip fracture are also reduced by about 25%).[9,22] The amount of calcium intake is generally recommended to be 1,000 mg for premenopausal women and 1,500 mg for postmenopausal women. Although dairy products are a common source of calcium, other options exist for those patients with lactose intolerance or a concern

Table 30-2 Nutritional Support for Osteoporosis

Substance	How Might It Work?	Dosage	Special Instructions	Contraindications and Possible Side Effects
Ipriflavone	Decreases bone turnover rate by inhibiting bone resorption.	200 mg capsule, 3 times/day.	Best taken with meals.	None at recommended dosage.
Calcium/magnesium/CitraMate	Most absorbable form of Ca/Mg. Calcium—reduces bone loss. Magnesium—enzyme responsible for conversion to active form of vitamin D is Mg-dependent.	1–3 capsules, 3 times/day.	Best taken with meals.	None at recommended dosage; however, increase in magnesium may cause diarrhea.
B6, B12, folic acid (homocysteine factors)	Decrease homocysteine (homocysteine contributes to defective bone matrix).	1 capsule, 2 times/day.	Best taken with meals.	None at recommended dosage.
Vitamin D3	Calcium absorption of 700—800 IM of D3			None at recommended dosage.

Note: These substances have not been approved by the FDA for the treatment of this disorder.

about the high cholesterol/calorie content of some +dairy products.

The debate over which calcium supplementation is best continues. Part of the prescription decision is clarified when considering the following:

- Those with lactase deficiency may not tolerate calcium lactate.
- Calcium carbonate is an acceptable choice because it is inexpensive and relatively effective; however, it may cause bloating or constipation.
- Supplements derived from bone meal or dolomite sometimes contain contaminants such as lead, mercury, and arsenic.[23]
- Calcium citrate is a good alternative and is available in some orange juices; however, some patients may not tolerate citric acid.

It is important that patients be educated about the misleading trappings of advertising. For example, although the product may be labeled as containing 1,500 mg of calcium carbonate, it may contain only 500 mg of elemental calcium.

African Americans, those with darker skin, and those using sunblock are less able to absorb sunlight and

therefore may have inadequate levels of vitamin D. In northern latitudes above 51°, and in the spring, summer, and fall, if an individual is exposed to sunlight for at least 15 minutes, two to three times per week adequate vitamin D can be made. However, in the winter at the same latitude, individuals may go three months without being able to make vitamin D; at 71° latitude it may take as long as five months.

Only recently, the value and need for vitamin D supplementation for osteoporosis has surfaced in the literature and guideline recommendations. As many as 64% to 69% of osteoporotic postmenopausal females are vitamin D deficient (<30 ng/ml).[24,25] Although the recommended minimally desirable serum concentration is 25(OH)D to 40 nmol/l, it is likely that the desirable level will be suggested as 75 nmol/l.[26] At this level, only one-third of seniors in the United States and even fewer European seniors will meet this requirement. To achieve this level, daily intake should be between 700–800 IU of D3 (cholecalciferol) with even higher doses recommended for osteoporotic females (1,000 IU/daily). Levels of up to 2,000 IU are considered safe. Treatment with 50,000 IU of D2 over several weeks is also considered safe and effective. Calcium intake should be a minimum of 1,200–1,500 mg/D. However, D2 (ergocalciferol) is clearly less effective with a potency of about one-third that of D3. Unfortunately, D2 (usually derived from plants) is the cheapest form used in milk and probably the majority of supplements. The oil-based gel cap packaging of D3 is the best absorbed.

Higher circulating homocysteine levels have been associated with increased fracture risk. Folic acid and B vitamin supplementation are being investigated to determine their effect, mediating this risk by decreasing homocysteine levels.

Estrogen replacement therapy (ERT) is controversial, yet it is the most effective treatment for postmenopausal osteoporosis.[27] Because of its demonstrated effectiveness in bone preservation, some physicians feel that all postmenopausal women should be placed on ERT; others feel that it should be a decision based on risk. There are some known contraindications to ERT, including the following:

- undiagnosed vaginal bleeding
- pregnancy
- breast cancer
- estrogen-dependent neoplasm
- active thromboembolic disorders or past history of thrombus related to estrogen

Relative contraindications include gallbladder and liver diseases and a history of menstrual migraines. To reduce the chance of uterine cancer, estrogen is combined with progesterone in women with an intact uterus.

Although it is clear that estrogen replacement therapy has a dramatic effect on BMD and bone turnover, there is increasing concern regarding the elevated risk of developing breast cancer, heart disease, stroke, and deep vein thrombosis. One recent study indicates that low-dose estradiol showed increased BMD of the spine, hip, and total body, as well as reduced bone turnover without any apparent increased occurrence of breast cancer.[28] A recent large randomized trial, the Women's Health Initiative (WHI) study, compared estrogen plus progestin to placebo in postmenopausal women to determine any differences in risks for various diseases.[29] Those women taking estrogen plus progestin had an increased risk compared to the placebo group for breast cancer (26%), coronary heart disease (29%), stroke (41%), and pulmonary embolism (113%). This is a monumental study that followed patients for 5.2 years, and due to its strong experimental design has stimulated serious concerns about the risks/benefits of HRT.

Although ERT and calcitonin have been the mainstay for the prevention of further bone loss in postmenopausal females, three new therapies are now becoming first-line approaches to management:

- Selective estrogen receptor modulators (raloxifene)
- Bisphosphonates (alendronate and risedronate)
- Parathyroid hormone

Both raloxifene and the bisphosphonates comprise a group of medications classified as antiresorptive. These medications inhibit bone resorption but eventually reduce bone formation due to a decrease in overall bone turnover. A standard intermittent treatment program with parathyroid hormone is intended to increase bone formation; however, it also increases bone resorption. The net effect, however, is bone formation. It is clear that prolonged exposure to parathyroid hormone, such as in hyperparathyroidism, causes osteoporosis. Intermittent use through daily subcutaneous injections has an anabolic effect, particularly with trabecular bone. The effect on cortical bone may be an increase in cortical porosity, yet most of this occurs at the endocortical surface (partially at the Haversian canals), having little mechanical effect (i.e., no increased risk of fracture). A recent study confirmed the effect of increased trabecular bone content in parathyroid treated patients versus combination treatment with alendronate and parathyroid.[30] A separate study in men confirmed the same effect. Additional findings indicate that any initial benefit of combined therapy changes over time, so that those treated with parathyroid hormone had higher bone mineral density than with combination therapy.[31] In fact, it appears that alendronate may reduce the beneficial effects of parathyroid treatment. The positive effect of parathyroid hormone therapy on reducing the risk of fracture has been demonstrated in one study.[32] Although it appears that 5-reductase inhibitors (statins) have been demonstrated to increase bone formation in vitro and in vivo in some studies, a recent study indicated that this had no effect on fracture risk for postmenopausal females.[33]

Calcitonin appears to have two effects. In addition to increasing bone density, it may reduce pain significantly in some patients. The infrequent complaints of nausea and flushing are usually managed by beginning with a low dose given at bedtime. Newer approaches that are being investigated are fluoride and parathyroid hormone use. **Table 30–3** lists the common medications used in the management of osteoporosis.

Table 30-3 Osteoporosis Medications

Drug Class	Examples	General Mechanism	Interactions/Side Effects
Bisphosphonates	**Ibandronate** Boniva	A nitrogen-containing bisphosphonate used in the management of osteoporosis. Bisphosphonates inhibit osteoclast-mediated bone resorption. Advantage over other similar medications is the once-per-month dosage. Requires adequate intake of calcium and vitamin D.	Upper GI problems such as esophagitis, dyspepsia, esophageal or gastric ulcers
	Alendronate Fosamax	Bisphosphonate; antiresorptive used in the treatment of osteoporosis and Paget's disease. These medications inhibit bone resorption but eventually reduce bone formation due to a decrease in overall bone turnover. A standard intermittent treatment program with parathyroid hormone is intended to increase bone formation; however, it also increases bone resorption. The net effect, though, is bone formation. It is clear that prolonged exposure to parathyroid hormone such as in hyperparathyroidism causes osteoporosis.	Hypocalcemia, GI effects include esophageal irritation/ulceration with abdominal pain, nausea, vomiting, diarrhea/constipation, arthralgias, myalgias, headache, and rash. Dairy products decrease absorption.
	Etidronate Didronel	Bisphosphonate; antiresorptive used in the treatment of osteoporosis and Paget's disease. Decreases vascularity of bone with Paget's. These medications inhibit bone resorption but eventually reduce bone formation due to a decrease in overall bone turnover. A standard intermittent treatment program with parathyroid hormone is intended to increase bone formation; however, it also increase bone resorption. The net effect, though, is bone formation. It is clear that prolonged exposure to parathyroid hormone such as in hyperparathyroidism causes osteoporosis.	May cause hypocalcemia, hyperphosphatemia, elevated serum phosphatase. GI effects include esophageal irritation/ulceration with abdominal pain, nausea, vomiting, diarrhea/constipation, arthralgias, myalgias, headache, and rash. Dairy products decrease absorption.
	Risedronate Actonel	Bisphosphonate; antiresorptive used in the treatment of osteoporosis and Paget's disease. These medications inhibit bone resorption but eventually reduce bone formation due to a decrease in overall bone turnover. A standard intermittent treatment program with parathyroid hormone is intended to increase bone formation; however, it also increases bone resorption. The net effect, though, is bone formation. It is clear that prolonged exposure to parathyroid hormone such as in hyperparathyroidism causes osteoporosis. Risedronate is believed to be more effective than other bisphosphonates at blocking bone dissolution.	Fewer GI side effects than other bisphosphonates
Selective estrogen receptor modulator	**Raloxifene** Evista	Selective estrogen receptor modulator; antiresorptive used in the treatment of osteoporosis. These medications inhibit bone resorption but eventually reduce bone formation due to a decrease in overall bone turnover. A standard intermittent treatment program with parathyroid hormone is intended to increase bone formation; however, it also increases bone resorption. The net effect, though, is bone formation. It is clear that prolonged exposure to parathyroid hormone such as in hyperparathyroidism causes osteoporosis. Raloxifene is believed to decrease total cholesterol and LDL cholesterol but does not raise HDL or lower triglycerides. Also, the selective estrogen receptor inhibition effect prevents tissue proliferation in the uterus and breasts.	May cause flu-like symptoms, also hot flashes, migraine headache, insomnia, depression, weight gain, vaginitis, breast pain, and vaginal bleeding.
Parathyroid hormone agonist	**Teriparatide** Forteo	A parathyroid hormone agonist used in the management of postmenopausal osteoporosis.	Pain, transient increases in calcium levels, headaches, dizziness, arthralgias, myalgias, leg cramps, rash, swelling

An interesting study measuring the long-term effects of exercise on risk for compression fracture in osteoporotic females determined that after a two-year program of back strengthening exercises (back pack with maximum manageable weight used for prone extension exercises), there was a difference in back strength between the exercise and control group but no significant differences in BMD.[34] However, after an eight-year follow-up, both back strength and BMD were increased. Also, at eight years' follow-up there was a 2.7 times greater risk for compression fracture in the control (non-exercise) group.

Exercise prescription for the osteoporotic patient should meet two goals. First, it is important to stimulate bone production and prevent loss. Second, it is important to strengthen muscles to provide support and to train the patient proprioceptively to prevent falls. The increases in bone mass seen with exercise are mild to modest, on the order of 1% to 3%. However, it must be kept in mind that simply preventing further bone loss is a major goal of an exercise prescription. The general rule of thumb for inducing a bone mass response is that the exercise must provide mechanical loading either through pull of muscle on bone or weight-bearing. Some important considerations are as follows:

- Walking alone does not seem to provide enough stimulation for increased bone mass; walking must be combined with resistance exercise.[35]
- Non-weight-bearing exercises including swimming and cycling are relatively ineffective approaches.[36]
- Resistance exercise must exceed that provided by daily activities.[37]
- The effects of exercise are site-specific (e.g., running does not provide stimulation for bone in the upper extremities).[38]
- Impact activities that apply relatively large loads on bone quickly are the most osteogenic and are the most risky; therefore, a progression of exercise up to the level of these types of activities is the ultimate goal.

The exercise prescription must take into account the degree of current bone loss, presence of compression fractures, the strength and balance level of the patient, accessibility to exercise equipment, and motivation of the patient. The response to exercise is dependent on type of exercise, diet, and, most important, hormonal status. In general, at least one hour of physical activity is needed to provide and maintain a response. Initial prescription would include some weight-bearing and mild resistance exercise progressing to more weight-bearing and more resistance slowly. Spinal exercises should focus on extension with avoidance of the compressive effects of flexion exercises. Also, initial high-impact and twisting should be avoided.

In addition to the prevention of further bone loss, it is equally important to prevent falls in the elderly. An assessment of physical risks that are the consequence of the individual's health status and those that are a consequence of the patient's living environment should be identified and utilized in patient education. Addressing the patient's balance, posture, and muscle strength, combined with modification of environmental hazards, can decrease the risk of falling by as much as 30%.[39]

An interesting approach is gaining some literature evidence for efficacy in improving BMD and strength. Devices on the market such as Power Plate vibrate at low frequency (20–90 Hz). Preliminary evidence in both animals and humans suggests a possible benefit.[40,41]

APPENDIX 30–1

References

1. Chrischelles EA, Butler CD, Davis CS, et al. A model of lifetime osteoporosis impact. *Arch Intern Med.* 1991;151(10):2026–2032.
2. Vidal EI, Coeli CM, Pinheiro RS, Camargo KR, Jr. Mortality within 1 year after hip fracture surgical repair in the elderly according to postoperative period: a probabilistic record linkage study in Brazil. *Osteoporos Int.* 2006;17(10):1569–1576.
3. Robbins JA, Biggs ML, Cauley J. Adjusted mortality after hip fracture: From the cardiovascular health study. *J Am Geriatr Soc.* 2006;54(12):1885–1891.
4. Sircar P, Godkar D, Mahgerefteh S, Chambers K, Niranjan S, Cucco R. Morbidity and mortality among patients with hip fractures surgically repaired within and after 48 hours. *Am J Ther.* 2007;14(6):508–513.
5. Bahl S, Coates PS, Greenspan SL. The management of osteoporosis following hip fracture: have we improved our care? *Osteoporos Int.* 2003;14(11):884–888.
6. Lindsay R. Sex steroids in the pathogenesis and prevention of osteoporosis. In: Riggs BL, Melton LI, eds. *Osteoporosis: Etiology, Diagnosis and Management.* New York: Raven Press; 1988:333–358.

7. Kanis JA, Melton LJ III, Christiansen C, et al. The diagnosis of osteoporosis. *J Bone Miner Res.* 1994;9(8):1137–1141.

8. Cauley JA, Hochberg MC, Lui LY, et al. Long-term risk of incident vertebral fractures. *JAMA.* 2007;298(23):2761–2767.

9. Dawson-Hughes B, Harris SS, Krall EA, et al. Effect of calcium and vitamin D supplementation on bone density in men and women 65 years of age or older. *N Engl J Med.* 1997;337(10):670–676.

10. Ahlborg HG, Johnell O, Turner CH, et al. Bone loss and bone size after menopause. *N Engl J Med.* 2003;349:327–334.

11. Moore NL, Kiebzak GM. Suboptimal vitamin D status is a highly prevalent but treatable condition in both hospitalized patients and the general population. *J Am Acad Nurse Pract.* 2007;19(12):642–651.

12. Snelling AM, Crespo CJ, Schaeffer M, Smith S, Walbourn L. Modifiable and nonmodifiable factors associated with osteoporosis in postmenopausal women: results from the Third National Health and Nutrition Examination Survey, 1988–1994. *J Womens Health Gend Based Med.* 2001;10(1):57–65.

13. Zimmerman SI, Girman CJ, Buie VC, et al. The prevalence of osteoporosis in nursing home residents. *Osteoporos Int.* 1999;9(2):151–157.

14. Eom CS, Park SM, Myung SK, Yun JM, Ahn JS. Use of acid-suppressive drugs and risk of fracture: a meta-analysis of observational studies. *Ann Fam Med.* May-Jun 2011;9(3):257–267.

15. Nativ A, Agostini R, Drinkwater B, Yaeger KK. The female athlete triad. *Clin Sports Med.* 1994;13:405–418.

16. Cobb KL, Bachrach LK, Greendale G, et al. Disordered eating, menstrual irregularity, and bone mineral density in female runners. *Med Sci Sports Exerc.* 2003;35(5):711–719.

17. Green AD, Colon-Emeric CS, Bastian L, Drake MT, Lyles KW. Does this woman have osteoporosis? *JAMA.* 2004;292(23):2890–2900.

18. Cummings SR, Bates D, Black DM. Clinical use of bone densitometry: scientific review. *JAMA.* 2002;288:1889–1897.

19. U.S. Preventive Services Task Force. Screening for osteoporosis in postmenopausal women; recommendations and rationale. *Ann Intern Med.* 2002;137:526–528.

20. Kellie SE. Diagnostic and therapeutic technology assessment (DATTA): measurement of bone density with dual-energy X-ray absorptiometry. *JAMA.* 1992;267:286–294.

21. Report of the U.S. Preventive Services Task Force. Screening for postmenopausal osteoporosis. In: *Guide to Clinical Preventive Services.* 2nd ed. Baltimore: Williams & Wilkins; 1996:509.

22. Chapuy MC, Arlot ME, Delmas PD, et al. Effect of calcium and cholecalciferol treatment for three years on hip fractures in elderly women. *Br Med J.* 1994;308(6936):1081–1082.

23. National Osteoporosis Foundation. *Boning Up on Osteoporosis: A Guide to Prevention and Treatment.* Washington, DC: National Osteoporosis Foundation; 1991:26.

24. Lips P, Hosking D, Lippuner K, et al. The prevalence of vitamin D inadequacy amongst women with osteoporosis: an international epidemiological investigation. *J Intern Med.* 2006;260(3):245–254.

25. Binkley N, Krueger D, Drezner MK. Low vitamin D status: time to recognize and correct a Wisconsin epidemic. *WMJ.* 2007;106(8):466–472.

26. Bischoff-Ferrari HA. How to select the doses of vitamin D in the management of osteoporosis. *Osteoporos Int.* 2007;18(4):401–407.

27. Breslau NA. Calcium, estrogen and progestin in the treatment of osteoporosis. *Rheum Dis Clin North Am.* 1994;8(1):23–62.

28. Prestwood KM, Kenny AM, Kleppinger A, Kulldorff M. Ultralow-dose micronized 17 β-estradiol and bone density and bone metabolism in older women: a randomized controlled trial. *JAMA.* 2003;290:1042–1048.

29. Writing Group for the Women's Health Initiative Investigators. Risks and benefits of estrogen plus progestin in healthy postmenopausal women: principal results from the Women's Health Initiative randomized controlled trial. *JAMA.* 2002;288(3):321–333.

30. Black DM, Greenspan SL, Ensrud KE, et al. The effects of parathyroid hormone and alendronate alone or in combination in postmenopausal osteoporosis. *N Engl J Med.* 2003;349:1207–1215.

31. Finkelstein JS, Hayes A, Hunzelman JL, et al. Effects of parathyroid hormone, alendronate, or both in men with osteoporosis. *N Engl J Med.* 2003;349:1216–1226.

32. Neer RM, Arnaud CD, Zanchetta JR, et al. Effect of parathyroid hormone (I-34) on fracture and bone mineral density in postmenopausal women with osteoporosis. *N Engl J Med.* 2001;344:1434–1441.

33. LaCroix AZ, Cauley JA, Pettinger M, et al. Statin use, clinical fracture, and bone density in postmenopausal

women: results from the Women's Initiative Observational Study. *Ann Int Med.* 2003;139:97–104.

34. Sinaki M, Itoi E, Walmer HW, et al. Stronger back muscles reduce the incidence of vertebral fractures: a prospective 10-year follow-up of postmenopausal women. *Bone.* 2002;30(6):836–841.

35. Cavanaugh DJ, Cann CE. Brisk walking does not stop bone loss in postmenopausal women. *Bone.* 1988;9(4):201–204.

36. Taffle DR, Snow-Harter C, Connolly DA, et al. Differential effects of swimming versus weight-bearing activity on bone mineral status of eumenorrheic athletes. *J Bone Miner Res.* 1995;10(4):586–593.

37. Dalsky GP. The role of exercise in the prevention of osteoporosis. *Compr Ther.* 1989;15(9):30–37.

38. Heinoren A, Sievanen H, Kamus P, et al. Effects of unilateral strength training and detraining on bone mineral mass and estimated mechanical characteristics of the upper limb bones in young women. *J Bone Miner Res.* 1996;11(4):490–501.

39. Tineti ME, Baker D, McAvay G, et al. A multifactorial intervention to reduce the risk of falling among elderly people living in the community. *N Engl J Med.* 1994;331:821–827.

40. Gusi N, Raimundo A, Leal A. Low-frequency vibratory exercise reduces the risk of bone fracture more than walking: a randomized controlled trial. *BMC Musculoskelet Disord.* 2006;7:92.

41. Garman R, Gaudette G, Donahue LR, Rubin C, Judex S. Low-level accelerations applied in the absence of weight bearing can enhance trabecular bone formation. *J Orthop Res.* 2007;25(6):732–740.

Gastrointestinal Complaints

Abdominal Pain

Context

Chiropractors are sometimes faced with a dilemma regarding whether or not to accept a patient. A patient may present with a chief complaint or secondary complaint of abdominal pain. The first concern is whether the pain is due to a visceral source; the second concern is whether the chiropractor can appropriately manage the patient. Delayed referral for appropriate diagnostic testing and care may have serious consequences for the patient (and inevitably for the chiropractor). Each year more than 3 million Americans seek medical care for abdominal pain[1] in hospital emergency departments. Inappropriate or unnecessarily early surgical referral may result in nonessential or inappropriate surgery with its consequences. At the core of this issue, for many chiropractors, is the belief or experience that management of apparently viscerally caused abdominal pain results in successful resolution under chiropractic care. A debate on whether spinal dysfunction is the cause of referred abdominal pain or an actual dysfunction of an organ still ensues. This issue is well addressed in a review by Nansel and Szlazak.[2] The reader is referred to this source for a more in-depth discussion. The issue is clouded when a patient presents with a back complaint associated with a "viscerally" associated symptom. Is the back pain the cause of the visceral symptom or is it the reverse? The remainder of this discussion is based on the assumption that serious, surgically treatable disease is the domain of the surgeon and will more likely present to the emergency department and rarely present in the chiropractic setting. The remaining conditions that do present may be in need of medical treatment, may respond to conservative measures, or are self-resolving. The task for the chiropractor is to determine which of these conditions the patient has.

General Strategy

Acute Abdominal Pain

Determine whether the condition requires referral:

- Determine the onset and severity of the pain (abrupt pain suggests rupture or blockage of a nonintestinal lumen such as a ureter [kidney stones] or the gallbladder [gallstones]).
- Determine whether other acquaintances of the patient have similar symptoms (gastroenteritis or food poisoning). (See **Table 31–1**.)
- Determine any relationship to ingestion of food (food poisoning).
- Determine, in women, recent history of sexual contact (pelvic inflammatory disease) and menstrual history (ectopic pregnancy).
- Determine whether there is any past history of surgery (postsurgical adhesions causing obstruction). (See Table 31–1.)
- Determine whether the patient maintains a position of relief (fetal position indicates pancreatitis; flexed hip position may indicate appendicitis).
- Attempt to localize the pain by patient description and palpation.
- Determine whether there are any peritoneal signs (pain with movement or jarring, central pain that has progressively localized, rebound tenderness, or rigid abdomen suggests appendicitis, perforated ulcer, or another peritoneal problem).
- Determine the timing of associated symptoms such as vomiting, constipation, or diarrhea.
- Attempt to narrow the differentials to a system, such as genitourinary (radiation from thoracolumbar

Table 31–1 Causes of Intestinal Obstruction

Type	Summary
Ileus	Two types: adynamic and obstructive. Adynamic is usually due to the side effects of CNS depression from anesthesia or narcotics and may also be related to pain-inhibition. Obstructive is due to mechanical blockages from atresia or stenosis, gallstones, fecaliths, or meconium (in infants with cystic fibrosis, adhesions secondary to surgery or peritonitis). May also be related to other causes of intestinal obstruction such as hernia, intussusception, or volvulus.
Hernia	Hernias result from a weakness or defect in the abdominal wall. Inguinal hernia is more common in males; femoral hernias more common in females. Other hernias include periumbilical (protrudes around the umbilicus), and diaphragmatic (hiatal) hernia.
Volvulus	Volvulus is a rotary twisting of the intestine leading to infarction and necrosis. This occurs most frequently in the small intestine or sigmoid colon.
Intussusception	A telescoping or invagination of one segment of the intestine into the other. The danger is vascular compromise, which may lead to necrosis. In children this occurs due to hyperperistaltic activity or enlargement of lymphoid tissue. In adults, the leading cause is tumor.
Adhesions	Adhesions are secondary to prior infection, peritonitis, and prior surgery.
Neoplasms	Neoplasms may entangle the intestines, causing a constricted area that prevents passage.

area to groin or associated dysuria, increased frequency, hesitancy, or hematuria), gastrointestinal (nausea, vomiting, constipation, diarrhea, or rectal bleeding), gynecologic (change in menstrual period, vaginal discharge or bleeding, or dyspareunia), or cardiovascular (history of hypertension, atrial fibrillation, or sickle cell disease).

- Determine whether laboratory tests (for acute infection or urinary tract involvement) or radiographic studies (free air or obstruction) are necessary.

Chronic, Recurrent Abdominal Pain

Determine the following:

- Determine whether the pain is associated with the timing of meals (empty stomach implies ulcer; full stomach implies reflux) or meal content (similar foods affect both ulcer and reflux).
- Determine whether the patient has traveled recently, locally on camping trips (giardiasis, amoebic dysentery), or abroad to a foreign country (parasitic infection).
- Determine whether there is a relationship to a woman's menstrual cycle (primary dysmenorrhea or endometriosis).
- Obtain the medication history of the patient (use of nonsteroid anti-inflammatory drugs [NSAIDs] or aspirin suggests gastric bleeding; use of antacids or

H2 receptor antagonists that help the pain suggests esophageal, gastric, or duodenal pathology).

- Ask about any associated diarrhea (inflammatory bowel disorders, parasitic infections, or a drug reaction) or alternating diarrhea and constipation (irritable bowel syndrome).
- Ask about any blood in the stool, weight loss, change in caliber of stool (colon or other cancer). (See **Table 31–2**.)

Relevant Anatomy and Physiology

Visceral pain is characteristically different from somatic pain. There may be overlaps, however. Visceral afferent receptors serve a function different from that of somatic receptors. Somatic receptors signal the brain about external threats and in so doing need to have a high degree of localization and reflex response capabilities. Visceral receptors are designed more to provide information that helps maintain homeostasis. In the abdominal area, the most important information for homeostasis is distention, constriction, and vascular status. Whether these nerve endings or specific nociceptors relay pain is still unknown. It is known, however, that the types of stimuli that will produce a sensation of pain are often extreme events of normal stimuli such as overdistention (e.g., gas in the intestine or a stone in a

Table 31–2 Some Gastrointestinal Cancers

Type	Summary Information
Carcinoma of the esophagus	• Accounts for 4% of all malignant neoplasms in U.S. Three times more common in African Americans, with a male-to-female ratio of 4:1 in the U.S.
	• 95% of patients die within 2 years.
	• In China, Iran, and South Africa, incidence is 10%–15% higher than U.S. due possibly to a carcinogen in the soil or food.
	• A large percentage of individuals have a history of chronic alcoholism and tobacco use.
	• Clinical presentation may be pain on swallowing, bad breath, dysphagia, and bleeding; being locally invasive, by the time symptoms/signs develop most tumors have spread into the lymph nodes; 90% are squamous cell carcinomas found in the middle or lower portions; 10% are adenocarcinomas originating from Barrett's esophagus.
	• Dx is by barium-swallow x-ray or esophagoscopy with biopsy.
	• Management is surgical resection.
Carcinoma of the stomach	• Incidence in U.S. is 10 per 1,000,000, which is 8 times lower than Japan or Chile.
	• Believed to be an environmental carcinogen, most likely in the food, specifically nitrosamines as is found in smoked fish. Also, processing of food in U.S. may decrease bacterial causes.
	• Some increased risk with atrophic gastritis, pernicious anemia, and gastric adenomatous polyps.
	• 60% found in distal stomach (pylorus and antrum); cardia in 25% of cases.
	• Four types: polypoid, fungating, ulcerating, and diffusely infiltrating (linitis plastica); histologically all adenocarcinomas; metastasis is through regional lymph nodes and the liver.
	• Symptoms are nonspecific with weight loss, anemia, weakness, and signs of local gastric irritation similar to peptic ulcer.
	• May have a supraclavicular lymph node involvement called a Virchow or sentinel node (may also metastasize to ovaries [bilateral involvement referred to as Krukenberg's tumor] and other distal sites).
	• Dx from gastroscopies with gastric brushing and cytologic examination.
	• The 5-year survival rate is only 10%–15%.
Carcinoma of the intestine	• 95% of malignant tumors of the intestine are adenocarcinomas.
	• Adenocarcinoma is 50 times more common in the large intestine.
	• Colorectal cancer is more common in the U.S. and other Western countries compared to Asia and Africa.
	• Incidence increases with age, with rectal cancer ratio of male to female 2:1; colonic ratios are equal.
	• Although most cancers appear insidiously, risk groups include those with familial predisposition such as hereditary nonpolyposis colorectal cancer (HNPCC), familial adenomatous polyposis (FAP), and Gardner's syndrome.
	• Findings vary, but most early cancer is asymptomatic. May have constipation; narrow, pencil-like feces; or blood in the stool. Hematochezia may also occur later in the disease profile.
	• Screening of those over age 50 years should include digital rectal examination, fecal occult testing, and colonoscopy and sigmoidoscopy (dependent on family risk and which is chosen).
	• Dx is via the screening methods mentioned above combined with barium enema and computed axial tomography using histologic evaluation of the suspected tissue for confirmation.
	• Staging morphologically is based on the Dukes system using four stages (A–D) with progressive involvement and decreasing risk for survival. Dukes A have an 85% 5-year survival; B have 55%; C have 30%; D have 10%.

(continues)

Table 31–2 Some Gastrointestinal Cancers (continued)

Type	Summary Information
Neoplastic polyps	• In addition to neoplastic polyps, there are some non-neoplastic lesions including hyperplastic, hamartomatous, and inflammatory or lymphoid polyps.
	• Neoplastic polyps occur usually as multiple lesions and are classified as tubular, villous, and tubulovillous. They are, as a group, considered premalignant because each has the possibility of progressing to adenocarcinomas; the highest risk is with tubulovillous and villous.
	• Incidence increases with age and is more common in males than females (2:1), with 70% located in the rectosigmoid colon.
	• Dx is with sigmoid and colonoscopic.
	• Endoscopic removal of precancerous has a high success rate; resection may be needed for some lesions dependent on degree of involvement.
Carcinoid	• These neuroendocrine tumors are malignant; however, less so than carcinomas.
	• The GI tract is where 90% of carcinoid tumors originate; specifically the intestines.
	• Typically located in the submucosa.
	• Metastasis is most common in tumors >2 cm located in the right colon, small intestine, or stomach.
	• The secretions from these tumors are detoxified by the liver; however, if they metastasize to the liver, the secretory products are released into the venous system producing a disease called carcinoid syndrome.
	• Symptoms of carcinoid syndrome include facial blushing, wheezing, diarrhea, and colic. This is likely due to the release of serotonin, bradykinin, and histamine.
	• Carcinoids are slow-growing, with a survival rate for treated patients of at least 80%.

nonintestinal lumen) or ischemia. This is in part due to the fact that nerve endings are located in muscular walls of the gut and organs such as the gallbladder and urinary bladder. Other irritating factors causing visceral pain are probably chemical in nature, such as pH changes or toxic irritation. This pain reaction is probably stimulated by local release of bradykinin, serotonin, histamine, and other substances. Also, the rate at which distention occurs often determines whether pain is felt at all. For example, gradual distention that occurs from malignancy (such as malignant biliary obstruction) may be painless, whereas acute blockage from cholelithiasis is painful. If the capsule of an organ such as the liver (Glisson's capsule) is involved, pain will be produced somatically. The organ itself, having no muscular component, is insensitive to pain. This is true not only of the liver, but also of the lungs, brain, kidneys, and intestines. Interestingly, the walls of most organs are insensitive to malignant involvement unless obstruction or ulceration also occurs.

The quality and location of visceral pain are in part determined by the neurology of the afferent supply. Localization to the center of the body is known to occur initially with most organ pain. Embryologically, the gastrointestinal tract and related structures originate as midline organs that receive bilateral innervation. Therefore, if a visceral afferent is activated, transmission occurs to both the right and the left sides of the spinal cord, making localization (lateralization) impossible. In other words, most stimulation is projected so that only a central recognition is possible. Overlapping of innervation to more than one organ and the multilevel input at the spinal cord make vertical localization difficult. For example, the lower esophagus, stomach, proximal duodenum, gallbladder, liver, and pancreas are innervated from the same levels of the spinal cord (T5-T10). (See **Table 31–3**.) This overlap in segmental innervation also accounts for the phenomenon of referred pain, either somatovisceral or viscerosomatic. About 75% of thoracic and lumbar dorsal horn neurons receive both somatic and visceral input. It appears that no specific group of spinal neurons responds to visceral input.[3]

The quality of pain is also a reflection of the neurologic logic behind a system designed for retreat and one for homeostasis. Somatic pain is often sharp and localized, with a reflex response of retreat. Visceral pain is usually due to an existing process such as inflammation

Table 31–3 Some Hepatobiliary Diseases

Condition	Summary Information
Immune disorders Autoimmune (lupoid) hepatitis	• A form of chronic hepatitis that is believed to be immune mediated. • Affects primarily females in the age group of 20–30 years. • ANA and other auto-antibodies are elevated.
Primary biliary cirrhosis	• An immune disorder involving T-cells that destroys the intrahepatic bile ducts, affecting females in the age group of 30–60 years. • Found in hepatic transplant patients and those having bone marrow transplantation. • An abrupt onset characterized by nonspecific complaints of fatigue, anorexia, and weight loss; also may have mild hemolytic anemia, atrophic gastritis, and thyroiditis, jaundice, and steatorrhea with small yellow subcutaneous lesions called xanthomas. • Dx with demonstration of antimitochondrial antibodies and with liver biopsy results. • Only chance for survival is liver transplantation.
Primary sclerosing cholangitis	• Found primarily in young males (ages 20–40 years), this immune disorder destroys both intra- and extrahepatic bile ducts via cell-mediated immune reaction. • A cellular phase followed by a fibrous stage that destroys bile ducts, leading to obstructive jaundice. • Some patients may also have inflammatory bowel disease with cholangiocellular carcinoma occurring in 10% of patients. • Treatment is with liver transplantation.
Carcinomas Liver cell adenoma	• These benign tumors resembling normal hepatocytes are almost exclusively seen in women. • There appears to be a relationship to the use of oral contraceptives. • Tumors are highly vascular and as a result may bleed, leading to death in some patients.
Hepatocellular carcinoma	• The male-to-female ratio is approximately 5:1, with the highest incidence in Asia and Africa (low in the U.S. and Europe); usually occurs in middle age (30–50 years of age). • Risk factors include those with cirrhosis secondary to hepatitis B, hepatitis C, hemochromatosis, and α1-antitrypsin deficiency. • Initial symptoms may be nonspecific, such as weight loss, loss of appetite, and nausea. • Further symptoms/signs may be related to several events: hepatomegaly with tenderness, bloody ascites and splenomegaly from portal hypertension, intravenous thrombosis (Budd-Chiari syndrome), various manifestations of paraneoplastic syndromes including insulin-like secretions leading to hypoglycemia, erythrocytosis from erythropoietin secretion, hyperestrinism, hypercholesterolemia, and hypercalcemia. • The diagnosis is made through liver biopsy and an assay for alpha-fetoprotein (AFP) for early detection. • The 5-year survival rate is 10%.
Cholangiocellular carcinoma	• A malignant adenocarcinoma tumor of the bile ducts; this tumor is rare in the U.S. • Associated with infection from the liver fluke, *C. sinensis*; primary sclerosing cholangitis is also a risk factor, although rare. • May originate from either intrahepatic or extrahepatic bile ducts, with the extrahepatic duct producing jaundice early on with a resultant increase in survival rate due to the early recognition. • 5-year survival for intrahepatic is 10%, whereas it is 35% for those involving the common bile duct and papilla of Vater.
Gallbladder carcinoma	• This carcinoma is more common in older patients and those with gallstones, such as Native Americans, with a female-to-male ratio of 2:1. • It appears that individuals with a body mass index (BMI) ≥ 25 kg/m² combined with low total physical activity have a higher risk, likely due to hyperinsulinemia. • Initially restricted to the gallbladder, symptoms are minimal. Extension into the liver may herald onset of jaundice or intestinal obstruction. • Late Dx leads to a poor prognosis with the opportunity for resection passed. • The 5-year survival rate is only 5%.

(continues)

Condition	Summary Information
Table 31–3 Some Hepatobiliary Diseases (continued)	
Hereditary disorders	
Gilbert's syndrome	• An autosomal dominant disorder of bilirubin metabolism involves an enzyme defect related to uptake of bilirubin from the blood to the liver; occurs in 5% of population.
	• More common in males, the only sign of disease is intermittent jaundice that appears around puberty.
	• Unconjugated hyperbilirubinemia is found.
	• No treatment is required.
Hemochromatosis	• An autosomal recessive defect in iron absorption leading to excess accumulation of iron in the liver and other organs.
	• Although the gene defect is found in 10% of the population, only 0.4 are homozygous and a small proportion of those individuals are symptomatic. Males are more commonly affected than females (10:1 to 20:1).
	• Triad includes bronze skin, liver cirrhosis, and diabetes mellitus.
	• When joints are affected there may be pain, stiffness, and swelling; usually bilateral, however, may begin in a single joint.
	• Laboratory includes elevated ESR and serum iron, increased saturation of plasma iron binding and liver biopsy findings.
	• Radiographically, usually bilateral involvement with osteoporosis, CPPD crystal deposition, and involvement of MCP joints.
	• Weekly phlebotomies are the treatment approach to prolong lives.
Wilson's disease	• An autosomal recessive disorder of copper metabolism producing lesions in the eye, brain, and liver; believed to be due to inability to excrete copper into bile.
	• Incidence is 3 in 100,000.
	• In eyes, copper deposition is seen as a Kayser-Fleischer ring (brownish discoloration of the iris).
	• In the brain, closely resembles basal ganglia disease.
	• Chelating agents are used such as D-penicillamine for prevention and management.

or infection. Given that an individual cannot escape from his or her body, the purpose seems more to provide a reflex splinting resulting in immobilization. The quality is often dull and aching (prior to peritoneal or capsular irritation), and there is no retreat response.

The afferent supply to internal organs follows a path similar to that of the sympathetic nervous system, often in close proximity to blood vessels. The nerve cell bodies are located in the dorsal root ganglion (similar to the somatic system). The fibers of these splanchnic nerves follow the sympathetic chains and enter the cord via the white rami communicants. The fibers enter the dorsal horn, and, through the tract of Lissauer, travel several segments cranially and caudally to end in laminae I and V. There are a small number of visceral fibers and receptors compared with those in the somatic system (such as the skin or even peritoneum). This sparse innervation often allows small, localized damage to be asymptomatic.

The stimulus must be strong enough to involve an area large enough to stimulate enough receptors to produce a conscious perception of pain.

Organ pain may become somatic pain and allow localization. This occurs when a somatic structure around an organ is stimulated, such as the peritoneum, pleura, pericardium, or capsule (liver and kidneys). These somatically innervated structures allow cortical or thalamic localization as a result of the unilateral innervation afforded by the spinal nerves of the thoracolumbar area and the phrenic nerve. Specifically, the phrenic nerve (C3-C5) innervates portions of the pericardium, the biliary tract, and the central zone of the diaphragm. The thoracic and upper lumbar spinal nerves innervate the parietal pleura, the parietal peritoneum, the outer diaphragm, and the roots of the mesentery of the intestines. The parietal peritoneum and the segmentally related dermatome (skin), sclerotome (bone), and

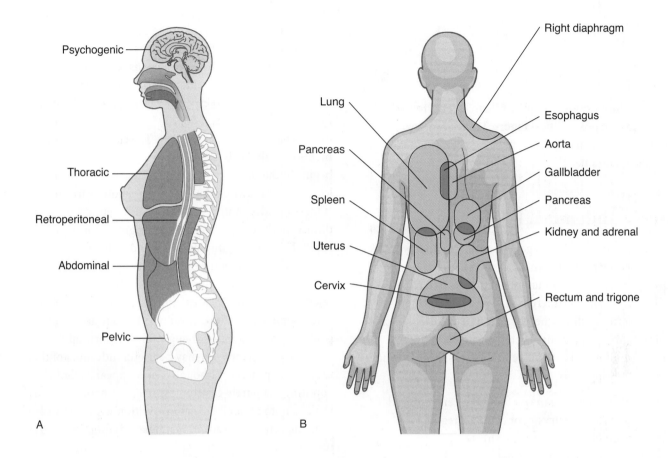

Basic considerations:
- Back pain may be the earliest manifestation of visceral disease.
- Pain due to metastatic lesions may be severe before x-ray confirmation.
- Visceral origin of back pain should be considered when there is an absence of muscular spasm, tenderness, and impaired mobility.
- Persistent backache due to extraspinal pathology is rare in children, common in adults.
- Backache may occur in any acute systemic infection.
- Myocardial infarction can cause back pain.
- Lumbar spasm may accompany the severe pain of certain retroperitoneal diseases.
- Radicular pain may occur with visceral lesions, as in sciatic radiation due to hypernephroma
- Just as visceral disease may suggest spinal pathology, so may the radiation of spinal lesions suggest a visceral origin of pain.
- Do not overlook the possibility of rectal and bladder lesions in persistent coccygodynia.

Figure 31–1 (A) Extraspinal causes of back pain: some basic considerations. (B) General visceral map in backache.

myotome (muscle) are truly overlapping. Irritation of one of these structures may refer pain to its segmentally related partner(s) (see **Figure 31–1**).

The appendix serves as a review of the above concepts. If the appendix is distended or inflamed, visceral afferents will be stimulated, usually leading to a perception of periumbilical, central pain. This is more likely to occur if the distention is rapid. If, however, the appendix were inflamed or distended enough to irritate the local peritoneum, somatic afferents would be stimulated, localizing the pain to the right lower quadrant (McBurney's point). Similar events could occur with the gallbladder, with referred pain to the right scapula due to a segmentally related overlap.

Evaluation

History

Pain localization is often quite valuable in narrowing down the possibilities. **Figure 31–2** summarizes some possible causes based on pain localization to a specific quadrant.

Acute Abdominal Pain

Acute abdominal pain is a generic term. In other words, a patient may present with a pain that began within a few seconds, a few minutes, or over hours to days; all are called acute. This distinction may be a relevant starting point in deciding whether or not to make a medical referral. Abrupt pain that begins within seconds to a matter of minutes is often due to a serious disorder, such as the following:

- rupture of an organ (perforated ulcer, ruptured abdominal aneurysm, or ectopic pregnancy)
- torsion (testicular or ovarian)
- blockage of a nonintestinal lumen (cholelithiasis, ureteral stone, and rarely acute appendicitis)
- vascular occlusion (mesenteric infarction in the elderly or sickle cell crisis)

The seriousness of the situation is not lost on the patient who calls 911 or rushes to the emergency department.

Pain that appears rather abruptly over minutes and builds over hours to a few days is characteristic of a number of processes such as cholecystitis, pancreatitis, appendicitis, pelvic inflammatory disease, food poisoning, and diverticulitis. Also, many of the conditions that become chronic and recurrent have their advent as an acute pain such as in peptic ulcer, endometriosis, diverticulitis, and inflammatory bowel disorders. Pain that grows slowly over days or longer suggests an underlying inflammatory process or intestinal obstruction.

Still, the majority of patients with pancreatitis, cholecystitis, and appendicitis will have a belated trip to the emergency department, not the chiropractor's office. If the chiropractor inadvertently is present at the time of onset (or has had a personal attack of acute abdominal pain), however, it is important to determine what was eaten within 24 hours, past history of similar attacks, alcohol ingestion, and any premonitory signs.

The quality and location of the pain are obviously important. Dull, aching central pain in the epigastric, umbilical, or hypogastric area is nonspecific, but it indicates visceral involvement. If this pain migrates to a specific quadrant, and especially if this is accompanied by a change in the quality of the pain, local peritoneal or capsular involvement is likely. The classic example, as mentioned above, is the sequence of appendicitis that begins in the central abdomen and localizes to the right lower quadrant when the local peritoneum is irritated. If the appendix ruptures into the peritoneum, a more diffuse, peritoneal response with a rigid abdomen will result. Pain that begins anteriorly and radiates to the back is often felt in a region segmentally related to the organ. For example, pain from a perforated ulcer is referred to the T6-T10 area; uterus, to the lumbopelvic area; esophagus, to the central midthoracic area; and gallbladder, to the inferior angle of the right scapula.

Associated symptoms may be useful indicators of the underlying process. Although it may appear as though vomiting is a purely gastrointestinal (GI) symptom, it is important to remember that in addition vagal stimulation, intracranial pressure, vestibular dysfunction, and metabolic processes (uremia, acidosis, chemotherapy, hypoxia, and toxins) may also induce vomiting. The timing of vomiting may be important. If vomiting occurs before abdominal pain, a "surgical" cause is less likely. Early gastroenteritis, food poisoning, and drugs may present this way. If vomiting relieves abdominal pain, peptic ulcer disease (less commonly upper intestinal obstruction) is often the cause in a patient with epigastric pain. Vomiting does not relieve the pain of many other acute abdominal conditions such as pancreatitis and cholecystitis. The content of vomit may indicate where the process is located in the alimentary tract. If the vomit contains undigested food, gastroesophageal obstruction is likely. If the vomit smells like feces, intestinal obstruction is high on the list. Coffee-ground vomit indicates GI bleeding.

Mallory-Weiss syndrome is the primary cause of hematemesis. It is due to excessive pressure that causes tearing of the gastric mucosa and the esophagus. There may be extreme bleeding. Alcoholics are one of the at-risk groups. Bleeding usually spontaneously resolves. Management with vasopressin or angiographic embolization may be necessary, with surgery used in only rare cases.

Constipation and diarrhea are less specific indicators. If constipation precedes abdominal pain, the rectum or colon is probably involved. However, abdominal pain

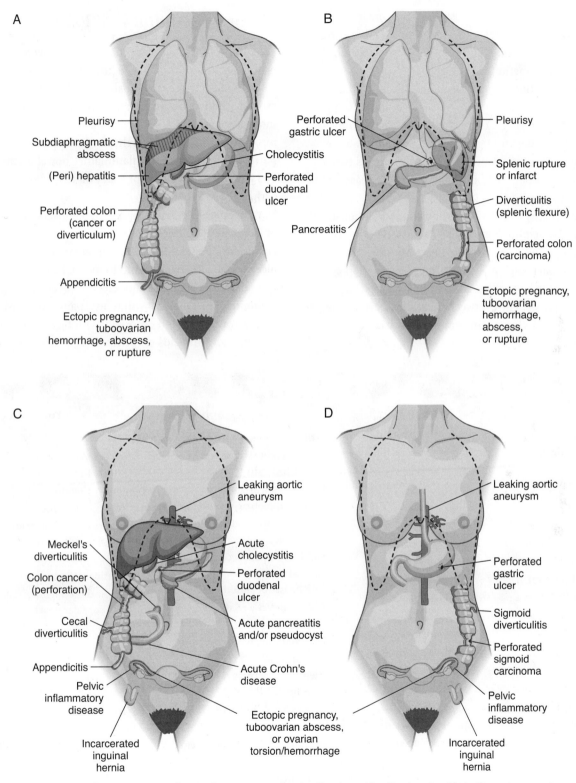

Figure 31–2 Common and uncommon conditions that may cause "parietal" pain and localized peritonitis in the various quadrants of the abdomen. (A) Right upper quadrant. (B) Left upper quadrant. (C) Right lower quadrant. (D) Left lower quadrant.

often causes a decrease in peristalsis; therefore, many patients with abdominal pain are constipated. For the same reason, anorexia is also nonspecific; however, if the patient has an appetite, serious disease is unlikely.

When the patient reports that family members or friends who shared a common meal have similar symptoms, food poisoning is likely. The onset of symptoms is highly variable depending on the underlying causative organism. This time frame varies from as little as two hours to as much as 48 hours; however, the average time is between four and eight hours.

In the female patient, the relationship to the menstrual cycle may be helpful. For example, a missed period or spotty last period may be a clue to ectopic pregnancy. Increase in pain during or soon after menstruation is suggestive of pelvic inflammatory disease in a sexually active female. Pain between menstrual periods may represent mittelschmerz, indicating an ovarian cyst or rupture.

Recurrent Abdominal Pain

When abdominal pain is recurrent, the differential list is decreased substantially. It is important to ask some general questions regarding alcohol abuse (pancreatitis, esophageal, hepatic, and gastric problems), medication intake (NSAIDs or other drugs causing gastric bleeding), predominance of diarrhea or constipation (irritable bowel syndrome versus inflammatory bowel disease), and a menstrual history (primary or secondary dysmenorrhea). (See **Table 31–4**.)

With epigastric pain, reflux esophagitis, peptic ulcer, or (much less commonly) pancreatitis is possible. Historical clues that help differentiate reflux from peptic ulcer include the relationship to meals. In general, food will relieve the pain of a duodenal ulcer (depending on the food type), whereas with reflux, pain is increased after a heavy meal and especially with tight garments or recumbency. Antacids may help both. It is important to

Table 31–4 History Questions for Recurrent Abdominal Pain

Primary Question	What Are You Thinking?	Secondary Questions	What Are You Thinking?
Is the pain in your upper abdomen?	Reflux esophagitis, peptic ulcer, pancreatitis, cholecystitis, or cholelithiasis	**Is the pain worse on an empty stomach?**	Duodenal ulcer likely
		Are you taking large doses of aspirin or other NSAIDs?	Gastric irritation, possible ulcer
		Do you drink alcohol often? (Perhaps use CAGE approach.)	Alcohol-related pancreatitis or ulcer irritation
		Do you feel worse after lying down after a heavy meal?	Reflux esophagitis
		Did a severe pain occur rather suddenly and last for several hours, associated with nausea or vomiting?	Biliary colic (cholecystitis)
			Possibly cholecystitis if severe; if epigastric and less severe consider reflux esophagitis
		Did you notice a relationship to fatty meals?	Peptic ulcer if it does; if it does not, consider pancreatitis or cholecystitis
		Does vomiting relieve the pain?	Food poisoning
		Did others in your family or did your friends also become sick after eating the same food?	
Is the pain lower in your abdomen?	Irritable bowel syndrome, inflammatory bowel diseases, dysmenorrhea, diverticulitis	**Do you have constipation that alternates with diarrhea?**	Irritable bowel syndrome likely
		Do you mainly have recurrent diarrhea?	Inflammatory bowel disease (most likely ulcerative colitis)
		(For females in reproductive years) Is the pain associated with your period?	Dysmenorrhea
		If the pain is related to your period, is it much worse than previously felt pain?	Secondary dysmenorrhea (most likely endometriosis)
		Lower left quadrant abdominal pain (in an older patient) with apparent change in stools?	Consider diverticulosis or colon cancer

question the patient regarding diet. Common foods may irritate a duodenal ulcer and increase reflux. Foods that lower the tone of the lower esophageal sphincter, leading to reflux, include chocolate, caffeine, fat, garlic, onions, and alcohol. Other substances include nicotine, theophylline, calcium channel blockers, and anticholinergic drugs.

Severe upper abdominal pain lasting for several hours and associated with nausea and sometimes vomiting is highly suggestive of cholelithiasis. A profile of female, fat, forty, and flatulent may be found; however, it is not an exclusive descriptor of the patient with biliary colic. The association of onset with a fatty meal also is not consistent. Alcoholic fatty liver is another possibility with upper right quadrant pain. Non-alcoholic fatty liver, also a cause of upper right pain, is becoming more common due to its association to obesity.

With the exception of menstrually related pain, recurrent lower abdominal pain generally can be grouped historically into those with bowel habit change and those without. Irritable bowel syndrome commonly causes alternating bouts of diarrhea and constipation. Usually constipation is the predominant symptom, with a characteristic passage of small, marble-sized stool in the morning that is associated with some mild diarrhea that may have mucus attached. The inflammatory bowel diseases often have diarrhea as a major complaint, often more than the abdominal pain with ulcerative colitis. Diverticulitis usually does not cause a change in bowel movement.

Recurrent cyclic pain in menstruating women is usually dysmenorrhea. Dysmenorrhea may be a "normal" problem that has established a baseline of pain for most females by their 20s. Any change in this pattern to a more severe menstrual pain is suggestive of secondary causes. High on this list is endometriosis.

Examination

Acute Abdominal Pain

With acute abdominal pain there are several clues with regard to the patient's posturing. Patients who are cautious to move for fear of increasing pain may have a peritoneal problem. Patients doubled over in pain or seeking relief by the fetal position are likely to have pancreatitis if the pain is upper abdominal. A patient who keeps the right leg in flexion and avoids extension may have appendicitis with irritation of the psoas muscle. Patients who cannot find a comfortable position and continue to move around or are writhing in pain will probably have a

ureteral stone (if associated with radiation into the groin) or cholecystitis (if the pain is upper abdominal).

Although a rare chiropractic office presentation, a patient with acute abdominal pain should be evaluated immediately for shock. Hypotension, tachycardia, impaired mentation, and oliguria are indications of volume loss from intra-abdominal bleeding or fluid loss. Shock requires an emergency department evaluation.

The yield on plain abdominal films (scout, kidney/ureter/bladder [KUB], flat plate) is usually quite low. Even in an emergency department setting, one study[4] indicated positive findings on only 10% of films. Most GI pathology is not visible on film. Free air from a perforated organ and bowel obstruction are the only nonstone indicators visible. Radiopacities indicating stones occur with gallstones, kidney stones, and fecaliths (with appendicitis). The yield is approximately 70% of the time with kidney stones, 10% to 15% with gallstones, and only 5% with fecaliths.[4] With gallstones, it is also important to recognize that finding stones does not always mean that the cause of the patient's abdominal pain has been found. There are significant numbers of asymptomatic patients with radiographic evidence of gallstones.

Laboratory studies may give general or very specific indications of an underlying process. On a general screen, a finding of leukocytosis with a shift to the left is an important indicator of an inflammatory reaction and, coupled with the history and location of pain, often will point to appendicitis or cholecystitis. Many acute inflammatory reactions may cause a similar finding, however. Acute pancreatitis also will raise the white blood cell (WBC) count and may have associated hyperglycemia, increased lactate dehydrogenase (LDH), and increased aspartate transaminase (AST) levels. With pancreatitis measurement of the specific isoenzyme p-amylase or, when measured later, lipase may assist in the diagnosis, but this is often performed in the hospital.

More specific are the urinalysis findings that may demonstrate an increase in red blood cells (RBCs) or WBCs. Microscopic hematuria (more than three cells per high-power field) is strong evidence of a ureteral stone in a patient with flank pain. Microscopic pyuria (more than five WBCs per high-power field) is suggestive of a urinary tract infection (UTI). Therefore, in a patient with pyuria, hematuria, and flank pain, pyelonephritis is likely. For patients with suspected ectopic pregnancy, a serum human chorionic gonadotropin (hCG), b-subunit test (pregnancy test) should be performed.

The abdominal examination is a sequential approach beginning with auscultation, progressing to percussion, then palpation.[5] The primary purpose of auscultation is to determine whether bowel sounds are present or absent. This may require up to three minutes. Complete absence is found with peritonitis and paralytic ileus. Although it may seem logical that bowel obstruction would also be a consideration, partial bowel obstruction often causes high-pitched rushes of bowel sounds. When bowel sounds are "hyperactive," gastroenteritis or intestinal bleeding should be considered. Percussion may be used to distinguish between air and fluid in the abdomen; however, it is more commonly used to detect referred tenderness. A positive rebound tenderness is often found at McBurney's point with appendicitis. Palpation is used to differentiate among masses that are superficial and deep. Superficial masses are still present with abdominal contraction. This is most common with incisions, umbilical hernias, or diastasis of the abdominals. Next, deeper palpation may distinguish among fat/feces, fluid, and masses that represent a tumor or fetus. In general, if there is lower abdominal tenderness that improves with a sustained pressure, feces or gas is likely the cause (especially when the patient reports relief with either passage of gas or a bowel movement).

The chiropractor should be conscious of the need for pelvic, testicular, and rectal examinations in patients with acute abdominal pain. If the chiropractor is unfamiliar or uncomfortable with these procedures, it is imperative that they be performed by a trained health professional. All indicators of pelvic inflammatory disease, testicular or ovarian torsion, and rectal masses indicating cancer will be missed without this portion of the examination.

Occasionally, mechanical testing will reproduce or exacerbate abdominal pain. Two apparently muscular responses may indicate underlying visceral irritating processes. The psoas sign is sometimes seen in patients with appendicitis.[6] The patient keeps the hip flexed and is reluctant to extend the leg. Resisted flexion or passive extension increases the pain. Another sign is the obturator sign. This is found more often with pelvic pathology in women. Internal rotation of the flexed hip may increase the abdominal pain in these patients.

Further evaluation with more sophisticated testing such as ultrasound, endoscopic ultrasound, transvaginal ultrasound, radionuclide scans, computed tomography (CT), ERCP, magnetic resonance imaging (MRI), or magnetic resonance cholangiopancreatography (MRCP) is dependent on one's underlying suspicion based on a thorough history and examination. In general, ultrasound is often used for appendicitis and cholelithiasis and, in women, to identify and differentiate among various pelvic processes such as tumors and ectopic pregnancy. Ultrasound is between 85% and 90% accurate for the diagnosis of gallstones.[7] Endoscopic retrograde cholangiopancreatography (ERCP) is often used diagnostically and therapeutically when there are stones, strictures, or dilatation of the bile or pancreatic ducts or sphincters. CT is reserved for abscess, tumors, or unexplained causes.

Recurrent or Chronic Abdominal Pain

The examination of chronic abdominal pain is often unrevealing. Laboratory testing is often necessary for upper right quadrant pain including liver function tests. Lower abdominal tenderness that is improved by slow sustained palpation pressure is suggestive of irritable bowel syndrome (IBS). A stool sample is important in the evaluation for parasites, occult blood, mucus, polymorphonuclear leukocytes (PMNs), and unprocessed food. Hemoccult testing must include three samples in an effort to increase the yield of the test.

Occult blood in the stool is not found with IBS but may be found with colon cancer and inflammatory bowel disease (IBD). Crohn's disease often has associated findings of fistulas and other anorectal disease. The stool sample will help differentiate between IBD and other causes of colitis such as parasitic infections (see Chapter 33).

Referral for sigmoidoscopy or colonoscopy is necessary with persistent diarrhea or suspicion of colorectal cancer or diverticulitis. Barium studies are occasionally used, but not during an acute attack of diverticulitis. Ultrasound may be helpful in the diagnosis of a number of disorders including, hepatobiliary, and genitourinary pathologies such as secondary dysmenorrhea, specifically with endometriosis. More recently, MRI with gadolinium may be used to accentuate the locations of endometrial implantation.

Management

A general rule of thumb is that if the pain has been present for two to three days and the physical examination shows no signs of abdominal distention, localized peritoneal irritation, or palpable masses, it is highly unlikely to be a "surgical" case.

Referral is still necessary when the pain is severe, or there are related signs of GI or genitourinary infection. Cases of gastroenteritis or food poisoning are often self-resolving, but the degree and abruptness of symptoms may cause the patient to seek medical attention.

The chiropractor's role in management of acute cases is to determine the need for referral for surgery or further investigation. The role in chronic or recurrent pain is to do the same; however, comanagement of patients with irritable bowel syndrome, inflammatory bowel syndromes, and diverticulitis may be appropriate. **Table 31–5** is a brief overview of common medications used in the management of some common chronic abdominal disorders. The focus of comanagement is the suggestion of or support of medical recommendations for lifestyle modifications and treatment of associated musculoskeletal complaints. These may include the following:

- high-fiber diet for diverticulosis
- avoidance of alcohol for pancreatitis
- avoidance or substitution for NSAIDs and other causes of gastric bleeding
- stress relaxation techniques and a balanced diet for patients with IBS
- avoidance of smoking, tight garments, high-fat meals, chocolate, and caffeine for reflux
- recommendation that the patient eat more frequent, smaller meals, and lose weight if necessary

An interesting phenomenon has developed with regard to management of peptic ulcer disease. Previously prescription-only medications, H₂ antagonists and proton-pump inhibitors are now available over the counter. The effectiveness of these medications in peptic disease and esophageal disease may make the patient reluctant to seek medical care. If the underlying cause of epigastric discomfort is peptic ulcer disease, however, the most effective treatment for long-term cure is a triple medication regimen that includes an antibiotic. Endoscopic evaluation is often suggested in patients over age 40 years or with an atypical pain presentation to rule out gastric carcinoma.

Algorithm

An algorithm for initial screening for abdominal pain is presented in **Figure 31–3**.

Table 31–5 GERD and Peptic Ulcer Medications

Drug Class	Examples	General Mechanism	Interactions/Side Effects
H2 Antagonists	Cimetidine Novo-Cimetidine Peptol Tagamet	An H2 (histamine) inhibitor blocking gastric acid secretion, raises pH of the stomach decreasing pepsin secretion. Used as an OTC medication in the management of ulcers, GERD, and Zollinger-Ellison syndrome.	May cause the usual GI symptoms, increase pain in joints for patients with pre-existing arthritis, rash, Stevens-Johnson syndrome, neutropenia, increase in uric acid, BUN, and creatinine, feminizing effects, and rarely aplastic anemia, or cardiac arrest.
	Famotidine Pepcid	An H2 (histamine) inhibitor blocking gastric acid secretion, raises pH of the stomach decreasing pepsin secretion. Used as an OTC medication in the management of ulcers, GERD, and Zollinger-Ellison syndrome.	May cause dizziness, headache, confusion, diarrhea, constipation, thrombocytopenia, rash, and may increase uric acid, BUN, and creatinine.
	Ranitidine Zantac	An H2 (histamine) inhibitor blocking gastric acid secretion. Used as an OTC medication in the management of ulcers and GERD.	May cause usually GI symptoms, dizziness, depression, reversible leukocytosis, thrombocytopenia, and possible decreases in liver enzymes.
Proton-pump inhibitors	Esomeprazole Nexium	Similar to omeprazole (isomer of Prilosec). A proton pump inhibitor, it inhibits H⁺K⁺-ATPase (acid production from parietal cells of stomach). Used for erosive esophagitis, GERD, and in concert with antibiotics for *H. pylori* infection with duodenal ulcer management.	May cause headache, nausea, vomiting, constipation, abdominal pain, and dry mouth.
	Omeprazole Prilosec Losec	A proton pump inhibitor, it inhibits H+K+-ATPase (acid production from parietal cells of stomach). Used for erosive esophagitis, GERD, and in concert with antibiotics (usually metronidazole and amoxicillin) for *H. pylori* infection with duodenal ulcer management.	May cause headache, nausea, vomiting, constipation, abdominal pain, and dry mouth.

(continues)

Table 31–5 GERD and Peptic Ulcer Medications (continued)

Drug Class	Examples	General Mechanism	Interactions/Side Effects
Other	**Sucralfate** Carafate Sulcrate	Used as part of GI ulcer therapy due to effects of creating a protective mucosal "paste" and inhibits pepsin, decreases bile absorption, and blocks back diffusion of H_+ ions. Valuable for smokers treated for duodenal ulcers.	Very few side effects. May cause constipation.

IBS Medications

Drug Class	Examples	General Mechanism	Interactions/Side Effects
Alosetron	Lotronex	Selective serotonin (5-HT3) receptor antagonist. These receptors are located throughout the myenteric plexus and have effect on distension perception, GI motility and secretions. Used in the control of abdominal pain and diarrhea with irritable bowel syndrome in women.	May cause constipation, ischemic colitis, urinary frequency, muscle cramps, weakness, and anxiety.
Tegaserod	Zelnorm	A serotonin 5-HT4 receptor agonist used in the management of constipation-predominant irritable bowel syndrome. The 5-HT4 receptor, a serotonin receptor, normalizes intestinal contractions. In addition, this medication acts to increase the pain threshold for distension of the colon.	May cause headache, dizziness, migraine, abdominal pain, nausea, flatulence, or back pain.

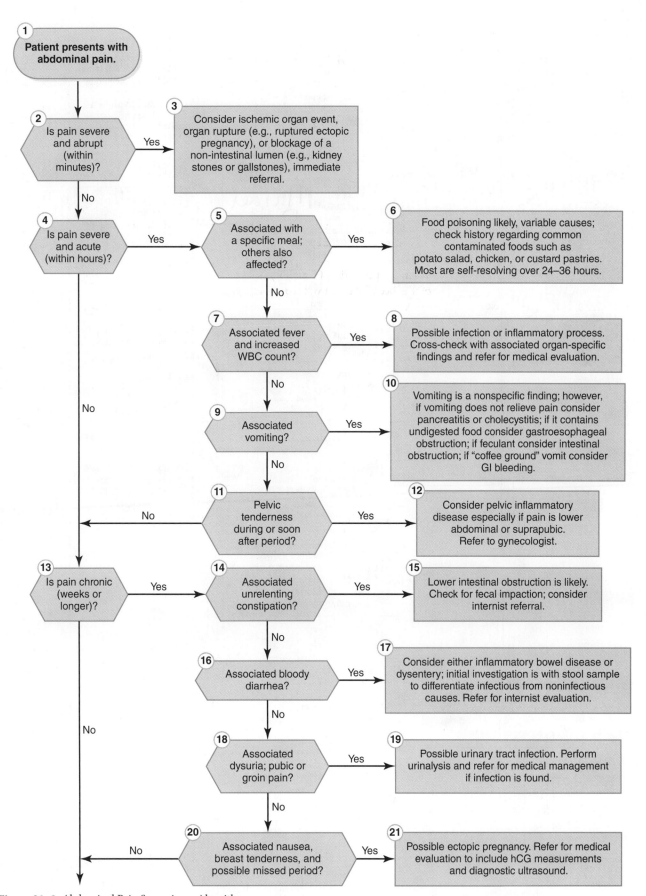

Figure 31–3 Abdominal Pain Screening—Algorithm

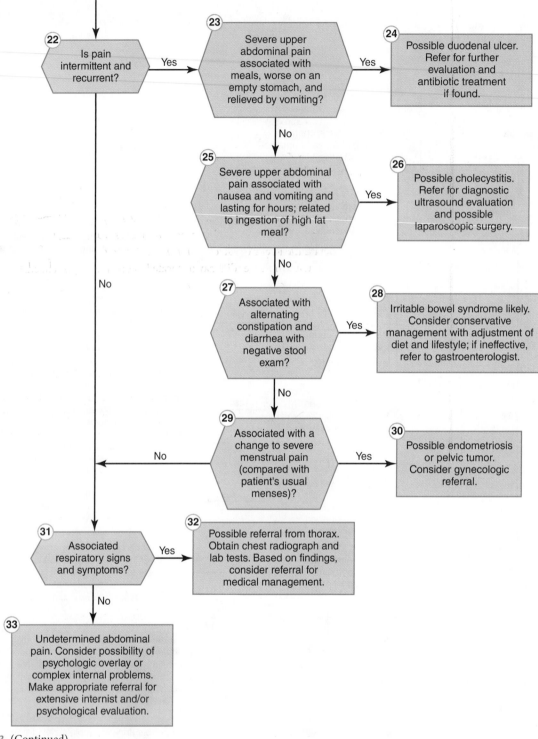

Figure 31–3 (Continued)

Reproduced from T. A. Souza, *Topics in Clinical Chiropractic*, Vol. 1, No. 1, pp. 68–69, © 1994, Aspen Publishers, Inc.

Selected Causes of Acute Abdominal Pain

Appendicitis

Classic Presentation

The classic presentation of acute appendicitis follows a sequence. The patient develops anorexia and poorly localized pain over the mid-abdomen that is followed by nausea or vomiting (75% of patients).[8] The pain then localizes to the right lower quadrant over the next 2 to 48 hours. At this point there is constant pain made worse by coughing or jarring. If the patient is not seen at this point, there may be a sudden relief of pain indicating rupture, usually followed by an increase in pain.

Cause/Occurrence

The cause of appendicitis is somewhat age-dependent. It is obstructed by inflammation (submucosal lymphoid hyperplasia) mainly in children and teens; by a fecalith in adults (most common), and by various other processes such as fruit seeds, worms, or tumor less often. It affects approximately 7% of the population, with the major occurrence in males between the ages of 10 and 30.[9] Atypical presentations occur in about 50% of cases; more often in adults. The appendix may be located in different areas, affecting the clinical presentation. It may lie anterior, posterior, medial, or lateral to the cecum or in the pelvis. Atypical presentation is most common with a pelvic or retrocecal location hidden from the overlying peritoneum.

Evaluation

In one literature review diagnostic information taken from the physical exam and special imaging were evaluated to determine the sensitivity and specificity for the diagnosis of appendicitis.[10] History findings that were most important were central pain migrating to right lower quadrant (RLQ) pain with anorexia and pain occurring before vomiting. There are two predictive scales used to diagnose appendicitis. One, the Alvarado score, was reviewed by Ohle et al.[11] who found that it was a useful "rule-out" approach if a cutoff score of 5 is used. However, its performance was inconsistent in children and overpredicted in women. To address the inconsistency in children, another scoring system, the Pediatric Appendicitis Score, was developed. Using the following eight variables, the Pediatric Appendicitis Score had a sensitivity of 1, specificity of 0.92, positive predictive value of 0.96, and negative predictive value of 0.99 with a score ≥6. Following are the variables with their respective positive predictive values.

1. Cough/percussion/hopping exacerbate pain in the right lower quadrant of the abdomen (0.96)
2. Anorexia (0.88)
3. Pyrexia (0.87)
4. Nausea/emesis (0.86)
5. Tenderness over the right iliac fossa (0.84)
6. Leukocytosis (0.81)
7. Polymorphonuclear neutrophilia (0.80)
8. Migration of pain (0.80)

Each of these variables was assigned a score of 1, except for physical signs (1 and 5), which were scored 2 to obtain a total of 10.

That being said, Schneider et al.[12] concluded that neither method provided sufficient positive predictive value to be used in the decision of whether surgery is needed or not. Also, using a single test such as rebound tenderness, which has an LR of 3.4, the prevalence is only around 5% to 7%, so that the post-test probability with a positive test is only about 20%.

In a review by Bundy et al.,[13] similar conclusions were drawn. They found that using likelihood ratios, fever was the single most sensitive sign associated with appendicitis, with a positive likelihood ratio (LR) of 3.4 and with no fever, a negative LR of 0.32. If a child appeared to have a classic clinical appearance, rebound tenderness provided an LR of 3.0, with no rebound tenderness resulting in a negative LR of 0.28. A white blood cell count of less than $10,000/\mu L$ decreases the likelihood of appendicitis with an LR of 0.22, as does an absolute neutrophil count of $6750/\mu L$ or lower with a negative LR of 0.06. As many as 40% of patients with appendicitis will have pyuria, hematuria, or bacteriuria. Urinary erythrocyte counts exceeding 30 cells per high powered field (PHPF), or leukocyte cell counts exceeding 20 cells PHPF suggest a urinary disorder.[14] Bowel sounds are not hyperactive as would be found with gastroenteritis. Because of the various locations of the appendix, some of the classic presentation and peritoneal findings may not be evident. If the appendix is retrocecal, it is hidden from the peritoneum, producing few peritoneal clues; however the psoas sign may be evident, where the patient cannot extend the right hip or resist hip extension without an increase in abdominal pain. The psoas sign is very specific, but not sensitive (not a good screening tool). If the appendix extends into the pelvis, it is less accessible to abdominal palpation and pain may be more easily provoked with a rectal examination or using the obturator sign where resisted rotation of the hip with the hip flexed 90° increases the abdominal pain.

In the elderly, only two-thirds of patients have RLQ pain.[15] Laboratory findings are nonspecific, indicating a mild leukocytosis. The diagnosis in female patients is complicated by possible gynecologic causes including ovarian cysts, ectopic pregnancy, and pelvic inflammatory disease among others. A pelvic examination should always be performed by an experienced professional on all women with abdominal pain of unknown origin. In one study[16] the false positive laparotomy rate was twice as high in women. This rate has been much improved, however, with the use of ultrasound.

The choice of imaging for appendicitis is based on cost, expediency, availability, and type of patient. The definitive diagnostic tool has for a long time been high-resolution, real-time ultrasonography (US).[17] Interpretation is operator-dependent though.[18] The specificity is about 81% with the sensitivity at around 86%. Currently, CT has been recommended. CT has been demonstrated to have a sensitivity of 91% to 98% and specificity of 95% to 99% with an overall accuracy of 98%.[19] CT with IV contrast has been shown to be as good as rectal or oral contrast without the delayed time to image.[20] CT with contrast is helpful in difficult cases because terminal ileitis can mimic appendicitis even radiographically (without contrast).[21] There is still concern, though, that for young patients, the amount of radiation is too high. MRI is growing in popularity for subgroups of patients—those who are pregnant, are allergic to contrast, or have renal failure. The newest experimental approach, radioisotope-labeled WBC scans, used for atypical presentations of appendicitis, uses leukoscintigraphy with sulesomab (antigranulocyte antibody Fab fragment). This technique has a high sensitivity and specificity in atypical cases. The negative predictive value in one study[22] was 97%, which would theoretically prevent unnecessary surgery in those cases.

Management

Laparoscopic appendectomy is the standard treatment. The most common abdominal operation performed in the United States is appendectomy, with as many as 250,000 performed annually.[23] In equivocal cases, most commonly in females, an exploratory laparotomy is performed, with 20% of those operated on having a normal appendix. In fact, with females and older patients, the error rate for managing pain in the right lower quadrant has approached 40% in some studies.[24] It has been recommended and demonstrated that for those who do not warrant immediate surgery, waiting 6 to 10 hours to observe and obtain further information has significantly decreased the rate of unnecessary surgery.[25]

A review by Andersson[25] suggests that spontaneous resolution of untreated appendicitis is more common than previously thought. He insists that patients can be managed by active observation in the hospital with a thorough diagnostic workup instead of a rush to surgery in an effort to avert perforation. Yet, treatment with only antibiotics will result in a recurrence of appendicitis within the first year of between 14% to 20%.[26] The rupture rate in pregnant females is 40%. In seniors the rupture rate is much higher at 67% to 90%. Also, a ruptured appendix will result in death about 3% of the time (those >60 years old account for 50% of deaths).

Cholecystitis/Cholelithiasis

Classic Presentation

A middle-aged or older woman complains of severe abdominal pain associated with nausea and vomiting that occurred rather abruptly after eating a fatty meal. The patient may report having had similar attacks in the past that resolved (60% to 75% of patients).[27]

Cause/Occurrence

The cause of cholecystitis (acute inflammation of the gallbladder) is blockage of the cystic duct by gallstones (90% of the time). Other causes may include pancreatitis or vascular abnormalities of the cystic duct. There are particular patient populations and risk factors to consider. Cholecystitis is more common in women.

Approximately 800,000 hospitalizations and 500,000 cholecystectomies occur each year.[28] Direct costs of over $2 billion and indirect costs approaching $5 billion are tied to gallbladder disease in the United States. Estimates are that 10% of men and 20% of women over age 65 years have gallstones; many are asymptomatic. Ethnic groups at high risk are Native Americans of both North and South America. Blacks are at less risk unless they have sickle cell disease. Patients who are obese, lose substantial weight, or take birth control pills or estrogen are at higher risk. Patients who are pregnant or who have Crohn's disease, cirrhosis, or diabetes are also at increased risk. Gallstones are usually classified as cholesterol stones or calcium bilirubinate stones. The cause for cholesterol stone development is suspected to be increased biliary secretion of cholesterol, delayed emptying of the gallbladder, or other factors that allow precipitation of cholesterol. Cholesterol stones account for 75% of all gallstones. Calcium bilirubinate stones are caused by the breakdown products of hemolysis.

Evaluation

Most patients will have an attack of severe pain with nausea and vomiting that lasts between 12 and 18 hours and then resolves. Twenty-five percent of patients are jaundiced, which represents a possible complication of common duct obstruction.

Tenderness is in the right upper quadrant (RUQ) with a positive Murphy's sign. This test involves gradually palpating under the lower right rib margins anteriorly and determining whether patient inspiration dramatically increases pain. The patient often has rebound tenderness in the RUQ (essentially the same as a Murphy's sign). The patient may also have referred pain to the inferior border of the scapula. The gallbladder may be palpable 15% of the time. Laboratory evaluation reveals a mild leukocytosis with a shift to the left. Higher ranges suggest gangrene or other complications. Alkaline phosphatase may also be elevated. Ultrasonography is the definitive diagnostic tool. Results from a review of the literature article indicated that no single clinical or laboratory test is able to establish or exclude cholecystitis without further evaluation with diagnostic ultrasound.[29] Highest on the list for specificity (rule-out) was the Murphy's sign and with laboratory evaluation, a combination of fever with leukocytosis. ALT, AST, alkaline phosphatase, and bilirubin were not very sensitive or specific. Diagnostic US has a specificity of 80% and sensitivity of 88%.

Decisions regarding imaging are now more complex but varied. Dependent on whether there are gallstones in the gallbladder versus in the ducts and whether there is concern regarding other abnormalities of the biliary ductal system, diagnostic approaches other than ultrasound may be utilized. ERCP uses a combination of endoscopy and fluoroscopy. ERCP is often used diagnostically and therapeutically when there are stones, strictures, or dilatation of the bile or pancreatic ducts or sphincters. In fact, given other imaging approaches such as MRCP and endoscopic ultrasound are safer and do not carry the radiation risk of fluoroscopy, ERCP is used less often unless there is a prior assumption that it will be used for both diagnostic and therapeutic purposes.

Management

There are several treatment options; however, the standard is laparoscopic cholecystectomy.[30] The patient is released in one day and returns to daily activities in a few days. A relatively common residual of cholecystectomy is persistent diarrhea.[31] Due to a decrease in colonic transit time, an increased defecation frequency and/or decreased stool consistency is found in as many as one-third of patients following surgery. Another treatment option is dissolution therapy with bile salts. The success rate is variable, and half of patients have recurrence within five years after stopping therapy. It may take up to two years for dissolution, and the medication often is expensive. Lithotripsy is available for patients with single stones less than 20 mm in size.[32]

Prevention is possible. Losing weight and keeping it off for obese patients will reduce their risk (ping-pong dieting or rapid weight loss over short periods of time will increase the risk). Several studies[33,34] have indicated that independent of obesity, for both men and women, the degree of physical activity is related to gallbladder disease. Men and women who exercise often are at much lower risk of developing symptomatic gallbladder disease. For men, one major study[35] indicated a decreased risk of gallstone development for those individuals who ingested consistently two to four or more cups of coffee per day regardless of which brewing method was used. The effect was not seen with tea or decaffeinated coffee. The proposed mechanism is cholecystokinin release, increased gallbladder motility, large bowel motility, inhibition of biliary cholesterol crystallization, or through cafestol (lipid component of coffee beans) that might affect bile cholesterol concentration.

Ureteral Stone

Classic Presentation

The patient reports a sudden onset of pain that is severe and often episodic. The pain is often felt at the costovertebral area of the lower ribs posteriorly, radiating anteriorly, often into the groin (testes in men, labia in women). There is associated nausea and vomiting.

Cause/Occurrence

Stones develop for two main reasons: lack of appropriate hydration and dietary factors. There are three common types of stones. The most common are calcium oxalate, uric acid, and cysteine. An environment for stone precipitation is created by excessive intake of calcium, oxalates, or protein.[36] This, in combination with insufficient water intake, sets the stage for stone formation in predisposed individuals. An environmental factor that may play a role is a humid, hot geographic area. Stones are more likely to form in the summer months. Other risk factors are family history of stones, white race, and a diet high in salt. About 80% of stones are composed of calcium salts. Urolithiasis develops in about 12% of the U.S. population each year with about a 75% recurrence, with about half occurring within five years.[37] Stone formation is much more common in men than women (4:1), usually occurring in the 30s or 40s. In the elderly, the ratio is almost even.

Evaluation

The patient is often constantly moving or writhing in pain, unable to find a position of relief. Prior to imaging, pain is addressed through the use of morphine or meperidine, or more recently some NSAIDs. The location of the pain, a urinalysis indicating hematuria, and a plain film of the abdomen indicating a corresponding radiopacity are often diagnostic. If not, noncontrast helical CT is the imaging tool of choice. The diagnostic accuracy is between 94% and 96%.[38] The advantages of helical CT are time (less than 1 minute), ability to detect all calculi regardless of composition, and differential diagnosis for other causes.

A check of creatinine, electrolytes, calcium, and phosphorus may be needed during the attack to determine if the obstruction is impairing renal function. An elevated WBC count may indicate a more serious involvement. After the attack has resolved, a laboratory search for cause may be appropriate. Elevated serum calcium or phosphorous may indicate primary hyperparathyroidism. Elevated uric acid may indicate gout. High cysteine levels may indicate cystinuria. Also, one to two 24-hour urine collections are recommended, with a third 24-hour urinalysis after dietary restrictions; a calcium load test is recommended to detect any calcium processing abnormality.

Management

The pain is usually severe enough to warrant an emergency department visit. About 80% of stones pass spontaneously, with about 20% of patients requiring hospitalization. Management is often symptomatic with follow-up monitoring. Stones that are 5 mm or less in diameter will likely pass without need of intervention. To assist the passage of stones, calcium channel-blockers are sometimes given. They have the effect of dilating the ureters. It is important to know that overhydration during an attack will not force the stones out. If the stone is large enough or is caught at an anatomic juncture, lithotripsy or ureteroscopic stone extraction is utilized.[39] Lithotripsy is contraindicated with pregnancy. Success rate with lithotripsy is about 85% and may require a second or third treatment.

The key to prevention is hydration and dietary management. The patient should be advised to double water intake; the patient should drink water between meals, with meals, and before going to bed at night. It is important that the patient understand that water intake is preferred at a level of about ten 10-oz glasses per day. A large retrospective study[40] of women suggests that coffee, tea, and wine, although acting as diuretics, do not seem to increase the chance of recurrence. Grapefruit juice should be avoided though. Interestingly, a high-calcium diet does not seem to predispose an individual to stone formation unless he or she has absorptive hypercalciuria (increased absorption of intestinal calcium). In fact, a low-calcium diet may increase urinary oxalate and increase risk of stone formation. Moderate dietary calcium intake is recommended for most patients. Fifty percent of those who do not follow this advice will have symptomatic stones again within five years. Patient adherence to hydration and dietary advice is generally quite low. Those with uric acid stones may have a return attack within months if therapy is not initiated and fluid advice is not heeded.[41] One herb that has been shown to decrease the formulation of kidney stone in rat studies is *Herniaria hirsuta*.[42] Further research on humans will be needed before knowing whether this medicinal Moroccan plant could be used as prophylaxis for those with recurrent stones.

Pancreatitis

Classic Presentation

The patient is often an alcohol abuser who develops a sudden onset of epigastric pain associated with nausea and vomiting. The pain often radiates to the back. The patient is in a bent-forward or fetal position to relieve pain.

Cause

Although the primary cause is alcohol abuse, there are a myriad of other possibilities including but not limited to:[43]

- Gallstones
- Many medications including ACE inhibitors, corticosteroids, statins, and diuretics, among others (the symptoms may not develop for weeks after initiating therapy)
- Sudden stoppage of medications for diabetes and hyperlipidemia
- Surgical procedures including ERCP
- Infection including most commonly, mumps

It appears that edema or obstruction of the ampulla of Vater causes a reflux of bile into the pancreatic ducts or acinar cells. The result is the release of pancreatic enzymes into the surrounding tissue. This sequence is often initiated by heavy alcohol intake.

Evaluation

There is often a mild fever, a tender and often distended upper abdominal region, and possible signs of hypotension. Because the pancreas is retroperitoneal, a palpable mass or rebound tenderness is not a common feature. Bowel sounds are often absent, and the patient may demonstrate a mild degree of jaundice. In rare cases, there may be hemorrhage, resulting in third-spacing, and clinically evident with flank discoloration (Grey Turner's sign) or discoloration surrounding the umbilicus (Cullen's sign). Although the laboratory may demonstrate mild leukocytosis, proteinuria and glycosuria (25%), hyperglycemia, and elevated bilirubin, the classic tests are serum amylase and lipase; both elevated more than three times normal. Although sensitive to pancreatitis, these tests are not always specific. The isoenzyme *p*-amylase is more specific. When transaminases rise dramatically, there is a 95% chance of bile duct obstruction as a cause of the pancreatitis. Imaging is not as valuable as with other abdominal problems. Plain films usually show indirect signs, including an air-filled small intestine or transverse colon. The sequence of imaging ordered is usually ultrasound followed by CT. CT is broadly the best tool because it can rule out other causes of abdominal pain, assess the damage associated with pancreatitis, and establish a baseline for follow-up imaging. Ultrasound is less valuable because of the artifact of gas distention but may still be helpful in evaluating gallbladder and stone involvement. MRCP is also used when available and can determine ductal changes. A grading system developed by Ranson is often used to estimate the prognosis with pancreatitis; however, its sensitivity is quite low at 40%.[44] The more positive criteria met, the higher the morbidity rate. In general, in an older patient with high glucose and elevation of liver enzymes, the prognosis is poorer. The APACHE II approach is more accurate but is considered more difficult to apply.[45]

Management

There are two main complications of acute pancreatitis: (1) hypovolemia secondary to intravascular fluid loss to the bowels, and (2) adult respiratory distress syndrome (ARDS). These usually occur within a few days to one week after the acute attack. In general the treatment for pancreatitis is bed rest with no food or fluids by mouth and pain medication. A nasogastric tube is often required. Follow-up imaging is usually necessary several weeks after the episode. Spontaneous resolution occurs in 85% to 90% of cases; mortality occurs in approximately 3% to 5%. After resolution, the preventive program is simply avoidance of the causative agent if medication- or alcohol -induced. Continued attacks may lead to chronic pancreatitis. This may be demonstrated on radiographs as pancreatic calcification. Also, being obese or overweight predicts severity of attacks if recurrent; therefore, dietary considerations should be discussed.[46]

Pelvic Inflammatory Disease

Classic Presentation

The patient is a woman of childbearing years who is sexually active (often with multiple partners) and who presents with a complaint of lower abdominal pain with associated chills and fever, dyspareunia (painful intercourse), and vaginal (cervical) discharge.

Cause

There are several major organisms that cause pelvic inflammatory disease (PID) of the upper genital tract in women. The primary organisms are *Chlamydia trachomatis* and *Neisseria gonorrhoeae*. Other organisms include *Haemophilus influenzae* and some enteric organisms. PID is more likely to occur in nonwhites and those who smoke or douche. Oral contraceptives or barrier methods of protection may help prevent infection. However, use of an intrauterine device (IUD) will increase the risk of PID for several months after insertion unless preinsertion counseling and proper selection of patients is followed.[47] Because vaginal douching is associated with bacterial vaginosis, PID, and ectopic pregnancy, and because there are no proven benefits, douching should be discouraged for adolescent girls and young women.[48]

Evaluation

The diagnosis may be difficult because many women are relatively asymptomatic. For asymptomatic, sexually active adolescent and young women, screening using urine-based ligase chain reaction (polymerase chain reaction [PCR] assay) is recommended as a cost-effective strategy to detect chlamydial and gonococcal genital infection, allowing early treatment and avoidance of the possible complications of PID, ectopic pregnancy, and bacterial vaginosis.[49] In acute scenarios, the differentiation of PID from appendicitis and other causes is sometimes necessary. The most predictive clues for PID are:[50]

- a history of the disorder
- a history of vaginal discharge
- vaginal discharge upon examination
- urinary symptoms and an abnormal urinalysis
- tenderness outside the RLQ
- tenderness upon cervical motion during pelvic examination

The patient may describe a slow onset of pain that begins during or soon after menstruation. The presentation of lower abdominal pain is relatively nonspecific; however, a pelvic examination will usually reveal adnexal and cervical motion tenderness or a palpable mass. Sometimes the presentation is bilateral lower abdominal pain and suprapubic pain. Laboratory testing is rarely helpful; however, if a woman with lower abdominal pain, adnexal tenderness, fever, and an elevated WBC count also presents with cervical discharge, PID is high on the list. Culdocentesis or Gram staining of discharge may reveal the underlying cause. Most patients will undergo ultrasound, which may help differentiate any masses felt on examination. The definitive diagnosis is with laparoscopy, but most women are treated with antibiotics with an assumption of PID. One study[51] indicated that the diagnoses of only 65% of women with PID were confirmed laparoscopically.

Management

Treatment is with appropriate antibiotics. Failure to recognize the diagnosis or to treat the disease may result in an ascending infection to the capsule of the liver called the Fitz-Hugh-Curtis syndrome. Also, the long-term consequences may include scarring that interferes with fertility or leads to an ectopic pregnancy. Chronic pelvic pain is also more likely in these patients.

Ectopic Pregnancy

Classic Presentation

The patient is a woman of childbearing years who complains of lower abdominal pain and a missed or "spotty" period over six to eight weeks prior to the pain onset.

Cause

Implantation of the ovum outside the uterine cavity occurs in approximately 1% of pregnancies. Ninety-eight percent of the time this is in the fallopian tubes. Predispositions include prior PID, IUD use (especially with progesterone), douching, progesterone-only contraceptives, endometriosis, or tubal ligation.[52]

Evaluation

The classic findings include adnexal tenderness on the pelvic examination coupled with a positive pregnancy test (b-hCG). The b-hCG level is higher than 5,000 to 6,000 mIU/mL with uterine pregnancies; ectopic pregnancy usually produces levels less than 3,000 mIU/mL. Also, if the test is followed over several days, the levels will rise slowly with an ectopic pregnancy, whereas they usually double with a normal pregnancy. A low b-hCG level (<1,500 mIU/mL) with an associated low progesterone level (<10 ng/mL) is highly supportive of an ectopic pregnancy.[53] For further differentiation, a transvaginal ultrasound examination is used in an effort to visualize an ectopic mass.

Management

Treatment is usually through laparoscopy. Recent studies indicate a role for methotrexate to destroy the placenta.[54]

Selected Causes of Recurrent Abdominal Pain

UPPER ABDOMINAL PAIN

Peptic Ulcer (Duodenal and Gastric)

Classic Presentation

Usually onset begins in a young man (teenage or the 20s; however, may occur from ages 30 to 50 years with duodenal ulcer; over age 50 years for gastric ulcer) and is felt as epigastric pain that is often reported as waking the patient from sleep. The pain is intermittent and recurrent. Antacids and over-the-counter (OTC) H2 antagonist or proton-pump inhibitors seem to provide relief. Classic presentations and classic relationships to pain on an empty stomach that is relieved by food are not consistent. Sixty percent of patients with complications such as bleeding or perforation have had no prior history of symptoms. As many as half of patients with NSAID ulcers are asymptomatic.

Cause

The major cause of gastric ulcers is NSAID use. The main cause of duodenal ulcer is *Helicobacter pylori* infection. Although gastric ulcers are due to a breakdown of the protective mechanisms in the stomach against acid and pepsin, the *H. pylori* role with duodenal ulcers is not yet defined. Ninety-five percent of duodenal ulcers occur at the bulb or pyloric channel. Benign gastric ulcers occur mainly at the antrum.

Evaluation

The physical examination is usually unrevealing. Laboratory testing may reveal anemia from blood loss or leukocytosis if the ulcer is perforated. Noninvasive testing for *H. pylori* infection includes office-based antibody testing, stool antigen testing, and nonendoscopic urease tests. Due to problems of false positives and the inability to distinguish between active disease versus those who have had infection in the past, stool *H. pylori* antigen testing (HpSA) and urea breath testing are the most commonly used tests.[55] Although the urea breath test is expensive, it is not as expensive as invasive testing. The urea breath test identifies urease, an enzyme produced by *H. pylori*. The most accurate diagnostic procedure is endoscopy with biopsy for *H. pylori* and cytologic brushings of ulcer margins for potentially (5%) malignant gastric ulcers. Endoscopy is generally reserved for those with recurrent symptoms. If an upper GI series is performed in lieu of endoscopy, any gastric lesions should be followed up with endoscopy in two to three months.

Management

There is now a general consensus that an antibiotic regimen to eradicate *H. pylori* is the most effective means of dealing with duodenal ulcer. Compared with standard therapy of H2 antagonists, antibiotic therapy demonstrated only a 5% recurrence (largely due to use of NSAIDs), compared with a 70% to 85% recurrence in the standard H2 group.[56,57] This "triple therapy" is a combination of omeprazole or lansoprazole (proton-pump inhibitor) with metronidazole (Flagyl) and amoxicillin (antibiotics). For gastric ulcers, discontinuing NSAIDs combined with a two- to three-month course of H2 antagonists or sucralfate (a drug that acts locally as a mucus bandage) is usually effective. Discontinuing smoking is often necessary. If the ulcers do not heal, Zollinger-Ellison syndrome is suspected.

One study[58] provides some preliminary support for the use of spinal manipulative therapy in the treatment of patients with ulcers. This small study indicated that clinical remission occurred 10 days earlier with spinal manipulation than with medical treatment. Cautions to interpretation must include that both groups were given an "ulcer diet" and that the medical treatment consisted of the now out-of-date use of H2 antagonists, sucralfate, antacids, etc. Also there was no clear description or apparent consistency in the manipulative treatment procedures.

Gastroesophageal Reflux

Classic Presentation

The patient is often an older, overweight individual complaining of epigastric pain after eating large meals and lying down.

Cause

The tone of the lower esophageal sphincter (LES) may decrease with age and also with ingestion of certain foods, including chocolate, caffeine, fat, and alcohol. In addition, smoking, theophylline, calcium channel blockers, and anticholinergic medications will decrease the tone of the LES, leading to reflux.[59]

Increased pressure from obesity, heavy meals, and recumbency may aggravate symptoms. In addition to overweight individuals, esophageal reflux is common in healthy athletes, such as conditioned runners, cyclists, and weightlifters.[60] Several mechanisms may account for this, including position, Valsalva, indirect effects of exercise and position on lower esophageal tone.

Evaluation

The diagnosis is mainly historical. The patient may report that by eating smaller, frequent meals, going to bed on an empty stomach, and avoiding chocolate, caffeine, and alcohol, the pain is better. Antacids or the newer OTC H2 antagonists (Tagamet, Zantac, etc.) usually help. A hiatal hernia may predispose the individual to a reduced LES tone. This may be seen on a chest or anterior-to-posterior thoracic film indicated by an air lucency above the diaphragm. Note that reflux is more common in asthmatics regardless of medication regimen. The main differential is peptic ulcer, Barrett's esophagus, and esophageal cancer. Patients with recurrent symptoms of GI reflux (especially those over age 50 years) should have upper GI endoscopy to detect Barrett's esophagus (potential precursor to esophageal adenocarcinoma).[61] For those with Barrett's, providing an acid-reduced environment (using high-dose proton pump inhibitors) allows endoscopic ablation using laser and nonlaser approaches. Otherwise, a high-risk attempt at removal of the distal esophagus is an option.

Management

Recommend to the patient that he or she avoid alcohol, caffeine, fatty meals, smoking, and eating large meals. Switching to smaller meals eaten more frequently and going to bed with a partially full stomach may help. If there is an associated hiatal hernia, chiropractic manipulation in the epigastric region may help reflexly. Weight loss is important for obese patients. Omeprazole (a proton pump inhibitor) is the standard for treatment of GI reflux. However, long-term use may lead to problems with absorption of calcium and other important nutrients. Most importantly, gastroesophageal reflux should not be confused with the temporary reflux with infants. A concern that has warranted strong editorial warnings is that medical doctors are prescribing proton-pump inhibitors for infants with reflux. The critics of this approach feel that this practice is more for the parents than the infant and may harm the infant with regard to important nutritional absorption and potentially increase risk for infection.

ABDOMINAL PAIN

Irritable Bowel Syndrome

Classic Presentation

Generally patients present with complaints of abdominal pain (usually lower left or suprapubic) and distention that is relieved with defecation. Patients often report early-morning constipation that results in the passage of small-sized feces. Signs and symptoms often begin in the late teens or 20s.

Clinical Categories Based on Presentation

IBS is often divided into three general classifications including an A type (alternating) that is a combination of diarrhea and constipation, a C type (constipation predominant), and a D type (diarrhea predominant). Classification systems have been developed including the Manning criteria, Kruis criteria, and the Rome criteria (I, II, and III). A JAMA review[62] found that the Kruis and Manning criteria have modest accuracy and that no single test is of value. Using the Rome criteria is a popular approach but only Rome I and II criteria have been evaluated extensively. A 2013 review[63] compared these criteria and found that for identifying patients with IBS, the sensitivities ranged from 61.9% for Manning criteria to 95.8% for the Rome I criteria, and specificities included 70.6% for Rome I and 81.8% for Manning. Positive LRs ranged from 3.19 (Rome II) to 3.39 (Manning), and negative LRs from 0.06 (Rome I) to 0.47 (Manning). Clearly, this performance is only modest in identifying patients with IBS, yet there are no laboratory tests to assist so that history findings are the only information available. Manning et al.[64] determined six symptoms that occur together more often in patients with IBS than in patients with other GI disorders. The other systems including the Rome criteria include these elements, and recent studies[65,66] confirm this observation and add that the likelihood increases with the number of positive criteria; the predictive value decreases with age and is less valuable with men. Also abdominal pain usually occurs two to three times per week for at least several months. These criteria are as follows:

- pain relief with bowel movement
- more frequent stools with the onset of pain
- looser stools with the onset of pain
- passage of mucus
- sensation of incomplete defecation
- abdominal distention sensed through tight clothing or visibly evident

Symptoms compatible with IBS are found in 10% to 22% of adults.[67, 68] Onset is as early as adolescence and tends to peak in the 30s and 40s; unlikely after age 50 years.[69] Only 14% to 50% of this group seek medical advice. Some studies[70,71] have classified patients into two subgroups: (1) abdominal pain predominant that seems to be related to meals and stress; (2) bowel habit predominant and usually constipation is the main complaint, but diarrhea may be; abdominal pain is not the chief complaint. Some studies describe a prototype patient who is often angry, depressed, or stressed.

Cause

The cause is unknown. However, there appears to be abnormal myoelectric activity in the intestines (and sometimes other structures) that results in a change in peristaltic activity. Studies indicate that a normal six-cycle-per-minute slow-wave rate is more often three cycles per minute in patients with IBS. Colonic spike activity peaks about 60 to 90 minutes after meals, which seems to correlate with a common complaint of pain after meals.[72] It also appears that patients may have a lower visceral pain threshold, perceiving what would be considered normal bowel distention as pain.[73]

IBS is viewed by many as a problem of central-modulated pain with what is termed the brain–gut axis where emotional stimulation may have a direct effect on gut motility but also the threshold of stimulation for pain. An emotional nociceptive area in the cingulate gyrus may be activated by stressful or aversive stimulus from internally in the body. It is proposed that preganglionic neurons from the parasympathetic nervous system may be tied to this response and instead of synapsing (or in addition to synapsing) on motor neurons in the intestinal wall, they synapse on interneurons related to visceral afferents. There may be a heightened sensitivity of nociceptors due to previous infection or perhaps an autoimmune response that causes hyperproliferation of enterochromaffin cells in the walls of the intestinal crypts and may also include mast cells in the lamina propria. Serotonin is released from enterochromaffin cells normally in response to distension, which then increases peristaltic activity. It is proposed that for patients with IBS, there is a stimulation also of nociceptors by serotonin, which in turn causes the release of substance P, which causes mast cells to release histamine, which then causes the release of more serotonin in a vicious cycle.

Patients with IBS may also have an increased colonic motor response to corticotrophin-releasing hormone (RH).[74–76] There are differences in CRH-R1 and CRH-R2. R1 is pro-inflammatory whereas stimulation of R2 is anti-inflammatory. Also, CRH-R1 is pronociceptive for visceral pain whereas CRH-R2 is antinociceptive.

Evaluation

IBS is largely a historical diagnosis and one of exclusion. The patient should have had symptoms for at least three to six months before considering IBS in the differential. Other causes of constipation should be screened historically, and education in proper fluid/fiber intake combined with proper bowel habits should be used initially for patients who are constipation predominant.[77] Patients with bowel-predominant symptoms should have a rectal and stool examination. Stool that is nonbloody (occult or frank) and free of fecal leukocytes, parasites, and ova suggests IBS. Mucus, seen as a stringy substance covering the stool, is often found in the stool of patients with IBS. In older patients, sigmoidoscopy is sometimes warranted if colon cancer is suspected.

Management

The patient should be counseled regarding the chronicity of IBS, and that there will be periods of exacerbation and remission. Primary conservative focus is on stress relaxation and dietary factors. Keeping a diary with relation to the onset of symptoms may be helpful. Chocolate milk products and alcohol are common triggers. Patients often benefit by avoidance of lactose, fructose, and sorbitol. In addition, gas-producing foods such as cabbage, cauliflower, raisins, grapes, raw onions, sprouts, coffee, red wine, and beer should be eliminated initially to determine effect. Many small meals throughout the day versus two or three large meals are recommended. A high-fiber diet may help, although if the fiber is bran, increased gas production may worsen symptoms. Exercise may be helpful as indicated by some uncontrolled studies.[78]

Pharmacologically, it is interesting that placebo agents result in improvement in up to 70% of patients. When medication is used, anticholinergic, antidiarrheal, or anticonstipation agents are sometimes prescribed. Also, there is a focus on calcium channel blockers, H2 antagonists, and 5-HT_3 receptor antagonists.[79,80]

Prescription is based on the type of IBS. If there is diarrhea dominance in the presentation, muscarinic receptor anticholinergics (M_3) or serotonin receptor antagonists (5-HT_3) (e.g., Alostrone) are used. Most recently, various forms of intestinal-specific calcium channel blockers such as pinaverium bromide (Dicetel), and trimebutine maleate (Modulon), are utilized to prevent smooth muscle contraction and therefore peristaltic activity. The purpose of this approach is to reduce pain and bloating with less of a focus on either diarrhea or constipation. For constipation, serotonin receptor agonists (5-HT_3) or cholinergics are prescribed. Obviously if the patient has the combination of diarrhea and constipation that alternates, prescription is a difficult if not impossible dilemma.

A study[81] published in 2013 compares the effect of Chinese manipulation to Dicetel in the management of IBS pain. The manipulation as described in the study appears similar to side-posture chiropractic manipulation. The study protocol utilized both thoracic and lumbar manipulation. The outcome measures included a visual analog pain scale and the bowel symptom scale (BSS). The results indicated a far superior effect for manipulation over the calcium-channel blocker at a ratio of 3:1.

Acupuncture has been proposed as an approach to IBS. Studies seem consistent with regard to a comparison of sham acupuncture to real acupuncture in relation to effect. Also, the time spent with the patient has an effect with increasing success rates related to longer time spent with the patient. Although acupuncture seems effective, a Cochrane review[82] summarized this effect by stating that acupuncture, whether real or sham, is significantly better than antispasmodic calcium channel blocking medications, yet given both real and sham acupuncture are effective, how to apply these findings is problematic. It would seem that if patients benefit, acupuncture should be utilized.

There is some evidence that hypnotherapy may also be beneficial.[83]

Diverticulitis

Classic Presentation

Usually, the patient will be elderly with complaints of left lower abdominal pain and tenderness and associated low-grade fever; bloody stool and/or nausea and vomiting may occur. Most patients will have symptoms mild enough that they will wait a few days before seeking medical attention. Patients with a large perforation will present with generalized abdominal pain and peritoneal signs.

Cause/Occurrence

Diverticula are herniations of the mucosa and submucosa into the colonic muscle wall at the site of mesenteric vessel penetration primarily in the sigmoid colon. Diverticular disease appears to be the result of years of colonic high pressure due to contracted segments of bowel that are undistended; thus it is believed that a chronic fiber-deficient diet is the cause. A high-fiber, low-fat diet increases stool volume, reduces intraluminal pressure in the colon, and decreases colonic transit time. The prevalence is higher in Western countries. Diverticular disease occurs in approximately 10% of individuals in the United States over age 40 years, 50% of individuals over age 60 years, and up to 66% of individuals in their 80s. Eighty percent to 85% of individuals with diverticulosis are asymptomatic. Patients become symptomatic when the diverticula become inflamed, accounting for more than 130,000 hospitalizations each year.[84] It should be noted that corticosteroid use or chronic NSAID use may mask symptoms of diverticular disease.

Evaluation

Lower-left abdominal tenderness with a palpable mass is a common finding. A low-grade fever, occult or frank blood, and a mild to moderate leukocytosis often are found. Abdominal and chest x-rays in the supine and upright positions may be used to determine free air (evidence of perforation) or obstruction in acute presentations. Referral for medical management will usually result in a limited hospitalization, followed 7 to 10 days later with either an outpatient barium study and sigmoidoscopy, or, more recently, CT. CT is the procedure of choice for the diagnosis of diverticulitis.

Management

In patients who have diverticular disease discovered incidentally, a high-fiber diet is recommended. Recommended levels range from 10 to 35 g/day of insoluble fiber. Bran is recommended because it improves oral glucose tolerance and increases fecal fat excretion. It is recommended to introduce fiber into the diet gradually to avoid cramping. For those with active diverticulitis, antibiotic therapy and intravenous fluids are initial approaches. Twenty percent to 30% of patients eventually will require surgery.

INFLAMMATORY BOWEL DISEASE

Ulcerative Colitis

Classic Presentation

Generally a younger patient presents with complaints of frequent bloody diarrhea, lower abdominal cramping, mild pain, and rectal urgency. Approximately 10% to 20% will complain of multiple joint pains. Variation in presentation is based on the number of bowel movements per day from less than four (mild) to more than six (severe).

Cause

The cause of ulcerative colitis (UC) is unknown. It appears that there may be some predisposition that somehow interacts with other factors to create varying degrees of inflammatory reaction. One theory is that a defect in the intestinal glycosaminoglycan (GAG) protective barrier allows penetration of infective agents, toxins, and antigenic protein moieties leading to a local inflammatory response cascading into a host of biochemical and immunologic changes (leaky-gut syndrome).[85] Individuals who have had Salmonella or campylobacter risk in the following year for developing IBD. Half of all patients with UC have involvement of the distal colon, 30% of patients have extension to the splenic flexure, with 20% of patients extending into the more proximal bowel.[86]

In many patients there is also an effect on the biliary system including fatty liver, cirrhosis of the liver, and sclerosing cholangitis. Patients with long-standing disease are at higher risk for colon cancer. An association with HLA-B27 explains the occurrence of peripheral arthropathies and uveitis in some patients. Oddly enough, smokers have half the risk of nonsmokers of developing UC (the opposite for Crohn's disease).

Evaluation

The patient with mild ulcerative colitis may have no more discriminating findings clinically than patients with other causes of colitis such as infection or antibiotic colitis. However, those with severe UC may also have signs of hypovolemia such as an increased pulse rate. Severe forms will also cause weight loss, a decreased hematocrit and albumin, and an increased erythrocyte sedimentation rate (ESR) and temperature. Anemia due to blood loss is usually iron-deficiency anemia.

For detecting UC and distinguishing it from Crohn's, the following single tests or combined tests in panels may be ordered:

- pANCA (perinuclear antineutrophil cytoplasmic antibody) for UC; found in about 50% to 85% of patients (only 5% to 20% of patients with Crohn's disease).
- Anti-I-2 (*Pseudomonas fluorescens* antibodies)

The diagnosis is established with sigmoidoscopy with characteristic findings of a granular mucosa with edema, erosions, and friability. Colonoscopy is reserved for patients who are not acutely ill to determine the extent of involvement. Laboratory testing of the stool is used to rule out other causes of colitis, usually infectious.

Management

Exacerbations seem related to stressful events, or may be activated by NSAIDs or aspirin, but they may occur without an obvious cause. The mainstay of medical management is similar to that for Crohn's disease, consisting of anti-inflammatory (sulfasalazine or mesalamine and corticosteroids), antidiarrheal, and immunosuppressive drugs used either to induce remission, such as infliximab, or for preventing relapse, such as azathioprine and 9-mercaptopurine (6-MP).

There are a number of dietary recommendations that to date do not have strong literature support but are nonetheless incorporated by most physicians. This includes decreasing the amount of meat and alcohol in the diet and increasing omega-3 fatty acids, cod liver oil, dietary lactulose, and wheat grass juice. Also, many patients report problems with chocolate, dairy products, fats, and artificial sweeteners.[87] The prognosis in most patients is good. Those acquiring the disease in infancy or after the age of 60 years have the poorest prognosis. Pregnancy often worsens UC; however, the use of medication does not seem to affect the fetus.

Crohn's Disease (Regional Enteritis)

Classic Presentation

The patient is often young with an insidious onset of intermittent bouts of right lower quadrant pain, some diarrhea, and a low-grade fever. In some patients, the initial presentation is with extra intestinal manifestations such as perianal fistulas, fissures, or abscesses. Eventually, the patient may appear anemic with weight loss.

Cause

The cause is unknown. It appears that some predisposition exists due to either genetically acquired sensitivity (e.g., Ashkenazy Jewish patients) and/or environmentally triggered reaction (e.g., live vaccines such as MMR, varicella, zoster) leads to varying degrees of inflammatory reaction. One theory is that a defect in the intestinal GAG protective barrier allows penetration of infective agents, toxins, and antigenic protein moieties leading to a local inflammatory response cascading into a host of biochemical and immunologic changes (leaky-gut syndrome).[85] Individuals who have had Salmonella or campylobacter are at higher risk in the following year for developing IBD. Specifically, it appears that there is an environment that allows chronic T-cell activation, which causes damage through secondary macrophage activation.[88] What activates the T-cells remains controversial. Current interest is in the role of measles and the measles vaccine as one potential instigator.[89,90] There is transmural involvement with extension possible through to the serosa. This patchy, segmental involvement is isolated to the ileum in about one-third of patients, with half of patients also having involvement of the colon. In 15% to 20% of cases only the colon is affected. The process may extend, however, from the mouth to the anus. The inflammatory reaction includes infiltration of lymphocytes and plasma cells. Fibrosis is often extensive, causing obstruction. Sarcoid-like granulomas occur in 30% to 40% of patients within involved intestinal segments. This involvement affects absorption of fat-soluble vitamins and B12, often leading to deficiencies. An association with HLA-B27 explains why some patients have peripheral arthropathies and uveitis.

Evaluation

Evaluation findings are contingent on the degree and location of involvement. The abdominal examination may reveal a tender right quadrant, anal-rectal disease, and weight loss. Laboratory examination is relatively nonspecific, showing an increase in ESR, macrocytic anemia (with terminal ileum involvement), leukocytosis, and occasionally decreased albumin. Stool examination for ova, parasites, and other pathogens is used to differentiate from other causes of diarrhea. Immunological evaluation for Crohn's includes tests that are not specific or sensitive enough to confirm the diagnosis but could be an initial step prior to colonoscopy. The ASCA test (*Saccharomyces cerevisiae* antibodies), IgG and IgA is positive in about 40% to 50% of patients with Crohn's. Using the Anti-CBir1 test (*Clostridium* species antibodies) about 50% of patients with Crohn's will have a positive test. Antiglycan antibody is found positive in about 75% of patients with Crohn's (only 5% with UC patients). The Anti-Omp C test (*Escherichia coli* antibodies) is used for rapidly progressing Crohn's disease.

Colonoscopy and barium studies are diagnostic. Colonoscopy allows direct visualization and biopsy. Barium studies may demonstrate "skip" lesions (areas of involvement adjacent to normal mucosa). Narrowing of the barium stream in involved areas may be referred to as the "string sign."

Management

In the National Cooperative Crohn's Disease Study, it appears that one-third of patients on a placebo went into remission within four months and remained in remission for two years.[91] This is important information for all who attempt to treat Crohn's disease with alternative approaches. Medical care varies based on patient presentation. In the armamentarium of medications the primary drugs are anti-inflammatory including strong NSAIDs such as 5-aminosalicylics (sulfasalazine and mesalamine), prednisone (also used to induce remission), and antidiarrheals. Immunosuppressive medications are used either to induce remission such as methotrexate or infliximab or for preventing relapse such as azathioprine and 9-mercaptopurine (6-MP). The two extremes of initial therapy are either to treat symptomatically prior to more aggressive therapy or the opposite end of the spectrum, beginning with immunomodulators and/or anti-TNF (tissue necrosis factor) agents.

Avoidance of potential risk factors includes cessation of smoking, which has been shown to increase frequency and severity of attacks. Diets high in refined sugars and animal protein have also been associated with a risk of recurrence. Also, many patients report problems with chocolate, dairy products, fats, and artificial sweeteners. Dietary management is important because of malabsorption. Vitamin supplementation is frequently necessary, often including parenteral vitamin B12. However, this does not appear to alter the disease course. Approximately 70% of all patients with Crohn's disease must have some surgery.

DYSMENORRHEA

Primary Dysmenorrhea

Classic Presentation

The patient is often one to two years postmenarchal with increasing pain associated with menses. The pain is felt in the lower abdomen and pelvis, sometimes radiating to the back or inner thighs.[92]

Cause

Pain is mediated via prostaglandins. The cause is a combination of vasoconstriction and myometrial contraction. Increased discomfort may be caused by fluid retention (estrogen causes salt retention).

Examination

No examination usually is necessary unless the pain is "new" or suddenly increased. Then a pelvic examination is warranted. With primary dysmenorrhea there are no obvious pathologic findings, but the examination may be more uncomfortable during menses.

Management

Medical management focuses on decreasing of certain prostaglandins. NSAIDs (ibuprofen, ketoprofen, naproxen) are usually helpful. One study[93] demonstrated chiropractic manipulation of the spine or pelvis to be effective in reducing pain and a prostaglandin F-2a metabolite. A follow-up study,[94] however, showed similar improvement with either manipulation or a low-force treatment intended to act as a placebo-like comparison. Future research may be able to indicate what is the effective element of the treatment episode. Stimulation of sacral and low-back reflex points through acupressure, electrical stimulation,[95] or acupuncture may provide relief.[96] Dietary formulas, including omega-3 polyunsaturated fatty acids,[97] and B12 may provide relief. One study[98] indicated benefit from the use of magnesium pidolate (4.5 mg/daily). There is mounting evidence that exercise is beneficial for primary dysmenorrhea.[99]

Secondary Dysmenorrhea

Classic Presentation

A female patient in her late 20s or 30s (as late as 40s) presents with a complaint that her menstrual pain is much worse than it had been previously. Suspicion is increased when the patient is infertile. Depending on sites of endometrial implantation, endometriosis may also cause dyspareunia and/or rectal pain with bleeding.[100]

Cause

The two most common causes are endometriosis (implantation of uterine tissue outside the uterus) and pelvic inflammatory disease (salpingitis). Endometriosis appears to be somewhat dependent on a dysfunction of cell-mediated immunity. One study[101] observed that women with endometriosis were more sensitive to the stimulatory effects of peripheral blood monocytes on proliferation of endometrial tissue. Other causes include submucous myoma, IUD use, and cervical stenosis (often post-induced abortion).

Examination

The pelvic examination may reveal pelvic tenderness or discrete nodules in the cul-de-sac (with endometriosis). Transvaginal ultrasonography is often used to identify lesion sites. However, the definitive diagnosis may rest on laparoscopy to differentiate between PID and endometriosis. Cervical stenosis should be suspected with a presentation subsequent to an induced abortion.

Management

The focus of management is to suspend ovulation for four to nine months. This is accomplished via a regimen similar to birth control pills or danazol (androgenic effects). This will usually result in a decrease in size of the endometrial implants.

Conservative management options for endometriosis that might be attempted and show some literature evidence, although weak evidence scientifically, include acupuncture,[102] Chinese herbal therapy,[103] and osteopathic manipulation.[104]

When extensive, surgery is often necessary. The approach is dictated by age and desire for reproductive function. Under age 35 years, resecting lesions and freeing adhesions laparoscopically allow fertility in about 20% of patients.[105] After age 35 years or for those not wishing to conceive, treatment involves bilateral salpingo-oophorectomy and hysterectomy if the disease is extensive.[106]

COLORECTAL CANCER

Classic Presentation

Patients are often asymptomatic. When symptomatic, an older patient complains of abdominal pain and cramping and notices narrowing of stool and possible blood in the stool.

Cause

Colorectal cancer (CRC) represents the second most commonly diagnosed cancer. It may result from the progression over years of high-risk polyps into cancer (i.e., multiple polyps, villous polyps, and large polyps). Contributing factors are both genetic and environmental. Smokers, those who are physically inactive, and those with a diet high in red meat and low in fruits and vegetables are at higher risk. Most patients are over the age of 50 years. Those patients with prior GI disorders such as inflammatory bowel disease are at higher risk as are African Americans. The lifetime risk is about 5.4% in the United States.

Exam

Recommendations vary dependent on the healthcare organization. The U.S. Preventive Services Task Force recommends screening men and women between the ages of 50 and 75 years with either fecal occult testing, sigmoidoscopy, or colonoscopy. The American Cancer Society has a broader and more prescriptive recommendation for this age group with fecal occult blood testing and fecal immunochemical testing (FIT) every year, stool DNA testing (sDNA), flexible sigmoidoscopy and double-contract enemas every five years and colonoscopy every 10 years. Screening at age 40 years is recommended for those with a family history of CRC or polyps. Screening for those genetically predisposed may begin in their 20s. Digital rectal exam alone is insufficient for screening.

Management

Patients with polyps discovered on colonoscopy have biopsy and follow-up. Even those with noncancerous lesions are evaluated more frequently. When discovered, imaging for metastasis is utilized including CT scanning, endoscopic US, and intraoperative US. The American Joint Commission on Cancer (AJCC) TNM criteria and Duke's criteria are the most commonly utilized staging tools. For TNM staging, Stages I through IB do not involve lymph nodes with Grade III with lymph node involvement but no distant sites involved, and Stage IV with distant sites involved. Surgical resection is the primary approach to CRC with chemotherapy for metastatic involvement. When there is metastatic involvement, chemotherapy may extend survival from 6 to 24 months. Other medications used include Avastin, a monoclonal antibody with the intent of inhibiting angiogenesis.

Prevention includes dietary changes to include increasing fruits and vegetables, decreasing red meat intake, reducing heavy alcohol intake, and possible increased intake of calcium, vitamin D, and folate. Increasing physical activity and smoking cessation are important lifestyle factors that many patients need to incorporate in their approach to cancer prevention.

CELIAC DISEASE

Classic Presentation

A young patient complains of chronic abdominal cramping, explosive flatulence, weight loss, and diarrhea.

Cause

Celiac disease (also called sprue and celiac sprue) is a malabsorption syndrome caused by sensitivity to gluten-containing foods such as wheat, barley, rye, and some oat-based products. Reaction is specifically to the gliadin portion of gluten and may be related genetically to HLA-DQ2 and/or DQ8. The estimated number of U.S. individuals with celiac disease is approximately 3 million. Signs and symptoms are related to malabsorption and its consequences of diarrhea and vitamin deficiencies.

Exam

Historically, in addition to abdominal cramping and diarrhea, consider celiac disease in pregnant females with anemia and in pediatric patients who have delayed growth or stature. On physical exam there may be abdominal distention, aphthous stomatitis and *dermatitis herpetiformis* manifesting as symmetrical papules and blisters of the elbows, knees, buttocks, or back.

Due to malabsorption, general lab testing would include a search for iron-deficiency anemia, elevated liver function tests, d-Xylose test for malabsorption, and decreases in protein, calcium, and vitamins A, D, C and folic acid (sometimes B12). There is also often a decrease in cholesterol and neutral fats with a >7% fat malabsorption wst.

For the evaluation/detection of celiac disease, the following tests have been utilized:

- IgA class of Anti-tissue Transglutaminase Antibody (anti-tTG): Anti-tTG, IgA is the most *sensitive* and *specific* blood test for celiac disease; however, it may be test negative in children under 3 years old who have celiac disease. For this group, Deamidated Gliadin Peptide (DGP) Antibodies, IgA, called the Anti-DGP test may prove useful.
- Anti-Gliadin Antibodies (AGA), IgG and IgA classes
- Quantitative Immunoglobulin A (IgA)
- Antiendomysial Antibodies (IgA)

Other tests that are either new or used less often for celiac disease include:

- Anti-Endomysial Antibodies (EMA), IgA class
- Anti-Reticulin Antibodies (ARA), IgA class
- Anti-Actin (F-actin), IgA class

Management

The key factor is avoidance primarily of wheat, barley, rye, and some oat products and substitution with rice, corn, and/or soybean flour. Many alternatives are now available at some stores and many restaurants for those with gluten intolerance. Patients will generally feel better with a week of a gluten-free diet, with most symptoms resolving over a two-month period. Refractory celiac disease is often treated as a typical autoimmune inflammatory disease with the utilization of prednisone or immunosuppressants.

APPENDIX 31–1

Web Resources

Inflammatory Bowel Disease

Crohn's & Colitis Foundation of America
www.ccfa.org

Celiac Disease

Celiac Disease Foundation
(818) 990-2354
www.celiac.org
Celiac Support Association
(402) 558-0600
www.csaceliacs.org

Liver and Hepatitis

Hepatitis Foundation International
(800) 891-0707
www.hepfi.org
American Liver Foundation
(800) GO-LIVER (465-4837)
www.liverfoundation.org

Gallstones

American College of Surgeons
(312) 202-5000
www.facs.org/public_info/operation/cholesys.pdf

GI Cancers

American Cancer Society
(800) 227-2345
www.cancer.org
National Cancer Institute
(800) 422-6237
**www.nci.nih.gov/cancer_information/cancer_type
/colon_and_rectal**
American Gastroenterological Association
www.gastro.org

APPENDIX 31–2

References

1. McCaig LF, Burt CW. National Hospital Ambulatory Medical Care Survey: 2002 emergency department summary. *Adv Data*. 2004(340):1–34.
2. Nansel D, Szlazak M. Somatic dysfunction and the phenomenon of visceral disease stimulation: a probable explanation for the apparent effectiveness of somatic therapy in patients presumed to be suffering from true visceral disease. *J Manipulative Physiol Ther*. 1995;18:379–397.
3. Foreman RD. Spinal substrates of visceral pain. In: Yaksh TL, ed. *Spinal Afferent Processing*. New York: Plenum Publishing; 1986.
4. Eisenberg RL, Heinekin P, Hedcock MW, et al. Evaluation of plain abdominal radiographs in the diagnosis of abdominal pain. *Ann Intern Med*. 1982;97:257–261.
5. Cope Z. *The Early Diagnosis of the Acute Abdomen*. 14th ed. London: Oxford University Press; 1972.
6. Vitello JM, Nyhus LM. The physical examination of the abdomen. In: Nyhus LM, Vitello JM, Condon RE, eds. *Abdominal Pain: A Guide to Rapid Diagnosis*. Norwalk, CT: Appleton & Lange; 1995:31–48.
7. Laing FC. Ultrasonography of the acute abdomen. *Radiol Clin North Am*. 1992;30:389–404.
8. Manning RT. Signs that point to appendicitis. *Diagnosis*. 1982;2:88–90.
9. Vitello JM. Appendicitis. In: Nyhus LM, Vitello JM, Condon RE, eds. *Abdominal Pain: A Guide to Rapid Diagnosis*. Norwalk, CT: Appleton & Lange; 1995:83–104.
10. Paulson EK, Kalady MF, Pappas TN. Suspected appendicitis. *N Engl J Med*. 2003;348(3):236–242.
11. Ohle R, O'Reilly F, O'Brien KK, Fahey T, Dimitrov BD. The Alvarado score for predicting acute appendicitis: a systematic review. *BMC Med*. 2011;9:139.
12. Schneider C, Kharbanda A, Bachur R. Evaluating appendicitis scoring systems using a prospective pediatric cohort. *Ann Emerg Med*. Jun 2007;49(6):778–784, 784 e771.
13. Bundy DG, Byerley JS, Liles EA, Perrin EM, Katznelson J, Rice HE. Does this child have appendicitis? *JAMA*. 2007;298(4):438–451.

14. Puskar D, Bedalov G, Fridrih S, Vuckovic I, Banek T, Pasini J. Urinalysis, ultrasound analysis, and renal dynamic scintigraphy in acute appendicitis. *Urology*. 1995;45(1):108–112.

15. Peltokallio P, Janhainen K. Acute appendicitis in the aged patient: study of 300 cases after the age of 60. *Arch Surg*. 1970;100:140–143.

16. Lews FR. Appendicitis: a critical review of diagnosis and treatment in 1,000 cases. *Arch Surg*. 1975:110:677–684.

17. Skane P, Amland PF, Nordshus T, et al. Ultrasonography in patients with suspected appendicitis: a prospective study. *Br J Radiol*. 1990;63:787.

18. Skane P, Schistad O, Amland PF, Solbeim K. Routine ultrasonography in the diagnosis of acute appendicitis: a valuable tool in daily practice? *Am Surg*. 1997;63:937–942.

19. Rao PM, Rhea JT, Noveline RA, et al. Effect of computed tomography of the appendix on treatment of patients and use of hospital resources. *N Engl J Med*. 1998;338:141–146.

20. Poortman P, Oostvogel HJ, Bosma E, et al. Improving diagnosis of acute appendicitis: results of a diagnostic pathway with standard use of ultrasonography followed by selective use of CT. *J Am Coll Surg*. Mar 2009;208(3):434–441.

21. Birnbaum BA, Jeffrey RB, Jr. CT and sonographic evaluation of acute right lower quadrant abdominal pain. *AJR Am J Roentgenol*. 1998;170(2):361–371.

22. Barron B, Hanna C, Pasalaqua AM, et al. Rapid diagnostic imaging of acute, nonclassic appendicitis by leukoscintigraphy with sulesomab, a technetium 99m-labeled anti-granulocyte antibody Fab' fragment. LeukoScan Appendicitis Clinical Trial Group. *Surgery*. 1999;125:288–296.

23. Owings MF, Kozak LJ. Ambulatory and inpatient procedures in the United States, 1996. *Vital Health Stat 13*. 1998(139):1–119.

24. Andersson RE, Hugander A, Thulin AJ. Diagnostic accuracy and perforation rate in appendicitis: association with age and sex of the patient and with appendectomy rate. *Eur J Surg*. 1992; 158(1):37–41.

25. Andersson RE. The natural history and traditional management of appendicitis revisited: spontaneous resolution and predominance of prehospital perforations imply that a correct diagnosis is more important than an early diagnosis. *World J Surg*. 2007;31(1):86–92.

26. Varadhan KK, Humes DJ, Neal KR, Lobo DN. Antibiotic therapy versus appendectomy for acute appendicitis: a meta-analysis. *World J Surg*. Feb 2010;34(2):199–209.

27. Diehl AK, Sugarek NJ, Todd KH. Clinical evaluation of gallstone diseases: usefulness of symptoms and signs in clinical diagnosis. *Am J Med*. 1990;89:29–34.

28. National Institute of Diabetes and Digestive and Kidney Diseases. *Digestive Disease Statistics*. Bethesda, MD: U.S. Dept of Health and Human Services; 1995. NIH publication 95–3873.

29. Trowbridge RL, Rutkoski NK, Shojania KG. Does this patient have acute cholecystitis? *JAMA*. 2003;289(1):80–86.

30. NIH Consensus Development Panel on Gallstones and Laparoscopic Cholecystectomy. Cholecystectomy: gallstones and laparoscopic cholecystectomy. *JAMA*. 1993;269:1018.

31. Fort JM, Azpiroz F, Casellas F, et al. Bowel habit after cholecystectomy: physiological changes and clinical implications. *Gastroenterology*. 1996;111:617–622.

32. Strasberg SM, Clavien PA. Cholecystolithiasis: lithotherapy for the 1990's. *Hepatology*. 1992;16:820.

33. Leitzmann MF, Giovannucci EL, Rimm EB. The relation of physical activity to risk for symptomatic gallstone disease in men. *Ann Intern Med*. 1998;128:417–425.

34. Leitzmann MF, Rimm EB, Willett WC, et al. Recreational physical activity and the risk of cholecystectomy in women. *N Engl J Med*. 1999;341:777–784.

35. Leitzmann MF, Willett WC, Rimm EB, et al. A prospective study of coffee consumption and the risk of symptomatic gallstone disease in men. *JAMA*. 1999;281:2106–2112.

36. Coe FL, et al. The pathogenesis and treatment of kidney stones. *N Engl J Med*. 1992;327:1141.

37. Van Drongelen J, Klemeney A, Debruyne RM, et al. Impact of urometabolic evaluation on prevention of urolithiasis: a retrospective study. *Urology*. 1998;52:384–391.

38. Chen MYM, Zagoria RJ. Can noncontrast helical computed tomography replace intravenous urography for evaluation of patients with acute urinary renal colic? *J Emerg Med*. 1999;17:299–303.

39. Assimos DG, et al. A comparison of anatrophic nephrolithotomy and percutaneous nephrolithotomy with and without extracorporeal shock wave lithotripsy for management of patients with staghorn calculi. *J Urol*. 1991;145:710.

40. Gurhan GC, Willett WC, Speizer FE, et al. Beverage risk and risk for kidney stones in women. *Ann Intern Med.* 1998;128:534–540.

41. Riese RJ, Sakhaee K. Uric acid nephrolithiasis: pathogenesis and treatment. *J Urol.* 1992;148:765.

42. Atmani F, Slimani Y, Mimouni M, Hacht B. Prophylaxis of calcium oxalate stones by *Herniaria hirsuta* on experimentally induced nephrolithiasis in rats. *BJU Int.* 2003;92(1):137–140.

43. Burns GP, Bank S. *Disorders of the Pancreas: Current Issues in Diagnosis and Management.* New York: McGraw-Hill; 1992.

44. Marshall JB. Acute pancreatitis: a review with an emphasis on new developments. *Arch Intern Med.* 1993;153:1185.

45. Gravante G, Garcea G, Ong SL, et al. Prediction of mortality in acute pancreatitis: a systematic review of the published evidence. *Pancreatology.* 2009;9(5):601–614.

46. Wang SQ, Li SJ, Feng QX, Feng XY, Xu L, Zhao QC. Overweight is an additional prognostic factor in acute pancreatitis: a meta-analysis. *Pancreatology.* 2011;11(2):92–98.

47. Canavan TP. Appropriate use of the intrauterine device. *Am Fam Physician.* 1998;58(9):2077–2084, 2087–2088.

48. Merchant JS, Oh K, Klerman LV. Douching: a problem for adolescent girls and young women. *Arch Pediatr Adolesc Med.* 1999;153(8):834–837.

49. Shafer MA, Pantell RH, Schachter J. Is the routine pelvic examination needed with the advent of urine-based screening for sexually transmitted diseases? *Arch Pediatr Adolesc Med.* 1999;153(2):119–125.

50. Rothrock SG, Green SM, Dobson M, Colucciello SA, Simmons CM. Misdiagnosis of appendicitis in non-pregnant women of childbearing age. *J Emerg Med.* 1995;13(1):1–8.

51. Jacobson L, Westron L. Objective diagnosis of acute pelvic inflammatory disease. *Am J Obstet Gynecol.* 1969;105:1088–1098.

52. Stabile I, Grudzinkas JG. Ectopic pregnancy: a review of incidence, etiology and diagnostic aspects. *Obstet Gynecol Surg.* 1990;45:335.

53. Vajaranant M. Acute pelvic pain in women. In: Nyhus LM, Vitello JM, Condon RE, eds. *Abdominal Pain: A Guide to Rapid Diagnosis.* Norwalk, CT: Appleton & Lange;1995:191–206.

54. Ory SJ. New options for diagnosis and treatment of ectopic pregnancy. *JAMA.* 1992;267:534.

55. Talley NJ. AGA technical review: evaluation of dyspepsia. *Gastroenterology.* 1998;114:582–591.

56. Graham DY, et al. Effect of treatment of *Helicobacter pylori* infection on the long-term recurrence of gastric and duodenal ulcer: a randomized controlled study. *Ann Intern Med.* 1992;116:705.

57. Graham DY, et al. Effect of triple therapy (antibiotics plus bismuth) on duodenal ulcer healing. *Ann Intern Med.* 1992;115:256.

58. Pikalov AA, Kharin VV. Use of spinal manipulative therapy in the treatment of duodenal ulcer: a pilot study. *J Manipulative Physiol Ther.* 1994;17:310–313.

59. Jackson SB. Gastroesophageal reflux disease. *Top Clin Chiro.* 1995;2(1):24–29.

60. Collings KL, Pratt P, Rodriguez-Stanley S, Bemben M, Miner PB. Esophageal reflux in conditioned runners, cyclists, and weightlifters. *Med Sci Sports Exerc.* 2003;35(5):730–735.

61. Sampliner RE. Practice guidelines on the diagnosis, surveillance, and therapy of early Barrett's adenocarcinoma. The Practice Parameters Committee of the American College of Gastroenterology. *Am J Gastroenterol.* 1998;93:1028–1033.

62. Ford AC, Talley NJ, Veldhuyzen van Zanten SJ, Vakil NB, Simel DL, Moayyedi P. Will the history and physical examination help establish that irritable bowel syndrome is causing this patient's lower gastrointestinal tract symptoms? *JAMA.* Oct 15 2008;300(15):1793–1805.

63. Ford AC, Bercik P, Morgan DG, Bolino C, Pintos-Sanchez MI, Moayyedi P. Validation of the Rome III criteria for the diagnosis of irritable bowel syndrome in secondary care. *Gastroenterology.* 2013 Aug, 28;1267–1268.

64. Manning AP, Thompson WP, Heaton KW, et al. Towards positive diagnosis of the irritable bowel. *Br Med J.* 1978;2:653.

65. Jeong H, Lee HR, Yoo BC, et al. Manning criteria in irritable bowel syndrome: its diagnostic significance. *Korean J Intern Med.* 1993;8:34.

66. Talley NJ, Philips SF, Melton MJ, et al. Diagnostic value of the Manning criteria in irritable bowel syndrome. *Gut.* 1990;31:77.

67. Crossman DA, Zhiming L, Andruzzi E, et al. US householder survey of functional gastrointestinal disorders: prevalence, sociodemography, and health impact. *Dig Dis Sci.* 1993;38:1569.

68. Jones R, Lydeard S. Irritable bowel syndrome in the general population. *Br Med J.* 1992;304:87.

69. Mertz HR. Irritable bowel syndrome. *N Engl J Med.* 2003;349(22):2136–2146.

70. Lynn RB, Friedman LS. Irritable bowel syndrome. *N Engl J Med.* 1993;329:1940.

71. Welgan P, Meshkinpour H, Beeler M. Effect of anger on colon motor and myoelectric activity in irritable bowel syndrome. *Gastroenterology.* 1988;94:1150.

72. Kellow JE, Phillips SF. Altered small bowel motility in irritable bowel syndrome is correlated with symptoms. *Gastroenterology.* 1987;92:1885.

73. Camilleri M, Prather C. The irritable bowel syndrome: mechanisms and a practical approach to management. *Ann Intern Med.* 1992;116:1001.

74. Rao SS, Hatfield RA, Suls JM, Chamberlain MJ. Psychological and physical stress induce differential effects on human colonic motility. *Am J Gastroenterol.* 1998;93(6):985–990.

75. Tayama J, Sagami Y, Shimada Y, Hongo M, Fukudo S. Effect of alpha-helical CRH on quantitative electroencephalogram in patients with irritable bowel syndrome. *Neurogastroenterol Motil.* 2007;19(6):471–483.

76. Fukudo S. Role of corticotropin-releasing hormone in irritable bowel syndrome and intestinal inflammation. *J Gastroenterol.* 2007;42 Suppl 17:48–51.

77. Vanner SJ, Depew WT, Paterson WG. Predictive value of the Rome criteria for diagnosing the irritable bowel syndrome. *Am J Gastroenterol.* 1999;94:2912–2917.

78. Colwell LJ, Prather CM, Phillips SF, Zinsmeister AR. Effects of an irritable bowel syndrome educational class on health-promoting behaviors and symptoms. *Am J Gastroenterol.* 1998;93(6):901–905.

79. Dave B, Rubin W. Inhibition of gastric secretion relieves diarrhea and postprandial urgency associated with irritable bowel syndrome or functional diarrhea. *Dig Dis Sci.* 1999;44:1893–1898.

80. Mangel AW, Northcutt AR. Review article: the safety and efficacy of alosetron, a 5-HT3 receptor antagonist, in female irritable bowel syndrome patients. *Aliment Pharmacol Ther.* 1999;13(suppl 2):77–82.

81. Qu L, Xing L, Norman W, Chen H, Gao S. Irritable bowel syndrome treated by traditional Chinese spinal orthopedic manipulation. *J Tradit Chin Med.* Dec 2012;32(4):565–570.

82. Manheimer E, Cheng K, Wieland LS, et al. Acupuncture for treatment of irritable bowel syndrome. *Cochrane Database Syst Rev.* 2012;5:CD005111.

83. Galovski TE, Blanchard EB. The treatment of irritable bowel syndrome with hypnotherapy. *Appl Psychophysiol Biofeedback.* 1998;23:219–232.

84. Gerda JJ, Hines C, Roberts PL. Diverticulitis: current management strategies. *Patient Care.* July 1997:170–186.

85. Russel AL. Glycoaminoglycan (GAG) deficiency in protective barrier as an underlying, primary cause of ulcerative colitis, Crohn's disease, interstitial cystitis, and possibly Reiter's syndrome. *Med Hypothesis.* 1999;52(4):297–301.

86. Podolsky DK. Inflammatory bowel disease. *N Engl J Med.* 1991;325:928–1008.

87. Joachim G. The relationship between habits of food consumption and reported reactions to food in people with inflammatory bowel disease-testing the limits. *Nur Health.* 1999;13(2):69–83.

88. MacDonald TT, Murch ST. Aetiology and pathogenesis of chronic inflammatory bowel disease. *Baillieres Clin Gastroenterol.* 1994;8:1–34.

89. Ekborn A, Wakefield AJ, Zack M, Adami HO. Perinatal measles infection and subsequent Crohn's disease. *Lancet.* 1994;344:508–510.

90. Thompson NP, Montgomery SM, Pounder RE, Wakefield NJ. Is measles vaccination a risk factor for inflammatory bowel disease? *Lancet.* 1995;345:1071–1074.

91. Singleton J, et al. The National Cooperative Crohn's Disease Study. *Gastroenterology.* 1979;7:53.

92. MacKay HT, Chang RJ. Dysmenorrhea. In: Rakel RE, ed. *Current Therapy 1993.* Philadelphia: WB Saunders Co; 1993.

93. Kokjohn K, Schmid DM, Triano JJ, Brenan PC. The effect of spinal manipulation on pain and prostaglandin levels in women with primary dysmenorrhea. *J Manipulative Physiol Ther.* 1992;15:279–285.

94. Hondras MA, Long CR, Brennan PC. Spinal manipulative therapy versus a low force mimic maneuver for women with primary dysmenorrhea: a randomized, observer-blinded, clinical trial. *Pain.* 1999;81: 105–114.

95. Kaplan B, Rabinerson D, Lurie S, et al. Clinical evaluation of a new model of a transcutaneous electrical nerve stimulation device for the management of primary dysmenorrhea. *Gynecol Obstet Invest.* 1997;44:255–259.

96. Helms JM. Acupuncture for the management of primary dysmenorrhea. *Obstet Gynecol.* 1987;69:51–56.

97. Harel Z, Biro FM, Kottenhahn RK, Rosenthal SL. Supplementation with omega-3 polyunsaturated fatty acids in the management of dysmenorrhea in adolescents. *Am J Obstet Gynecol.* 1996;174:1335–1338.

98. Benassi L, Barletta FP, Baroncini L, et al. Effectiveness of magnesium pidolate in the prophylactic treatment of primary dysmenorrhea. *Clin Exp Obstet Gynecol.* 1992;19:176–179.

99. Golomb LM, Solidum AA, Warren MP. Primary dysmenorrhea and physical activity. *Med Sci Sports Exerc.* 1998;30:906–909.

100. Olive DL, Swartz LB. Endometriosis. *N Engl J Med.* 1993;24:1759.

101. Dmowski WP, Gebel HM, Braun DP. The role of cell-mediated immunity in the pathogenesis of endometriosis. *Acta Obstet Gynecol Scand Suppl.* 1994;159:7–14.

102. Giudice LC. Clinical practice. Endometriosis. *N Engl J Med.* 2010;362(25):2389–2398.

103. Flower A, Liu JP, Lewith G, Little P, Li Q. Chinese herbal medicine for endometriosis. *Cochrane Database of Systematic Reviews* 2012, Issue 5. Art. No.: CD006568. DOI: 10.1002/14651858.CD006568.pub3.

104. Chadwick K, Morgan A. The efficacy of osteopathic treatment for primary dysmenorrhea in young women. *The AAO Journal.* 1996;6(3):15–17.

105. Jacobson TZ, Duffy JMN, Barlow D, Farquhar C, Koninckx PR, Olive D. Laparoscopic surgery for subfertility associated with endometriosis. *Cochrane Database of Systematic Reviews* 2010, Issue 1. Art. No.: CD001398. DOI: 10.1002/14651858.CD001398.pub2.

106. Witt BR, Barad DH. Management of endometriosis in women older than 40 years of age. *Obstet Gynecol Clin North Am.* 1993;20:349.

Constipation

Context

There is a wide range of reported prevalence of constipation, from 2% to 27% in Western countries.[1] Although considered a benign problem that generally self-resolves, it is interesting to note that constipation accounts for at least 2.5 million office visits to physicians and 92,000 hospitalizations per year in the United States.[2]

Although many patients complain of constipation, it is important to remember that constipation is a relative term. Most physicians would classify a normal bowel movement as one bowel movement per day without straining; others may find passage every three to five days acceptable. The answer lies in the patient's history. If the patient has always had bowel movements every three days, this may likely be his or her normal pattern. A clear definition of constipation is difficult given the wide variation of "normal" patterns. Several factors may be included in the definition of constipation, including:

- Hard stools
- Infrequent stools (fewer than three per week)
- Need for excessive straining
- A sense of incomplete bowel evacuation
- Excessive time defecating

More formal criteria are presented with the Rome II criteria[3] which, in essence, includes the above for at least 12 weeks in the preceding year for at least 25% of bowel movements. In one study that used the criteria of no more than two bowel movements per week and/or straining on more than one in four bowel movements, only 62% of self-reporters met the criteria, although 47% of all patients reported constipation.[4] Self-reporters took twice as many laxatives as those who did not report constipation. The self-reported rate of constipation is as high as 60% among the elderly. Thirty percent of healthy elderly persons report using laxatives, although the majority of these patients have never gone more than three days without a bowel movement ($400 million per year in cost for laxatives).[5]

Most causes of constipation are benign and are the result of external or internal influences that are easily identifiable. In the context of chiropractic practice, it is a common observation that patients with low back pain are also constipated. The assumption is that this is due to either increased pain with bearing down or simply neural inhibition without straining. In either case, it is important for the chiropractor to rule out more serious causes. When not present, assist the patient with what may be an aggravating factor to his or her low back pain.

General Strategy

History

Careful questioning of the patient during the history taking can lead to appropriate management (**Table 32–1**).

- Determine the patient's definition of constipation.
- Determine the degree of constipation and whether it is acute or chronic.
- Determine any additional signs or symptoms that may indicate a systemic disorder such as hypothyroidism or diabetes.
- Determine the patient's current medication history, including over-the-counter (OTC) drugs.
- Determine the amount of dietary fiber and fluid intake and also iron supplementation.
- Determine whether laxatives are being used if so, and how often.

Table 32–1 History Questions for Constipation

Primary Question	What Are You Thinking?	Secondary Questions	What Are You Thinking?
How often do you have a bowel movement?	Determine what is normal for the individual.	How long have you had constipation? Did it occur over the last few weeks, months, or years?	Determine in an older patient whether there is a gradual decrease in the frequency of bowel movements as opposed to a recent change.
Is it painful to defecate?	Local pathology is causing pain; pain is increased due to muscle contraction or increase in intrathecal pressure.	Do you have hemorrhoids or other local problems around the anorectal area? Does bearing down cause local back pain? Does bearing down cause pain radiating into the legs?	Pain inhibits defecation urge or there is conscious inhibition due to fear of pain. Muscle spasm or other local irritation. Consider intrathecal pressure increase indicating disc lesion or tumor.
Do you take medications?	Direct action of medication or medication indicates underlying medical condition associated with decreased bowel function.	Have you been diagnosed with diabetes, irritable bowel syndrome, depression, or hypothyroidism (based on medication prescribed)? Did you have constipation before or after starting the medication? Are you taking medications with codeine in them (e.g. Percocet or Oxycontin) or iron supplementation?	Underlying disease may be cause of constipation. Many medications may cause constipation as a side effect. Many seniors take laxatives out of habit, not necessarily because they need them; also some laxatives can cause constipation.
What are your eating and drinking habits?	Low-fiber diet.	What do you eat on an average day?	Get a sense of dietary fiber intake.
(For children) Do you go to the bathroom when you feel the urge?	Too busy, does not like bathroom facilities, defecation hurts.	Does it hurt to go to the bathroom?	Either too little fiber or hydration causes hard stools; or an anal fissure causes local pain.

- Note whether the patient is pregnant.
- Determine the patient's status with regard to abdominal muscle tone; immobilized, incapacitated, or sedentary individuals may have less propulsive ability.
- Determine whether there is any soiling of undergarments (may be more suggestive of constipation than fecal incontinence).

Evaluation

- On physical examination determine whether any anorectal disease is present and the status of the rectum (empty or impacted); 25% of colorectal cancer may be found on rectal examination.
- Testing for occult blood is often warranted; referral for sigmoidoscopy is warranted in chronic constipation.

Management

- If the bowel is impacted, use digital disimpaction or an enema, or refer for disimpaction.
- Educate the patient on proper bowel habits, including proper fluid and dietary fiber intake, mild exercise, avoidance of laxatives, strengthening pelvic/abdominal musculature, allowing enough time for bowel movement, and avoiding inhibition of gastrocolic reflex.

Relevant Anatomy and Physiology

For the regular, unstrained passage of stool, it is necessary to have the proper balance of fluid, dietary fiber, and normal motility and transit time. The colonic mucosa usually absorbs 95% of intestinal sodium and water.[6] Interestingly, this function is usually normal in constipated patients. Increased desiccation, however, may occur as a result of increased mucosal contact due to slowed colonic transport time.[7] It would seem logical that this would be due to a decrease in colonic motor activity; however, investigators have actually found contraction of the pelvic colon to be increased.[8] The colonic myoelectric activity of patients with idiopathic constipation is usually normal, but this activity seems to be abnormally responsive to several outside stimuli, such as emotional stimulation, eating a meal, and hormonal stimulation. The intestinal smooth muscle cells have an inherent property that results in cyclic depolarization and repolarization. This occurs at what is referred to as a slow wave rate. There are two observed rates of six and three cycles per minute. Although normal individuals have an almost exclusive six-cycle-per-minute frequency in the colon and rectum, patients with irritable bowel syndrome have almost half the contractions occurring at three cycles per minute.[9]

Diseases that affect the central nervous system (CNS), spinal cord, and autonomic nervous system may have an effect on intestinal motility. A common example is the ileus that develops after abdominal surgery. This is due to effects of anesthesia (CNS depression) and manipulation of the organs. Diabetes may also affect bowel movements through dysfunction of the autonomic nervous system.

Most cases of constipation can be assigned to two general problems: ineffective filling and ineffective emptying. Ineffective filling is most often due to inadequate amounts of fluid and/or dietary fiber. Other common causes are CNS depression, which is usually the effect of medications, or clinical depression.

Another classification of cause is to divide constipation into four broad categories in relationship to colon transport time and defecation:[10]

1. Normal transit through the colon (accounts for 50%): Symptoms usually respond to increased dietary fiber or the addition of an osmotic-type laxative.
2. Slow transit through the colon (accounts for 13%): Most common in young women beginning around puberty and associated with bloating, abdominal pain, and an infrequent urge to defecate. Colonic inertia is a related disorder that is characterized by slow colonic transit. In this condition there is no response of increased motor activity with either a meal or medication stimulation.
3. Disorders of defecatory or rectal evacuation (accounts for 25%): Most commonly due to pelvic-floor dysfunction or anal sphincter dysfunction. Structural problems include anal fissures or hemorrhoids and, less commonly, rectal intussusception, rectocele, and excessive perianal descent. If defecation dysfunction is suspected, defecography may be ordered. Reduced descent of the perineum (less than 1 cm) and a reduced change in the anorectal angle (usually less than 15°) are found on simulated defecation.
4. Combination of defecatory disorder and slow transit (accounts for 3%).

For patients with slow transit problems, studies have shown that there is often a problem of several regulatory mechanisms:[11, 12, 13]

- Fewer number of mymetric plexus neurons producing the neurotransmitter substance P that acts as a stimulator for transit.
- Abnormalities in vasoactive intestinal peptide and nitric oxide that are inhibitory transmitters.
- A reduction in the number of interstitial cells of Cajal that help regulate GI motility.

An extreme example of slow transit is Hirschsprung's disease whereby ganglion cells in the distal bowel are absent. This is due to a failure of neural-crest cells to migrate caudally during embryonic development.

The main stimulus to defecate is distention of the rectum by the colon contents. This initiates the recto-anal inhibitory reflex and internal sphincter relaxation.[14] The resultant urge to defecate is voluntarily controlled. Through contraction of the external sphincter and pelvic musculature, defecation can be prevented. To defecate, a combination of intra-abdominal pressure through bearing down and external sphincter and pelvic floor muscle relaxation is voluntarily employed. Ineffective emptying is usually due to suppression of the defecation urge. This suppression may be due to painful anorectal disorders or circumstantial detractors. For example, children who are playing rarely want to interrupt their play to go to the bathroom. Additionally, they may find a restroom away from home unpleasant, which causes them to suppress the urge to defecate. In adults, commuting at the time of the defecation urge, being in a meeting, exercising, and a host of other interferences may be a reason to suppress the urge. Unfortunately, in all cases, this suppression becomes a habit, which then eventually decreases the sense of urge.

Evaluation

History

For most cases of constipation a simple line of questioning will quickly uncover the cause. Determining a patient's dietary fiber, fluid, and medication intake often will reveal the problem. Most patients do not understand that coffee, tea, and sodas do not have the same hydrating effect as water and often result in a diuretic effect. Dietary fiber is harder to determine; however, the amounts of fruits, vegetables, and fiber substitutes will give a general indication of inadequacy. Medications may cause or aggravate constipation through several mechanisms. Many drugs, such as anticholinergics, anticonvulsants, antidepressants, antiparkinsonians, and tranquilizers, act as central or peripheral neural depressants. Nonsteroid anti-inflammatory drugs (NSAIDs) may inhibit motility through prostaglandin blockade. Diuretics decrease the water content of stool. Calcium channel blockers and angiotensin-converting enzyme (ACE) inhibitors decrease smooth muscle contraction. Several laxative types (especially anthraquinones) may cause megacolon and decreased response to distention; sometimes with damage to the intramural nerve plexuses (**Table 32–2**).

The next avenue of investigation is the degree to which the urge to defecate is suppressed. Children, in particular, will avoid defecation, although adults may be found to have similar habits. Usually this falls into three categories: (1) too busy or having too much fun to stop to go to the bathroom, (2) unpleasant bathroom environment (while traveling or at school), and (3) painful defecation. Overriding the defecation reflex will eventually lead to a habit that is difficult to reestablish. If defecation is painful, questions regarding the aggressive use of rough toilet paper can often expose the cause of anal fissures.

Examination

- Determine whether there is any anorectal disease that might suppress the urge to defecate.
- Determine whether there is an empty rectum (ineffective filling disorders) or a full rectum and whether this is impacted.
- Laboratory testing is usually not necessary unless there is a suspicion of either an ionic imbalance or

Table 32–2 Laxatives	
Type	**Important Considerations**
Bulk—psyllium, husk, methylcellulose	Natural and semisynthetic polysaccharides and cellulose derivatives. Form emollients and gels when mixed with intestinal water. May produce colonic gas (especially bran), causing distention and pain. Risk of impaction if fluid intake is not increased.
Lubricants—mineral oils	Nonabsorbable hydrocarbons lubricate the colon, allowing easier passage. These have limited use because chronic use may decrease absorption of fat-soluble vitamins or cause perianal inflammation.
Osmotic—two types: saline cathartics (Milk of Magnesia) and synthetic disaccharides (lactulose)	Salts or nonabsorbable sugars act to draw fluid into the intestines. Lactulose is safe, but sorbitol is less expensive. Both are considered safe for the elderly. The saline cathartics also stimulate the release of cholecystokinin (CCK). Watch electrolyte levels, especially calcium and magnesium. Magnesium and phosphate laxatives should be avoided with renal insufficiency.
Stimulants and surface active—castor oil, anthraquinones (senna; Senokot), diphenylmethane derivatives, docusate	Decrease colonic absorption and increase secretion. Stimulate adenylate cyclase and synthesis of prostaglandin E, inhibit sodium-potassium absorption, and alter mucosal permeability. Castor oil may cause cramping. Docusate is a stool softener and is usually only effective when patients must avoid straining (postsurgically). Docusate side effects are largely due to an increased absorption of toxic drugs (gastritis with aspirin ingestion).
Enemas—glycerin, bisacodyl, tap water, saline, or soapsuds (castile soap)	Must be watchful of electrolyte losses, mucosal damage with repeated use of soaps, and hyperphosphatemia with abuse of Fleet enemas.

a specific underlying disorder such as diabetes or hypothyroidism.

- If radiographs are taken for low back pain, determine whether there is evidence of gas and fecal stasis.

Although generally it has been assumed that constipation leads to hemorrhoids, which then prolong the constipation, a recent study suggests that constipation is not a risk factor for hemorrhoids, but diarrhea may be.[15]

Special testing may be ordered for those patients unresponsive to increased dietary fiber, hydration, or laxatives and may include the following:

- Patients over age 50 years with chronic constipation should undergo colonoscopy or sigmoidoscopy with barium enema to screen for colorectal cancer.
- Colonic transit testing: Colonic transit is usually less than 72 hours. An approach to measuring transit time is through abdominal radiography 120 hours after the patient ingests radiopaque markers. Retention of more than 20% of the markers indicates prolonged transit. Suggestion of a defecatory disorder is retention of the markers in the lower-left colon and rectum.
- Anorectal manometry: Detects pressure of the anal sphincter at rest and maximal voluntary contraction, detection of absence of relaxation of the internal sphincter, rectal sensation, and the ability of the sphincters to relax during straining. Generally, patients with defecatory disorders have an inappropriate contraction of the anal sphincter both at rest and when bearing down. A high anal pressure suggests anal fissure, anismus. Rectal hyposensitivity is indicated by an increase in the volume of balloon distention needed to induce a sense of urgency, which suggests a neurologic source.
- Balloon expulsion: A latex balloon is inserted into the rectum, with 50 ml of water or air placed into the balloon. The patient is then asked to expel the balloon into the toilet. Either inability to expel the balloon or inability to do so within two minutes suggests a defecatory disorder.
- Defecography: A radiographic procedure performed using a special commode after instilling a thickened barium into the rectum. This study is able to detect the anorectal angle and perineal descent, the degree of emptying,

and certain structural abnormalities such as a rectocele, internal mucosal prolapse, or intussusception.

Management

- Bowel habit education for all patients.
- Diet recommendations for fiber and fluid intake.
- Referral if significant anorectal pathology is evident.
- Referral if indicators of colon cancer are present.
- Patients with defecatory disorders unresponsive to dietary fiber increases should undergo retraining of defecation with biofeedback.
- Patients with impaction should have manual disimpaction performed.
- Medications may be prescribed with a variety of mechanisms. Generally, osmotic laxatives are used. They take several days to a week to work. Stimulant laxatives work faster but may cause abdominal cramping. Newer approaches are Tegaserod, which is a colonic prokinetic agent (causes stimulation of $5\text{-}HT_4$ receptors, which increases peristalsis) used for women with irritable bowel syndrome who predominantly have constipation.
- Surgery is reserved for refractory cases and may include colonic resection or, more rarely, anal surgery.

The approach to management is usually conservative. When it appears that there is no evidence of a secondary cause such as medication, laxative abuse, or anorectal disease, patient education regarding proper bowel habits is usually effective. Fluid intake should be at least 1.5 L/d. It is important to define "fluid" as water and not coffee, tea, and sodas, which act more as diuretics and will usually worsen the problem. At least 30 g of fiber should be included in the daily diet. This is preferably provided by bran and vegetables. If the patient admits to a sedentary lifestyle or has been bedridden, activity and exercise (when appropriate) should be encouraged. With inactivity or illness, it is also likely that the tone of abdominal and pelvic musculature is weak. Abdominal exercises need not be strenuous. With the patient lying supine, ask her or him to bend the knees and place the feet flat on the floor or table. Then the patient is asked to lightly press the palms of the hands against his or her thighs. This is enough to give a starting contraction of the abdominals. Sit-ups are the next step, but they are not necessary if the patient is elderly, overweight, or frail.

It is imperative that patient education include a discussion of how important timing and relaxation are to proper bowel movements. The patient should understand the importance of comfort, privacy, sufficient time to defecate, and the need to "heed the call" of the defecation urge. Setting aside a regular time for bowel movements is helpful. Elevating the legs while on the toilet may also assist.[16]

When medication appears to be the culprit, referral back to the prescribing physician with a note regarding the suspected connection to the patient's constipation complaint should be made.

If fecal impaction is evident, an attempt at digital removal or recommendation for an enema is usually sufficient. If not, referral to a medical doctor for use of medications or surgery is warranted. When there is evidence of painful but mild anorectal disease (hemorrhoids or anal fissures), correction of dietary habits and bowel habits is usually sufficient; however, referral for medical management is recommended when the patient is noncompliant or the changes are ineffective.

Laxative abuse is certainly an example of too much of a good thing. Although laxative use occasionally may be needed, it is not a recommended method of bowel control. Apparently half of patients who use laxatives chronically would establish a normal bowel habit if the laxative

Table 32–3 Constipation

Drug Class	Examples	General Mechanism	Interactions/Side Effects
Bisacodyl	Apo-Bisacodyl Bisacolax Deficol Dulcolax Fleet Laxit Theralax	Used in the management of constipation. It increases intestinal fluid volume through increasing epithelial permeability.	May cause mild cramping or nausea. May cause mild electrolyte disturbances.
Docusate	PMS Docusate Surfak Dialose Colace Regulax Therevac	Used as a stool softener. Through detergent action, lowers surface tension allowing water and fats to penetrate stool.	May cause mild abdominal cramps, diarrhea, bitter taste, and throat irritation.
Psyllium	Hydrocil Instant Karasil Konsyl Metamucil Modane bulk Perdiem Plain Reguloid Serutan Silbin Syllact V-Lax	A bulk-producing laxative made from colloid of psyllium seed. Promotes peristalsis. Used for constipation.	May cause eosiniphilia, nausea, abdominal cramps, and GI tract strictures (using dry form).
Senna (sennosides)	Black Draught Gentlax Senexon Senokot Senolax	Dried leaf preparation that is converted to glycone, which causes an increase in peristalsis. Used for acute constipation.	May cause abdominal cramping, flatulence, diarrhea, weight loss, and associated loss of electrolytes.

use was discontinued.[17] The effects of laxatives generally can be divided into several categories. **Tables** 32–2 and **32–3** list these categories and give examples of various agents and their effects. Bulk-forming agents act similarly to fiber. When ingested, these agents form emollients and gels when they mix with intestinal water, expanding their size. This distention increases peristaltic activity. One side effect with these agents is that they may contribute to gas production, causing distention and discomfort. Lubricants (i.e., mineral oils) are of limited value. Chronic use may impair fat-soluble vitamin absorption and lead also to a chronic perianal inflammatory response. Salts are used for their osmotic effects of drawing in fluid and increasing reflex colon contractions. They are usually the sulfate or phosphate salts of sodium and magnesium ions (saline cathartics). A similar action occurs with lactulose; however, lactulose has no effect on the small bowel. Another group of agents is referred to as surface-active agents. They act to decrease colonic absorption and increase secretion. Stimulation of adenylate cyclase and prostaglandin E, inhibition of sodium absorption, and alteration in mucosal permeability are all possible mechanisms of these agents. Castor oil is an example of a surface-acting agent.

Rectal enemas or suppositories are usually in the form of glycerin, bisacodyl, water (tap and saline), and soaps (usually castile). These should be reserved for the patient with impaction. Chronic use may lead to colitis.

Pregnancy often results in a complaint of constipation. Although this may be multifactorial, an increase in progesterone has an effect of decreased gut motility. Aggravating this may be the increased weight, which may result in hemorrhoids. Finally, iron supplementation, which often is used in pregnancy, will have a constipating effect.

Algorithm

An algorithm for evaluation and management of constipation is presented in **Figure 32–1**.

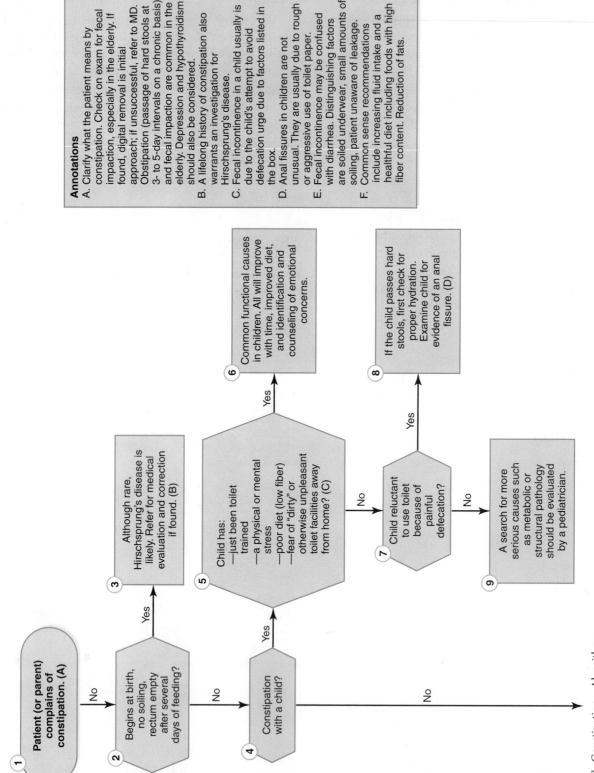

Annotations

A. Clarify what the patient means by constipation. Check on exam for fecal impaction, especially in the elderly. If found, digital removal is initial approach; if unsuccessful, refer to MD. Obstipation (passage of hard stools at 3- to 5-day intervals on a chronic basis) and fecal impaction are common in the elderly. Depression and hypothyroidism should also be considered.

B. A lifelong history of constipation also warrants an investigation for Hirschsprung's disease.

C. Fecal incontinence in a child usually is due to the child's attempt to avoid defecation urge due to factors listed in the box.

D. Anal fissures in children are not unusual. They are usually due to rough or aggressive use of toilet paper.

E. Fecal incontinence may be confused with diarrhea. Distinguishing factors are soiled underwear, small amounts of soiling, patient unaware of leakage.

F. Common sense recommendations include increasing fluid intake and a healthful diet including foods with high fiber content. Reduction of fats.

Figure 32–1 Constipation—Algorithm

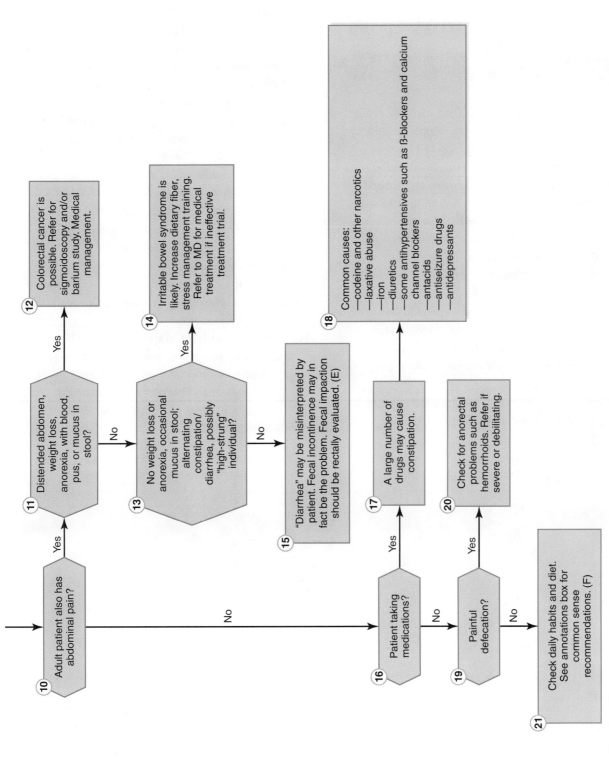

Figure 32–1 (Continued)

APPENDIX 32–1

References

1. Lembo A, Camilleri M. Chronic constipation. *N Engl J Med.* 2003;349:1360–1368.

2. Sonnenberg A, Koch TR. Physician visits in the United States for constipation: 1958–1986. *Dig Dis Sci.* 1989;34:606–611.

3. Thompson WG, Longstreth GF, Drossman DA, et al. Functional bowel disorders and functional abdominal pain. *Gut.* 1999;45: Supplement 2:11–43:11–47.

4. Harari D, Gurwitz JH, Avorn J, et al. Constipation assessment and management in an institutionalized elderly population. *J Am Geriatr Soc.* 1994;42:947–952.

5. Harari D, Gurwitz JH, Minaker KL. Constipation in the elderly. *J Am Ger Soc.* 1993;41:1130–1140.

6. Schultz SG, Frizzel RA, Nellans HN. Ion transport by mammalian small intestine. *Annu Rev Physiol.* 1974;36:51–91.

7. Devroede G, Soffe M. Colonic absorption in idiopathic constipation. *Gastroenterology.* 1973;64:552–561.

8. Connell AM. The motility of the pelvic colon, 2: paradoxical motility in diarrhea and constipation. *Gut.* 1962;3:342–448.

9. Snape WJ Jr, et al. Evidence that abnormal myoelectric activity produces colonic motor dysfunction in the irritable bowel syndrome. *Gastroenterology.* 1977;72:383.

10. Nyan DC, Pemberton JH, Ilstrup DM, Rath DM. Long-term results of surgery for constipation. *Dis Colon Rectum.* 1997;40:259–263.

11. Travella K, Riepel RL, Klauser AG, et al. Decreased substance P levels in rectal biopsies from patients with slow transit constipation. *Eur J Gastroenterol Hepatol.* 1996;8:207–211.

12. Cortesini C, Cianchi F, Infantino A, Lise M. Nitric oxide in enteric nervous system in idiopathic chronic constipation. *Dig Dis Sci.* 1995;40:2450–2455.

13. He CL, Burgart L, Wang L, et al. Decreased intestinal cells of Cajal volume in patients with slow-transit constipation. *Gastroenterology.* 2000;118:14–21.

14. Usbach TJ, Tobon F, Hambrecht T, et al. Electrophysiological aspects of human sphincter function. *J Clin Invest.* 1970;49:41–48.

15. Johanson JF, Sonnenberg A. Constipation is not a risk factor for hemorrhoids: a case-control study of potential etiological agents. *Am J Gastroenterol.* 1994;89:1981–1986.

16. Bueono-Miranda F, Cerull M, Schuster MM. Operant conditioning of colonic mobility in irritable bowel syndrome. *Gastroenterology.* 1976;70:867.

17. Zimring JG. High fiber diet versus laxatives in geriatric patients. *N Y State J Med.* 1978; 78(14):2223-2224.

Diarrhea

# CHAPTER 35

Context

Diarrhea is second only to respiratory infections as a health complaint in the United States.[1] However, the vast majority of patients have a self-limited, familiar problem that does not warrant enough concern to seek the advice of a doctor. Self-treatment with over-the-counter (OTC) medications is used effectively by many patients with acute diarrhea. Diarrhea is more a nuisance, and only when it becomes disruptive or life-threatening are answers sought by the patient or parent. Diarrhea is a concern when it is chronic and/or when it occurs in a frail individual, infants and immunocompromised patients in particular.

Diarrhea is considered acute when it lasts less than two weeks; it is considered chronic when it lasts more than two weeks. Common culprits with acute diarrhea are infections, lactose (and other deficiencies), and medications. Less commonly, but more important, diarrhea may represent part of a syndrome with gastrointestinal (GI) disease such as inflammatory bowel disease, dysentery, irritable bowel syndrome, or cancer. One helpful distinguishing factor is whether blood is present in the stool.

General Strategy

History

Determine the following according to **Exhibit 33–1**:

- Determine whether diarrhea is acute (<2 weeks), chronic (>2 weeks), or recurrent.
- Determine whether there are associated signs of infection (i.e., fever, abdominal pain, vomiting) and whether any family members or friends have

similar symptoms (viral gastroenteritis likely). (See **Table 33–1**.)

- Determine the volume and consistency of the stool (large-volume, watery stool suggests small bowel problem; small-volume stool indicates colon problem).
- Determine whether the diarrhea is bloody (consider inflammatory bowel disease, dysentery, and cancer).
- Determine any recent ingestion of medications; in particular, antibiotics or magnesium-containing antacids (a side effect with some antibiotics is overgrowth of *Clostridium difficile*).
- Determine whether there is a history of lactose intolerance (more common in patients with Mediterranean and African ancestry, in the elderly, and after acute gastroenteritis transiently).
- Determine whether diarrhea persists if the patient fasts (if present after fasting, secretory diarrhea is likely).
- Determine whether the patient has traveled to a foreign country (*Escherichia coli* or parasitic infection).

Evaluation

If chronic, check patient for electrolyte loss with lab testing and have stool evaluated for blood, mucus, fecal leukocytes (enteroinvasive bacteria), undigested food (pancreatic or small-bowel disease), and ova or cysts (parasites).

Management

- If diarrhea is in an infant, recommend electrolyte substitution drink, avoidance of milk, and cold

Exhibit 33–1 Diarrhea

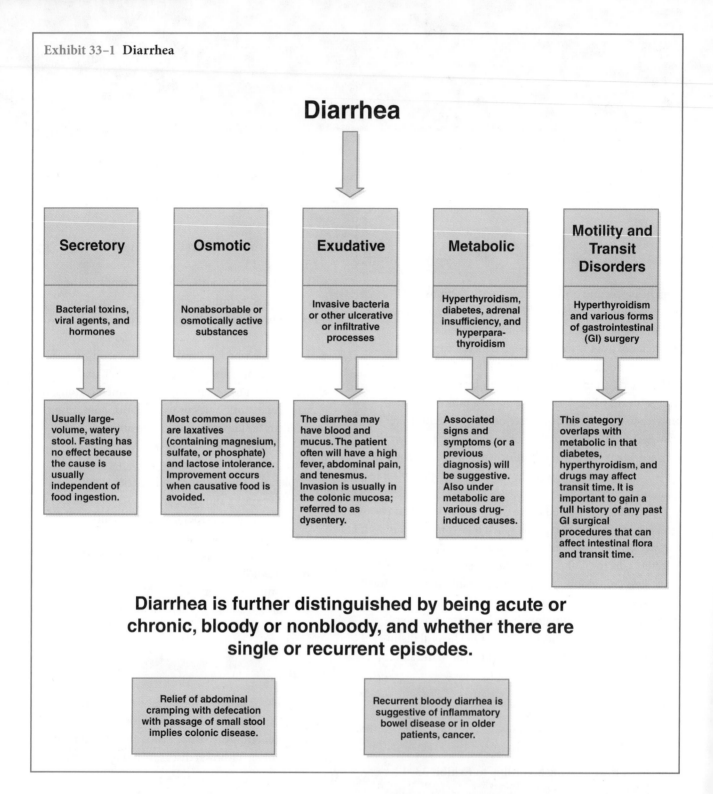

Diarrhea

Secretory	Osmotic	Exudative	Metabolic	Motility and Transit Disorders
Bacterial toxins, viral agents, and hormones	Nonabsorbable or osmotically active substances	Invasive bacteria or other ulcerative or infiltrative processes	Hyperthyroidism, diabetes, adrenal insufficiency, and hyperpara-thyroidism	Hyperthyroidism and various forms of gastrointestinal (GI) surgery
Usually large-volume, watery stool. Fasting has no effect because the cause is usually independent of food ingestion.	Most common causes are laxatives (containing magnesium, sulfate, or phosphate) and lactose intolerance. Improvement occurs when causative food is avoided.	The diarrhea may have blood and mucus. The patient often will have a high fever, abdominal pain, and tenesmus. Invasion is usually in the colonic mucosa; referred to as dysentery.	Associated signs and symptoms (or a previous diagnosis) will be suggestive. Also under metabolic are various drug-induced causes.	This category overlaps with metabolic in that diabetes, hyperthyroidism, and drugs may affect transit time. It is important to gain a full history of any past GI surgical procedures that can affect intestinal flora and transit time.

Diarrhea is further distinguished by being acute or chronic, bloody or nonbloody, and whether there are single or recurrent episodes.

Relief of abdominal cramping with defecation with passage of small stool implies colonic disease.	Recurrent bloody diarrhea is suggestive of inflammatory bowel disease or in older patients, cancer.

unfiltered juices. If not effective after two days, refer to pediatrician.

- For adults, recommend Imodium or other OTC medication coupled with elimination of milk products and cold, unfiltered juices to determine effectiveness. If ineffective, refer to medical doctor for further work-up such as with proctosigmoidoscopy.

Relevant Anatomy and Physiology

Motility of the GI tract is dependent on an intact and functioning autonomic nervous system, appropriate digestive tract flora, an appropriate transit time, and an appropriate diet. Additionally, the osmotic balance

Table 33–1 Some Causes of Gastroenteritis

Onset and Type	Summary Information
Minutes to 2 hours	
Monosodium glutamate	Sometimes referred to as Chinese restaurant syndrome, there is some debate as to whether this condition exists. If it does, it may cause a burning sensation in the abdomen, head, neck, or extremities, and may cause chest pain.
Fish toxins	There are a number of sources for fish toxins, including scombrotoxin, shellfish toxin, puffer fish toxin, and ciguatoxin (for which symptoms may take up to 24 hours to appear). Source of toxin and some symptoms for each follow: • Scombrotoxin: tuna, mahi-mahi, mackerel, skipjack, or bonito; symptoms include those of a histamine reaction with flushing headache and dizziness; may require hospitalization • Shellfish toxin: found in mussels, clams, oysters, and scallops; neurologic symptoms such as paresthesias, dizziness, and occasionally paralysis • Puffer fish toxin: puffer fish; symptoms, including paresthesias, are common • Ciguatoxin: barracuda, red snapper, grouper, and amberjack; symptoms include paresthesias, painful teeth, visual disturbances, arthralgias, itching, and a metallic taste in the mouth
Heavy metals	Usually due to a carbonated or acidic beverage, causing a metallic taste and vomiting without fever. If possible, drink should be tested for specific metal.
Mushrooms	Found with mushrooms that have not been processed commercially. May develop into encephalopathy with an altered mental state and visual disturbances. Also, hepatitis may result. Mushrooms should be tested for specific toxin such as muscarine or psilocybin.
2 hours ≥ 8 hours	
Staphylococcus aureus	Caused by ham, poultry, cream-filled pastries, and mixed salads; the predominant sign is vomiting without fever. Usually lasts less than 24 hours. Organism may be isolated from food.
Bacillus cereus	There is an emetic and a diarrhea form. Both are caused by fried rice or macaroni-and-cheese mixes. The enteric form is characterized by vomiting with no fever and lasts less than 24 hours, whereas the diarrhea form is characterized more by diarrhea and abdominal cramps with no fever and lasting less than 2 days. Organism may be isolated from food.
Clostridium perfringens	Caused by meat or poultry, it is characterized by vomiting with no fever and lasts less than 24 hours. Organisms may be isolated from food and/or stool.
12 hours to days	
Enterotoxigenic	
Escherichia coli	Rarely reported, thereby difficult to identify vehicle. Characterized by abdominal cramps and watery diarrhea that may last up to one week. Organism can be isolated in stool. Also test for enterotoxin production.
Vibrio cholerae	Rare in the U.S. Characterized by abdominal cramps and watery diarrhea that may last up to one week. Organisms may be isolated from food and/or stool.
Invasive *E. coli*	No clear vehicle for organism. Characterized by a prolonged course of fever, diarrhea, and/or dysentery. Organism may be isolated from stool. Test also for enteroinvasiveness (e.g., increase in fecal leukocytes).
Shigella	Found with fish or mixed salads. Characterized by a prolonged course of fever, diarrhea, and/or dysentery. Culture organisms in stool or food.
Salmonella	Found after ingestion of meat, poultry, dairy products, eggs, and various salads such as macaroni or potato. Characterized by a prolonged course of fever, diarrhea, and/or dysentery. Culture organisms in stool or food.
Vibrio parahaemolyticus	Found after ingestion of seafood. Characterized by a prolonged course of fever, diarrhea, and/or dysentery. Culture organisms in stool or food.
Campylobacter	Found after ingestion of poultry, meat, or unpasteurized milk. Characterized by a prolonged course of fever, diarrhea, and/or dysentery. Culture organisms in stool or food.
Clostridium botulinum	Serious problem due to cranial nerve palsies, paralysis, and ventilatory failure. Diarrhea also found. Found after ingesting contaminated house-canned foods. Botulinum toxin may be found in food, stool, or serum. Hospitalization is required.

is important in maintaining a proper fluid ratio in the stool. Two general causes of diarrhea are osmotic imbalance and secretory stimulus. Osmotic diarrhea occurs when material is nonabsorbable, acting as a fluid magnet. Examples include lactose, sorbitol, mannitol, and magnesium-containing antacids. Secretory diarrhea is due to irritation of the intestinal wall by bacterial toxins and viruses. Exudative diarrhea indicates mucosal ulceration, exudation, and bleeding. A common cause is direct bacterial invasion by organisms such as shigella and salmonella. Parasites, most commonly *Entamoeba histolytica,* also should be considered.

Insufficient time for absorption of nutrients may be caused by intestinal bypass operation, gastric surgery, hyperthyroidism, and vagotomy. These may speed up transit time. Generally, diarrhea that is due to involvement of the small intestine or the proximal colon will be more profuse, watery, and usually nonbloody. With large amounts of fluid loss, electrolytes are also lost, causing particular concern in the young and the elderly. Because of interference in digestion and absorption, the stool may contain undigested food or be greasy and foul smelling. When the pathology is in the distal colon or rectum the defecation reflex is activated, often releasing frequent, small volumes of stool that often are accompanied by flatulence. The stool is not usually foul smelling, but it may contain mucus or blood.

Evaluation

History

Usually a well-elicited history will quickly pinpoint the general cause of acute diarrhea (**Table 33–2**). More specific delineation requires laboratory evaluation of the stool; this is rarely indicated, however, unless the diarrhea is chronic or recurrent. From a historical perspective, determination of an offending substance or organism is gained by the distinction of the amount of stool, the presence of blood or mucus, and a detailed ingestion inventory.

Combinations of findings suggest a cause. For example, if the patient has large amounts of diarrhea (high fluid content) that is unrelieved by fasting, it is likely that the patient has a secretory diarrhea most commonly caused by bacterial toxins, viruses, laxative abuse, and hormones. Toxin-mediated diarrhea is usually due to small-bowel irritation. Bacterial and viral etiologies will usually have accompanying symptoms such as fever, abdominal pain, vomiting, and other symptoms. Hormonal causes are often linked to cancers. This type is rare in the chiropractic office. Laxative abuse may not be elicited on the history, but laboratory testing may uncover a surreptitious cause.

Infectious diarrhea is primarily due to colonic mucosal invasion referred to as dysentery (tenesmus, fever, abdominal pain, and bloody stools). This type of diarrhea is also characterized by early-morning rushes of diarrhea. The stool is often soft and contains mucus.

With acute diarrhea it is important to determine whether other individuals have similar symptoms (i.e., diarrhea, vomiting, or abdominal pain). Food poisoning is likely when the same food was eaten. When the diarrhea is not associated with same-food eating, but occurs in the same family or daycare facility, a viral cause is likely. Traveler's diarrhea is common, with reports of incidents affecting from 10% to 50% of those traveling abroad depending upon location, particularly in underdeveloped countries. Approximately 70% of cases are due to enterotoxigenic *Escherichia coli* (*E. coli*). Other causes include *Shigella, Salmonella,* and *Giardia.* Prophylaxis is often attempted. The primary recommendations are large doses of Pepto-Bismol (2 oz. 4 times a day (qid) for 2 to 3 weeks). Antibiotic prophylaxis occasionally may help, such as use of tetracycline (doxycycline); however, resistance has developed and has made this a less effective approach. Also, side effects include photosensitivity and candida vaginitis, among others.

It is always important to obtain a complete drug history, including prescription and nonprescription drugs. Many drugs can cause diarrhea. The primary drugs are magnesium-containing antacids, antibiotics, β-blockers, digitalis, methyldopa, alcohol, phenothiazine, and high doses of pain medications (unless a sedative). Laxative abuse should be suspected when other historical clues are negative or in the unlikely event the patient volunteers the information. Some patients may be unaware of the abuse and feel that it is necessary for "normal" bowel movements (see Chapter 32). Antibiotics can also allow overgrowth of *C. difficile,* which then produces irritating toxins. The timing of drug ingestion is often helpful, for example, if the diarrhea began after the initiation of a drug regimen. With antibiotics, however, there is often a delayed response.

Table 33-2 History Questions for Diarrhea

Primary Question	What Are You Thinking?	Secondary Questions	What Are You Thinking?
Is the diarrhea of recent onset?	Viral gastroenteritis, foreign travel (parasites), drug reaction or side effect.	**Did others in your family or did your friends have similar symptoms?** **Have you just returned from a trip to another country or back from a camping trip?** **Do you take magnesium containing antacids, laxatives, antibiotics, β-blockers, digitalis, or high doses of pain medication?**	Viral gastroenteritis is likely. Parasitic infection, or "traveler's diarrhea." All may cause diarrhea.
Do you have recurrent bouts of diarrhea?	Irritable bowel disease, inflammatory bowel disease, lactose intolerance.	**Do you have alternating bouts of constipation and diarrhea, especially in the morning?** **Do you have recurrent bouts of bloody diarrhea often associated with stress?** **Have you noticed an association with dairy products and have associated complaints of bloating and gas?** **Ask CAGE questions for alcoholism.** **Do you have any diagnosed conditions?**	Irritable bowel syndrome likely. Ulcerative colitis is possible, especially with an onset in the 20s or 30s. Lactose intolerance likely. Alcohol-related. Diabetes, hyperthyroidism, cancer.

When a patient has a complaint of chronic diarrhea, the separation of bloody from nonbloody types is an important first step. Bloody diarrhea that is constant or recurrent is highly indicative of inflammatory bowel disease. The historical distinction between ulcerative colitis (UC) and Crohn's disease is not always clear.[2] Both often begin at a young age (<30 years of age). It is more likely, because of the small-bowel involvement usually found with Crohn's disease, that there will be associated weight loss and, because of the obstruction, perianal fistulas. Patients with Crohn's disease usually have more persistent symptoms and are more likely to have a fever. Bloody diarrhea is possible but less common than with UC. UC is more likely to present with bloody diarrhea. Stressful life events tend to activate the process.[3] Abdominal pain is more common with Crohn's disease than with UC. The final determination is made with barium studies and colonoscopy.

Patients who complain of early-morning constipation (marble-sized stool) and subsequent diarrhea that is recurrent are likely to have irritable bowel syndrome (IBS). It is important, though, that as many other clues be obtained as possible prior to jumping to this conclusion. These patients often have difficulty with specific foods that they can identify for the doctor. The stool is nonbloody, but it may have mucus. If there are associated hemorrhoids, the stool may be blood-tinged.

Other clues may suggest less common causes such as venereal-related diarrhea and diarrhea secondary to other diseases:

- Patients with known diabetes or complaints of numbness/tingling in the extremities, frequent vaginal yeast infections, or orthostatic hypotension should be evaluated for diabetic autonomic involvement.
- Patients with a history of hyperthyroidism or having complaints of heat intolerance, exophthalmos, or fine hand tremors should be evaluated for the secondary effects of hyperthyroidism on increased metabolism.
- Patients involved in unprotected sex, in particular anal sex, should be evaluated for possible venereal disease with diarrhea as part of the symptom complex. Also these patients are at higher risk for acquired immunodeficiency syndrome (AIDS).

- Foul-smelling, light-colored stool that floats is suggestive of pancreatic disease, small-bowel disease, or post-cholecystectomy.
- A cause of malabsorption with associated diarrhea, found primarily in Caucasians (especially those of European descent), is celiac sprue. Also called nontropical sprue and gluten-sensitive enteropathy, celiac sprue involves an allergic response to gliadin, part of gluten that is found in wheat, rice, barley, and, to a lesser degree, oats. It is unknown whether this antibody (IgA antigliadin and antiendomysial) response is preexisting or acquired. Apparently a combination of factors, including environmental, genetic, and immunologic elements, contributes to the development of celiac sprue. Symptoms may appear at any age, with the first appearance possible when an infant is introduced to cereals in the diet. A remission from childhood onset is not uncommon during the twenties. Symptoms include diarrhea, steatorrhea, weight loss, and the outcome of nutrient deficiencies, primarily anemia. Suspicion is high when symptoms are eliminated through avoidance of gluten-containing foods. Confirmatory diagnosis requires a small intestine biopsy. Celiac sprue is also associated with insulin-dependent diabetes and dermatitis herpetiformis. Approximately 90% of patients will respond to gluten restriction in their diet. The remainder should avoid soy, lactose, and/or include fat restriction. If ineffective, other medical approaches may be considered, including corticosteroids.

Examination

The majority of important indicators are historical. With acute diarrhea, an abdominal examination should be performed to determine acute inflammatory processes. A rectal examination should be performed in patients with chronic diarrhea.

Laboratory testing to determine the cause of diarrhea includes both serologic testing and stool sample testing. Serologic testing should be performed based on the suspected cause; however, it may include any or all of the following:

- For general inflammation, ESR (erythrocyte sedimentation rate) and/or CRP (C-reactive protein)
- For anemia, infection, and some cancers, CBC (complete blood count)

- TSH (thyroid stimulating hormone) to check for thyroid dysfunction as a cause

For detecting and distinguishing inflammatory bowel disease, the following single tests or combined tests in panels may be ordered:

- pANCA (perinuclear antineutrophil cytoplasmic antibody) for UC; found in about 50% of patients (only 5% to 20% of patients with Crohn's disease).
- ASCA (*Saccharomyces cerevisiae* antibodies), IgG and IgA. For Crohn's disease found in about 40% to 50% of patients. For UC, this test is not very definitive, with ASCA IgG found in only about 20% and with ASCA IgA found in less than 1%.
- Antiglycan antibodies. Elevated in 75% of patients with Crohn's versus only 5% of patients with UC.
- Anti-CBir1 (*Clostridium* species antibodies). For Crohn's, found in about 50% of patients.
- Anti-Omp C (*Escherichia coli* antibodies). For rapidly progressing Crohn's disease.
- Anti-I-2 (*Pseudomonas fluorescens* antibodies)

For the evaluation/detection of celiac disease, the following tests have been utilized:

- IgA class of anti-tissue transglutaminase antibody (anti-tTG): Anti-tTG, IgA is the most *sensitive* and *specific* blood test for celiac disease; however, it may be negative in children under age 3 years who have celiac disease. For this group, deamidated gliadin peptide (DGP) antibodies, IgA, called the Anti-DGP test, may prove useful.
- Anti-gliadin antibodies (AGA), IgG and IgA classes
- Quantitative immunoglobulin A (IgA)

Other tests that are either new or used less often for celiac disease include:

- Anti-endomysial antibodies (EMA), IgA class
- Anti-reticulin antibodies (ARA), IgA class
- Anti-actin (F-actin), IgA class

Stool testing is important to find the underlying cause. Stool samples are tested for blood and for polymorphonuclear leukocytes (PMNs) (e.g., Calprotectin and Lactoferrin).

Fecal PMNs are highly suggestive of an enteroinvasive bacterial cause such as *Campylobacter, Shigella,* or enteroinvasive *E. coli.*[4] When fecal PMNs are found, the laboratory should be instructed to culture the stool in an effort to identify the causative organism. Given that the isolation rate of bacteria in stool cultures is under 3% with acute diarrhea, it is unnecessary and expensive to order stool culture in those patients. When giardiasis is suspected, the laboratory should be instructed to look for cysts.

Patients with chronic diarrhea should be screened historically for identifiable causes prior to resorting to laboratory evaluation.

- If medications appear to be the culprit, discontinue if OTC or refer the patient back to the prescribing physician.
- If the patient has a diagnosis of diabetes, hyperthyroidism, pancreatic disease, or other conditions that may cause diarrhea, refer the patient to the primary provider without further laboratory testing.
- If the patient is suspected of having lactose intolerance, recommend a lactose-free diet or an OTC lactase product prior to further laboratory testing.

When a patient is suspected of having an inflammatory bowel disorder, refer to a physician for GI imaging studies or proctosigmoidoscopy. If the patient is suspected of having a metabolic disorder, order laboratory tests specific to the disorder (i.e., serum glucose for diabetes, supersensitive thyroid stimulating hormone [TSH] for thyroid disorders). If maldigestion is evident in the history (i.e., weight loss, vitamin deficiency, and osmotic diarrhea), quantification of fecal fat should be ordered; fatty acids suggest malabsorption.

Management

Antibiotic treatment is needed only in selected cases. In those patients who are immunosuppressed, antibiotics may protect against complications of a bacterial-caused diarrhea. Most acute diarrhea resolves in two days and therefore does not need antibiotic management. Viral and bacterial toxin-mediated diarrhea is not responsive to antibiotics. Antibiotic therapy is recommended for shigellosis and for any patient with severe enteroinvasive diarrhea.[5] Infections with parasites such as *Giardia* and *E. histolytica* often require metronidazole (Flagyl).

The OTC drug approach to diarrhea is often effective. However, it is important to remember that diarrhea is often the body's attempt to rid itself of infectious agents. Using these agents too early in the course may be counterproductive and may prolong the infection. There are generally three types of medications available:[6]

1. Antimotility drugs—Loperamide (Imodium) is the most common type and quite effective (codeine is an effective prescription drug).
2. Antisecretory drugs—Bismuth subsalicylate (Pepto-Bismol) reduces diarrhea through prostaglandin inhibition (aspirin has some effect).
3. Absorbents—Kaopectate (mainly clay and pectin from apples/citrus fruits) bulks up the stool.

Table 33–3 lists common medications and their side effects. The primary goal of treatment is to maintain proper glucose and electrolytes. Sports drinks are not

Table 33–3 Antidiarrheal Medications

Drug Class	Examples	General Mechanism	Interactions/Side Effects
Bismuth	Pepto-Bismol	Hydrolyzed to salicylate which inhibits inflammatory prostaglandins. Used as an antidiarrheal both prophylactic and treatment. Also for temporary relief of indigestion.	May cause temporary darkening of stool, a metallic taste in the mouth, a bluish gum line, and possible bleeding tendencies.
Kaolin-Pectin	Kaopectate Kaospan Kolain w/Pectin	Kaolin as an aluminum silicate may have adsorbent and demulcent actions. Pectin may help to consolidate stool. Used for mild to moderate diarrhea.	May cause mild constipation.
Loperamide	Imodium Maalox antidiarrheal Pepto Diarrhea Control	Synthetic piperidine derivative that inhibits GI peristaltic activity. OTC medication used in the treatment of acute diarrhea or chronic diarrhea associated with inflammatory bowel disease.	Toxic megacolon with overuse, may cause drowsiness, CNS depression, dizziness, bloating, constipation, or abdominal pain.

appropriate because the fluid must be hypo-osmolar. For infants, several OTC drinks are available, such as Pedialyte. A simple home concoction is a mixture of ½ tsp salt, 1 tsp baking soda, 8 tsp sugar, and 8 oz of orange juice diluted in water to produce 1 L of liquid.[7]

Persons traveling to foreign countries should pack an antidiarrheal compound and, if concerned, ask their physicians about newer antibacterial agents such as Xifaxan (rifaximin).[8]

A common problem for senior patients is *C. difficile*. This is the result of antibiotic treatment that allows the overgrowth of *C. difficile* due to the destruction of much of the normal flora of the digestive tract. Difficult to treat and with recurrence high, this form of infection kills 14,000 Americans each year. A novel approach is now being used for recalcitrant cases. It involves taking a sample of stool from a healthy individual and through a process of preparation, giving this to a patient with *C. difficile*. It is referred to as a fecal transplant and has shown some success warranting its consideration.[9,10]

For prophylaxis, commercially available probiotics generally contain combinations of strains or species, generally from two to eight. Most contain lactic acid-producing *Bifidobacterium* or *Lactobacillus* species and strains. The available evidence for probiotics to support many of the commercial claims is not strong. What is available are some studies indicating some success in managing prevention of antibiotic-associated diarrhea in adults, acute infectious diarrhea, and prevention of necrotizing enterocolitis in premature infants.[11]

Algorithms

Algorithms for evaluation and management of acute and chronic diarrhea are presented in **Figures 33–1** and **33–2**.

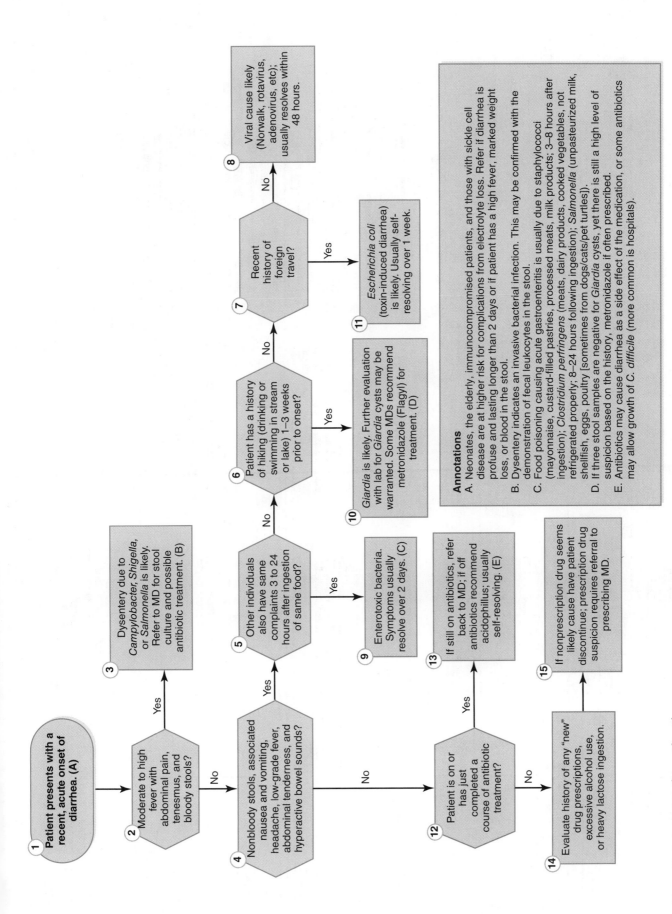

Figure 33–1 Acute Diarrhea—Algorithm

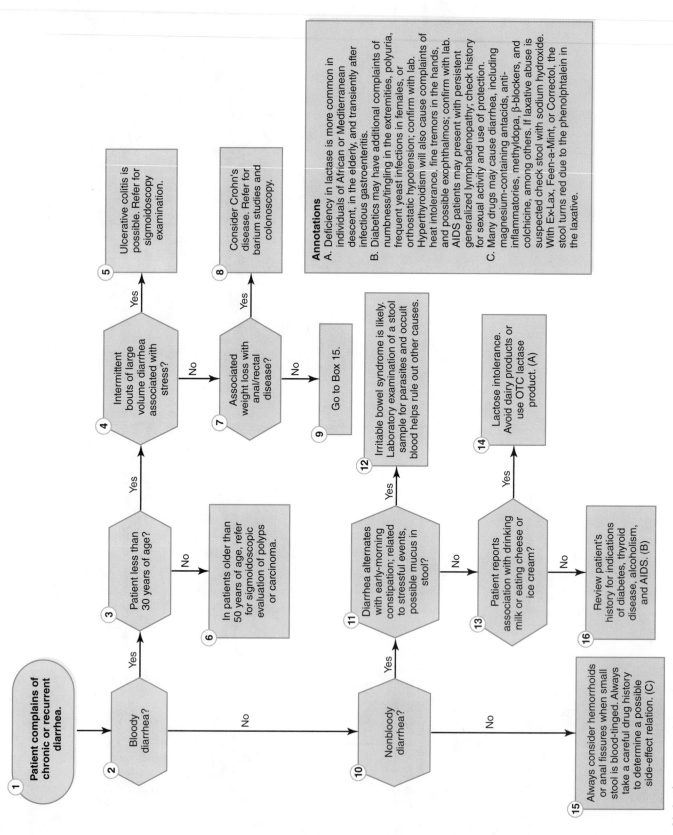

Figure 33–2 Chronic Diarrhea—Algorithm

Annotations

A. Deficiency in lactase is more common in individuals of African or Mediterranean descent, in the elderly, and transiently after infectious gastroenteritis.

B. Diabetics may have additional complaints of numbness/tingling in the extremities, polyuria, frequent yeast infections in females, or orthostatic hypotension; confirm with lab. Hyperthyroidism will also cause complaints of heat intolerance, fine tremors in the hands, and possible exophthalmos; confirm with lab. AIDS patients may present with persistent generalized lymphadenopathy; check history for sexual activity and use of protection.

C. Many drugs may cause diarrhea, including magnesium-containing antacids, anti-inflammatories, methyldopa, β-blockers, and colchicine, among others. If laxative abuse is suspected check stool with sodium hydroxide. With Ex-Lax, Feen-a-Mint, or Correctol, the stool turns red due to the phenolphtalein in the laxative.

1 **Patient complains of chronic or recurrent diarrhea.**

2 Bloody diarrhea?

3 Patient less than 30 years of age? — Yes

4 Intermittent bouts of large volume diarrhea associated with stress? — Yes

5 Ulcerative colitis is possible. Refer for sigmoidoscopy examination.

6 In patients older than 50 years of age, refer for sigmoidoscopic evaluation of polyps or carcinoma.

7 Associated weight loss with anal/rectal disease? — Yes

8 Consider Crohn's disease. Refer for barium studies and colonoscopy.

9 Go to Box 15.

10 Nonbloody diarrhea?

11 Diarrhea alternates with early-morning constipation; related to stressful events, possible mucus in stool? — Yes

12 Irritable bowel syndrome is likely. Laboratory examination of a stool sample for parasites and occult blood helps rule out other causes.

13 Patient reports association with drinking milk or eating cheese or ice cream? — Yes

14 Lactose intolerance. Avoid dairy products or use OTC lactase product. (A)

15 Always consider hemorrhoids or anal fissures when small stool is blood-tinged. Always take a careful drug history to determine a possible side-effect relation. (C)

16 Review patient's history for indications of diabetes, thyroid disease, alcoholism, and AIDS. (B)

APPENDIX 33–1

References

1. Baldassano RN, Liacouras CA. Chronic diarrhea: a practical approach for the pediatrician. *Pediatr Clin North Am.* 1991;38:667–687.

2. Farmer RG. Differentiating Crohn's disease from ulcerative colitis. *Diagnosis.* 1987;7:66–74.

3. Levenstein Sprantera C, Varvo V, et al. Psychological stress and disease activity in ulcerative colitis: a multi-dimensional cross-sectional study. *Am J Gastroenterol.* 1994;89:1219–1225.

4. Ritka P, Banwell JG. Laboratory workup of the patient with diarrhea. *Diagnosis.* 1986;12:22–38.

5. Park SI, Gianella RA. Approach to the adult patient with acute diarrhea. *Gastroenterol Clin North Am.* 1993;22:483.

6. Reilly BM. Diarrhea. In: *Practical Strategies in Outpatient Medicine.* 2nd ed. Philadelphia: WB Saunders; 1991:856.

7. McQuaid KR. Alimentary tract: acute diarrhea. In: Tierney LM Jr, McPhee SJ, Papadakis MA, eds. *Current Medical Diagnosis & Treatment 1995.* 3rd ed. Norwalk, CT: Appleton & Lange; 1995:485.

8. Scarpignato C, Rampal P. Prevention and treatment of traveler's diarrhea: a clinical pharmacological approach. *Chemotherapy.* 1995;41:48–81.

9. Burke KE, Lamont JT. Fecal transplantation for recurrent *Clostridium difficile* infection in older adults: a review. *J Am Geriatr Soc.* 2013;61(8):1394–1398.

10. van Nood E, Dijkgraaf MG, Keller JJ. Duodenal infusion of feces for recurrent *Clostridium difficile. N Engl J Med.* 2013;368(22):2145.

11. Guarner F, Khan AG, Garisch J, et al. World Gastroenterology Organisation Global Guidelines: probiotics and prebiotics October 2011. *J Clin Gastroenterol.* Jul 2012;46(6):468–481.

Genitourinary Complaints

Urinary Incontinence and Voiding Dysfunction

Context

Although 10 million individuals in the United States have urinary incontinence, it often remains a secret to loved ones and the patients' doctors.[1] It is estimated that in the elderly, 15% to 30% who live at home have urinary incontinence. This percentage increases in the acute-care setting to one-third, and up to one-half of all the elderly in extended-care facilities are incontinent.[2]

Because of the associated embarrassment, the patient rarely volunteers information about incontinence if it is not a chief complaint. It is important, especially in the elderly and in women over age 40 years, to question the patient about loss of bladder control. It is unfortunate that many women consider incontinence as "normal."

For the chiropractor, it is important to realize that a full evaluation involves examination of the genital and perianal regions in both males and females. This scenario may not be a comfortable one for the chiropractor if his or her training is not extensive for this area of investigation. Historical clues, though, can narrow down the diagnosis to the type of incontinence (or whether there is incontinence) and facilitate proper referral. For those who perform a thorough examination, it is important to realize that a complete evaluation for some types of incontinence requires ultrasound and/or urodynamic studies. These fall within the domain of the urologist.

General Strategy

History

Determine the following:

- Whether the patient has signs of irritative bladder (urgency, increased frequency, nocturia,

dysuria) or obstructive bladder (decreased stream, dribbling, hesitancy, or intermittent stream) dysfunction
- Whether the patient has any known diseases such as Parkinson's disease, diabetes, multiple sclerosis, or others, including other urinary tract diseases (see **Table 34–1**)
- What, when, and how much fluid the patient drinks (large intake of diuretic fluids such as coffee, tea, colas, alcohol, or large amounts of water [especially before bed] may cause nocturia)
- Whether the patient is taking any over-the-counter or prescription medications that may influence micturition (loop diuretics, α-adrenergic blockers, calcium channel blockers, cold capsules or nasal decongestants, haloperidol, or others)
- Whether there are positions in which the incontinence is most likely to occur (stress incontinence usually occurs while standing [unless patient laughs], nycturia occurs while recumbent)
- Whether coughing, sneezing, laughing, exercising, or jumping causes loss of small amounts of urine (common with stress incontinence)
- Whether the patient's mental state or mobility is a factor
- Whether there is a history of past surgeries or radiation therapy

Examination

- Determine whether the patient has any signs of neurologic dysfunction; test for perianal reflex and lower extremity reflexes.
- Evaluate the perianal area for signs of fistulas or prolapse.

Table 34–1 Some Urinary Tract Diseases*

Type	Summary Information
Kidney	
Polycystic kidney disease	A bilateral autosomal dominant disease where numerous fluid-filled cysts are formed (from obstructed tubules) causing the kidneys to be enlarged in size and weight (as much as 20 times heavier). Impairment of renal function leads to early renal failure at around 30–40 years of age. Other congenital disorders, including cystic renal dysplasia, generally affect only one kidney.
Glomerulopathies	**Acute Glomerulonephritis:** Usually secondary to streptococcal infection, occurring 1–2 weeks after antibodies form antigen-antibody complexes that activate complement resulting in inflammation. Rare in the United States. Clinically presents as nephritic syndrome with proteinuria and hematuria, with resulting edema and hypertension. Usually resolves, with 1%–2% having acute renal failure and in <10% of cases, chronic glomerulonephritis.
	Crescentic Glomerulonephritis: A rare condition occurring after focal necrosis of the glomerular capillaries as in Goodpasture's syndrome, which is an autoimmune disease forming antibodies to the basement membrane both in the kidneys and lungs (collage type IV). May also be caused by Wegener's granulomatosis, polyarteritis nodosa, or poststreptococcal glomerulonephritis. Capillary loops are blocked, leading to glomerular filtration failure. Survival requires dialysis or renal transplantation.
	Membranous Nephropathy: An immune disorder causing thickening of the glomerular basement membrane, leading to nephrotic syndrome. Idiopathic in 85% of cases. Known causes include hepatitis B virus or Treponema pallidum. Proteinuria is found for years, which progresses in about 40% of patients with eventual need of dialysis or renal transplantation.
	Lipoid Nephrosis (minimal change disease or nil disease): A disease of unknown etiology that leads to nephritic syndrome (most common in children). Responds to corticosteroid treatment.
	Chronic Proliferative Glomerulonephritis: Immune-mediated disorders (e.g., Berger's disease—IgA nephropathy) and with autoimmune disorders, most commonly systemic lupus erythematosus (SLE). Leads to either nephritic or nephrotic disorder with variable results, including possible hematuria and proteinuria with or without symptoms. Some are responsive to corticosteroid treatment.
	End-stage Nephropathy: For many immune-mediated glomerulonephropathies, progression to hyalinization of glomeruli leads to shrunken kidneys and end-stage kidney disease.
	Diabetic Nephropathy: Diabetes causes a number of changes in the kidneys, including diffuse glomerulosclerosis (thickening of the basement membrane), arteriolar hyalinization and thickening, and papillary necrosis. Membrane permeability leads to proteinuria and chronic renal insufficiency. Diabetic kidneys are also prone to infection.
Pyelonephritis	Infection of the kidneys may be conveyed through the blood or retrograde through the ureters (most common). In children, 30%–50% may be due to vesicoureteral reflux or congenital abnormalities. Females are far more affected than males. Usually bacterial (e.g., *E. coli, Proteus, Klebsiella, Pseudomonas*) and rarely parasitic, yeast, or protozoal. Onset is often acute, with fever, flank pain with radiation into the groin, nausea, and vomiting. There is kidney tenderness upon palpation and a positive kidney punch sign. Symptoms of a lower UTI occur in about 33% of patients. Lab findings include leukocytosis, pyuria, and bacteria cultured from urine. Treatment is with antibiotics specific to the organism.
Renal cell carcinoma	The most common kidney neoplasm. Males are affected twice as often as females. There may be a higher risk for smokers to develop renal cell carcinoma. Only 10% of patients are symptomatic, with flank pain, hematuria, and a palpable mass. Fifty percent are discovered incidentally on computed tomography. Nonspecific clinical complaints are more common, including weight loss, fever, or hypertension. Paraneoplastic findings occur in about 20% of patients. Surgical excision results in a 5-year survival of 40%.
Wilms' tumor	Also called a nephroblastoma, it is the most common solid tumor of infants and young children. May be associated with a syndrome that includes anindia (lack of iris), general malformations, and mental retardation. The tumor, composed of immature cells, is present at birth but is not apparent until 2–4 years of age, usually detected as an abdominal mass by the parent or doctor. The tumor is quite malignant but responds well to chemotherapy and/or surgery, with an 85% cure rate.

Table 34–1 Some Urinary Tract Diseases* (continued)

Type	Summary Information
Bladder	
Cystitis	Infection of the bladder is via a number of different organisms including bacterial (e.g., *E. coli*, *Proteus*, *Klebsiella*, *Pseudomonas*) and yeast (e.g., candida). Females are far more often affected than males. The onset of symptoms is acute, with common irritative complaints of urgency, frequent urination of small amounts of urine (including nocturia), and burning upon urination. Other complaints include suprapubic pain/tenderness and low back pain. Laboratory evaluation reveals gross hematuria with bacterial cystitis. Pyuria and culture of midstream catch reveals causative organisms. Common to recur in many patients, especially those with diabetes, benign prostatic hypertrophy, and those with calculi. Drinking cranberry juice may be preventive.
Carcinoma	Occurring in the elderly, urinary bladder carcinoma is three times more common in males than females. The primary risk factor is smoking, directly proportional to the amount of smoking during a lifetime. An unusual cause is *S. haematobium*, a parasite in Egypt. Symptoms usually occur early with dysuria, lower abdominal pain, and hematuria. Diagnosis is confirmed with cystoscopy with histologic examination of biopsied specimen. Response to surgery, chemotherapy, and immunotherapy such as *bacillus Calmette-Guerin* (BCG) is 98% for local tumors that have not metastasized; those that have are usually deadly.
Male Genital (for females, see Table 55-4 in Chapter 55)	
Cryptorchidism	Undescended testicles are usually due to the inguinal canal being obliterated. Descent usually occurs by the time of birth with only a few (3%–4%) having retractile testes where the cremasteric muscle may pull them through the inguinal canal. Only 1% after the first year of life have undescended testicles. Surgical repositioning is an effective treatment. However, some complications include atrophy and hypospermatogenesis, leading in later life to infertility. Also, cryptorchid testes are more likely to develop carcinoma (10-fold greater risk). Early correction reduces this risk.
Testicular cancer	Accounting for only 1% of neoplasms in males, these germ cell tumors occur around ages 30–40 years. There are various types, including seminomas, teratomas, embryonal carcinomas, endodermal sinus tumor, and choriocarcinoma. Metastasis is through the periaortic lymph nodes in the abdomen, potentially spreading to the liver, lungs, and brain. Diagnosis is usually first made with the detection of a scrotal mass. Radioimmunoassay for α-fetoprotein and β-human chorionic gonadotropin are the lab markers for tumor. Chemotherapy is quite successful, with a 90% cure rate.

*Not covered in "Selected Causes" section.

- Perform or refer for a prostate examination on men; a vaginal examination on women.
- Perform a urinalysis on all patients in an attempt to determine renal function or indicators of urinary tract infection (UTI).
- Refer for urodynamic testing by a urologist if incontinence is severe.

Management

- For patients with stress incontinence, prescription of exercises and behavioral training may be effective; if not, refer for medication or, in rare cases, surgery.
- For patients with diabetes mellitus, comanage with the medical doctor.

- For patients with prostate hypertrophy, manage with behavioral training and some dietary recommendations; if ineffective, refer for medication or possible surgery.

Relevant Anatomy and Physiology

Bladder control is an intricate balance among several neural systems. The tension within the bladder that is generated by filling must be balanced by restriction of outflow at the bladder neck. The primary innervation of the body of the bladder is parasympathetic (pudendal nerve S2-S4). Therefore, parasympathetic stimulation facilitates urination by causing contraction of the body of the bladder (detrusor muscle) and urinary sphincter relaxation. Sympathetic innervation is via the hypogastric nerve plexus with nerve cell bodies at T11-L2. β-adrenergic (sympathetic) stimulation causes detrusor muscle relaxation during filling. α-Adrenergic (sympathetic) stimulation at the bladder neck (which acts as an internal urethral sphincter) acts to prevent urination.

The micturition center is located in the pons and acts to inhibit urination. Cortical override occurs through connections from the frontal lobe, corpus callosum, and cingulate gyrus, which generally inhibit the pontine micturition center.

Various forms of dysfunction can affect this intricate balance. Involuntary contractions of the detrusor muscle may occur as a result of irritation or neurologic disease. This hyperreflexia is referred to as detrusor instability, or an unstable bladder. A different type of dysfunction occurs when the force of contraction of the bladder is too weak to expel all the urine, leading to residual retention and subsequent irritation or infection. This condition also may occur with any bladder outlet obstruction, such as prostatic hypertrophy or urethral stricture, when the ability to overcome this added resistance from obstruction is exceeded. When there is pelvic floor weakness and secondarily hypermobility of the urethra, an unequal pressure is created. Maneuvers that increase intra-abdominal pressure cause bladder pressure to exceed urethral sphincter resistance, and urine is lost.

Urinary incontinence has been divided into several major types,[3] as follows:

- Urge incontinence—A sudden, uncontrollable urge to void is created by bladder irritation or neurologic dysfunction with urge incontinence. The most common cause is benign prostatic hypertrophy or urinary tract infection.
- Stress incontinence—Stress incontinence occurs when actions such as laughing, coughing, sneezing, or jumping cause loss of a small amount of urine. The most common cause is pelvic floor weakness in women.
- Mixed incontinence—This is a combination of urge and stress incontinence, often occurring in the elderly. Also, two-thirds of men with prostatic hypertrophy have obstruction and detrusor hyperactivity.
- Overflow incontinence—Overflow incontinence occurs when an overdistended bladder exceeds the resistance of the urethral sphincter, and urine is

lost. This is often due to detrusor weakness and/or outflow obstruction.

- Total incontinence—Total incontinence is the loss of urine at all times regardless of body position. Rarely would it be seen undiagnosed in the chiropractic setting. It is usually due to serious neurologic or structural abnormalities.

Evaluation

History

The distinction between irritative and obstructive symptoms may give valuable clues to an underlying etiology. For example, if the patient complains of dysuria, urgency, increased frequency, and nocturia, an irritative cause is likely. Further investigation with urinalysis for a UTI is essential. For patients complaining of a decreased stream, hesitancy, dribbling, and a sense of incomplete emptying, an obstructive problem is likely. With men the most common problem is prostate hypertrophy, warranting a digital rectal examination.

For obstructive symptoms in males, the standard questionnaire in use is the American Urological Association (AUA) Symptom Index for Evaluation of Benign Prostate Hyperplasia.[4] It consists of seven questions with the possibility of the following responses for each: not at all, less than 1 time in 5, less than half the time, about half, more than half, and almost always. The questions all begin with "over the past month" and continue with:

- How often have you had a sensation of not emptying your bladder completely after you finished urinating?
- How often have you had to urinate again less than two hours after you had finished urinating?
- How often have you found you stopped and started again several times when you urinated?
- How often have you found it difficult to postpone urination?
- How often have you had a weak urinary stream?
- How often have you had to push or strain to begin urination?
- How many times do you most typically get up to urinate from the time you went to bed at night until you got up in the morning?

Each question can result in 0 to 5 points with a total score from 0 to 35 possible. Patients scoring 0 to 7 are considered mildly symptomatic, 8 to 19 moderately symptomatic, and 20 to 35 severely symptomatic.

With a complaint of incontinence, the timing of incontinence onset with regard to childbirth, surgery, radiation therapy, low back pain, or medication ingestion often will provide valuable clues. Important clues to differentiation among the various types of incontinence are the amount of fluid lost and the position or circumstances surrounding the loss. Patients who have problems only with increased abdominal pressure from laughing, sneezing, coughing, or jarring and subsequently void small amounts are likely to have stress incontinence. If patients are unable to stop voiding in midstream, stress incontinence is suggested. Patients who have a sense of uncontrollable urge without regard to body position are likely to have urge incontinence. A large amount of fluid loss associated with a large fluid intake is highly suggestive of diabetes, although some nondiabetic patients believe that an intake of more than eight glasses of water a day is necessary for optimal health.

If the patient complains mainly of nocturia it is critical to determine when the patient goes to bed, how often he or she actually gets up at night, how much is voided, and what his or her fluid intake is prior to going to bed. Patients who report voiding large amounts of fluid after one to two hours of recumbency are more likely to have nycturia. This reflects a shift in fluid from a lower extremity interstitial site to intravascular incorporation assisted by recumbency. This is seen with patients having right-sided heart failure, liver disease, or chronic venous insufficiency. Nocturia is often the continuation of a daily voiding problem caused by diabetes or renal failure.

If the patient is elderly, it is important to remember that there is a natural tendency to void most fluid after 9 p.m. In younger patients, most fluid is voided prior to 9 p.m. In addition, the bladder capacity is reduced in the elderly.[5] If patients ingest water or beverages with xanthine, such as coffee, tea, and sodas, they will likely have to void more often.

Male patients who complain of irritative bladder symptoms that appear to be evidence for a UTI may have an aseptic inflammation of the prostate, referred to as prostatosis. Approximately one-third of male patients who appear to have a UTI do not respond to antibiotic therapy. The belief is that some stimulus for inflammation causes a protracted course lasting approximately nine months to one year. During this time, male patients are likely to seek second and third opinions without any satisfactory answer or solution. If the patient is responsive to an elimination approach, he may have prostatosis.

Elimination or avoidance of alcohol, spicy foods, citrus drinks, and caffeine will usually cause a dramatic decrease in symptoms and in some cases resolve the problem. Reassurance that this is a self-resolving condition is important psychological counseling as the patient may become very frustrated.

Examination

General examination findings that might suggest an underlying cause for incontinence are lower extremity edema, mental status abnormalities, decreased reflexes, or sensory abnormalities. An elderly patient's ability to ambulate should be evaluated as an indicator of the ability to reach the bathroom when needed.

Specific focus is on the genital/rectal area. As mentioned previously, this may be uncomfortable for the chiropractor and especially the patient. If performed in the chiropractic setting, it is important to have a same-sex (as the patient) witness (if opposite sex doctor). The examination begins with an examination of the urethra in an effort to detect possible signs of infection. Rectal examination is used to determine prostate status in men and possible fecal impaction in both men and women. A pelvic examination in women may reveal a cystocele or a prolapse and the estrogen status (atrophic vaginitis). A urethrocele may be evident by bulging of the urethra with coughing. Another similar approach (for women) is to insert a cotton-tipped swab into the urethra and watch for movement of more than 30° from the horizontal with coughing or straining. This indicates a hypermobile urethra, which is associated with stress incontinence.

If the patient is cooperative, the doctor may watch the patient void (especially helpful in men) to determine the degree of hesitancy, the amount of stream, and the consistency of flow. With women it may be helpful to have the patient cough with a full bladder to determine whether there is any leaking. If there is immediate leaking, stress incontinence is likely. If there is a delay of a few seconds, detrusor instability is more likely. The bladder should be palpated in an effort to determine distention, although this may be difficult in many patients because of obesity or muscularity.

Neurologic status should also be checked, including rectal sphincter tone, by stroking the perianal area, looking for an anal "wink" that indicates an intact S2-S4 spinal cord level.

An essential in-office evaluation of urine is important to detect signs of UTI, renal dysfunction, or possible bladder cancer. A laboratory finding of greater than five white blood cells per high-power field is suggestive of a UTI, especially when accompanied with bacteriuria. A culture should be ordered. Glucosuria, proteinuria, or yeast suggests diabetes. Hematuria may indicate bladder cancer if associated with suprapubic pain. Total and free prostate-specific antigen (PSA) should be included for males with suspicion of prostate cancer.

Special testing may be performed in a urologic setting. Urodynamic studies combine uroflowmetry and cystometry and/or videofluoroscopy. These studies are briefly listed as follows:

- Uroflowmeter—measures the urine flow in millimeters per second and is used in combination with postvoid residual (PVR) urine volume to differentiate between obstruction and weak detrusor tone.
- Cystoscopy—allows a direct visualization of the bladder and is used to determine any obstruction to outflow.
- Cystometry—used to measure capacity and compliance, assess bladder sensation, and determine any voluntary or involuntary detrusor contractions.
- Ultrasonography—used to measure PVR urine volume.

PVR urine volume is often used to differentiate among the various types of incontinence. If the PVR volume is greater than 100 mL, impaired detrusor contraction is suspected. If the PVR volume is greater than 300 mL, overflow incontinence is likely. If the PVR volume is under 100 mL, stress or urgency incontinence is likely. If the uroflowmeter measurement is normal and the PVR volume is normal, obstruction is unlikely.

Management

Conservative nondrug, nonsurgical options may be helpful in patients with detrusor instability or stress incontinence. The basis of these behavioral approaches is bladder training for detrusor instability and Kegel (pelvic floor) exercises for stress incontinence. Additional approaches include biofeedback training, electrical stimulation, and vaginal cones. Conservative approaches require a compliant and highly motivated patient. The success rate with these conservative approaches is rather good when both cure rate and improved rate are combined. For urge incontinence, one study[6] indicated a "success" rate of 87% (12% cured; 75% improved). For stress incontinence the success rate with pelvic floor exercises was also 87% (12% cured; 75% improved); with bladder training, the success rate was 70% (16% cured; 54% improved).

Bladder Training

Bladder training sets timed intervals for voiding. The patient is instructed to postpone voiding until the scheduled time. Starting with one-hour intervals during the day, the patient is asked to increase the time interval gradually (over days) by 15 to 30 minutes. Over weeks, the patient should set a goal of 2½- to 3-hour intervals. In supporting this attempt, it is important to have the patient keep a diary. Another important factor is to have the patient time his or her drinking habits. Avoidance of intake of large amounts of water, coffee or tea, or carbonated drinks may help. A variation on this technique is timed voiding. With timed voiding the patient sets a schedule that fits his or her natural schedule instead of rigid timed intervals.

Pelvic Floor Exercises

Although women with stress incontinence traditionally use Kegel exercises, they also may be helpful with urge incontinence and for men with incontinence after prostate surgery. The purpose of the exercises is to strengthen the pubococcygeus muscle and increase control over the periurethral and pelvic muscles. One reason for failure (other than noncompliance) is improper performance. In essence, the patient makes the mistake of performing a Valsalva maneuver. It is crucial to explain clearly and give written instructions on the performance of these exercises (or direct patient to Help for Incontinent People [HIP]). The patient must understand that the contractions are localized without concomitant contraction of the abdominal, gluteal, or thigh muscles. A good beginning exercise is to ask the patient to stop voiding in midstream. This can be accomplished only with the proper muscle recruitment. With the same focus, the patient should perform the exercise off the toilet and hold the contraction for approximately 10 seconds. The exercises should be performed religiously and often as many as 100 times per day. An adjunctive approach is to use vaginal cones for females. The cone is inserted and the patient attempts to hold it in place by contracting the pelvic floor muscles. This is performed twice a day for 15 minutes using multiple repetitions lasting for 20 to 30 seconds each.

Augmented Voiding

For residual urine, it may be helpful to have the patient strain at the end of voiding or to have the patient press suprapubically in an attempt to add pressure to the bladder (Credé's maneuver). This technique also may be helpful with urge incontinence.

Other Options

Both biofeedback and electrical stimulation have been used for incontinence. Pelvic floor electrical stimulation (PFES) has been used for half a century as a treatment approach to stress incontinence. PFES stimulates pudendal nerve afferents, activating pudendal and hypogastric nerve efferents and resulting in contraction of smooth and striated periurethral muscles and the striated pelvic floor muscles. Researchers in a recent randomized controlled trial assigned women to one of three groups: an eight-week behavioral training program, behavioral training plus PFES, or reading a self-help booklet.[7] There was significant improvement in those treated with behavioral training (69%) or behavioral training plus PFES (72%), but no significant difference between the two groups. Those using the self-help booklet also had improvement (52%).

Two devices have been approved for use as a mechanical block to urine flow. One is a short balloon-catheter device that, after insertion into the urethra, is inflated to block urine flow. The other is a shield device for women that cups over the vaginal area.

For the elderly it is important to focus on mobility issues. The proximity of bathroom facilities and the ease of arising from bed play important roles in preventing bed-wetting. A semirecumbent position, a walking device, rail support at the toilet, and the location of the bed may all assist in decreasing the time it takes to reach the bathroom, avoiding "accidents." Recommendation for protective pads or adult diapers may be needed.

When patients are unresponsive to conservative management or the incontinence is socially disabling, it is important to refer for medical approaches to care. The primary focus with medication is to select drugs that are specific to the cause. In other words, drugs that are helpful for one problem may have no effect or even aggravate incontinence due to another cause. For detrusor instability or hyperactivity, drugs that have anticholinergic effects are used. These block bladder contractions and therefore may be contraindicated in patients with obstructive problems. Anticholinergics may also cause dry mouth, mental confusion, or constipation. The two classes of drugs that are used include tricyclic antidepressants (may cause orthostatic hypotension in the elderly) and propantheline. A number of new medications that are muscarinic receptor antagonists are used to manage detrusor instability (overactive bladder). One of these is VESIcare (solifenacin). **Table 34–2** lists these commonly used medications.

For stress incontinence, the rationale is to access medically the α-adrenergic control of the bladder neck and proximal urethra. An α-adrenergic agonist such as phenylpropanolamine hydrochloride is often used. Oral and topical estrogens are also used. Topical estrogen is particularly useful for women with atrophic vaginitis because it reduces the incidence of infection and dysuria.

Surgical options include retropubic suspension and needle suspension for stress incontinence. For women with intrinsic sphincter deficiency, bulking with Teflon or collagen, a pubovaginal sling, and an artificial urinary sphincter replacement are options. It is extremely important that prior to these approaches a conservative approach with or without medication be attempted first. Also a thorough urodynamic evaluation preoperatively is important for input in decision-making regarding the best procedure.

Although it is often assumed that the primary cause of bladder outlet obstruction with prostate hypertrophy is mechanical blockage, a dynamic component based on increased sympathetic tone is probably the primary cause in many males. As a dynamic cause, the degree of obstruction and resulting symptoms vary based on external factors such as exposure to cold, overfilling of the bladder, anticholinergic medication (common ingredient in decongestants), and resulting reflexes that affect urethral tension and stress. Symptoms may then vary and often improve during periods of less stress or during warm weather. The medical approach to this sympathetic effect is to use sympathetic blockade as a strategy. The most common medications are alpha-1 adrenergic blockers.[8]

Although not always a cause of voiding dysfunction, it is important to mention prostate cancer. Prostate cancer is quite common in older males. The ethnic risk is more with African Americans and less with Asians.

Table 34–2 Medications for Incontinence and Prostate Hypertrophy

Drug Class	Examples	General Mechanism	Interactions/Side Effects
Prostate Hypertrophy			
5-Reductase inhibitors	**Dutasteride** Avodart	Blocks the conversion of testosterone to 5 alpha DHT (responsible for prostate hypertrophy). Inhibits both type 1 and 2 5-alpha reductase inhibitors.	Gynecomastia, ejaculation dysfunction, impotence, decreased libido.
	Finasteride Propecia Proscar	A 5-reductase inhibitor of the enzyme necessary for conversion of testosterone into DHT. Used in the management of benign prostatic hypertrophy and male pattern baldness.	Decreased libido, impotence, or decreased volume of ejaculation.
Alpha-1 blocker	**Tamsulosin** Flomax	Used in the management of prostate hypertrophy, this is an antagonist to alpha 1A adrenoceptors in the prostate.	Orthostatic hypotension, priapism, allergic-type reactions, constipation, and vomiting.
	Terazosin Hydrin	An alpha-1-adrenergic blocker used in the management of hypertension in combination with a beta-adrenergic blocker and thiazide diuretic. Also used in the management of benign prostatic hypertrophy.	Weakness, dizziness, headache, weight gain, or syncope.
Neurogenic Bladder (Unstable Bladder)			
Muscarinic receptor antagonists	**Solifenacin** VESIcare	A muscarinic receptor antagonist used in the management of overactive bladder (detrusor instability).	Dry mouth, constipation, blurred vision.
	Oxybutynin Chloride Ditropan Ditropan XL	A synthetic amine used for neurogenic bladder or detrusor instability (unstable bladder). Effects are antispasmodic through inhibition of muscarinic effect of acetylcholine on smooth muscle.	May cause drowsiness, blurred vision, dry mouth, constipation, urinary hesitation, dizziness, weakness, or skin rash.
	Tolterodine Detrol Detrol A	A synthetic amine used for neurogenic bladder or detrusor instability (unstable bladder). Effects are antispasmodic through inhibition of muscarinic effect of acetylcholine on smooth muscle.	Drowsiness, blurred vision, dry mouth, constipation, urinary hesitation, dizziness, weakness, or skin rash.
	Oxybutynin Oxytrol	Antispasmodic, anticholinergic, transdermal medication used to control overactive bladder (now available OTC).	Allergic reactions, dry mouth, dizziness, blurred vision, constipation, headaches.
Other	**Fluoxetine** Prozac	A selective serotonin reuptake inhibitor (SSRI) making more serotonin available in the CNS. Used in the treatment of depression and obsessive-compulsive disorders.	About 15% of patients discontinue use due to nausea, anxiety, diarrhea, insomnia, or headache.

Factors that have been identified include a genetic predisposition and potentially some dietary factors. A high-fat diet increases the risk of prostate cancer.[9] Possible protective factors such as vitamins C, D, and E, beta-carotene, cadmium, and zinc are still being studied at this time.[10]

Beginning in their 40s, males with a high familial predisposition and African American males should have an annual digital rectal examination (DRE) and PSA measurement. For those not at high risk, annual DRE and PSA should begin at age 50 years.

Algorithm

An algorithm for evaluation and management of urinary incontinence in adults is presented in **Figure 34–1**.

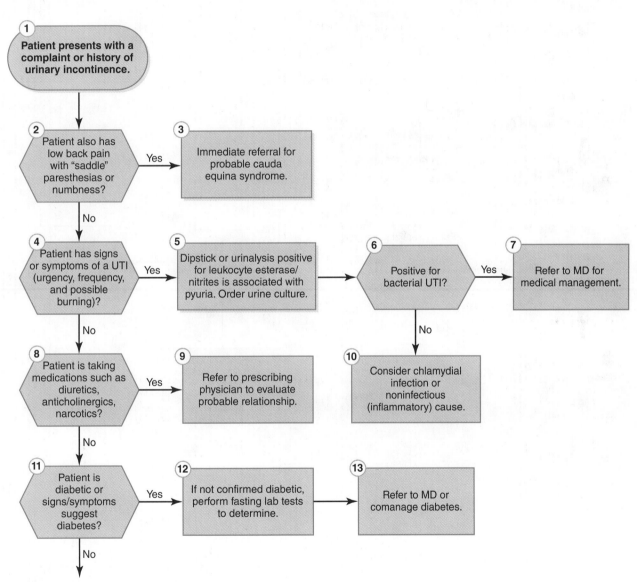

Figure 34–1 Urinary Incontinence in Adults—Algorithm

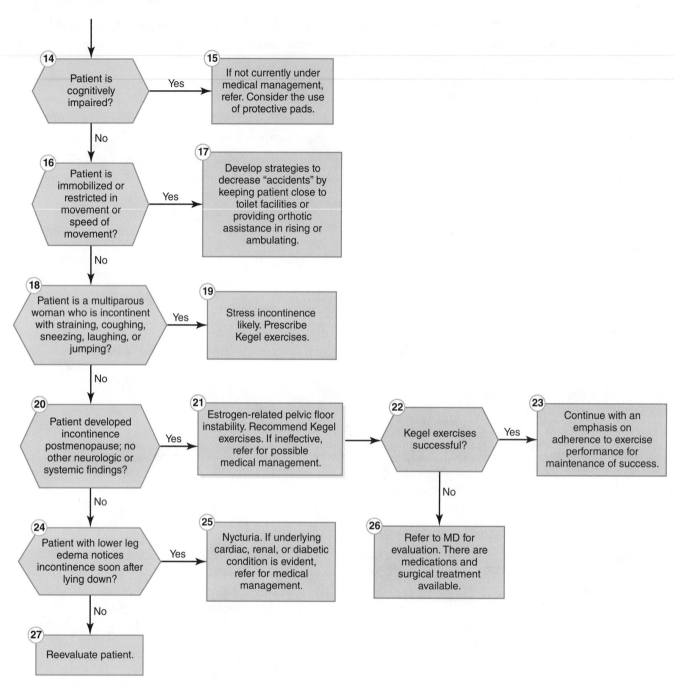

Figure 34–1 (Continued)

Selected Causes of Voiding Dysfunction or Pain

Urinary Tract Infection

Classic Presentation

A female patient presents with complaints of urinary frequency, a sense of urgency, and painful urination (dysuria). Although this is the classic presentation, there are many possibilities, dependent on site of infection and cause. Note: The classic presentation of UTI is not common in the elderly with UTI. Their signs/symptoms are generally behavioral including confusion, memory loss, agitation, hallucinations, or social inappropriateness. Also common are dizziness and falls.

Cause/Occurrence

The cause differs dependent on age and gender. Boys who have recurrent infection may have an anatomic abnormality such as posterior urethral valves that allow vesicoureteral reflux with subsequent kidney involvement. In most cases of UTI (>95%) the infecting organism is a gram-negative aerobic bacteria. Most often the cause is one of the following: member of *Enterobacteriaceae, Pseudomonas aeruginosa,* enterococci, and, in young women, *Staphylococcus saprophyticus.* In addition to a first infection, UTIs are classified into unresolved bacteriuria and bacterial persistence. Unresolved bacteriuria is usually due to patient noncompliance to medication, bacterial resistance, and mixed infection. Bacterial persistence often indicates another site of infection or abnormality including various kidney malformations, infected stones, chronic bacterial prostatitis, and fistulas, among others. Protection from infection includes a low pH and high osmolality, an intact glycosaminoglycan (GAG) protective barrier, full emptying of the bladder (no neurologic or other bladder dysfunction), and estrogen. Risk factors include diabetes, douching, tampon use, catheters, diaphragm use, infrequent voiding, pregnancy, renal failure, and bladder outlet obstruction from various causes.

Evaluation

The primary confusion in making a diagnosis of urinary tract infection is the overlap with other infections with similar signs and symptoms. The three primary infectious considerations are vaginal infections (e.g., *Gardnerella, Candida albicans,* and *Trichomonas*), sexually transmitted diseases that lead to possible pelvic inflammatory disease (e.g., *Chlamydia trachomatis, Neisseria gonorrhoeae*), and other sexually transmitted diseases (e.g., Herpes simplex virus). This distinction is important because the organisms are different, and the management approach is different for each category. The primary difference between other local infections and UTI is that STDs and vaginal infections are usually associated with vaginal discharge and vaginal irritation.

Although the relative weighting of risk factors for UTI is not known, there are three risk factors for acute UTI in young women that appear important: recent sexual intercourse, use of spermicide (on condoms or with diaphragms during intercourse), and history of UTI (especially a maternal history of UTI or history of childhood onset of UTI). A combination of symptoms is highly suggestive of a UTI. Dysuria and frequency of urination without vaginal discharge or irritation raise the probability of a UTI to over 90%.[11] Dipstick testing can be used in the chiropractor's office as a quick screen in patients with a high likelihood of a UTI. Dipstick or urinalysis indicators for UTI include nitrites for bacteria and leukocyte esterase. However, these tests do not rule out or confirm a UTI because nitrites may be negative with staph and strep. UTIs and vaginal discharge and bleeding may cause a false positive for leukocyte esterase. A positive result increases that likelihood and should result in a referral for further medical evaluation and possible treatment. However, if the dipstick test is negative, the probability of a UTI is still 23% and should therefore be taken together with presenting symptoms in making the decision for medical referral. For patients with complicating factors such as a history of polycystic renal disease, nephrolithiasis, neurogenic bladder, pregnancy, diabetes, immunosuppression, or recent urinary tract catheterization or instrumented testing, referral for medical evaluation and management is imperative.

The patient is evaluated with a urinalysis. Urinalysis includes a microscopic evaluation of clean-catch urine for bacteria and pyuria (pus in the urine). Pyuria and colony counts greater than 100,000 bacteria/mL of urine are found in most infected patients. In symptomatic patients pyuria and colony counts of 100 to 100,000 bacteria/mL establish infection, most often lower UTI. The urine is cultured if bacteria are found. Generally, the isolation of two or more bacterial species on culture indicates a contaminated specimen. Patients with pyuria without bacteriuria may have chlamydial urethritis, gonococcal urethritis, or gram-positive cocci infection. Gross hematuria strongly suggests cystitis. Men with urethritis and purulent discharge often have *N. gonorrhoeae* infection; men with a whitish mucoid discharge have a nonspecific infection. Yeast infections are most common in diabetics and patients who have had a course of antibiotic treatment. For urethritis in females, see Chapter 55.

Management

For a conventional UTI, antibiotic treatment with amoxicillin/clavulanate, a cephalosporin, a fluoroquinolone, nitrofurantoin, or trimethoprim/sulfamethoxazole is prescribed. For pyelonephritis, more aggressive therapy including hospitalization with intravenous antibiotics is often recommended. Asymptomatic infections should be treated if there is underlying vesicoureteral reflux, stone, diabetes, or pregnancy or if the patient is an immunosuppressed individual. Prevention may be possible with changes in pH through the use of cranberry juice. A 2008 Cochrane review[12] of the preventive value of cranberries (cranberry juice) concluded that it may reduce the number of symptomatic UTIs over a one-year period especially for women with recurrent UTIs. This was confirmed in a 2013 prospective study.[13]

Benign Prostate Hypertrophy

Classic Presentation

A male patient presents with complaints of decreased force of urine stream, hesitancy, dribbling, and a sense of incomplete bladder emptying.

Cause/Occurrence

There is a direct relationship between age and benign prostate hypertrophy (BPH). There is histologic evidence of BPH in 50% of men at age 60 years, which increases to 90% by age 80 years.[14] The relationship between glandular enlargement and symptoms is not always present. Symptoms of BPH are usually due to a combination of causes including: (1) enlargement of glandular nodules causing urethral blockage (androgens are primary cause), (2) smooth muscle tone of the posterior capsule and bladder neck (α-1-adrenergic stimulation), and (3) impaired bladder contractility and detrusor instability (involuntary "spasms" of the bladder). Although BPH increases with age, the symptoms do not necessarily follow this pattern.

Evaluation

A digital prostate examination is required. In an effort to rule out other causes of symptoms or complications of BPH, order a urinalysis to evaluate for UTI or indicators of bladder cancer (hematuria requires an immediate urologic referral). Yearly serum creatinine measurement is recommended to screen for possible involvement of the upper urinary tract.

Management

Patients with mild symptoms may be managed with watchful waiting, with recommendations of decreasing sympathetic stimulation (i.e., decreasing stress, decreased caffeine, etc.) and phytotherapy. Men who smoke more than 35 cigarettes/day and have high alcohol intake are at higher risk.[15] Men who are more physically active have a lower frequency of symptoms.[16] Those with more disruptive symptoms or risk of upper urinary tract involvement may need medical or surgical treatment.

Prostate growth is governed by hormonal influences. Testosterone is converted to 5-alpha-dihydrotestosterone (DHT) in the prostate. This is accomplished through an enzyme 5-α-reductase. The medical approach to reducing DHT is to block the conversion of testosterone to DHT through the use of 5-alpha-reductase inhibitors (e.g., finasteride [Proscar]). In this way the levels of testosterone are not affected. α-1-adrenergic blocking agents such as terazosin (Hytrin) and doxazosin (Cardura) are often prescribed to reduce smooth muscle tone. Table 34–2 lists common medications and their side effects.

Recently, an association between low 25-OH vitamin D, calcium, and high-density lipoprotein cholesterol and an enlarged prostate has been demonstrated.[17] Studies still need to be conducted on whether correction of these associated low factors will decrease the occurrence of prostatic hypertrophy.

These medical options are being used more frequently in place of transurethral resection of the prostate (TURP). Other surgical options include open prostatectomy, balloon dilation, stents, and newer techniques including laser ablation and microwave hyperthermia. Surgery should be reserved for those who do not respond to conservative or medical management or those with serious complications.

Although initially promising, the clinical value of saw palmetto is being questioned. A study in 2006 by Bent et al.[18] found no symptom or objective measure difference between placebo and saw palmetto using an extract of 160 mg twice per day. A review by Avins and Bent[19] suggests that as larger studies are conducted, the current conflict in report will likely be resolved. It is postulated that saw palmetto reduces levels of DHT. A recommended dose is 320 mg of standardized extract per day. Symptoms may improve within one month.[20]

Prostate Cancer

Classic Presentation

A male patient is usually asymptomatic in the early stages. Later, local growth may cause the patient to present with complaints of decreased force of urine stream, hesitancy, dribbling, and a sense of incomplete bladder emptying. Later presentations with metastasis may include back or pelvic pain.

Cause/Occurrence

There is a higher incidence of prostate cancer in African American males in the United States and lower rates for Asian males while in Asia. Rates increase for Asian males when they immigrate to the United States, indicating an environmental influence. The development of prostate cancer is related to an interaction of genetic predisposition, dietary factors, and lifestyle. Two genes, RNASEL and MSR1, may increase the risk of prostate cancer in relation to infection.[21] It is now believed that prostatic inflammation, either septic (as in sexually transmitted infection) or aseptic, may progress to proliferative inflammatory atrophy. Loss of π-class glutathione-S-transferase (GSTP1) enzyme caretaker function then allows the development of cells of prostatic intraepithelial neoplasia and prostate cancer cells. The findings from one large study indicate that approximately 42% of cases of prostate cancer are related to inheritance, with the remainder most likely due to environmental factors.[22] Possible dietary relationships include:

- A diet high in animal fats and meats may increase the risk of prostate cancer (especially meats cooked at high temperature or grilled/broiled, which form heterocyclic aromatic amine and polycyclic aromatic hydrocarbon carcinogens).[23]
- Low vegetable intake: High intake of the antioxidant carotenoid lycopene, found in tomatoes, may be associated with a reduced risk of prostate cancer.[24] Also, high intake of cruciferous vegetables containing isothiocyanate sulforaphane may reduce risk of prostate cancer.[25]
- Supplementation with vitamin E and selenium may reduce risk of prostate cancer.
- Although zinc supplementation may be protective at low levels, one study indicated that zinc supplementation above 100 mg/day might increase the risk of prostate cancer.[26]

Adenocarcinoma of the prostate is only second to lung cancer as a cause of cancer-related death in men. Incidence increases with age so that by age 65 years and older, 75% have some prostate cancer.[27]

Most prostate cancers do not progress to metastasis and death. However, those with local disease and high tumor grade tend to progress. Although the incidence does not increase, the risk of fatal prostate cancer increases with smoking, tallness, high calcium intake, and is inversely related to physical activity.[28–30]

Evaluation

There is still considerable controversy regarding the use of prostate-specific antigens as a screening approach for prostate cancer. Factors including a high false-positive rate, numbers needed to treat, and the effect of obesity on interpretation have made definitive recommendations for threshold levels difficult. Among others, the American College of Preventive Medicine concluded in 2008[31] that there is insufficient evidence to recommend routine screening with digital rectal examination or PSA. African American men and those with positive family histories cause a higher level of concern, and therefore suggest the use of these screening tools.

For those at high risk (familial predisposition or African Americans), an annual DRE and PSA screen should begin at age 40 years.[32] For men not at high risk, annual screening with DRE and PSA should begin at age 50 years.[32] PSA values in the 4 to 10 ng/mL range have a 25% positive predictive value. PSA values higher than 10 ng/mL have a 67% positive predictive value. Also, the measurement of free and total PSA may help. The proportion of free-to-total PSA is higher for men with BPH and lower in men with prostate cancer. Other available testing includes PSA density, PSA velocity, and PSA age-specific ranges, although their value has not been established. An elevated PSA and an abnormal DRE will usually result in transrectal ultrasound-guided prostate biopsy. Four to six samples are often recommended to increase the yield. The grading system for prostate cancer is the Gleason system. This is divided into five grades based on degree of differentiation. The reality is that the debate continues; the U.S. Preventive Task Force acknowledges that it does save lives for men between around 50 to 65 years of age, but the change in mortality overall does not seem affected. It still is a complex decision to be made with the patient.[33]

Management

Patients who are over 70 years old or have less than 10 years' life expectancy are usually not treated. Options for those in need of treatment include radical prostatectomy, radiation therapy, or hormonal therapy. As noted above, patients who smoke and have a high calcium intake are at higher risk for fatal cancer. Those who are more physically active, have a high fruit intake, and supplement their diet with zinc and vitamins C and E may have a lower risk for fatal prostate cancer.[34,35]

APPENDIX 34–1

References

1. Consensus Conference. Urinary incontinence in adults. *JAMA*. 1992;251:2685–2690.

2. Jolleyes J. Urinary incontinence. *Practitioner*. 1993;237:630–633.

3. Urinary Incontinence Guideline Panel. *Urinary Incontinence in Adults. Clinical Practice Guidelines.* Rockville, MD: U.S. Dept of Health and Human Services, Public Health Service, Agency for Health Care Policy and Research; 1992. AHCPR publication 92-0038.

4. Barry MJ, Fowler FJ, Jr, O'Leary MP, et al. The American Urological Association Symptom Index for benign prostatic hyperplasia. *J Urol*. 1992;148:1549–1552.

5. Hopkins TB. Dysfunctional voiding. In: Greene HL, Fincher RME, Johnson WP, et al., eds. *Clinical Medicine*. 2nd ed. St. Louis, MO: Mosby-Year Book; 1996:339–343.

6. Fantl JA, Wyman JF, McClish DK, et al. Efficacy of bladder training in older women with urinary incontinence. *JAMA*. 1991;265:609–613.

7. Goode PS, Burgio KL, Leoher JL, et al. Effect of behavioral training with or without pelvic floor electrical stimulation on stress incontinence in women: a randomized controlled trial. *JAMA*. 2003;290:345–352.

8. Cooper JW, Piepho RW. Cost-effective management of benign prostatic hyperplasia. *Drug Benefit Trends*. 1995;7:10–48.

9. Kolonel LN. Nutrition and prostate cancer. *Cancer Causes Control*. 1996;7:83–94.

10. Giovannucci E. How is individual risk for prostate cancer assessed? *Hematol Oncol Clin North Am*. 1996;10:537–548.

11. Bent S, Nallamothu BK, Simel DL, Fihn SD, Saint S. Does this woman have an acute uncomplicated urinary tract infection? *JAMA*. 2002;287:2701–2710.

12. Jepson R, Craig J. Cranberries for preventing urinary tract infections. *Cochrane Database Syst Rev*. 2008(1): CD001321.

13. Burleigh AE, Benck SM, McAchran SE, et al. Consumption of sweetened, dried cranberries may reduce urinary tract infection incidence in susceptible women—a modified observational study. *Nutr J* 2013,12:139–146.

14. Berry SJ, Coffey DS, Walsh PC, et al. The development of human benign prostatic hyperplasia with age. *J Urol*. 1984;132:474–479.

15. Platz EA, Rimm EB, Kawachi I, et al. Alcohol consumption, cigarette smoking, and risk of benign prostatic hyperplasia. *Am J Epidemiol*. 1999;149(2):106–115.

16. Platz EA, Kawachi I, Rimm EB, et al. Physical activity and benign prostatic hyperplasia. *Arch Intern Med*. 1998;158(21):2349–2356.

17. Haghsheno MA, Mellstrom D, Behre CJ, et al. Low 25-OH vitamin D is associated with benign prostatic hyperplasia. *J Urol*. Aug 2013;190(2):608–614.

18. Bent S, Kane C, Shinohara K, et al. Saw palmetto for benign prostatic hyperplasia. *N Engl J Med*. 2006;354(6):557–566.

19. Avins AL, Bent S. Saw palmetto and lower urinary tract symptoms: what is the latest evidence? *Curr Urol Rep*. 2006;7(4):260–265.

20. Murray M. Saw palmetto vs Proscar. *Am J Natural Med*. 1994;1(1):8–9.

21. Nelson WG, DeMarzo AM, Isaacs WB. Prostate cancer. *N Engl J Med*. 2003;349:366–381.

22. Lichtenstein P, Holm MV, Verkasolo PK, et al. Environmental and heritable factors in the causation of cancer—analysis of cohorts of twins from Sweden, Denmark, and Finland. *N Engl J Med*. 2000;343:78–85.

23. LeMarchand L, Kolonel LN, Williams LR, et al. Animal fat consumption and prostate cancer: a prospective study in Hawaii. *Epidemiology*. 1994;5:276–282.

24. Chen L, Stacewitcz-Sapantzakis M, Duncan C, et al. Oxidative DNA damage in prostate cancer patients consuming tomato-sauce-based entrees as a whole-food intervention. *J Natl Cancer Inst*. 2001;93:1872–1879.

25. Cohen JH, Kristal AR, Stanford JL. Fruit and vegetable intakes and prostate cancer risk. *J Natl Cancer Inst*. 2000;92:61–68.

26. Leitzman MF, Stampfer MJ, Wu K, et al. Zinc supplement use and risk of prostate cancer. *J Natl Cancer Inst*. 2003;95(3):2004–2007.

27. Hahnfeld LE, Moon TD. Prostate cancer. *Med Clin North Am*. 1999;83(5):1231–1245.

28. Giovannucci E, Rimm EB, Ascherio A, et al. Smoking and risk of total and fatal prostate cancer in United States health professionals. *Cancer Epidemiol Biomarkers Prev*. 1999;8(4, pt 1):277–282.

29. Giovannucci E, Rimm EB, Stampfer MJ, Colditz GA, Willett WC. Height, body weight, and risk of prostate cancer. *Cancer Epidemiol Biomarkers Prev*. 1997;6(8):557–563.

30. Giovannucci E, Rimm EB, Wolk A, et al. Calcium and fructose intake in relation to risk of prostate cancer. *Cancer Res.* 1998;58(3):442–447.

31. Lim LS, Sherin K. Screening for Prostate Cancer in U.S. Men ACPM Position Statement on Preventive Practice. *Am J Prev Med.* 2008;34(2):164–170.

32. VonEschenbach A, Ho R, Murphy GP, et al. American Cancer Society guidelines for the early detection of prostate cancer. Update June 10, 1997. *Cancer.* 1997;80:1805–1807.

33. Screening for prostate cancer: draft recommendation statement. Rockville, MD: U.S. Preventive Services Task Force, October 7, 2011 (http://www.uspreventiveservicestaskforce.org/draftrec3.htm).

34. Giovannucci E, Leitzmann M, Spiegelman D, et al. A prospective study of physical activity and prostate cancer in male health professionals. *Cancer Res.* 1998;58(22):5117–5122.

35. Kristal AR, Stanford JL, Cohen JH, et al. Vitamin and mineral supplement use in association with reduced risk of prostate cancer. *Cancer Epidemiol Biomarkers Prev.* 1999;8(10):887–892.

Enuresis

Context

Nocturnal enuresis is a distressing disorder for parents and children. Approximately 5 to 7 million children in the United States are affected. It is more common in boys than in girls. Girls are more likely to have daytime incontinence, more often associated with bacteriuria. In a large study in Sweden, 2.9% of girls and 3.8% of boy school entrants reported bed-wetting once per week.[1]

Parents are often unaware of the natural history of continence development and expect their child to be continent at a relatively early age. One study indicated that between 30% and 70% of parents punish their children for bed-wetting.[2] Ironically, there is a strong genetic component. Children whose parents both have a history of enuresis as a child have a 77% chance of bed-wetting, 44% chance if only one parent has a positive history, and only 15% chance if neither did.[3]

Parents seeking a nondrug, nonparent-intensive approach to bed-wetting seek a chiropractor's advice. The chiropractor may perform the initial evaluation to determine known causes such as urinary tract infection or diabetes. The nonpathologic, neurodevelopmental type of enuresis may be managed with conservative approaches. When these fail, referral for medication may be warranted.

Enuresis has been defined by the American Psychiatric Association as bed-wetting occurring in a child at age 5 years or above (and mental age of 4 years). The frequency is defined as two or more incontinent occurrences in a month between the ages of 5 and 6 or one or more occurrences after age 6 years in children who do not have an associated physical disorder such as urinary tract infection (UTI), diabetes, or seizures.[4] At age 5 years, approximately 20% of children have enuresis, which decreases to 10% at age 10 years and 1% at age 15 years.[5, 6]

Enuresis is often categorized into primary and secondary causes. Primary causes include both functional and structural causes. Secondary enuresis is defined as the presence of a prior history of continence for more than a six-month period. These patients often have a regression due to a stressful emotional event in the early years of life. Approximately 80% to 90% of childhood enuresis is the primary type.[7, 8]

When not due to a structural cause, enuresis seems to follow a natural spontaneous remission. This natural history must be taken into account when it appears that a child is responding to a specific therapy. Without any specific therapy the natural history indicates that 50% of patients will become continent within four years. The prevalence of enuresis decreases with age at a rate of 10% to 20% per year after age 6.[9]

General Strategy

History

- Determine whether the patient fits the criteria for nocturnal enuresis.
- Determine identifiable causes such as a history or indications of diabetes, seizures, or other neuromuscular contributors.
- Determine the family history of enuresis.
- Determine the environmental and social history of the child with regard to changes in living environment, stresses, any psychologic problems, and parental punishment for enuresis.
- Determine any other treatment methods that have been attempted, and the patient/parent compliance.

Evaluation

- Evaluate the neurologic status of the child with emphasis on peripheral sensation and reflexes, genital sensation and perianal reflexes, and a search for any indications of congenital abnormalities such as clubfoot, spina bifida, or other.
- If there are associated complaints of frequent urination or irritation while urinating, obtain a urinalysis.
- Referral for specialized studies such as diagnostic ultrasound or cystourethrograms should be reserved for those patients who have daytime incontinence or signs of frequent UTI.

Management

- If chiropractic management is suggested to the patient, discuss the rationale and literature support and other conservative options, including their advantages and disadvantages.
- If food allergies are the cause of detrusor instability, advise the parents to eliminate dairy products, colas, chocolate, and citrus juices for several weeks to determine the effect.
- The bell-and-pad urine alarm method is probably the most effective approach.
- For those children with persistence and failure of conservative approaches, medical options may be considered; the natural course of enuresis, however, should be discussed with the parents.

Relevant Anatomy and Physiology

Bladder control is an intricate balance among several neural systems. The tension within the bladder that is generated by filling must be balanced by restriction of outflow at the bladder neck. The primary innervation of the body of the bladder is parasympathetic (pudendal nerve S2-4). Therefore, parasympathetic stimulation facilitates urination by causing contraction of the body of the bladder (detrusor muscle) and urinary sphincter relaxation. Sympathetic innervation is via the hypogastric nerve plexus with nerve cell bodies at T11-L2. β-adrenergic (sympathetic) stimulation causes detrusor

muscle relaxation during filling. α-adrenergic (sympathetic) stimulation in the bladder neck (which acts as an internal urethral sphincter) acts to prevent urination.

The micturition center is located in the pons and acts to inhibit urination. Cortical override occurs through connections from the frontal lobe, corpus callosum, and cingulate gyrus, which generally inhibit the pontine micturition center.

There is a normal micturition maturation that occurs, paralleling changes in bladder capacity and neural development. In the first two years, a child has little control over urination, yet senses when the bladder is full. By the age of 3 years, a child should have some development of daytime control. By ages 4 and 5 years, the child should be able to control urination in mid-stream with starting and stopping at will. A delay in this normal maturation and a small bladder capacity (less than 50% of normal in 85% of enuretic children) seem to be the primary factors.[3] Another treatment-based theory centers around an abnormal diurnal rhythm of antidiuretic hormone (ADH) secretion.[10]

If there is a decrease or absence during sleep, excessive amounts of unconcentrated urine accumulate.[11] This mechanism may account for enuresis in older children, given that one study found the bladder capacity of these children to be normal.[12]

Evaluation

History

First, it is necessary to determine whether the child fits the criteria for enuresis. The child may, in fact, be too young or have infrequent occurrences. When these criteria are met, it is important to screen the child's history via the parent with regard to underlying psychiatric disorders or systemic disorders such as diabetes. If such disorders are not found, performing a review of systems should identify any suspicions with regard to urinary tract infections or diabetes.

Because of the strong familial tendency, it is crucial to identify a family history of enuresis. As mentioned above, the number of relatives (especially parents) with a history of enuresis has an effect on the tendency of a child to have enuresis. Beyond this observation, Ferguson et al.[13] noted that the number of first-order relatives with enuresis correlated with when a child would attain continence. Those with two or more first-order relatives were 1.5 years late in attaining control, compared with those with no family history.

Examination

The physical examination is often unrevealing. However, it is important to check genital sensation, perianal reflexes, and peripheral sensation and reflexes. Observation of voiding may be helpful in determining control, caliber of stream, and any associated discomfort.

A host of studies may be performed on the enuretic child, but urine screening tests may help obviate the need for further testing. Measurement for bacteriuria, glucose, blood, casts, and a first-morning urine sample for specific gravity will help disclose whether diabetes, renal disorders, or disorders of urine concentration, respectively, are involved in the patient's enuresis.

Further evaluation using voiding cystourethrograms, renal and pelvic ultrasound, or intravenous pyelograms should be reserved for those with daytime incontinence and associated signs of UTI. These tests are expensive and often are ordered prematurely in cases of primary nocturnal enuresis.

Management

The reality of primary nocturnal enuresis management is that no treatment has been found to be significantly superior to the natural history on a consistent basis.[14] Most forms of therapy may have an initially high success rate, yet relapse is extremely common. Methods that do work seem to be most effective in older children. Primary care physicians apparently rely more on a pharmacologic approach than a conditioning approach, with as many as 50% of them prescribing medication; 5% prescribe urine-alarm systems.[15]

The role of manipulative therapy has yet to be defined. Few studies have been performed. One or two case studies and two large studies have been published.[16–19] It is difficult to conclude that chiropractic manipulative therapy is effective, given the limitations of these studies. Unfortunately, most studies suffered for lack of long-term follow-up evaluation to determine maintenance of continence or relapse. In generalizing, the two larger studies indicated 15.5% and 25% improvement rates in the treatment groups. Given that the annual remission rate is between 10% and 20% per year, it does not appear that manipulation provides a significant effect over the natural history of the disorder. The one advantage may be that the effect may occur sooner than it would with natural history. Larger studies with longer follow-up periods are required to define more clearly chiropractic manipulation's role in enuresis management. One other difficulty is that the studies that have been performed and the textbooks that recommend specific treatment for enuresis are consistently inconsistent about which spinal levels to address. A side note is that some researchers have attempted to identify a relationship between spina bifida occulta and diurnal enuresis in children. This association seems related only when other clinical findings of neurologic abnormalities are apparent that suggest underlying lipoma or a tethered cord.[20]

It is generally agreed that the most effective therapy is conditioning therapy using a bell-and-pad urine alarm. The alarm system has been studied extensively and is consistently better than medication, desmopressin, and behavioral treatment.[21] Success rates average between 50% and 80% in children over 8 years of age if there is strict compliance for four to six months.[22] Unfortunately, the relapse rate is between 15% and 47%. Noncompliance occurs in at least 20% of cases. The intention of the alarm approach is to signal the child to awaken through an alarm that is set off by moisture sensors attached to the pajamas. The child is then instructed to finish voiding in the bathroom, change clothes and bedding, and reset the alarm.

It has been suggested that food allergies may play a role in detrusor instability.[23] Unfortunately, the studies have failed to identify specific foods or to use control groups to compare effect. Foods that have been suggested are dairy products, cola, chocolate, and citrus juices.[24] One study attempted to individualize the treatment approach by starting subjects on an oligoantigenic (few foods) diet.[25] When enuresis was improved, introduction of a single food at a time allowed identification of the antigenic food. This study focused on enuretic children with migraine or hyperkinetic behavior. Elimination diets have been proposed by others in the broader group of enuretic children.[26]

When conservative approaches fail, referral for medical management may be warranted. Two approaches are used. One is the administration of a tricyclic antidepressant, imipramine hydrochloride, for two to three months followed by gradual reduction over the following three to four months. The success rate is between 25% and 40% after withdrawal. Some studies have shown less dramatic success.[3, 6, 9] It is believed that the medication lightens sleep and improves voluntary control of the urethral sphincter with an associated increase in bladder capacity. The major concern with imipramine is side effects and—as one review paper suggests—accidental overdose.[27] The main side effects are dry mouth, blurred vision, lethargy and headaches, abdominal pain, mood and sleep disturbances, and in rare cases syncope and cardiac arrhythmias.[28]

Although intranasal ADH (desmopressin) has been advocated as a viable treatment option for enuresis, studies indicate that the numbers of children who improve are relatively small and that the relapse rate is quite high.[29] Additionally, the cost is high. When desmopressin is effective, it is usually evident within two weeks. The short-term success is as high as 70%; however, this is decreased to between 17% and 41% with drug withdrawal. Some studies indicate a higher success with older children. Most side effects are related to the portal of delivery. Nasal irritation, epistaxis, and headaches are the most common. Water intoxication may occur rarely and can be prevented with a serum electrolyte measurement taken at one week after therapy is initiated.

Algorithm

An algorithm for evaluation and management of enuresis in children is presented in **Figure 35–1**.

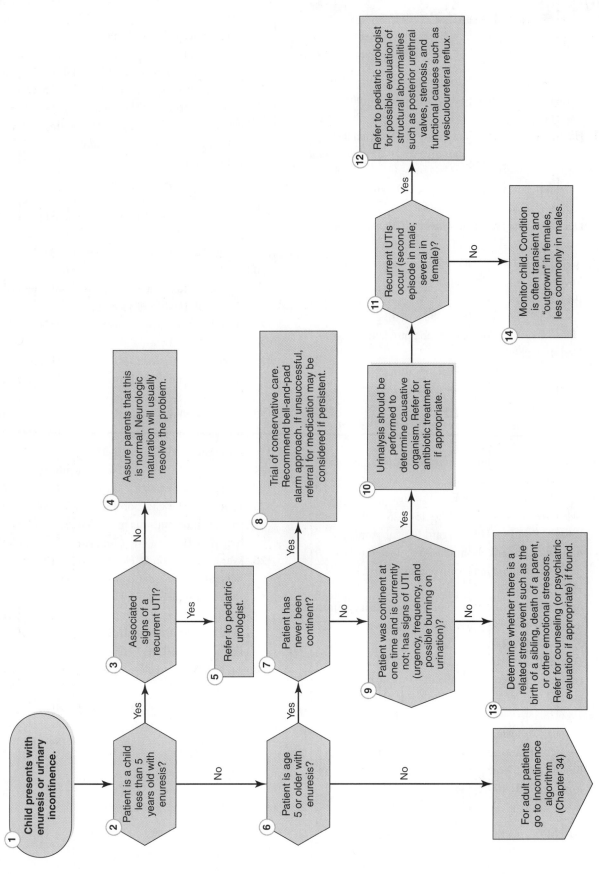

1 Child presents with enuresis or urinary incontinence.

2 Patient is a child less than 5 years old with enuresis?

— Yes → **3** Associated signs of a recurrent UTI?

3 → No → **4** Assure parents that this is normal. Neurologic maturation will usually resolve the problem.

3 → Yes → **5** Refer to pediatric urologist.

2 → No → **6** Patient is age 5 or older with enuresis?

6 → Yes → **7** Patient has never been continent?

6 → No → **13** For adult patients go to Incontinence algorithm (Chapter 34)

7 → Yes → **8** Trial of conservative care. Recommend bell-and-pad approach. If unsuccessful, referral for medication may be considered if persistent.

7 → No → **9** Patient was continent at one time and is currently not; has signs of UTI (urgency, frequency, and possible burning on urination)?

9 → Yes → **10** Urinalysis should be performed to determine causative organism. Refer for antibiotic treatment if appropriate.

9 → No → **13** Determine whether there is a related stress event such as the birth of a sibling, death of a parent, or other emotional stressors. Refer for counseling (or psychiatric evaluation if appropriate) if found.

10 → **11** Recurrent UTIs occur (second episode in male; several in female)?

11 → Yes → **12** Refer to pediatric urologist for possible evaluation of structural abnormalities such as posterior urethral valves, stenosis, and functional causes such as vesiculoureteral reflux.

11 → No → **14** Monitor child. Condition is often transient and "outgrown" in females, less commonly in males.

Figure 35–1 Enuresis in Children—Algorithm

APPENDIX 35–1

References

1. Hjalmas K. Functional daytime incontinence: definitions and epidemiology. *Scand J Urol Nephrol Suppl.* 1992;141:39–46.
2. Haque M, Ellerstein NS, Grandy JH. Parental perceptions of enuresis: a collaborative study. *Am J Dis Child.* 1981;135:809–811.
3. Friman PC. A preventative context for enuresis. *Pediatr Clin North Am.* 1986;33:871–876.
4. *Diagnostic and Statistical Manual of Mental Disorders.* 3rd rev. ed. Washington, DC: American Psychiatric Association; 1983:84–85.
5. Mann EM. Nocturnal enuresis. *West J Med.* 1991;155:520–521.
6. Rosenfeld J, Jerkins GR. The bed-wetting child: current management of a frustrating problem. *Postgrad Med.* 1991;89:63–70.
7. Himsi KK, Hurwitz RS. Pediatric urinary incontinence. *Urol Clin North Am.* 1991;18:283–293.
8. Priman PC, Warzak WJ. Nocturnal enuresis: a prevalent, persistent, yet curable parasomnia. *Pediatrician.* 1990;17:38–45.
9. Novello AC, Novello JR. Enuresis. *Pediatr Clin North Am.* 1987;34:719–733.
10. Toffler WL, Weingarten F. A new treatment of nocturnal enuresis. *West J Med.* 1991;154:326–330.
11. Rittig S, Knudsen UB, Norgard JP, et al. Abnormal diurnal rhythm of plasma vasopressin and urinary output in patients with enuresis. *Am J Physiol.* 1989;256:664–671.
12. Norgard JP, Rittig S, Djurhuus JC. Nocturnal enuresis: an approach to treatment based on pathogenesis. *J Pediatr.* 1989;114(suppl):705–710.
13. Ferguson DM, Horwood LJ, Shannon FT. Factors related to the age of attainment of nocturnal bladder control: an eight-year longitudinal study. *Pediatrics.* 1986;78:884–890.
14. Monda JM, Jusmann DA. Primary nocturnal enuresis: a comparison among observation, imipramine, desmopressin acetate and bed-wetting alarm systems. *J Urol.* 1995;154:745–748.
15. Rushton HG. Nocturnal enuresis: epidemiology, evaluation, and currently available treatment options. *J Pediatr.* 1989;114:691–696.
16. Reed WR, Beavers S, Reddy SK, Kern G. Chiropractic management of primary nocturnal enuresis. *J Manipulative Physiol Ther.* 1994;17:596–600.
17. Leboeuf C, Brown P, Herman A, et al. Chiropractic care of children with nocturnal enuresis: a prospective outcome study. *J Manipulative Physiol Ther.* 1991;14:110–115.
18. Gemmel HA, Jacobson BH. Chiropractic management of enuresis: time series descriptive design. *J Manipulative Physiol Ther.* 1989;12:386–389.
19. Blomerth PR. Functional nocturnal enuresis. *J Manipulative Physiol Ther.* 1994;17:335–338.
20. Ritchey ML, Sinha A, DiPietro MA, et al. Significance of spina bifida occulta in children with diurnal enuresis. *J Urol.* 1994;152:815–818.
21. Alon US. Nocturnal enuresis. *Pediatr Nephrol.* 1995;9:94–103.
22. Devlin JB, O'Cathain C. Predicting treatment outcome in nocturnal enuresis. *Arch Dis Child.* 1990;65:1158–1161.
23. Zaleski A, Shokeir HK, Gerrard JW. Enuresis: familial incidence and relationship to allergic disorders. *Can Med Assoc J.* 1972;106:30–31.
24. Harrison A. Allergy and urinary infections: is there an association? *Pediatrics.* 1971;48:66–69.
25. Egger J, Carter CH, Soothill JF, Wilson J. Effect of diet treatment on enuresis in children with migraine or hyperkinetic behavior. *Clin Pediatr.* 1992;31:302–307.
26. Warady BA, Alon U, Hefferstein S. Primary nocturnal enuresis: current concepts about an old problem. *Pediatr Ann.* 1991;202:246–255.
27. Kreitz BG, Aker PD. Nocturnal enuresis: treatment implications for the chiropractor. *J Manipulative Physiol Ther.* 1994;17:465–473.
28. Ng KH. Nocturnal enuresis. *Singapore Med J.* 1994;35:198–200.
29. Evans JH, Meadow SR. Desmopressin for bed wetting: length of treatment, vasopressin secretion, and response. *Arch Dis Child.* 1992;67:184–188.

Vaginal Bleeding

Context

A patient would rarely present to a chiropractor with a chief complaint of vaginal bleeding. However, with directed questioning on a review of systems, a complaint of abnormal bleeding may surface. The chiropractor's role in this scenario is to narrow the list of possibilities to determine whether there is a cause for concern and what that concern may be. Narrowing the list is primarily a historical process; however, some chiropractors trained in pelvic examination may extend the search through physical examination, adding more information to the referral.

General Strategy

History

- Determine the patient's staging with regard to her menstrual cycle.
- Determine whether the bleeding appears to be ovulatory or anovulatory.
- Determine whether there are any indicators of thyroid disease.
- Determine whether the patient is taking medications that interfere with menstrual function.
- Determine the patient's use of contraceptives, including an intrauterine device (IUD).
- Determine whether the patient might be pregnant.
- Determine whether the patient has any secondary signs of bleeding loss, such as anemia or iron deficiency.

Evaluation

For those chiropractors who have training and experience, perform a thorough pelvic examination.

Management

Refer the patient to her gynecologist with a letter or phone call explaining relevant findings.

Relevant Anatomy and Physiology

Menarche is not a fully matured occurrence. Maturation of the central nervous system (CNS)-hypothalamic-pituitary axis is the result of a complex triggering of hormonal release that, when not complete, may cause bleeding. The endometrium is the target site for the effect of this hormonal interplay. Phases in the growth and subsequent degeneration of the endometrium are based on hormonal dominance. In the proliferative phase (days 5 to 14 of the cycle), the ovarian follicle secretes estrogen, which stimulates the growth of the endometrium. The secretory phase (days 15 to 28 of the cycle) is dominated by progesterone, which is released from the corpus luteum. Progesterone stops the development of the endometrium and stimulates differentiation to a secretory epithelium. Both progesterone and estrogen levels drop if conception does not occur by about day 23. This is due to the degeneration of the corpus luteum. The dramatic decrease in progesterone and estrogen triggers the release of follicle-stimulating hormone (FSH). FSH stimulation of ovarian follicle growth causes a concomitant rise in estrogen from the follicle. At the midcycle, a sudden rise in estradiol causes a rise in FSH and a surge of luteinizing hormone (LH), which leads to the formation of the corpus luteum. Without this LH surge, ovulation does not occur.

During adolescence, ovulation does not occur initially. Gonadotropin levels must reach a level high enough to stimulate development of ovarian follicles, which in turn produces estrogen, which in turn leads to the necessary LH surge leading to ovulation. This LH surge may not occur until as late as five years postmenarche.[1] Approximately 75% of abnormal bleeding in the adolescent is due to immaturity of this system.[2]

Dysfunctional bleeding occurs in the perimenopausal (before menopause) woman because of the decreased sensitivity of the ovary to FSH and LH. The resulting decrease in estrogen prevents the LH surge necessary for ovulation. However, similar to the adolescent, there is still enough estrogen being produced to stimulate endometrial growth. Without the balance of progesterone that would normally be produced by the corpus luteum, the endometrium becomes extremely vascular and friable, leading to intermittent sloughing. This type of bleeding is often referred to as estrogen withdrawal bleeding. Estrogen breakthrough bleeding may be due to (1) constant low levels of estrogen, causing portions of the endometrium to degenerate (often seen with low-dose oral contraceptive use); and (2) high levels of estrogen, which allow the endometrium to become hyperplastic and outgrow its blood supply, leading to degeneration and often profuse bleeding. Another type of hormonal imbalance bleeding is progesterone withdrawal and breakthrough bleeding. This is usually the result of exogenous administration of progesterone.

Evaluation

Vaginal bleeding is usually due to uterine bleeding. The causes of vaginal bleeding are limited and are usually the result of trauma or atrophic vaginitis found in elderly women. Uterine bleeding should be correlated with the woman's menstrual history in an attempt to place her in a stage of menstrual development. Chronologically, a woman's reproductive system's development may be divided into the following five stages:[3]

1. premenarchal
2. menarche
3. the reproductive years

4. perimenopausal
5. postmenopausal

This categorization is useful in considering the most likely causes in each stage of development. Bleeding in stages 1 and 5 is abnormal and warrants investigation. In premenarchal years, the most common cause is direct trauma and/or sexual abuse. In postmenopausal years, any bleeding that appears to be uterine should be suspected to be cancerous in origin. Irregular bleeding during menarche and perimenopausal stages is often the natural consequence of fluctuations in hormonal balance. However, one-fifth of abnormal bleeding during menarche is due to a bleeding diathesis. During the reproductive years, the major concerns are that there may be excessive bleeding and there may be bleeding during pregnancy. Alterations in the degree and timing of bleeding related to the menstrual cycle are defined by specific terms as follows:

- polymenorrhea—more frequent than every 20 days
- oligomenorrhea—less often than every 42 days
- menorrhagia—bleeding lasting longer than 8 days
- metrorrhagia—bleeding between periods

The time limits listed above are generalizations and may vary with other text definitions by a few days.

The major differential pivot point is whether bleeding is ovulatory or anovulatory. Ovulatory bleeding is cyclic and is associated with dysmenorrhea and some premenstrual symptoms. In general, the cause is usually a pelvic lesion such as endometriosis, fibroids, an IUD, pelvic inflammatory disease (PID), or pelvic tumors. Anovulatory bleeding is irregular and usually painless; it is often heavy. Endocrine dysfunction or contraceptive use is often the cause. Anovulation often is due to lack of production of LH during the midcycle. The type of bleeding may suggest an underlying cause. If bleeding is bright red with associated clots, a nonmenstrual flow is suggested.

The examination is limited to determination of endocrine causes or a bleeding tendency. An evaluation for thyroid dysfunction is prudent. Pelvic examination should be performed by chiropractors with training in a search for a bleeding source such as tumors. Laboratory evaluation may be helpful in determining whether the patient is anemic.

Management

After performing a thorough history and brief examination, the patient should be given an explanation as to the different types of bleeding and what is specifically suggested in her case. Referral should be made with a letter explaining the doctor's rationale or recommendations.

If a structural lesion is not found to be the source of bleeding, an attempt at controlling the bleeding and normalizing the cycle is made. The standard form of treatment is prescription of oral contraceptive pills (OCPs) or nonsteroid anti-inflammatory drugs (NSAIDs). Both OCPs and NSAIDs can reduce bleeding by up to 50%

(NSAIDs usually are a little less effective).[4, 5] NSAIDs have a strong vasoconstrictive effect. A side benefit is possible reduction of any associated dysmenorrhea. A small number of women may have an increase in bleeding.

Algorithm

An algorithm for evaluation and management of vaginal bleeding is presented in **Figure 36–1**.

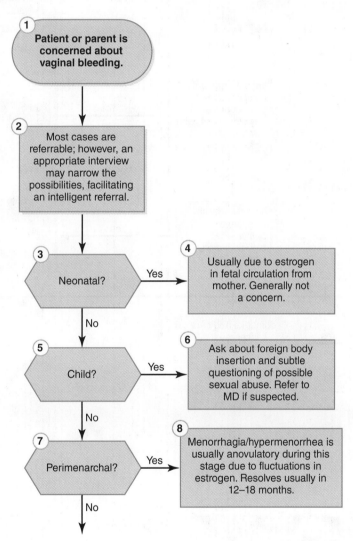

Figure 36–1 Vaginal Bleeding—Algorithm

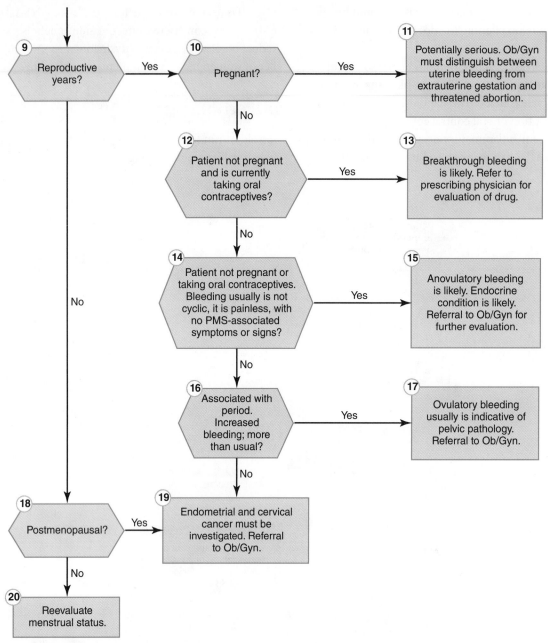

Figure 36–1 (Continued)

APPENDIX 36–1

References

1. Hertweck SP. Dysfunctional uterine bleeding. *Obstet Gynecol Clin North Am.* 1992;19:129–148.
2. Neinstein LS. Menstrual dysfunction in pathophysiologic states. *West J Med.* 1985;143:476–484.
3. Deprez DP. Abnormal vaginal bleeding. In: Greene HL, Fincher RME, Johnson WP, et al., eds. *Clinical Medicine.* 2nd ed. St. Louis, MO: Mosby-Year Book; 1996:821.
4. Nilsson L, Rybo G. Treatment of menorrhagia. *Am J Obstet Gynecol.* 1971;110:713–720.
5. van Eijkeren MA, Cristiaens GC, Scholten PC, et al. Menorrhagia: current drug treatment concepts. *Drugs.* 1992;43:201–209.

Cardiopulmonary Complaints

Syncope/Presyncope

Context

Syncope is the cause of approximately 3% of emergency department visits and 6% of hospital admissions; however, it generally represents a benign clinical entity in and of itself.[1] In the Framingham study, it was found that about 3% of individuals will have an episode of fainting. Syncope was not associated with an increased risk of stroke, myocardial infarction, or sudden death.[2] In 40% of cases, the cause is not identified and up to 30% of individuals have recurrent episodes. Certainly in the senior population the list of possible causes increases with increasing medication use, atherosclerosis, and dysfunctional neurogenic reflexes.

Although it is not a common primary complaint in the chiropractic setting, syncope is often a secondary concern or is evident on a past history review. Generally, the patient will ignore an infrequent sense of almost fainting (presyncope); however, he or she will be quite concerned with actual fainting if not obviously associated with a stressful, painful, or "sickening" scenario.

The most common cause in younger individuals is vasovagal faint. In the elderly, cardiac dysfunction and carotid sinus hypersensitivity are high on the list of causes.

General Strategy

History

- Determine whether the patient has actually fainted or has almost fainted (syncope versus presyncope).
- If the patient did faint, determine whether he or she or a witness can answer questions regarding how long the loss of consciousness (LOC) lasted and whether there were accompanying convulsions or any significant warning symptoms or postfaint signs or symptoms (distinguish between syncope and seizure).
- Determine the frequency of these events.
- Determine the patient's medication history (alcohol, diuretics, vasodilators, antidepressants, sedatives, or sympatholytic drugs).
- Determine whether there was an associated historical trigger such as heat (vasodilation), prolonged standing (pooling effect), sudden pain, emotional stress, tight collar (carotid sinus syndrome), turning the head to one side (carotid sinus syndrome), exercise (hypertrophic subaortic stenosis or vascular pooling), coughing (cough syncope), urinating (micturition syncope), a frightening/nauseating situation (vasovagal), or anxiety (hyperventilation).

Evaluation

- Test the patient with supine and standing blood pressure measurements (orthostatic hypotension).
- Perform or refer for electrocardiogram (ECG).
- Evaluate the patient with laboratory tests to determine whether anemia or diabetes is present.
- When the diagnosis is not clear, consider referral for tilt-table testing (vasovagal syncope).

Management

- If triggers are avoidable, give the patient advice regarding a defensive approach.

- Give the patient strategy options for when the sensation of fainting first recurs.
- Refer cases that seem to be medication-related or are unexplained/frequent episodes.

Relevant Physiology

There are several important cardiovascular reflexes that may be influenced by medications, structural abnormalities, and emotional and environmental factors. There are two broad classifications of receptors that participate in these reflexes based on location and function. First are high pressure receptors. These are found in the walls of arteries, specifically in the carotids and the aortic bodies. The second is a low pressure receptor with two different types. First is the atrial stretch type and second the ventricular type (Bezold–Jarisch reflex). The atrial stretch receptors participate in two reflexes, the atrial stretch reflex and the Bambridge reflex.

Syncope or presyncope is often the result of a pooling effect of either prolonged standing or extreme heat, or the vasodilative effects of many medications. Interference with the normal functioning of cerebral blood pressure may be the result of a dysfunctional neuronal reflex. This occurs in the elderly, those with diabetes, and those with a dysfunctional adrenal gland. With the elderly, a combination of hypersensitivity of the carotid sinus and decreased neuronal conduction may contribute to a decrease in blood pressure upon rising, referred to as orthostatic hypotension. This may be potentiated by certain medications known to blunt the sympathetic response, such as β-blockers. Also, patients with volume depletion caused by diuretics, vomiting, or diarrhea may develop orthostatic hypotension.

Patients with orthostatic syncope appear to have neurocardiogenic dysfunction due to autonomic dysfunction. They demonstrate β-adrenergic hypersensitivity.[3] Patients who become faint with exercise or fasting may have vasodepressor syncope. This has been shown to occur following a rise in β-endorphin concentration just before syncope. These endogenous opiates have an inhibitory effect on sympathetic tone.[4] Another suggested cause in exercise-induced presyncope or syncope is inappropriate peripheral vasodilation due to ventricular mechanoreceptor stimulation. This was found in patients who had no discernible cardiac structural abnormalities.[5] These two theories obviously may overlap. Another theory to consider is that these individuals have a failure to decrease parasympathetic tone.[6] In addition to syncope, other autonomic nervous system dysfunction signs and symptoms may be related to hypermobility syndromes.[7] Presyncope, palpitations, chest discomfort, fatigue, and heat intolerance appear to be more common in patients with hypermobility. In particular, orthostatic hypotension was found in 78% of patients diagnosed with joint hypermobility syndrome who fulfilled the 1998 Brighton criteria.

Obviously, any decrease in blood supply to the head is a potential syncope cause. Therefore, a consideration of the pulmonary and cardiovascular systems structurally, functionally, and physiologically is needed. Blockage of outflow due to aortic (or subaortic) stenosis will decrease blood supply to the brain. Severe atherosclerosis is also a consideration. Functionally, the heart must pump effectively to maintain cerebral perfusion. Arrhythmias and heart block may result in hypoxia and syncope in some patients. Anemia is rarely a cause of syncope; with severe blood loss or severe anemia due to other causes, however, exertional syncope may occur. In particular with chronic obstructive pulmonary disease, decreased perfusion or oxygenation may result in a relative cerebral hypoxia.

Evaluation

History

The initial focus of the history is to attempt to differentiate between syncope and seizure (**Table 37–1**). This is not as clear-cut as first assumed. One study demonstrated that, when syncope was induced through a combination of hyperventilation, Valsalva maneuver, and orthostasis, myoclonic activity occurred in 90% of those who fainted. Additionally, head turns, automatisms, and righting movements were observed in 79% of patients who fainted.[8] An important clue is the length of LOC. With a simple faint, the patient is often conscious within seconds. This may be extended in some instances, such as with hypoglycemia. When an epileptic seizure is the cause of LOC, the patient is usually unconscious for much longer; when there is convulsive activity, it usually lasts for several minutes. With a simple (vasovagal) faint, most patients have a warning with prodromal symptoms such as nausea, yawning, or belching with accompanying symptoms of lightheadedness, sweatiness, and cold hands. After fainting, the patient with vasovagal syncope is usually able to become functional in a short period

Table 37–1 History Questions for Syncope

Primary Question	What Are You Thinking?	Secondary Questions	What Are You Thinking?
What position were you in when you fainted ?	Recumbent suggests cardiac. Upright suggests vasovagal. Rising suggests orthostatic hypotension.	**Were you doing anything just before fainting? How did you feel after fainting?**	Twisting/turning head suggests subclavian steal syndrome. Coughing suggests Valsalva response. Urinating suggests micturition syncope.
How did you feel just prior to fainting?	Sweating, lightheadedness, or queasiness suggests vasovagal. Visual, auditory, or olfactory prodrome suggests an aura (seizure). Vision "closing in" or going dark suggests cardiac or orthostatic.	**How did you feel after fainting?**	Confusion with possible incontinence suggests seizure rather than vasovagal or cardiac syncope.
How quickly did you regain consciousness?	Less than 1 minute suggests vasovagal. Five to 15 minutes is more common with epilepsy.	**Were there witnesses?**	Try to determine whether there was seizure activity.
Are you taking any medications?	Medications that vasodilate (antihypertensives), deplete fluid (diuretics), or cause nervous system depression (sedatives) are high on the list.	**Have you been diagnosed with a condition for which medication was prescribed, but you do not take the medication?**	Diabetes. Arrhythmia.
Is this related to exertion?	Cardiopulmonary dysfunction. Extreme exertion with volume depletion or in extreme heat.	**Did the fainting occur with exertion or after exertion?**	With exertion, cardiopulmonary status should be checked; aortic stenosis, anemia, or pulmonary hypertension. After a strenuous event, rule out dehydration or heat exhaustion, then consider hypertrophic cardiomyopathy.
Were you emotionally stressed?	Most common cause is simple (vasovagal) faint. Anxiety-related hyperventilation.	**Were there symptoms prior to fainting?**	Nausea, lightheadedness, sweating/clamminess, and cold hands suggest simple faint. Numbness, paresthesias, and cold hands suggest hyperventilation.

of time. Those with seizure-associated LOC take much longer to regain function and often are disoriented after regaining consciousness. In addition, there may be signs of incontinence, extreme tiredness, and general body aching after a seizure episode (postictal). Eyewitnesses often are necessary to document the length of LOC and the associated patient activity during the attack.

A determination of whether the patient was standing, sitting, or lying down at the time of syncope is often revealing. Patients who faint when lying down are almost always suffering from a cardiac condition such as an arrhythmia or heart block. If the patient faints when in an upright position, vasovagal syncope is the most likely cause. This may be precipitated by prolonged standing, causing pooling of blood in the lower half of the body, or by heat, causing vasodilation. If the patient reports the occurrence only when rising from a recumbent position, orthostatic hypotension is most likely the mechanism. The normal sympathetic response from lying to standing causes splanchnic vasoconstriction (mainly venous) to prevent venous pooling in the abdominal area and increases the force of contraction of the heart. If the sympathetic effect is blocked by some medications or the autonomic nervous system is dysfunctional, this protective response is blunted. The most common drugs involved are those that decrease fluid volume (diuretics), cause vasodilation (many antihypertensives and erectile dysfunction medications), decrease the nervous system response (sedatives and sympatholytics), and antidepressants and antipsychotic medications. Some simple physiologic causes should also be suspected with ortho-static hypotension, such as prolonged recumbency or prolonged standing, the augmenting effects of pregnancy (vascular pooling), and volume depletion from pro-longed vomiting or diarrhea and possibly an associated sodium depletion.

The relationship of syncope to exercise may also be an important clue. If fainting occurs with exertion, severe aortic stenosis (particularly in the elderly) or pulmo-nary hypertension should be suspected. If the syncope is postexertional (particularly in a young man) subaortic hypertrophic cardiomyopathy should be investigated. If the syncope occurs after a prolonged endurance event, many other factors, such as volume depletion and heat exhaustion, must be taken into account.

Exertional syncope in athletes is of particular concern due to the known incidence of sudden death. Syncope in athletes often indicates cardiac structural abnormali-ties. Athletes have a host of what would appear to be cardiac pathology based on ECG abnormalities includ-ing sinus bradycardia, first- or second-degree AV block, increased voltage of R- or S-waves, and incomplete right bundle branch block. It is best to refer to recommenda-tions by the 36th Bethesda Conference to determine the appropriate course of action and athletic participation criteria for athletes with indications of cardiac involve-ment.[9] Although generally benign, mitral valve prolapse syndrome combined with a history of syncope and mitral valve regurgitation may indicate an individual at risk for sudden death.[10]

There appear to be a few neurally mediated causes of syncope that are rare but worth mentioning because of strong historical clues. If syncope occurs with coughing, an exaggerated vagal response is likely. If syncope occurs post-urination a similar mechanism may be in effect. This type usually occurs in elderly men at night. If syn-cope is associated with facial pain provoked by swallow-ing or yawning, glossopharyngeal syncope is likely, due to a reflex mechanism. If the patient notices that syncope occurs while wearing a tight collar or when turning the head, carotid sinus syndrome is likely.

If the patient appears anxious or volunteers an associa-tion of presyncope with anxiousness, ask about associ-ated symptoms such as numbness, paresthesias, and coldness in the extremities. Similar symptoms may occur with hypoglycemia; therefore, it is important to ask about the relation to meals, use of insulin, or use of hypoglyce-mic medications.

Examination

Initial evaluation involves a search for cardiopulmonary disease through auscultation for carotid bruits, heart murmurs, or indications of congestive heart failure. Often the physical examination is unrevealing in those with a complaint of fainting or near-fainting. Most valu-able is a search for orthostatic hypotension. The patient's blood pressure is taken supine and then standing after three minutes. A decrease of greater than 20 mm Hg in the systolic blood pressure or 10 mm Hg in the diastolic blood pressure is suggestive of orthostatic hypotension and warrants an investigation into volume depletion and neuronal dysfunction due to adrenal, medication, or diabetic causes. Carotid sinus sensitivity is often tested with carotid massage. This is probably not prudent in the chiropractor's office in the event of complications. Many times this potential cause may be suspected from a historical report of tight collar or neck rotational provo-cation. Laboratory testing may be helpful in detecting an underlying problem with anemia, hyponatremia, diabetes, or more specific testing for endocrine dysfunc-tion. Electrocardiographic evaluation or Holter moni-toring may uncover an underlying arrhythmia as the cause, especially in those with a concomitant complaint of palpitations or in patients who faint while lying. In patients who faint after exertion it is important to obtain an echocardiogram to evaluate subaortic hypertrophic cardiomyopathy. If the patient appears to have a his-tory of anxiety-related presyncope or syncope, perform a hyperventilation test whereby the recumbent patient hyperventilates for approximately one minute while the examiner appears to be auscultating the chest. If the patient becomes faint, a suspicion of hyperventilation as the cause is appropriate unless the patient has underlying cardiopulmonary disease.

Recently, upright tilt testing has been increasingly utilized for evaluation of vasovagal syncope. This test incorporates varying degrees of tilt for varying amounts of time to provoke syncope. A comprehensive litera-ture review of upright tilt testing suggests that although isoproterenol is often used to augment the effect, its use is usually unnecessary, adding to cost, complexity, and a higher associated false-positive response. The recom-mended protocol is passive testing at 60° for 45 to 60 minutes. This approach seems to have a higher overall specificity than other methods.[11]

Management

Referral is warranted for patients who appear to have any of the following:

- epilepsy
- a cardiac or pulmonary cause
- medication-induced syncope

For patients with orthostatic hypotension unrelated to medication, for patients who have an underlying disease that is managed by a medical doctor, or for patients with vasovagal syncope the following suggestions may be helpful:

- Avoid dehydration, fever, excessive heat, prolonged standing, prolonged recumbency, large meals, skipping meals, alcohol and unnecessary drugs, and quick standing.
- Rise slowly from a lying or sitting posture, maintain adequate fluid and salt intake, maintain physical conditioning, and support the lower extremities with elastic garments if venous insufficiency is a contributing factor.

APPENDIX 37–1

References

1. Goldschlager N, Epstein AE, Grubb BP, et al. Etiologic considerations in the patient with syncope and an apparently normal heart. *Arch Intern Med.* 2003;163(2):151–162.

2. Savage DD, Corwin L, McGee DL, Kannel WB, Wolf PA. Epidemiologic features of isolated syncope: the Framingham Study. *Stroke.* 1985;16(4):626–629.

3. Balaju S, Oslizlok PC, Allen MC, et al. Neurocardiogenic syncope in children with a normal heart. *J Am Coll Cardiol.* 1994;23:779–785.

4. Wallbridge DR, MacIntyre HE, Gray CE, et al. Increase in plasma beta endorphins precedes vasodepressor syncope. *Br Heart J.* 1994;71:446–448.

5. Sneddon JF, Scalia G, Ward DE. Exercise induced vasodepressor syncope. *Br Heart J.* 1994;71:554–557.

6. Lippman N, Stein KM, Lerman BB. Failure to decrease parasympathetic tone during upright tilt predicts a positive tilt-table test. *Am J Cardiol.* 1995;75:591–595.

7. Gazit Y, Nahir AM, Grahame R, Jacob G. Dysautonomia in the joint hypermobility syndrome. *Am J Med.* 2003;115:33–40.

8. Lempert T, Bauer M, Schmidt D. Syncope: a videometric analysis of 56 episodes of transient cerebral hypoxia. *Ann Neurol.* 1994;36:233–237.

9. Shah AM, Estes NA 3rd, Weinstock J, Homoud MK, Link MS. Treatment of athletes with cardiac disease or arrhythmias. *Curr Treat Options Cardiovasc Med.* 2006;8(5):353–361.

10. Kligfield P, Devereux RB. Is the mitral valve prolapse patient at high risk of sudden death identifiable? *Cardiovasc Clin.* 1990;21(1):143–157; discussion 158–160.

11. Kapoor WN, Smith MA, Miller NL. Upright tilt testing in evaluating syncope: a comprehensive literature review. *Am J Med.* 1994;97:78–88.

Chest Pain

Context

Chest pain can be a frightening event. Patients often associate chest pain with the heart and experience enough concern to see a medical physician. The majority of patients with chest pain who present to a chiropractic office setting suspect that their pain is musculoskeletal or know from past diagnoses that their pain is cardiac and are being managed by a medical doctor. However, with some patients, there may be few historical clues or the pain is mild, leaving the patient unaware of an underlying problem of a potentially serious nature. Without a clear history of musculoskeletal cause, the assumption should be cardiac until proven otherwise. Conversely, noncardiac pain may be frighteningly convincing as a cardiac impersonator. The primary role of the chiropractor as a first-contact physician is to differentiate between cardiac (ischemic) pain and noncardiac pain. This is also often the difference between a referable condition and a nonreferable condition. It is crucial, however, that the chiropractor be aware of the important role he or she can play in the long-term comanagement of the patient with angina. The long-term quality of a patient's life and perhaps his or her prognosis may be affected through a lifestyle management approach with emphasis on diet, exercise, and stress management for which the chiropractor can play a supportive role.[1]

In the emergency department, the diagnostic distinction must first be whether or not the patient has acute coronary syndrome (ACS). Acute coronary syndrome represents coronary occlusion and subsequent damage. This is differentiated from stable angina where no damage occurs. There are three primary types of ACS, each representing about one-third of all ACS patients:

1. ST elevation myocardial infarction (STEMI)
2. Non-ST elevation myocardial infarction (NSTEMI)
3. Unstable angina

High-risk patients are usually identified using a version of the Thrombolysis in Myocardial Infarction (TIMI) score.[2] Included are older age (>65 years), use of aspirin without relief, known cardiac disease, ECG abnormalities (ST segment), elevated cardiac biomarkers, and other risk factors (among other indicators), which are each given a point score and then the total is stratified based on risk. ACS represents only about 5% to 6% of all admissions to emergency departments in Europe and the United States,[3] and only 20% to 25% of admissions to the ED for *chest pain* are caused by ACS.[4]

Recently, clinical prediction approaches have demonstrated the ability to take low-risk patients and through a series of testing, which includes no high-risk factors on admission in the emergency department coupled with testing with serial cardiac troponins and electrocardiography, and exercise tolerance testing (ETT) if indicated, successfully identify 82% of patients as not having cardiac chest pain.[5] In another recent study,[6] only one-third of patients with chest pain and known coronary disease, but with negative ECG, and biomarkers were subsequently found to have adverse cardiac events.

Chest pain that appears to be cardiac may in fact be from another source. Studies indicate that 30% of patients who have catheterization for angina-like pain have no abnormalities angiographically. Of these patients, 50% may have pain due to esophageal disorders. The remainder may have microangiographic involvement not visible on angiography (syndrome X). It is estimated that musculoskeletal causes of chest pain account for approximately 13% to 30% of cases.[7,8]

Recurrent episodes of chest pain are estimated to affect 50% to 90% of patients with noncardiac chest pain.[9] Even though patients are told they do not have cardiac disease, only 30% to 50% feel reassured and as many as 50% remain on cardiac medication and 75% continue seeing a physician.[10]

General Strategy

History

- Attempt to distinguish between cardiac and noncardiac pain (**Exhibit 38-1** and **Table 38-1**).
- Use the history to develop a high level of suspicion for cardiac pain—diffuse, substernal pain with radiation into the arm (medial) or jaw, lasting between 10 and 60 minutes (**Table 38-2**).
- In those suspected of having angina, check the history for risk factors, triggers, and other indicators.
- Check the drug history of all patients to determine use of cocaine or other stimulants, and response to nitroglycerin in patients who previously have been diagnosed with angina; some patients do not take their medication properly.

Evaluation

- Attempt to distinguish among the various causes of noncardiac chest pain—visceral, musculoskeletal, skin, psychogenic, referred, or local.
- Auscultate, obtain a screening electrocardiogram (ECG), and consider a chest radiograph when cardiac causes are suggested.
- With suspicion of musculoskeletal conditions, incorporate a mechanical challenge (stretch, compression, and palpation) in an attempt to reproduce the complaint.

Management

- Refer cardiac-caused pain for comanagement (input on proper diet and exercise if pain is anginal).
- Manage musculoskeletal causes conservatively based on the tissue involved.

Relevant Anatomy and Physiology

Cardiac pain is essentially ischemic pain. The degree of ischemia extends from mild, transient decrease of coronary blood flow to life-threatening infarction. Decrease in coronary artery blood flow (CABF) is generally due to vasospasm. Prinzmetal's (variant) angina is also possible as a pure or overlapping cause. CABF is also dependent on the status of the heart and its ability to pump an adequate supply of blood.[11] Specifically, the status of the aortic valve is important. If the aortic valve is stenotic, less blood leaves the heart. This is also true with aortic incompetence, where blood that would normally drain to the coronaries is allowed to return to the left ventricle. This in turn places a high demand on the heart to pump blood from a double source. Over 50% of patients with calcific aortic stenosis and angina have significant coronary artery disease.[12] Hypertrophic obstructive cardiomyopathy (HOCM) is a rare problem that in effect blocks off the aortic exit from the heart, often leading to sudden death. While it is developing it may give a prewarning with chest pain due to ischemia. Through a somewhat similar mechanism, mitral valve prolapse syndrome may cause atypical chest pain because of ischemia. Additionally, anemia may be a factor due to the decreased oxygen-carrying capacity of the blood. Other stimulators are increased sympathetic activity from mechanical or environmental stresses such as anxiety, cold, and exercise.

Differentiating between Cardiac Pain and Noncardiac Pain

Chest pain is rarely lung pain because the sensitivity of the lungs to pain has been delegated to the endemic vasculature and surrounding pleura. This is why a patient may have bronchogenic carcinoma or other lung processes such as chronic obstructive pulmonary disease (COPD) without any signal of pain until late in the process.

Pleural pain illustrates an important concept with regard to pulmonary conditions. Processes that affect the pleura such as pleurisy, pneumothorax, pulmonary embolism, and cancer cause pain that is relatively well localized. This is because the parietal pleura is a somatic structure and therefore is innervated by unilateral spinal nerves, making possible localization in vertical and horizontal planes. This also explains why positions such as side bending and lying on the involved side may increase the pain. The pericardium may also react similarly and cause a more localized, left-sided chest pain.

Visceral chest pain is often central, reflecting the embryologic arrangement of most thoracic and abdominal organs. As organs migrate during development, the brain does not receive their forwarding address. As originally midline structures, these organs have a bilateral

Exhibit 38–1 **Differentiating between Cardiac Pain and Noncardiac Pain**

Patient presents with a complaint of chest pain

Differentiate between cardiac and noncardiac causes

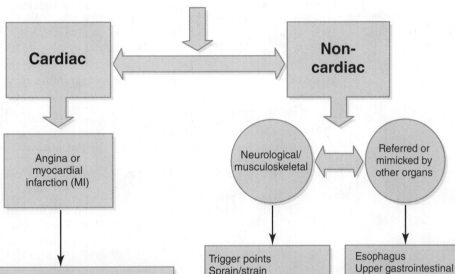

Cardiac

Non-cardiac

Angina or
myocardial
infarction (MI)

Neurological/
musculoskeletal

Referred or
mimicked by
other organs

Angina
Pain is described as gripping, squeezing, or
pressure in the chest.
The location is substernal or precordial.
Pain may be exertion related.
The pain may last from 10 to 30 minutes and is
relieved by nitroglycerin.
MI
Same as above but more severe; pain is
described as crushing. Radiation into the
medial left arm or jaw is common.

Trigger points
Sprain/strain
Subluxation
Rib fracture
Tietze's syndrome
Intercostal neuritis
Herpes zoster (shingles)
Slipped rib or subluxation

Esophagus
Upper gastrointestinal
(GI)
Cervical spine
Pleura

ECG and cardiac enzymes are studies initially
indicated. For angina, ST depression is seen. For
MI, T wave inversion, significant Q waves, and axis
deviation away from the side are often seen. Lab
elevations are initially cardiac-specific tropinin,
creatine kinase, and later lactate dehydrogenase.

Pain is often brief or
continuous; reproduced
by movement, position,
or contraction of
specific muscles; the
location is rather
specific. With
intercostal neuritis, rib
fracture, or shingles,
pain is along
dermatome (rib).

Esophagitis and GI
disorders have
associated GI complaints
such as difficulty
swallowing
(unfortunately, the vagal
component of cardiac
pain also causes GI
symptoms).
Pleurisy should have
associated respiratory
signs including
auscultatory indications
of involvement.
With cervical spine
involvement, there is
usually associated
osteoarthritis with
reproduction using
standard orthopaedic
tests.

Table 38–1 Differentiating Noncardiac Causes of Chest Pain

Cause	Significant History Findings	Provocative Maneuvers, Special Exams
Visceral		
Pleural	History may include pneumonia, pneumothorax, tuberculosis, bronchogenic carcinoma, etc.; pain is sharp	Deep breathing, bending toward same side may aggravate complaint; auscultate/radiograph
Esophageal	May or may not have dysphagia; pain is substernal or radiates to central back	Hot or cold food may trigger pain; manometry/barium x-ray may be necessary
Neuromusculoskeletal		
Nerve		
Herpes zoster	Often unilateral, dermatomal pattern; hypersensitivity followed vesicle formation; burning, sharp pain; recurrent	Hypersensitive to palpation
Intercostal neuritis	Similar to herpes presentation without vesicles; common causes include osteophytes and diabetes	May reproduce on rib separation or compression of intercostal space
Bone		
Rib fracture	Usually history of trauma	Reproduce on compression anterior-to-posterior (if posterolateral); tuning fork, oblique radiographs
Joint		
Costochondral junction	Tietze's syndrome found in older women; higher ribs; unilateral; sharp pain	Direct pressure of junction or between ribs
Costovertebral or costotransverse	May or may not be traumatic; pain radiates along rib	Pressure over affected joint causes radiation
Cervical spine	Referral from osteophytic involvement; usually in older patients	Compression/distraction tests
Muscle		
Sprain	Possible history of overuse or trauma; usually, pectorals, serratus anterior, or intercostals	Stretch, contract, combine
Trigger point	Many causative factors, including visceral referral zone; possible autonomic nervous system changes; no neurologic changes; sternocleidomastoid, pectorals, scalenes, sternalis all possible	Sustained pressure on trigger points
Other		
Anxiety related	Patient may appear anxious or depressed; pain is often over heart and is often either quick/stabbing (seconds) or "heavy"/constant	Psychologic evaluation may be necessary; may be aggravated by deep breathing

Reproduced with permission from T.A. Souza, *Topics in Clinical Chiropractic*, Vol.1, No.1, p. 2, 1994, Aspen Publishers, Inc.

Table 38–2 History Questions for Chest Pain: Cardiac or Noncardiac?

Primary Question	What Are You Thinking?	Secondary Question	What Are You Thinking?
Can you point to where it hurts?	If they can, it is unlikely that there is a cardiac cause.	Were you hit in the chest, back, or side?	Possible rib fracture, especially if worse with deep breathing or lying on the same side.
		Have you had a chest cold or flu?	Pleurisy possible, especially in elderly.
		Is it worse with arm movements; especially overhead or trunk bending?	Muscular cause is more likely; pleurisy is possible with trunk bending.
Is it more diffuse or hard to pinpoint?	Cardiac or esophageal, especially if substernal or precordial. Pressure-type pain often described.	Did it occur after exertion and was it relieved with rest?	Stable angina likely.
		Does it occur at rest?	Unstable or Prinzmetal's (variant) angina.
		Does it radiate down your inner arm or to your jaw?	Angina or pre-myocardial infarction likely.
		Does it radiate along your rib?	Intercostal neuritis, diabetes, shingles (with skin lesions), thoracic osteoarthritis.
		Does it radiate to your back?	Esophageal pathology or aortic aneurysm.
How long does it last?	Distinguish among brief, continuous, or a timed period.	Is it continuous (all the time)?	Cardiac unlikely.
		Does it last less than half an hour?	Cardiac more likely.
		Is it a split-second jab (sharp) pain?	Cardiac unlikely; probably short muscle spasm.
Is it relieved by nitroglycerin?	Angina or esophageal spasm.	How long does it take after taking nitroglycerin?	Should take a few minutes, not seconds to relieve angina.
		Do you have difficulty swallowing at times?	Esophageal spasm possible.
Do you smoke?	Lung cancer.	How long have you smoked?	Years of heavy smoking are usually needed.
Any other associated complaints?	Depression/anxiety, collagen/vascular disorders, osteoarthritis.	Do you find your relationships and hobbies still exciting?	Depression.
		Any past diagnosis of collagen diseases?	Lupus, sarcoidosis.
		Is there any neck pain?	Osteoarthritis.

innervation not capable of providing localizing information. Therefore, a painful stimulus of an organ is not perceived as being on the right or the left. Confounding this natural neural bias is the fact that there is an overlap of sensory innervation to organs that are geographically related (see **Figure 38–1**). For example, the upper two-thirds of the esophagus, the lungs, trachea, bronchi, and heart are innervated by thoracic spinal cord segments T1 through T4 or T5. Overlap continues, with the lower third of the esophagus, stomach, duodenum, liver, gallbladder, pancreas, and part of the small intestine all being innervated by the segments from T5 through T10. Therefore, pathology in one structure is difficult to localize from others when interpreted by the brain at the conscious level. Visceral afferent receptors primarily serve the goal of gathering information about function in an effort to maintain homeostasis. Therefore, information about distention and blood supply governs responses that help maintain normal functioning of these systems. The same pain-producing stimuli for somatic structures apparently do not elicit pain in deep visceral structures. Pain in somatic structures is a stimulus for survival, avoiding the external, potential risk of damage or death. So, although cutting, burning, stabbing, or pinching of somatic structures causes pain, it is not perceptible when applied to deep organs. Pressure, and in particular ischemia, however, do cause pain (see **Table 38–3**).

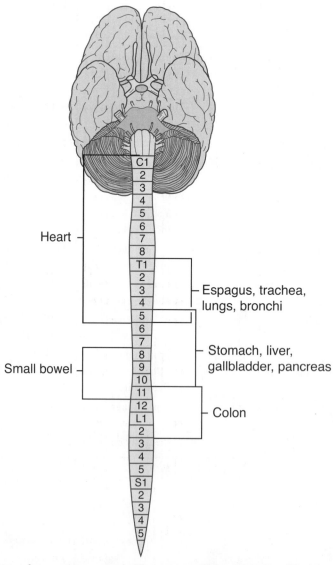

Figure 38–1 Segmental overlap in visceral sensory nerve supply. The poor correlation between referred pain and its site of origin necessitates a thorough history and a careful screening of the differential possibilities. Cardiac ischemic pain (A) is transmitted via the upper four to five thoracic spinal segments (as well as cervical levels). Sensory impulses from the lungs and bronchi (B) as well as the esophagus, aorta, and body walls (C), however, share the same spinal segments, making the diagnosis difficult in many cases.

Table 38–3 Differentiation of Somatic and Visceral Pain Based on General Characteristics

Character	Superficial Somatic	Deep Somatic	Visceral
Neurology	Spinal nerves (unilateral innervation)	Spinal nerves (unilateral innervation)	Visceral affronts (bilateral innervation)
Structures	Skin, superficial fasciae, tendon sheaths, periosteum	Muscles, fasciae, tendons, joint capsules, ligaments, periosteum	Hollow organs, parenchymatous organs
Quality	Sharp	Aching, dull	Aching, dull
Localization	Yes (lateralizes)	Fairly good; refers often	Difficult; perceived away from organ site; often central
Main stimuli	Cutting, compression, burning	Cutting, compression, burning ischemia	Distention, inflammation, ischemia
Movement	Pain often increases	Pain often increases	Activity often has no effect

Reproduced with permission from T.A. Souza, *Topics in Clinical Chiropractic*, Vol. 1, No. 1, p. 2, 1994. Aspen Publishers, Inc.

Esophageal causes of chest pain are thought to be due to a dysfunction in visceral sensory perception.[13] Either motility or acid sensitivity may play a role in a hypersensitivity reaction or a lowering of the pain sensitivity threshold. The motility disorders are represented by the nutcracker esophagus (NCE) and esophageal spasm. NCE is an occurrence of high-amplitude peristaltic contractions. Esophageal spasm is due to simultaneous contractions of the esophagus. Some theorize that these disorders and acid hypersensitivity do not cause chest pain but are markers for a propensity toward a dysfunctional visceral sensory system.[12]

Referred pain from the cervical or thoracic spine is possible. Biliary disorders such as cholelithiasis and cholecystitis also can cause pain in the chest. Finally, any irritation of the pleura and the distention by gas of the hepatic or splenic flexures of the colon may cause chest pain.

Evaluation

History

The presentation with cardiac pain is often one of concern. Usually, the severity of the pain and the incapacitation with myocardial infarction will result in an emergency department visit or a 911 call. Therefore, most cardiac pain in an ambulatory setting is anginal. The characteristic attributes of cardiac pain are as follows:

- substernal or precordial in location
- diffuse (patient cannot point to a discrete spot)

- a dull, squeezing, or pressure sensation
- radiation to the medial side of the left arm or to the jaw
- relieved by rest
- pain usually lasts between 10 and 60 minutes
- body position has no obvious effect on improving or increasing the pain (with the possible exception of angina, where many patients are often reluctant to be recumbent)
- ischemic pain is usually relieved by nitroglycerin

Cardiac pain is often the result of coronary artery occlusion caused by atherosclerosis or vasospasm. Given that atherosclerosis is a slowly accumulating process, it is logical to assume cardiac disease in older patients who have chest pain. The classic presentation of an older man with retrosternal pain relieved by 5 to 15 minutes of rest is so characteristic of coronary heart disease (CHD) that the patient has a 94% probability of having at least 75% occlusion of one coronary artery on angiography.[14] The opposite is also true; a young woman with chest pain that is not typical cardiac pain has a less than 1% chance of coronary artery occlusion.

Musculoskeletal and somatic chest pain has a broader range of attributes; however, it often presents as follows:

- localized pain
- pain that is often stabbing or sharp; but deep, dull, aching pain is also possible
- no radiation unless along a rib or between ribs (dermatomal)
- pain is either brief, lasting as little as a few seconds, or continuous

- the pain is made worse by specific body positions that stretch, contract, or compress the involved area
- a history of overuse or trauma may be found

When a history of trauma is given (fall or blow to the chest), a suspicion of rib fracture is high. Rib fractures generally feel worse with deep inspiration, coughing, sneezing, and while lying supine. Rib fractures may be the result of abuse, and eliciting a clear history is often difficult. Instead, the patient may claim an "accident." It is important to look for other clues of abuse during the examination, such as bruises and scars or radiographically for past fractures.

Overuse may be obvious, such as starting a new exercise or workout routine, or as subtle as doing housework, yard work, or helping someone move furniture. If the pain is sharp and felt unilaterally at the costosternal junction, Tietze's syndrome should be considered. Other causes include repeated coughing or vomiting.

By focusing on the standard approach to history of a chief complaint questioning, a rather accurate distinction can usually be made between cardiac and noncardiac pain. Further distinction between cardiac and other visceral sources may be more clouded. Substernal pain is also possible with esophageal disorders such as reflux or esophageal spasm.[15] Questions pertaining to swallowing and relationship to meals are often revealing. If swallowing is difficult, it is important to ask about the relationship to hot, cold, solid, and liquid foods. If the pain begins after drinking or eating very hot or cold foods and is associated with difficulty swallowing both solids and liquids, esophageal spasm must be considered a likely possibility. Pain that is worse with recumbency, especially after meals or with wearing a tight belt, is indicative of reflux. Reflux may also be associated with the ingestion of certain foods such as chocolate, fats, caffeine, orange juice, onions, and garlic. It is important to note, however, that patients with cardiac pain often have associated epigastric complaints.

The distinction between superficial and deep pain helps first to distinguish between cardiac and noncardiac pain. It also helps in distinguishing among various noncardiac sources of pain. If the patient complains of a superficial sensation of burning or hypersensitivity along a patch of skin, herpes zoster (shingles) should be suspected. This is confirmed within a few days with the appearance of a vesicular rash roughly following a dermatome (not necessarily the entire dermatome). This same superficial sensation may be the result of irritation

from osteophytic impingement of a thoracic nerve root or may be due to diabetes. Another rare possibility is Mondor's disease. This occurs in women as a superficial thrombophlebitis of the thoracoepigastric vein. The patient feels a tender cordlike swelling beneath the breast.

Chest pain associated with difficulty breathing is common. If there are no indicators of an underlying respiratory infection, several possibilities to consider are the following:[16]

- A sudden onset of chest pain associated with dyspnea and fever suggests a pulmonary embolism, especially in a patient who was immobilized, is taking oral contraceptives, or has antecedent calf pain. Immediate referral is necessary.
- Dyspnea preceding chest pain and associated with lightheadedness, dizziness, or syncope, especially in a younger male athlete, suggests HOCM.[17] Referral for ECG or ultrasound evaluation is necessary.
- Sharp pains localized to the posterior chest that are made worse with respiration, there is no history of trauma, and there are no signs of infection suggest the possibility of spontaneous pneumothorax, especially if the patient is young and tall with a history of an exerting activity such as backpacking or exercise. Chest films are necessary.

A psychogenic cause should be suspected in patients with multiple body complaints that appear unrelated, in patients with a past or current psychiatric diagnosis (especially depression), and in those who appear to have anxiety reactions to stressful situations. It is important not to "excuse" the complaint without a thorough evaluation. Hyperventilation is often found with anxious patients.

Examination

Cardiac involvement is discovered largely through the history. Signs of cardiac involvement are rarely found when the patient is asymptomatic. These signs, when present, would largely be found on an ECG. Changes in the ST segment may reflect underlying ischemia. Depending on severity, either ST elevation or ST depression may be indicative of an ischemic cardiac problem. Given that a resting ECG can provide information only over a short period of time, a Holter monitor (portable recording unit) is often prescribed in an attempt to match the patient's symptoms to a recorded ECG abnormality. Further monitoring with a stress ECG should be done through referral and consultation with a cardiologist. Prediction of recurrent coronary artery disease may be possible, as indicated by a recent study.[18] Using several biomarkers, the researchers were able to accurately predict risk of recurrence of CAD. These markers included natriuretic peptide, cystatin C, albuminuria, C-reactive protein, interleukin-6, and fibrinogen.

Indirect implications are generated through auscultatory findings such as murmurs or lung congestion. Hypertension also may be an indirect indicator of systemic atherosclerosis suggesting coronary involvement. Other indicators of atherosclerotic involvement are signs of intermittent claudication in the lower or upper extremities. This is characterized by pain and weakness/tiredness when exercising the extremity that is promptly relieved by rest.

Musculoskeletal involvement may be exposed, reproducing mechanically the patient's complaint with regard to location and quality. Muscles are challenged through a procedure involving contraction, stretch, and contraction in a stretched position. Palpation is used to localize tenderness and in a search for nodules or referred pain upon palpation of specific trigger points. The most common muscles that can cause chest pain are those that are geographically situated in close proximity: the pectoralis major, pectoralis minor, serratus anterior, and intercostals. Following are positions and contraction patterns that may stretch or contract these structures:

- The pectoralis muscles are stretched by elevation of the arms coupled with horizontal abduction (arms brought behind the back); contraction from this position with the patient attempting to adduct the arms horizontally is sufficiently specific to elicit pain when these muscles are involved.
- The serratus anterior can be stretched with the arm abducted and the trunk passively stretched to the opposite side; contraction is accomplished through either protraction maneuvers such as wall pushups or high arm elevation against resistance.
- The intercostals can be challenged by having the patient seated, arms overhead, while the examiner contacts each rib individually and passively stretches the patient away from and to the involved side in an effort to stretch and compress the area.

Rib involvement is challenged by anterior-to-posterior and transverse pressure to the chest, being careful not to apply direct pressure at the painful area. Additional testing may involve the use of a tuning fork. Using a nonvibrating tuning fork, tenderness is checked in areas along the rib distal to the main site of pain. With this baseline reading, applying the vibrating probe of the tuning fork to the same area may cause a jump reaction due the vibrating fracture area. Radiographs for rib fractures must include oblique views because of the overlap that occurs on regular anterior-to-posterior and lateral views.

Chest films should be reserved for cases of suspected pneumothorax, pleurisy, congestive heart failure, and rib fracture. Following are some guidelines:

- Patients with suspected rib fracture should have a posterior-to-anterior (PA) chest film ordered in search of an associated pneumothorax, and oblique films localized to the area of complaint if fracture is not seen on the PA view.
- Patients with suspected pleurisy should have a PA chest film and a lateral recumbent view ordered in search of an air-fluid level.
- With a posterior chest pain complaint, it is important for the chiropractor not to rely on a collimated thoracic anterior-to-posterior view because significant pathology may be obscured.

Management

Although cardiac-caused pain should be referred for medical evaluation, comanagement may be helpful when attempting to change the patient's lifestyle, including diet, exercise, and stress management.[19] Noncardiac causes are managed based on the underlying tissue involved. See Selected Causes of Chest Pain, later in this chapter, for more detailed recommendations for listed conditions.

Reduction in cardiovascular risk can save lives and improve the quality of life for those living longer. Recommendations in 2013 have included decreasing cardiovascular risk through reduction in LDLc and blood pressure (BP).[20] A synopsis of these recommendations is based on diet and exercise as follows:

- Consume a diet with emphasis on vegetables, fruits, and whole grains including low-fat dairy products, poultry, fish, legumes and nontropical vegetable oils and nuts; decrease sugars and meats. This can be accomplished without a plan or using the DASH diet, the USDA Food Pattern or the AHA Diet. Reduce percent of calories from saturated fats and trans fat.

- For BP lowering add advice to lower sodium intake, consuming no more than 2,400 mg of sodium/day.
- For both groups, it is recommended to exercise aerobically three to four times per week, 40 minutes per session, involving moderate to vigorous activity.

The following are recent changes to the American Heart Association (AHA) guidelines and proposed recommendations[21] for use of CPR, automated electronic defibrillator (AED) units, and the Heimlich maneuver in emergency situations.[22]

A. Automated Electronic Defibrillator (AED) Units

1. AED protocols have changed based on research of their usage. Studies have found that patients who receive multiple shocks have a low likelihood of survival and a high incidence of significant brain damage if they do survive. The thought is that this is likely due to long periods of anoxia while AED is processing, analyzing, and checking for need for subsequent shocks.
2. Even when the AED is successful in resetting the electrical output of the heart, the hypoxic heart muscle does *not* get reset, thus resulting in insufficient contractions and potentially further anoxia.
3. Based on these two findings, the following protocol changes have been put in place for AED units:
   a. When a nonresponsive adult patient is found, 911 should be called immediately via a hard-line phone (infants and children commonly have respiratory causes; thus, CPR is applied first for two minutes (five cycles), then 911 is called).
      - For a single rescuer, the ratio of compressions to ventilations is 30:2 for all patients.
      - For two rescuers, the ratio is 30:2 for adults, and 15:2 for infants and children.
      - Compression rate should be 100 comp/min.
      - Five cycles (30 compressions/2 ventilations) should be completed in two minutes.
   b. Continue with compressions while the AED pads are applied and machine is going through the initial processes.
   c. Stop compression *only* to allow the application of a pad (if necessary) and when the machine advises you that it is "analyzing."
   d. Once the machine has "analyzed" the patient, it will suggest either a shock will be delivered, or advise you to continue CPR. If the latter, then continue one- or two-responder CPR. If a shock is to be delivered, then continue with step "e."
   e. While the shock is being delivered, change responsibilities for two-person CPR (ventilations to compressions and vice versa).
   f. Upon completion of the shock, *immediately* begin delivery of chest compressions (30:2) regardless of what the machine says ("analyzing" for repeat shock).
      - *Do not* be concerned if the patient's electrical rhythm is restored; the compressions are still helpful in assisting the heart muscle in the pumping of blood.
   g. Have the person providing ventilations unplug the pads from the AED unit (leave pads attached to the patient).
   h. Provide five cycles of CPR (30:2).
   i. Plug AED pads back into the unit; unit will pick up where it left off and analyze the need to apply another shock.
   j. Continue to apply compressions until AED unit begins to "analyze."
   k. Repeat steps "d–k" until emergency response personnel arrive.

B. Effect of Ventilations

1. Research has found that chest compressions alone are as good as, if not better than, compressions plus ventilations. The compression of the chest itself helps drive air into and out of the lungs.
2. This research has yet to result in a change of the protocols. However, this is likely to be the next major change.
3. In situations where there is no ventilation mask available (or other barrier):
   a. Provide compressions only (100/min).
   b. Ventilation via compressions is improved if airway is maintained; therefore, if there is a second responder, have him/her perform head tilt and chin lift; if a single responder, place shoe or object under neck to improve head tilt.

C. Cricoid Pressure

1. Studies have recently found that applying AP pressure on the cricoid significantly improves CPR outcomes by minimizing gastric distension and episodes of vomiting. Patients who vomit during CPR have significantly worse outcomes than those who do not.

2. When a second rescuer is present and ventilations are being provided, the second rescuer should apply cricoid pressure by using the thumb and forefinger to capture the cricoid and then press the cricoid cartilage posterior until the point of resistance. This helps collapse the esophagus while maintaining the airway, minimizing gastric distension.

D. Heimlich Maneuver

1. The abdominal thrust on patients who become unconscious due to choking has been eliminated.
2. Blind sweeps have also been eliminated.
3. Once a patient becomes unconscious during the course of rendering the Heimlich maneuver, the following protocol is followed:
   a. Perform one cycle of compressions (30).
   b. Prior to ventilations, check for visible blockage and if found, remove with finger sweep.
   c. If no object is seen, attempt ventilations (if first ventilation does not work, remember to reposition head; lift/chin tuck to ensure adequate airway).
   d. Repeat compressions for one cycle.
   e. Repeat steps "b–e" until emergency personnel arrive.

Algorithm

An algorithm for initial screening of chest pain is presented in **Figure 38–2**.

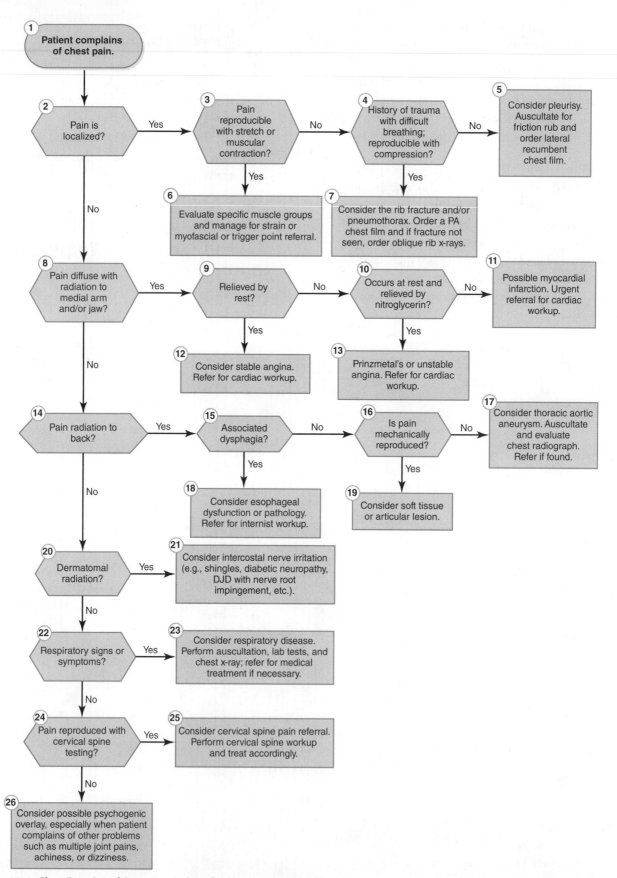

Figure 38–2 Chest Pain: Initial Screening—Algorithm

Selected Causes of Chest Pain*

CARDIAC

Angina

Classic Presentation

The patient complains of a squeezing or pressure sensation in the chest. It came on rather suddenly after exertion. The patient said that after resting for several minutes the sensation went away. This was not the first time it had happened. He or she also noticed that there was an aching pain felt down the left inside arm to the fingers.

Cause

Angina is usually due to atherosclerosis; however, a variant of angina is related to vasospasm that may occur in isolation or with atherosclerosis (Prinzmetal's angina). Patients with Prinzmetal's angina often have an atypical presentation in that they may be women under age 50 years with angina that occurs at night (involves the right coronary artery most often). Another entity is called syndrome X, in which there is no apparent coronary atherosclerosis. It is believed that there are microvascular abnormalities in these patients.[23] The threshold for an angina attack may be decreased by factors such as anemia, valvular disorders (especially aortic stenosis), or conduction problems. Cocaine may also provoke an attack.[24] When atherosclerosis is excessive, angina may occur at rest without provocation (unstable angina). These attacks tend to be longer and may be a portent of impending myocardial infarction.

Evaluation

The history of a pressure or squeezing pain lasting for several minutes to 30 minutes with possible radiation to the arm or jaw is characteristic of angina. If the pain occurs at rest or without provocation, unstable angina is likely, indicating more occlusion. Given that it is rarely possible to examine a patient during an attack, most findings such as hypertension are indirect indicators of underlying atherosclerosis. Valvular abnormalities such as aortic stenosis in older patients and mitral valve prolapse in younger patients may be found. ECG findings are nonspecific except during the attack, when either ST depression or, with more severe ischemia, ST elevation is found. Provocation with exercise testing includes an ECG. Based on these findings scintigraphic or echocardiographic studies may be added.[25] Ambulatory monitoring with a Holter device may be used, especially if an underlying arrhythmia is suspected. Coronary angiography should be used in selected patients only.

Management

Nitroglycerin is used for symptomatic management of angina. It decreases contraction of the heart and causes vasodilation. It is usually taken sublingually and takes a minute or two to work. Other medications may be prescribed such as calcium channel blockers. With more fulminant involvement of the coronary arteries, angioplasty or surgery may be suggested to the patient. It is important to advise patients with mild symptoms that supervised lifestyle changes including a healthful diet and exercise may decrease the need for nitroglycerin and, in some patients, reverse the underlying process. It is a comanagement scenario in which the medical doctor, chiropractor, and patient work together.

Myocardial Infarction

Classic Presentation

Not all patients with myocardial infarction (MI) are unconscious or in severe pain, although the majority of patients have pain severe enough to warrant a trip to the emergency department or a 911 call. It is possible to have a patient complain about pain that is often preceded by a history of angina. The substernal pain is more severe and often builds up over a few minutes. Nitroglycerin does not help. The pain lasts longer than 30 minutes. Twenty percent of individuals die before reaching the hospital. Approximately 25% of infarctions are silent, apparent only on an ECG.[26]

Cause

Usually MI is due to coronary thrombus or vasospasm. Blockage of a specific coronary artery causes damage to the area supplied. For example, blockage of the anterior descending branch of the left coronary artery causes infarction of the anterior left ventricle and interventricular septum. The extent of damage is subendocardial with some transmural extension evident in most cases. Extension of infarcted tissue increases after the occlusion and may be diminished by prompt thrombolytic therapy.

* See also Chapter 39, Palpitations, and Chapter 40, Dyspnea.

Evaluation

Evaluation is performed in the hospital with a check for associated arrhythmias. There are large variations at presentation with regard to heart rate, adventitial respiratory sounds, and general status of the patient. Laboratory testing performed within the first few hours will reveal an elevation of creatine kinase (CK) that peaks in about 12 to 24 hours. The isoenzyme CK-MB (myocardial band) is specific for the heart. The level of CK elevation correlates to the degree of damage. The new laboratory approach to detecting cardiac damage after an MI is the use of cardiac-specific troponin T (cTnT) and cardiac-specific troponin 1 (cTn1). cTn1 levels are elevated for at least one week following MI (an advantage over creatinine phosphokinase [CPK-MB]), and cTnT levels are elevated from 10 to 14 days following MI. This has led to the use of these tests in place of the older method of measuring lactate dehydrogenase (LDH) isoenzyme levels in patients who present after 48 hours or are assessed after this time. Cardiac troponins are also valuable in detecting small MIs that are not detectable by CPK-MB levels. LDH, especially the isoenzyme 1, may still be elevated five to seven days later. ECG findings involve a sequence of hyperacute T-waves, progressing to ST elevation, to Q-wave development, to T-wave inversion. When found, Q-waves are diagnostic for MI; however, 30% to 50% of patients do not have them.[27] A new approach is the use of myeloperoxidase as an early indicator of risk for myocardial infarction as well as adverse cardiac events in the following one- to two-month period in individuals presenting to an emergency department with chest pain.[28] In this way, it is likely to be a better predictor than measurement of troponin, CPK, or LDH—measures that indicate what has happened but not necessarily what will happen. Another possible predictor of adverse cardiovascular events evaluated in patients with CAD is glutathione peroxidase 1 activity.[29] It has been found that there is an inverse relationship to glutathione peroxidase 1 activity and lowered risk. In other words, the lower the activity level, the higher the risk. For older men, evaluating Lp(a) lipoprotein levels has been shown to be an independent predictor of stroke, death from vascular disease, and, actually, death from any cause in men but not in women.[30]

Management

It is important for chiropractors to maintain cardiopulmonary resuscitation (CPR) certification (or knowledge). Although rare, it may be necessary to perform CPR in or out of the office. Initial treatment is crucial for survival and to diminish the extent of damage. Thrombolytic therapy must be given within the first one to three hours for best results.[31] This includes streptokinase, tissue plasminogen activator (t-PA), or anistreplase. Post-MI it is important for the chiropractor to work closely with the patient and cardiologist to maintain a program of prevention, including diet and exercise.

Pericarditis

Classic Presentation

The patient usually complains of chest pain and difficulty breathing that is worse with lying down; it is better seated. The pain is substernal, often radiating to the neck or shoulder. There may be a history of a preceding respiratory infection, renal failure, or cancer.

Cause

The pericardium is the double-layered sac covering and stabilizing the heart. Infiltration with infections or other inflammatory processes decrease the available space and movement of the heart. Viral organisms such as Coxsackie virus, Epstein-Barr virus, mumps, varicella, or human immunodeficiency virus (HIV) may be the cause. It can also be associated with hepatitis, tuberculosis, uremia from kidney failure, neoplasms, post-MI, or radiation treatment.[32]

Evaluation

The presentation may be very similar to that of an acute MI. The characteristic finding is a pericardial friction rub heard on auscultation. ECG findings are similar to those of an MI, including ST elevation or T-wave inversion. A pericardial friction rub is found in 85% of cases and is described as a scratchy, leather-like, or Velcro-like sound.[33] It does wax and wane and may not be constant. Pericardial effusion is a common finding, and when it reaches a critical stage (which may be acute or slowly developing) pericardial tamponade will occur. This is a combination of cardiac output failure, systemic hypotension, and shock. Findings include hypotension, tachycardia, anxiety, muffled heart sounds, and pulsus paradoxus. Jugular vein distension may also be present. If systolic blood pressure decreases more than 10 mm Hg on inspiration or disappears, pericardial tamponade is likely the cause.

Management

Management is dependent on the underlying cause; however, it should be managed medically. Aspirin or nonsteroid anti-inflammatory drugs (NSAIDs) are given for viral etiologies, antitubercular therapy for tuberculosis, and chemotherapy for neoplastic causes. For pericardial effusion, a pericardial window is created between the ribs to aspirate the fluid and take samples of the pericardial tissue.[34] For known causes, the underlying disease is addressed. In addition, and for idiopathic recurrent cases, a combination of NSAIDs, colchicine, and corticosteroids is used.[35]

Hypertrophic Cardiomyopathy

Classic Presentation

The patient may be a young athlete complaining of exercise-induced chest pain and difficulty breathing. More important, there may be a report of postexercise syncope. Unfortunately, the first presentation may be sudden death.

Cause

Hypertrophic cardiomyopathy (HCM) is a nonfunctional ventricular wall enlargement (not due to increased pressure or volume of blood). This enlargement can involve mainly the interventricular septum, causing an outflow blockage during systole. This diminished outflow leads to ischemia with syncope as the clearest indicator. HCM may be inherited as an autosomal-dominant trait. HCM is one of the leading causes of sudden death in young athletes.[36] It may also occur in the elderly.

Evaluation

The evaluation begins as a preventive measure on preparticipation screenings. Although it is still difficult to identify susceptible individuals, a history of chest pain, dyspnea, and/or syncope related to exercise and a family history of HCM or sudden death in a close relative are indicators for further evaluation. The only physical examination finding that is suggestive of HCM is a systolic murmur that is made worse with a Valsalva maneuver; it is improved with squatting. However, this is found only with patients having an outflow tract obstruction, who are the minority. ECG changes usually show ventricular hypertrophy. The echocardiogram is the definitive tool demonstrating asymmetric left ventricular hypertrophy.

Management

Management depends on the degree of involvement. β-blockers or calcium channel blockers may be used for symptom relief. More severe problems may require excision of part of the enlarged myocardium.

NONCARDIAC, MUSCULOSKELETAL

Muscle Strain

Classic Presentation

The patient usually will recall a single event or repetitive overuse event. This may include weight lifting or, in many patients, cleaning the house or moving furniture.

Cause

Exceeding the limits of a muscle's ability to withstand a given load or overstretching the muscle may cause damage to the muscle or tendon.

Evaluation

Evaluation of muscle injury involves palpation for tender areas and referral zones from these areas, contraction in midrange and in a stretched position, and stretching the muscle passively. The main muscles to consider in the chest are the pectoralis major and minor, the serratus anterior, and the intercostals.

Management

Myofascial work in the form of trigger point massage and myofascial release techniques are most appropriate. Gradual retraining of the muscle should proceed from isometrics to isotonics and, depending on the need, isokinetics.

Rib Fracture

Classic Presentation

The patient will report either a direct blow to the chest or a fall onto the chest. The most common location of fracture is posterolateral.

Cause

Direct trauma is needed to break the ribs in adults. In seniors and those with underlying disease processes that result in osteoporosis or lytic processes, minor events may cause a fracture. The rib may be only partially fractured and is referred to as a "cracked" rib. Associated with complete rib fractures is pneumothorax, in which air enters the pleural space.

Evaluation

The patient has guarded respiration and finds it more difficult to lie supine. Pressure directed anterior-to-posterior or transversely (taking care not to apply pressure directly to the site of involvement) will often cause a sharp increase in pain. Tuning fork application may increase the pain dramatically. It is important to apply a nonvibrating tuning fork first to ascertain a baseline level for tenderness. Applying the vibrating tuning fork should be at a site along the rib away from the suspected fracture site. Radiographs should include a PA chest film and if the rib fracture is not seen, order oblique films of the painful area. The PA chest film is necessary to evaluate for a coexisting pneumothorax. Radiographic evidence of fracture is often subtle and may take two to three weeks for callus formation to uncover the site. With cracked ribs, this may not be apparent.

Management

Multiple rib fractures are best managed medically. Cracked ribs or small single fractures can be managed conservatively with rest, pain medication, recommendations to avoid sleeping on the back, laughing, coughing, and sneezing. Immobilization with a rib belt or taping is not recommended because of the inhibitory effect it may have on breathing. Gradual stretching should be introduced to avoid contracture and its effect on respiration. Slow, deep breathing should be attempted when possible. Pain is often present for approximately one to two months. In sports, intercostal blocks are often used to allow the player to return to play. This is a medical decision that carries with it possible medicolegal consequences.

Tietze's Syndrome

Classic Presentation

The patient is often a woman over age 50 years who complains of a moderate to severe pain in the upper part of the chest on one side. She points to the second and third costochondral junctions.

Cause

The cause is unknown. There appears to be an inflammatory reaction at the costochondral and, occasionally, chondrosternal, sternoclavicular, or manubriosternal areas. There may be an overexertion history of prolonged coughing or exertion such as moving furniture. It is bilateral in 30% of cases.[37]

Evaluation

The area (usually upper chondrocostal junction) is tender, as is the adjacent intercostal area. There is swelling but no associated warmth or erythema.

There are no radiographic findings; however, in the differential diagnosis of rheumatoid conditions, radiographs may be needed. In rare cases, a bone scan may show abnormal uptake at the involved site. Chiropractic evaluation of rib and rib articulation movement is important.

Management

The condition is benign and self-resolves in about six months. During the symptomatic period, chiropractic mobilization or adjusting may help (or aggravate) the condition. Failure to respond may require medical referral for an anesthetic/corticosteroid injection, which is 90% effective. This condition may be recurrent.

Costochondritis

Classic Presentation

The patient is usually young, with a complaint of anterior chest pain that is bilateral and affects the middle ribs close to the sternum.

Cause

The cause is unknown. This term is also used to describe Tietze's syndrome; however, costochondritis appears to be a distinct entity because of the more common bilateral involvement of multiple rib articulations.[38] Trauma is suspected as the underlying cause. There are no consistent pathologic findings.

Evaluation

Tenderness without swelling is found at the costal junction of ribs two through five most commonly. A "crowing rooster" position with the patient's cervical spine extended and his or her flexed elbows extended upward behind the body may stretch the involved area and increase pain. Another position that may increase pain is forced horizontal adduction of the shoulder while the patient turns the head to the ipsilateral side. Chiropractic evaluation of the rib and rib articulation are important aspects of the evaluation.

Radiographs are unrevealing and usually unnecessary. Laboratory testing is reserved for those individuals suspected of having an underlying rheumatoid etiology.

Management

Moist heat and NSAIDs may help in this self-resolving, benign condition. It may be necessary to refer for an anesthetic and/or corticosteroid injection.

Slipped Rib
Classic Presentation

The patient complains of a popping or clunking sensation in the lower ribs, usually associated with an exertion maneuver such as a bench press or other lifting maneuver. The patient may report that the rib pops in and out with a specific type of maneuver.

Cause

Loosening of the lower costal cartilages, often due to direct trauma or constant overcontraction of the chest muscles, allows the rib tip to curl upward. Chest pain may result if this impinges on the superior rib or intercostal nerve.[39]

Evaluation

Palpation of the involved area is usually unrevealing unless the patient can reproduce the problem with a specific maneuver. Chiropractic evaluation of costovertebral accessory motion may indicate involvement.

Management

Avoidance of the causative maneuver is important for stabilization. Adjustment of the involved ribs may help the patient temporarily; however, in most cases the condition is recurrent if the patient continues the inciting activity.

Fibromyalgia
Classic Presentation

The patient is often a woman (5:1) and complains of an aching, fatigued, and stiff sensation in multiple muscle groups.

Cause

The cause is unknown. It is believed that there is some relationship to a disturbance in nonrapid eye movement (NREM) sleep.[40] Cold, damp weather, fatigue, a sedentary position or overexertion, mental stress, and poor posture may make it worse.

Evaluation

The standard evaluation is to find a minimum of 11 of 18 bilateral tender areas designated by the American College of Rheumatology.[41]

Management

The conservative approach is to use local application of dry heat, mild to moderate exercise, and stress reduction. It may be necessary to refer for Lyrica (pregabalin) or a trial of minidosing of tricyclic antidepressants, which are believed to assist in restoring normal NREM sleep.

Intercostal Neuritis
Classic Presentation

The patient complains of pain that is unilateral, extending in a band around the chest.

Cause

Intercostal neuritis may be idiopathic, or the result of herpes zoster (shingles), diabetes, osteophytic encroachment, or rib subluxation. Herpes zoster is due to a varicella virus infection. The organism's residence is the dorsal root ganglion. During periods of emotional or mechanical stress the organism becomes active.

Evaluation

In a diabetic patient with poor glycemic control, diabetic neuropathy is likely. For patients with shingles, the pain is followed in three to five days by a vesicular rash along part of the dermatome. Rib subluxation may be determined by palpation of the movement of the rib and at the costotransverse articulation.

Management

For shingles, avoidance of emotional and mechanical stresses is recommended. When the infection is active, the use of lysine and the avoidance of caffeine may help. For more involved or resistant cases, acyclovir may be prescribed by a medical doctor. Rib subluxations should be adjusted. Patients with suspected osteoarthritic involvement should be adjusted cautiously. Low-force techniques may be more appropriate. Adjusting also may be beneficial for the idiopathic and diabetic cases. Control of the underlying diabetes is the long-term goal.

NONCARDIAC, VISCERAL

Pleurisy

Classic Presentation

The patient presents with sharp pains in the chest that seem related to coughing, sneezing, and positions such as bending to the same side or lying on the involved side. The patient often will have a coexisting or recent history of a respiratory infection.

Cause

Pleurisy is usually associated with pleural effusion. Effusion is categorized as a transudate or exudate based mainly on the protein content. Transudates are more the result of congestive heart failure or hypoalbuminemia (loss of oncotic pressure). Exudates are usually due to bacterial pneumonia or cancer. Other causes include empyema (direct infection of the pleural space), hemothorax (blood in the pleural space), or chyliform (chyle in the pleural space).

Evaluation

Physical examination findings (and symptoms) are dependent on the underlying cause and the degree of effusion. A pleural friction rub may be heard. With large effusion there may be a decreased fremitus, dullness to percussion, and an increase or decrease in breath sounds. Chest films may reveal large pleural effusions. Smaller effusions are visible with a lateral recumbent view.

Management

Small, transudate effusions are often managed conservatively. Larger effusions may require thoracentesis. When cancer is suspected, biopsy is often indicated. Treatment of the underlying condition is the primary feature of management.

Pulmonary Embolism

Classic Presentation

A middle-aged male has sudden chest pain after having had pain in his calf. The pain is severe, appearing similar to a myocardial infarction (heart attack).

Cause

Most often, in the ambulatory population patients develop deep vein thrombophlebitis with subsequent migration to the lungs, causing either embolism or progression to full infarct and death. Approximately 600,000 episodes of pulmonary embolism occur each year in the United States, with approximately one-third resulting in death.[42] It is estimated that 20% to 30% are due to hemodynamic impairment. The remainder may be prevented with elimination of recurrence of embolism.

Evaluation

Chest pain that is "pleuritic" in nature without dyspnea is a strong indicator of pulmonary embolism; a low-grade fever may be present also, more commonly with infarction. There are several clinical guidelines used to determine the patient who has enough of a clinical profile to warrant special imaging investigation. These include the American Thoracic Society and the European Society of Cardiology. The primary difference is the use of D-dimer testing (degradation products of cross-linked fibrin; nonspecific test for venous thromboembolism). In essence, the path of investigation for patients suspected of a pulmonary embolism includes either helical CT angiography scanning or ventilation perfusion scanning as the initial study. If the perfusion scanning is negative, pulmonary embolism is ruled out. If CT and perfusion testing are negative, further testing would include duplex ultrasonography of the lower legs; however, this is not sensitive, so with a negative test, pulmonary angiography would be used to further evaluate the patient.[43]

Management

Acute management involves the use of thrombolytic agents such as streptokinase, urokinase, and tPA; then anticoagulant medication is used to prevent further recurrence.

Esophageal

Classic Presentation

The patient may complain of substernal chest pain associated with recumbency, dysphagia, and heartburn.

Cause

Convergence of afferent nerve fibers for both the heart and esophagus may explain why esophageal pain may be a cardiac imitator. There are numerous theories and categories of esophageal dysfunction. Currently there is much disagreement as to the cause and relative importance of these conditions. The three syndromes suggested are an acid-sensitive esophagus including gastroesophageal reflux disease (GERD) (20% of patients), a mechanosensitive esophagus (including motility disorders such as esophageal spasm) (15% of patients), and an irritable esophagus seen as a combination of the other groups (25% of patients).[44] Chest pain of undetermined origin is believed to be due to esophageal disorders in 50% to 60% of patients.[45] Approximately 85% of patients with manometrically demonstrated esophageal abnormalities have a psychiatric abnormality.[46] A connecting hypothesis is that the esophageal disorders may represent a marker for individuals who have a dysfunctional visceral sensory mechanism wherein physiologic or pathophysiologic events may trigger pain, perhaps by lowering the threshold.[47]

Evaluation

After cardiac diseases have been evaluated and ruled out, evaluation for esophageal disorders is begun, and is varied depending on the suspected underlying dysfunction. Some physicians use a proton-pump medication as an initial test for GERD, looking for relief as a positive test. The most sensitive test for GERD is 24-hour pH monitoring. Further testing may involve using balloon distention, the Bernstein acid perfusion test, or endoscopy. If esophageal motility is the underlying problem, manometry is often indicated.[48]

Management

Conservative treatment for GERD consists mainly of dietary and positional advice. It would seem logical that patients with motility disorders would improve with the use of smooth muscle relaxants or calcium channel blockers; however, even though often they are objectively improved with manometry, symptoms do not abate. These patients are usually reassured that they have a benign problem and often are given similar advice to that given the GERD patient, including stress relaxation approaches. Patients with an underlying psychiatric problem may benefit from psychiatric counseling or medication.

APPENDIX 38–1

Web Resources

American Heart Association
(888) 694-3278
http://www.heart.org
National Heart, Lung, and Blood Institute
(301) 592-8573
http://www.nhlbi.nih.gov
National Coalition for Women with Heart Disease
(202) 728-7199
http://www.womenheart.org

APPENDIX 38–2

References

1. Ornish DM, Scherwitz LW, Doody RS, et al. Effects of stress management training and dietary changes in treating ischemic heart disease. *JAMA*. 1983;249:54–59.
2. Bonaca MP, Wiviott SD, Braunwald E, et al. American College of Cardiology/American Heart Association/European Society of Cardiology/World Heart Federation universal definition of myocardial infarction classification system and the risk of cardiovascular death: observations from the TRITON-TIMI 38 trial (Trial to Assess Improvement in Therapeutic Outcomes by Optimizing Platelet Inhibition With Prasugrel-Thrombolysis in Myocardial Infarction 38). *Circulation*. 2012;125(4):577–583.

3. Nawar EW, Niska RW, Xu J. National Hospital Ambulatory Medical Care Survey: 2005 emergency department summary. *Adv Data.* 2007(386):1–32.

4. How J, Volz G, Doe S, Heycock C, Hamilton J, Kelly C. The causes of musculoskeletal chest pain in patients admitted to hospital with suspected myocardial infarction. *Eur J Intern Med.* 2005;16(6):432–436.

5. Mazhar J, Killion B, Liang M, Lee M, Devlin G. Chest pain unit (CPU) in the management of low to intermediate risk acute coronary syndrome: a tertiary hospital experience from New Zealand. *Heart Lung Circ.* Oct 8 2012.

6. Conti A, Poggioni C, Viviani G, et al. Short- and long-term cardiac events in patients with chest pain with or without known existing coronary disease presenting normal electrocardiogram. *Am J Emerg Med.* 2012;30(9):1698–1705.

7. Levine RP, Mascette AM. Musculoskeletal chest pain in patients with angina: a prospective study. *South Med J.* 1989;82:580.

8. Lee TH, Cook EF, Weisberg M. Acute chest pain in the emergency room: identification and examination of low risk patients. *Arch Intern Med.* 1985;145:65.

9. Panju A, Farkouh ME, Sackett DL, et al. Outcome of patients discharged from a coronary care unit with a diagnosis of "chest pain not yet diagnosed." *CMAJ.* 1996;155(5):541–546.

10. Chambers J, Bass C. Chest pain with normal coronary anatomy: a review of natural history and possible etiologic factors. *Prog Cardiovasc Dis.* 1990;33(3):161–184.

11. Masseri A. Mechanisms and significance of cardiac ischemic pain. *Prog Cardiovasc Dis.* 1992;35:1.

12. Lombard JT, Selzer A. Valvular aortic stenosis: a clinical and hemodynamic profile of patients. *Ann Intern Med.* 1987;106:292.

13. Fennerty MB. Esophageal causes of noncardiac chest pain. *Hosp Med.* 1995;10:15–24.

14. Diamond GA, Forrester JS. Analysis of probability as an aid in the clinical diagnosis of coronary artery disease. *N Engl J Med.* 1979;300:1350.

15. Anselmino M, Clark GWB, Hinder RA. Esophageal chest pain: state of the art. *Surg Annu.* 1993;25 (pt 1):193–210.

16. Wasserman K. Dyspnea on exertion: is it the heart or the lungs? *JAMA.* 1982;248:2039.

17. Louie EK, Edwards LC. Hypertrophic cardiomyopathy. *Prog Cardiovasc Dis.* 1994;36:275.

18. Shlipak MG, Ix JH, Bibbins-Domingo K, Lin F, Whooley MA. Biomarkers to predict recurrent cardiovascular disease: the Heart and Soul Study. *Am J Med.* 2008;121(1):50–57.

19. Ornish D. *Dr. Dean Ornish's Program for Reversing Heart Disease.* New York: Ivy Books; 1996.

20. Eckel RH, Jakicic JM, Ard JD, et al. 2013 AHA /ACC Guideline on Lifestyle Management to Reduce Cardiovascular Risk: A Report of the American College of Cardiology/American Heart Association Task Force on Practice Guidelines. Circulation. 2013 (epub ahead of print).

21. Hazinski MF, Nolan JP, Billi JE, et al. Part 1: Executive summary: 2010 International Consensus on Cardiopulmonary Resuscitation and Emergency Cardiovascular Care Science With Treatment Recommendations. *Circulation.* 2010;122(16 Suppl 2): S250–275.

22. Jacobs I, Sunde K, Deakin CD, et al. Part 6: Defibrillation: 2010 International Consensus on Cardiopulmonary Resuscitation and Emergency Cardiovascular Care Science With Treatment Recommendations. *Circulation.* 2010;122(16 Suppl 2):S325–337.

23. Cannon RD. Microvascular angina: cardiovascular investigations regarding pathophysiology and management. *Med Clin North Am.* 1991;75:1097.

24. Gitter MJ. Cocaine and chest pain: clinical features and outcome of patients hospitalized to rule out myocardial infarction. *Ann Intern Med.* 1991;115:277.

25. Shub C. Stable angina pectoris, 1: clinical patterns; 2: cardiac evaluation and diagnostic testing. *Mayo Clin Proc.* 1990;65:233,243.

26. Reeder GS, Gersh BJ. Modern management of acute myocardial infarction. *Curr Probl Cardiol.* 1993;18:81.

27. Schweitzer P. The electrocardiographic diagnosis of acute myocardial infarction: the thrombolytic era. *Am Heart J.* 1990;119:642.

28. Brennan ML, Penn MS, Van Lente F, et al. Prognostic value of myeloperoxidase in patients with chest pain. *N Engl J Med.* 2003;349:1595–1604.

29. Blankenberg S, Rupprecht HJ, Bickel C. Glutathione peroxidase 1 activity and cardiovascular events in patients with coronary artery disease. *N Engl J Med.* 2003;349:1605–1613.

30. Ariyo AA, Thach C, Tracy R. Lp(a) lipoprotein, vascular disease, and mortality in the elderly. *N Engl J Med.* 2003;349:2108–2115.

31. Anderson HB, Willerson JT. Thrombolysis in acute myocardial infarction. *N Engl J Med.* 1993;329:703.

32. Shabetai R. Disease of the pericardium. *Cardiol Clin.* 1990;8:579.

33. Spodick DH. Acute pericarditis: current concepts and practice. *JAMA.* 2003;289(9):1150–1153.

34. Rashed A, Vigh A, Alotti N, Simon J. The etiology, differential diagnosis and therapy of pericardial effusion. *Orv Hetil.* 2007;148(33):1551–1555.

35. Brucato A, Brambilla G, Adler Y, Spodick DH, Canesi B. Therapy for recurrent acute pericarditis: a rheumatological solution? *Clin Exp Rheumatol.* 2006;24(1):45–50.

36. Maron BJ, Epstein SE, Roberts WC. Causes of sudden death in competitive athletes. *J Am Coll Cardiol.* 1986;204:214.

37. Kaye BR. Chest pain: not always a cardiac problem. *J Musculoskel Med.* 1993;10:37.

38. Mukerji B, Alpert MA, Mukerji G. Musculoskeletal causes of chest pain. *Hosp Med.* 1994;11:26–39.

39. Heinz GJ, Javala DC. Slipped rib syndrome: diagnosis using the "hooking maneuver." *JAMA.* 1977;237:794.

40. Bennet RM. Nonarticular rheumatism and spondyloarthropathies—similarities and differences. *Postgrad Med.* 1990;87:97–104.

41. Wolfe F, Smyth HA, Yunus MB, et al. The American College of Rheumatology 1990 criteria for the classification of fibromyalgia: report of the Multicenter Criteria Committee. *Arthritis Rheum.* 1990;33:160–172.

42. Carson JL, Kelley MA, Duff A, et al. The clinical course of pulmonary embolism. *N Engl J Med.* 1992;326:1240–1245.

43. Fedullo PF, Tapson VF. The evaluation of suspected pulmonary embolism. *N Engl J Med.* 2003;349:1247–1256.

44. Janssens JP, Vantrappen G. Irritable esophagus. *Am J Med.* 1992;92(5A):27S.

45. Assey ME. The puzzle of normal coronary arteries in the patient with chest pain: what to do? *Clin Cardiol.* 1993;16:170.

46. Clouse RE, Lustman PJ. Psychiatric illness and contraction abnormalities of the esophagus. *N Engl J Med.* 1983;309:1337.

47. Lynn RB. Mechanisms of esophageal pain. *Am J Med.* 1992;92:11S.

48. Browning TH, Earnest DL, Balint JS. Diagnosis of chest pain of esophageal origin: a guideline of the Patient Care Committee of the American Gastroenterology Association. *Dig Dis.* 1990;35:289.

Palpitations

# CHAPTER 39

Context

Although patients may not describe their complaints as palpitations, they may describe an uncomfortable awareness of the heart pounding, fluttering, stopping, skipping a beat, or racing. It is important to note that, although this would logically suggest a structural heart problem, the majority of cases represent physiologic reactions or normal fluctuations perceived as abnormal, or are augmented by psychologic overlay.[1] One study suggests that approximately 16% of outpatients present with a complaint of palpitations.[2] This percentage is likely less in the chiropractic setting. The role of the chiropractor is somewhat limited if an electrocardiogram (ECG) is not available in-office; however, defining the patient's concerns often may reveal an obvious benign cause or suggest the appropriate referral for further evaluation.

There is great variation in an individual's ability to perceive heart rate and rhythm. Common augmenting effects of normal heart activity include a quiet environment (more obvious when going to bed), lying on the left side with the ear against the mattress (sound transmitted through the mattress), and a conduction hearing problem (augments sound in the involved ear). Conditions that cause an increased stroke volume, such as regurgitant murmurs, functional hyperfunction as occurs with anemia, thyrotoxicosis, and hypertension, may augment the sensation of a palpitation due to cardiac movement. Although it may seem logical that an arrhythmia could be perceived as a palpitation, many patients do not "feel" the arrhythmic occurrence. When patients with palpitations were monitored over 24 hours with an ECG, an arrhythmia was found in a range of 39% to 85% of patients.[3–7] Only about 15% of patients' arrhythmias correlate with a complaint of palpitations. When not correlated, palpitations are unlikely to be due to cardiac pathology.

General Strategy

History

- Obtain a more defined description of the complaint (heart racing, pounding, stopping, etc.).
- Determine the timing and frequency with relation to exercise, stress, medication intake, and environment (e.g., more in a quiet place versus any other environment).
- Determine whether there are any related symptoms or signs (chest pain, presyncope, syncope, diaphoresis).
- Determine any past evaluation or diagnosis of the complaint and any coexisting diagnoses (i.e., diabetes, hyperthyroidism, coronary artery disease, anemia, depression, panic disorder).

Evaluation

- Evaluate through auscultation, blood pressure measurement, and a 12-lead ECG.
- Laboratory testing should be reserved for patients suspected of having an underlying electrolyte, anemic, hypoglycemic, or endocrine abnormality.

Management

- Referral for further testing should be made with symptomatic patients (chest pain, syncope/

presyncope) or asymptomatic patients who are suspected of having an underlying conduction or structural cardiac abnormality.

- The remainder of patients, therefore, will have an identifiable benign problem that can be modified or eliminated, such as by eliminating caffeine use or recreational drug use, or will have no identifiable problem. Psychologic referral may be necessary for some of the remaining patients.

Relevant Anatomy and Physiology

Normal transmission of the pacemaking impulse from the sinoatrial (SA) node to the atrioventricular (AV) node and continuing propagation to the bundle of His and Purkinje fibers is reliant on autonomic nervous system integrity, proper electrolyte balance, proper blood supply, absence of accessory neural pathways, and nonpathologic cardiac structure. Generally, dysfunctional transmission is due to disorders of impulse formation/automaticity, abnormal conduction, re-entry, and "triggered" activity. Cardiac cells have an inherent ability to act as a pacemaker. When this occurs, ectopic generation of impulses is possible, leading to flutter, fibrillation, and re-entry phenomena. Impulse blockage, often due to organic disease, electrolyte imbalance, or the effects of medication, leads to various degrees of heart block in which impulse propagation from the AV node to the ventricles is prevented.

Re-entry is one of the most common causes of arrhythmias, causing tachycardias, premature beats, and atrial flutter. Re-entry occurs when an impulse is transmitted to a neural fork in the road, which allows travel down one path only. The signal participates in normal activation yet continues to travel in a circuit back to (retrograde transmission) the blocked path. Since blockage is antegrade only, this circle-around-the-back impulse is able to re-enter the original open path and cause restimulation.

Evaluation

History

Identify the patient who needs further work-up, such as the following:

- any patient with symptoms such as chest pain or syncope/presyncope

- any patient who has frequent attacks or attacks with exercise
- any patient with known cardiac disease or an immediate family member who died of cardiac disease before age 50 years

Also determine the following:

- any relationship to eating, exercise, or stress/anxiety
- any relationship to medications or ingestion of stimulants
- whether the patient has been diagnosed with or has symptoms of metabolic disorders involving diabetes, hypo- or hyperthyroidism, or depression/anxiety

Patients may describe their concerns many different ways. One study indicated that when patients used the descriptors *racing* or *pounding,* it was unlikely that there was an underlying associated arrhythmia.[8] When patients described the sensation as heart stopping, however, there was a high correlation with an ECG documentation of preventricular premature contractions. A description of an irregular heartbeat or fluttering was often associated with an associated arrhythmia. Neck palpitations or poundings are caused by simultaneous contraction of the atria and ventricles, which leads to reflux into the superior vena cava. This occurs with some forms of supraventricular and ventricular tachycardias. Ventricular tachycardias are more likely to cause symptoms such as syncope; palpitations are not often reported, probably because of the associated small stroke volume.

It is often difficult for the patient to describe palpitations with respect to regularity or rate. As few as one-third of patients were able to do so in a study by Reid.[9] His solution was to have the patient tap out what is felt. Harvey,[10] however, suggests that the examiner simulate different arrhythmias in a sequential manner on the patient's chest. He starts with a quick tap followed by a pause to simulate a premature beat. If this does not represent the patient's sensation, a simulation of bigeminy or trigeminy is attempted. Failure to reproduce the correct simulation sequences requires further simulation of other tachycardias. The first is a simulated sinus tachycardia, similar to what occurs with normal stress. The tapping is gradually accelerated to about 100 beats per minute, keeping the rhythm regular. The examiner describes this to the patient as the sensation he or she might feel in an anxious scenario. If this is not the correct simulation, faster tapping is employed, first with a regular rhythm, then an irregular rhythm, in an attempt to simulate paroxysmal sinus tachycardia and atrial fibrillation, respectively. There are no studies to indicate the reliability or validity of this approach, yet it would seem to assist in narrowing the myriad possibilities in some patients.

A fruitful avenue of questioning is whether there is overuse of drugs such as alcohol, caffeine, tobacco (smoking or snuff), amphetamines, over-the-counter cold/sinus/allergy medications (ephedrine), or illicit stimulants such as cocaine. Ironically, antiarrhythmic medication can eliminate or facilitate arrhythmias. Facilitation may occur with class I agents, which prolong the Q-T interval, predisposing the patient to ventricular tachycardias. Other cardiac or antihypertensive agents may precipitate bradycardia or tachycardias. It is important to warn patients that sudden withdrawal from these medications may cause arrhythmias and to consult with the prescribing physician before attempting to discontinue medication.

General assumptions may be helpful in discriminating between benign and clinically significant causes of palpitations. Often information by which to make these assumptions is not available at the time of evaluation; however, a well-trained patient may be able to provide these data with any future events.

- If a tachycardia is a possible cause have the patient palpate the pulse during an attack. If the pulse is regular with a rate greater than 160 beats per minute, it is likely to be supraventricular.
- If a tachycardia is a possible cause have the patient perform a Valsalva maneuver or press lightly over the carotid sinus to determine whether it abates an attack. If it does, the cause is likely supraventricular (the patient may report that induced vomiting eliminates the tachycardia, also suggestive of a supraventricular origin).

The relationship to eating may be helpful. If the arrhythmias occur several hours after eating (often late afternoon and early evening) reactive hypoglycemia is possible and can be evaluated via glucose tolerance testing. A similar presentation with diabetic use of insulin occurs at the time of maximum insulin activity. Both types of hypoglycemic responses often are accompanied with sweating and tremors and are often supraventricular in origin. A somewhat similar presentation may occur in the anxious patient, who often complains of difficulty breathing, dizziness, and paresthesias of the hands or face. These are associated with hyperventilation, which may or may not be apparent to the patient.

The relationship to exercise may also be a helpful discriminator with premature ventricular contractions. Palpitations that increase with exercise are likely to be cardiac in origin and require stress testing. Those that decrease with exercise are generally benign. ECG documentation and echocardiography is warranted, however, if the "palpitations" are frequent, to rule out hypertrophic cardiomyopathy and other life-threatening conditions.

When otherwise healthy patients describe palpitations as rare or infrequent and there are no associated symptoms, the patient probably is not in need of further work-up. At this point in the evaluation, the patient may be reassured that it is unlikely that any significant problem exists. Patient monitoring of the problem; keeping a diary of events with the recommendation to return if the frequency of occurrence increases or to seek medical attention if there are any associated symptoms such as chest pain, dizziness, or fainting; and taking the pulse at the time of the next attack are usually sufficient.

Examination

It is unlikely that the patient will have the sensation of palpitations at the time of examination. If palpitations do occur, palpation for heart rate and rhythm and, if possible, an ECG would be helpful discriminators between cardiac and noncardiac causes. Some common findings on ECG are listed in **Table 39–1**. If the heart rate, rhythm, and ECG are normal, a cardiac condition is unlikely. Atrial fibrillation may be suspected if the heart rate is grossly irregular and a pulse deficit or auscultated beat that fails to present peripherally is detected. Examination of the jugular venous pulse is subtle; however, it may provide information regarding dissociation (atrial and ventricular activation are independent of each other). If the atria and ventricle contract simultaneously, blood is refluxed by atrial contraction against a closed tricuspid valve, which results in a large or cannon A-wave at the jugular vein. This may occur with ventricular tachycardia. In patients with a slow heart rate, cannon A-waves may suggest heart block. Large A-waves with each heartbeat occur with retrograde AV, junctional, or ventricular tachycardia. No A-waves are present during atrial fibrillation because of inefficient atrial contraction.

The physician is more often indirectly evaluating cardiovascular function in a patient who is not at the time of presentation symptomatic, in an attempt to identify

Table 39–1 Arrhythmias

Classification/Pathology	ECG Findings	Treatment
Arrhythmias Originating in the Atrium		
Sinus Bradycardia:		
Increased parasympathetic (vagal) tone causes heart to beat at < 60 beats per minute. Depolarization originates from sinoatrial node (hence the name sinus).	Slow, but regular rate on rhythm strip.	Not treated if asymptomatic. If patient develops angina, hypotension, heart failure, or other symptoms, treated with: Atropine Isoproterenol Epinephrine (Each of these drugs induces sympathetic predominance.)
Sinus Tachycardia:		
Increased sympathetic tone causes heart to race (100–160 beats per minute). Depolarization originates from sinoatrial node.	Rapid but regular rate on rhythm strip.	Not treated if asymptomatic. If treatment is necessary: Propranolol (It decreases catecholamine-induced firing rate of SA node and slows conduction through AV node.)
Multifocal Atrial Tachycardia:		
Depolarization originates from several atrial foci at irregular intervals. Rate is rapid (100–200 beats per minute) and irregular.	P-waves are present, but are morphologically different from one another. P-R interval varies.	Correct precipitating factor(s). Once underlying cause is corrected, may initiate: Verapamil Quinidine (Both slow conduction velocity of cells that are abnormally pacing.)
Premature Atrial Depolarization:		
Heart beats prematurely because a focus of atrial cells fires spontaneously before the SA node is ready to fire.	Interruption of regular rhythm by an early P-wave. P-wave may be followed by a normal QRS if the SA node and ventricle have had time to repolarize.	Not treated if asymptomatic. If symptomatic, treated with Class Ia anti-arrhythmics: Quinidine Procainamide Disopyramide
Atrial Flutter:		
Ectopic focus of atrial cells generates 250–350 impulses per minute. The ventricle responds to every second or third impulse. Both atrial and ventricular rhythm are regular.	Series of 2–4 closely spaced P-waves followed by a normal QRS complex.	1. Control ventricular response by suppressing AV node conduction. Suitable agents are: Digoxin Propranolol Verapamil 2. Convert atrial rhythm to sinus rhythm: IV Procainamide
Atrial Fibrillation:		
Multiple ectopic foci of atrial cells generate 350–450 impulses per minute. The ventricle responds to an occasional impulse. Both atrial and ventricular rhythm are irregular.	P-waves cannot be discerned. Baseline is irregular with unevenly spaced QRS complexes.	1. If hemodynamically stable, control ventricular response by suppressing AV node: Digoxin Propranolol Verapamil 2. Convert to sinus rhythm: Class Ia anti-arrhythmics IV Procainamide

Table 39–1 Arrhythmias (continued)

Classification/Pathology	ECG Findings	Treatment
Arrhythmias Involving the AV Junction		
AV Re-entry:		
AV node is split into a pathway that conducts toward the ventricle and a pathway that conducts the impulse back to the atrium. Re-entry of the impulse into the atrium causes the atrium and ventricle to contract simultaneously.	Generally normal QRS complexes following normal P-waves. The inverted P-wave (retrograde atrial contraction) is buried in the QRS. Rate is 150–250/minute.	Carotid sinus massage may suppress tachycardia by increasing vagal tone. Alternatively: Verapamil Propranolol Digoxin
Wolff-Parkinson-White:		
A strip of conducting tissue (other than the AV node) connects the atrium and ventricle. Impulses reaching the ventricle via the AV node circle back to the atrium via the accessory pathway. Alternatively, the circuit may be reversed.	Each P-wave is followed rapidly by a QRS. A "delta wave" leads into the QRS. Rate can exceed 300 beats/minute.	If symptomatic, either slow AV conduction with: Verapamil Propranolol Digoxin or slow accessory pathway conduction: Lidocaine Procainamide
Arrhythmias Originating in the Ventricle		
Ventricular Premature Depolarization:		
Spontaneous depolarization of ectopic focus in the ventricle. Considered benign if fewer than six per minute.	Wide, tall QRS complexes that are not associated with a P-wave. A prominent T-wave often points in the opposite direction as the QRS complex.	Usually not treated if asymptomatic. If treatment is necessary: IV Lidocaine IV Procainamide Long-term suppression may be achieved with: Class I agents
Ventricular Tachycardia:		
Usually secondary to re-entry circuit. Both AV re-entry and Wolff-Parkinson-White may progress to ventricular tachycardia.	Wide QRS complexes with abnormal S-T segment and T-wave deflections (opposite in direction to QRS). AV dissociation and right bundle branch block are often associated.	Acute treatment involves one of the following: IV Lidocaine IV Procainamide IV Bretylium Oral drugs are used for chronic therapy: Quinidine Procainamide Disopyramide Flecainide, Encainide, Tocainide, Mexiletine
Ventricular Fibrillation:		
Erratic discharge from many ectopic foci in the ventricle. Rate is 350–450 beats/minute. Rhythm is irregular.	Completely erratic. Cannot distinguish normal waves or complexes.	Life-threatening. If cardioversion fails, epinephrine is given prior to defibrillation. If this fails, combine IV Lidocaine and defibrillation. Either additional doses of lidocaine or Bretylium can then be used with defibrillation.

Reproduced with permission from J. Olson, *Clinical Pharmacology Made Ridiculously Simple*, pp. 74–75, © 1994, MedMaster.

a potential cause of the patient's complaint. When other systemic problems are suggested by the history, a search for clues to hyperthyroidism, anemia, or sick sinus syndrome should be followed.

Laboratory testing is valuable when a specific suspicion is generated by the history. The following are examples:

- hypoglycemia—five-hour glucose tolerance testing
- diabetes—serum glucose testing (> 126 mg/dL on two lab tests)
- illicit drug use—drug screen
- thyroid dysfunction—ultrasensitive thyrotropin (ultra-TSH)
- anemia—complete blood count (CBC) or anemia panel
- volume depletion from vomiting, diarrhea, or diuresis—electrolyte panel

When the initial evaluation is unrevealing, it is necessary to evaluate with a Holter monitor. The doctor attempts to correlate any symptom complaints temporally with any abnormal electrophysiologic events. If no correlation is found, the patient's problem presumably is not cardiac. For patients with less frequent yet troublesome events, a cardiac event recorder is given to the patient for a period of one month. The patient is taught to activate the device any time he or she feels symptoms. The information can be transmitted or stored for analysis. Some devices will store information just prior to activation to catch premature events.

Patients who have historical or physical examination clues of mitral valve prolapse or structural problems often will be referred for echocardiography. Those patients with exertion-induced palpitations are sent for stress testing. Invasive electrodiagnostic studies are rarely needed to diagnose the cause of palpitations; however, patients with suspected anomalous pathways or underlying cardiac structural abnormalities may be candidates.

Atrial fibrillation (AF) is the most common chronic arrhythmia in adults and is associated with an increased risk of stroke and death. More than two million adults in the United States have AF and with the increase in the senior population, this is likely to increase dramatically. Even at the current rate, approximately one in four adults has an overall risk of developing AF. Identifiable risk factors include older age, an increase in systolic blood pressure, diabetes, hypertension, heart failure, valvular disease, obesity, and past myocardial infarction. The association with obesity is higher than previously believed.[11] There have now been studies that demonstrate progressive atrial restructuring and electrical remodeling occurring secondary to obesity.[12] For those with nonrheumatic AF, echocardiographic findings include left atrial enlargement, left ventricular thickness, and decreased ventricular systolic function. A randomized controlled trial[13] in 2013 demonstrated that when patients were put on a weight management program, there were significant reductions in both atrial fibrillation and actual atrial remodeling. One study indicates that there is an associated risk with increased pulse pressure (systolic BP/diastolic BP), which indicates increased aortic stiffness.[14] This risk is beyond that associated with other identifiable factors. Stroke associated with AF is often the result of cardioversion when the heart returns to normal sinus rhythm due to a thrown thrombus.

Management

If the chiropractor does not have direct access to ECG with medical interpretation or if there is evidence of underlying systemic or cardiovascular disease, referral to a cardiologist is recommended. A number of medications are used in the management of arrhythmias, with some commonly prescribed drugs listed in **Table 39–2**.

The mechanism of action for medications used to treat arrhythmias is generally to slow transmission through sodium and potassium blockade or through smooth muscle relaxation through calcium channel blockers or sympathetic blockers (i.e., beta blockers). These are important for ventricular tachycardias, AF, and supraventricular tachycardia. Examples include:

- Sodium channel blockers—Examples include flecainide (Tambocor), propafenone (Rythmol), quinidine, procanbid, and lidocaine. Avoid Ca and K supplements and grapefruit, and maintain sodium.
- Beta blockers (B1)—Commonly used is Propranolol. Avoid alcohol, calcium, sodium, and licorice supplements.
- Potassium channel blockers—Examples are amiodarone (Cordarone or Pacerone) and sotalol (Betapace). Taken with food due to increased absorption with fat. Avoid St. John's wort, and grapefruit.
- Calcium channel blockers—Example is Cardizem. Avoid Ca supplements, decrease salt intake, limit caffeine, and high-dose vitamin D (2,000 IU).

Table 39–2 Cardiovascular Medications

Drug Class	Examples	General Mechanism	Interactions/Side Effects
Anti-arrhythmic			May cause dizziness, headache, syncope, bradycardia, nausea, vomiting, and postural hypotension.
Adrenergic blocker	**Bretylium tosylate** Bretylol Bretylate	An adrenergic blocker having an effect on ventricular fibrillation and also a peripheral vascular effect which initially leads to postural hypotension. Used specifically for re-entry arrhythmias.	
Calcium channel blocker	**Verapamil HCL** Calan Covera Isoptin Verelan	A calcium channel blocker that decreases vasoconstriction (especially coronaries) and slow conduction at SA and AV nodes. Used in the management of Prinzmetal (variant) angina and various arrhythmias.	May cause headache, AV block, hypotension, constipation, elevated liver enzymes, or syncope.
Anesthetic	**Lidocaine** Alestacon Dilocaine L-caine Lidopen Octocaine Nervocaine Xylocaine Xylocard	Acts as both a local anesthetic and also anti-arrhythmic blocking automaticity of His-Purkinje system. Used both for rapid control of ventricular arrhythmias and also as an injectable local anesthetic.	May cause difficulty breathing, anaphylaxis, respiratory depression, numbness, paresthesias, confusion, disorientation, or cardiovascular collapse in rare cases.
Sodium channel blockers	**Flecainide** Tambocor	A sodium channel blocker used in the treatment of supraventricular tachycardias, AV nodal re-entrant tachycardia, and Wolf-Parkinson-White (WPW) syndrome	Not to be used if there is structural damage such as past MI. Also there is a risk of proarrhythmia.
	Procainamide Procan Procanbid Pronestyl	Used as an anti-arrhythmic especially for atrial fibrillation and flutter. Decreases excitability of myocardium and increases refractory time with possible peripheral vasodilatation effect.	May cause SLE-type syndrome, polyarthralgias, ventricular fibrillation, or agranulocytosis with prolonged use.
	Propafenone Rythmol	A sodium channel blocker used in the treatment of supraventricular tachycardias, ventricular tachycardias, and atrial fibrillation.	May cause SLE-type syndrome, polyarthralgias, ventricular fibrillation, or agranulocytosis with prolonged use.
Potassium channel blockers	**Amiodarone** Cordarone Pacerone	Prolongs phase 3 of the cardiac action potential. A potassium channel blocker used in the treatment of supraventricular tachycardias, ventricular tachycardias, and atrial fibrillation. Also has beta-blocker-like effects.	May cause blue-grey discoloration of skin, spots on cornea, thyroid dysfunction, and pulmonary fibrosis.
	Sotalol Betapace Betapace AF	Prolongs phase 3 of the cardiac action potential. A potassium channel blocker used in the treatment of supraventricular tachycardias, ventricular tachycardias, and atrial fibrillation. Also has beta-blocker-like effects.	Dizziness, lightheadedness, risk of heart failure, and allergic reactions.
Congestive heart failure (CHF)	**Spironolactone** Aldactone Novospiroton	Blocks action of aldosterone by competing with receptor sites in distal renal tubules. Used as a diuretic without an effect of hyperglycemia or hyperuricemia. A potassium-sparing diuretic. Used in the management of CHF and other forms of edema, and as adjunct therapy for hypertension.	May cause confusion, lethargy, rapid weight loss, gynecomastia, electrolyte imbalances, elevated BUN, gout, decreased glucose tolerance, or SLE.

(continues)

Table 39–2 Cardiovascular Medications (continued)

Drug Class	Examples	General Mechanism	Interactions/Side Effects
	Triamterene Dyrenium	Blocks action of aldosterone by competing with receptor sites in distal renal tubules. Used as a diuretic. It has direct effects on distal renal tubules to prevent excretion of potassium. Decreases glomerular filtration rate and increases BUN. Used in the management of CHF, and other forms of edema, and as adjunct therapy for hypertension.	May cause hyperkalemia and other electrolyte imbalances, anaphylaxis, some blood dyscrasias, GI disturbances, gout, rash, or hypotension.
	Milrinone Primacor	A new type of drug which is an isotropic/vasodilator inhibitory against cyclic-AMP phosphodiesterase. Increases cardiac output while decreasing pulmonary wedge pressure. Used in the short-term management of CHF.	May cause arrhythmias such as PVCs, supraventricular and ventricular tachycardias, or hypotension.
Anti-thrombotic	**Clopidogrel** Plavix	An inhibitor of platelet aggregation acting by inhibition of ADP binding to its receptor. Used to prevent atherothrombotic events after recent MI (especially ST-segment elevation-related), stroke, or with peripheral artery disease, acute coronary syndrome.	Bleeding major and minor, abnormal liver function tests, hepatitis, confusion, hallucinations, taste disorders, angioedema, bronchospasm, hypotension and other autonomic nervous system events.

There is a general consensus that medical treatment of arrhythmias is not warranted with the following asymptomatic presentations:

- unsustained supraventricular tachycardia
- unsustained ventricular tachycardia in the absence of structural cardiac disease
- Wolff-Parkinson-White syndrome

Algorithms

Algorithms for evaluation of pulse rate, ECG for palpitations, and palpitations in general are presented in **Figures 39–1** and **39–2**.

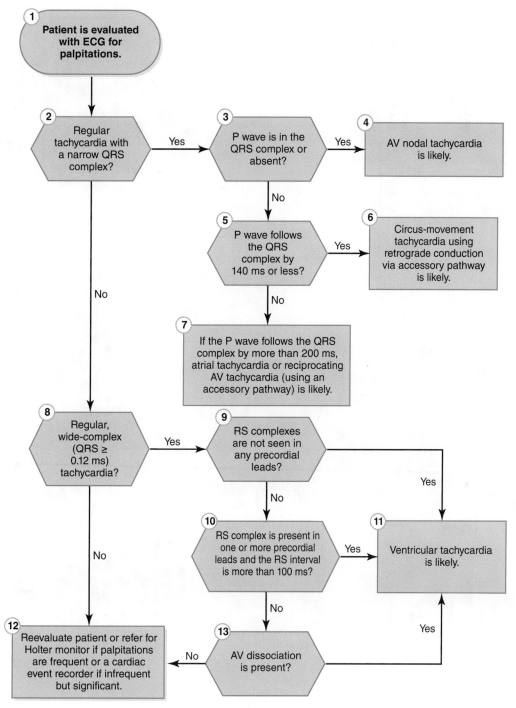

Figure 39–1 12-Lead Resting ECG Evaluation for "Palpitations"—Algorithm

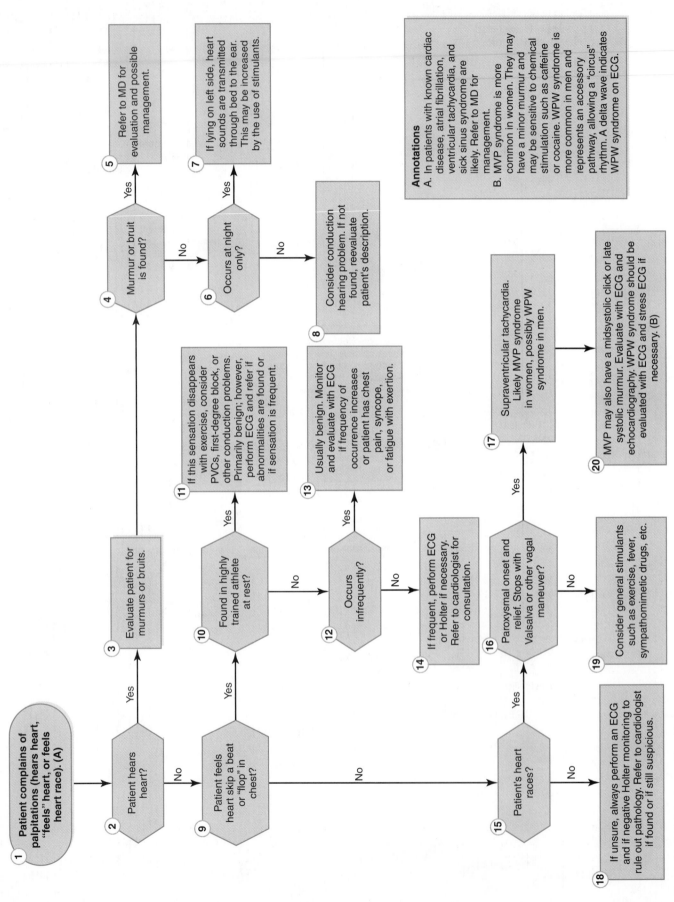

Figure 39-2 Palpitations—Algorithm

Possible Causes of Palpitations

Intra- and Para-Atrioventricular Tachycardia (Narrow QRS Tachycardias)

Classic Presentation

Patients report a sudden, unprovoked onset of a racing heart. This split-second onset lasts for 15 minutes to several hours and just as suddenly stops. Other symptoms may be lightheadedness, dyspnea, or weakness; syncope is rare. Depending on the cause and length, atypical chest pain may be felt. Patients are often young, with no cardiac pathology. Heart rate is regular and occurs at 160 to 220 beats per minute.

Cause

There are several names for intra- and para-atrioventricular tachycardia, including supraventricular tachycardia (SVT). The incidence of SVT is about 35 cases per 100,000 per year.[15] Generally, there is no structural heart disease; however, accessory pathways often exist. There are important distinctions between SVT and other tachycardias:

- Sinus tachycardia—a progressive onset that is not sudden with normal ECG findings due to sympathetic stimulation or increased cardiac demand.
- Ventricular tachycardia—similar to SVT in that the onset and termination of regular palpitations occurs. However, the patient's initial onset of tachycardia is in the over 50 years age group and in someone with known ischemic heart disease. ECG findings may differentiate by the findings of pathological Q-waves. Ventricular tachycardia is associated with MI and sudden death.
- Atrial fibrillation or flutter—generally the onset is in patients older than 60 years of age with existing heart disease and cardiovascular risk factors. The palpitations are irregular and ECG demonstrates left ventricular or left atrial hypertrophy.
- Paroxysmal SVT—occurs at any age; however, the heart is generally normal with the only ECG finding during asymptomatic periods being pre-excitation.

The most common reason for paroxysmal attacks is re-entry, which ironically can be initiated or abated by a premature atrial contraction (PAC) or a premature ventricular contraction (PVC). This anomalous circuit may involve the SA, AV, or accessory pathways. Approximately 33% of patients have these accessory bundles in the ventricles. Mainly in men, Wolff-Parkinson-White (WPW) syndrome should be considered. WPW syndrome may also cause atrial fibrillation or flutter. In women, consideration of mitral valve prolapse syndrome is warranted. In the elderly, sick sinus syndrome should be considered, where a "tachy-brady syndrome" is possible.

Evaluation

It is difficult to catch these often short-lived attacks clinically. ECG evidence is often absent, but WPW syndrome may demonstrate a delta wave or other combination of findings. Mitral valve prolapse (MVP) syndrome usually has no associated findings. Echocardiography for MVP and stress testing for WPW may be necessary.

Management

Management is largely dependent on the underlying cause. MVP and WPW are often monitored if there are no associated symptoms or findings of underlying cardiac pathology. Sick sinus syndrome or drug-induced paroxysmal tachycardia is managed medically.

Mitral Valve Prolapse Syndrome

Classic Presentation

Although MVP may occur at any age and in either sex, most commonly the patient is a woman of childbearing years who complains of palpitations, easy fatigability, or dyspnea. On rare occasions chest pain may be felt. The patient is often thin; more than half of patients may have associated chest wall deformities, including scoliosis, straight back (loss of kyphosis), or pectus excavatum.

Cause

The cause is unknown. However, there is usually one of several features, including redundant mitral valve leaflets, elongated chordae tendineae, an enlarged mitral annulus, and an abnormal ventricular wall motion. MVP is associated with other conditions such as Marfan's syndrome, atrial septal defect, and coronary artery disease. Apparently, MVP patients have decreased parasympathetic and increased α-adrenergic tone.[16]

Evaluation

As mentioned above, thoracic cage abnormalities may be evident on observation. The cardiac exam may reveal midsystolic click(s) and a late systolic murmur best heard at the apex. These findings are often intermittent; they are not consistent. Maneuvers that may help reveal clicks are standing (decreased ventricular size), which moves the click and murmur closer to S1, and hand gripping or squatting (increased ventricular size), which moves the click and murmur toward late systole. A combination of M-mode and two-dimensional echocardiography will usually demonstrate abnormal valve movement.

Management

Patients who are asymptomatic or have infrequent attacks of tachycardias are usually watched, but not medically managed. The only recommendation is prophylactic antibiotics for dental work to avoid the risk of subacute bacterial endocarditis. Those with chest pain are sometimes given β-blockers.

Wolff-Parkinson-White Syndrome

Classic Presentation

The WPW syndrome is similar in presentation to MVP, except the patient is more often male. The patient presents with a complaint of palpitations that occur suddenly and without provocation. Twenty percent to 30% of patients have atrial flutter or fibrillation.[1]

Cause

Anomalous pathways connecting the atria to ventricles (Kent bundles) allow re-entry-based tachycardias.

Evaluation

The primary diagnostic tool is the ECG, which may demonstrate a delta wave. ECG criteria based on the QRS complex morphology seem to be a more sensitive approach. St. George's and Skeberi's methods are the most accurate.

Management

Given the natural history of WPW syndrome in most patients, ablation of the anomalous pathways is reserved for those with severe disease reflected in symptomatology and ECG criteria. Narrow-wave (antegrade conduction through the node) re-entry WPW syndrome is managed pharmacologically, whereas patients with atrial flutter or fibrillation with RR cycle length are at risk for sudden death and are treated with radiofrequency catheter ablation therapy. This approach is 90% effective with antegrade conduction. Failure of ablation therapy forces surgical correction of the problem.[17]

APPENDIX 39-1

References

1. Weitz HH, Weinstock PJ. Approach to the patient with palpitations. *Med Clin North Am.* 1995;79:449–456.
2. Kroenke K, Arrington M, Mangelsdorff A. The prevalence of symptoms in medical outpatients and the adequacy of therapy. *Arch Intern Med.* 1990;150:1685–1689.
3. Clark P, Glasser S, Spoto E. Arrhythmias detected by ambulatory monitoring. *Chest.* 1980;77:722–725.
4. Goldberg A, Rafferty E, Cashman P. Ambulatory ECG records in patients with transient cerebral attacks of palpitations. *Br Med J.* 1975;4:569–571.
5. Goodman R, Capone R, Most A. Arrhythmia surveillance by transtelephonic monitoring. *Am Heart J.* 1979;98:459–464.
6. Lipski J, Cohen L, Espinoz J, et al. Value of Holter monitoring in assessing cardiac arrhythmias in symptomatic patients. *Am J Cardiol.* 1976;37:102–107.
7. Zeldis S, Levine BJ, Michelson EL, et al. Cardiovascular complaints: correlation with cardiac arrhythmias on 25-hour ECG monitoring. *Chest.* 1980;78:456–462.
8. Barsky A, Cleary P, Barnett M, et al. The accuracy of symptom reporting by patients complaining of palpitations. *Am J Med.* 1994;97:214–221.
9. Reid P. Indications for intracardiac electrophysiologic studies in patients with unexplained palpitations. *Circulation.* 1987;75(suppl 3):154–158.
10. Harvey W. Cardiac pearls. *Dis Mon.* 1994;40:41–113.
11. Abed HS, Samuel CS, Lau DH, et al. Obesity results in progressive atrial structural and electrical remodeling: implications for atrial fibrillation. *Heart Rhythm.* Jan 2013;10(1):90–100.
12. Abed HS, Wittert GA. Obesity and atrial fibrillation. *Obes Rev.* Nov 2013;14(11):929–938.
13. Abed HS, Wittert GA, Leong DP, et al. Effect of weight reduction and cardiometabolic risk factor management on symptom burden and severity in patients with atrial fibrillation: a randomized clinical trial. *JAMA.* 2013;310(19):2050–2060.
14. Mitchell GF, Vasan RS, Keyes MJ, et al. Pulse pressure and risk of new-onset atrial fibrillation. *JAMA.* 2007;297(7):709–715.
15. Delacretaz E. Clinical practice. Supraventricular tachycardia. *N Engl J Med.* 2006;354(10):1039–1051.
16. Fontana ME. Mitral valve prolapse and the mitral valve prolapse syndrome. *Curr Probl Cardiol.* 1991;16:311.
17. Arai A, Kron J. Current management of the Wolff-Parkinson-White syndrome. *West J Med.* 1990;152:383.

Dyspnea (Difficulty Breathing)

Context

Difficulty breathing (dyspnea) is usually a chronic complaint in the context of a chiropractic office setting. Patients are more likely to present with "acceptable" nondisabling dyspnea or a past history of paroxysmal dyspnea suggestive of asthma. Acute distressing dyspnea is usually due to a severe asthma attack, anaphylaxis, myocardial infarction, or pulmonary embolism. These patients are in need of emergency medical attention.

Although there are a number of disorders that have dyspnea as one of the complaint symptoms, two-thirds of patients with dyspnea as the main complaint have either a pulmonary or a cardiac disorder.[1] It is important then to differentiate cardiopulmonary disease from other causes in an effort to determine referable disorders from those that are manageable or comanageable.

General Strategy

History

Determine the following:

- what the patient means when he or she complains of difficulty breathing: painful inspiration, tightness in the chest, unable to catch breath, etc. (**Exhibit 40–1**)
- whether the difficulty is positionally related: worse while lying, lying on the side, or standing
- whether it is related only to exertion, the degree of exertion, and the general fitness level of the patient
- whether there was an antecedent respiratory infection
- whether the patient has a diagnosis or signs of depression

- whether the patient was in a setting that produced anxiety prior to the onset of dyspnea
- whether the patient had any previous calf pain and whether he or she was either immobilized for a long period or is taking birth control pills

Evaluation

- Auscultate the heart and lungs and listen for any murmurs or adventitial sounds (rales, rhonchi, or wheezes).
- Order a posteroanterior (PA) chest film; if rib fracture is suspected order anteroposterior (AP) and PA rib views, if no fracture is seen but suspected order oblique views of the involved area.
- Perform spirometry, if available, to determine pulmonary function (a simple, yet less accurate, monitoring approach is a peak flow meter).
- Order a general screening lab test to determine whether the red blood cell (RBC)/hematocrit (anemia), blood gas, and glucose (diabetes) levels are normal.

Management

- Refer the patient if pulmonary embolism, pneumothorax, pulmonary hypertension, pleurisy, infection, or tumor is suspected. (See **Table 40–1**.)
- Possible comanagement conditions include asthma, emphysema, congestive heart failure, and rib fractures or the myofascial/subluxation–related elements of these conditions.
- Manage "cracked" ribs (rest and time), vertebral or rib subluxations (chiropractic manipulation), and myofascial disorders (myofascial-release techniques or massage and stretching).

Exhibit 40–1   Clarification of Difficulty Breathing

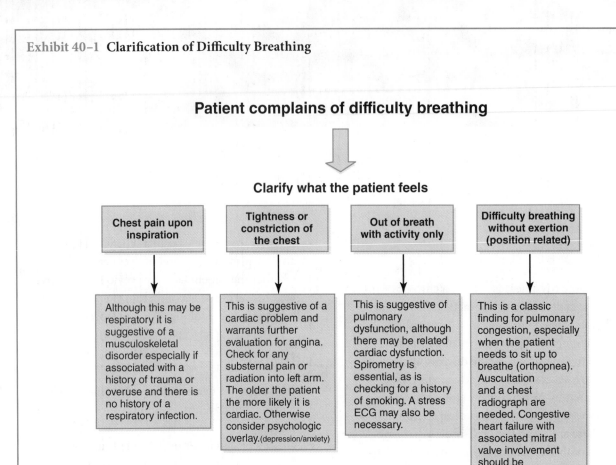

Patient complains of difficulty breathing

Clarify what the patient feels

Chest pain upon inspiration	Tightness or constriction of the chest	Out of breath with activity only	Difficulty breathing without exertion (position related)
Although this may be respiratory it is suggestive of a musculoskeletal disorder especially if associated with a history of trauma or overuse and there is no history of a respiratory infection.	This is suggestive of a cardiac problem and warrants further evaluation for angina. Check for any substernal pain or radiation into left arm. The older the patient the more likely it is cardiac. Otherwise consider psychologic overlay.(depression/anxiety)	This is suggestive of pulmonary dysfunction, although there may be related cardiac dysfunction. Spirometry is essential, as is checking for a history of smoking. A stress ECG may also be necessary.	This is a classic finding for pulmonary congestion, especially when the patient needs to sit up to breathe (orthopnea). Auscultation and a chest radiograph are needed. Congestive heart failure with associated mitral valve involvement should be investigated.

Recurrent paroxysmal attacks of breathing difficulty are characteristic of asthma and hyperactive airway disease. Both should be evaluated with spirometry and possibly bronchoprovocation challenge if necessary.

A sudden onset of difficulty breathing associated with chest pain is suggestive of pulmonary embolism, myocardial infarction, or pneumothorax (spontaneous). This demands immediate medical evaluation.

Table 40–1 Pulmonary Disorders*	
Type	**Summary Information**
Atelectasis	Atelectasis occurs when a portion of the lungs collapses, usually alveolar collapse. There are a number of causes and types, including lack of surfactant in infants, compression atelectasis due to pressure from fluid accumulation in the pleural cavity as is seen with heart failure, tumors, and other causes of pleural effusion. Resorptive atelectasis occurs in the distal bronchi due to an obstructed bronchus. Most often the obstruction is a mucous plug, tumor, or aspirated foreign material. Air in the distal alveoli is resorbed and the alveoli collapse. Atelectasis is usually amenable to treatment if the underlying cause is eliminated.

Table 40–1 Pulmonary Disorders* (continued)

Type	Summary Information
Adult-respiratory distress syndrome (ARDS)	ARDS may develop secondary to a number of insults to the body or lungs, including trauma, burns, acute heart failure, pneumonias, toxic fumes, or near-drowning (latent affect). Generally, there is damage to either the pulmonary capillaries or alveolar cells leading to increased permeability and the accumulation of both fluid and blood, with the consequent plasma-derived hyaline clots. Associated disseminated intravascular coagulation (DICS) occurs secondary to shock when intra-alveolar hemorrhages are associated with microthrombi in the pulmonary vasculature. Usually symptoms develop within 24 hours of the causative event. Progression to respiratory failure is rapid with the need for ventilatory support. Mortality is high, with 66% of patients dying within weeks (33% within days).
Pneumoconiosis	The chronic inhalation of mineral dusts, fumes, and other organic or nonorganic particulate matter may cause a chronic inflammatory process that leads to, among other problems, fibrosis and even cancer. These very small particles are not cleared by the normal protective clearance with mucus. Entering the alveoli, these small particulates may cause damage through macrophage release of cytokines. There are several varieties, with the most common being coal-workers' lung disease, also known as black lung disease, involving chronic inhalation of carbon and/or silica. Silicosis may also occur in those performing stone cutting and sand blasting. The exposure to silica dust is usually at least 10 to 20 years. There is no treatment for either disease, with symptoms and severity related to the degree of destruction and fibrosis. Chronic exposure to asbestos also may lead to fibrosis, but can also be causative for pleural fibrosis, lung cancer, and mesothelioma. Asbestos exposure was common at one time, specifically with house and building construction, particularly insulation, and also found with car brake lining. Symptoms are restrictive, with dyspnea persisting for years.
Sarcoidosis	An autoimmune disorder of unknown etiology that affects blacks more often, especially females. Lymph node involvement primarily in the lungs includes predominately CD4+ helper cells (outnumbering CD8-suppressor cells) with a reduction of circulating CD4+ cells. In addition to the mediastinal involvement, lymph nodes in the neck, liver, and salivary and lacrimal glands are also affected in many patients. There is a proliferation of granulomas and effusions that may affect any part of the body. These are unlike fungal granulomas in that they are noncaseating (no necrotic center). About half of patients are asymptomatic when diagnosed after a routine physical examination identifies lymphadenopathy. When symptoms develop, they may be generalized, such as low-grade fever, fatigue, and anorexia. The laboratory diagnosis is nonspecific; however, elevated serum levels of angiotensin converting enzyme (ACE) are found in over half of patients. Also, some patients have hypercalcemia. Radiographically, hilar lymph adenopathy may be visible; confirmation is with biopsy of lymph nodes. Approximately 70% of patients recover spontaneously; however, those with symptoms lasting more than 2 years may have a poor prognosis.
Fungal diseases (mycoses)	Fungal infection of the body is primarily related to immunocompromise as would occur with patients with AIDS, diabetes, and long-term corticosteroid use. Also found with lung disorders such as emphysema, bronchiectasis, and tuberculosis, among others that compromise the body's defense mechanisms. Primary fungal disease in the lungs is often geographically related with the most common being coccidioidomycosis (San Joaquin Valley fever); histoplasmosis, mainly in the east and midwest; blastomycosis in North America and Africa; and paracoccidioidomycosis (South American blastomycosis). Symptoms are often nonspecific; however, a combination of low-grade fever, chills, night sweats, anorexia, and malaise coupled with prolonged respiratory symptoms is suggestive. Radiographic findings of diffuse granulomatous lesions are sometimes seen. Diagnosis is through confirmation of the organism in sputum, urine, blood, or bone marrow. Treatment incorporates very potent medications such as amphotericin B fluconazole, and itraconazole as first-line treatment with other medications used as adjunctive if primary treatment is ineffective.
Hypersensitivity pneumonitis	Hypersensitivity may be induced by mold and fungi such as on hay or tree barks, in contaminated air-conditioning equipment; also, bird droppings, animal dust, and wood dust may induce hypersensitivity. The allergen causes the formation of antigen-antibody complexes, activating complement-causing symptoms within several hours after exposure. With the chronic type, a cell-mediated reaction occurs, often leading to alveolar granulomas. Common examples are farmer's lung (moldy hay or grain), bagassosis (sugar cane), maple bark disease, mushroom worker's lung, humidifier lung, pigeon-breeder lung, and furrier's lung (animal pelts). With the acute form, avoidance of the antigen is sufficient. With the chronic type, a progressive destructive process may occur leading to the need for lung transplantation.

*Not covered in the "Selected Causes" section.

- Be advised that management of asthma is controversial, but some practitioners report control with chiropractic manipulation; serious issues are medication changes in those diagnosed with asthma and unavailability of medication in the event of an acute attack with those who have not received medical evaluation and prescription.

Relevant Anatomy and Physiology

Dyspnea is a conscious sensation and as such is a variable impression based on an individual's comparison to what is considered normal. In other words, although someone may feel an increased workload going up a flight of stairs, he or she would not report this as dyspnea unless it was felt to be an "unexpected" amount of effort. A variety of tissues with different receptors may convey information that is eventually interpreted as dyspnea; however, it is not clear how much each contributes. It does seem clear that respiratory muscle contractions play a predominant role. Some possible factors follow.

Acid–base balance serves as the primary stimulus for ventilation; however, it is not clear how much decrease in oxygen or increase in partial pressure of carbon dioxide (Pco_2) contributes to the sensation of dyspnea.[2] The carotid bodies sense pH and oxygen/carbon dioxide levels and stimulate breathing when levels are perceived as unbalanced. However, hypercapnia associated with breath holding can be eliminated as a stimulus for breathing by neuromuscular blockade.[3] This allows discomfort-free breath holding.

Several intrapulmonary receptors play a role. Irritant and C-fiber receptors react to chemical and physical irritants.[4] Slowly adapting pulmonary stretch receptors respond to large increases in lung volume. This afferent information is carried via autonomic pathways. These receptors may be partially blocked by lidocaine or morphine, decreasing some of the severity of dyspnea.[5] However, patients with heart-lung transplantation (denervated lungs) can still sense dyspnea. Also, bilateral vagal block does not totally eliminate the perception of dyspnea.[6]

The key may lie in the sensory receptors of respiratory muscles. Muscle spindles and tendon organs are found mainly in the intercostal muscles. The diaphragm contains mainly tendon organs. These sensory organs are sensitive to increased muscle work. It appears that acid–base balance and irritant receptor stimulation play a contributory role through stimulation of muscular contraction. The increased muscular effort conveys the sense of dyspnea.[2, 3]

Blockage to inspiration occurs with extrathoracic (upper airway) disorders. Blockages by inflammation acutely with anaphylaxis and subacutely associated with mononucleosis or pertussis are serious causes requiring immediate treatment. Blockage due to foreign body aspiration is also a common serious cause in children and in the immunocompromised. With upper airway obstruction, stridor is often heard if the blockage is not complete. Intrathoracic obstruction has more of an effect on expiratory effort. Blockages from bronchoconstriction, mucosal edema, and mucus production are seen primarily with asthma with some overlapping with other chronic obstructive pulmonary disease (COPD) such as chronic bronchitis and emphysema. When both inspiration and expiration are affected, restrictive lung disorders should be considered. These include intrinsic lung disorders such as pneumonia, fibrotic lung disease, and pulmonary hypertension/edema. Extrathoracic causes of restriction include musculoskeletal disorders such as severe kyphoscoliosis, pectus excavatum, flail chest, and muscular dystrophy. Neurologic depression from central (tumor or stroke) or peripheral (Guillain-Barré, poliomyelitis, or myasthenia gravis) nervous system dysfunction also may cause dyspnea. Myasthenia gravis may simulate cardiac or lung disorders in some patients.[7]

Asthma is certainly one of the most common chronic causes of dyspnea. It is surprising that a 180-degree change in thinking regarding allergic contribution and natural history of asthma has occurred over the last twenty years. Growing evidence, still controversial, suggests that the traditional theory of avoidance of allergens is probably an extrapolation that did not take into account timing of immune response and reactivity. From observations in mice, it is believed that there are two types of CD4+ T-cells. These may be somewhat reciprocally inhibitory to each other. It is believed that type 1 helper T (Th1) cells are important for cellular defense, producing interleukin-2 and interferon-γ. Type 2 helper T (Th2) cells mediate allergic inflammation through the production of cytokines (interleukins-4, 5, 6, 9, and 13). A new "hygiene hypothesis" posits that there is an imbalance between these two cells that is environmentally specific, with timing of exposure as the crucial variable. It is known that newborn infants are more Th2-cell dominant immunologically, and it is hypothesized that the infant needs appropriate exposure to environmental stimulus to create a balance between Th1 and Th2 responses. Therefore, microbial products may play a crucial role in the maturation of a child's immune response, resulting in tolerance to other components of environmental exposure, such as pollen and animal dander, due to the balance of Th1 and Th2 responses. As a result of new research, there is a focus on developing a prevention approach timed to the individual's age (primarily before age 6 years) based on exposure to specific stimulators of Th1 response coupled with knowledge of an individual's "asthma genes" (inherited tendencies). Added information about the "natural" history of asthma from childhood to adulthood suggests that approximately 25% of children had wheezing that was relapsing or persistent into adulthood, predicted by early age of onset, female gender, airway hyper-responsiveness, sensitization to house mites, and smoking. Yet the damage done at least in reference to lung function did not appear to progress through adulthood.[8]

New evidence suggests the following:[9]

- There is an increase in the Th2 helper-cell response in children with asthma that may be related to the following factors:
  1. widespread use of antibiotics
  2. western lifestyle
  3. an urban environment
  4. diet
  5. sensitization to dust mites and cockroaches
- There is an increase in the Th1 helper-cell response in children who do not have asthma that may be related to the following factors:
  1. the presence of older siblings[10]
  2. early exposure to day care (within first six months of life for children without a maternal history of asthma)[11]
  3. tuberculosis, measles, or hepatitis A infection
  4. a rural environment

Further, it has been demonstrated in some studies that exposure to dogs or cats in the first year of life may reduce subsequent risk of reaction to allergens.[12] An association between the development of an IgG response to certain foods (i.e., wheat, rice, soybeans, peanuts, egg whites, cow's milk, meat, oranges, and potatoes) and an increased risk for development of IgE antibodies to inhaled allergens was studied recently. The researchers did find that an increased IgG antibody level to a mixture of wheat-rice or oranges occurred in children who subsequently developed an IgE response to cats, dogs, and/or dust mites.[13] A recent study indicates that there is mast-cell infiltration of airway smooth muscle, which differentiates asthma patients from others with allergic disorders.[14]

There is growing evidence that allergy risk (allergy and extrinsic asthma are related) is in large part related to maternal influence and age of exposure to allergens. One recent study indicates that in children with a hereditary tendency toward atopy, breastfeeding for a minimum of three months protected against it.[15, 16] Interestingly, in those children without atopic heredity, it increased the risk of atopy. Also of interest is that although milk products are often suspected as being a cause or activator of asthma, the results from a recent study indicate that there was a reduced risk for asthma in preschool children who consumed products with milk fat.[17]

Evaluation

History

It is important to distinguish between general fatigue and dyspnea. Of course, these two possibilities may overlap; however, with chronic fatigue, depression, or metabolic/endocrine disorders, the patient will likely feel a more constant, yet nonthreatening, sense of dyspnea unless associated with anxiety or hyperventilation.

A patient's description of what he or she means by difficulty breathing, coupled with the context of when this occurs, is often the compass point needed for directing further evaluation.

- Painful breathing—Patients who feel that breathing is difficult solely because of painful restriction on inspiration are likely to have a somatic problem such as a musculoskeletal cause or pleurisy (parietal pleural irritation). This is differentiated by determining whether there is a history of trauma or respiratory infection, respectively. Rib subluxations are often nontraumatic, whereas rib fractures are usually due to direct chest trauma. If the patient has no history of a respiratory infection or trauma, spontaneous pneumothorax should be considered. This disorder occurs without warning and appears to be more common in young, tall men, often after exertion (although it may occur at rest). This disorder is also a possibility in those patients with COPD who develop a sudden, sharp, unilateral chest pain that is worse with inspiration. These same patients may have a rib subluxation due to chronic coughing. Relatively recent additions to the literature are reports of diaphragmatic spasm.[18] This condition will present with an abrupt onset of chest pain and dyspnea with no obvious provocation or triggering event. Some patients will report the ability to eliminate the pain and dyspnea with a forced, full expiratory effort.

- Chest tightness—If a patient complains of chest tightness and/or substernal discomfort or pain, angina should be considered as a strong possibility, especially if relieved by rest (or nitroglycerin). Patients who appear depressed or anxious may complain of a similar sensation. Further questioning regarding emotional context is important.
- Dyspnea at night—Difficulty breathing while sleeping suggests congestive heart failure (CHF)/ pulmonary hypertension, or asthma. Patients with CHF often are awakened with dyspnea (paroxysmal nocturnal dyspnea) and find they have to prop themselves up with pillows (redistributes blood and decreases visceral compression on the diaphragm). Patients with asthma may have attacks at around 12 AM to 4 AM because of changes in sympathetic activity and cortisol levels.
- Dyspnea with exertion—Difficulty breathing with exertion suggests cardiopulmonary or pulmonary disease (especially asthma or hyperactive airway disease). With CHF or pulmonary hypertension, minor effort is enough to bring on shortness of breath. With asthmatics, dyspnea usually occurs after 10 to 15 minutes of intense exercise and/or after exercise in general. The recovery period with CHF and pulmonary hypertension would generally take longer.

If dyspnea appears to be position-related, a clue to underlying causes may be found. Common terms used and conditions associated with position-related dyspnea include the following:

- Trepopnea—occurs in one lateral position; if lying on the involved side improves breathing a pleural effusion or internal lung disorder is likely because of the increased perfusion created by gravity; if breathing is made worse by lying on the same side,

a somatic problem such as rib fracture or pleurisy is more likely.
- Orthopnea—occurs when lying supine; it is usually relieved by sitting up and is characteristic of left ventricular failure and sometimes with COPD or weakness of the respiratory muscles.
- Platypnea—occurs in the standing position, is relieved by lying down; this is suggestive of right-to-left shunt in the heart or pulmonary vascular shunting of venous blood.

A history of prolonged immobilization, use of birth control pills, or prior calf pain suggests the possibility of pulmonary embolism, especially in a patient with a mild fever. A history of prolonged smoking would steer the investigation toward COPD. An associated history of a chronic productive cough suggests chronic bronchitis. If the patient appears to be in respiratory distress, having to lean forward to breathe through pursed lips and using the secondary muscles of respiration (like someone who has just finished a race), emphysema is likely. A history of smoking with a recent history of weight loss warrants a suspicion of lung cancer. It is important to determine prolonged occupational exposure to various dust particulates in an effort to uncover a possible pneumoconiosis such as asbestosis or silicosis.

When dyspnea is gradual and constant, progressive cardiac or pulmonary disease is likely. Other possibilities include deconditioning and obesity. When dyspnea is characterized by recurrent attacks with resolution into symptom-free periods, asthma is likely. Questioning regarding family history of asthma or allergies and any triggering events or substances (allergens, drugs, or pollutants) is important. Cold and dry environments are more likely to trigger an asthmatic reaction, especially in an athlete. Allergies to pollen, pets, dust mites, foods, clothing, and medications (aspirin or nonsteroid anti-inflammatory drugs [NSAIDs]) are common in asthmatics. Emotional triggering with stressful events is known to occur with asthma.

Most other causes are due to conditions that have enough premonitory signs or symptoms prior to dyspnea that the diagnosis is already made. For example, a patient with Guillain-Barré syndrome will almost always present with an ascending weakness starting in the legs. This usually gives ample time for the diagnosis and preparation for ventilation support. The same is true of polio (associated muscle weakness), myasthenia gravis (weakness of cranial muscle first with repetitive use), and other disorders.

Examination

Although there are classic examination techniques recommended in the evaluation of pulmonary and cardiac conditions, a review of a large literature base on sensitivity, specificity, and reliability is disappointing. One common examination technique is percussion, used to detect various lung pathologies and in estimating heart size and diaphragmatic excursion.[19] Although factors such as the speed of the stroke of the plexor finger, the speed at which the finger is withdrawn, and the degree of force (light or heavy) are determinants of the sensitivity and accuracy of percussion, it appears that their value has been overestimated. It is generally believed that percussion travels several centimeters through the body, and the result is a sound whose pitch and quality reflect the density of tissue directly under the percussion. There is poor literature support for this belief. In several studies,[20,21] chest percussion revealed large pleural effusions; however, smaller lesions such as granulomas or deep nodules went undetected.

Traditionally, chest percussion is used to evaluate diaphragmatic excursion. Several difficulties with this approach exist. There is a high interexaminer disagreement,[22] and radiographically, differences between bedside percussion and chest film measurements are as much as 3 cm.[23,24] This means that the difference between rating a patient normal or abnormal with percussion is often not possible.

As long ago as 1899, the accuracy of percussion for delineating cardiac size was challenged. Through comparisons with cardiac weight at autopsy it was discovered that only about half of moderately enlarged hearts and less than one-third of mildly enlarged hearts had been discovered and noted by clinicians. More recent studies indicate a generally good correlation between a displaced left-sided heart border detected by percussion and an enlarged cardiothoracic ratio on a chest radiograph.[25] The only problem is that patient outcome is poorly correlated with this measure. Other factors are more predictive of patient outcome, such as left ventricular end-diastolic volume and left ventricular mass. Percussion was sensitive (0.91) to these two measures, but not specific (0.30).[26]

A chest radiograph is important in the evaluation of cardiac size and the status of the lungs. Following are some classic findings and associated disorders:

- Haziness of vascular markings with an associated cardiomegaly may be evident with CHF.
- Diffuse granulomatous involvement of the lungs may suggest a fungal disorder and, if more apical, tuberculosis.
- Decreased markings suggest emphysema.
- Hyperlucency (no markings) and/or shifting of the trachea suggest pneumothorax.
- Lobar consolidation suggests pneumonia.
- Evidence of an air–fluid line would suggest pleural effusion.
- Perihilar opacities may suggest sarcoidosis or lung cancer.

Pulmonary function testing is essential in patients with a complaint of dyspnea. Peak expiratory flow rate (PEFR) can be measured using a peak flow meter. This is an inexpensive device that measures the patient's ability to expire. It is an acceptable monitoring device; however, it is effort-dependent, and decreases are found with many disorders. Age-, gender-, and height-matched standards are used as optimal comparison values. Spirometry is more sophisticated and may give more specific clues. If the forced expiratory volume in one second (FEV_1) or maximum midexpiratory flow rate (FEF 25%–75%) is decreased, COPD is likely. If this response is reversed with a bronchodilator or made worse by a bronchoconstrictor (methacholine challenge), asthma is likely. Measurements of lung volume or diffusing capacity are expensive and should be reserved for the specialist. When a pulmonary embolism is suspected, referral for lung perfusion scanning or digital subtraction angiography is needed.

Laboratory testing is usually unnecessary unless anemia, diabetes, or endocrine disorders are suspected. In children with asthma, it is important to obtain skin-allergy test results. This may direct the development of an avoidance program if necessary.

Management

Management of the acutely dyspneic patient is better delegated to medical personnel in an effort to provide any supportive emergency efforts when needed. The patient with a more chronic or mild complaint may be amenable to comanagement. Specific management approaches are discussed under Selected Causes of Dyspnea. Medical management of COPD is often based on an approach to decrease inflammation and stimulate the sympathetic nervous system during acute attacks. These medications are listed in **Table 40–2**. In general, the chiropractic

Table 40–2 Respiratory Medications

Drug Class	Examples	General Mechanism	Interactions/Side Effects
Allergy Medications			
Antihistamines	**Fexofenadine** Allegra	An antihistamine H1 receptor antagonist used for the management of seasonal allergic rhinitis and chronic urticaria	Headache, nausea, fatigue, dyspepsia, nausea, throat irritation
	Diphenhydramine HCL Allerdryl Banophen Belix Ben-Allergin Benadryl Benahist Benylin Diahist Nordryl Nytol with DPM Valdrene Many others	An H1 receptor antagonist used in the treatment of many varied conditions. Has significant anticholinergic effects and seems to prevent reuptake of dopamine. As a result it is used for allergic conditions, partial management of Parkinson's, as a non-narcotic cough suppressant, and as a sleep aid for those with intractable insomnia.	May cause dizziness, drowsiness, tachycardia, thickening of bronchial mucus with associated wheezing, anaphylaxis, dry mouth, and hypersensitivity.
	Hydroxyzine Vistaril Atarax Vistacon Vistaject	An antihistamine with anticholinergic and sedative properties. Tranquilizing effect mainly due to depression of hypothalamus and brainstem reticular formation. Primarily used to treat allergic reaction and to relieve nasal congestion and other symptoms.	May cause drowsiness, dizziness, headache, urticaria, dyspnea, wheezing, rash, or hypotension.
	Loratadine Claritin Claritin RediTab	An antihistamine used in the treatment of allergies, hives (urticaria), and other allergic inflammatory conditions. A long-acting selective peripheral H1 receptor blocker (prevents release of histamine).	May cause dry mouth, dizziness, fatigue, changes in salivation, flushing, hypotension, palpitations, tachycardia, arthralgias, myalgias, blurred vision, rash, and photosensitivity.
Steroid	**Fluticasone** Flonase Flovent Cutivate	A synthetic corticosteroid used for the management of nasal symptoms for allergic and nonallergic rhinitis.	Nose bleeds, nasal sores, nasal or oral fungal infection, glaucoma, cataracts.
COPD Medications			
Epinephrine	**Epinephrine** Bronkaid Mist Epi E-Z Pen Epinephrine Primatene Mist Bromitin Mist Asthmahaler AsthmaNefrin Epitrate	Both synthetic and prepared from animal adrenal glands. Used in the treatment of asthma. Effects are to cause bronchial arterial constriction, bronchodilation (smooth muscle relaxation), and inhibit histamine release. Also used for anaphylactic shock, restoring sinus rhythm, for open-angle glaucoma, and to reduce uterine contractions.	Causes sympathetic effects of nervousness, tremor, palpitations, tachycardia, anorexia, urinary retention, etc. Also may cause pulmonary edema, ventricular fibrillation, or MI.

Table 40–2 Respiratory Medications (continued)

Drug Class	Examples	General Mechanism	Interactions/Side Effects
Beta-agonists	**Salmeterol xinafoate** Serevent	Similar to albuterol, it is a long-acting beta2 receptor agonist. Effects include reduction of bronchospasm, increased motility of cilia, and decrease in inflammatory mediators such as histamine. Used in the treatment of asthma and hyperactive airway disease. Not used to treat acute bronchospasm.	May cause dizziness, headache, tremor, palpitations, and in rare cases, acute respiratory arrest.
	Metaproterenol Alupent	Beta2 agonist used in the treatment of asthma. Causes bronchodilation without secondary vascular and cardiac effects.	May cause anorexia, tachycardia, nausea, arrhythmias, tremor, hypertension, muscle cramps, convulsions, weakness, hallucinations, or postural hypotension.
	Albuterol Ventolin Proventil	Beta2 agonist used in the treatment of asthma. Causes bronchodilation without secondary vascular and cardiac effects.	May cause anorexia, tachycardia, nausea, arrhythmias, tremor, hypertension, muscle cramps, convulsions, weakness, hallucinations, or postural hypotension.
	Isoproterenol Isuprel Dispose-a-Med	Used primarily as a bronchodilator with asthma. A beta1 adrenergic agonist that causes increased expectoration, increased ciliary motility, and bronchodilation with increase in cardiac output and strength. Also used for cardiac stimulation with cardiac arrest, and various arrhythmias.	May cause anorexia, tremors, palpitations, tachycardia, flushing, or ventricular arrhythmias.
Xanthines	**Theophylline** Bronkodyl Elixophyllin Pulmophylline Slo-Bid Slo-Phyllin Somophyllin Theo-Dur Theospan Uni-Dur	A xanthine derivative that causes the relaxation of smooth muscle, stimulates the medullary respiratory center, and stimulates myocardium. Used primarily in the management of bronchospasm and prophylactic and acute attacks of asthma. Also may be used for edema associated with CHF.	May cause gastric upset, irritability, anorexia, abdominal pain, dizziness, headache, drug-induced seizures, palpitations, tachycardia, albuminuria, fever, dehydration, and rarely respiratory arrest.
Leukotriene receptor antagonists	**Montelukast** Singulair	Used as prophylactic treatment of chronic asthma, exercise-induced bronchospasm, and allergic rhinitis.	Sinusitis, nausea, diarrhea, dyspepsia, otitis, viral infection, and laryngitis.
	Zafirlukast Accolate	An oral leukotriene receptor antagonist. Leukotrienes are pro-inflammatory chemicals derived from arachidonic acid. Blocks the binding of leukotriene types D4 (LTD4) and E4 (LTE4). Used in the treatment of asthma; decreasing the inflammatory aspect of asthma.	May cause headache, GI distress, and in older patients an increase in respiratory infection.
Combination meds	**Fluticasone propionate with salmeterol** Advair	An inhaled medication for the treatment of asthma and chronic bronchitis. A combination of a long-acting beta-2 agonist (salmeterol) and oral corticosteroid. Not used for acute asthma attacks.	May increase the risk of asthma-related deaths. Dizziness, headache, palpitations, sinus tachycardia, respiratory arrest, long-term steroid use effects.

(continues)

Table 40–2 Respiratory Medications (continued)

Drug Class	Examples	General Mechanism	Interactions/Side Effects
	Triamcinolone	A corticosteroid with anti-inflammatory and antirheumatic effects. Aerosol version commonly used in the management of asthma. A spacer is used with the inhaler to prevent possible candida infection of the mouth. With the inhaled version the usual side effects associated with long-term glucocorticoid use are not seen, partially due to the clearance on first pass through the liver.	With injectable type may have Cushing's-like features, growth retardation, hyperglycemia, carbohydrate intolerance, nausea, vomiting, headache, euphoria, muscle weakness, osteoporosis, aseptic necrosis of bone, and delayed wound healing.
	Aristocort		
	Atolone		
	Kenacort		
	Kenalog-E		
	Aristospan		
	Cenocort		
	Triam-Forte		
	Articulose		
	Trilone		
	Tristoject		
Mast cell stabilizer	Cromolyn	A prophylactic medication used in the management of asthma; specifically extrinsic or allergic-related asthma. Stabilizes sensitized mast cells preventing the release of histamine and SRS-A (slow reacting substance of anaphylaxis). May also be used ophthalmologically for allergic ocular disorders.	Side effects mainly due to method of administration. Includes nasal stinging and burning, irritation of throat, nausea, rarely angioedema and bronchospasm.
	Intal		
	Disodium cromoglycate		
	Fivent		
	NasalCrom		
	Gastrocrom		
	Rynacrom		
	Vistacrom		
Anticholinergic	Tiotropium	A once-a-day inhaled anticholinergic specific for muscarinic receptors used in the management of bronchospasm associated with COPD.	Dry mouth, constipation, increased heart rate, blurred vision, glaucoma, urinary difficulty.
	Spiriva		
Smoking Cessation			
Nicotinic receptor agonist	Varenicline	Used in the management of smoking cessation. It is a partial agonist for alpha-1, beta-2 nicotinic acetylcholine receptors.	Nausea, sleep disturbance, constipation, flatulence, and vomiting.
	Chantix		

approach may include cervical or thoracic manipulation, myofascial work, stretching, and breathing exercises.

A controversial issue is the management of asthma or asthma-like conditions with chiropractic manipulation. The current literature support is still slim; however, there is a suggestion that there is a possible subjective benefit.[27, 28] More research is needed prior to making claims of consistent success. Like many conditions, there are multifactorial causes, and therefore multiple aspects of management. The approach to many conditions is avoidance of triggers. This is certainly part of chiropractic management as well. In addition, there may be reflex mechanisms that either simulate or worsen an asthma

attack. Perhaps these are important aspects that can be addressed through chiropractic manipulation. The major concern with sole management of asthma is the unavailability of abortive medication in the event of a severe attack. Attacks occur without warning, or with little warning, and the opportunity to get to the chiropractor (or the emergency department if severe) in time may be unrealistic. Therefore, comanagement is a safer approach for the patient. There are, however, many younger patients with either cough-variant asthma or minor episodes, solely related to upper respiratory infections, for whom dyspnea is not the prominent component. Initial management of these cases over several weeks of an actively symptomatic period may be appropriate. If there appears to be no improvement, especially in peak-flow or spirometry measurement, comanagement or referral is suggested.

The underlying mechanism with asthma appears to be a chronic inflammatory process. The medical approach is to reduce this underlying inflammation through the use of anti-inflammatory medications (e.g., aerosol corticosteroids) in an effort to decrease this predispositional state. The medical literature also seems to support an earlier resolution in asthma patients. In other words, those treated seemed to recover entirely from their asthma at an earlier age with fewer complications.[29]

Algorithm

An algorithm for evaluation and management of dyspnea is presented in **Figure 40-1**.

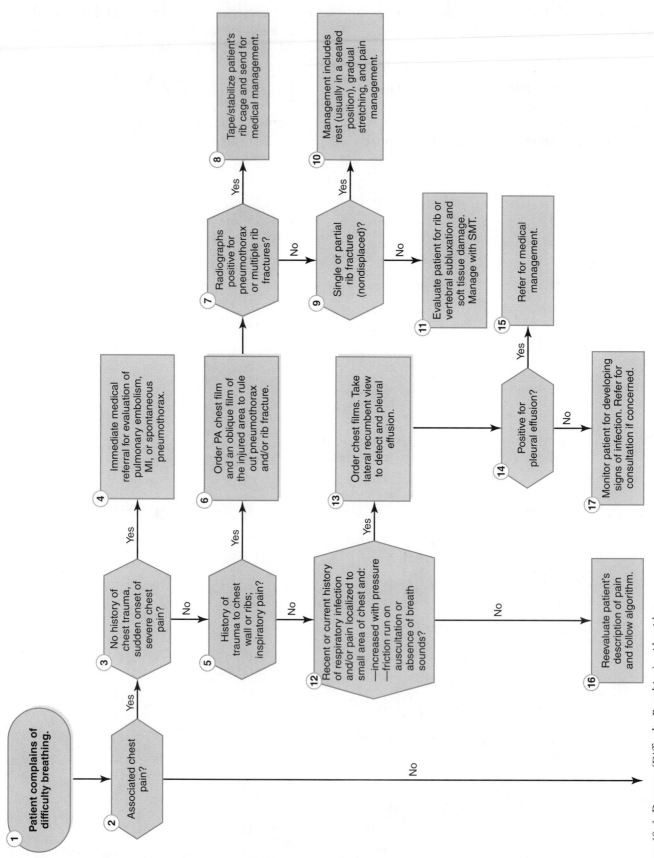

Figure 40–1 Dyspnea (Difficulty Breathing)—Algorithm

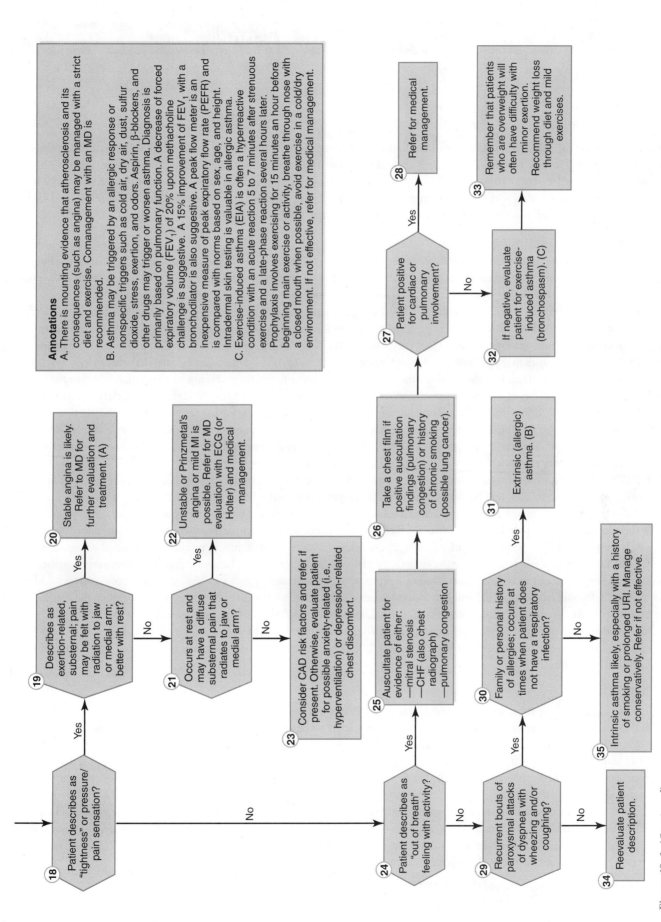

Annotations

A. There is mounting evidence that atherosclerosis and its consequences (such as angina) may be managed with a strict diet and exercise. Comanagement with an MD is recommended.

B. Asthma may be triggered by an allergic response or nonspecific triggers such as cold air, dry air, dust, sulfur dioxide, stress, exertion, and odors. Aspirin, β-blockers, and other drugs may trigger or worsen asthma. Diagnosis is primarily based on pulmonary function. A decrease of forced expiratory volume (FEV_1) of 20% upon methacholine challenge is suggestive. A 15% improvement of FEV_1 with a bronchodilator is also suggestive. A peak flow meter is an inexpensive measure of peak expiratory flow rate (PEFR) and is compared with norms based on sex, age, and height. Intradermal skin testing is valuable in allergic asthma.

C. Exercise-induced asthma (EIA) is often a hyperreactive condition with an acute reaction 5 to 7 minutes after strenuous exercise and a late-phase reaction several hours later. Prophylaxis involves exercising for 15 minutes an hour before beginning main exercise or activity, breathe through nose with a closed mouth when possible, avoid exercise in a cold/dry environment. If not effective, refer for medical management.

Figure 40-1 (Continued)

Selected Causes of Dyspnea*

Asthma

Classic Presentation

The presentation is variable depending on type. In a child with an allergic form of asthma, the presentation will be one of recurrent episodes of wheezing, cough, dyspnea, and a feeling of chest tightness. These attacks may be related to exposure to an environmental allergen or may be aggravated by stress or exercise. The patient may notice attacks occurring in the early morning. In an adult, it is more common to have a patient with similar symptoms; however, the patient will not be aware of allergies. There is often a history of a prolonged respiratory infection, exposure to occupational toxins, and/or a history of smoking.

Cause/Occurrence

Approximately 17 million individuals in the United States have asthma, according to a forecasted state-specific estimate made by the Centers for Disease Control and Prevention (CDC).[30] The prevalence of self-reported asthma increased 75% from 1980 to 1994 in the United States. Asthma onset occurs by age 6 to 7 years in 80% of patients.[31] During the past 15 to 20 years there has been an increase in both incidence and prevalence of severe asthma.[32, 33] Alarming is the recent finding that among school-aged children in Hartford, Connecticut, 19% had asthma.[34] Given the increase in the number of asthma cases diagnosed each year over the last two decades, theories of cause have been developed. One obvious conclusion is that pollution has increased, which then increases either asthma or the response of asthmatics to the pollution. In a recent study, researchers found evidence of an association between low-level ozone and respiratory symptoms in children with asthma.[35] Other findings were that there was not an association with fine particles as was hypothesized. The level of ozone exposure that would trigger symptoms was lower than levels set as protective standards by the Environmental Protection Agency (EPA). Remission or significant improvement during late teenage years is likely in those with mild asthma. It is believed that those with moderate to severe asthma have an underlying epithelial inflammatory condition and suffer damage to the epithelium and mechanisms of airway defense. The rationale for medical control is to decrease this underlying continuous inflammatory response.

It is believed that asthma is due to an underlying subacute inflammatory disease of the airways. Early-phase response occurs when allergens or irritants cross-link immunoglobulin E (IgE) receptors on mast cells, activating them to release histamine and other inflammatory mediators. A subgroup of helper T-cells helps orchestrate the inflammatory response by secreting cytokines. With the allergic form, there are sensitized mast cells that degranulate releasing histamine, bradykinin, and other factors that lead to acute-phase and late-phase reactions.[29] During an attack, bronchoconstriction, mucus production, mucosal edema, and underlying inflammation join together to cause wheezing with associated dyspnea. In addition to this immediate response, there is often a late response four to six hours later. During this phase, the inflammatory process causes sections of the epithelium and mucociliary transport system to slough off. This leads to the exposure and sensitization of irritant receptors priming the area to be hyperresponsive to normal stimuli. There are many triggers, including cold/dry air (e.g., exercise induced), allergens, dusts and sulfur dioxide fumes, emotional stress, upper respiratory infections, and medications such as aspirin, β-blockers, NSAIDs, and angiotensin-converting enzyme (ACE) inhibitors. In about 25% of patients, the primary complaint is coughing. This is referred to as cough-variant asthma.

Evaluation

An investigation for historical clues such as family history of allergies (extrinsic asthma), triggers to attacks, and severity of attacks is helpful to establish a high index of suspicion. Auscultation may detect wheezes. Simple pulmonary function testing with a hand-held device such as a peak flow meter may detect a decrease in peak expiratory flow rate when compared with age-, sex-, and height-matched values. Spirometry testing focuses on detecting a decrease in forced expiratory volume in one second (FEV_1). If there is no decrease, two other functional tests are possible. The first is a provocation test, often with methacholine (a bronchoconstrictor). A hyperresponsive reaction will significantly reduce expiratory measurements (e.g., a decrease of 20% or greater in FEV_1). The opposite approach is the use of a bronchodilator to measure improvement in pulmonary function (improvement of 15% or greater in FEV_1).[36] Ancillary tests include laboratory evaluation of sputum to detect Curschmann's spirals, eosinophils, or Charcot-Leyden crystals. Skin testing for allergens is particularly helpful in younger patients with extrinsic asthma. Radioallergosorbent (RAST) testing is usually too expensive and less sensitive than skin allergen testing.

*See also Chapter 38, Chest Pain, and Chapter 41, Cough.

Management

There are anecdotal reports of success with chiropractic management. Some studies and a literature review provide mixed results but suggest the need for further research.[27, 28, 37, 38] What is consistent between two randomized studies is that when chiropractic manipulation is used in conjunction with medical management, there is no apparent benefit.[39, 40] However, it is also interesting to note that these two studies incorporated "sham" manipulation phases or groups. Both the sham and true-manipulated groups of patients showed decreases in β-agonist use and symptom severity decreased or quality of life increased. These findings must be interpreted with caution given that patients were always on medication during chiropractic care and therefore direct treatment of asthma with manipulation was not tested. Second, a further research question is created: What aspect of "sham" treatment is "common" with true manipulation and can this be utilized to help reduce symptoms and medication usage? A study[41] on patients who were highly susceptible to hypnosis is perhaps related. There were marked improvements in airway responsiveness and symptoms. In addition, two small osteopathic studies evaluated the effectiveness of using a full array of osteopathic techniques. One study by Guiney et al.[42] incorporated techniques such as rib "raising," muscle energy for the ribs, and myofascial release. The other study by Bockenhauer et al.[43] utilized traditional techniques such as bilateral ligamentous tension in the occipito-atlantoid and cervicothoracic junctions, "upward displacement" of the first rib, and diaphragmatic release. The studies both attempted to determine if there was an improvement in respiration as measured by a peak flow meter. The strength of the studies was the use of a sham treatment control group. The difficulties with the studies are the small number of patients in each, and the use of peak flow meter measurement instead of the more accurate and standardized forced expiratory volume measured with spirometry. In the Guiney study there were improvements in peak flow measurement. In the Bockenhauer study there was no statistically significant improvement in peak flow measure; however, measurements of upper and lower thoracic forced respiratory excursion, and subjective measure of asthma symptoms both indicated improvement after treatment with osteopathic manipulative techniques. In a study[44] that was unblinded but randomized and controlled, patients who practiced yoga experienced improvements in respiratory function and symptom reduction.

It is important to realize that the chiropractor cannot make recommendations to parents or patients on medication regarding a change in the prescribed use; consultation with the prescribing physician is necessary. If a treatment trial is initiated, it is extremely important to use spirometry or a peak flow meter to measure function when the patient is not symptomatic to establish a comparative baseline. Comanagement or referral is recommended in cases where asthma is moderate to severe or the patient is unresponsive.

Medication is used to abort an attack and manage acute reactions, and another group of medications is used as prophylactics. β-agonist medications such as albuterol (Ventolin) are used during an attack. Newer drugs such as longer acting β-2 agonists (e.g., salmeterol or formoterol) or leukotriene receptor antagonists (e.g., Zafirlukast) have been suggested as "preventive" approaches taken at low dosages daily. The benefits and risks of this approach are still being debated. Anti-inflammatory drugs, such as aerosol corticosteroids, are used to control the underlying inflammation that exists between attacks. Combination therapy with corticosteroid and beta-2 agonist are now popular (e.g., Advair). A mast cell stabilizer (cromolyn sodium) is used to prevent degranulation and release of histamine and other mediators. The general recommendation from the National Institutes of Health is to use cromolyn sodium and monitor response for several weeks. If unsuccessful, an inhaled corticosteroid at the lowest dose possible using a large-volume spacer (to avoid local oral candidiasis) is recommended.[45]

One recent study[46] indicated that patients with moderate to severe asthma who wrote about their stressful life experiences demonstrated clinically significant improvements in their health status compared to those who did not. The literature is complex and mixed on the contribution of diet to either the development of asthma or the effect of diet on existing asthma. Several themes have developed:

- The consumption of apples and fish may have a protective effect on the development of childhood asthma or allergies.[47]
- The consumption of apple juice from concentrate (not apples) and bananas may protect against wheezing in children.[48]
- Another study found that apples and pears may be protective against asthma.
- Contrary to prior belief, whole milk may protect against current asthma and conversely, soy beverages may increase risk of current asthma.[49]
- Women who have a high intake of tomatoes, carrots, and leafy vegetables have a lower prevalence of asthma.[50]
- There were similar findings in a study on the Mediterranean diet, which appears to be protective for allergic rhinitis and asthma symptoms.[51] The diet studied contained mainly fruits, vegetables, and nuts.

Emphysema

Classic Presentation

The patient has a history of smoking and has noticed gradual difficulty breathing. If the emphysema is advanced the patient will appear barrel chested and will demonstrate the use of accessory muscles of respiration, or breathing through pursed lips. When advanced, the patient is often thin and frail.

Cause

Destruction of alveolar walls due to the release and deregulation of proteases released from neutrophils and macrophages leads to a decrease in the available cross-sectional area available for gas exchange. The cause appears to be smoking and, in a small percentage of patients, a deficiency in α-1-antiprotease (an inhibitory enzyme for proteases). As a result of the destruction of the elastin portion of the lung matrix, the natural elastic recoil response with expiration is lost, forcing the patient to work hard to expel air. The inefficient expiratory effort leads to an increase in residual air in the lungs. The patient is forced to expend 25% of his or her total body energy just for breathing and often will become a respiratory cripple. It is common to find chronic bronchitis and emphysema coexisting in patients.

Evaluation

The patient's appearance is characteristic when presenting in the later stages. This is often referred to as a "pink-puffer" (breathing through pursed lips to create a positive back pressure, opening the airways and making breathing less laborious). The patient in the later stages will have hyperresonant lungs on percussion coupled with diminished breath sounds on auscultation. The chest radiograph will reveal diminished markings in the periphery with associated low and flat hemidiaphragms.

Management

The patient must cease smoking. This may require outside support. In addition, referral to a respiratory therapist is necessary to prevent the cycling of decreased function that leads to the "respiratory cripple." Chiropractic management of associated musculoskeletal complaints would be likely beneficial.

Pulmonary Embolism

Classic Presentation

Although it is unlikely that a patient will present to a chiropractor with an acute attack of pulmonary embolism, the patient would be in distress with chest pain, dyspnea, cough, and diaphoresis.

Cause

Thrombi that develop in the lower extremity, particularly in the calves, travel to the lungs and cause vascular blockage and/or infarction. About one to two out of 1,000 individuals will be diagnosed with a pulmonary embolism in the United States annually.

Evaluation

The difficulty with the presentation of a patient with pulmonary embolism is the wide variation. Typically, chest pain and dyspnea are part of the presentation but cough, hemoptysis, or fainting are less often part of the clinical picture. Risk factors, together with presentation, may be helpful. Several studies have indicated that, although the clinical picture is inaccurate, patients can be categorized as low-, moderate-, and high-risk.[52] High-risk indicators include unexplained hypoxemia ($SaO_2 < 95\%$ in a patient who is not a smoker, asthmatic, or has another COPD), hemoptysis, or recent surgery (within last four weeks). Also of concern would be individuals with a shock index >1 (HR/SBP), or those age 50 years and older.

Physical exam findings that may be suggestive are tachycardia, tachypnea, and an accentuated pulmonary component of the second heart sound (S2). Other findings that have been suggested in the past are of little value, such as jugular distention, and S3 or S4 heart sound, or hepatomegaly. D-dimer is a specific fibrin degradation product that indicates the presence of venous thromboembolism. It can be helpful in ruling out a pulmonary embolism; however, there are several different types of assays each with their own sensitivity and specificity. To date, the most sensitive is the Organon–Teknika assay. If still in question, a pulmonary lung perfusion is performed. If equivocal, a compression ultrasonography is the next evaluation, followed by pulmonary angiography if negative or equivocal.

Management

Antithrombotic therapy with streptokinase, urokinase, or recombinant tissue plasminogen activator (TPA) is used in an acute event. Preventive therapy incorporates anticoagulant therapy with heparin or warfarin.[53]

Pneumothorax

Classic Presentation

There are different types of pneumothorax, each with a different patient presentation. The patient with spontaneous pneumothorax (SPT) is often a tall, thin male between 20 and 40 years of age with an acute onset of sharp, unilateral chest pain with dyspnea. It often occurs at rest or when sleeping. Traumatic pneumothorax is often the consequence of rib fracture. The presentation would be one of someone who presents with a blow or a fall to the chest. Pneumothorax can also occur as a consequence to COPD, asthma, cystic fibrosis, or tuberculosis (TB).

Cause

Pneumothorax is an accumulation of air in the pleural space. With SPT, it appears that subpleural apical blebs rupture spontaneously. Traumatic pneumothorax is usually due to outside air entering the pleural space. This may progress to tension pneumothorax if air is allowed in with each respiration, but on expiration air is trapped (check-valve mechanism).

Evaluation

The patient with SPT may have complaints mild enough to wait several days before being evaluated. The patient may have a family history of SPT or a history of smoking. Unilateral, sharp chest pain without a history of trauma, no recent or current signs of a respiratory infection, and no signs of other pulmonary disease should raise the suspicion of spontaneous pneumothorax. Severe tachycardia and mediastinal or tracheal shift are not likely to occur unless the pneumothorax is massive, as may occur gradually in tension pneumothorax. Also, the signs of decreased fremitus and breath sounds are detectable only in a large pneumothorax. Chest films may reveal a visceral pleural line (especially on expiration). If a film is taken supine, a "deep sulcus" sign may be evident as an unusually radiolucent costophrenic sulcus. If thoracic films are used for chiropractic evaluation, it is important not to collimate out the lungs.

Management

It is important to distinguish SPT from a rib subluxation. Because the pain of SPT is pleuritic, it may be reproducible mechanically. If the patient is found to have a large pneumothorax, he or she is hospitalized and monitored. If the pneumothorax is small (< 15%) the air is often absorbed over time. However, if it is larger, tube thoracotomy is performed.

Congestive Heart Failure

Classic Presentation

The patient complains of bilateral leg edema. He or she has associated complaints of difficulty breathing with exertion or lying fully supine at night (orthopnea).

Cause

Right-sided heart failure may be isolated or more often secondary to left-sided failure, which may be due to mitral valve dysfunction. Pressure increases into the venous system, delaying return to the heart from the lower extremities. Fluid backup results in liver congestion, ascites, and lower leg edema.

Although mortality related to coronary artery disease and stroke has been declining over the last decade, there is an increase in those dying from CHF. In the United States, the total is 4.7 million annually. There appears to be a relationship between a high-sodium diet and an increase in congestive heart failure for those individuals who are overweight.[54]

Evaluation

The edema is reduced by elevation of the legs. Rales are often apparent on auscultation. Hepatojugular reflux may be evident with the patient lying in a position where the highest level of venous pulsation is evident in the lower half of the neck. Exerting sustained pressure (30 to 60 seconds) in the patient's right upper quadrant may increase the level of pulsation by 1 cm or more when CHF is present. The chest radiograph provides important confirmation of cardiac failure with a demonstration of cardiomegaly, dilation of the upper lobe veins, haziness of vessel outlines, and interstitial edema. Electrocardiography may reveal associated arrhythmias or hypertrophy. Laboratory testing may reveal proteinuria.

Management

Comanagement is recommended. The standard approach is the use of diuretics for early-stage failure. However, long-term management should include a change to a strict, low-fat diet, with gradual supervised exercise. Recent studies[55, 56] showed marked improved in respiratory function in patients who performed moderate aerobics. Exercising at this level of intensity was both safe and effective even in patients with severe congestive heart failure. A recent Cochrane review[57] evaluated the benefit of hawthorn extract for treating CHF. This systematic review indicates there is significant value in symptomatic control and physiologic outcomes when hawthorn extract is used as an adjunctive treatment for CHF.

APPENDIX 40–1

Web Resources

National Institute of Allergy and Infectious Diseases
http://www.niaid.nih.gov/factsheets/westnile.htm
Environmental Protection Agency
http://www.epa.gov/pesticides/
National Pesticide Information Center
(800) 858-7378
http://www.npic.orst.edu
American Lung Association
(212) 315-8700
http://www.lung.org
National Heart, Lung, and Blood Institute
(301) 592-8573
http://www.nhlbi.nih.gov
Centers for Disease Control and Prevention
(888) 246-2675
http://www.cdc.gov
American Cancer Society
(800) 227-2345
www.cancer.org
National Cancer Institute
(800) 422-6237
**www.nci.nih.gov/cancer_information/cancer_type/
colon_and_rectal**

APPENDIX 40–2

References

1. Gillespie DJ, Staats BA. Unexplained dyspnea. *Mayo Clin Proc.* 1994;69:657–663.
2. Wasserman K, Casaburi R. Dyspneic physiological and pathophysiological mechanisms. *Annu Rev Med.* 1988;39:503–515.
3. Killian KJ, Jones NL. Respiratory muscles and dyspnea. *Clin Chest Med.* 1988;9:237–248.
4. Tobin MJ. Dyspnea: pathophysiologic basis, clinical presentation, and management. *Arch Intern Med.* 1990;150:1604–1613.
5. Schwartzstein RM, Manning HL, Weiss JW, et al. Dsypnea: a sensory experience. *Lung.* 1990;4:185–199.
6. Burki NK. Dyspnea. *Lung.* 1987;165:269–277.
7. Hopkins LC. Clinical features of myasthenia gravis. *Neurol Clin.* 1994;12:243–261.
8. Sears MR, Greene JM, Willan AR, et al. A longitudinal, population-based cohort study of childhood asthma followed to adulthood. *N Engl J Med.* 2003;349:1414–1422.
9. Mackay IR, Rosen FS. Asthma. *N Engl J Med.* 2003;344:350–362.
10. Ball TM, Castro-Rodriguez JA, Griffith KA, et al. Siblings, day-care attendance, and the risk of asthma and wheezing during childhood. *N Engl J Med.* 2000;343:538–543.
11. Celdon JC, Wright RJ, Litonjua AA, et al. Day care attendance in early life, maternal history of asthma, and asthma at the age of 6 years. *Am J Critical Care Med.* 2003;167:1239–1243.
12. Ownby DR, Cole Johnson C, Peterson EL. Exposure to dogs and cats in the first year of life and risk of allergic sensitization at 6 to 7 years of age. *JAMA.* 2002;288:963–972.
13. Eysink PE, Bindels PJ, Stapel SO, et al. Do levels of immunoglobulin G antibodies to foods predict the development of immunoglobulin E antibodies to cat, dog and/or mite? *Clin Exp Allergy.* 2002;32:556–562.
14. Brightling CE, Bradding P, Symon FA, et al. Mast-cell infiltration of airway smooth muscle in asthma. *N Engl J Med.* 2002;346:1699–1705.
15. Sears MR, Greene JM, Willan AR, et al. Long-term relation between breastfeeding and development of atopy and asthma in children and young adults: a longitudinal study. *Lancet.* 2002;360:901–907.
16. Siltanen M, Kajosaari M, Poussa T, et al. A dual long-term effect of breastfeeding on atopy in relation to heredity in children at 4 years of age. *Allergy.* 2003;58:524–530.
17. Wijga AH, Kerkhof M, deJongste JC, et al. Association of consumption of products containing milk fat with reduced asthma risk in pre-school children: the PIAMA birth cohort study. *Thorax.* 2003;58:567–572.
18. Wolf SG. Diaphragmatic spasm: a neglected cause of dyspnea and chest pain. *Integr Physiol Behav Sci.* 1994;29:74–76.
19. McGee SR. Percussion and physical diagnosis: separating myth from science. *Dis Mon.* 1995;10:641–692.
20. Bohadana AB, Coimbra FTV, Santiago JRF. Detection of lung abnormalities by auscultatory percussion: a comparative study with conventional percussion. *Respiration.* 1986;50:218–225.
21. Bourke S, Nunes D, Stafford F, et al. Percussion of the chest revisited: a comparison of the diagnostic value of

auscultatory and conventional chest percussion. *Ir J Med Sci.* 1989;158:82–84.

22. Badgett RG, Tanaka DJ, Hunt DK, et al. Can moderate chronic obstructive pulmonary disease be diagnosed by historical and physical findings alone? *Am J Med.* 1993;94:188–196.

23. Williams TJ, Ahmad D, Morgan WKC. A clinical and roentgenographic correlate of diaphragmatic movement. *Arch Intern Med.* 1981;141:878–880.

24. Cole MB, Hummel JV, Manginelli VW, Lawton AH. Bedside versus laboratory estimations of timed and total vital capacity and diaphragmatic height and movement. *Dis Chest.* 1970;38:519–521.

25. Karnegis JN, Kadri N. Accuracy of percussion of the left cardiac border. *Int J Cardiol.* 1992;37:361–364.

26. Heckerling PS, Wiener SL, Moses VK, et al. Accuracy of precordial percussion in detecting cardiomegaly. *Am J Med.* 1991;91:328–334.

27. Ziegler R, Carpenter D. The chiropractic approach to the treatment of asthma: a literature review. *J Chiro.* 1992;29:71.

28. Renand CI, Pichette D. Chiropractic management of bronchial asthma: a literature review. *Amer Chiroprac Assoc J.* 1990;27:25–26.

29. McFadden ER, Jr, Gilbert IA. Asthma (current concepts). *N Engl J Med.* 1992;327:1928.

30. Rapport S, Boodram B. Forecasted state-specific estimates of self-reported asthma prevalence—United States, 1998. *MMWR.* 1998;47:1022–1025.

31. Cropp GJ. Special features of asthma in children. *Chest.* 1985;87:55S–62S.

32. Yunginger JW, Reed CE, O'Connell J, et al. A community-based study of the epidemiology of asthma: incidence rates 1964–1983. *Am Rev Respir Dis.* 1992;146:888–894.

33. Mannino DM, Homa DM, Pertoswki CA, et al. Surveillance for asthma—United States, 1960–1995. *MMWR CDC Surveil Summ.* 1998;47(SS1):1–11.

34. Cloutier MM, Wakefield DB, Hall CB, Bailit HL. Childhood asthma in an urban community. *Chest.* 2002;122:1571–1579.

35. Gent JF, Triche EW, Holford TR, et al. Association of low-level ozone and fine particles with respiratory symptoms in children with asthma. *JAMA.* 2003;290:1859–1867.

36. National Asthma Education Program, National Heart, Lung, and Blood Institute. Executive summary. *Guidelines for the Diagnosis and Management of Asthma.* Bethesda, MD: National Institutes of Health; 1991. NIH publication 91–3042A.

37. Jameson JR, Lescovec K, Leport S, Hannan P. Asthma in a chiropractic clinic: a pilot study. *J Aust Chiro Assoc.* 1986;16:137–143.

38. Bronfort G. Asthma and chiropractic. *Euro J Chiro.* 1996;44:1–7.

39. Nielsen NH, Bronfort G, Bendix T, et al. Asthma and chiropractic treatment: a randomized clinical trial. *Clin Exp Allergy.* 1995;25:80–84.

40. Balon J, Aker PD, Crowther ER, et al. A comparison of active and simulated chiropractic manipulation as adjunctive treatment for childhood asthma. *N Engl J Med.* 1998;339:1013–1020.

41. Ewer TC, Stewart DE. Improvement in bronchial hyper-responsiveness in patients with moderate asthma after treatment with a hypnotic technique: a randomized controlled trial. *Br Med J.* 1986;293:1129–1132.

42. Guiney PA, Chou R, Vianna A, Lovenheim J. Effects of osteopathic manipulative treatment on pediatric patients with asthma: a randomized controlled trial. *J Am Osteopath Assoc.* 2005;105(1):7–12.

43. Bockenhauer SE, Julliard KN, Lo KS, Huang E, Sheth AM. Quantifiable effects of osteopathic manipulative techniques on patients with chronic asthma. *J Am Osteopath Assoc.* 2002;102(7):371–375;discussion 375.

44. Nagaratha R, Nagendra HR. Yoga for bronchial asthma: a controlled study. *Br Med J.* 1985;291:1077–1079.

45. Holgate ST, Frew AJ. Choosing therapy for childhood asthma. *N Engl J Med.* 1997;337:1690–1692.

46. Smyth JM, Stone AA, Hurewitz A, Kaell A. Effects of writing about stressful experiences on symptom reduction in patients with asthma or rheumatoid arthritis. *JAMA.* 1999;281:308–309.

47. Willers SM, Devereux G, Craig LC, et al. Maternal food consumption during pregnancy and asthma, respiratory and atopic symptoms in 5-year-old children. *Thorax.* 2007;62(9):773–779.

48. Okoko BJ, Burney PG, Newson RB, Potts JF, Shaheen SO. Childhood asthma and fruit consumption. *Eur Respir J.* 2007;29(6):1161–1168.

49. Woods RK, Walters EH, Raven JM, et al. Food and nutrient intakes and asthma risk in young adults. *Am J Clin Nutr.* 2003;78(3):414–421.

50. Romieu I, Varraso R, Avenel V, Leynaert B, Kauffmann F, Clavel-Chapelon F. Fruit and

vegetable intakes and asthma in the E3N study. *Thorax.* 2006;61(3):209–215.

51. Chatzi L, Apostolaki G, Bibakis I, et al. Protective effect of fruits, vegetables and the Mediterranean diet on asthma and allergies among children in Crete. *Thorax.* 2007;62(8):677–683.

52. Chunilal SD, Eikelboom JW, Attia J, et al. Does this patient have pulmonary embolism? *JAMA.* 2003;290(21):2849–2858.

53. Hirsh J. Oral anticoagulant drugs. *N Engl J Med.* 1991;324:1865.

54. He J, Ogden LG, Bazzano LA, et al. Dietary sodium intake and incidence of congestive heart failure in overweight U.S. men and women. *Arch Int Med.* 2002;162(14):1619–1624.

55. Coats AJS. Exercise training for heart failure: coming of age. *Circulation.* 1999;99(9):1138–1140.

56. Sturn B, Quittan M, Weisinger GF, et al. Moderate-intensity exercise training with elements of step aerobics in patients with severe chronic heart failure. *Arch Phys Med Rehabil.* 1999;80:746–750.

57. Pittler M, Guo R, Ernst E. Hawthorn extract for treating chronic heart failure. *Cochrane Database Syst Rev.* 2008(1): CD005312.

Cough

CHAPTER 41

Context

Everyone coughs at some time. Coughing is a natural defense mechanism used to clear the airways. Most individuals accept this as a naturally occurring component to most respiratory infections and assume that it is self-limiting to a week or two. When the cough is persistent, individuals are more likely to seek attention. In a primary care setting, cough is the fifth most common presenting complaint in adults.[1] This accounts for 30 million office visits per year. In children, the numbers may be higher.[2] As a common complaint, it is not surprising that approximately $600 million is spent per year in the United States alone on prescription and over-the-counter (OTC) cough medications.[3]

Chiropractors are probably more inadvertently involved in the evaluation of a patient with cough. Most patients would first seek medical consultation with a chronic cough. However, the chiropractor is well positioned to evaluate and diagnose a patient with cough and offer suggestions regarding conservative approaches that may benefit. Patients with chronic cough may also have musculoskeletally related complaints due to the constant strain on the chest and thoracic spine and musculature.

The majority of acute cough is due to viral infection or smoking.[4] Other causes include bacterial pneumonias, inhaled irritants, allergies, and medications. Chronic cough is most often due to one of a short list of causes.[5, 6] The following is a hierarchical list of these causes:

1. postnasal drip—40% of cases (87% in one study)
2. asthma—25% to 35% of cases (cough is the only presenting complaint in up to 25% of asthmatics)[7]
3. gastroesophageal reflux (GER)—20% of cases
4. chronic bronchitis—5% to 10% of cases
5. bronchiectasis—4% of cases

However, it is important to consider that smoking may be the underlying initiator of many of the above causes. Most important, a history of chronic smoking should raise the concern of bronchogenic carcinoma. Tuberculosis (TB) should also be considered when a low-grade upper respiratory infection (URI) seems to persist or there is known exposure to a TB carrier. Rarer causes of chronic cough are subdiaphragmatic abscess or tumors.

General Strategy

Acute Cough (<3 weeks)

Determine the following:

- whether the patient has been exposed to any chemicals—occupational or home cleaning solutions
- whether the patient could have aspirated food or liquid—infants, seniors, alcoholics, or sedated individuals
- whether the patient has additional signs of a URI and possible history of exposure to others with similar symptoms—viral infection most common; consider TB also
- whether the patient smokes or is exposed to a smoker
- whether the patient is taking medications that may provoke cough—angiotensin-converting enzyme (ACE) inhibitors, other antihypertensives, and some antiasthmatic medications such as albuterol (Ventolin) or cromolyn (drying of airways)
- response to OTC drugs—often ineffective, yet patient overutilizes
- whether the cough is positionally related—cough that increases with recumbency indicates postnasal drip, pulmonary vascular congestion, or asthma (if at night)

- whether there are any associated complaints such as fainting, incontinence, rib or chest pain, headaches, nausea/vomiting, hernias, or low back pain with radicular symptoms

Chronic Cough

Determine the following:

- whether initial signs of a URI resolved within two weeks, but cough is persistent—possible viral infection, superinfection with bacteria, or TB
- whether the cough is recurrent and appears to be either seasonal or associated with eye itching or stuffy nose—allergies, possible postnasal drip
- whether the patient has to clear the throat often—postnasal drip
- whether the patient is a smoker or is exposed to a smoker—chronic bronchitis
- whether the cough is worse with recumbency and is associated with a tickling in the upper throat—postnasal drip
- whether the cough is worse when recumbent and possibly associated with epigastric discomfort or a sour taste in the mouth—GER
- whether the cough is worse with exertion or associated with shortness of breath—cough-variant asthma
- whether there are any associated complaints such as fainting, incontinence, rib or chest pain, headaches

Evaluation

- Auscultate for wheezes, rales, or other adventitial sounds.
- If TB, congestive heart failure, fungal infection, pleurisy, or lung cancer is suspected, order a chest film.
- Laboratory testing may help differentiate bacterial causes from viral causes.
- Pulmonary function testing is particularly important when asthma or chronic bronchitis is suspected.

Management

- Depending on underlying cause, hydration and brief OTC medication are all that are needed for acute cough.

- When GER is suspected, changes in the types of food eaten, quantity of food, avoidance of lying down after large meals, and loss of weight will all be of benefit.
- For chronic bronchitis, smoking cessation is most important.
- A short course of manipulative therapy may be applied for uncomplicated asthma; comanagement is suggested.

Relevant Anatomy and Physiology

Cough receptors are ubiquitous. They are found in the nose, pharynx, larynx, trachea, bronchi, pleura, diaphragm, stomach, esophagus, also in the tympanic membrane and external auditory canal. Within the tracheobronchial tree there are several types of receptors: (1) slowly adapting stretch receptors; (2) rapidly adapting, irritant receptors; (3) pulmonary C-fiber receptors (J receptors); and (4) bronchial C-fibers.[8] The stretch and irritant receptors are myelinated. The rapidly adapting receptors are probably the main group associated with coughing. The C-fiber receptors are sensitive to inflammation and toxins or other noxious substances. Receptors in the external auditory meatus are sensitive to hair or cerumen and may be the cause of cough in some individuals.

The medullary cough center modulates the cough reflex via afferent vagal, glossopharyngeal, trigeminal, and phrenic nerves and efferent vagal, phrenic, and spinal accessory nerves.[9] Coughing is a rather violent act requiring several simultaneous participants. First, inspiration prior to coughing stretches the lungs, taking advantage of an elastic recoil effect. Next, a Valsalva maneuver occurs with closing of the glottis and contraction of the muscles of the abdomen, chest, and diaphragm. This is followed by an expiratory blast occurring with abduction of the glottis. This is then followed by a deep inspiration. During the cough phase, flow rate is as high as 600 L/min at speeds of up to 500 miles/h.[10]

Interference of coughing may be caused by position, weakened musculature, pain, or an overwhelmed mucociliary ladder. The inability to expel foreign material or mucus can result in atelectasis and/or infection. Chronic smoking is known to inhibit the mucociliary ladder and cause metaplasia of the cells in the smaller bronchioles. Normally, the cells of the smaller airways secrete a clear, nonviscous fluid. Chronic smoking causes these cells to transform into mucus-producing cells called Clara cells. It is much more difficult to clear the smaller airways except through coughing.

Sometimes associated with cough is a tendency toward thoracic flexion. This is an important consideration in older osteoporotic patients who may cause a compression fracture while coughing.

Evaluation

History

The history will provide a high level of suspicion in most cases (Table 41–1). A search for external irritants should include smoking, exposure to smoke, occupational dust

exposure, apparent pet allergies, and smog. Given that the most common cause of acute cough is a viral infection, questioning regarding associated signs of fever, runny or stuffy nose, and lethargy is helpful. In older patients and immunocompromised patients, a concern for the possibility of an underlying pneumonia is warranted.

A drug history, especially in those with a diagnosis of hypertension or asthma, is often revealing. ACE inhibitors are known as potential cough stimulators in some patients.[11] This is believed to be due to either stimulation of C-fibers through an ACE inhibitor effect of accumulation of kinins (i.e., bradykinin) or secondarily through production of a postnasal drip. Unfortunately, the association may not be clearly evident because the reported reaction may occur three to four weeks and as much as one year following initial usage. ACE inhibitor

Table 41–1 History Questions for Cough

Primary Question	What Are You Thinking?	Secondary Question	What Are You Thinking?
Algorithm	Consider common causes such as viral or bacterial URI, bronchitis, or pneumonia.	Is there someone you have been in contact with who has similar symptoms? Associated signs of sore throat, low-grade fever, stuffy nose, malaise? Associated signs of high-grade fever, chills, or rigors (shaking, teeth chattering) in addition to above list?	Determine contact's symptoms. Common infection likely. Viral cause likely. Bacterial cause likely. Does the patient have other predisposing conditions such as AIDS, diabetes, chronic obstructive pulmonary disease (COPD)?
Does the cough occur only with or soon after exertion?	Asthma, hyperactive airway disease, and cardiopulmonary causes.	Worse in dry, cold environment?	Asthma and hyperactive airways disease more likely. Look for auscultation findings if cardiopulmonary cause is suspected.
Have you had the cough longer than 3 weeks?	Causes of chronic cough include postnasal drip, COPD, esophageal reflux, and bacterial complication of viral disorder.	Is the cough worse when you are lying down at night? Is the cough productive? Do you smoke?	Consider postnasal drip; if associated with difficulty breathing, orthopnea (cardiopulmonary); with meals, consider esophageal reflux. A productive cough would suggest bacterial infection. COPD; with isolated wheeze consider bronchogenic carcinoma.
Does the cough occur intermittently (off and on)?	Occupational or environmental exposure. Also consider medications such as ACE inhibitors, beta-blockers, and some asthma medications.	Does the cough happen without other signs/symptoms? Does it occur only at work? Does it occur after returning home but before bed?	Probably environmental. Ask about occupational exposure, relationship to eating, etc. May be allergic if patient lives in rural area and works in urban area.

cough may also be worse in the supine position, probably related to the above-mentioned secondary effect.[12] Other medications include β-blockers (especially nonselective) that may, through a bronchoconstricting effect, irritate an asthmatic or those with hyperresponsive airways.[13] Ironically, asthmatics taking β-agonists such as albuterol or cromolyn sodium (Intal) or corticosteroids may develop a nonproductive cough due to irritation or drying of the bronchial membranes.[14]

If the cough is present only under stressful circumstances, both cough-variant asthma and psychogenic cough should be considered, especially in the adolescent. If the cough is provoked by exertion, exercise-induced asthma should be considered.[15]

If the cough appears or is made worse by recumbency, consider the following:

- Chronic cough occurring after lying down after a large meal and/or association with epigastric discomfort is probably GER.
- Recurrent cough occurring while lying flat and improved by support of the body or head at an angle is suggestive of postnasal drip or congestive heart failure (pulmonary vascular congestion).
- If the cough is worse while lying flat and is associated with dyspnea (orthopnea), congestive heart failure is more likely.
- Chronic cough that becomes worse in the middle of the night and is not always position-dependent is likely to be asthma.

The distinction between a productive and a nonproductive cough is helpful. Productive coughs usually imply infection. Nonproductive coughs are often the result of irritation such as with the underlying inflammation of asthma, postnasal drip, and external irritants such as from allergies or smoke. Questions regarding the color and consistency of phlegm are traditionally asked; however, they probably contribute little to the diagnosis. The typical assumption is that yellow or green phlegm is found often with bacterial or viral infections. A clear or mucus-like phlegm is suggestive of allergy or viral infection. Blood in the sputum (hemoptysis) is an indication of erosion or trauma from coughing found with pulmonary infarct, TB, bronchiectasis, and bronchogenic carcinoma.

Patients with a productive cough on the majority of days for three consecutive months occurring over two or more consecutive years are likely to have chronic bronchitis. This is particularly true in chronic smokers.

Examination

The primary focus of the examination is observation of the nose and throat and auscultation of the lungs. A cobblestone appearance of the oropharyngeal mucosa or direct visualization of mucoid secretions may be seen with postnasal drip.

Auscultation for wheezes may provide clues to an underlying chronic obstructive pulmonary disease (COPD) such as asthma, chronic bronchitis, or emphysema. A localized wheeze is suggestive of bronchogenic carcinoma in a patient who is a chronic smoker. Always check for a prominent supraclavicular lymph node (sentinel or Virchow's node). Extrathoracic wheezing—stridor—is associated with whooping cough (pertussis) in infants and children. This must be differentiated from blockage by a foreign object. When further testing is requested, supportive historical and/or physical examination findings must be present, as follows:

- Only when suspicion is high for pneumonia, TB fungal infection, or cancer does a chest film need to be ordered.
- When perinasal tenderness, positionally related nose stuffiness, or transillumination of the sinuses is positive, skull radiographs for sinus infection should be considered.
- If asthma is suggested by the history, spirometry testing with a focus on forced expiratory volume should be performed or ordered (peak flow meter evaluation is an inexpensive, but less sensitive measurement tool).
- Laboratory studies are rarely needed. The most common scenarios are with the suspected asthmatic patient in whom skin testing or pulmonary function testing is needed. A search for eosinophilia is not warranted given the nonspecificity of this finding. Sputum evaluation for Charcot-Leyden crystals or Curschmann spirals is rarely performed or needed.

Management

Conservative management of cough should be pursued in both a generic and specialized approach. The generic approach focuses on environmental factors that are modifiable, including the following:

- Ensure adequate hydration—8 oz of water every waking hour. Use of a humidifier/vaporizer may be helpful, but some asthmatics respond poorly to humidified air. Humidifiers must be thoroughly and properly cleaned to avoid spread of other allergens or infectious agents.

- Avoid smoking or being in a smoke-filled environment.
- Ensure that the house environment is clean. Change or clean furnace filters regularly. Use a vacuum cleaner that does not recycle room air.
- Avoid any potential allergens including grasses, plants, animals, or foods.
- Avoid supine positions; elevate the head of the bed or prop up the head and upper trunk with pillows.
- Consider supplementation with antioxidants such as vitamins A (β-carotene 20,000 IU/day), C (100 mg/waking hour), and E (400 to 800 IU/day).

Specific musculoskeletal approaches may include the following:

- Perform spinal and costovertebral adjusting to allow unrestricted movement while breathing.
- Perform deep trigger point work or myofascial release to the trapezius, serratus anterior, intercostals, pectorals, and midscapular muscles, and cervical spine musculature when the need is determined.
- Educate the patient to breathe through use of the diaphragm, and to breathe through the nose when possible; breathing should be deep and relaxed.

When GER is the cause, avoidance of large, heavy meals and foods such as chocolate, caffeine, alcohol, fat, onions, garlic, and orange juice will usually help. Avoidance of a supine position, especially after eating, is a requisite.

Pharmacologic treatment of cough should be tempered with the knowledge that, initially, cough serves a protective function. Inhibition of this function should be considered in patients only under the following conditions:

- when it interrupts sleep (which is necessary for recovery of an underlying infection)
- when there is the potential of damage, such as in osteoporotic patients or postsurgery
- in those patients with spinal pain and radicular symptoms
- in patients with hernias, stress incontinence, or syncope
- when the cough is incapacitating

Pharmacologic treatment is based on several approaches. Interruption of the cough reflex may occur peripherally, by acting on sensory receptors, or centrally,

by acting on the cough center in the medulla and nucleus tractus solitarius. Antitussive (anticough) medications are generally divided into (1) central suppressants, (2) expectorants, (3) mucolytics, and (4) peripheral anesthetics (benzonatate). The primary prescription suppressant is codeine, a narcotic. Because it is so effective, OTC (nonnarcotic) medications pale in comparison. OTC medications are a confusing array of mixtures with unproven effectiveness. When looking for or recommending an effective OTC antitussive, check for one of two ingredients: dextromethorphan or diphenhydramine. The combination of antihistamines, cough suppressants, and expectorants is probably useless or counterproductive.

Expectorants theoretically stimulate submucosal gland fluid secretion, rendering mucus less viscous and easier to clear. The primary approach to accomplishing this task is proper hydration, orally and via a humidifier. When ineffective, OTCs with guaifenesin (glycerol guaiacolate) or iodinated glycerol are sometimes effective. It is interesting to note that there is no evidence that these medications are any more effective than home remedies such as garlic, horseradish, pepper, or chicken soup. In patients with thicker sputum unresponsive to expectorants (rarely seen in a chiropractic office) a mucolytic agent, N-acetylcysteine, may be prescribed.

The common OTC approach of using cough lozenges is probably no more effective than sucking on candy. However, the psychologic effect of the sensation provided by camphor, menthol, or eucalyptus oil is soothing enough to continue sales.

Preventive measures should be encouraged when an infectious cause of cough is suspected. This includes washing one's hands after sneezing, nose blowing, or coughing. Use disposable tissues rather than handkerchiefs. Coughing into a flexed elbow or sleeve may also prevent direct spread through hand contact with others.

Patients suspected of having ACE inhibitor-provoked cough should be referred back to the prescribing physician. It is important to note that switching to another ACE inhibitor usually is not effective. Therefore, a switch to another antihypertensive is usually necessary.

Sinusitis may benefit from myofascial work over the temporal and masseter muscles, acupressure perinasally, or moist heat over the sinuses. Congestion-provoking positions should be avoided. Diathermy may be helpful in some cases. Patients suspected of having a sinus infection based on clinical examination and radiographs usually require referral for a decongestant and antibiotics. Some chiropractors employ a nasal-specific balloon therapy to drain the sinuses. It is anecdotally reported to be effective when performed by a chiropractor trained specifically in this approach.

Algorithm

An algorithm for evaluation and management of chronic cough is presented in **Figure 41–1**.

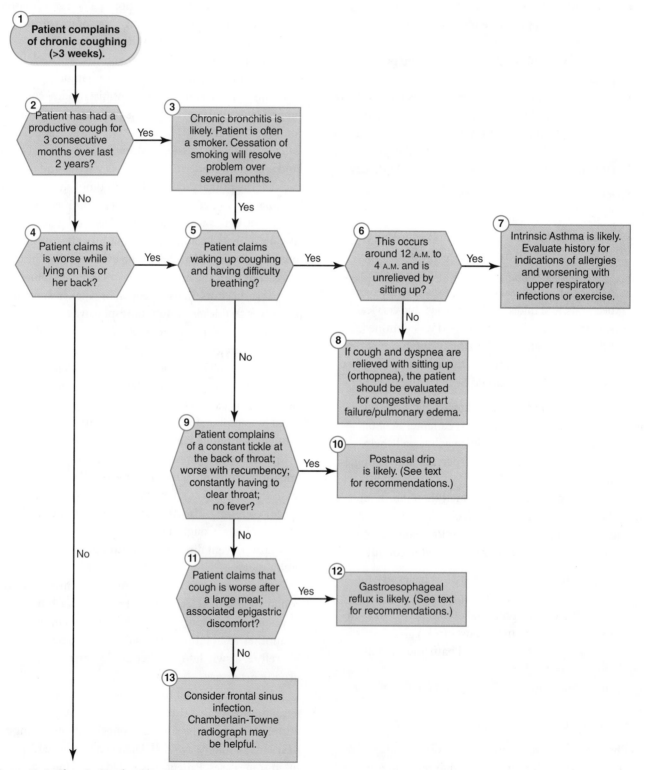

Figure 41–1 Chronic Cough—Algorithm

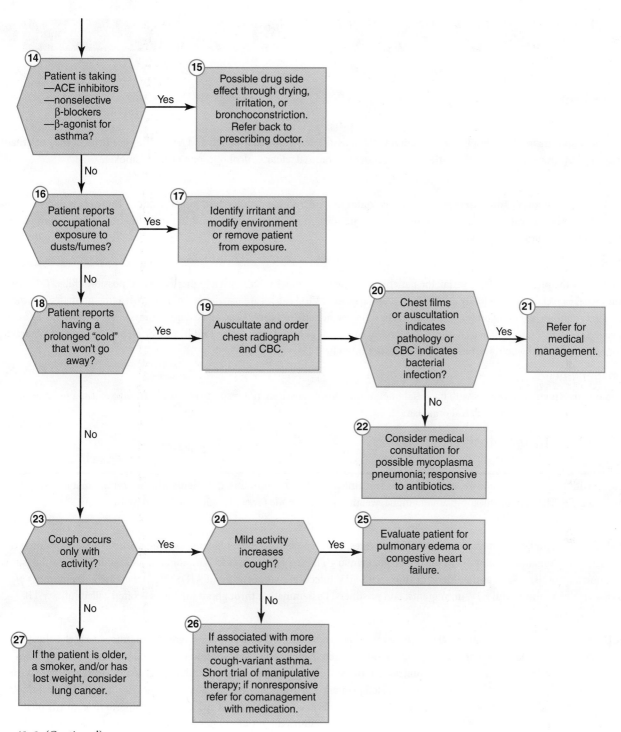

Figure 41–1 (Continued)

Selected Causes of Cough*

Pneumonia

Classic Presentation

The patient appears to have a respiratory infection with an associated productive cough and fever. The specificity of the presentation is increased by knowing whether the patient is immunocompromised, elderly, alcoholic, or a chronic smoker.

Cause

Inhalation or aspiration of oropharyngeal secretions containing microorganisms leads to lung infection. There are numerous causes, each with its own clinical presentation and treatment. Generalization will be made to assist in the distinction of pneumonia from other causes of respiratory infection.

Evaluate

In general, if the pneumonia is bacterial, the patient will appear to be more sick, with a higher fever and possibly chills. This is not always true, especially in the elderly and immunocompromised. Viral causes are usually more mild with a low-grade fever; however, the symptoms are more prolonged. Radiographs may be helpful, but there is no consistent pattern in all cases of any one cause. However, abnormal findings on a chest radiograph, such as lobar consolidation, patchy infiltrates, or pleural effusion, are characteristic of pneumonia and would warrant referral. Rales are often heard.

Management

Antibiotic treatment is necessary with bacterial pneumonia. Viral causes are not responsive. However, mycoplasma pneumonia may be responsive because it is an atypical organism.

Pulmonary Tuberculosis

Classic Presentation

Patients with primary infection are often asymptomatic unless immunocompromised. Patients who are symptomatic usually have reactivated TB. The patient will complain of fatigue, weight loss, low-grade fever, chronic cough, and night sweats.

Cause

Inhalation of mycoplasma tuberculosis will result in widespread lymphatic or hematogenous spread and an immune response that results in granulomatous walling-off of the organism. Primary TB rarely progresses to symptomatic presentation unless the patient is immunocompromised, such as the elderly or those with HIV infection (with or without AIDS).[16] An increase in the number of TB cases is due to those with HIV, immigrants, and prisoners. Dissemination throughout the lungs is often called miliary TB.

Evaluation

The patient presentation is not always classic. Patients known to be infected with HIV, immigrants, and the elderly should always be monitored for the development of pulmonary or other organ involvement. Auscultation may reveal post-tussive apical rales. Radiographs may demonstrate nodules or infiltrates in the apical or posterior segments in the upper lobes. However, there is much variation. Calcified areas (Ghon lesion) indicate healed primary TB. The definitive diagnostic tool is sputum stain (Kinyoun or Ziehl-Neelsen) and culture. Fiberoptic bronchoscopy may be necessary if not enough sputum is available. Skin testing is unable to distinguish active, current disease from past infection. The tuberculin skin test (TST) has been the standard test for diagnosing latent tuberculosis infection (LTBI). It involves measurement of the delayed type hypersensitivity response 48 to 72 hours after intradermal injection of purified protein derivative (PPD). Interferon-gamma release assays (IGRAs) are diagnostic tests used to detect an immune response to TB infection. The most commonly used is QuantiFERON, also known as QFT. It is an ELISA-based, whole-blood test that utilizes three TB antigens (ESAT-6, CFP-10, and TB7.7). The most recent as of the publication of this text is the Gold In-Tube (QFT-GIT). It is important to note that the TST and QFT measure different aspects of the immune response for latent TB and are not interchangeable. With TST, prior BCG vaccination can produce false-positive test results.

Management

Referral for medical management is necessary. All cases demonstrating positive findings and those in whom there is a high suspicion must be reported to local and state public health departments. This is best left to the treating physician. Because of the development

---

*See also Chapter 40, Dyspnea, for asthma and Chapter 38, Chest Pain, for gastroesophageal reflux.

of TB-resistant organisms, the Centers for Disease Control and Prevention has developed a new strategy that involves multiple drug application and monitoring. Isoniazid and rifampin are supported by other medications such as pyrazinamide and streptomycin.

Postnasal Drip

Classic Presentation

The patient complains of a chronic cough that seems worse while lying down (supine). The patient reports a dry or nonproductive cough. He or she may also notice a persistent tickle at the back of the throat, requiring frequent clearing of the throat.

Cause

There is a variety of causes, including upper respiratory infection, sinusitis, allergies, drugs (e.g., ACE inhibitors), smoking, and environmental pollutants. Chronic irritation of the pharyngeal and tracheal membranes initiates the cough reflex. Postnasal drip is by far the most common cause of chronic cough.

Evaluation

Classically, there will be a cobblestone appearance of the posterior mucosa; however, this is a nonspecific finding. Primarily, it is necessary to identify the underlying cause through a history. If there is associated nasal congestion, a suspicion of sinusitis warrants sinus evaluation with skull radiographs.

Management

The patient is instructed to avoid any identifiable triggering stimuli. OTC nasal decongestants or antihistamines used for a short course may be effective. If a prescribed medication is the suspect, such as an ACE inhibitor, referral back to the prescribing physician is necessary. Failure to respond to conservative measures requires referral for prescribed decongestants or antihistamines. An evaluation of sinusitis is warranted if this treatment trial fails. There is a nasal-specific technique used by some chiropractors for the treatment of sinusitis; however, it should be used only by those with special training and experience. Physicians often will use a trial of antibiotics first before more invasive procedures.

Chronic Bronchitis

Classic Presentation

The patient complains of a chronic productive cough for three months or more in at least two consecutive years. The patient is a smoker.

Cause

Airway blockage occurs as a result of metaplasia of cells, smooth muscle hypertrophy, and increased mucus production. It appears that chronic cigarette smoking is the major risk factor. However, air pollution, respiratory infections, and allergies have all been implicated as contributory. Chronic bronchitis and emphysema often coexist in the later stages of COPD.

Evaluation

Initially, the patient is asymptomatic. Unlike the purely emphysematous patient, the patient with chronic bronchitis is often overweight and may show some degree of cyanosis. Dyspnea is primarily exertion related. The prominent feature at presentation is a chronic productive cough. Auscultation often will reveal rhonchi or wheezes. Chest films may show an increase in markings with an associated cardiomegaly. ECG changes may indicate right ventricular hypertrophy.

Management

The primary treatment is the same for prevention: cessation of smoking and avoidance of any known irritants such as dusts or other pollutants. Complications such as associated asthmatic reaction or infections warrant comanagement with a medical physician.

Bronchogenic Carcinoma

Classic Presentation

The patient is older than 40 years of age, has a history of smoking, and complains of a persistent cough, hemoptysis, weight loss, and anorexia.

Cause

Primary lung cancer is due most often to cigarette smoking. Additional causes include exposure to therapeutic radiation, heavy metals, or industrial toxins such as asbestos. Bronchogenic carcinoma is classified according to cell type, including squamous cell, adenocarcinoma, small cell, and large cell carcinomas. In general, squamous cell and small cell carcinomas are more central in location, demonstrating a tendency for widespread metastasis. Adenocarcinoma and large cell carcinoma are usually more peripherally located in the lungs. Because the lungs themselves are insensitive to pain, widespread involvement may occur without symptoms. Until bronchi are compressed or eroded or the pleura is involved, the patient is usually asymptomatic.

Evaluation

By the time obvious symptoms and signs are evident, the cancer has often reached a stage that is not amenable to treatment. About one-fifth of cases may demonstrate lymphadenopathy, splenomegaly, and clubbing of the fingers.

Horner's syndrome (miosis, ptosis, and anhidrosis) from a Pancoast (apical) tumor is seen in a small number of cases (< 5%). Auscultation may reveal a solitary wheeze or nothing at all. Laboratory tests may reveal nonspecific but incriminating evidence of metastasis, including increased calcium, alkaline phosphatase, or anemia. Sputum cytologic examination will confirm the diagnosis in over half of cases if the cancer is centrally located. Chest radiographs usually will demonstrate nonspecific yet important clues, including hilar masses, atelectasis, pleural effusions, or mediastinal widening. If suspicious findings are evident, computed tomography or magnetic resonance imaging is helpful in determining the degree of involvement and may suggest the type based on location and pathologic process viewed.

Management

Treatment includes surgery, chemotherapy, and radiation therapy based on the type and staging of disease. Although the overall five-year survival rate is less than 15%, patients with early squamous cell cancer may have a much higher rate (35% to 40%).[17] Chiropractors treating patients with lung cancer or other cancers that metastasize should be concerned about spinal or joint pains. These may indicate metastasis and warrant first a radiograph of the area and then possible referral for bone scan coordinated with the patient's oncologist.

APPENDIX 41–1

References

1. Irwin RS, Curley FJ, French CL. Chronic cough: the spectrum and frequency of causes, key components of the diagnostic evaluation, and outcomes of specific therapies. *Am Rev Respir Dis.* 1990;141:640.

2. Kamei RK. Chronic cough in children. *Pediatr Clin North Am.* 1991;38:593–604.

3. Corrao WM. Chronic cough: an approach to management. *Comp Ther.* 1986;12:14.

4. Irwin RS, Rosen MJ, Braman SS. Cough: a comprehensive review. *Arch Intern Med.* 1977;137:1186–1191.

5. Pratter MR, Bartter T, Akers S, et al. An algorithmic approach to chronic cough. *Ann Intern Med.* 1993;119:977–983.

6. Irwin RS, Curley FJ. The diagnosis of chronic cough. *Hosp Pract.* 1988;11:82.

7. Seaton A. The management of cough in clinical practice. *Scott Med J.* 1977;22:99.

8. Adcock JJ. Peripheral opioid receptors and the cough reflex. *Respir Med.* 1991;85(suppl A):43–46.

9. Korpas J, Widdicombe JG. Aspects of the cough reflex. *Respir Med.* 1991;85:3–5.

10. Fuller RW. Physiology and treatment of cough. *Thorax.* 1990;44:425.

11. Sesoko S, Kaneko Y. Cough associated with use of captopril. *Arch Intern Med.* 1985;145:1324.

12. Karlberg BE. Cough and inhibition of the reninangiotensin system. *J Hypertens.* 1993;11:549–552.

13. Braman SS, Corao WM. Cough: differential diagnosis and treatment. *Clin Chest Med.* 1987;8:177.

14. Zervanos NJ, Shute KM. Acute, disruptive cough. *Postgrad Med.* 1994;95:153.

15. Johnson D, Osborne LM. Cough-variant asthma: a review of the clinical literature. *J Asthma.* 1991;28:85–90.

16. Barnes PF, Barrows SA. Tuberculosis in the 1990's. *Ann Intern Med.* 1993;119:400.

17. Matthay RA. Lung cancer. *Clin Chest Med.* 1993;14:1.

Head and Face Complaints

Eye Complaints

Context

The prevalence of undetected vision problems appears to be between 5% and 10% in preschool children.[1] Of these, approximately 2% to 5% have amblyopia, "lazy eye."[2] Left uncorrected, vision loss may be permanent. Of school-age children, 90% to 95% have "normal" eyesight.[3] The majority of the children with eyesight problems have refractory errors.

In the elderly, vision loss is more common. In one large study[4] approximately 70% of the nursing home residents over the age of 65 years had good vision. Approximately 15% had adequate vision (15/50 to 15/70) and 15% had poor vision of 15/100 or worse (1% had no light perception). Sixty percent of people over the age of 65 years have some opacification of the ocular lens, although they are not necessarily impaired. Past the age of 75 years, 5% of all individuals have exudative macular degeneration (another 25% have the dry, less severe form)[5] and 5% have glaucoma.[6] Approximately 50% have significant cataracts (higher frequency in women). Whites have a higher incidence of macular degeneration, whereas blacks have a higher incidence of untreated cataract, open-angle glaucoma, and diabetic retinopathy.[7] Up to 25% of those wearing glasses had inappropriate visual correction.[8]

Vision loss in the elderly can be a significant factor in fatal car crashes. States that require vision testing for those over the age of 65 years have a lower incidence.[9] It is also important to recognize the increased risk of falling when eyesight is poor. Proprioceptive compensation is often diminished in the elderly; therefore, maneuvering in dimly lit areas places the low-vision senior at risk.

Eye complaints may reflect local pathology in the eye, a reaction to systemic infection or metabolic abnormalities, or vascular/neurologic pathology (**Figure 42–1**). Most causes of visual loss that are not congenital are treatable or curable. To facilitate an organized approach, each eye complaint is discussed separately under each section. A list of common patient complaints and possible causes follows:

- Loss of vision—may be due to vascular disease (local cause due to retinal infarct; central processes such as stroke are usually associated with other findings), increased intraocular pressure (glaucoma), increased opacification of the lens (cataract), retinal detachment (trauma, vitreoretinal traction, or neovascularization), tumors (distinguished by type of visual field defect and associated cranial nerve findings)
- Blurred vision—refractory error (near- or farsightedness), cataracts
- Diplopia—monocular (cataract or refractory error), binocular (cranial nerve problem due to tumor, drugs, myasthenia gravis, diabetes, or drugs)
- Flashing lights—migraine prodrome, vitreoretinal detachment, epilepsy
- Floaters—usually benign; sudden onset of many may indicate retinal detachment
- Photophobia—certain medications, migraine, corneal inflammation, iritis, albinism, fever
- Dry eyes—aging, medications (diuretics and anticholinergics), Sjogren's syndrome, Bell's palsy
- Eye pain—acute-angle glaucoma, foreign body
- Red or pink eye—conjunctivitis, iritis, or uveitis
- Itchy eyes—allergies

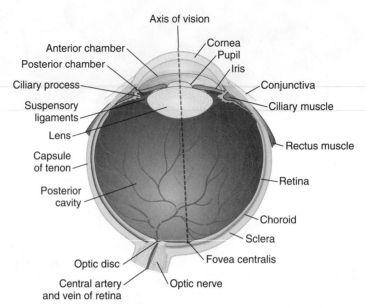

Figure 42–1 Anatomy of the eye, as seen in cross-section.

Review of General Terminology

- Accommodation—to focus on near objects the eyes "accommodate" through contraction of the ciliary muscles, increasing the curvature (convexity) of the lens
- Presbyopia—loss of accommodation with aging
- Amblyopia—loss of vision due to disuse ("lazy eye")
- Myopia—nearsighted; the eye is longer; light rays focus in front of the retina (requires a concave or diverging lens to move the focal point back)
- Hyperopia—farsighted; the eye is shorter; light rays focus at a point behind the retina (if they could pass through; requires a convex or converging lens to move the focal point forward)
- Astigmatism—the refractory errors in the vertical and horizontal axes differ, requiring a cylindrical lens for correction
- Strabismus—deviation of the eye; esotropia = internal deviation; exotropia = external deviation (strabismus may lead to permanent vision loss through cortical suppression of the weak eye)
- Exophthalmos—abnormal protrusion of the eye usually caused by hyperthyroidism due to proteinaceous buildup behind the eye
- Nystagmus—a rhythmic beating movement of the eyes comprised of a fast and slow movement

General Strategy

History

Vision Loss

Determine whether
- The vision loss is acute (often vascular or traumatic) or chronic (macular degeneration, presbyopia), transient (amaurosis fugax, multiple sclerosis, papilledema) or permanent (macular degeneration, retinitis pigmentosa, stroke).
- The vision loss is painful (traumatic or acute-angle glaucoma) or painless (macular degeneration, cataract, open-angle glaucoma, amaurosis fugax). If the vision loss is painless, does the patient have indicators of hypertension, diabetes, or a history of smoking (amaurosis fugax, diabetic retinopathy)?
- The vision loss is unilateral (vascular or neurologic; may eventually become bilateral) or bilateral (usually glaucoma or cataracts).
- The vision loss is central (cataract or macular degeneration [slow onset] or retinal detachment [sudden onset usually]) or peripheral (glaucoma in initial stages or retinitis pigmentosa).

- The vision loss is associated with a headache (migraine [transient prior to headache usually] or temporal arteritis [permanent]).

Blurred Vision

Determine whether

- Blurriness is in one or both eyes
- Onset is sudden or gradual
- The patient is diabetic (in addition to diabetic retinopathy, diabetics have an increased risk of glaucoma and cataract formation)
- Distant or near vision is affected
- Corrective lenses have improved vision (last change in prescription)

Diplopia

Determine whether

- Patient has monocular (refractory error or cataract) or binocular (vascular, cranial tumor, myasthenia gravis, drug effect, or multiple sclerosis) diplopia
- Binocular, whether patient has indicators of tumor, diabetes, or multiple sclerosis

Flashing Lights and/or Floaters

Determine whether

- Flashing lights are associated with a headache
- Floaters are acute (possible retinal detachment if sudden onset of many) or chronic (usually benign)

Photophobia

Determine whether

- There are associated complaints such as redness or itchiness or headache
- The patient is taking any medications that may cause photophobia
- The patient has a fever

Dry or Gritty Eyes

Determine whether

- The patient has indicators of hyperthyroidism (exophthalmos may prevent proper lubrication)
- The patient has indicators of Sjogren's syndrome

Eye Pain (without Vision Loss)

Determine whether

- It is felt superficially (local pathology) or behind the eye (referred pain from headache or tumor)
- There are accompanying signs or symptoms such as a urinary tract infection (Reiter's syndrome)

Red or Pink Eye

Determine whether

- The redness occurred suddenly without associated itching or pain (subconjunctival hemorrhage from coughing or sneezing)
- There is associated debris and itching (conjunctivitis)
- There are associated signs of allergies

Examination

- Observe and inspect for redness, dryness, eye deviation, lid lag, and exophthalmos.
- Perform a battery of tests to check for extraocular muscle weakness, symmetry of the eyes, and use a cover test.
- Test for pupillary reaction and accommodation.
- Test for visual acuity with a Snellen eye chart or Jaeger chart with adults; with children, picture cards or oriented E charts are valuable.
- Test for color perception in male children and those not previously tested.
- Examine the anterior chamber with a temporally positioned light.
- Refer for slit-lamp or fluorescein stain if corneal abrasion or foreign body is suspected.
- Refer for further testing when glaucoma is suspected.

Evaluation

History

Vision Loss

Although it may appear that simply asking the patient whether he or she has difficulty seeing would be an effective screen for vision loss, studies have shown that it is not. It is estimated that 1 million individuals have glaucoma and are unaware of significant vision loss. When adult patients were asked, "Do you have difficulty seeing distant objects?" the sensitivity for detecting vision worse than 20/40 was only 28%.[10] The question, "Can you see well enough to recognize a friend across the street (while wearing glasses)?" had a sensitivity of only 48%.[11]

When vision loss is sudden, a vascular cause is likely. When there are other associated neurologic signs, a site proximal to the eye is the cause. When vision loss is the only neurologic sign and its appearance is without pain, amaurosis fugax (microembolism from carotid arteries) or retinal detachment is likely. The patient will often describe either occurrence as "like a curtain was pulled down over my eye." The difference is that amaurosis fugax usually lasts only for minutes, while vision loss from retinal detachment does not improve without treatment. The vision loss from temporal arteritis is also painless and often sudden or over a few days due to infarction of the optic nerve head. Associated signs of temporal arteritis are a temporal headache, neck and upper trunk myopathy (polymyalgia rheumatica), and general arthralgia prior to the loss of vision.

Other than trauma, acute, painful loss of vision is usually due to acute-angle glaucoma. Associated indicators are age over 60 years, a family history, nausea and vomiting, provocation from prolonged periods in a dark environment, and drugs that cause dilation of the pupils, such as anticholinergics (antiparkinsonian drugs, antidepressants, and some gastrointestinal drugs).

Gradually developing vision loss or blurriness is common with progressive refractory errors, glaucoma, cataracts, diabetic retinopathy, and macular degeneration.

- Diabetes mellitus is the leading cause of blindness in the United States in patients between the ages of 20 years and 74 years.
- Age-related macular degeneration is the leading cause of legal blindness for individuals 60 years and older.
- Glaucoma is the second-leading cause of blindness in the United States and is thought to be the leading cause among African Americans.
- Cataracts are the most common cause of treatable vision loss in the elderly.

With chronic open-angle glaucoma, the patient often will have a bilateral peripheral vision loss (often in the nasal field). Historical indicators of predisposition to glaucoma include a family history (occasionally), topical or systemic corticosteroid use, prior surgery or trauma to the eye, and diabetes. Cataracts are also seen in the elderly, producing a gradual loss of central vision. Associated indicators include a change in color vision and halos around lights, affecting the patient's ability to drive at night. There are different types of cataracts; however, with nuclear cataracts, some patients report an improvement with near vision early in the course of the disorder. Macular degeneration is usually bilateral with progressive central vision loss.

Red Eye

Patients complaining of itchy eyes, a foreign-body sensation, tearing, and eyelid edema likely have bacterial or viral conjunctivitis, especially if the symptoms first occurred in one eye and over the following two days involved both eyes. When the complaint is bilateral from the onset, allergic conjunctivitis is more likely. The discharge is purulent and more profuse with a viral or bacterial cause and more watery with allergic conjunctivitis.

Examination

Some initial observational clues that are helpful include the following:

- Groping, squinting, or craning of the neck often will indicate loss of vision.
- Eye deviation (strabismus), unequal or absent movement of the eyes, ptosis (Horner's or oculomotor nerve), or inability to close the eyes (facial nerve) are indicators of nerve damage.
- Exophthalmos or lid lag indicates hyperthyroidism.
- Loss of the outer eyebrows indicates hypothyroidism; scaling of the eyebrows indicates seborrhea.
- Red or pink eyes with discharge suggest conjunctivitis; without discharge and with pain suggest acute uveitis.

A general screen for the eye should include visual acuity testing, extraocular muscle function, tests for eye position with a pen light and cover card, pupillary reflex, a corneal status check with a flashlight, accommodation, and color vision testing in male children or those not tested in the past. A brief discussion of each follows:

- Extraocular muscle function is tested in several ways. By shining a light about 1 ft away from the patient's eyes the corneal light reflex (Hirschberg test) determines whether the light shines on the same spot on each eye. If not, there is deviation of one of the eyes. Next, the cover test is performed. Have the patient look straight ahead and cover one eye. With the macular image suppressed, the covered eye will drift into a relaxed position. If, when the examiner uncovers the eye, a jump is noted it indicates that a weakness is present and the eye needed to reestablish fixation. Finally, test the six cardinal positions of gaze by holding an object such as a pencil approximately 1 ft away and having the patient track movement into up-and-out, straight-lateral, and down-and-out paths on both sides. Third-nerve palsy is indicated by deviation that is generally down and out. With complete involvement there is paralysis of the eyelid; the examiner must lift the lid to see the deviation. Esotropia and inability to abduct the eye are indicative of sixth nerve involvement. The patient may rotate his or her head to the weak side. A torsional or oblique deviation with head tilt away from the involved side is found with fourth-nerve palsy. In general, when a muscle is weak, the image separation will be greatest while looking into the normal direction of action. Many of these nerve palsies are associated with diplopia. In particular the diplopia will be binocular, meaning that diplopia is present with both eyes open and disappears when either eye is covered. Diplopia that is monocular, meaning that it is present only when the involved eye is open and disappears when it is closed, indicates a refractive error in most cases.

- The pupillary light reflex tests the function of both the second and third cranial nerves. By having the patient look into the distance, normal eyes will have pupils that dilate. By shining a light from the side, two reactions should occur: (1) pupillary constriction on the side tested, and (2) constriction on the opposite side (consensual reflex). If a pupil is large and poorly reactive, a third-nerve palsy is likely. If it is small and poorly reactive, a Horner's syndrome may be present. Fixed and constricted pupils (meiosis) are seen with glaucoma treatment, use of narcotics, or damage to the pons. Fixed and dilated pupils (mydriasis) are seen with severe brain damage or deep anesthesia. Unequal pupils seen without light stimulation that react equally to light are probably anisocoria, a normal variant.

- Accommodation is tested by having the patient look in the distance and then introducing an object into his or her field of gaze. The normal response is pupillary constriction and convergence of the eyes.
- A simple test to observe the anterior chamber is to shine a light from the side across the eye. A nasal shadow across the iris due to a shallow anterior chamber may be seen with glaucoma. Diffuse redness indicates conjunctivitis. On occasion, a corneal lesion or scarring may be seen. For a complete evaluation, referral for slit-lamp evaluation and fluorescein stain is necessary.
- Color blindness affects about 8% of white males (only 4% of black males). Females are affected only 0.4% of the time. Testing should be performed on boys age 4 years to 8 years with an Ishihara test comprising a series of polychromatic cards. The child must identify a pattern made up of a single color of dots against a multicolored background.

A fundoscopic examination is more difficult for the chiropractor because tropicamide dilation drops cannot be used. However, with careful observation, some abnormalities may still be visible. A list of possible findings follows:

- Disc pallor—optic nerve atrophy
- Papilledema—increased intracranial pressure
- Vessel nicking, narrowed arteries, silver-wire arteries, and copper-wire arteries—usually due to hypertension
- Microaneurysms—seen with diabetes
- Soft exudates (cotton-wool patches)—fluffy and irregular; seen with diabetes, hypertension, lupus, subacute bacterial endocarditis, and papilledema
- Fatty exudates—well defined, small, regular, and often seen in clusters; found in diabetic and hypertensive retinopathy
- Hard exudates (drusen)—normal with aging

Visual Acuity Testing

Screening tests for children between the ages of 3 and 5 years should include inspection, the cover test, visual acuity tests, and stereovision assessment. Taken together, an estimated negative predictive value of 99% for amblyopia, strabismus, and/or high refractive problems may be achieved.[12, 13] Unfortunately, stereovision testing is not available in most chiropractic offices. For children, the Snellen eye chart is relatively insensitive (25% to

37%).[14] Other visual acuity tests include the Landolt C, the Tumbling E, Allen picture cards (familiar objects or animals), and others.[15] The advantage of these tests is that the ability to read is not tested as much as the ability to determine orientation of a letter or recognition of an object or animal.

Snellen eye charts should always be used as the initial screening for visual acuity in adults. With the Snellen eye chart test, the patient is expected to read with one eye at a time, covering the other with a card. The patient should keep his or her glasses (unless they are reading glasses) or contacts on. Encourage patients to read to the smallest line possible. The recorded measurement includes two numbers. The first number represents the distance the patient was standing (20 = 20 ft) and the second number indicates the distance at which a normal eye could read that specific line (letter size = 20 micrometers; 20 = a normal eye could see this line at 20 ft). For patients who have difficulty reading, a hand-held version such as the Jaeger card may be used. In the United States, an individual is legally blind if vision is 20/200 or less in the better eye with correction. If peripheral vision is reduced to 10° or less in both eyes (tested on perimetry) the patient is also considered legally blind even if his or her central vision is better than 20/200.

A simple test for visual acuity that tests for refractory errors is the pinhole test. Repeating the Snellen test with the patient looking through a 2-mm pinhole in a card will improve performance if the cause is a refractory error. The patient may state that the image is dimmer (this is due to less light being allowed into the eye).

Confrontation testing is used to test for visual field defects. All fields are the same for the examiner (except in the temporal field). Therefore, when a patient is asked to say "now" when a finger or object enters his or her visual perception, the examiner should see it at the same time. With a temporal field examination, it is necessary to start with the finger or object behind the patient and advance it forward. The patient should see it at approximately 90°. Visual field testing may indicate where the problem is in the vision relay system. A brief, generalized list follows:

- Central scotoma—optic nerve involvement
- Nasal quadrant deficits—glaucoma is a common cause
- Bilateral temporal field deficits—compression at the optic chiasma (often from a tumor)

- Homozygous hemianopic deficit (same side in both eyes)—optic tract to the calcarine cortex

Red or Pink Eye

When there is purulent discharge associated with eyelid involvement with crusted material and no associated preauricular lymph node involvement, the patient will probably have a bacterial conjunctivitis requiring referral. When crusting of the eyelids is a predominant finding, a blepharitis (bacterial infection of the sebaceous follicles and meibomian glands) has occurred through extension of the conjunctival infection. When the conjunctivitis is more watery or mucus-like, with no crusting, and associated with preauricular node involvement, a viral cause (usually adenovirus) is likely. Other conditions, such as corneal abrasion or infection, often are associated with pain, impaired vision, light sensitivity, and unequal pupils. These added findings dictate referral to an ophthalmologist for further evaluation. Also, patients with eye inflammation who have had prior eye surgery, wear contact lenses, or have a history of herpes simplex keratitis should be referred to an ophthalmologist.

A similar presentation may occur with the use of eye drops (prescribed or over-the-counter [OTC] products). This is usually bilateral and is a diagnosis of exclusion. Referral back to the prescribing physician for evaluation or discontinuation of an OTC eye drop is usually effective.

Management

Immediate referral to an ophthalmologist is needed in the following cases:

- Acute glaucoma
- Abrasion of the cornea or foreign body implantation
- Temporal arteritis
- Retinal detachment or vitreoretinal traction
- Suspicion of bacterial conjunctivitis
- Acute cerebrovascular event

Nonemergent referral to an ophthalmologist is needed in the following cases:

- Suspicion of open-angle glaucoma, age-related macular degeneration, cataracts
- Cases where there is progressive loss of vision without a known cause

- Patients interested in radiokeratotomy or laser ablation therapy

Referral to an optometrist (with the possibility of comanagement) should be made in the following cases:

- Children age 4 years and over with vision of 20/40 or worse in either eye or a difference between two eyes of one line or more on the Snellen eye chart
- All patients with indication of diabetic retinopathy (to determine need for ophthalmologic referral)
- Patients who wear glasses but have lost the corrective ability of the lenses

Recommendations for prevention of vision loss include the following:

- All children between the age of 3 and 4 years should have a visual screening.
- All individuals over age 40 years (particularly blacks) should have a tonometry and ophthalmoscopic examination every three to five years to detect glaucoma.
- All diabetics should be closely monitored for any vision changes and have a minimum of an annual eye examination; emphasis on control of diabetes is crucial to the prevention of diabetic retinopathy.
- All hypertensive patients should be educated regarding the higher probability of vision loss with chronic hypertension and should strictly adhere to a program to reduce hypertension.

Therefore, the chiropractor may act as a screening source for many eye problems. Although there are anecdotal and in some cases paper presentations of recovery of eyesight with chiropractic care, it is too early to recommend this approach as an isolated attempt.[16] Comanagement with an optometrist or ophthalmologist is highly suggested for purposes of both patient safety and documentation. Although older theories focused on a proposed sympathetic nervous system irritation, a more convincing theory suggests cerebral hibernation as a cause, with manipulation "reviving" the quiescent nerve cells. The theory is based on an observation that when cerebral blood flow is deprived from an area of the brain, cell death occurs. However, if the vascular reduction is less than that causing death, a protective cellular hibernation with no apparent electrical activity occurs. When the blood flow or neural stimulation is returned to the area, cellular function returns.[17] One study[18] claims such a response in cerebral blood flow following manipulative

therapy. With regard to lesser vision problems such as phorias and tropias, there is a theory that the relationship between cervical input into the vestibular nuclei and other connections may have an effect on cranial nerves or extraocular muscle function. There have been two small studies[19, 20] of patients without glaucoma who demonstrated a reduction in intraocular pressure after spinal manipulation. Unfortunately, tonometry is known to be quite variable, and the results might be flawed by this deficiency.

New refractive surgical procedures are commonly used for the correction of myopia and, in some cases, astigmatism. Due to the fact that the cornea provides approximately two-thirds of the eye's refracting ability (the remainder is provided by the lens), and given that currently the length of the eye cannot be altered, these new refractive techniques attempt to make changes in the cornea that allow refocusing of an image onto the retina. The results of these surgeries can be rather dramatic; however, they are based on the degree of myopia and associated astigmatism. There are three procedures:[21]

1. Radial keratotomy (RK)—with anesthetic eye drops, a thin diamond surgical instrument is used to make a series of radial incisions that causes a relative flattening of the cornea.
2. Photorefractive keratotomy (PRK)—with anesthetic eye drops, an excimer laser is used to remove specific, small amounts of corneal tissue.
3. Laser in situ keratomileusis (LASIK)—with anesthetic eye drops, a flap of corneal tissue is made with a microkeratome; an excimer laser is also used to remove corneal tissue, and then the flap is returned to its original position.

Prior to an individual being considered a candidate for these refractive surgical procedures, certain inclusion and exclusion criteria are used:

- Must be 18 years of age or older
- Must not be pregnant or nursing
- Must be able to demonstrate stable lens correction for at least one year
- Must discontinue use of soft lenses for one week and rigid lenses three to four weeks before the surgical procedure
- Must be free of medical conditions that might contraindicate surgery or specifically surgery of the cornea; ocular conditions include severe dry eye, corneal scarring, severe uveitis, severe untreated blepharitis, or kerataconus; also

exclusionary are medical conditions such as collagen vascular diseases, keloid formation, or an immunocompromised status (relative contraindication)

Generally, patients with up to –6.00 diopters of myopia may benefit from RK and PRK, whereas patients with visual acuity less than –6.00 diopters will have better results with LASIK. Newer options in development are implantation of an intrastromal corneal ring and the use of intraocular lens (lens implantation).

These surgeries are not entirely without risks, and some have not withstood the test of time and large retrospective studies. Compared to LASIK, recovery from PRK takes slightly longer and the patient may have some discomfort due to healing of the corneal surface. Glare and halos may develop but usually diminish over time. It appears that patients with brown eyes may have this temporary side effect more often than those with blue eyes.[22]

Patients who are classified as legally blind are not able to obtain a driver's license and have some restrictions in contact or vehicle-operated sports. These individuals are eligible for assistance with education, visual aids, and seeing-eye dogs.

Algorithm

An algorithm for evaluation and management of vision problems in the elderly is presented in **Figure 42–2**.

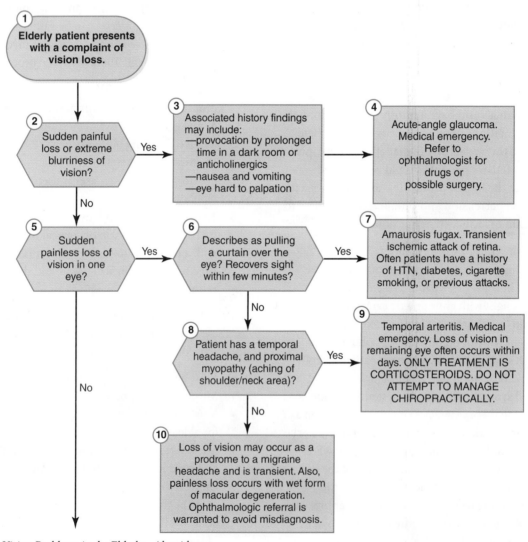

Figure 42–2 Vision Problems in the Elderly—Algorithm

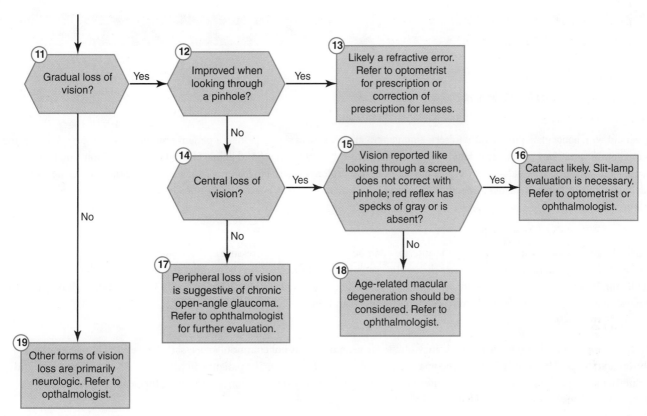

Figure 42–2 (Continued)

Selected Causes of Vision Loss

Acute Angle-Closure Glaucoma

Classic Presentation

A patient with acute glaucoma is likely to seek emergency care because of severe pain. If a patient presents to a chiropractic office, the presentation would be eye pain associated with a complaint of apparent halos around lights, blurred unilateral vision, and possibly nausea and vomiting. The patient may report having been in a prolonged dark environment such as a movie theater, during stress, or having had his or her eyes dilated for medical purposes. The patient is usually a senior with a positive family history for acute angle-closure glaucoma.[6]

Cause

Blocked outflow of aqueous humor from the anterior chamber causes increased pressure and severe pain. The "angle" is formed between the cornea and the root of the iris. The outflow canal that is blocked consists of a trabecular network and the canal of Schlemm. Preexisting narrow angles are found in the elderly (due to lens enlargement), patients with hyperopia (farsighted), and Asians.[7] Fortunately, acute-angle glaucoma accounts for less than 10% of all glaucoma cases.

Evaluation

Because the patient is likely to see an emergency physician, examination is not commonly necessary. However, if less acute, the chiropractor should be aware of acute glaucoma as a possible cause of eye pain. The patient will have eye redness (ciliary flush) and a cloudy-looking cornea. The depth of the anterior chamber can be assessed with a penlight. Shining the penlight from the side, a shadow will be visible over the nasal half of the iris. The eye is hard to palpation.

Management

This is a medical emergency. A permanent correction may be accomplished with laser peripheral iridectomy. Left untreated, the patient will have permanent vision loss in three to five days.

Open-Angle Glaucoma

Classic Presentation

Unfortunately, a patient with early open-angle glaucoma has no warning symptoms. If asymptomatic, a patient would present with a complaint of a peripheral visual field "cut," usually the nasal half.

Cause

The cause is unknown; however, a surfacing theory is that glaucoma is an optic nerve disease that may be related to specific vascular changes.[23] In addition, these vascular changes may be caused by free radicals (as in stroke or similar diseases). The intraocular pressure is chronically elevated in patients with this type of glaucoma, yet the cause is unknown. It is usually bilateral and seen earlier in blacks than other ethnic groups. The patient may be genetically predisposed to an adverse reaction to topical or oral corticosteroids, leading to the development of glaucoma. Past eye surgery or trauma may also predispose the patient.

Evaluation

The evaluation for glaucoma in the chiropractic setting is difficult. There would have to be a high level of suspicion (given most patients are asymptomatic) and the tools and expertise to perform a comprehensive examination. These include tonometry (the measurement of intraocular pressure), ophthalmoscopic visualization of specific changes, and visual field testing. The measurement of intraocular pressure increase is not a reliable indicator. Required is inspection of the anterior chamber angle with a special lens (goniolens) with the slit-lamp biomicroscope. Two screening tools have been advocated: (1) frequency-doubling perimetry, and (2) oculokinetic perimetry. Future studies will determine their usefulness. If the glaucoma is advanced, visual field testing may reveal an upper nasal field cut. Ophthalmoscopic changes include cupping of the disc and nasal displacement of the vessels.

Management

Ophthalmoscopic referral is necessary. Initial treatment is with medication. Failure to improve usually requires a referral for laser trabeculoplasty.

Cataracts

Classic Presentation

The patient is usually a senior complaining of progressive, painless, central vision loss or blurred vision. Ironically, some patients may report an improvement in close vision in the initial stages of cataract formation.

Cause

Cataracts are the leading cause of blindness in the world.[24] Cataract surgery is the most commonly performed surgical procedure in the United States, with 1.5 million operations annually.[25] More than half of individuals over the age of 65 years will develop age-related cataracts. A cataract is due to opacification of the lens. There are several different types and causes, including congenital (often due to rubella and cytomegalovirus intrauterine infection) and secondary to diabetes, chronic corticosteroid use, or uveitis. However, the most common type of cataract is the one associated with heredity and aging—senile cataract.

Some different types of cataracts are described below.

- Nuclear cataracts are found in the central part of the lens and are the most common type of age-related cataracts. Older age, female gender, and smoking are risk factors. Potential risk factors are diet, estrogen levels, and cardiovascular factors.
- Cortical cataracts are found surrounding the central lens and are more common in black individuals.
- Posterior subcapsular cataracts are found behind the lens and are associated with sunlight exposure as a risk factor. They are more common in white individuals, especially those taking corticosteroids.
- Mixed cataracts are a combination of the above types.

Cataracts are also secondary to ocular trauma, diabetes, alcohol use, and with some medications including corticosteroids (associated with the posterior subcapsular type). Chronic ultraviolet light exposure appears to be the main cause with aging. Most patients over the age of 50 years have some degree of lens opacification, yet not all have a visual impairment. Risk factors include cigarette smoking or alcohol abuse.[26, 27]

Evaluation

The vision loss is central and not improved by looking through a pinhole. There is a normal pupillary reaction. Ophthalmoscopic examination may reveal flecks of gray appearing with the red reflex, or obliteration of the red reflex in advanced cases. Visualization of the opacity is possible in later stages, but a slit-lamp examination is necessary to locate it (and therefore the type of cataract).

Management

Prevention of nuclear cataracts may be in part due to attention to adequate protein, vitamin A and niacin, thiamin, and riboflavin.[28] The decision to have cataracts removed must be a weighted process, taking into account the age of the patient, the degree of cataract formation, and, most important, the effect on function. For example, an 80-year-old patient confined to bed may not have the same benefits as a younger, more active patient. Surgery involves one of two procedures: (1) extracapsular surgery, and (2) phacoemulsification. Extracapsular surgery leaves the posterior capsule of the lens intact, providing a firm anchoring for the implant. Phacoemulsification, called no-stitch surgery, involves fractionation of the lens with sound waves. The surgical management includes removal of the lens and placement of a permanent artificial lens called an intraocular lens (IOL). The most prevalent practice is to use an ultrasonic probe that emulsifies the lens through vibration. The lens is removed and an IOL is inserted. New improvements will include alternatives to ultrasonic energy, such as laser photolysis, and new technology that allows for rapid dispersion of heat with a smaller incision.[29] Foldable silicone implants have been developed that can be inserted through smaller incisions and with newer techniques can be implanted with no sutures. Bifocal or multifocal lenses are also available in some locations.[30]

Age-Related Macular Degeneration

Classic Presentation

The patient may present differently based on the underlying type. A patient with atrophic (dry) degeneration will complain of slowly developing, painless, central vision loss. A patient with the disciform (wet) degeneration presents with sudden, painless loss of vision. Prior to loss the patient may notice parts of words missing or straight lines appearing crooked.

Cause

Age-related macular degeneration (ARMD) is the leading cause of blindness in the geriatric population. It affects up to 30% of the elderly to varying degrees. Ninety percent of cases are the dry, slowly progressive form.[5] Associated risk factors include smoking and a family history of ARMD. Asians have a very low risk; whites have a higher risk. Individuals with light blue or green irises or exposure to intense blue light are also at risk. The layer between the retinal pigmented epithelium and choriocapillaris is called Bruch's membrane. Degeneration of this membrane and the retinal pigmented epithelium results in the atrophic form. This degeneration, specifically the lipofuscin aggregation, is due to oxidative damage that is both light and oxygen dependent. Damage to Bruch's membrane by drusen allows an angiogenic stimulant to promote ingrowth of new vessels (neovascularization) and the exudative or wet form occurs.

Evaluation

Fundoscopic findings include drusen (yellow-white spots) and hyper- or hypopigmentation of the fundi with the atrophic form. Hemorrhages and exudates are seen. Patients at risk for ARMD are often told to use a straight line or Amsler grid to detect any new distortion, which would require immediate consultation with an ophthalmologist.

Management

There is no treatment for the dry form of ARMD, but low-vision aids and adaptation to gradual loss are usually sufficient to allow mobility. Patients with the wet form of ARMD often require laser photocoagulation to ablate the neovascular membrane. The location of the membrane affects the success of the laser ablation. In some cases, restoration of some central vision may reduce general vision, yet, ironically, prevent blindness. Up to 60% of patients need repeat treatment because of regrowth. Obana et al.[31] evaluated the carotenoid levels of the retina in patients with ARMD and found them to be lower than patients without ARMD. Smoking is a well-established risk factor for ARMD in patients with a genetic predisposition.[32]

Morris et al.,[33] evaluating the relationship between zinc and antioxidant intake and ARMD, found that intake of alpha- and beta-carotene, lycopene, total retinal A, total vitamin A, and total vitamin E were significantly inversely related to the prevalence of pigmentary abnormalities (PA). Specifically, consuming foods high in alpha- or beta-carotene lowered the odds of PA. It appears that a diet high in vitamin A and antioxidants, in particular beta-carotenes (large amounts of fruits and vegetables), may reduce the risk of developing ARMD.[34] An important new treatment method for wet ARMD is with intravitreal bevacizumab. This approach, based on anticancer treatment, targets the neovascularization aspect of the wet-type of macular degeneration. It is a monoclonal antibody drug designed to block the growth of new blood vessels. An injection into the eye, usually followed by one per month for two months, causes significant anatomical and functional improvement.[35, 36] This new approach has strong literature support but only for a one-year follow-up. Long-term efficacy is still being evaluated. Specific recommendations include the following amounts taken daily: 200 mg of selenium, 1,000 mg vitamin C, 400 IU of vitamin E, and 25,000 IU of natural beta-carotene. There are mixed reports regarding zinc supplementation as a prevention for ARMD.

Retinitis Pigmentosa

Classic Presentation

The patient is often a youngster who notices (or a parent notices) poor night vision.

Cause

This disorder is hereditary, with recessive, autosomal-dominant, and X-linked modes identified. It may also occur as part of Bassen-Kornzweig syndrome or Laurence-Moon-Biedl syndrome. Degeneration of the retina, particularly the retinal rods, occurs. This is why night vision loss is one of the earliest signs. A peripheral-ring scotoma usually expands to include some central vision loss by middle age.

Evaluation

Fundoscopic examination will reveal dark pigmentation in the equatorial region of the retina, often associated with a yellow, waxy disk. Definitive diagnosis requires specialized testing that includes dark adaptation, electroretinography, and electrooculography.

Management

No treatment is currently effective. Genetic counseling is recommended for those affected. Retinoid supplementation is advocated by many, yet the results have not been clearly reproducible. There appears to be a possible role for vitamin A and taurine (amino acid).[37] In the future it is hoped that genetic engineering may allow replacement of the defective gene. Retinal transplantation is currently being researched. Currently, "retinal glasses" are being used as a means for patients to retain some degree of functional eyesight.

Amaurosis Fugax

Classic Presentation

The patient is usually over the age of 50 years and complains of an episode of vision loss in one eye that lasted a few minutes and then the vision returned. The patient often describes the loss and recovery of vision like a shade being pulled down and raised, respectively. There is often a history of diabetes, hypertension, or smoking.

Cause

Emboli originating in the ipsilateral internal carotid travel to the retina via branches of the ophthalmic artery, causing a "fleeting blindness," amaurosis fugax. The same risk factors for atherosclerosis are found, such as hypertension, diabetes, and chronic cigarette smoking.

Evaluation

An ipsilateral carotid bruit may be heard. Fundoscopic examination will usually reveal signs of hypertensive disease. In addition, whitish emboli and/or refractive cholesterol emboli may be seen. Patients should be sent for Doppler studies and possibly angiography to determine the extent of stenosis.

Management

After an attack, the patient should be warned of a predisposition to stroke or loss of vision if a subsequent attack occurs (16% of patients).[38] Aspirin and antiplatelet drugs are used in patients with mild stenosis. Endarterectomy has a high success rate in patients with severe stenosis. There is a subgroup of patients who are younger and have no signs of atherosclerosis or stenosis. The belief is that these patients may suffer from retinal artery spasm. These patients will be placed on a calcium channel blocker. For obvious reasons, patients who have had an attack of amaurosis fugax are probably at somewhat greater risk with cervical adjustments. Other techniques should be employed.

Optic Neuritis

Classic Presentation

The patient presents with an abrupt loss of vision in one eye. Central vision is affected and may progressively worsen over the next two days. If the patient presents two to three weeks later the vision often has returned to normal. However, now the patient has some eye pain associated with eye movement.

Cause

Inflammation of the optic nerve is usually due to demyelinating disorders, specifically multiple sclerosis (MS). It may occur less commonly with a host of other problems such as infection (mumps, measles, influenza, or varicella virus), autoimmune disorders (lupus), bee sting, meningitis, or infarction from temporal arteritis.

Evaluation

Ophthalmoscopic evaluation by a specialist is required.

Management

In the past, oral prednisone was used; however, it has been discovered that this approach, in addition to not being effective, doubles the risk of recurrence in the following two years in the same or opposite eye.[39] Currently, intravenous methylprednisolone sodium succinate, followed by oral prednisone, effects a quicker recovery and has a fortuitous side effect of delaying the onset of MS in some patients.[40]

APPENDIX 42–1

Web Resources

National Eye Institute
(301) 496-5248
www.nei.nih.gov
American Academy of Ophthalmology
(415) 561-8500
www.aao.org
American Society of Cataract and Refractive Surgery
(703) 591-2220
www.ascrs.org
Lighthouse International
(800) 829-0500
http://www.lighthouse.org

APPENDIX 42–2

References

1. National Center for Health Statistics. *Refraction Status and Motility Defects of Persons 4–74 Years, 1971–1972. US Vital Health Statistics,* Series II; 1978.

2. Ehrlich MI, Reinecke RD, Simons K. Preschool vision screening for amblyopia and strabismus: programs, methods, guidelines. *Surv Ophthalmol.* 1983;28:145–163.

3. Hevlston EM, Weber JC, Miller K, et al. Visual function and academic performance. *Am J Ophthalmol.* 1985;99:346–355.

4. Tielsch JM, Javitt JC, Coleman A, et al. The prevalence of blindness and visual impairment among nursing home residents in Baltimore. *N Engl J Med.* 1995;332:1205–1209.

5. Klein R, Klein BE, Linton KL. Prevalence of age-related maculopathy: the Beaver Dam eye study. *Ophthalmology.* 1992;99:933–943.

6. Klein BE, Klein R, Sponsel WE, et al. Prevalence of glaucoma: the Beaver Dam eye study. *Ophthalmology.* 1992;99:1499–1504.

7. Sommer A, Tiesch JM, Katz J, et al. Racial differences in the cause-specific prevalence of blindness in East Baltimore. *N Engl J Med.* 1991;325:1412–1417.

8. Stults BM. Preventive health care for the elderly. *West J Med.* 1984;141:832–845.

9. Nelson DE, Sacks JJ, Chorba TI. Required vision testing for older drivers. *N Engl J Med.* 1992;326:1784–1785.

10. Stone DH, Shannon DJ. Screening for impaired vision in middle age in general practice. *Br Med J.* 1978;2:859–861.

11. Haase KW, Bryant EE. Development of a scale designed to measure functional vision loss using an interview technique. *Proc Am Stat Assoc.* 1973;(SS):274–279.

12. De Becker I, MacPherson HJ, LaRoche GR, et al. Negative predictive value of a population-based preschool vision screening program. *Ophthalmology.* 1992;99:998–1003.

13. MacPherson H, Braunsetin J, LaRoche GR. Utilizing basic screening principles in the design and evaluation of vision screening programs. *Am Orthopt J.* 1991;41:110–121.

14. Lieberman S, Cohen AH, Stolzberg M, Ritty JM. Validation study of the New York State Optometric Association (NYSOA) vision screening battery. *Am J Optom Physiol Optics.* 1985;62:165–168.

15. Fern KD, Manney RE. Visual acuity of the preschool child: a review. *Am J Optom Physiol Optics.* 1986;63:319–345.

16. Terrett A J, Gorman RF. The eye, cervical spine, and spinal manipulative therapy: a review of the literature. *Chiro Tech.* 1995;7:43–54.

17. Astrup J, Siesjo BK, Symon L. Thresholds in cerebral ischemia: the ischemic prenumbra. *Stroke.* 1981;12:723–725.

18. Zhang C, Wang Y, Lu W, et al. Study on cervical visual disturbance and its manipulative treatment. *J Tradit Chin Med.* 1984;4:205–210.

19. Cipolla VT, Dubrow CM, Schuller EA. Preliminary study: an evaluation of the effects of osteopathic manipulative therapy on intraocular pressure. *J Am Osteopath Assoc.* 1975;74:147–151.

20. Beckenstein L. Glaucoma: detection and management. *J Chiro.* 1969;6:525–527.

21. Schartw BH, Zageibaum BM. Refractive surgery for active patients. *Physician Sports Med.* 1999;27:72–86.

22. Tabbara KF, El-Sheikh HF, Sharara NA, Aabed B. Corneal haze among blue eyes and brown eyes after photorefractive keratectomy. *Ophthalmology.* 1999;106:2210–2215.

23. Drance SM. Glaucoma: changing concepts. *Eye.* 1992;6:337.

24. Yorston D. A perspective from a surgeon practicing in the developing world. *Surv Opthamol.* 2000;45:51–61.

25. Munoz B, West SK, Ruben GS, et al. Causes of blindness and visual impairment in a population of older Americans: the Salisbury Eye Evaluation Study. *Arch Ophthamol.* 2000;118:819–825.

26. Ritter LL. Alcohol use and lens opacities in the Beaver Dam eye study. *Arch Ophthalmol.* 1993;111:113.

27. Christin WG. A prospective study of cigarette smoking and risk of cataract in men. *JAMA.* 1992;268:989.

28. Head KA. Natural therapies for ocular disorders, part one: diseases of the retina. *Altern Med Rev.* 1999;4(5):342–359.

29. Solomon R, Domenfeld ED. Recent advances and future frontiers in treating age-related cataracts. *JAMA.* 2003;200:248–251.

30. Sher NA, Trobe JD, Weingeist TA. New options for vision loss. *Patient Care.* 1995;9:55–76.

31. Obana A, Hiramitsu T, Gohto Y, et al. Macular carotenoid levels of normal subjects and age-related maculopathy patients in a Japanese population. *Ophthalmology.* 2008;115(1):147–157.

32. Klein R. Overview of progress in the epidemiology of age-related macular degeneration. *Ophthalmic Epidemiol.* 2007;14(4):184–187.

33. Morris MS, Jacques PF, Chylack LT, et al. Intake of zinc and antioxidant micronutrients and early age-related maculopathy lesions. *Ophthalmic Epidemiol.* 2007;14(5):288–298.

34. Seddon JM, Ajani UA, Sperduto RD, et al. Dietary carotenoids: vitamins A, C, and E, and advanced age-related macular degeneration. *JAMA.* 1994;272:1413–1420.

35. Chang TS, Bressler NM, Fine JT, Dolan CM, Ward J, Klesert TR. Improved vision-related function after ranibizumab treatment of neovascular age-related macular degeneration: results of a randomized clinical trial. *Arch Ophthalmol.* 2007;125(11):1460–1469.

36. Bashshur ZF, Haddad ZA, Schakal A, Jaafar RF, Saab M, Noureddin BN. Intravitreal bevacizumab for treatment of neovascular age-related macular degeneration: a one-year prospective study. *Am J Ophthalmol.* 2007.

37. Cumming RG, Mitchell P, Smith T. Diet and cataract: the Blue Mountains Eye Study. *Ophthalmology.* 2000;10(7):450–456.

38. Li L. Vision problems in the elderly. In: Greene HL, Fincher RME, Johnson WP, et al., eds. *Clinical Medicine.* 2nd ed. St. Louis, MO: Mosby-Year Book; 1996;678–682.

39. Beck RW, Cleary PA, Anderson MM, Jr, et al. A randomized, controlled trial of corticosteroids in the treatment of acute optic neuritis. *N Engl J Med.* 1992;326:581–588.

40. Beck RW, Cleary PA, Trobe JD, et al. The effect of corticosteroids for acute optic neuritis on the subsequent development of multiple sclerosis. *N Engl J Med.* 1993;329:1764–1769.

Facial Pain

Context

Initial distinction between facial pain and headache is necessary. Facial pain may arise from several anatomic sources, including the ears, oral cavity, sinuses, cervical spine, and eyes. Although there is obvious overlap and the possibility of referral, patient localization and associated findings are usually revealing.[1] Facial pain is best approached from a temporal perspective. Sudden onset with recurrent attacks is typical of several neuralgias. Deep, boring, aching pain is more characteristic of oral, ear, eye, and sinus problems and intracranial pathology. Dental causes are often distinguished by oral stimuli such as cold, hot, sweetness, or pressure.

General Strategy

History

- Distinguish among facial, ear, eye, oral, and headache pain.
- Determine whether the onset is sudden and recurrent (neuralgic) or chronic (intracranial or eyes, ears, nose, and throat [EENT]).
- Determine the quality of pain; sharp, lancinating pain of relatively short duration suggests neuralgias; deep, boring pain is more characteristic of dental, sinus, and intracranial masses.

Neuralgias

- Determine whether the pain is acute or chronic.
- If acute, determine whether there are any triggers such as shaving, cold, eating, or other (trigeminal neuralgia).

- Determine whether the pains are sharp and stabbing in the mouth and awaken the person at night (possible glossopharyngeal neuralgia).
- Determine whether there are any associated neurologic symptoms (neuralgia secondary to other processes such as multiple sclerosis).

Oral Cavity

- Determine whether there has been any recent prolonged dental work and/or last dental examination.
- Determine whether pain is related to eating cold, hot, or sweet foods.

Sinus

- Determine whether there is a prior or current history of an upper respiratory infection.
- Determine whether there are positional exacerbations of the pain (i.e., bending forward or lying down).

Temporomandibular Joint

- Determine whether opening the mouth increases the pain.
- Determine whether there is a history of grinding teeth.
- Determine whether there is a history of popping or clicking at the temporomandibular joint (TMJ).

Myofascial

- Determine whether the pain location includes the periaural or temporal area.

- Determine whether the pain is in the region of the masseter (cheeks) and associated with prolonged opening of the mouth or movement of the jaw.

Psychologic

- Determine whether the patient may be depressed or have periods of stress, drug addiction, or a dysfunctional home environment.
- Determine whether there is a family history of similar complaints.

Evaluation

- Examine the eyes, ears, nose, throat, and TMJ for any obvious pathology with a focus on dental abnormalities.
- When a sinusitis is suspected, transillumination or specific skull radiographs may be helpful in determining involvement.
- When a diagnosis is not clear, referral for special imaging is warranted.

Management

- If tolerable, patients with neuralgias may benefit from a trial treatment with manipulative therapy; if unresponsive after two to three weeks, referral for medical management is suggested.
- Sinus pain is often self-resolving, but the patient may benefit from facial massage, cervical adjustments, and physical therapy; over-the-counter decongestants have some value with limited use; failure to respond is suggestive of a sinus infection that may require antibiotic management.

Relevant Neurology

The trigeminal nerve is responsible for general sensation of the head and face. The skin of the face and forehead is supplied by three divisions of the trigeminal nerve. The nose, forehead, and scalp to the vertex of the skull are supplied by the ophthalmic (V1) division; the cheek and below the nose to the lip are supplied by the maxillary (V2) division; the jaw to the front of the ear is supplied by the mandibular (V3) division. The trigeminal nerve

also supplies the mucosa of the oral and nasal cavities, the perinasal sinuses, the teeth, and most of the dura. The angle of the jaw and scalp of the back of the head are supplied by C2 and C3. Bogduk and Marsland[2] demonstrated that referral pain overlapping the V1 division of the trigeminal nerve may be due to facet irritation in the upper cervical region.

Evaluation

History

Neuralgias

Generally, neuralgias are differentiated by a classic onset in older patients (after age 50 years) with a description of sharp, excruciating jolts of facial (or oral) pain that are recurrent and often progressive. The same presentation in a younger patient would suggest other conditions such as multiple sclerosis, a trigeminal neuroma, and, more rarely, an acoustic neuroma.

Trigeminal neuralgia is the most common facial neuralgia. The short, sudden, electric shock–like pains usually follow either the second or third trigeminal branch. Trigger areas may be reported by the patient. Even light touch to, for example, the nasolabial fold or upper lip may trigger an onset if the maxillary branch is involved. An area lateral to the lower lip may trigger an attack with mandibular division involvement.

When the less common glossopharyngeal neuralgia is the cause, pain is felt deep in the oral cavity and palate. Pain often occurs during the night, awakening the patient. Triggers involve relatively common benign activities such as talking, swallowing, yawning, or eating. It appears that salty, spicy, or bitter foods may be triggers. Postnasal drip is occasionally found as a trigger for some patients. Patients may also report having fainted upon coughing or yawning.[3]

Dental

When dental pulp is inflamed (pulpitis) as a result of caries, trauma, or dental surgery, pain is provoked by hot or cold foods and sweets. When the pulp undergoes necrosis, local gas is produced, which, when expanded by heat, increases pressure and causes pain. Cold decreases the gas pressure and relieves the pain. There are apical foramina that connect the pulp to the periodontal ligament and periapical alveolar bone. Infection or inflammation may spread through this connection, leading to a tooth that is sensitive to compressive pressure from chewing or percussion. This is also found with a cracked tooth.

Myofascial

Myofascially related temporomandibular problems are often evident from a history of early-morning jaw pain or if the patient is aware of grinding the teeth throughout the night or day. Other indicators may be pain upon opening the mouth. The pain is often felt at the pretragus area or temporalis muscle and may radiate into the face (see Chapter 3).

Sinus

In many cases there may be a history of an upper respiratory problem currently or preceding the development of facial pain. It may be possible to localize which sinuses are involved by questions regarding positional exacerbation or relief. The pain from frontal sinus involvement is relieved by standing or sitting. It is likely that the patient will report worse pain at night or when lying down and improvement after arising in the morning or as the day progresses. Those patients with maxillary sinus involvement may report the opposite: relief when lying down, which allows better drainage. Sphenoid sinusitis is unusual in that it may refer to the vertex of the skull, the eye, or the neck.

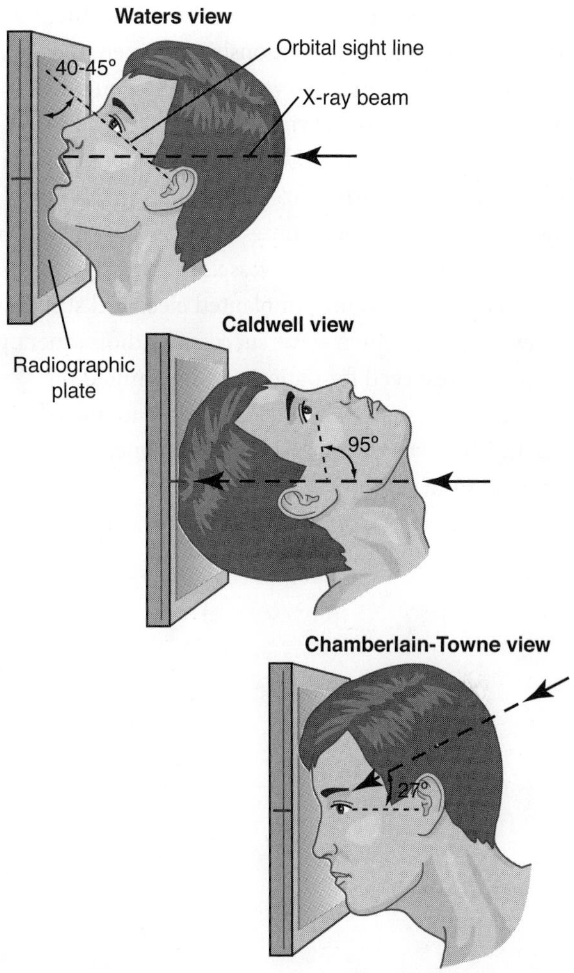

Figure 43–1 Radiographic views of the maxillary, ethmoid, and frontal sinuses.

Examination

The examination for facial pain should focus on a detailed examination of the mouth, paying particular attention to dental status and any oral lesions. The examination continues with palpation of facial structures in an attempt to reproduce pain. Patients with neuralgias may have their pain triggered by light touch around the mouth or cheek areas. Palpation of the TMJ while the patient opens and closes the mouth will usually localize the problem. Further evaluation is discussed in Chapter 3.

Acute sinusitis is usually quite obvious, with localized tenderness to either palpation or percussion over the involved sinus. Bending forward may increase pressure and therefore pain in the sinus. When the maxillary sinus is involved, referral to the teeth may produce a complaint of toothache, and percussion of the maxillary teeth may produce discomfort. Transillumination of the sinuses may be decreased. Radiographic evaluation of the sinuses includes the following views (**Figure 43–1**):[4]

- Waters view for maxillary sinuses
- Caldwell view for ethmoid sinuses
- Chamberlain-Towne view for frontal sinuses

Management

Chiropractic management of facial pain is based entirely on the suspected source. If there is a dental source, referral to a dentist is appropriate. If the patient appears to have one of the neuralgias, such as trigeminal neuralgia, a brief treatment trial of chiropractic care may be attempted if the patient is amenable; however, there are no studies indicating success with the facial neuralgias in the chiropractic literature. The rationale for this approach is the anatomic relationship between the spinal nucleus of the trigeminal nerve and the upper spinal nerves in the trigeminocervical nucleus. Medical management of trigeminal neuralgia is with an antiseizure medication such as carbamazepine (Tegretol). If this is unsuccessful, surgical decompression may be effective in cases where anomalous blood vessels are pressing on the trigeminal nerve. Recently, implanted electrical stimulation devices have shown some success.[5] Radiofrequency rhizotomy is reserved for patients with a limited life expectancy. Glossopharyngeal neuralgia is managed similarly. Microvascular decompression appears to be very successful.[6]

Sinusitis pain is often self-resolving. This may be aided by moist heat and possibly aided through facial massage. Cranial manipulation is advocated by some osteopaths and chiropractors. When there is an underlying infection, conservative measures to reduce sinus pressure will often fail and require medical referral for antibiotics and in rare cases drainage.

The reader is referred to Chapter 3 for appropriate patients.

Algorithm

An algorithm for evaluation and management of facial pain is presented in **Figure 43–2**.

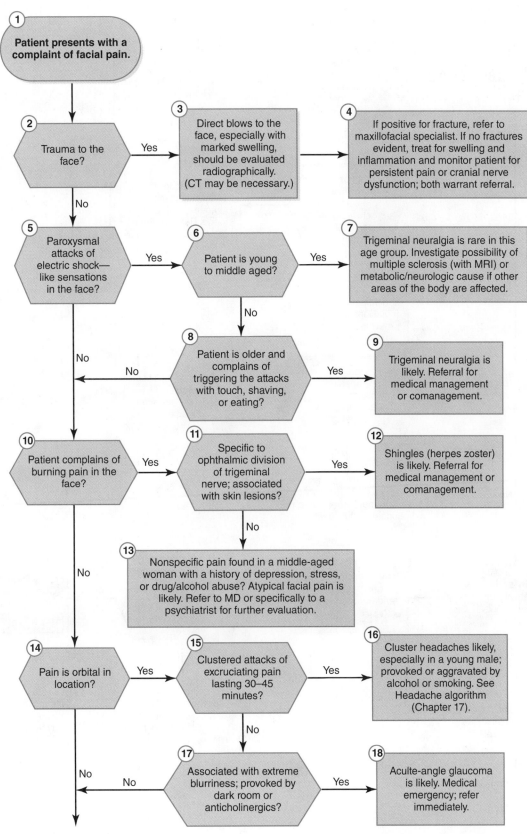

Figure 43–2 Facial Pain—Algorithm

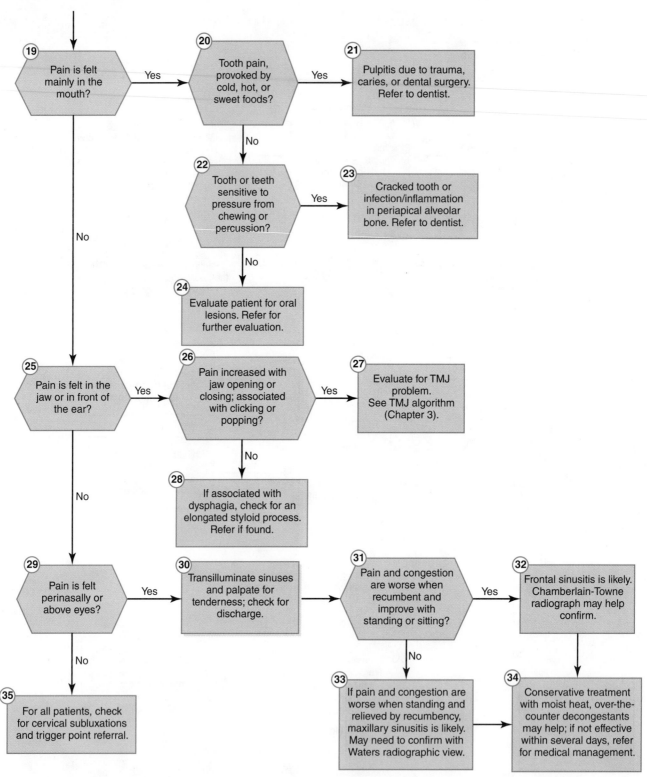

19 Pain is felt mainly in the mouth? — Yes → **20** Tooth pain, provoked by cold, hot, or sweet foods? — Yes → **21** Pulpitis due to trauma, caries, or dental surgery. Refer to dentist.

20 No → **22** Tooth or teeth sensitive to pressure from chewing or percussion? — Yes → **23** Cracked tooth or infection/inflammation in periapical alveolar bone. Refer to dentist.

22 No → **24** Evaluate patient for oral lesions. Refer for further evaluation.

19 No → **25** Pain is felt in the jaw or in front of the ear? — Yes → **26** Pain increased with jaw opening or closing; associated with clicking or popping? — Yes → **27** Evaluate for TMJ problem. See TMJ algorithm (Chapter 3).

26 No → **28** If associated with dysphagia, check for an elongated styloid process. Refer if found.

25 No → **29** Pain is felt perinasally or above eyes? — Yes → **30** Transilluminate sinuses and palpate for tenderness; check for discharge. → **31** Pain and congestion are worse when recumbent and improve with standing or sitting? — Yes → **32** Frontal sinusitis is likely. Chamberlain-Towne radiograph may help confirm.

31 No → **33** If pain and congestion are worse when standing and relieved by recumbency, maxillary sinusitis is likely. May need to confirm with Waters radiographic view. → **34** Conservative treatment with moist heat, over-the-counter decongestants may help; if not effective within several days, refer for medical management.

32 → **34**

29 No → **35** For all patients, check for cervical subluxations and trigger point referral.

Figure 43–2 (Continued)

Facial Pain Caused by Neuralgias

Trigeminal

Classic Presentation

Usually a middle-aged or older (>50 years) patient (usually female) presents with a complaint of sharp, electric shock–like pains that start at the mouth and shoot toward the ear, eye, or nose on the same side. The attacks are recurrent and often progressively become more frequent. The patient is often distraught and may be considering suicide.

Cause

The cause is unknown. Triggers include sensory stimulation from touch, the wind, shaving, or eating.

Evaluation

The neurologic examination is negative. If positives are found, especially in a younger patient, suspect multiple sclerosis. Other causes include trigeminal neuroma and other tumors. If suspected, referral for imaging studies may be necessary.

Management

Current medical management includes carbamazepine (Tegretol). Surgical decompression may be effective if anomalous blood vessels are pressing on the trigeminal nerve. Radiofrequency rhizotomy is reserved for those individuals with limited life expectancy. Acupuncture is often tried as an alternative. Implanted electrical stimulation devices may be of benefit.[5]

Glossopharyngeal

Classic Presentation

Patient presents with a complaint of deep, stabbing, or electric shock–like pain in the mouth (tongue, tonsils, throat, or sometimes ear). It may awaken the patient at night. There may be a history of syncope from coughing.

Cause

The cause is unknown. Triggers may include swallowing, yawning, talking, or chewing.

Evaluation

Neurologic examination is negative.

Management

Management is the same as for trigeminal neuralgia—carbamazepine. Surgical microvascular decompression appears to be an effective treatment.[6]

Atypical Face Pain

Classic Presentation

A middle-aged woman (between 30 and 50 years of age) complains of constant facial pain that is described as burning. The woman often will have a history of psychiatric problems, depression, drug addiction, high-stress personal life, and a positive family history (60% of patients).

Cause

The cause is unknown.

Evaluation

Neurologic examination is negative. If suspected, evaluation for depression may be appropriate.

Management

Cervical spine manipulation theoretically may be of benefit, but there are no reports in the literature. Analgesics should be considered; if not effective, referral for stronger medication.

APPENDIX 43–1

References

1. Green DB. Orofacial and craniofacial pain: primary care concerns. *Postgrad Med.* 1992;57:64.

2. Bogduk N, Marsland A. The cervical zygapophyseal joints as a source of neck pain. *Spine.* 1988;13:610.

3. Aminoff MJ. Nervous system. In: Tierney LM, McPhee SJ, Papadakis MA, eds. *Current Medical Diagnosis & Treatment.* 34th ed. Norwalk, CT: Appleton & Lange; 1995:831.

4. Yochum TR, Rowe LJ. *Essentials of Skeletal Radiology.* 2nd ed. Baltimore: Williams & Wilkins; 1996;1:12–19.

5. Young RF. Electrical stimulation of the trigeminal nerve root for the treatment of chronic facial pain. *J Neurosurg.* 1995;83:72–78.

6. Resnick DK, Jannetta PJ, Bissonnette D, et al. Microvascular decompression for glossopharyngeal neuralgia. *Neurosurgery.* 1995;36:64–68.

Ear Pain

Context

A complaint of ear pain usually raises the concern of an ear infection. It is interesting to note that although commonly a cause in children, in adults, one study[1] indicated that ear pain was referred in 60% of patients. Even more interesting is that 80% of those with referred pain were found to have temporomandibular (TMJ), cervical spine, or a dental (50%) pathology or dysfunction. Therefore, it appears that ear pain is often best evaluated and treated by one of three specialists: the chiropractor, the pediatrician, or the dentist.

Otitis media is the most common diagnosis in children and the second most common diagnosis in medicine; approximately two-thirds of all children in the United States are affected by age 2 years.[2, 3] Depending on the type (acute otitis, recurrent acute otitis, otitis media with effusion, chronic otitis media), management may include antibiotics, decongestants, tympanostomy tubes, or other surgical procedures. The major medical concern with otitis media with effusion is that it is believed that associated hearing loss in infants can impair language development.[4, 5] Other studies have criticized the methodology used in studies that claim risk.[6] Most cases of hearing loss associated with otitis media with effusion resolve spontaneously in six to eight weeks.[7]

General Strategy

History

- Determine whether the pain is due to trauma (lacerations, hematoma, temporal bone fracture).
- Determine whether the pain is superficial (skin lesions) or deep (otitis externa, media, or cholesteatoma).

- Determine whether the pain is unilateral or bilateral (bilateral is more common with otitis externa).
- Determine whether there are associated auditory or vestibular symptoms (otitis media, labyrinthitis, cholesteatoma).
- Determine whether there are associated signs or symptoms of infection (acute otitis media).
- Determine whether there are any oral, TMJ, cervical spine, or facial symptoms.

Evaluation

- Evaluate the outside of the ear and palpate for tenderness; otoscopically evaluate the ear.
- Examine the TMJ, cervical spine, and mouth.

Management

- Refer for obvious cases of bacterial infection.
- Follow Agency for Healthcare Research and Quality guidelines[8] with regard to otitis media with effusion.
- Refer to dentist for dental pathology.
- Manage TMJ and cervical spine problems initially; refer if unsuccessful.

Relevant Anatomy and Physiology

The external ear is innervated by several sensory nerves, as follows:

- Arnold's nerve (sensory branch of the vagus)
- Jacobson's nerve (sensory branch of the glossopharyngeal)

- Auriculotemporal nerve (sensory branch of the trigeminal; V3)
- A branch of the facial nerve
- Greater auricular and lesser occipital nerves (C2 and C3)

However, the common end-point for central projections from the primary neurons of the above nerves is in the spinal nucleus of cranial nerve V. This spinal nucleus merges with the dorsal horn of C1 through C3 in the trigeminocervical nucleus. This convergence explains why referred pain to the ear is so common.

A central concept in ear complaints and disorders is dysfunction of the eustachian (auditory) tube. The eustachian tube is extremely important in that it provides a drainage and ventilation source for the middle ear via a communication with the nasopharynx.[9] Normally, the eustachian tube remains closed except when swallowing or yawning. Through swallowing, the middle ear is ventilated about three to four times per minute. Narrowing or blockage of the tube may occur through tube lining edema. This is often due to viral infections or allergies. Congenital narrowing of the canal may also occur. In children, the canal is usually narrow and more horizontal than it is in adults, leading to an age-related predisposition to eustachian tube involvement. A temporal sequence of dysfunction may occur. If the blockage is temporary or partial, air in the middle ear is trapped and absorbed, with a resultant negative pressure. This may be visible otoscopically as a retracted tympanic membrane. If transient, yawning, swallowing, or autoinflation (forced exhalation through closed nostrils) will cause a popping or crackling sound with some relief. If more chronic, the negative pressure will draw fluid into the ear, causing a serous otitis media. If the fluid becomes infected, the patient may develop acute otitis media.

Evaluation

History

The history can quickly determine whether the cause is due to barotrauma effects; infection; or referral from the teeth, TMJ, or cervical spine (**Table 44–1**). Bilateral pain is uncommon and often indicates external otitis. Other clues include whether the person has recently gone swimming, cleans the ears by overinserting cotton swabs, or sticks other foreign objects in the ears, such as pencils.

Young children with signs of an upper respiratory infection with fever may have a bacterially caused, acute otitis media. Associated temporary conductive hearing loss is common. Left untreated, the pain may migrate to behind the ear when the mastoid air cells become involved. The pain is often severe and causes disruption of sleep. Infants may constantly grab their ears. If ear pain is associated with vertigo and hearing loss, consider labyrinthitis. If the pain is better with swallowing, chewing, or yawning, barotrauma or serous otitis media is possible. If the pain occurs with air travel only or diving, barotrauma is likely the cause. With air travel the pain is often worse on descent. Sharp, stabbing pains are felt deep in the ear.

Pain made worse with chewing or yawning is suggestive of a TMJ disorder. Associated complaints will include clicking or popping of the jaw or occasional locking of the jaw. The pain is often unilateral. Dental pathology is also a possible cause of referral. When dental pulp is inflamed (pulpitis) as a result of caries, trauma, or dental surgery, pain is provoked by hot or cold foods and sweets. When the pulp undergoes necrosis, local gas is produced, which, when expanded by heat, increases pressure and causes pain. Cold decreases the gas pressure and relieves the pain. There are apical foramina that connect the pulp to the periodontal ligament and periapical alveolar bone. Infection or inflammation may spread through this connection, leading to a tooth that is sensitive to compressive pressure from chewing or percussion. This is also found with a cracked tooth.

Examination

A general screen of the patient with ear pain consists of the following:

- Observe the area for lacerations, skin lesions, or discharge from the ear canal.
- Take the patient's temperature.
- Otoscopically evaluate the canal for inflammation, obstruction, infection, or fluid distention.
- Screen for possible TMJ referral pain.
- Screen the cervical spine with palpation, compression, and distraction.
- Evaluate the teeth and palpate/percuss for tenderness, especially in the molar region.

Otoscopic evaluation of the ear will often reveal an underlying cause. Some classic otoscopic appearances follow:

- Otitis externa—erythema and edema of the ear canal with a purulent discharge

Table 44–1 History Questions for Ear Pain

Primary Question	What Are You Thinking?	Secondary Question	What Are You Thinking?
Did the pain occur after being hit in the ear?	Lacerations, fracture, hematoma, perforated ear drum, perilymphatic fistula.	Any fluid leaking from the ear? Pain associated with dizziness or tinnitus?	Fracture. Perilymphatic fistula or perforated ear drum.
Did the pain occur after or during flying or scuba diving?	Barotrauma, eustachian tube dysfunction.	Severe pain felt mainly on the descent?	Eustachian tube dysfunction, especially in a patient with an upper respiratory infection or allergies.
Was the pain felt after swimming?	Otitis externa, ruptured tympanic membrane.	Past history of severe or recurrent ear infections? Ear is painful to touch and/or itchy?	Ruptured tympanic membrane. Otitis externa.
Do you have a cough or fever and/or other signs of a respiratory infection?	Acute otitis, labyrinthitis.	Are you also dizzy or have any hearing loss? Is the pain associated with a fullness with a "blocked" ear sensation?	Labyrinthitis more likely (rare). Acute otitis more likely.
Do you insert anything into your ears such as paper clips, pencils, cotton-tipped swabs, towel tips?	Foreign body, otitis externa.	Is your ear tender to touch or itchy?	Otitis externa likely.
Is the pain made worse with jaw motion?	TMJ, dental problem, elongated styloid.	Is the pain worse when eating cold, hot, or sweet foods? Is the pain worse with biting down? Is the pain worse with opening the mouth wide or associated with popping and clicking of the jaw? Is the pain in front of the ear and worse while opening?	Cavity or pulpitis likely. TMJ or cracked tooth. TMJ likely. Elongated styloid.
Is the pain worse with neck movement?	Cervical spine dysfunction.	Do you have associated neck pain?	Cervical spine arthritis or subluxation.

- Acute otitis media—absent or distorted light reflex indicating bulging of the tympanic membrane; the tympanic membrane may be hypomobile with pneumatic challenge
- Serous otitis media—tympanic membrane may appear yellow-amber in color; air-fluid level or air bubbles may be evident
- Chronic otitis media—diminished or absent landmarks on the tympanic membrane; perforation is often seen

Numerous skin lesions may affect the ear. A list of some of the more common includes:

- Furuncles from infected hair follicles may appear.

- Polyps due to granulomatous processes may appear in the ear canal.
- Keloid is an overgrowth of scar tissue that is often the result of trauma (often due to ear piercing), more commonly seen in blacks.
- Sebaceous cysts are more common behind the lobule of the ear; they have a central black punctum (indicates blocked sebaceous gland).
- Tophi are small, whitish-yellow nodules found on the helix or antihelix in individuals with gout; they are usually hard and nontender.
- Chondrodermatitis presents as painful nodules on the rim of the helix.

When results of the otoscopic examination and outer inspection of the ear are normal, referral pain is likely. Focus on a thorough examination of the teeth, TMJ, and cervical spine.

Management

There is much debate with regard to the management of otitis media. Regarding chiropractic management, it is common practice for many chiropractors to use manipulation and other mechanical maneuvers to improve otitis media, but a recent review[10] found no evidence to support or refute this approach. Interestingly a review in 2013[11] reflected a major shift in opinion by the medical profession regarding the initial management of otitis media. The authors from an international otolaryngology organization stated that management should begin with watchful waiting. They recommended that herbal eardrops or homeopathic treatments may help decrease pain and even lead to faster resolution, and those that fail to improve with observation or CAM (after 48–72h) should be treated with antibiotics and, in some cases, surgical intervention. They go on to recommend a preventive strategy that includes elimination of risk factors such as second-hand smoke, and encouraging breast feeding and discouraging bottle-feeding, and maintaining proper nutrition and vaccinations. They also suggested that probiotics and xylitol may be helpful.

With acute otitis, it is generally accepted that antibiotics are warranted because of the bacterial etiology. If the otitis is in fact viral (recurrent otitis or otitis media with effusion), however, the approach is not clear. It is known that otitis media with effusion will self-resolve in six to eight weeks. However, when recurrent, it is often suggested to use drainage tubes (tympanostomy tubes). The evidence for their effectiveness has come under criticism. One study[12] indicated that more than half of these procedures were either inappropriate or had equivocal clinical indications. Clarification has come from recommendations for otitis media with effusion made by the Agency for Healthcare Research and Quality (AHRQ) guidelines of 1994.[8] If the child has no craniofacial or neurologic abnormalities or sensory deficits, the AHRQ panel recommends initial treatment to consist of observation or antibiotic treatment. The panel recommends against myringotomy with or without tympanostomy tubes. After three months, antibiotics or tubes are recommended in children with a bilateral hearing deficit of 20-dB hearing threshold level or worse. One environmental influence that can be modified includes avoidance of exposure to cigarette smoking. There also appears to be an association with daycare facilities and bottle-feeding in infants. The panel also found that decongestants and/or antihistamines, corticosteroids, and tonsillectomy were ineffective treatments for otitis media with effusion.

There are many anecdotal reports of the benefits of chiropractic treatment. However, only one recent study[13] showed a benefit. This well-designed study used otoscopic and tympanographic data to evaluate the effectiveness of chiropractic adjusting on acute otitis, chronic serous otitis, and a mixed typed. Preliminary results are encouraging. More research is needed.

The following are brief recommendations for ear pain based on condition.

Barotrauma

- Swallow, yawn, and autoinflate often during a flight descent.
- Take decongestants several hours before arrival.
- Use nasal spray one hour before arrival.
- Do not sleep during the descent phase (leads to markedly negative pressure).
- Warn individuals who have tympanic membrane perforation that diving is not allowed because the unbalanced thermal stimulation may lead to vertigo.
- Advise individuals with normal hearing in only one ear to avoid diving because of the risk of otologic injury to the good ear.
- Caution patients with upper respiratory infections to avoid diving.

Otitis Externa

- Patients should be instructed to keep the ear dry, avoid overinsertion or cleaning with cotton swabs, and avoid scratching the ears.
- Patient should be warned not to swim in potentially contaminated water.

There is a belief among some chiropractors that otitis media is best managed conservatively with cervical spine manipulation and/or massage and diet recommendations. The effectiveness of chiropractic manipulation requires research. Articles by Hendricks and Larkin-Thier,[14] Hobbs and Rasmussen,[15] and Philips[16] review these concepts.

Algorithm

An algorithm for evaluation and management of ear pain is presented in **Figure 44–1**.

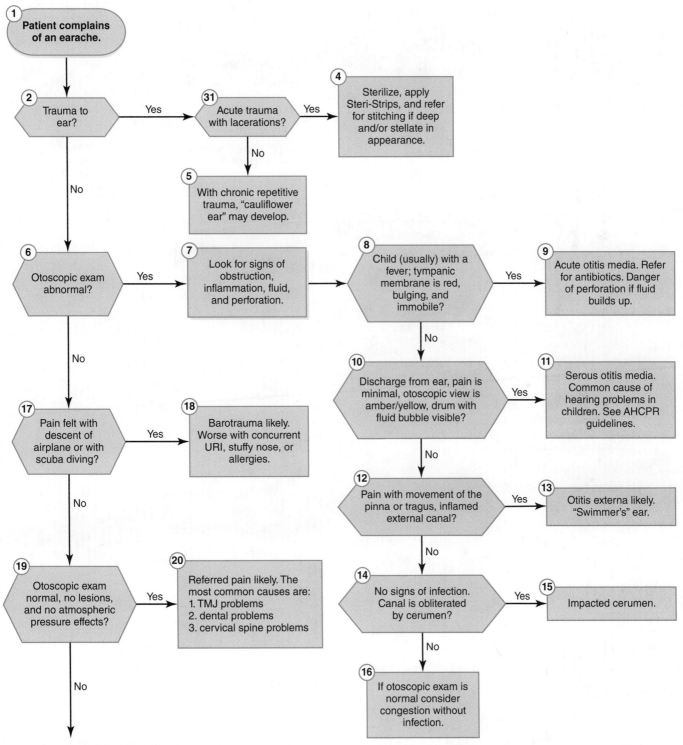

Figure 44–1 Ear Pain—Algorithm

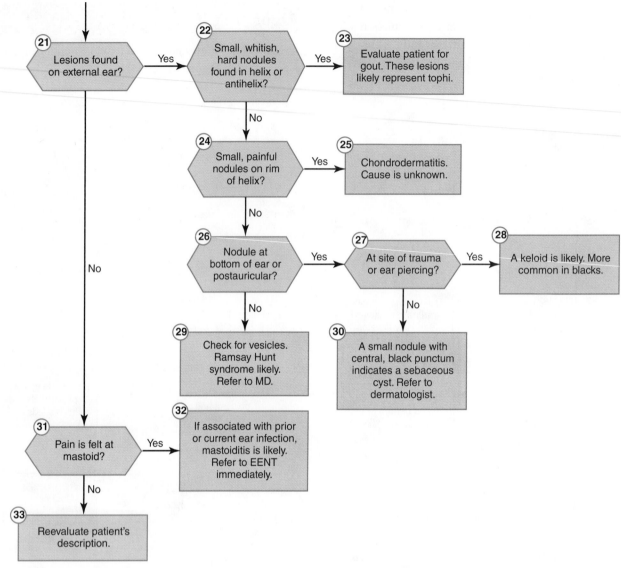

Figure 44–1 (Continued)

Selected Causes of Ear Pain

Barotrauma

Classic Presentation

The patient complains of severe ear pain on airplane descent. A sharp, stabbing pain in the ear may be felt. Another presentation is a patient who feels a similar sharp pain with underwater diving. The pain is usually felt within the first 15 ft of descent.

Cause

The cause is failure of equalization of pressure in the middle ear by a narrowed eustachian tube. This is usually due to mucosal edema from an upper respiratory infection or allergy or from a congenitally narrowed tube. Vascular congestion, specifically venous congestion, may also occur but be more prolonged symptomatically.

Evaluation

Otoscopic evaluation should be performed to determine whether there is any associated rupture of the tympanic membrane or otitis externa or media.

Management

Suggestions to the airplane traveler are to use frequent yawning, swallowing, and autoinflating (forced exhalation against closed nostrils) during the descent. If unsuccessful, the use of a systemic decongestant several hours before descent and a nasal decongestant one hour before descent is usually successful. In recalcitrant cases, myringotomy or the insertion of ventilating tubes is necessary, or the avoidance of flying altogether. Serous otitis media may follow an episode of barotrauma.

Serous Otitis Media

Classic Presentation

A patient presents with a complaint of fullness for several weeks, and possible hearing loss or pain associated with past history of upper respiratory infection, an episode of acute otitis, or barotrauma.

Cause

A persistently closed eustachian tube allows a negative pressure to develop in the middle ear, which then causes transudation of fluid into the middle ear space. This is more common in children because of a more horizontal canal, and in both adults and children because of infection, allergy, or barotrauma.

Evaluation

Otoscopic evaluation will reveal a dull, hypomobile tympanic membrane. Occasionally, bubbles may be visible. Hearing loss, if present, is conductive.

Management

Although a short course of corticosteroids or antibiotics is often prescribed, there appears to be little long-term benefit. Medical recommendations for tympanostomy tubes for the treatment of recurrent otitis have been questioned. It is estimated that the recommendations in more than half of cases are either inappropriate (23%) or based on equivocal indications (35%).[12] (The reader is directed elsewhere[14-16] for a discussion of chiropractic management.) In adults, persistent otitis media may be an indication of nasopharyngeal carcinoma.[17]

Acute Otitis Media (AOM)

Classic Presentation

The patient is often a child or infant (although adults are affected) with fever who complains of deep ear pain, a pressure sensation, and decreased hearing.

Cause

Potential risk factors for AOM include:

- Younger than 2 years old (eustachian tube is shorter and angled less)
- Male gender
- Daycare attendance
- Fall or winter season
- Exposure to cigarette smoke
- Genetic factors
- Prior history of AOM

Recurrence of AOM is common. A recent study[18] examined the contribution of a number of suspected factors and concluded that the use of pacifiers, less breastfeeding, infants of older age, the winter season, upper respiratory tract infections and adenoid hypertrophy all increase risk of recurrence. Exposure to secondhand smoke did not seem to be a factor in this study.

In primary care, AOM accounts for 30 million patient visits in the United States, costing an estimated $5 billion annually.[19] Seemingly straightforward, the diagnosis of AOM is actually difficult. Some studies have indicated that 40% of the time doctors are uncertain of their diagnosis.[20,21] There are varying criteria, making the diagnosis even more ambiguous; however, the Agency for Healthcare Research and Quality (AHRQ) standard is probably the most accepted.[22] The criteria, in essence, states that in addition to signs of a middle ear effusion, there must be rapid onset (over 48 hours) plus an additional sign or signs including otalgia (pulling of ear in an infant), otorrhea, irritability (in infant or toddler), and/or fever. One study indicated that if these criteria were used, there would be a reduction in the diagnosis of AOM by more than 20%.[23] Co-infection with viruses is common, although in less than 10% of cases viruses are the only cause. Ironically, most ear infections resolve without any treatment, so the role of bacteria or viruses is unclear.

Acute otitis often represents the next stage after serous otitis with eustachian tube involvement. Viral infections and other causes of eustachian tube inflammation cause blockage and subsequent negative pressure development. Middle ear fluid resulting from a negative pressure provides a culture medium for bacteria. Also, migration of microorganisms along the eustachian tube mucosa may occur without blockage. Common organisms are *Moraxella catarrhalis, Streptococcus pneumoniae, Haemophilus influenzae,* and *Streptococcus pyogenes.* Episodes are more common in the fall, winter, and spring. More than 66% of children under age 3 years have at least one episode. There is mounting evidence that there is a strong genetic component to the length of time one has middle ear effusion and the number of episodes.[24]

Evaluation

The patient will often have a fever. The tympanic membrane will appear erythematous and be hypomobile. Bullae may also be seen. When empyema occurs, the tympanic membrane may bulge, indicating impending perforation. The diagnostic value was measured in a meta-analysis in 2010.[25] For tympanic membrane bulging there was a positive likelihood ratio of 51 (95% confidence interval {CI}, 36-73) and for redness a positive likelihood ratio of 8.4 (95% CI, 7-11). Mobility of the tympanic membrane is tested using the pneumatic attachment to the otoscope (bulb), sometimes referred to as insufflation. One study indicated that only 10 to 15 mm of pressure is needed to assess drum mobility and that most bulb attachments can generate up to 1,000 mm or more.[26] For children older than 18 months, a soft-tipped speculum should be used to provide an adequate seal. It is crucial that the otoscope is checked on a regular basis given the findings of one emergency department study indicating that 22% of the time there was a worn bulb or a weak battery.[27] A recent study evaluated the ability of the physician to diagnose AOM and found that, although many studies have been limited by bias, the most helpful indicator is a cloudy, bulging, immobile tympanic membrane.[28] An additional indicator is the color of the tympanic membrane: A normal color makes AOM highly unlikely, whereas a red membrane substantially increases the likelihood.

Management

Referral for further evaluation and determination of the need for antibiotic treatment is warranted because of the seriousness of potential complications. However, it should be noted that in a 2010 *JAMA* review and meta-analysis,[25] the conclusion was that antibiotics are only modestly more effective than no treatment. They add that the concern about use is that antibiotics cause adverse effects in 4% to 10% of children. Although the introduction of a vaccine to prevent recurrent AOM occurred a number of years ago, the use of pneumococcal conjugate vaccine (PCV), in particular PCV7, is not recommended based on the conclusions of a 2009 Cochrane review.[29] Also, the use of this vaccine caused a decrease of *S. pneumonia* cases and an increase in *H. influenzae* cases. The concern by medical physicians, though, is that left untreated there may be complications that include labyrinthitis, meningitis, mastoiditis, hearing loss, and facial paralysis. One to several weeks of untreated or inadequately treated acute otitis can lead to these serious consequences. Clues of complication may include the development of a headache, sudden hearing loss, vertigo, or fever with chills.

Chronic Otitis Media

Classic Presentation

The patient presents with a history of recurrent acute ear infections. Currently, he or she complains of ear discharge that is worse with colds and swimming. There is little pain, but often a complaint of some hearing loss.

Cause

Chronic infection of the middle ear and mastoid may lead to perforation of the tympanic membrane and degeneration of the tympanic membrane or ossicles. This results in a conductive hearing loss. Common organisms include *Pseudomonas aeruginosa*, *Proteus*, and *Staphylococcus aureus*.

Evaluation

Otoscopy often reveals perforation of the tympanic membrane and discharge. Tests for hearing reveal a conductive hearing loss.

Management

Initial treatment consists of antibiotic drops to the ears, systemic antipseudomonal antibiotics, removal of infected debris, and either avoidance of swimming or the use of ear plugs. Surgery eventually may be necessary to reconstruct the tympanic membrane.

Cholesteatoma

Classic Presentation

The patient presents similarly to the patient with chronic otitis media; however, the patient may have more dizziness or pain.

Cause

With a chronic dysfunction of the eustachian tube, negative pressure pulls the upper tympanic membrane inward to form a sac, which can grow and become infected. If the cholesteatoma enlarges it may erode or compress the tympanic membrane, ossicles, or the mastoid.

Evaluation

Otoscopic evaluation may reveal a retraction pocket and exudate. Hearing loss is conductive.

Management

The treatment of choice is surgical removal and sometimes a surgically created connection between the ear canal and mastoid.

Otitis Externa

Classic Presentation

The patient is often a swimmer complaining of ear pain, itching, and discharge. The patient is more likely to present during warm, humid weather.

Cause

Infection of the ear or ear canal is caused by exposure to infected water or is caused by scratching or overaggressive use of cotton applicators. The infection is usually due to bacteria such as *Pseudomonas* or *Proteus* or fungi such as *Aspergillus*. The fungal growth is assisted by excessive moisture in the ear.

Evaluation

Pain is produced by pulling on the ear. The ear canal demonstrates erythema and edema, associated sometimes with a purulent discharge.

Management

Referral for antibiotic drops is necessary. Additional preventive advice includes keeping the ear dry and avoiding cotton swabs or other mechanical trauma (e.g., pencils) in the ear canal.

APPENDIX 44–1

Web Resources

Otitis Media
American Academy of Pediatrics
http://www.aap.org/en-us/Pages/Default.aspx

APPENDIX 44–2

References

1. Thaller SR, Thaller JL. Head and neck symptoms: is the problem in the ear, face, neck, or oral cavity? *Postgrad Med.* 1990;87:75–77,83–86.

2. Lohr KN, Beck S, Kamberg KJ, et al. *Measurement of Physiologic Health for Children: Middle Ear Disease and Hearing Impairment.* Santa Monica, CA: Rand Health Experiment Series; 1983.

3. Shappert SM. *Office Visits for Otitis Media: United States, 1975–1990: Advance Data.* Hyattsville, MD: National Center for Health Statistics; 1992:214.

4. Teele DW, Klein JO, Rosner RA, et al. Greater Boston Otitis Media Study Group: otitis media with effusion during the first three years of life and development of speech and language. *Pediatrics.* 1984;74:282–287.

5. Rach GH, Ziethuis GA, VanBaarle PW, et al. The effect of treatment with ventilating tubes on language development in preschool children with otitis media with effusion. *Clin Otolaryngol.* 1991;16:128–132.

6. Paradise JL. Otitis media during early life: how hazardous to development? A critical review of the evidence. *Pediatrics.* 1981;68:869–873.

7. Cross AW. Health screening in schools. *J Pediatr.* 1985;107(pt 1):487–494.

8. Stool SE, Berg AO, Berman S, et al. *Managing Otitis Media with Effusion in Young Children: Quick Reference Guide for Clinicians.* Rockville, MD: Agency for Health Care Policy and Research, Public Health Service, U.S. Dept of Health and Human Services; 1994. AHCPR publication 94-0623.

9. Bluestone CD, Doyle WJ. Anatomy and physiology of eustachian tube and middle ear related to otitis media. *Allerg Clin Immunol.* 1988;81:997.

10. Pohlman KA, Holton-Brown MS. Otitis media and spinal manipulative therapy: a literature review. *J Chiropr Med.* 2012;11(3):160–169.

11. Levi JR, Brody RM, McKee-Cole K, Pribitkin E, O'Reilly R. Complementary and alternative medicine for pediatric otitis media. *Int J Pediatr Otorhinolaryngol.* 2013;77(6):926–931.

12. Kleinmann LC, Kosecoff J, Dubois R, Brook RH. The medical appropriateness of tympanostomy tubes proposed for children younger than 16 years in the United States. *JAMA.* 1994;271:1250–1255.

13. Fallon JM. The role of the chiropractic adjustment in the care and treatment of 332 children with otitis media. *J Clin Chiro Pediatr.* 1997;2(2).

14. Hendricks CL, Larkin-Thier SM. Otitis media in young children. *Chiro J Chiro Res Study.* 1989;2:9–13.

15. Hobbs DA, Rasmussen SA. Chronic otitis media: a case report. *J Chiro.* 1991;28:67–68.

16. Philips NJ. Vertebral subluxation and otitis media: a case study. *Chiro J Chiro Res Study.* 1992;8:38–39.

17. Sham JST. Serous otitis media: an opportunity for early recognition of nasopharyngeal carcinoma. *Arch Otolaryngol.* 1992;118:794.

18. Salah M, Abdel-Aziz M, Al-Farok A, Jebrini A. Recurrent acute otitis media in infants: analysis of risk factors. *Int J Pediatr Otorhinolaryngol.* 2013;77(10):1665–1669.

19. Rosenfeld R, Bluestone C. *Evidence-Based Otitis Media.* St. Louis, MO: BC Decker, 1999.

20. Steinbach WJ, Sectish TC. Pediatric resident training in the diagnosis and treatment of acute otitis media. *Pediatrics.* 2002;109:404–408.

21. Steinbach WJ, Sectish TC, Benjamin DK Jr. Pediatric residents' clinical diagnostic accuracy of acute otitis media. *Pediatrics.* 2002;109:993–998.

22. Marcy M. *Management of Acute Otitis Media.* Rockville, MD: Agency for Healthcare Research and Quality, May 2001:1–159.

23. Rosenfeld RW. Diagnostic certainty for acute otitis media. *Int J Pediatr. (International Journal of Pediatrics Otorhinolaryngology).* 2002;64:89–95.

24. Casselbrant ML, Mandel EM, Fall PA. The heritability of otitis media: a twin and triplet study. *JAMA.* 1999;282:2125–2130.

25. Coker TR, Chan LS, Newberry SJ, et al. Diagnosis, microbial epidemiology, and antibiotic treatment of

acute otitis media in children: a systematic review. *JAMA.* 2010;304(19):2161–2169.

26. Cavanaugh RM Jr. Pediatricians and the pneumatic otoscope: are we playing it by ear? *Pediatrics.* 1989;84:362–364.

27. Barriga F, Schwartz RH, Hayden GF. Adequate illumination for otoscopy: variation due to power source, bulb, and head and speculum design. *AIDC.* 1986;140:1237–1240.

28. Rothman R, Owens T, Simel DL. Does this child have acute otitis media? *JAMA.* 2003:290:1633–1640.

29. Jansen AG, Hak E, Veenhoven RH, Damoiseaux RA, Schilder AG, Sanders EA. Pneumococcal conjugate vaccines for preventing otitis media. *Cochrane Database Syst Rev.* 2009(2):CD001480.

Hearing Loss

# CHAPTER 45

Context

Hearing loss is a frightening occurrence, which, when sudden, would cause most patients to seek the attention of a medical doctor or emergency department. The acuteness and degree of loss would be steering factors that would influence a patient's decision to seek immediate attention. Mild to moderate loss, especially over time, or if assumed to be related to congestion from a respiratory infection, post-airline flight, or cerumen would allow most patients to adopt a "wait-and-see" attitude for at least several days. Another context is the patient who is not aware of the degree of loss because of the chronicity of the problem or he or she assumes that it is related to aging. The chiropractor is more likely to see these patients with chronic, mild loss or those unaware of loss. If a screening examination for hearing loss is conducted on patients complaining of loss and on the elderly, most cases can be discovered. Although some cases of hearing loss are nonrecoverable, sudden loss often spontaneously recovers over 7 to 10 days.[1, 2]

Although chiropractic was launched from an anecdotal reporting of hearing recovery, it is unfortunate that the literature is barren of any significant case reports or large studies. Nonetheless, there are still anecdotal reports, often given at seminars and among colleagues, warranting at least a consideration for study.

Hearing loss in the infant or child is most often due to congenital causes or acquired secondary to infection. In older adults, hearing loss is often age-related due to degeneration of hair cells in the organ of Corti. Following osteoarthritis and hypertension, hearing loss is the third most common chronic condition in seniors.[3] Estimates of prevalence are about 25% to 40% in patients 65 years and older.[4] After 75 years of age the prevalence increases to between 40% and 66%, and then to 80% after age 85 years. It is important to note that there is a strong correlation between hearing loss and depression in the older patient. Although hearing loss in the elderly is primarily due to presbycusis, up to 30% of the elderly have hearing loss secondary to cerumen impaction and chronic otitis media.

General Strategy

History and Examination

- Determine whether the hearing loss was sudden (trauma, viral, or vascular) or chronic/insidious.
- Determine if associated with dizziness.
- Determine whether there are any underlying systemic or whole-body processes such as diabetes, multiple sclerosis, or Paget's disease.
- Determine whether there was an associated event such as trauma or infection.
- Differentiate between conductive and sensorineural loss with simple tuning fork tests.
- Refer for audiologic or imaging studies when hearing loss is evident.

Management

- Refer to otolaryngologist or neurologist when appropriate. Some examples include the following:
  1. ear infection or mastoid involvement
  2. suspected medication-induced hearing loss from prescribed ototoxic medication
  3. possible acoustic neuroma or other tumor
  4. perilymphatic fistula that is interfering with patient's lifestyle

- Refer for hearing aid if the following circumstances apply:
  1. patient has a diagnosis of presbycusis and hearing loss is interfering with lifestyle
  2. patient has had surgical correction for otosclerosis and now suffers some sensorineural loss
- Use a trial treatment with chiropractic manipulative therapy (CMT) when it appears that a complex of symptoms such as post-whiplash syndrome is apparent or when medical management offers no clear-cut solution.

Relevant Anatomy and Physiology

Hearing is a remarkable sense that performs a transformation of mechanical vibration into electric potentials that are then processed and integrated into a composite impression of one's environment. The interface of this transformation is the fluid environment of the middle ear. The structural components of this system are the ear canal, the eardrum, and the bony ossicles. The efficiency of this impedance-matching system may be compromised, leading to a decrease in the perception of loudness but leaving the quality of the sound unaffected. This is referred to as a conduction hearing loss. Dampening of sound may occur with blockage of the ear canal by cerumen or a foreign body, or by middle ear effusion. If the ossicles are sclerotic (otosclerosis) or damaged due to trauma/pathology, sound is not transmitted efficiently.

Pathology of the hair cells of the organ of Corti, the cochlear nerve, or in rarer cases, the central transmission of these sound signals will result in a sensorineural loss that is clinically represented by both a decrease in loudness and a distortion of sound quality.

Hearing is not only a function of loudness threshold and frequency perception; a patient's individual requirements (e.g., a musician), the ability to concentrate, environmental distraction, and central processing are also factors. The audible range of frequencies is between approximately 16 and 16,000 Hz, with the majority of speech limited to 300 to 3,000 Hz. The overtones that affect the quality of speech, however, are above 3,000 Hz. Loudness is measured in decibels (dB). This is a logarithmic scale, not linear. Therefore, a 20-dB tone carries 100 times the energy of a 1-dB tone; a 30-dB tone, 1,000 times that of a 1-dB tone. The threshold level is an important indicator of hearing loss. Normally, a whisper can be heard, indicating a hearing threshold of between 0 and 20 dB. Normal speaking is between 40 and 60 dB; a shout is 80 dB or above. A 10- to 15-dB threshold loss is often not noticed. Generally, a loss averaging between 20 and 25 dB between 300 and 3,000 Hz (speech frequencies) is noticed by the patient. A loss exceeding 30 to 40 dB is a significant handicap for conversation.

Evaluation

History

In obtaining the history (**Table 45–1**), determine the following:

- whether the patient has had a sudden or insidious loss and whether it is bilateral
- whether there has been any specific event onset such as past infection or trauma, including head trauma and barotrauma from scuba diving or airplane travel
- whether the patient has been prescribed any ototoxic medications
- whether there is past or current history of occupational or recreational noise exposure
- the extent of functional impact on patient's life (social and occupational)
- whether there are any previous diagnoses or treatment, including hearing aids or surgeries

Age of onset, acuteness of onset, and associated signs are extremely valuable in narrowing the diagnosis. Hearing deficits in an infant or young child should suggest congenital deafness or the sequelae to infection or ototoxic medication. Known ototoxic medications include:

- Antibiotics, including aminoglycosides, erythromycin, vancomycin
- Anticancer medications, including cisplatin, carboplatin, and vincristine sulfate
- Loop diuretics, including furosemide and ethacrynic acid
- Anti-inflammatory medications, including aspirin and quinine

Although the daily intake of aspirin that can cause hearing loss is not known, it is believed that 80 mg per day is safe. In most cases of aspirin-induced hearing loss, the patient will regain hearing after discontinuing

Table 45-1 History of Questions for Hearing Loss

Primary Question	What Are You Thinking?	Secondary Question	What Are You Thinking?
Was the hearing loss sudden?	Trauma, vascular, or viral infection.	**Was there an injury to the head?** **Was there trauma to the ear?** **Is there a recent history of coronary bypass surgery or a history of stroke or transient ischemic attacks?** **(If appropriate) Did the hearing loss resolve within 10 days?**	Fracture of the temporal bone. Barotrauma to the tympanic membrane or a perilymphatic fistula. Vascular infarction of cochlear nerve (usually would involve other areas with other signs or symptoms). Viral infection likely.
Does the hearing loss fluctuate (come and go)?	Ménière's, recurrent otitis media, cerumen impaction, eustachian tube dysfunction.	**Hearing loss associated with recurrent bouts of dizziness?** **Recurrent ear infections?** **History of allergies and/or extreme pain with airplane descent, bilateral?**	Ménière's disease is likely. Chronic otitis media. Auditory tube dysfunction.
Is the hearing loss chronic?	Presbycusis, otosclerosis, congenital acoustic neuroma, ototoxicity, noise pollution.	**Is it difficult to hear on the phone?** **No problem in noisy rooms?** **(With an older patient) Difficulty carrying on a conversation in crowded rooms or understanding women's voices or those with accents?** **Are you taking high doses of aspirin or other "pain killers," chemotherapy, or antibiotics (aminoglycosides)?** **Do you or have you worked with loud power tools or in a loud machinery environment?**	Otosclerosis is likely. Presbycusis is likely. Ototoxicity is likely. Sensorineural loss due to hair cell trauma (organ of Corti).

aspirin. In one study[5] evaluating almost 27,000 men for hearing loss related to analgesic use, researchers concluded that regular use of aspirin, NSAIDs, or acetaminophen increases the risk of hearing loss in men, with the highest risk group being those 50 years of age and younger. A similar association was found for women in a study[6] published in 2012; however, the researchers found no association with aspirin but there was an association with ibuprofen and acetaminophen. In all studies, the relationship is dose-dependent with those chronically taking these medications more than twice per week.

Insidious onset in the middle-aged patient is suggestive of otosclerosis. In the elderly patient, various forms of presbycusis are the first suspicion. When sudden and associated with signs of infection, transient benign processes that are viral are suggested. When the hearing loss is more profound and permanent, a bacterial etiology is more likely. Accumulated otologic trauma from

environmental noise should be sought in the middle-aged and elderly. Common sources are loud machinery and loud music (concerts or headphones). Hearing loss may be a complication of many disorders; especially noted are collagen vascular diseases, vasculitis, multiple sclerosis, osteogenesis imperfecta, and compression from Paget's disease.

Conductive hearing loss generally does not interfere with speech discrimination. The patient even may be able to hear better in noisy environments. This is due to the blockage of low-frequency sounds. This phenomenon is analogous to wearing earplugs, when the general loudness is attenuated, but the distinctness of the sound may be increased because of the blockage of other frequencies. The patient with a sensorineural deficit usually will have difficulty with speech discrimination. Patients often note that women's voices and British accents pose more of a problem. They especially find it difficult to screen out ambient noise in a noisy environment. Their hearing loss is generally in the higher ranges, whereas most environmental noise is low frequency, the range they hear best.

Sudden loss with accompanying vertigo is suggestive of labyrinthine etiology. If the attacks are recurrent with progressive hearing loss, Ménière's disease is suspected. If the vertigo gradually improves over several weeks, bacterial labyrinthitis is most likely.

Examination

- Examine the ear for signs of lesions, cerumen impaction, or infection.
- Screen with tuning fork tests, including Weber and Rinne tests.
- Use an otoscope/audiometer combination, if available, to screen for loss within speech frequency ranges.
- Refer for audiologic testing if a deficit is found.

Examination of the ear with an otoscope focuses on a search for signs of impacted cerumen, otitis media, vesicles (Ramsay Hunt syndrome), cotton swab injury, cholesteatoma, and any other obvious pathology. Patients who express a concern about hearing loss or patients with findings of hearing loss on either the whispered-voice test or audioscope test should be sent for further audiologic testing. A literature review by Bagai et al.[7] on the accuracy and precision of the clinical examination for hearing loss indicates that the best screening test for hearing loss for the elderly patient is the whispered-voice test. In-office audiologic testing with an audioscope may be performed as an alternative to the whispered-voice test or as an additional test to objectify findings of the whispered-voice test. The reviewers conclude that the Rinne and Weber tests should not be used for screening for hearing loss, and in fact these tests are designed only to discriminate between sensorineural versus conductive hearing loss.

The whispered-voice test is prefaced by explaining to the patient how the test will be performed. Standing behind the patient (out of patient's field of vision) the examiner gently occludes and rubs the external auditory canal of the nontested ear while whispering three letters and three numbers in no perceivable sequence. The patient is then instructed to repeat the letters and numbers heard. A pretest screen can be performed by repeating "99" loudly to determine if the patient understands and is able to repeat.

Type of hearing loss may be tested with two tuning fork tests, Weber and Rinne, to attempt to differentiate between conductive and sensorineural loss. Recommended are 512-Hz and 1,024-Hz tuning forks. The Weber test is performed several ways. The vibrating tuning fork is applied to the middle forehead, glabella, or middle incisors (some authors have the patient bite on the vibrating handle). With a conduction loss, the sound is heard more loudly in the affected ear. It is heard equally in both ears with normal patients and in patients with bilateral sensorineural loss (e.g., presbycusis). A conductive loss of only 5 dB will cause sound to localize to the "bad" ear.

The Rinne test evaluates bone versus air conduction. The vibrating tuning fork is applied to the patient's mastoid. The patient is instructed to indicate when the sound disappears. At this point the examiner places the tines of the tuning fork approximately 1 cm from the patient's ear. The sound should now be audible for about twice as long as when applied to the mastoid (bone). Air conduction is usually twice as long as bone conduction. Masking of the opposite ear with a noise box or any other external sound source such as compressed air or suction may help. A conductive loss of at least 20 dB is necessary to cause a negative response; sound is not longer with air conduction. Therefore, less severe hearing loss is not detectable with the Rinne test.

An in-office audiologic evaluation may be performed with an otoscope containing a built-in audiometer. Audioscopes produce pure tones at 500, 1,000, 2,000, and 4,000 Hz at 20, 25, and 40 dB. The patient is instructed to identify a test tone at the lowest decibel level of 20 dB. If not audible, a second test at 25 dB, and a third, if necessary at 40 dB, is used to determine the patient's threshold. When the threshold is identified, a start button sequences the instrument through the various frequencies in apparent random order. The patient is instructed to raise a finger each time he or she hears a tone. Missing even one tone warrants referral to an audiologist for further evaluation. A normal test is good at ruling out loss of hearing in the frequencies of speech. However, if a deficit is detected, it may be a false positive. The sensitivity for detecting hearing loss is 94%. Interestingly, the specificity is 72% in a standard physician's office and 90% in an audiologist's office.[8]

Through the use of an audioscope and a self-administered questionnaire, the Hearing Handicap Inventory for the Elderly Screening Version (HHIE-S), older patients can be reliably screened for hearing loss.[9] The HHIE-S is a ten-item, five-minute questionnaire that focuses on the degree of social and emotional handicap created by hearing loss.[10] A hearing handicap of >8 on the HHIE-S is relatively sensitive for a hearing loss of 40 dB. More serious hearing loss does not seem to change the scoring. If no hearing handicap is detected on the HHIE-S, there is only a marginally decreased probability of hearing impairment (not good for ruling out hearing loss). The ten questions are:

1. Does a hearing problem cause you to feel embarrassed when meeting new people?
2. Does a hearing problem cause you to feel frustrated when talking to members of your family?
3. Do you have difficulty hearing when someone speaks in a whisper?
4. Do you feel handicapped by a hearing problem?
5. Does a hearing problem cause you difficulty when visiting friends, relatives, or neighbors?
6. Does a hearing problem cause you to attend religious services less often than you would like?
7. Does a hearing problem cause you to have arguments with family members?
8. Does a hearing problem cause you difficulty when listening to TV or radio?
9. Do you feel that any difficulty with your hearing limits or hampers your personal or social life?
10. Does a hearing problem cause you difficulty when in a restaurant with relatives or friends?

The patient is instructed to answer yes (4 points), sometimes (2 points), or no (0 points) to each question. Scores may range from 0 (no handicap) to a maximum of 40. General use delineates probability of impairment through the following categorization:

- 0–8 = 13% probability
- 10–24 = 50% probability
- 26–40 = 84% probability

Audiologist referral is helpful when a hearing loss has been detected or in the case of infants and others unable to communicate effectively.

Referral to an audiologist results in a standard series of tests performed in a soundproofed environment. These tests include:

- Pure-tone audiometry: assesses the patient's threshold of hearing for low frequency (250 Hz) and high frequency (8 kHz)
- Word recognition testing: determines the percentage of monosyllabic words that a patient can recognize/repeat (speech discrimination score)

- Speech reception threshold measurement: measures the lowest decibel level at which a patient can repeat at least 50% of spondaic words (i.e., 2-syllable words that have equal emphasis on each syllable, such as baseball)
- Bone-conduction testing: tests for otosclerosis, acoustic reflexes for acoustic neuromas, and tympanometry for otitis media

Loss of speech discrimination ability is highly suggestive of a central cause of hearing loss. Additional testing to differentiate between central and peripheral causes of hearing loss consist of the following:

- Small-tone increment discrimination—Small differences in frequency are appreciated with more sensitivity with a peripheral cause than in the normal ear.
- Tone decay—When a tone is played over earphones, the tone appears to diminish in intensity when, in fact, it remains the same; this occurs with a central cause.
- Recruitment—Loud sounds are heard normally. This occurs with a peripheral cause.

Further testing not requiring a patient response is the brainstem auditory-evoked potential (BAEP). Surface electrodes are placed over the scalp and ears. A high-frequency click at a fixed rate and intensity is delivered and the electrical responses are measured. Seven short-latency waves can be measured within 10 milliseconds of the click. The latency of response may be used to localize the lesion site. For acoustic neuroma the true-positive rate is high at 98% (false-positive about 1%).

Management

- If there is a buildup of cerumen, suggest over-the-counter ear wax dissolvers; if ineffective, refer to primary care physician for ear lavage.
- If an acoustic neuroma, tumor, infection, or systemic process is suspected as the cause, refer to appropriate specialist for management.
- For those patients with persistent chronic otitis media, surgical management may include myringotomy (a small incision in the tympanic membrane) and tubes placed in the ear to normalize pressure by aspirating contents and aerating the middle ear. This will usually restore hearing immediately. Otolaryngologists should

determine any underlying condition that might cause eustachian tube obstruction, such as allergic disease and nasopharyngeal carcinoma.

- There are varying degrees of tympanic membrane perforations. Small perforations, usually due to either trauma or otitis media, may heal spontaneously whereas larger perforations may require surgical repair with a fascial graft (tympanoplasty).
- Another conductive hearing problem, ossicular chain discontinuities, may result from trauma or chronic, persistent ear infections. Surgical treatment includes reconstruction of the ossicular chain using implants or transposed ossicles.
- Cholesteatomas are cystic masses that form usually secondary to chronic ear infections. This mass may be limited to the middle or extend to the mastoid cavity. Otoscopic signs include superior and posterior tympanic membrane perforation and white keratinaceous debris. Although there is no medical treatment, surgical management may be suggested. The standard is a mastoidectomy to remove the cholesteatoma.
- Treatment may be warranted when there are associated signs of headache, dizziness, and neck pain post-whiplash (assuming more serious causes have been ruled out).
- Comanagement with an audiologist is appropriate when hearing loss is affecting lifestyle, all serious causes have been ruled out, and the patient is likely to have presbycusis.

Management will vary depending on scope of practice restrictions and interest. Referral is often necessary.

However, if the hearing loss is either the result of cerumen impaction or a transient phenomenon from a whiplash injury with concomitant headache, dizziness, and/or neck pain, the chiropractor may be helpful.

For pediatric hearing loss, dependent on cause, cochlear implants are now in common use. As of 2013, more than 300,000 cochlear implant surgeries have been performed.[11] Pioneered in the 1960s, major breakthroughs occurred in the 1990s so that currently mainstream schooling is the norm, reducing the number of "deaf schools." These implants are worn at ear level and consist of an implanted element that contains a receiver and electronic array that are placed within the cochlea. External components include a microphone, a speech processor, and a transmitter coil. Bilateral devices are now being utilized so that sound localization and hearing in noisy environments are improved. Cochlear implants are not perfect. They do not restore normal hearing and their function is limited by ambient noise. Music perception is also limited although these limitations are currently being researched for viable improvements.

With presbycusis, comanagement with an audiologist for prescription of a hearing aid is appropriate. For those who do not benefit from standard hearing aids, implantable hearing aids are now available. Although speech recognition and quality of life were greater with the implants, one study[12] found that two devices, the Esteem and the Carina, had problems including taste disturbance and device failure.

Algorithm

An algorithm for evaluation and management of hearing loss is presented in **Figure 45-1**.

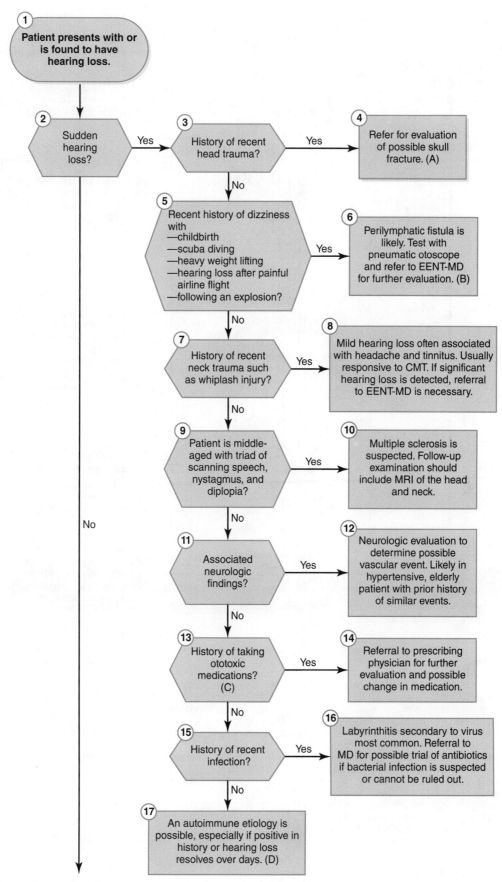

Figure 45–1 Hearing Loss—Algorithm

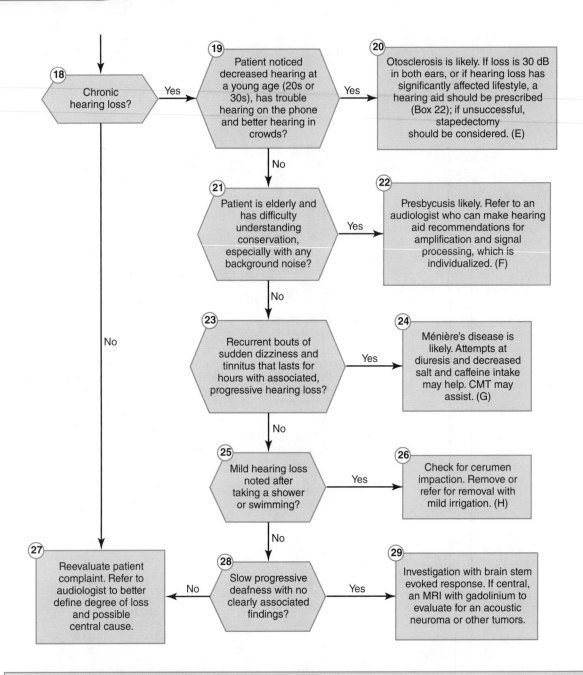

18 Chronic hearing loss? — Yes → **19** Patient noticed decreased hearing at a young age (20s or 30s), has trouble hearing on the phone and better hearing in crowds? — Yes → **20** Otosclerosis is likely. If loss is 30 dB in both ears, or if hearing loss has significantly affected lifestyle, a hearing aid should be prescribed (Box 22); if unsuccessful, stapedectomy should be considered. (E)

No ↓ (from 19)

21 Patient is elderly and has difficulty understanding conservation, especially with any background noise? — Yes → **22** Presbycusis likely. Refer to an audiologist who can make hearing aid recommendations for amplification and signal processing, which is individualized. (F)

No ↓

23 Recurrent bouts of sudden dizziness and tinnitus that lasts for hours with associated, progressive hearing loss? — Yes → **24** Ménière's disease is likely. Attempts at diuresis and decreased salt and caffeine intake may help. CMT may assist. (G)

No ↓

25 Mild hearing loss noted after taking a shower or swimming? — Yes → **26** Check for cerumen impaction. Remove or refer for removal with mild irrigation. (H)

No ↓

27 Reevaluate patient complaint. Refer to audiologist to better define degree of loss and possible central cause. ← No — **28** Slow progressive deafness with no clearly associated findings? — Yes → **29** Investigation with brain stem evoked response. If central, an MRI with gadolinium to evaluate for an acoustic neuroma or other tumors.

(18) No ↓ → 27

Annotations
A. Hearing loss subsequent to fracture is usually due to a transverse fracture of the temporal bone.
B. A perilymphatic fistula is a defect in the round or oval window that allows communication between the inner and middle ear. Surgery is often necessary.
C. Some common ototoxic drugs include salicylates, aminoglycosides, loop diuretics, and some anticancer medications.
D. A short course of corticosteroids is often used with acute hearing loss.
E. Otosclerosis is a progressive, conductive hearing loss disorder characterized by sclerosis of the bony capsule and ear ossicles, leading to a conductive hearing loss.
F. Presbycusis is a progressive sensory hearing loss that is age related. There is a selective deterioration of high-frequency hearing with an associated loss of hair cells of the organ of Corti.
G. Ménière's is a disease characterized by an increase in endolymphatic fluid pressure. There is a selective loss of low frequencies early in the course of the disease.
H. Cerumen (wax) absorbs water and expands, causing a conductive hearing loss. With swimmers check for otitis externa (swimmer's ear); often in need of antibiotic drops.

Figure 45–1 (Continued)

Selected Causes of Hearing Loss*

Otosclerosis

Classic Presentation

A patient in his or her 20s or 30s presents with a complaint of difficulty hearing on the telephone. He or she notices that there is no difficulty hearing a conversation in a noisy room or environment. The patient may note a similar history in a parent. The difficulty hearing is usually bilateral.

Cause

The cause is unknown; however, there is a familial tendency with onset occurring in the late teenage years to the 30s. There is a progressive sclerosis of the bony capsule and ear ossicles with a consequent decreased mechanical transmission of sound, producing a conductive hearing loss. The stapes is often the first bone to be affected, with the foot plate being fixed to the oval window. However, if the lesions are large enough to compress the cochlea, a sensory hearing loss will occur that is often permanent. Some practitioners feel that otosclerosis is caused by an inflammatory reaction to the measles virus.[13]

Examination

Evaluate for other causes of obstruction such as cerumen or exostoses/osteomas, which may block the ear canal. With the Rinne test, bone conduction is louder and longer than air conduction. The Weber test will localize to the involved ear if unilateral. Referral for audiologic testing is important.

Treatment

Although 10% of the white population has some degree of otosclerosis, only a small percentage develop appreciable hearing loss. Those who do may benefit from microsurgical techniques. Stapedectomy or stapedostomy are usually performed if the patient has significant hearing impairment. Others decide to live with the problem.

Presbycusis

Classic Presentation

An elderly patient presents with a complaint of hearing difficulty. He or she may notice that hearing is worse in noisy environments such as crowded rooms. Other complaints may be difficulty hearing women's voices or people with British or other accents. There may also be an associated increase in tinnitus.

Cause

It is believed that there is damage to the hair cells of the organ of Corti, producing a selective high-tone frequency hearing loss, usually bilateral. The contribution of noise trauma to presbycusis varies among individuals. It is particularly hard to hear consonants.

Evaluation

Standard Rinne and Weber testing may demonstrate a conductive hearing loss if there is cerumen or a middle ear effusion. However, the hearing loss from presbycusis is a sensorineural loss. Referral for audiologic testing is warranted if the hearing loss is a concern.

Management

There are numerous types of hearing aids available. With newer technology, some of the previous complaints have been decreased or eliminated. It is important that the patient work with the audiologist to develop a strategy for determining the degree of amplification and signal processing needed. New programmable devices allow for more sound filtering and can be set for different environmental scenarios.[14]

Although most patients with sensorineural hearing loss live with the dysfunction or use a hearing aid, those who are profoundly affected (> 80 dB loss on the better ear) may benefit from cochlear implants. Although implants have been used primarily in the pediatric population, it appears that they are a reasonable and successful option for those patients with severe hearing loss.

---

*See also Chapter 18, Dizziness, and Chapter 44, Ear Pain.

Acoustic Neuroma

Classic Presentation

A patient in their 50s or 60s presents with a complaint of mild but constant hearing loss and dizziness sometimes with associated tinnitus. The onset is gradual and may be ignored initially. There are rarely acute attacks.

Cause

A benign schwannoma of the vestibular nerve is called an acoustic neuroma. It is located in the cerebellopontine angle, where other cranial nerves are susceptible to compression. Most commonly this involves the facial nerve. As the tumor grows it may cause brainstem compression. Ninety-five percent of the time these are unilateral (bilateral may occur with neurofibromatosis). Risk factors may be smoking, pregnancy, and epilepsy.

Evaluation

Unless the tumor is large and pressing on other cranial nerves, there are likely to be no additional clinical findings. Auditory testing may reveal poor speech discrimination. Hearing loss is sensorineural. Stacked auditory brainstem response (ABR) is 95% sensitive and 88% specific for lesions < 1 cm (standard ABR only for lesions > 1 cm). When the suspicion is high, an MRI should be ordered. It is the definitive diagnostic tool.

Management

Age and growth rate need to be considered prior to a decision for surgical excision. Growth is about 5 mm in the first year of detection but less than 1 mm in the fourth year following detection.[15] Fifty-seven percent of neuromas shrink and 70% of extracanalicular lesions grow less than 2 cm per year.[16,17] Preservation of hearing is better with conservative management than with radiotherapy or surgery. A distinguishing factor is speech discrimination. Sixty-nine percent of patients with 100% speech discrimination on initial detection maintain their hearing 10 years after detection.[18] Options that are nonconservative include gamma-knife single-dose stereotactic surgery and three standard surgical approaches including retromastoid/retrosigmoid, middle cranial fossa, and translabyrinthine that use microscopic approaches.

APPENDIX 45–1

Web Resources

Hearing

National Institute on Deafness and Other
Communication Disorders (NIDCD)
(800) 241-1044
http://www.nidcd.nih.gov
American Academy of Pediatrics
(847) 434-4000
http://www.aap.org
American Academy of Otolaryngology–Head and
Neck Surgery
http://www.entnet.org
American Speech-Language-Hearing Association
http://www.asha.org
American Academy of Audiology
http://www.audiology.org/consumer

APPENDIX 45–2

References

1. Grandis JR. Treatment of idiopathic sudden sensori-neural hearing loss. *Am J Otol.* 1993;14:183.
2. Farrior JB. Sudden hearing loss. *Emerg Med.* 1994;2:60–74.
3. Cruickshanks KJ, Wiley TL, Tweed TS, et al. Prevalence of hearing loss in older adults in Beaver Dam, Wisconsin: the epidemiology of hearing loss study. *Am J Epidemiol.* 1998;148:879–886.
4. Rueben D, Walsh K, Moore A, et al. Hearing loss in community-dwelling older persons: national prevalence data and identification using simple questions. *J Am Geriatr Soc.* 1998;46:1008–1011.
5. Curhan SG, Eavey R, Shargorodsky J, Curhan GC. Analgesic use and the risk of hearing loss in men. *Am J Med.* 2010;123(3):231–237.
6. Curhan SG, Shargorodsky J, Eavey R, Curhan GC. Analgesic use and the risk of hearing loss in women. *Am J Epidemiol.* 2012;176(6):544–554.
7. Bagai A, Thavendiranathan P, Detsky AS. Does this patient have hearing impairment? *JAMA.* 2006;295(4):416–428.
8. Katz MS, Gerety MB, Lichtenstein MJ. Gerontology and geriatric medicine. In: Stein JH, ed. *Internal Medicine.* St. Louis, MO: Mosby-Year Book; 1994:2834.
9. Yueh B, Shapiro N, MacLean CH, Shekelle PG. Screening and management of adult hearing loss in primary care: scientific review. *JAMA.* 2003;289:1976–1985.
10. Weinstein BE. Validity of a screening protocol for identifying elderly people with hearing problems. *ASHA.* 1986;28:41–45.
11. O'Donoghue G. Cochlear implants - science, serendipity, and success. *N Engl J Med.* 2013;369(26): 2564–2566.
12. Klein K, Nardelli A, Stafinski T. A systematic review of the safety and effectiveness of fully implantable middle ear hearing devices: the carina and esteem systems. *Otol Neurotol.* 2012;33(6):916–921.
13. Niedermeyer HP, Arnold W. Otosclerosis: a measles virus associated inflammatory disease. *Acta Otolaryngol (Stockh).* 1995;115:300–303.
14. Gantz BJ, Schindler RA, Snow JB. Adult hearing loss: some tips and pearls. *Patient Care.* 1995;9:77.
15. Battaglia A, Mastrodimos B, Cueva R. Comparison of growth patterns of acoustic neuromas with and without radiosurgery. *Otol Neurotol.* 2006;27(5):705–712.
16. Smouha EE, Yoo M, Mohr K, Davis RP. Conservative management of acoustic neuroma: a meta-analysis and proposed treatment algorithm. *Laryngoscope.* 2005;115(3):450–454.
17. Stangerup SE, Caye-Thomasen P, Tos M, Thomsen J. The natural history of vestibular schwannoma. *Otol Neurotol.* 2006;27(4):547–552.
18. Stangerup SE, Thomsen J, Tos M, Caye-Thomasen P. Long-term hearing preservation in vestibular schwannoma. *Otol Neurotol.* Feb 2010;31(2):271–275.

Tinnitus

Context

Tinnitus is a relatively common symptom, with approximately 6.4% of the population affected.[1] Although the most common presentation is a patient who complains of "ringing" in the ears, there are numerous sounds that a patient may complain of that fit under the umbrella term *tinnitus*. These include clicking, rushing, echoing, fluttering, and hissing. Ringing in the ears is a ubiquitous symptom and is unavoidable, yet the question for the chiropractor is whether it is temporary or permanent, and whether there are any clear clues as to its cause. Additionally, distinguishing among the other sounds the patient may be hearing may lead to an identifiable vascular, toxic, cochlear, small muscle spasm, or cervicogenic etiology.

Tinnitus may be categorized by some simple differentiations. First, is the tinnitus localized to an ear or ears or is it more central and diffuse? *Tinnitus cerebri* is the term used for the latter and may represent organic pathology. Therefore, referral for medical evaluation is appropriate. The localization to one or both ears is called tinnitus aurium and is further divided into subjective and objective. Are the patient's hearing sounds appreciable only by him or her or are they sounds that are audible to the examiner? Subjective tinnitus is audible only to the patient and is probably the most common (99% of patients), yet the most difficult type to identify as to cause. Objective tinnitus may sometimes be appreciated by the examiner and usually represents various vascular sounds.

General Strategy

- Have the patient describe what he or she is hearing.
- Determine whether the patient hears the sounds in the ears or as central or diffuse sounds in the head.

- Determine whether the patient has associated hearing loss or vertigo.
- Determine whether the patient is taking salicylates or indomethacin.
- Determine whether the patient is taking any ototoxic medications such as aminoglycoside antibiotics.
- Determine whether the patient has been exposed to environmental noise such as machinery, loud music, or earphones.
- Determine whether the patient has been diagnosed with any endocrine, vascular, neurologic, or otologic diseases.
- Determine whether the patient experienced trauma to the head or ear.

Relevant Anatomy and Physiology

Although the ear is designed to monitor the external environment, it is capable of perceiving internal "noise," especially when the outside environment is muted or eliminated. Most objective tinnitus is due to this phenomenon and requires a search for the internal sound source. Most of these sounds are the result of vascular turbulence or small muscle spasm in close proximity to the ear.

Subjective tinnitus of neural origin is extremely difficult to explain and to cure. Although it would seem logical to assume that part of the labyrinth system or the neural connections to the cortex are damaged, labyrinthectomy or cochlear division may still leave a patient with subjective tinnitus.[2] This phantom aural sensation has no known anatomic or physiologic substrate. Theoretically, the auditory epithelium, basilar membrane, or endolymph may be damaged or altered in a way to send a continuous stream of mechanical stimulus, which is interpreted as a high-frequency background hiss, yet this has not been demonstrated. This is, in fact, the theory behind excessive loud noise exposure, when the basilar membrane is forced to vibrate continuously beyond its normal amplitude.[3] The result is that there is a spontaneous discharge in the high-frequency range. It is known that patients who develop hearing loss often have accompanying tinnitus. Other theories focus on a decrease in vertebral artery blood flow[4] and, most recently, a proposed deficiency or dysfunction of serotonin.[5] It is known that serotonin acts as a sensory "suppressor," preventing hypersensitivity to light and sound.

Although a sympathetic nervous system dysfunction with consequent vertebral blood flow reduction has seemed attractive, the findings of Bogduk et al.[6] significantly decrease this possibility as a consideration. A spinal connection to tinnitus may be the relationship of the trigeminal nerve to the ear and the upper cervical spinal segments.

Evaluation

History

Subjective tinnitus is by far the most common type. When related to systemic causes such as medications or the aging process, it is often continuous, high-pitched, and bilateral. Questioning with regard to medication is helpful when the latter description is a relatively recent phenomenon. When long-standing, otosclerosis or presbycusis should be suspected, especially when associated with bilateral hearing loss. Unilateral tinnitus with associated hearing loss and recurrent vertigo should suggest Ménière's disease or multiple sclerosis. When unilateral, continuous, and associated with hearing loss, an acoustic neuroma is more likely.

There are some characteristic descriptions that may identify the underlying cause when objective tinnitus is suspected, as follows:

- pulsating or rushing—vascular (cardiac murmurs, bruits, arteriovenous malformations [AVM], glomus tumors)
- humming—venous (cervical venous hum)
- low-pitched clicking or fluttering—muscular spasm (stapedius, tensor tympani, or tensor palati)

Examination

Physical examination of the patient with tinnitus centers on the ear and auscultation for a vascular etiology. It is likely that the examination will reveal few if any clues as to the patient's complaint, yet an attempt is made to determine whether secondary causes or primary ear pathology may be contributing. When the patient complains of local ear pain, vertigo, or hearing loss, a thorough investigation of the ear should be performed, including standard Rinne and Weber hearing tests and a search for the following:

- cerumen impaction
- otitis media
- otosclerosis

Physical examination for the source of objective tinnitus centers on auscultation for the following:

- orbital, cranial, or carotid bruits
- cardiac murmurs
- venous hum

By connecting the tubing of one stethoscope to another, the doctor can hear what the patient hears if the cause is objective. Additional examination procedures include evaluating the palate for spasm and checking the temporomandibular joint for clicking or popping. A pulsatile type of tinnitus relieved by pressure on the jugular vein confirms a venous hum.

Management

When other auditory and other sensory stimuli are reduced, the tinnitus may be unbearable for some patients. These patients often attempt sensory distraction by leaving the radio or television on when trying to sleep. Other solutions include biofeedback, which appears to have a relatively good initial response rate, and the use of a tinnitus masker (worn like a hearing aid).[7] Patients with hearing loss often find that the tinnitus improves with the use of a hearing aid. If the tinnitus is post-whiplash (acceleration/deceleration injury to the neck) or associated with other indicators of vertebrogenic vertigo, chiropractic manipulative treatment may be helpful in resolving the complaint.[8]

Although a number of drugs are used in the treatment of tinnitus, there is little consistent evidence of success.

Patients with intractable tinnitus often undergo surgical procedures. When the tinnitus is associated with vertigo or hearing loss, surgery may be helpful.[9] Cochlear nerve section is used for those with isolated or intractable tinnitus, with the obvious trade-off of permanent hearing loss.[2] However, for some patients who are so disabled

that suicide is considered, this surgery may be an attractive alternative.

Algorithm

An algorithm for evaluation and management of tinnitus is presented in **Figure 46–1**.

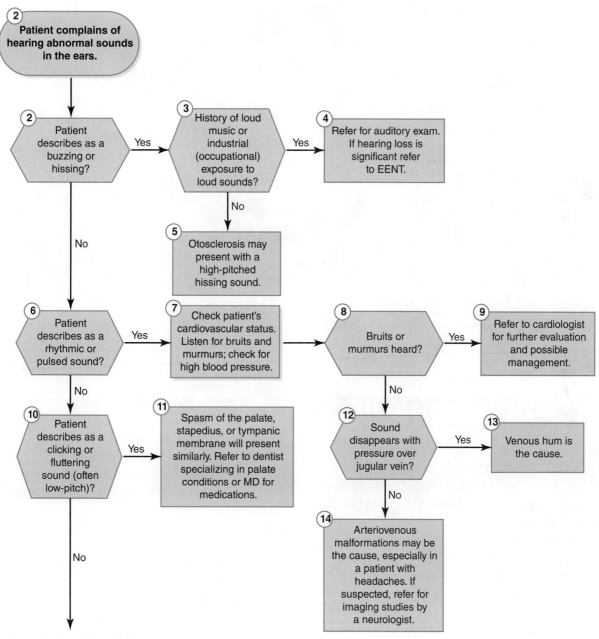

Figure 46–1 Tinnitus—Algorithm

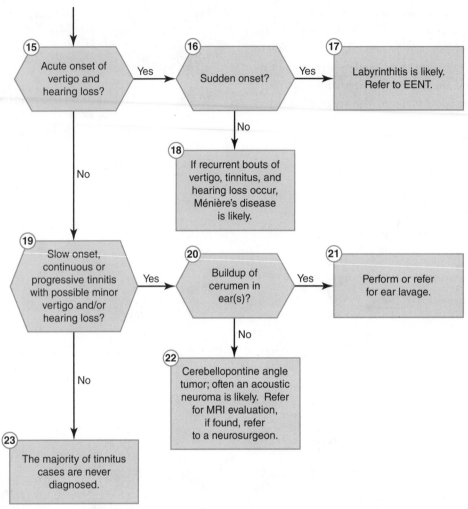

Figure 46–1 (Continued)

APPENDIX 46–1

References

1. Hughes JP. Tinnitus. In: Greene HL, Fincher RME, Johnson WP, et al., eds. *Clinical Medicine.* 2nd ed. St. Louis, MO: Mosby-Year Book; 1996:791.

2. Pulec JL. Cochlear nerve section for intractable tinnitus. *Ear Nose Throat J.* 1995;74:468–476.

3. Mitchell CR, Creedon TA. Psychophysical tuning curves in subjects with tinnitus suggest outer hair cell lesions. *Otolaryngol Head Neck Surg.* 1995;113:223–233.

4. Koyuncu M, Celik O, Luleci C, et al. Doppler sonography of vertebral arteries in patients with tinnitus. *Auris Nasus Larynx.* 1995;22:24–28.

5. Marriage J, Barnes NM. Is central hyperacusis a symptom of 5-hydroxytryptamine (5-HT) dysfunction? *J Laryngol Otol.* 1995;109:915–921.

6. Bogduk N, Lambert G, Duckworth JW. The anatomy and physiology of the vertebral nerve and its relation to cervical migraine. *Cephalalgia.* 1981;1:1–14.

7. Anderson RG. Tinnitus. In: Holt GR, et al., eds. *Decision Making in Otolaryngology.* Toronto: BC Decker; 1984.

8. Terrett AGJ. Tinnitus, the cervical spine, and spinal manipulative therapy. *Chiro Tech.* 1989;1:41–45.

9. Henrich DE, McCabe BF, Gantz BJ. Tinnitus and acoustic neuromas: analysis of the effect of surgical excision on postoperative tinnitus. *Ear Nose Throat J.* 1995;74:462–466.

Epistaxis (Nosebleed)

Context

Nasal bleeding (epistaxis) is a common, usually benign, phenomenon that warrants little concern. Occasionally, however, patients seek help when bleeding is severe and uncontrollable or when it is recurrent. Approximately 25% of the time, epistaxis cannot be tied to a specific etiology.[1] Most benign causes are easily identifiable, often due to drying, irritation, or inflammation of the vessel-rich nasal mucosa. These are probably more often seen in children, in whom nose blowing, wiping, and picking account for 95% of common initiators.[2] Another common cause is the drying effect of house heating during winter months. Trauma from a blow to the nose is quite obvious and often benign; however, if the severity of trauma is significant, underlying fracture should be investigated. A particular concern is the hypertensive patient who presents with nosebleeds. These are often profuse and poorly controlled without medical management. More rarely, bleeding dyscrasias may present with nasal bleeding. A major concern in children is the possibility of acute leukemia. This is manifested by a recently sick child with epistaxis and gingival and subcutaneous bleeding.

General Strategy

Acute and Profuse

If significant trauma occurred, consider radiographs to rule out an associated fracture. If simple measures to control bleeding are not effective, referral for medical management is important. This will usually involve the use of silver nitrate sticks or electro-coagulation and packing.

Acute with Minimal Bleeding

- Control with slight pinching of the nose with the head held in neutral, not extended. In extension, blood may be swallowed, leading to nausea and/or vomiting.

History of Recurrent Nose Bleeds

- Determine the frequency, amount of bleeding, and length of attacks.
- Determine whether there are any obvious causes with respect to allergies or nasal trauma from picking, blowing, or wiping; or whether the patient lives in a house where home heating produces a low-humidity environment (especially when the heater runs all night).
- In adults, determine whether the patient is hypertensive.
- Evaluate the patient for any other signs of bleeding tendencies, such as easy bruising.
- If recurrent and no obvious cause can be identified, lab tests may indicate any underlying blood dyscrasia.
- Refer if the suspected underlying cause is hypertension, mitral stenosis, a bleeding disorder, or drug related (chemotherapy, anticoagulant therapy for thrombophlebitis, etc.).

Relevant Anatomy

Nasal bleeding is rather common because of an abundant and redundant blood supply and the vulnerability of the nose to trauma. Both the internal and external carotid arteries supply branches that feed the nasal mucosa. Epistaxis is classified as either anterior or posterior. Bleeding is most common anteriorly because of the abundance of vessels in Kiesselbach's plexus. Bleeding posteriorly is less common and more likely to be profuse. The blood vessels are quite superficial and vulnerable to various environmental factors as a result of allergies, infections, low humidity, and trauma.

Evaluation

History

A focused history addresses common causes associated with nasal trauma, such as chronic blowing of the nose, nose picking or wiping, and direct trauma from blows. It is particularly important to determine the humidity of the patient's living or working environment. Specifically, when heating is used all night in the winter months, the nasal mucosa dries and leaves the area susceptible to bleeding from minor trauma.

A drug history is important. The use of anticoagulant or antiplatelet drugs, such as warfarin sodium (commonly used for deep vein thrombosis) or aspirin on a long-term basis, may predispose the patient. Drug-induced thrombocytopenia may occur with chemotherapy. Use of cocaine will cause nasal vasospasm and eventual tissue necrosis leading to bleeding (ironically, cocaine may be used in the acute management of nasal bleeding due to the vasoconstrictive effects). A family history of bleeding may indicate a rare hereditary hemorrhagic telangiectasia (Rendu-Osler-Weber syndrome). Determine whether the patient has a history of hypertension that is poorly controlled. Also investigate any possibility of advanced liver disease.

Examination

At the time of bleeding it is important to distinguish anterior from posterior bleeding.[3] This is often difficult because of the amount of bleeding. Posterior bleeding is classically profuse and difficult to control without silver nitrate sticks or electrocoagulation and nose packing. If trauma was involved, a close check for nasal or facial fracture is warranted. Radiographs or computed tomography may be needed to determine the extent of a facial fracture. For patients with recurrent or profuse bleeding, the evaluation should include the following:

- nasal mucosa inspection
- blood pressure measurement

- a complete blood cell count to determine thrombocytopenia (more extensive testing, including liver function tests, should be reserved for those suspected from history) or pancytopenia

Management

- Patients with thrombocytopenia or pancytopenia have serious disease and require immediate medical referral.
- Nasal hygiene is important to convey to children and their parents to eliminate common benign causes. When house humidity is suspected as the cause, two suggestions should be given. First, reduce the thermostat at night so that the heater is not used as much during the evening. Second, apply a lubricant such as Vaseline around the nose before going to bed, which helps to moisten incoming air.
- For children who do not have a nasal hygiene cause, it may help to address the possibility of dairy product allergies through a trial of elimination for several weeks if the bleeding is recurrent.
- Persistent epistaxis with associated signs of bruising, fatigue, or weight loss may suggest an underlying leukemia warranting further medical evaluation.
- For patients with hypertension, referral for medical management is imperative. This type of bleeding may be potentially life-threatening if the underlying hypertension is not controlled.

APPENDIX 47–1

References

1. Hughes JP. Nose bleed (epistaxis). In: Greene HL, Fincher RME, Johnson WP, et al., eds. *Clinical Medicine.* 2nd ed. St. Louis, MO: Mosby-Year Book; 1996:793.
2. Davis WE. Epistaxis. In: Holt GR, et al., eds. *Decision Making in Otolaryngology.* Toronto: BC Decker; 1984.
3. Josephson JD, Codley FA, Stierna P. Practical management of epistaxis. *Med Clin North Am.* 1991;75:1311.

Sore Throat

# CHAPTER 48

Context

Sore throat is the third most common presenting complaint for primary care physicians totaling approximately 3% to 4% of all visits.[1] Although sore throat is one of the five most common complaints in a primary care setting,[2] presentation in a chiropractic setting is far less common. This is largely based on an assumption by the patient that antibiotics will be given for his or her problem and that drug prescription is not within the scope of chiropractors. The rationale for antibiotic treatment of pharyngitic sore throat, however, is not so much to treat for cure of the primary infection (there is no strong evidence indicating improvement of the sore throat with antibiotic treatment beyond the natural history), but to prevent the serious complication of streptococcal throat infection—rheumatic fever. It is interesting to note, though, that fewer than 15% of adults and 40% of children with sore throat have group A β-hemolytic *Streptococcus pyogenes* infection, the main cause of "strep" throat.[3] Viral causes account for about 50% of pharyngitis. Therefore, it is important to distinguish the patient with a nonstrep cause from the patient who is likely to have a viral (nonantibiotic treatable) cause of sore throat.

The two primary management issues with the indiscriminate use of antibiotics for sore throat (accounts for 50% of antibiotic prescription in outpatient clinics) are the inappropriate use of antibiotics, resulting in resistant bacterial strains, and the cost.[4] It would seem that such a common complaint as sore throat would have a clear-cut gold standard for evaluation or at least a classic presentation that would nail down the diagnosis. However, presentation varies, and the distinction between viral and bacterial pharyngitis is not always clear. There is no gold standard for the diagnosis of *S. pyogenes*. With a suggestive history and examination coupled with the appropriate use of a rapid screen for antibodies to group A streptococcus and/or throat culture, the diagnosis should be evident in the majority of patients. Ironically, one study indicated that although primary care physicians who were educated regarding probabilities of strep throat improved in their diagnosis (decreased overestimation tendencies), they had a slight trend toward increasing prescription of antibiotics.[5] The study concludes that it is difficult to change treatment tendencies even with an improved ability to make treatment decisions.

In general, those patients at high risk for *S. pyogenes* or its complications should be referred for antibiotic treatment. Others may be managed for symptoms and monitored for symptom persistence and severity. Failure to improve (or if the patient worsens) warrants referral for further testing or antibiotic treatment. As a potential first-contact doctor, chiropractors should have available the ability to perform a rapid antigen test for strep in an effort to save the patient from an unnecessary visit to his or her medical doctor.

General Strategy

History

Determine whether the patient has the following:
- indicators of high risk for *S. pyogenes* or its complications (diabetes, prior rheumatic fever, strep throat in a close-contact individual)
- recurrent attacks that are relatively mild (allergic pharyngitis)

- history of orogenital sex or other indicators of gonorrhea

Examination

Perform the following:

- Determine whether the patient has a fever and/or rash
- Determine whether the patient has signs of a respiratory infection
- Examine sinuses for indication of infection (transilluminate)
- Determine whether the patient has associated anterior or posterior lymph node involvement (anterior suggests bacterial, posterior suggests viral)
- Determine whether there are any lesions in the mouth or oropharynx (examine the teeth and gums, tongue, palate, and pharynx)
- Check the thyroid gland
- Perform a rapid determination for streptococcus antigen if patient appears to have either strep or viral pharyngitis; if negative, yet history and exam are highly suggestive, perform a throat culture
- Perform a screening lab test for patients suspected of having mononucleosis (monospot in two weeks if still unsure)

Management

- Refer patients who are at high risk for strep.
- Refer patients who have a positive strep antigen test or throat culture for group A β-hemolytic strep.
- Manage patients symptomatically who have mononucleosis (unless extremely painful on swallowing or difficulty breathing).
- Manage patients for symptoms if a viral cause is suspected; monitor for worsening or persistence.

Evaluation

History

The focus of the history is to determine whether patients have been exposed to strep throat and those who may be predisposed. Children are more likely to acquire strep throat than adults. A positive history of exposure to a schoolmate or a family member is often found.

It is important to confirm that the contact individual has had positive tests for streptococcus and was not simply treated with antibiotics as a gunshot approach. It is also important to determine whether the patient has had prior rheumatic fever or a current history of diabetes; both predispose the individual to streptococcal infection.

The next step is to determine whether there are historical indicators of other causes of sore throat.

- With diabetics, the immunosuppressed, or those taking oral corticosteroids (inflammatory diseases) or inhaled corticosteroids (asthma) there is a higher risk for candidiasis.
- Patients (in particular homosexual men) who engage in orogenital sex are more likely to acquire oral gonorrhea.
- Patients who report a mild sore throat that is recurrent and unassociated with a fever are likely to have allergic pharyngitis (unless following a more severe initial attack). There is often an associated complaint of a chronic cough or sinus congestion.
- Patients who have had extensive dental procedures who complain of difficulty swallowing and an associated sore throat may have a retropharyngeal abscess (visible only with a lateral cervical spine radiograph).

Examination

One of the key findings is a pharyngeal exudate. Unfortunately, taken alone, this is a relatively nonspecific finding, occurring in as many as 65% of patients with viral pharyngitis and 40% of patients with mycoplasma infection. Following are some classic descriptions for various causes of exudates (it is recommended to examine a color atlas to gain better recognition):

- Streptococcal—tonsils are covered with a loose yellow exudate; tonsils are swollen.
- Herpangina—due to coxsackie virus infection; there are multiple, small (1 to 2 mm), painful ulcerations (often in children) of the soft palate and pharynx (a similar condition called hand-foot-and-mouth disease is caused by coxsackie virus but also involves the palms and soles of the feet).
- Herpes simplex—similar to herpangina in appearance; there are multiple, small (1 to 2 mm)

vesicles that rupture in a few days to produce painful ulcerations; however, they may involve the lips, gingivae, or palate.

- Herpes zoster—the lesions are usually unilateral, involving the lip, tongue, or buccal mucosa; lesions are usually larger (2 to 4 mm) and go through vesiculation.
- Candidiasis—usually produces white, curdy patches on the tongue or mucosa.
- Mononucleosis—palatine petechiae are virtually diagnostic with small, red lesions with small, white bases.
- Vincent's angina (necrotizing ulcerative gingivostomatitis)—caused by fusobacterium or *Borrelia vincetii;* begins as a fulminant gingivitis with bleeding, ulcerations, and a grayish covering that spreads to the posterior pharynx; there is an associated foul breath.
- Stomatitis is not an exudate but an inflammation of the oral mucosa that may occur far enough posteriorly that it causes painful swallowing and may appear to the patient to be a sore throat. Stomatitis is caused by various entities, including infections (such as herpes and gonorrhea), medications (including methotrexate and similar immune-altering medications), and trauma.

In addition to examination of the mouth and throat, it is important to palpate for lymphadenopathy. Anterior lymph node enlargement is suggestive of a bacterial cause of pharyngitis. Posterior lymph node involvement suggests a viral source. Regional node enlargement in the axillary and inguinal regions in association with posterior neck involvement suggests mononucleosis. With a suspicion of mononucleosis it is always important to check for splenomegaly. In patients with no obvious oral involvement, palpation of the thyroid gland should be included. A scarlatiniform rash is strong evidence for streptococcal infection.

A temperature greater than 38.3°C (101°F) is found more commonly with a streptococcal infection or a complication, peritonsillar abscess, involving unilateral swelling of a tonsil (a referral condition). Mild fever is more suggestive of a viral infection.

Unfortunately, the classic findings of fever, pharyngeal exudate, and anterior adenopathy without cough are not always found in all patients with strep throat (found in only 56% of patients). These findings are also nonspecific, occurring with other causes of pharyngitis.

This, taken together with expediency issues, leads to a tendency toward overestimation of strep throat when the patient presents with pharyngitis. Reliance on clinical impression alone leads to an overestimation rate of between 80% and 95% by experienced clinicians.[6] For this reason laboratory evaluation is necessary.

Pharyngitis is caused by a number of infectious and noninfectious causes. Infections may be viral or bacterial, including *Chlamydia, Mycoplasma, Neisseria gonorrhoeae, Haemophilus influenzae* type b, Candidiasis, Diphtheria, and others. Other noninfectious causes include gastroesophageal reflux, allergic rhinitis, postnasal drainage, acute thyroiditis, persistent cough, and sinusitis, among others. Concerns regarding group A β-hemolytic streptococcal pharyngitis are the suppurative complications and rheumatic fever. This tends to cause an overreaction, by both patients and physicians, to treat with antibiotics as a "shotgun" approach to all sore throat presentations. Rheumatic fever is now quite rare, occurring in only 1 per million of the U.S. population.[7] Researchers recently evaluated the likelihood ratios for the history and physical examination of patients with sore throat in an attempt to determine various components or cluster of components in detecting strep throat.[8] Their findings follow:

- Tonsillar exudates, pharyngeal exudates, or exposure to strep throat infection in the previous two weeks (positive likelihood ratios of 3.4, 2.1, and 1.9 respectively)
- Absence of tender anterior cervical lymph nodes, no tonsillar enlargement, or no exudate (negative likelihood ratios of 0.60, 0.63, and 0.74 respectively)

They conclude that there is no single element of the history or physical examination that can sufficiently diagnose or exclude the diagnosis of strep throat. However, by following an algorithmic approach, patients can be categorized into high-, moderate-, and low-risk categories. Those at high risk (combination of tender anterior lymph nodes, pharyngeal exudates, and/or recent exposure to strep throat) should be treated with antibiotics because they likely have strep throat. Those at moderate risk (absence of the high-risk elements but with a recent cough and oral temperature of ≥ 38.3°C [101°F]) should have further diagnostic evaluation (rapid antigen test or throat culture). Those at low risk should be managed symptomatically and are likely not to have strep throat. One study of 30,000 patients found that by encouraging the use of a rapid antigen test only, there was a decrease from 65% to 13% in the number of patients receiving a throat culture, with no change in the number of suppurative complications.[9]

There are two general approaches to detection of group A streptococcus. First is an in-office (or referral) check for rapid strep antigen. This approach has an estimated sensitivity of 79% to 88% and a specificity of about 95%.[6] Newer optical methods approach the 94% to 96% sensitivity level. Specificity was similar to that in the older methods. Based on these generalizations, it is suggested that patients with a positive test be referred for antibiotic treatment. The difficulty is the patient who appears to have strep throat, yet has a negative rapid antigen test. Most physicians would still order a culture, but would not treat until the results indicated infection with *S. pyogenes*. Given the high specificity, some physicians would not culture. This is based solely on a cost-effectiveness decision.

In a patient with mononucleosis a complete blood count will demonstrate a lymphocytosis greater than 50% or atypical lymphocytes greater than 10%. A monospot test should be ordered for confirmation after one week, or three weeks if the first test is negative.

Management

- Refer patients who are at high risk for streptococcal infection.
- Refer patients who have a positive strep antigen test or throat culture for group A β-hemolytic streptococci.
- Manage patients symptomatically who have mononucleosis (unless extremely painful on swallowing or difficulty breathing).
- Manage patients for symptoms if a viral cause is suspected; monitor for worsening or persistence.

Symptomatic management includes hydration and throat lozenges; cervical adjusting and massage may help with lymphatic drainage.

APPENDIX 48–1

References

1. National Center for Health Statistics. *1995 National Ambulatory Medical Care Survey* (CD-ROM Series 13, No. 11). Hyattsville, MD: National Center for Health Statistics, 1995.
2. Winters TH. Sore throat. In: Greene HL, Fincher RME, Johnson WP, et al., eds. *Clinical Medicine.* 2nd ed. St. Louis, MO: Mosby-Year Book; 1996:794.
3. Vukmir RB. Adult and pediatric pharyngitis: a review. *J Emerg Med.* 1992;10:607–616.
4. Pichichero ME. Explanations and therapies for penicillin failure in streptococcal pharyngitis. *Clin Pediatr.* 1992;31:642.
5. Poses RM, Cebul RD, Wigton RS. You can lead a horse to water: improving physicians' knowledge of probabilities may not affect their decisions. *Med Decis Making.* 1995;15:65–75.
6. Pichichero ME. Group A-streptococcal tonsillopharyngitis: cost-effective diagnosis and treatment. *Ann Emerg Med.* 1995;25:390–403.
7. Ebell MH, Smith MA, Barry HC, Ives K, Carey M. Does this patient have strep throat? *JAMA.* 2000;284:2912–2918.
8. Centers for Disease Control and Prevention. Summary of notifiable diseases, United States, 1997. *CDC Serveil Summ.* 1998;46:1–87.
9. Webb KH, Needham CA, Kurtz SB. Use of a high-sensitivity rapid strep test without culture confirmation of negative results. *J Fam Pract.* 2000;49:34–38.

Special Conditions

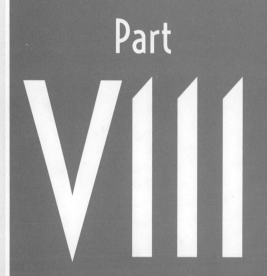

Part

VIII

Diabetes Mellitus

Context

Diabetes mellitus (DM) is a disorder that results in chronic hyperglycemia due to absence of insulin, decreases in insulin, and/or decreased sensitivity of insulin receptors. DM generally is evident in two major forms: type 1, insulin-dependent diabetes mellitus (IDDM), and type 2, non-insulin-dependent diabetes mellitus (NIDDM). Type 1 diabetes becomes apparent in childhood or adolescence, while type 2 diabetes is generally not evident until later in life (over the age of 40 years). There is an ethnic distinction in that Scandinavians have a much higher proportion of individuals with type 1 diabetes (20%). In Japan and China, only 1% of diabetic patients have type 1 diabetes.

The two types of diabetes are not always clearly defined by age, with some older patients developing type 1 diabetes and some younger patients developing type 2 diabetes. Recent evidence suggests that type 2 diabetes is increasingly being found in children and adolescents.[1, 2] Of diabetics in the United States, 90% to 95% have type 2 diabetes.[3] Type 2 diabetes may affect as many as 20% of the senior U.S. population (ages 65 to 74 years). In the United States about 1.9 million individuals were newly diagnosed with diabetes in 2010. Approximately 7 million adults in the United States have undiagnosed type 2 diabetes. A study[4] performed in 2003 attempted to predict the lifetime likelihood of developing diabetes. The researchers estimated that for individuals born in the United States in 2000, the lifetime probability of being diagnosed with diabetes for males was 33% and for females 39%. It is important to also note that the lifetime risk for African Americans and Hispanics is 50%.

Because of the dramatic increase in cases of type 2 diabetes, the American Diabetes Association and the National Institute of Diabetes and Digestive and Kidney Diseases issued a position statement urging that patients be evaluated for prediabetes and managed prior to the development of diabetes and its associated health consequences.[5] They focus on a new category referred to as prediabetes. Estimates are that at least 20.1 million people in the United States (approximately 21% of the population) from age 40 years to 74 years have prediabetes. The belief is that long-term damage occurs in this prediabetic state (especially to the cardiovascular system) prior to the full development of diabetes. In the past, the threshold level for the diagnosis of diabetes on a fasting plasma glucose (FPG) level had been lowered from 140 mg/dL to 126 mg/dL. With the introduction of the prediabetes category, the level for intervention has been lowered to 100 mg/dL for a FPG and 140 mg/dL for an oral glucose tolerance test (OGTT).

The major complications of a chronic hyperglycemic state (and associated abnormalities) are macrovascular and microvascular disease. As a result, several complications of diabetes make it an extremely important disease to control. The major complications include the following:

- Death—DM significantly increases the risk of atherosclerosis-related death (seventh leading cause of death in the United States).[6] Seventy-five percent of DM-related deaths are due to this macrovascular manifestation. Two-thirds of adult patients with DM have hypertension.
- Blindness—DM is the leading cause of blindness in the United States in patients between the ages of 20 years and 74 years.[7]
- Renal failure—DM is the leading cause of end-stage renal disease in the United States; 25% to 30% of patients receiving some form of renal replacement therapy are diabetic.[8]

- Neuropathy—DM is the most common cause of neuropathy, affecting between 70% to 80% of individuals, and polyneuropathy, affecting 50% of all diabetics within 25 years.[9]
- Gangrene of the feet—Diabetics have an incidence 20 times higher than the nondiabetic population. This may lead to amputation. Smoking increases the risk.

Because of these and other complications, the estimated total annual price tag for the United States alone is $174 billion.[10]

The Diabetes Complication and Control Trial (DCCT)[11] studied patients with type 1 diabetes and demonstrated a reduction in microvascular complications in patients who were tightly controlled (hyperglycemia controlled). These included diabetic retinopathy, nephropathy, and neuropathy. A recent study[12] indicated, however, that intensive treatment of type 2 diabetes over a 10-year period did not decrease illness or death from macrovascular causes.

The chiropractor will often have diabetic patients present with various musculoskeletal and neurologic complaints. It is important to place the evaluation and management of these complaints in the context of a diabetic patient. In other words, if a diabetic patient presents with numbness, tingling, or pain in the lower extremity associated (or not associated) with low back pain, the question is whether the lower extremity problem is a complication of the diabetes or due to some other nondiabetic etiology. More important, only half of patients with diabetes are aware of their disorder.[13] This means that if a patient complains of symptoms of a neuropathy and no history of a diabetes diagnosis, the chiropractor could be unaware of an important component for decision making in the patient's management and prognosis.

Therefore, the chiropractor who uses laboratory facilities is in an advantageous position to detect the diabetic patient. In addition, if a patient is discovered to have NIDDM, comanagement with a strong emphasis on dietary and exercise control should be the focus of the chiropractor's involvement. Diabetic management is complex and difficult with regard to patient compliance, given that many patients may be asymptomatic. If the patient has a supportive network, including the chiropractor, the medical doctor, and the family, his or her chances for conservative control of NIDDM are increased.

General Strategy

History

Determine whether

- the patient has risk factors, such as:
  1. older than 45 years
  2. obese (the single most important risk factor) BMI > 35 kg/m²
  3. a family history of diabetes
  4. ethnic background (type 1 more common in Scandinavians; type 2 more common in African Americans, Hispanic Americans, American Indians, Asian Americans, and Pacific Islanders)
  5. a history of polycystic ovary disease
  6. signs and symptoms such as blurred vision or numbness and tingling in the extremities; or polyphagia, polyuria, or polydipsia
  7. the patient has a history of high cholesterol or triglyceride levels
  8. the patient has a history of smoking
  9. the patient is physically active or not
  10. the patient has a history of gestational diabetes or delivered a baby weighing more than 9 lb
  11. the patient has a low level of circulating vitamin D—25(OH)D: an inverse association between low levels of vitamin D and incident type 2 diabetes.[14]
- the patient has a history or signs and symptoms of other disorders that may cause hyperglycemia (Cushing's disease, pheochromocytoma) or whether he or she is taking medications that may cause hyperglycemia or worsen diabetes (corticosteroids, diuretics causing hypokalemia)
- the patient is a known diabetic—ascertain whether the patient is taking medication (insulin or a hypoglycemic agent), following a dietary program, following an exercise program, monitoring his or her blood glucose level, being monitored with a glycosylated hemoglobin

Evaluation

- Pay particular attention to weight, blood pressure, and vision (patients with type 2 diabetes are often overweight and hypertensive).

- Check for secondary signs of diabetes, including an ophthalmoscopic examination, a check of the skin and nails, and a neurologic check for vibration or sensory deficits.
- Screen high-risk patients (see risk factors above), preferably with a fasting laboratory test; if not being performed by primary caregiver, screen for gestational diabetes in pregnant women between weeks 24 and 28, using a one-hour glucose tolerance test.
- Use a glycosylated hemoglobin in known diabetics to check control of diabetes (coordinate with medical doctor if necessary).

Management

- Type 1 diabetes should be managed by the patient's medical doctor; however, the chiropractor can provide a supportive role with the medical doctor to better guarantee tight glycemic control and prevention of complications.
- Type 2 diabetes can be comanaged with a strong emphasis on a specific dietary and exercise program.
- Given the time and resources necessary, referral to an American Diabetes Association certified diabetes self-management program is often the most reasonable approach.
- Monitor all patients for glycemic control and clinical indicators of progressive macrovascular and microvascular complications.
- Understand the management of acute diabetic ketoacidosis in emergency settings.

Relevant Physiology

Glycemic metabolism is controlled by the interaction of insulin (which has mainly a hypoglycemic function) and hormones that are referred to as counter-regulatory. These counter-regulatory hormones include glucagon, epinephrine/norepinephrine (catecholamines), cortisol, and growth hormone. In general, these hormones act to stimulate glycogenolysis and gluconeogenesis. Catecholamines, in particular, suppress insulin secretion and stimulate hepatic glucose production. The hypoglycemic function of insulin is the result of several mechanisms, including promoting the uptake of glucose by mainly muscle and adipose tissue, inhibiting the breakdown of glycogen (promotes glycogen stores), and inhibiting the production of other sources of energy such as from free fatty acids. Both chromium and potassium are needed for the proper functioning of insulin.

There are two circadian effects that influence diabetes.[15] The Somogyi effect begins with a nocturnal hypoglycemia that occurs with type 1 diabetes. This may stimulate an overproduction of counter-regulatory hormones leading to hyperglycemia by 7:00 A.M. Another effect is called the dawn phenomenon.[16] This phenomenon occurs in most diabetic and nondiabetic individuals with a reduced tissue sensitivity to insulin between 5:00 A.M. and 8:00 A.M. These effects and exercise may have an effect on the timing and need for insulin.

During exercise, insulin need is diminished. This is due to the enhanced insulin binding at receptor sites, so that glucose uptake is increased without an increase in insulin (insulin demand reduced). Also, because the amount of circulating plasma glucose is quite small and unable to meet the demands of exercise, the inhibitory effects of insulin on liver glucose production are inhibited by the counter-regulatory hormones, in particular, glucagon and the catecholamines.

Patients with a level of plasma glucose high enough to exceed the renal threshold for glucose will have a spillover into the urine. This causes an osmotic diuresis (polyuria) leading to dehydration. This will lead to increased thirst—polydipsia. When glucose uptake in the peripheral sites is decreased, patients will often feel a lack of energy or feel fatigued. This relative "cell starvation" may lead to a desire to eat—polyphagia.

Type 1 diabetes is due to the failure of the beta cells of the pancreas to produce and secrete insulin. The destruction of islet cells is a variable process, with the onset occurring within the first year of life through young adulthood. It is currently believed that this is due to an autoimmune response that is genetically predetermined. It is proposed that either through an infectious or toxic environmental stimulus, the body produces an autoimmune response against either altered pancreatic beta cell antigens or against part of the beta cell that resembles a viral protein. As a result, 85% of patients with type 1 diabetes have circulating islet cell antibodies, with the majority having anti-insulin antibodies detected. Islet cell autoimmunity (IA) has also been associated with specific foods and the introduction of these foods to the infant. One proposed relationship has been between cow's milk and an increased risk of IA. Out of four cohort studies that use the presence of IA tested serologically, three studies showed no effect.[17-19] In two recent studies, researchers examined a possible relationship between gluten and IA.[20,21] This investigation was prompted by the observation that there is an increased association between type 1 DM and celiac disease.[22] It was found that exposing an infant before the age of 3 months and after 7 months or older increased IA frequency, especially in those with the HLA genotype HLA-DRB1*03/04, DQB8. This implies a possible relationship to cereal feeding (gluten, specifically) and the timing of exposure in genetically predisposed individuals. It must be made clear though that these studies focused on the construct of islet cell autoantibodies and not diagnoses of type 1 DM. These studies also involved a small group of individuals. It is likely that the combination of genetics and exposure to a multitude of environmental factors will be identified as causal factors in the future, versus a single stimulator of autoimmunity. Some of the suspected viral causes are the mumps and coxsackie B4 virus. With type 1 diabetes, patients may become ketotic and subsequently develop life-threatening metabolic acidosis. With diabetes, there is a switch from oxidative aerobic glycolysis to anaerobic glycolysis resulting in excess lactic acid formation. This combined with inadequate utilization of fats coupled with lipogenesis leads to the accumulation of fatty acids which are oxidized to ketones, another cause of acidosis.

Type 2 diabetes represents a range of glycemic disorders that are due mainly to tissue insensitivity to insulin, a blunted beta-cell response to glucose, and an increase in hepatic production of glucose. These patients usually have enough insulin to prevent ketoacidosis, but do not have enough to prevent the consequences of chronic hyperglycemia. The increase in liver production appears to be due to an increased circulating level of glucagon. Most patients in the United States with type 2 diabetes are obese. Sudden weight loss is sometimes the hallmark of an onset of diabetes for some individuals. Those who are not obese may represent a subcategory of type 1 because they often eventually need insulin. There appears to be a pattern of autosomal dominant inheritance with type 2 diabetes.

The relationship to obesity appears to be predominantly associated with an abdominal fat distribution. Apparently, fat that is in the extremities or distributed superficially in the abdomen has less of an effect on hepatic production of glucose than does fat that is "visceral."[23] This visceral type of fat is distributed mainly in the omental and mesenteric regions. Both insulin resistance and hepatic glucose production are increased with this type of obesity.

The relationship between type 2 diabetes and associated hypertension, hyperlipidemia, hyperglycemia, and hyperinsulinemia has led to a proposed syndrome called insulin resistance syndrome, syndrome X, or CHAOS.[24] CHAOS is an acronym for coronary artery disease, hypertension, atherosclerosis, obesity, and stroke. This acronym represents the clinical consequences of insulin resistance. It is known that the conditions associated with syndrome X are interdependent to some degree and that a reduction in one of them will have a beneficial effect on reducing risk for CHAOS by reducing other related factors.

Gestational diabetes is diabetes that is first detected during pregnancy. It carries with it the risk of fetal abnormalities, including neural tube deficits (folic acid helps), macrosomia, and fetal death. A well-controlled blood glucose level (mainly through diet) can substantially reduce the risk.

Clinical Manifestations

Diabetic neuropathy presents in various clinical forms, including poly- and mononeuropathies (**Exhibit 49-1**). Primarily, there are four main types:

1. Symmetrical distal—The patient complains of bilateral numbness, tingling, pins and needles (dysesthesias), pain with normal sensory stimuli (allodynia), sometimes a burning sensation. Mononeuropathy of thoracic and lumbar nerves may lead to pain in supplied areas that mimics angina or myocardial infarction, cholecystitis, or even appendicitis.

2. Asymmetrical, cranial—The patient usually has a complaint of diplopia due to involvement of the oculomotor nerve.

3. Diabetic amyotrophy—Usually involves large nerve such as the femoral or median nerve involving a deep pain with weakness and atrophy of muscles in the area. Carpal tunnel syndrome is difficult to distinguish from amyotrophy in diabetic patients.

4. Autonomic—Leads to a myriad of complaints and problems such as orthostatic hypotension (splanchnic blood vessels), arrhythmias, diarrhea, incontinence, erectile dysfunction.

The loss of sensory input to joints may lead to damage (Charcot joint) with progressive, painless destruction,

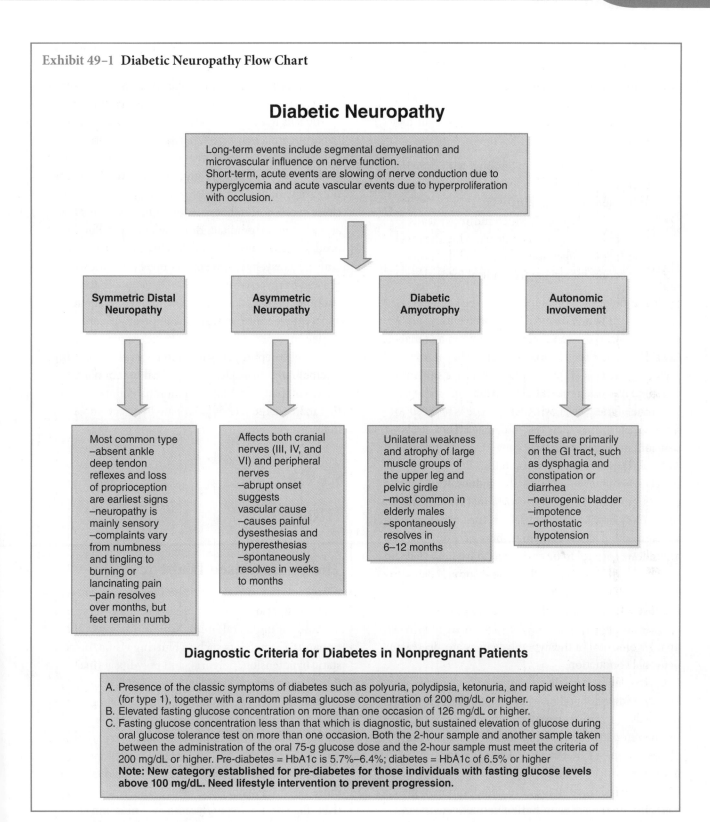

Exhibit 49–1 Diabetic Neuropathy Flow Chart

Diabetic Neuropathy

Long-term events include segmental demyelination and microvascular influence on nerve function.
Short-term, acute events are slowing of nerve conduction due to hyperglycemia and acute vascular events due to hyperproliferation with occlusion.

Symmetric Distal Neuropathy	Asymmetric Neuropathy	Diabetic Amyotrophy	Autonomic Involvement
Most common type –absent ankle deep tendon reflexes and loss of proprioception are earliest signs –neuropathy is mainly sensory –complaints vary from numbness and tingling to burning or lancinating pain –pain resolves over months, but feet remain numb	Affects both cranial nerves (III, IV, and VI) and peripheral nerves –abrupt onset suggests vascular cause –causes painful dysesthesias and hyperesthesias –spontaneously resolves in weeks to months	Unilateral weakness and atrophy of large muscle groups of the upper leg and pelvic girdle –most common in elderly males –spontaneously resolves in 6–12 months	Effects are primarily on the GI tract, such as dysphagia and constipation or diarrhea –neurogenic bladder –impotence –orthostatic hypotension

Diagnostic Criteria for Diabetes in Nonpregnant Patients

A. Presence of the classic symptoms of diabetes such as polyuria, polydipsia, ketonuria, and rapid weight loss (for type 1), together with a random plasma glucose concentration of 200 mg/dL or higher.
B. Elevated fasting glucose concentration on more than one occasion of 126 mg/dL or higher.
C. Fasting glucose concentration less than that which is diagnostic, but sustained elevation of glucose during oral glucose tolerance test on more than one occasion. Both the 2-hour sample and another sample taken between the administration of the oral 75-g glucose dose and the 2-hour sample must meet the criteria of 200 mg/dL or higher. Pre-diabetes = HbA1c is 5.7%–6.4%; diabetes = HbA1c of 6.5% or higher
Note: New category established for pre-diabetes for those individuals with fasting glucose levels above 100 mg/dL. Need lifestyle intervention to prevent progression.

and the loss of proprioception may lead to imbalance when in dimly lighted areas or at nighttime.

The underlying cause is uncertain. However, with acute onset of symptoms, the suspicion is that there is an infarction of one or several branches of the vaso nervorum (the arteries feeding the nerves), so the cause is actually vascular. When progression is slower it is believed that there is a gradual deterioration that causes the sensory aberrations seen in many long-term or poorly controlled diabetics. The cause appears to be excess glycosylation of proteins, specifically, sorbitol accumulation in Schwann cells or nerve trunks in reaction to chronic hyperglycemia.

The following represent some of the proposed effects of chronic hyperglycemia that lead to neuronal dysfunction:

- Non-enzymatic covalent bonding with proteins alters their structure and may lead to dysfunction
- Activation of protein kinase C
- Depletion of NADPH, which indirectly leads to lower levels of nitric oxide blocking the vasodilation effect and decreased glutathione production increasing free radical formation

Alteration of the polyol pathway is the primary basis through which many of these problems result. A sequence occurs related to the hyperglycemia of diabetes. Cells that do not require insulin include hepatocytes, erythrocytes, cells of the peripheral nervous system, intestinal mucosa, renal tubules, retina, and cornea. For some of these cells, whether glucose is reduced to sorbitol determines their risk of damage. Those cells that contain aldose reductase convert excess glucose to sorbitol. These include the lens, retina, Schwann cells of the peripheral nervous system, the kidney, RBCs, hepatocytes, and cells of the ovaries, seminal vesicles and placenta. Only hepatocytes and cells of the ovaries, seminal vesicles, and placenta contain sorbitol dehydrogenase. This allows sorbitol to be converted to fructose that can then escape the cell. For cells without sorbitol dehydrogenase, sorbitol is trapped and cannot be converted to fructose. These cells become glycosylated. The Na^+/K^+ ATPase pump may be affected by a decrease in intracellular myoinositol in the hyperglycemic state, decreasing neuronal conduction.

Glycosylation partially explains the damage to the eye, kidney, and peripheral nervous system. Pathologically, this leads to the microvascular changes seen in retinopathy, nephropathy, and neuropathy. Diagnostically, the glycosylation of RBCs can be taken advantage of with hemoglobin $HA1_c$ testing.

Diabetic retinopathy is due to deterioration of glycosylation to the retina, resulting in microaneurysms. Tight glycemic control may decrease the rate of these microaneurysms. The microaneurysms may progress to the development of exudates and punctate hemorrhages, together called background retinopathy. Although relatively stable, background retinopathy may progress to large hemorrhages with subsequent scarring. Following

scarring, angiogenesis factor released by the ischemic retina leads to a proliferation of new blood vessels called neovascularization. As these contract into the vitreous, the retina may become detached, causing blindness.

The lens is also affected in many diabetics. Chronic hyperglycemia may lead to a change in lens shape, resulting in visual acuity that fluctuates. It usually takes six to eight weeks of tight glycemic control to correct the problem. In addition, chronic hyperglycemia may cause excess sorbitol deposition in the lens. This creates an osmotic gradient, drawing in extracellular waste products and leading to the development of a cataract. Unfortunately, tight glycemic control does not seem to prevent or reverse this process. Glaucoma is also more common in diabetics (occurring in 6% of diabetics), apparently because of scar formation at the canal of Schlemm.

Diabetic nephropathy leads to hyperfiltration and microalbuminuria. Decreasing renal function leads to glomerulopathy and subsequent renal failure. Factors that increase the rate of failure are hypertension and a high-protein diet.

Evaluation

History

The Undiagnosed Diabetic

A high level of suspicion is raised when a patient with a family history of diabetes presents with a complaint of bilateral (or unilateral) numbness or tingling in the feet or hands. Complaints such as blurring vision, orthostatic hypotension, polyuria, and polydipsia (increased thirst) in an older patient with associated weight gain are also highly suggestive. Symptoms of hypoglycemia following meals or simply generalized fatigue in an older patient warrant evaluation for diabetes. Hypertension, obesity, hyperlipidemia, and smoking are important as potential risk factors (or possibly associated factors). A thorough drug history is crucial to determine a contributing effect to hyperglycemia or unmasking effect on diabetes. Included are glucocorticoids, furosemide, thiazides, estrogen-containing products, beta-blockers, and nicotinic acid.

One of the first signs of type 2 diabetes in women is pruritus or signs of vaginitis. Frequent candida (yeast) infections are also suggestive. Women who have given birth to large babies (greater than 9 lb) or who have experienced preeclampsia or unexplained fetal death also should be screened for diabetes. Pregnant women should be questioned regarding gestational diabetes screening.

The Diagnosed Diabetic

Type 1 Diabetes—Assuming that the patient is presenting with a neuromusculoskeletal complaint, it is important to determine how well the type 1 diabetes patient is controlled. It may well be that a complaint of radicular pain into the extremities or localized in the extremities may be a manifestation of diabetic neuropathy. This will strongly influence interpretation of examination findings, management, and prognosis (many are self-resolving). History questions regarding age at diagnosis, type of insulin, frequency of visits to the physician, development of diabetic complications, exercise and diet history, and current medication history are necessary to gauge where a patient stands with regard to risk.

Type 2 Diabetes—The main concern with the type 2 diabetes patient is adherence to a diet/exercise regimen. Questions regarding general well-being and/or the development of any diabetes-related neurovascular problems should be included. It is important to determine whether the patient has been given all the available patient information provided by the American Diabetes Association. It is also important to determine how often the patient is being evaluated for glycosylated hemoglobin. The chiropractor may provide this service if more convenient or cost effective than through the patient's primary physician.

Examination

The physical examination of all patients with diabetes or suspected diabetes should focus first on the associated comorbidity problems of obesity (in type 2 diabetes), hypertension, retinopathy, and neuropathy. Therefore, blood pressure measurement (supine and standing); an ophthalmoscopic examination; deep tendon reflexes; and distal vibration, proprioception, and touch should be evaluated. In known diabetics, it is important to screen the status of the teeth/gums, toes/toenails (in particular between the toes), and skin (especially skin injection sites).

Although the gold standard for neurological testing is nerve conduction studies, in-office evaluation should include Semmes-Weinstein monofilament testing for

sensory evaluation (specificity of 96%; +LR of 10.2) [25] and vibration testing using two approaches: the on–off and timed vibration testing, both using a 128-Hz tuning fork. For the on–off approach apply the tuning fork to the bony prominence of the dorsum of the first toe (proximal to the nail bed), repeating twice on each foot. Point values are generated by adding one point for each successful recognition by the patient of when the tuning fork was felt to vibrate and also correctly identifying when the vibration stops with a total possible of eight points. An abnormal test would be a score of three or less, which has a strong likelihood ratio (LR) of 26.6, strongly suggesting neuropathy. The timed test, again using a 128-Hz tuning fork, involves a comparison between the examiner feeling the vibration stopping and the patient's perception. Applying the tuning fork at the same location as the on–off test, the patient indicates when he or she feels the vibration stops. The examiner compares this on their thumb and records the time when the vibration stops for them. A point value is obtained by determining the number of times the patient's perceived time was less than the examiner's. Generally, if there were three or fewer correctly perceived times, the positive LR was 18.5, strongly suggesting neuropathy. Also, testing for superficial pain has a sensitivity of about 97% and a +LR of 9.2. The absence of ankle reflexes has a sensitivity of only 60% (–LR of 0.44) but a specificity of 90% (+LR of 6). In one study [26] three clinical criteria were compared to a gold standard and revealed that if two out of the three findings were present, the +LR was 10.8 with a sensitivity of 87% and specificity of 91%.

Diabetic Neuropathy

Laboratory Testing

Screening of all patients for diabetes has not been recommended by most national guidelines, including those of the U.S. Preventive Services Task Force.[27] However, some associations such as the American Diabetes Association[28] and the Canadian Diabetes Association[29] recommend screening high-risk patients. The Canadian Diabetes Association makes its recommendation based on expert opinion, not literature evidence.

The laboratory evaluation for the determination of diabetes in undiagnosed patients is currently being debated with regard to the best test and the threshold level for diagnosis. The criteria set by the American

Diabetes Association[28] are generally accepted. The categories and criteria for diabetes are:

Prediabetes FIX

- HbA$_{1c}$ is 5.7%–6.4% (39–46 mmol/mol)
- a fasting plasma glucose at 100 mg/dL
- at 40 mg/dL for an oral glucose tolerance test (OGTT).

Diabetes

- HbA$_{1c}$ is 6.5% (47 mmol/mol) or higher
- a fasting plasma glucose (FPG) level of 126 mg/dL or higher
- a two-hour plasma glucose (2 h PG; glucose tolerance test) of 200 mg/dL or higher
- patients with apparent signs and symptoms of diabetes with a random plasma glucose concentration of 200 mg/dL or higher

Normoglycemia is indicated by an FPG of less than 110 mg/dL or a 2 h PG of less than 140 mg/dL. Impaired fasting glucose is indicated by an FPG level of 110 mg/dL up to 125 mg/dL. Impaired glucose tolerance is indicated by a 2 h PG of 140 mg/dL up to 199 mg/dL.

The disagreement regarding these criteria revolves around two key issues. First, it appears that if the FPG is used as the only indicator, it identifies a different group than identified by the 2 h PG. In fact, it appears that many patients with an abnormal 2 h PG have normal levels of FPG.[30] The concern is that those patients would be missed if using the FPG only. Patients with impaired glucose tolerance have a much higher rate of cardiovascular disease and a higher mortality rate compared to those with impaired fasting glucose. Second, there is concern that the lowered threshold from 140 to 126 mg/dL for FPG will falsely identify individuals not at risk. This concern is based on a study[31] that found 60% of patients with an FPG of between 126 and 139 mg/dL had normal glycosylated hemoglobin levels. A simple solution to the latter concern is simply to check patients in this borderline group with a glycosylated hemoglobin.

Recommendations have changed regarding the need for oral glucose tolerance testing to identify persons at high risk for type 2 DM. A recently published review summarizes the recommendations made by the authors based on the use of a receiver-operating characteristic (ROC) curve used to determine the value of adding a two-hour glucose tolerance test to the predictive value of a fasting plasma glucose level.[32] The difference was minimal; therefore, the group suggested that due to the

time, cost, and inconvenience, plasma glucose levels are sufficient to identify the majority of individuals at risk.

When checking for gestational diabetes, a one-hour glucose tolerance test between weeks 24 and 28 should be ordered.

Additional laboratory findings suggestive of diabetes are as follows:

- glucosuria
- proteinuria (albumin)
- ketonuria
- budding yeasts on urinalysis
- hyperlipidemia

In the known diabetic, it is not necessary or desirable to test for a fasting glucose level. Diabetics self-monitor their blood glucose levels often. It is more important to gain a sense of whether or not there is glycemic control. This is accomplished with a nonfasting test called glycosylated hemoglobin. Because glycosylated hemoglobin is a measure of the amount of glycosolation of red blood cells (RBCs), it gives a good estimate of glycemic status over the preceding 8 to 12 weeks (the life of the RBC). Adequate control of glucose is indicated by an average glucose level of 150 mg/dL or a hemoglobin A$_{1c}$ of 7% to 8%.[33] Levels above 10% indicate poor control and a greater risk of developing complications.

Management

Management of the diabetic patient is a complex, time-consuming program for both the patient and the doctor. For type 1 diabetic patients, control through injection is required. Medical instruction in delivery with regard to timing and injection site is necessary. Newer delivery systems are in development including an intranasal insulin spray. Self-monitoring of blood glucose is essential in determining insulin needs. Currently, the test is through a finger-prick test. This may soon be replaced by a noninvasive device that uses iontophoresis to extract glucose from the skin and measure it with an electrochemical-enzymatic sensor.[34]

Instructions on proper care of the feet to avoid gangrenous complications are also necessary. The patient usually is sent to a dietitian, who explains a comprehensive diet, including the American Diabetic Association exchange lists, the need for fiber, and artificial sweeteners as a substitute for table sugar.

For type 2 diabetic patients, the focus is on diet and exercise. The main role of the diet is to reduce weight in type 2 diabetic patients. Unfortunately about half of all diabetics do not follow their diets.[35] Given the complexity of management, a stratified approach may be more feasible. For those patients who are prediabetic or newly diagnosed diabetics with no visible end-organ damage (i.e., retinopathy or lab indicators of kidney involvement) a three- to six-month trial of diet and exercise advice may be appropriate monitoring with HbA_{1c}. This staged approach could include a progressive walking program that starts with 5 to 10 minutes of walking per day and gradually increasing this amount by 5 minutes every week to arrive at a daily program of between 30 to 45 minutes. Simple diet changes can include adding a green leafy vegetable to each major meal and switching two lunches per week to low-fat yogurt and fruit. Combine that with a cup of coffee and the effect may be augmented. For those willing to commit more, convince your patient to join a gym and go through an exercise-training program. Provide and encourage your patient to use web sources to find healthy recipes and/or join a weight loss program. This also may be accomplished through outsourcing to an American Diabetes Association certified diabetes self-management program.

For patients with signs of end-organ damage or for those unable to adhere to or benefit from a conservative approach, medical management is necessary. The patient should be reminded though that even with medication, diet and exercise are requisite to avoid the progression to insulin dependence. Thus medical management should be combined with an American Diabetes Association certified diabetes self-management program.

For type-1 DM, insulin is given by subcutaneous self-injection in the arms, abdomen, thighs or buttocks by pen injections or pump delivery systems. There are many factors affecting insulin requirements and absorption when injected including colds, fever, infections, illness, surgery, stress, and exercise. Side effects are related mainly to hypoglycemia, but also include allergic reactions, and lipodystrophy at the injection site. Some contraindicated supplements include melatonin, chaparral, tobacco, herbal tea, broccoli, cabbage, charbroiled meats, shiitake mushrooms, and turmeric. There is some hope for an intranasal insulin option which is also being proposed for the treatment of Alzheimer's.

Medical management of type 2 diabetes includes the use of the following drugs prior to resorting to insulin:

- Sulfonylureas (e.g., glipizide [Glucotrol], glyburide [Glynase, Micronase, DiaBeta], glimepiride [Amaryl], chlorpropamide [Diabinese])—close energy-sensitive potassium channels on beta cells causing influx of calcium and subsequent release of insulin.

- Biguanides (e.g., Glucophage [metformin])—hypoglycemic action is based on its effect of decreasing glucose production from the liver.

- Thiazolidinones (e.g., pioglitazone [Actos], rosiglitazone [Avandia])—attach to nuclear receptors in cells to cause an increase in production of cellular proteins that facilitate glucose transport. Note Avandia has been taken off the market in Europe since fall of 2010 and restricted in the United States to patients who do not respond to other medications due to its associated increase in cardiovascular risk.

- Alpha-glucosidase inhibitors (e.g., Acarbose [Precose], Miglitol [Glyset])—reduce the rate of digestion of carbohydrates by competitive inhibition of enzymes needed to digest carbohydrates.

- Dipeptidyl peptidase 4 inhibitors (e.g., sitagliptin [Januvia])—increase incretin levels that inhibit glucagon, which allows increase in insulin secretion. Incretins are a group of proteins secreted by the GI tract along with glucose that enhance insulin secretion in the pancreas. These include glucagon-like peptide-1 (GLP-1) and gastric inhibitory peptide (GIP). GLP-1 also inhibits glucagon secretion and delays gastric emptying.

- GLP-1 receptor agonist injectables—exenatide (Byetta) and liraglutide (Victoza). Soon to be released is a GLP-1 receptor agonist that is delivered intranasally not requiring injection.

- SGLT2 inhibitors (e.g., canagliflozin (Invokana®) dapagliflozin (Farxiga®)—act by blocking the kidneys' reabsorption of glucose. The result is decreased plasma glucose due to loss in the urine.

Self-monitoring is important for known diabetics. There are many new products that allow better control of this monitoring process. Target levels that are influenced by the type of patient, but in general:

- Before meals—between 70 and 130 milligrams per deciliter (mg/dL), or 4 and 7 millimoles per liter (mmol/L)
- One to two hours after meals—lower than 180 mg/dL (10 mmol/L)
- Fasting at least eight hours—between 90 and 130 mg/dL (5 and 7 mmol/L)

For those using insulin, there are new approaches beyond the traditional approach of injection using a vial. One is a pen that uses an insulin cartridge with disposable needles. This obviates the need of filling a syringe. Another device is a continuous subcutaneous insulin infusion pump, which requires a catheter that must be changed every few days. **Table 49–1** summarizes the most commonly used medications for diabetes.

Although medical treatment of type 2 diabetes decreases some of the microvascular complications, it does not seem to decrease the risk of macrovascular disease.[12] Treatment of hypertension or hyperlipidemia does appear to decrease this risk.[36,37]

A separate list of medications is utilized for those patients with diabetic neuropathy. These include but are not limited to:

- Some antidepressants including tricyclics (e.g., amitriptyline [Elavil], nortriptyline, desipramine) and selective serotonin norepinephrine reuptake inhibitors (e.g., Cymbalta [duloxetine], Effexor [venlafaxine])
- Anticonvulsants such as Lyrica (pregabalin) and Neurontin (gabapentin)
- Methylcobalamin (mecobalamin, MeCbl, or MeB$_{12}$) or form of B$_{12}$ taken orally or injected

Other approaches to peripheral neuropathy include the following:

- Topical or transdermal lidocaine, or in some cases capsaicin
- Cold laser (photo energy therapy) devices—there are a number of different devices and intensities. Those that emit near infrared light (NIR therapy) are typically at a wavelength of 880 nm. NIR is believed to stimulate the release of nitric oxide causing vasodilation of small blood vessels increasing circulation and improving symptoms[38,39]

Physical activity is extremely important for the management of type 2 diabetes. It is also clear that the associated problems of hypertension and obesity are affected by exercise. For patients taking medication, there may be a fall in blood sugar with exercise, leading to hypoglycemia that lasts as long as 12 hours. This affects the injection site for diabetics using insulin. Exercise, though, increases levels of glucagon and catecholamines that may counter these medication effects. Recent studies have demonstrated a decrease in risk for type 2 diabetes in men and women who exercise.[40] A recent study[41] indicated that the level of activity is also important, demonstrating that vigorous activity is more beneficial than mild physical activity.

Following is a summary of new information regarding lifestyle and diabetes:

- Results from a monumental study by the Diabetes Prevention Program Research Group comparing

the effect of lifestyle versus metformin versus placebo in the reduction of incidence of type 2 diabetes instigated a recommendation from the American Diabetes Association, among other groups, for change.[42] The surprise was that the reduction of the incidence of diabetes was 58% for those on the lifestyle intervention compared to 31% for those using metformin. Although this is similar to other findings, such as the Finland[43] and China[44] reports, the effects were more dramatic. The researchers suggest that the primary reason may be the individualized approach used in their study. In addition to a low-carbohydrate, low-fat diet, participants engaged in physical activity of moderate intensity (such as brisk walking) for at least 150 minutes per week. They also participated in a 16-hour curriculum designed to support the changes in diet, exercise, and behavior modification. The goal was to maintain a weight reduction of at least 7% of the initial body weight.

- A 12-year follow-up study of over 42,000 males involved a comparison between two dietary regimens and the relative risk of type 2 diabetes. The researchers concluded that a Western dietary pattern (i.e., high in red meat, fat, refined grains, and sweets/desserts) combined with low physical activity or obesity substantially increased the risk of type 2 diabetes compared to a "prudent" dietary pattern (i.e., high consumption of vegetables, fruit, fish, poultry, and whole grains).[45] Another more recent study estimated the lifetime risk for type 2 diabetes in the United States. The researchers estimated that for individuals born in the United States in 2000, the lifetime probability of being diagnosed with diabetes for males was 33% and for females 39%.[4]
- Among many studies emphasizing the need for exercise in reducing the morbidity of diabetes, some indicate minor lifestyle changes may affect mortality. One such study indicated that if diabetic patients were convinced to walk two hours per week, the rate of death would decrease by one per year for every 61 people.[46] A similar outcome was found with women who performed an eight-week walking program of 10,000 steps/day, with benefits of improved glucose tolerance and a reduction in blood pressure.[47]

In a study[48] comparing physical activity levels with BMI and waist circumference and relationship to diabetes, researchers found that for both lean and obese

Table 49-1 Diabetes Medications

Drug Class	Examples	General Mechanism	Interactions/Side Effects
Thiazolidinones	Rosiglitazone maleate Avandia	An oral medication used as adjunct therapy with diet and exercise for type 2 diabetes. It acts primarily by increasing insulin sensitivity but is not related to sulfonylureas, the biguanides, or the alpha-glucosidase inhibitors.	Not to be used with nitrates. Hypoglycemic symptoms, edema, exacerbation of congestive heart failure (CHF). Note Avandia has been taken off the market in Europe since fall of 2010 and restricted in the U.S. to patients who do not respond to other medications due to its associated increase in cardiovascular risk.
	Pioglitazone Actos	Attaches to nuclear receptors in cells to cause an increase in production of cellular proteins that facilitate glucose transport.	As thiazolidinones, Actos can worsen CHF. Also reported are stomach pain, nausea, blood in the urine, dysuria, blurred vision, chest pain, and swelling.
Sulfonylureas	Glipizide Glucotrol Glucotrol XL	A sulfonylurea hypoglycemic agent used in the initial management of type 2 diabetes after dietary management without medication has failed. Has the effects of sensitizing functioning pancreatic beta cells to release insulin, and indirectly, increasing the number and sensitivity of insulin receptors.	May cause hypoglycemia, heartburn, pruritus, nausea/vomiting, hepatic porphyria, hypersensitivity, and visual disturbances.
	Glyburide DiaBeta Glynase Micronase Euglucon	A sulfonylurea hypoglycemic agent used in the initial management of type 2 diabetes after dietary management without medication has failed. Has an effect of sensitizing functioning pancreatic beta cells to release insulin.	May cause hypoglycemia, heartburn, pruritus, nausea, or vomiting.
Biguanides	Metformin Glucophage Glucophage XR	Biguanide hypoglycemic agent (not a sulfonylureas). Does not increase insulin production, but helps bind insulin to insulin receptors and potentate insulin activity. Used in the treatment of type 2 diabetes. Sometimes in combination with sulfonylureas.	May cause abdominal complaints of pain, nausea, or vomiting. May interfere with absorption of folic acid and B_{12} or amino acids. Patient may complain of a bitter or metallic taste. Caution for lactic acidosis.
Insulin	Insulin (many types) NovoLog (RCA) Lantus (RCA) Humulin Novolin Iletin II Humalog (RCA)	These are recombinant human analogs (RCA) extracted from pork, used in the treatment of diabetes. Affects are to lower blood sugar levels by increasing peripheral uptake in muscle and fat, and promoting of conversion of glucose to glycogen (and inhibiting reverse).	Side effects related to hypoglycemia, profuse sweating, hunger, tremors, palpitations; also coma is possible.
Alpha-glucosidase inhibitors	Acarbose [Precose] Miglitol [Glyset]	Reduces the rate of digestion of carbohydrates by competitive inhibition of enzymes needed to digest carbohydrates	Reported are abdominal pain, bloating, gas, and diarrhea. Caution for patients who have kidney or liver disease.
Dipeptidyl peptidase 4 inhibitor	Sitagliptin [Januvia]	Increases incretin levels which inhibit glucagon which allows increase in insulin secretion	Cough, sore throat, body aches, ear congestion, difficulty breathing, and abdominal pain.

men or women there was a benefit to physical activity in the reduction of diabetes. A reduction in the incidence of diabetes was found with even a modest increase in daily physical activity. An increase in activity equal to approximately 460 and 365 kJ/day in men and women, respectively, was independently associated with a 13% (HR 0.87, 95% CI 0.80, 0.94) and 7% (HR 0.93, 95% CI 0.89, 0.98) relative reduction. Beginning with general recommendations, the American Diabetes Association recommends a fiber-rich diet with a maximum of 30% fat (primarily mono- and polyunsaturated fats) and 50% to 60% complex carbohydrates. Specifically, foods that improve insulin sensitivity include:[49]

- broccoli, cabbage, Brussels sprouts, cauliflower
- green leafy vegetables, beans, legumes
- vegetable protein (e.g., soy, peas)
- fiber including rice, oat bran, guar gum, psyllium
- foods rich in omega-3s

Complex carbohydrates are slowly digested so that the rise in blood sugar is more gradual. The advantage of vegetable proteins is that they contain soluble fiber, which decreases the insulin response. Also, protein simulates the release of glucagon.

There are several strategies to help diabetic patients make decisions about which foods to eat. These include the exchange approach, the glycemic index, and the glycemic load. With the exchange approach, foods are grouped into categories such as starches, fruits, milk products, meats, vegetables, and fats. Each "exchange" means that foods and portions listed within each category can be substituted for each other. The substitutions represent generally the same caloric content and similar makeup of carbs, proteins, and fats. For example, each meat "exchange" choice contains 45 to 100 calories, 7 g of protein and 0 g to 8 g of fat. The basic currency of this program is a serving size of carbohydrates, which equals 15 grams. There is also a diabetes food pyramid, which suggests number of servings for each category of food. The glycemic index (GI) is an indicator of how quickly a consumed carbohydrate affects postprandial serum glucose levels. The value is based on a scale of 100, represented by glucose (or white bread). The lower the better. The problem with this approach is that some foods with a high glycemic index are actually in percent of total content low in sugar content, and the portion of the food determines the total glycemic effect. An example would be watermelon, which is primarily water but has a high glycemic index. The glycemic load (GL) attempts to correct for the glycemic index issues and

adds in the feature of a "typical" serving portion of the food so that foods that may have a high glycemic index may have a smaller impact based on the glycemic load, based on portion size, giving a more accurate measure of their glycemic effect in total. By combining these approaches, patients may find it easier to develop meal plans that are healthy and sustainable.

A number of foods have been evaluated for their role in controlling diabetes and hypertension. Although studies on humans are still pending, there is some evidence that these foods have either a high phenol content or have an effect on enzymes involved in glucose metabolism. Foods include yogurt (in particular, soy and fruit yogurts), pumpkins, cranberries, and fenugreek.[50–52] Taken together, this data seem to indicate that a diet including more fruits, vegetables, soy, and perhaps yogurt may be beneficial, especially in substitution for other commonly consumed foods in the traditional American diet. On the opposite end of the spectrum are the concerns of refined carbohydrates which tend to spike blood sugar levels, and more recently, meat intake. In recent studies,[53,54] reducing meat intake decreased the risk of diabetes. In one of these studies,[53] reducing intake by 0.5 servings per day decreased the risk of diabetes by about 14%.

Coffee consumption, up to six cups per day, has been shown in several studies and reviews to have an inverse effect on diabetes.[55] This is likely not related to the caffeine content because in some studies decaffeinated coffee also has an effect. The effects may be due to the high level of antioxidants and chlorogenic acid. One study[56] indicated that timing may be important. The results of this study indicated that coffee ingested at lunch had the largest effect. Tea may have a similar effect. In one study,[57] people who drank at least four cups of tea per day had a 16% lower risk of developing type 2 diabetes than non-tea drinkers.

A study by Norris et al.[58] evaluated the effects of omega-3 polyunsaturated fatty acid intake on islet cell autoimmunity in children with an increased risk for type 1 diabetes. These included those with the genetic biomarkers, or with parents or siblings with type 1 diabetes. The outcome measures were being positive for insulin, glutamic acid decarboxylase, or insulinoma-associated antigen 2 autoantibodies on two consecutive visits, or diabetes at the last follow-up visit. Based on these outcomes, it appears there is a decreased risk for those children with a high omega-3 diet.

In addition to the recommendations of eating a healthy diet and keeping weight down, some specific dietary supplements and herbs have been suggested in the scientific literature (**Table 49–2**):

- alpha-lipoic acid[59]
- vitamin E[60,61]
- vitamin C[62]

- vitamin B_6 (pyridoxine alpha-ketoglutarate)[63]
- biotin[64]
- chromium[65]
- gymnema[66]
- Asian ginseng[67]
- aloe vera[68]

Table 49–2 Nutritional Support for Diabetes

Substance	How Might It Work?	Dosage	Contraindications and Possible Side Effects
Vitamins C & E	May improve glucose tolerance in the elderly and in those with non-insulin-dependent diabetes (NIDDM).	900 IU vitamin E daily 1–3 g vitamin C daily	Side effects for vitamin E are rare. Diarrhea may occur at high doses of vitamin C. Also ensure adequate copper intake with high doses of vitamin C.
Specific form of B_6 (pyridoxine alpha-ketoglutarate)	May improve glucose tolerance.	1,800 mg/day	At very high levels, damage to sensory nerves leading to numbness in the distal extremities may occur. Caution patient to stop supplementation if symptoms appear.
Biotin	May improve glucose tolerance and reduce pain from diabetic neuropathy.	9 mg/day	None due to excretion in urine.
Chromium	May improve glucose tolerance.	200 to 800 mcg/day	At very high levels (> 1,000 mcg/day) severe liver or kidney disease is possible. For those using brewer's yeast, some people have allergies.
Magnesium	May improve insulin production.	300–400 mg/day	Some individuals develop diarrhea even at low doses. Individuals with kidney disease should consult physician.
Coenzyme Q10	Assists in carbohydrate metabolism.	120 mg/day	If patients have congestive heart failure, they should not suddenly discontinue taking.
Evening primrose oil	May improve diabetic neuropathy.	4–6g/day	None reported.
Alpha-lipoic acid	Antioxidant that may improve diabetic neuropathies.	600 mg/day	Skin rash and hypoglycemia are possible. Possible interference with biotin.
Inositol	May help improve diabetic neuropathy.	500 mg taken two times daily	None reported; however, individuals with chronic renal failure may have elevated levels.
Gymnema	May assist the pancreas in insulin production.	400 mg of gymnema extract daily	The safety of gymnema with pregnancy and lactation has not been determined.
Asian ginseng	May increase production of insulin and increase number of insulin receptors.	200 mg of ginseng extract per day	May cause overstimulation or insomnia. Patients with hypertension should consult with physician. Long-term use may result in menstrual abnormalities and breast tenderness. Not recommended during pregnancy or lactation.
Aloe vera juice	May lower blood sugar levels.	1 tablespoon twice daily	If used as a laxative, aggravation of constipation is possible.
Capsaicin (*Capsaicin frutescens* or *annuum*)	A cream applied topically to deplete substance P at nerve endings in an attempt to relieve pain.	Cream base containing 0.025% to 0.075% capsaicin applied	Stings when first applied. Apply 4–5 times/day for at least 4 weeks to determine effectiveness.

Note: The above substances have not been approved by the Food and Drug Administration for the treatment of this disorder. None should be used in place of insulin and for those patients on hypoglycemic agents, consultation with prescribing MD is required.

Note: High levels (several grams/day) of niacin may impair glucose tolerance.

There is still debate as to whether supplementation with beta-carotene or magnesium is useful in the management or prevention of type 2 diabetes.[69-71] Refer also to Chapters 24, 29, and 51 for recommendations related to associated hypertension, weight gain, and hyperlipidemia.

Recent attention has been focused on the relationship between vitamin D and many chronic disorders. With regard to diabetes, a recent meta-analysis[72] published in *Diabetes Care* summarizes the studies to date as of 2013. As a generalized summary, low levels of 25(OH)D, resulted in a relative risk for type 2 diabetes of 0.62 (95% CI 0.54-0.70). Most importantly, this risk occurred regardless of gender, study size, or diabetes criteria. There was a relationship that was linear. For each 10 nmol/L increment in 25(OH)D levels there was associated 4% lower risk of type 2 diabetes (95% CI 3-6; P for linear trend < 0.0001).

For medical doctors managing type 2 diabetic patients, it is important to keep in mind that correction of hypertension may raise lipid levels if diuretics or β-blockers are used, or if, in an attempt to correct hyperlipidemia, a prescription for niacin is given. This could lead to an increased insulin resistance. Niacinamide (Inositol) may be an alternative. Women who are pregnant or on birth control pills may benefit from vitamin B_6 supplementation.

Specific complications of diabetes and their management are as follows:

- Diabetic nephropathy—To prevent progressive deterioration, a low-protein diet, combined with hypertension control using an angiotensin-converting inhibitor, has been proven effective.
- Diabetic retinopathy—Good glycemic control, management of hypertension, and avoidance of smoking may help prevent the development of retinal changes. If neovascularization occurs, photocoagulation with an argon laser is sometimes effective.
- Diabetic neuropathy—Good glycemic control and avoidance of smoking are essential. Most of the poly- and mononeuropathies will self-resolve in 6 to 12 months. Nutritional recommendations include vitamins B_{12}, biotin, and inositol.

Algorithm

An algorithm for evaluation and management of the diabetic patient is presented in **Figure 49–1**.

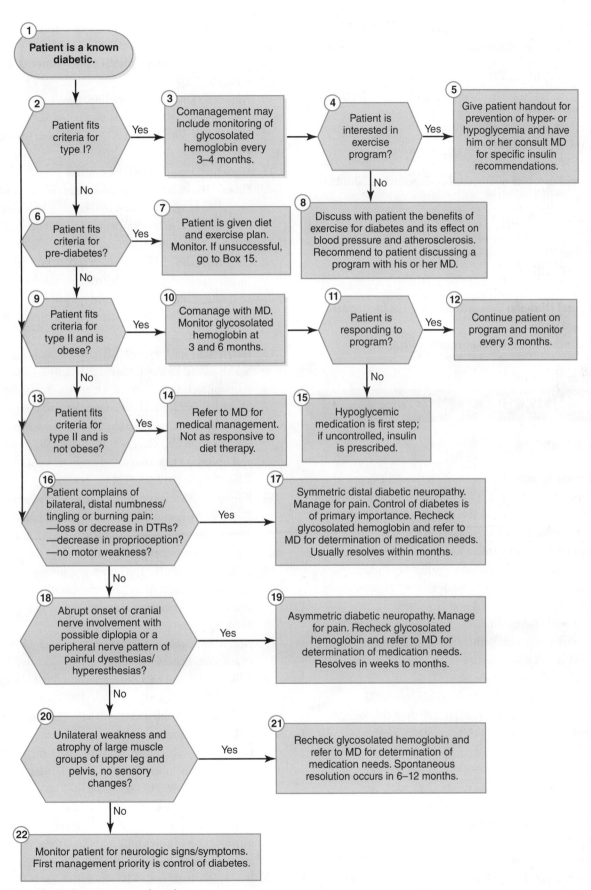

Figure 49-1 The Diabetic Patient—Algorithm

APPENDIX 49–1

Web Resources

Diabetes/Kidney/Urologic
American Diabetes Association
(800) DIABETES (342-2383)
http://www.diabetes.org
National Institute of Diabetes & Digestive & Kidney
Diseases
(800) 891-5390
http://www.niddk.nih.gov
National Kidney Foundation
(800) 622-9010
http://www.kidney.org
**National Diabetes Education Resource for Health
Professionals**
http://ndep.nih.gov/resources/health.htm

APPENDIX 49–2

References

1. Pinhas-Hamiel O, Standiford D, Hamiel D, et al. The type 2 family: a setting for development and treatment of adolescent type 2 diabetes mellitus. *Arch Pediatr Adolesc Med.* 1999;153:1063–1067.
2. Pinhas-Hamiel O, Dolan LM, Daniels SR, et al. Increased incidence of non-insulin-dependent diabetes mellitus among adolescents. *J Pediatr.* 1996;128:608–615.
3. National Diabetes Information Clearinghouse. *Diabetes Statistics.* Bethesda, MD: National Institute of Diabetes and Digestive and Kidney Diseases; 1994. NIH Publication 94–3822.
4. Venkat Narayan KM, Boyle JP, Thompson TJ, Sorensen SW, Williamson DF. Lifetime risk for diabetes mellitus in the United States. *JAMA.* 2003;290:1884–1890.
5. American Diabetes Association. The prevention or delay of type 2 diabetes. *Diabetes Care.* 2002;25:742–749.
6. American Diabetes Association. *Diabetes—1996 Vital Statistics.* Alexandria, VA: American Diabetes Association; 1995.
7. Centers for Disease Control and Prevention. Public health focus: prevention of blindness associated with diabetic retinopathy. *MMWR.* 1993;42:191–195.
8. Breyer JA. Diabetic nephropathy in insulin-dependent patients. *Am J Kidney Dis.* 1992;20:533–547.
9. Harati Y. Diabetic peripheral neuropathies. *Ann Intern Med.* 1987;107:546–559.
10. American Diabetes Association. *Direct and Indirect Costs of Diabetes in the United States in 1992.* Alexandria, VA: American Diabetes Association; 1993.
11. Diabetes Complication and Control Trial Research Group. The effect of intensive treatment of diabetes on the development and progression of long-term complications in insulin-dependent diabetes mellitus. *N Engl J Med.* 1993;329:977.
12. UK Prospective Diabetes Study (UKPDS) Group. Intensive blood-glucose control with sulphonylureas or insulin compared with conventional treatment and risk of complications in patients with type 2 diabetes (UKPDS-33). *Lancet.* 1998;352:837–853.
13. Harris MI. Undiagnosed NIDDM: clinical and public health issues. *Diabetes Care.* 1993;16:642–652.
14. Forouhi NG, Ye Z, Rickard AP, et al. Circulating 25-hydroxyvitamin D concentration and the risk of type 2 diabetes: results from the European Prospective Investigation into Cancer (EPIC)-Norfolk cohort and updated meta-analysis of prospective studies. *Diabetologia.* 2012;55(8):2173–2182.
15. Karam JH. Diabetes mellitus and hypoglycemia. In: Tierney LM, McPhee SJ, Papadakis MA, eds. *Current Medical Diagnosis and Treatment.* 34th ed. Norwalk, CT: Appleton & Lange; 1995:1022.
16. Bolli GB, Gerich JE. The "dawn phenomenon"—a common occurrence in both non-insulin-dependent and insulin-dependent diabetes. *N Engl J Med.* 1984;310:746.
17. Norris JM, Beaty B, Klingensmith G, et al. Lack of association between early exposure to cow's milk protein and beta cell autoimmunity. *JAMA.* 1996;276:609–614.
18. Hummel M, Fuchtenbusch M, Schenker M, Ziegler AG. No major association of breast feeding, vaccinations, and childhood with diseases with early islet autoimmunity in the German BABYDIAB study. *Diabetes Care.* 2000;23:969–974.
19. Couper JL, Steele C, Beresford S, et al. Lack of association between duration of breastfeeding or introduction of cow's milk and development of islet autoimmunity. *Diabetes.* 1999;48:2145–2149.
20. Norris JM, Barriga K, Klingensmith G, et al. Timing of initial cereal exposure in infancy and risk of islet autoimmunity. *JAMA.* 2003;290:1713–1720.

21. Ziegler AC, Schmid S, Huber D, et al. Early infant feeding and risk of developing type 1 diabetes-associated autoantibodies. *JAMA*. 2003;290: 1721–1728.

22. Cronin CC, Shanahan F. Insulin-dependent diabetes mellitus and celiac disease. *Lancet*. 1997;349:1096–1097.

23. Bjorntorp P. Metabolic implications of body fat distribution. *Diabetes Care*. 1991;14:1132.

24. Karam JH. Type II diabetes and syndrome X: pathogenesis and glycemic management. *Endocrinol Metab Clin North Am*. 1992;21:329.

25. Olaleye D, Perkins BA, Bril V. Evaluation of three screening tests and a risk assessment model for diagnosing peripheral neuropathy in the diabetes clinic. *Diabetes Res Clin Pract*. 2001;54(2):115–128.

26. Perkins BA, Olaleye D, Zinman B, Bril V. Simple screening tests for peripheral neuropathy in the diabetes clinic. *Diabetes Care*. 2001;24(2):250–256.

27. U.S. Preventive Services Task Force. *Guide to Clinical Preventive Services*. 2nd ed. Baltimore: Williams & Wilkins; 1996:193–208.

28. American Diabetes Association. Report of the Expert Committee on the Diagnosis and Classification of Diabetes Mellitus (Committee Report). *Diabetes Care*. 1999;22 (suppl 1):S5–S19.

29. Meltzer S, Leiter L, Danman D, et al. 1998 clinical practice guidelines for the management of diabetes in Canada. *Can Med Assoc J*. 1998;159(8, suppl): 1S–29S.

30. The DECODE study group (European Diabetes Epidemiology Group). Glucose tolerance and mortality: comparison of WHO and American Diabetes Association diagnostic criteria. *Lancet*. 1999;354:617–621.

31. Davidson MB, Schriger DL, Peters AL, Lorber B. Relationship between fasting plasma glucose and glycosylated hemoglobin: potential for false-positive diagnoses of type 2 diabetes using new diagnostic criteria. *JAMA*. 1999;281:1203–1210.

32. Stern MP, Williams K, Haffner SM. Identification of persons at high risk for type 2 diabetes mellitus: do we need the oral glucose tolerance test? *Ann Intern Med*. 2002;136:575–581.

33. Fore WW. Non-insulin-dependent diabetes mellitus: the prevention of complications. *Med Clin North Am*. 1995;79:287–298.

34. Tamada JA, Garg S, Jovanovic L, et al. Noninvasive glucose monitoring: comprehensive clinical results. *JAMA*. 1999;282:1839–1844.

35. Wing R, Venditti E, Jackicic J, et al. Lifestyle intervention in overweight individuals with a family history of diabetes. *Diabetes Care*. 1998;21:350–360.

36. UK Prospective Diabetes Study Group. Tight blood pressure control and risk of macrovascular and microvascular complications in type 2 diabetes. UKPDS 38. *Br Med J*. 1998;317:703–713.

37. Thorgeirsson G, for the Scandinavian Sinvastatin Survival Study (45) Group. Cholesterol lowering with sinvastatin improves prognosis of diabetic patients with coronary heart disease. *Diabetes Care*. 1997;20:614–620.

38. Leonard DR, Farooqi MH, Myers S. Restoration of sensation, reduced pain, and improved balance in subjects with diabetic peripheral neuropathy: a double-blind, randomized, placebo-controlled study with monochromatic near-infrared treatment. *Diabetes Care*. 2004;27(1):168–172.

39. Prendergast JJ, Miranda G, Sanchez M. Improvement of sensory impairment in patients with peripheral neuropathy. *Endocr Pract*. 2004;10(1):24–30.

40. Lynch J, Helmrich SP, Lakka TA, et al. Moderately intense physical activities and high levels of cardiorespiratory fitness reduce risk of non-insulin dependent diabetes mellitus in middle-aged men. *Arch Intern Med*. 1996;156:1307–1314.

41. Mayer-Davis EJ, D'Agustino R, Jr, Karter AJ, et al. Intensity and amount of physical activity in relation to insulin sensitivity: the Insulin Resistance Atherosclerosis Study. *JAMA*. 1998;279:669–674.

42. Diabetes Prevention Program Research Group. Reduction in the incidence of type 2 diabetes with lifestyle intervention or metformin. *N Engl J Med*. 2002;346:393–401.

43. Tuomilehto J, Lindsrohm J, Erikson JG, et al. Prevention of type 2 diabetes mellitus by changes in lifestyle among subjects with impaired glucose tolerance. *N Engl J Med*. 2001;344:143–150.

44. Pan XR, Li GW, Hu YH, et al. Effect of diet and exercise in preventing NIDDM in people with impaired glucose tolerance. The Da Qing IGT and Diabetes Study. *Diabetes Care*. 1997;20:537–544.

45. Van Dam RM, Rimm EB, Willett WC, et al. Dietary patterns and risk for type 2 diabetes mellitus in U.S. men. *Ann Intern Med*. 2002;136:201–209.

46. Cregg EW, Gerzoff RB, Caspersen CJ, et al. Relationship of walking to mortality among U.S. adults with diabetes. *Arch Internal Med*. 2003;163:1440–1447.

47. Swartz AM, Strath SJ, Bassett DR, et al. Increasing daily walking improves glucose tolerance in overweight women. *Prev Med*. 2003;37:356–362.

48. Interact Consortium. Physical activity reduces the risk of incident type 2 diabetes in general and in abdominally lean and obese men and women: the EPIC-InterAct Study. *Diabetologia.* 2012;55(7):1944–1952.

49. Cooper AJ, Forouhi NG, Ye Z, et al. Fruit and vegetable intake and type 2 diabetes: EPIC-InterAct prospective study and meta-analysis. *Eur J Clin Nutr.* 2012;66(10):1082–1092.

50. Apostolidis E, Kwon YI, Shetty K. Potential of cranberry-based herbal synergies for diabetes and hypertension management. *Asia Pac J Clin Nutr.* 2006;15(3):433–441.

51. Kwon YI, Apostolidis E, Kim YC, Shetty K. Health benefits of traditional corn, beans, and pumpkin: in vitro studies for hyperglycemia and hypertension management. *J Med Food.* 2007;10(2):266–275.

52. Kwon YI, Apostolidis E, Shetty K. in vitro studies of eggplant (*Solanum melongena*) phenolics as inhibitors of key enzymes relevant for type 2 diabetes and hypertension. *Bioresour Technol.* 2008 May;99(8):2981–8.

53. Pan A, Sun Q, Bernstein AM, Manson JE, Willett WC, Hu FB. Changes in red meat consumption and subsequent risk of type 2 diabetes mellitus: three cohorts of US men and women. *JAMA Intern Med.* 2013:1–8.

54. InterAct Consortium. Association between dietary meat consumption and incident type 2 diabetes: the EPIC-InterAct study. *Diabetologia.* 2013;56(1):47–59.

55. Huxley R, Lee CM, Barzi F, et al. Coffee, decaffeinated coffee, and tea consumption in relation to incident type 2 diabetes mellitus: a systematic review with meta-analysis. *Arch Intern Med.* 2009;169(22):2053–2063.

56. Sartorelli DS, Fagherazzi G, Balkau B, et al. Differential effects of coffee on the risk of type 2 diabetes according to meal consumption in a French cohort of women: the E3N/EPIC cohort study. *Am J Clin Nutr.* 2010;91(4):1002–1012.

57. InterAct Consortium. Tea consumption and incidence of type 2 diabetes in Europe: the EPIC-InterAct case-cohort study. *PLoS One.* 2012;7(5):e36910.

58. Norris JM, Yin X, Lamb MM, et al. Omega-3 polyunsaturated fatty acid intake and islet autoimmunity in children at increased risk for type 1 diabetes. *JAMA.* 2007;298(12):1420–1428.

59. Ziegler D, Ametov A, Barinov A, et al. Oral treatment with alpha-lipoic acid improves symptomatic diabetic polyneuropathy: the SYDNEY 2 trial. *Diabetes Care.* 2006;29(11):2365–2370.

60. Paolisso G, D'Amore A, Galzerano D, et al. Daily vitamin E supplements improve metabolic control but not insulin secretion in elderly type II diabetic patients. *Diabetes Care.* 1993;16:1433–1437.

61. Paolisso G, D'Amore A, Galzerano D, et al. Pharmacologic doses of vitamin E improves insulin action in healthy subjects and non-insulin dependent diabetic patients. *Am J Clin Nutr.* 1993;57:650–656.

62. Paolisso G, Balbi V, Volpe C, et al. Metabolic benefits deriving from chronic vitamin C supplementation in aged non-insulin dependent diabetics. *J Am Coll Nutr.* 1995;14:387–392.

63. Passariello N, Fici F, Gingliano D, et al. Effects of pyridoxine alphaketoglutarate on blood glucose and lactate in type I and II diabetes. *Int J Clin Pharmacol Ther Toxicol.* 1983;21:252–256.

64. Maebashi M, Makino Y, Furukawa Y, et al. Therapeutic evaluation of the effect of biotin on hyperglycemia in patients with non-insulin dependent diabetes mellitus. *J Clin Biochem Nutr.* 1993;14:211–218.

65. Lee NA, Reasner CA. Beneficial effect of chromium supplementation on serum triglyceride levels in NIDDM. *Diabetes Care.* 1994;17:1449–1452.

66. Barkaran K, Almath BK, Shammugasumdaram KR, Shammugasumdaram ERB. Antidiabetic effect of a leaf extract from *Gymnema sylvestre* in non-insulin dependent diabetes mellitus patients. *J Ethnopharmacol.* 1990;30:295–305.

67. Sotaniemi EA, Haopaloski E, Rautio A. Ginseng therapy in non-insulin dependent diabetic patients. *Diabetes Care.* 1995;18:1373–1375.

68. Yongchaiyudha S, Rungpitarrangsi V, Bumyapraphastura N, Chokeshaijaroenpora O. Antidiabetic activity of aloe vera juice. Clinical trial in new cases of diabetes mellitus. *Phytomed.* 1996;3:241–243.

69. Ford ES, Will JC, Bowman BA, Venkat Narayan KM. Diabetes mellitus and serum carotenoids: findings from the Third National Health and Nutrition Examination Survey. *Am J Epidemiol.* 1999;149:168–176.

70. Liu S, Ajani U, Chae C, et al. Long term beta-carotene supplementation and risk of type 2 diabetes mellitus. *JAMA.* 1999;282:1073–1075.

71. Kao WHK, Folsom AR, Nieto FJ, et al. Serum and dietary magnesium and the risk for type 2 diabetes mellitus: the Atherosclerosis Risk in Communities Study. *Arch Intern Med.* 1999;159:2151–2159.

72. Song Y, Wang L, Pittas AG, et al. Blood 25-hydroxy vitamin D levels and incident type 2 diabetes: a meta-analysis of prospective studies. *Diabetes Care.* 2013;36(5):1422–1428.

Thyroid Dysfunction

Context

Patients with thyroid dysfunction often have signs and symptoms that are suggestive of other disorders, including fatigue, depression, or other metabolic problems. Determination of the appropriate patient to screen for thyroid disease is based on either a clinical presentation of overt disease or high-risk categories for asymptomatic patients. There is a general consensus that screening all patients for thyroid dysfunction is not cost-effective because of the low yield and the difficulty with sorting out small increases and decreases that may reflect a euthyroid state (temporary change with no thyroid pathology).[1,2] Thyroid dysfunction is found in approximately 1% to 4% of the adult population of the United States with an annual incidence of 0.08% for hypothyroidism and 0.05% for hyperthyroidism.[2] Epidemiologic studies have determined several groups of patients who are at higher risk. Those patients who are symptomatic often will have a constellation of signs of symptoms; however, there are a number of individuals who are subclinically dysfunctional. A percentage of these patients will progress to overt hypo- or hyperthyroidism. These categories include the following:

Those with a risk 20 times that of the general population:[3]

- patients who have had radioisotope or radiation therapy
- patients with other autoimmune disorders
- patients with first-degree relatives with thyroid disease
- patients taking amiodarone hydrochloride

Those with a risk eight times that of the general population:[4-6]

- the elderly

Those with a risk four times that of the general population:[7]

- women over age 40 years

Consideration for screening in patients with minor risk:

- psychiatric patients[8]
- those patients taking lithium or who have a quickly fluctuating bipolar disorder

Neonatal testing is required in all states. This is due less to the risk (1 of 3,500 to 4,000 births) than to the devastating effects of not detecting what will become cretinism with its associated mental retardation and other neuropsychological effects.

Although there are a number of thyroid disorders and even temporal sequencing of hyper- and hypothyroidism with the same named condition, the majority of patients fit into two categories: (1) hyperthyroidism—most often due to Graves' disease, and (2) hypothyroidism—most often due to Hashimoto's disease. Hypothyroidism also may be due to treatment for hyperthyroidism with either radioactive iodine therapy or surgery. There are also age-related changes in thyroid physiology, which is why patients over age 65 years, especially women, must be considered for screening. Thyroid dysfunction may also be due to secondary (pituitary) and tertiary (hypothalamic) disorders. Specific thyroid disorders and how they differ are listed under Selected Thyroid Disorders.

General Strategy

History

- Determine whether the patient has been diagnosed with a thyroid disorder or has had treatment for a thyroid disorder.

- Determine whether the patient has any complaints of fatigue, intolerance to heat or cold, tremors, or eye problems.

Evaluation

- Determine whether a goiter is present.
- Determine whether there are secondary signs of hypothyroidism, including dry skin, loss of outer third of eyebrows, weight gain, slow speech, a decrease in deep tendon reflexes, or the more classic facial appearance of cretinism.
- Determine whether there are secondary signs of hyperthyroidism, including increased pulse rate and blood pressure, increased respiration, increase in deep tendon reflexes, detection of a fine tremor, exophthalmos, or lid lag.
- Screen asymptomatic patients at higher risk based on the above-listed categories.
- Run an ultrasensitive thyrotropin (uTSH) or thyroid panel on patients believed to have a thyroid disorder.

Management

- Refer patients who fit classic laboratory criteria for overt thyroid disease.
- Educate patients who have subclinical thyroid disease about the pros and cons of treatment and refer to a medical doctor for a second opinion.

Relevant Physiology

A feedback loop controls thyroid hormone production. When circulating thyroid hormone levels are low, pituitary thyrotroph cells are stimulated by hypothalamic thyrotropin-releasing hormone (TRH). TSH (thyrotropin) is then secreted from the pituitary to initiate several steps in the production of active thyroid hormone. Iodine is trapped and linked to tyrosine by peroxidase. Next, coupling of monoiodotyrosine and diiodotyrosine form T_3 (triiodotyrosine) and T_4 (thyroxin). The thyroid gland then secretes T_4 and a very small amount of T_3. T_3 is the most active form of thyroid hormone. Most of the circulating T_3 is, in fact, produced via peripheral deiodination of T_4 in the liver. Reverse T_3, an inactive form, is also produced. Thyroid-binding globulin (TBG) binds 99.95% of thyroid hormones. Therefore, any condition that affects protein levels will affect total thyroid hormone levels. These conditions include liver disease, pregnancy, estrogen levels, starvation, and acute or chronic illness. With severe illness the peripheral conversion of T_4 to T_3 is reduced even though there is no thyroid organ pathology.

Evaluation

History

Signs and symptoms suggestive of hyperthyroidism include nervousness, irritability, tremor, muscle weakness, heat intolerance, change in appetite, decreased or dysfunctional menstrual flow, and increased frequency of bowel movements. Many of these complaints are the result of increased metabolism. The patient may also notice a change in appearance, such as a neck mass, enlarged or more prominent eyes and associated eye irritation. Only 5% to 10% develop severe eye changes. Lymphocytic infiltration is the cause of exophthalmos and occasionally diplopia when the extraocular muscles become entrapped by infiltrates.

Patients with hypothyroidism may have complaints similar to those with hyperthyroidism. Complaints include weakness, tiredness, fatigue, depression, weight gain (true obesity is unusual), cold intolerance, dry skin, hoarseness, impaired mental function, joint pains and muscle cramps, and menstrual difficulties such as anovulatory bleeding and infertility. An enlarged gland may be apparent to the patient.

Examination

The physical examination focuses on possible enlargement of the thyroid gland and the secondary effects of thyroid dysfunction on skin/hair, weight, myxoid deposition, and the cardiovascular system. The first aspect of evaluation of thyroid size and contour is inspection. Viewing the patient from the front and having him or her extend the neck often provides a better visualization of the thyroid. Cross-lighting may be helpful to better delineate contour. Next, viewing from the side, determine if there is any protrusion between the cricoid cartilage and the suprasternal notch. Palpation of the thyroid has been described many different ways. Some of the variations are whether to palpate from behind or in front of the patient and whether to use the ipsilateral or opposite hand. No studies indicate any specific method as superior. The location of the thyroid gland is determined in relation to the thyroid and cricoid cartilage. Normally the thyroid gland is palpable on either side of the distal half of the thyroid cartilage down to the upper trachea. Palpation is facilitated by relaxing the sternocleidomastoids. This is accomplished by having the patient flex and rotate the head to the ipsilateral side of palpation. It is often recommended that having the patient swallow may assist in determining size and possibly reveal a low-lying gland. It is important to have the patient swallow a sip of water, only because the larger the amount of water, the more the excursion, the more difficult the task of discrimination from other structures.

Some individuals are difficult to palpate. These include the obese, the elderly, and those with chronic pulmonary disease, where the neck is relatively short. Errors may occur due to misinterpretation in the following patients:[9]

- overestimation of size in thin individuals or those with long, slender necks (Modigliani syndrome)
- overestimation due to a more superior location (normal variant)
- misidentification of a fat pad in the anterior and lateral neck as a goiter (pseudogoiter) found in the obese and those of normal weight (in particular young women) (the fat pad does not move with swallowing and the texture is different from that of the thyroid)
- underestimation due to a low-lying thyroid (can be retrosternal)
- underestimation due to sternocleidomastoid interference

Interexaminer agreement on the detection of a goiter and whether individual lobes are enlarged has been demonstrated to be very good.[10, 11]

Additional maneuvers such as measuring neck circumference and determining mobility, modularity, and texture are more subtle and not necessarily consistently rated by examiners. Auscultation for bruits may provide a clue to a hyperfunctioning gland. It is important to remember that a goiter may appear with either hyper- or hypothyroidism and does not help to distinguish between them. It is also possible to have no enlargement and have either disorder.

Patients with hyperthyroidism may have a widened pulse pressure and tachycardia. Approximately 10% to 25% of patients will have atrial fibrillation. Confirmation with an electrocardiogram is needed. In postmenopausal women, bone loss is increased and may be confirmed with dual x-ray absorptiometry.

Laboratory Testing and Management

Laboratory testing for thyroid dysfunction can be extremely confusing. However, in the context of chiropractic practice, most cases of dysfunctional thyroid can be detected by running a uTSH test.[12] The advantages of this test are that it can discriminate between euthyroidism (increased levels due to an underlying disorder/disease), which is transient, and overt thyroid dysfunction. When the TSH is elevated, it should be rerun adding FT_4 and a thyroid autoantibody panel. If the TSH is high and the FT_4 is low, the patient is hypothyroid. If there is an elevation of anti-thyroperoxidase (anti-TPO) antibodies, it is likely the patient has Hashimoto's disease. If the TSH is high and the FT_4 is normal, the patient is considered to be subclinically hypothyroid. Recommendations are to recheck TSH levels every three to six months for the first year and every six to twelve months thereafter. Referral for medical management is suggested by some practitioners, especially when there is a high level of autoantibodies.

When the TSH is low, rerun with FT_4 and FT_3 with a thyroid autoantibody panel. If the TSH is low and either the FT_4 or FT_3 is elevated, the patient is hyperthyroid. If there is an elevation of thyroid antibodies, specifically thyroid-stimulating immunoglobulin (TSI) antibodies, and activating thyrotropin receptor antibodies (TRAbs), it is likely that the patient has Graves' disease. If the TSH is low and the FT_3 and FT_4 are normal, the patient is considered subclinically hyperthyroid. If the TSH is low, or if it is minimally high or normal with a low T_4, a search for hypothalamic or pituitary disease is necessary. It is important to note that thyroid function tests are often abnormal in hospitalized and severely ill patients. This may represent a temporary dysfunction and cannot be viewed with the same degree of trust as with the ambulatory patient.

Additional findings with hypothyroidism include macrocytic anemia, increased creatinine phosphatase, and hyperlipidemia. Hyperthyroidism may also demonstrate hypercalcemia, increased alkaline phosphatase, anemia, and decreased granulocytes.

Algorithm

An algorithm for thyroid lab evaluation is presented in **Figure 50–1**.

Table 50–1 Thyroid Medications

Drug Class	Examples	General Mechanism	Interactions/Side Effects
Levothyroxine sodium	Eltroxin Synthroid Levoxyl Levothroid Unithroid	A synthetic version of thyroxine (T_4) used to treat hypothyroidism and to suppress thyroid hormone release with cancerous thyroid nodules.	May cause similar effects of hyperthyroidism related to increased metabolism including palpitations, hypertension, agitation, insomnia, heat intolerance, weight loss, leg cramps, arrhythmias, headache, menstrual irregularities such as anovulatory bleeding.
Liothyronine (T_3)	Cytomel Triostat	Replaces T_3 in hypothyroid patients. Used in the 3 suppression test. Main use is for those patients who do not respond to levothyroxine (Synthroid).	Overdose effects are signs/symptoms of hyperthyroidism.
Methimazole	Tapazole	Blocks transformation of inorganic iodine to organic iodine. Blocks conversion of T_4 and T_3. Often used to produce a euthyroid state prior to radiation or surgery. Long-term use may produce euthyroid state in half of patients.	May cause headache, vertigo, nausea, vomiting, hepatitis, myelosuppression, leucopenia, and rarely agranulocytosis. May elevate prothrombin time and liver enzymes.
Propylthiouracil (PTU)	Propyl-Thyracil	Blocks transformation of inorganic iodine to organic iodine. Often used to produce a euthyroid state prior to radiation or surgery. Long-term use may produce euthyroid state in half of patients.	May cause headache, vertigo, nausea, vomiting, hepatitis, myelosuppression, leucopenia, and rarely agranulocytosis. May elevate prothrombin time and liver enzymes.

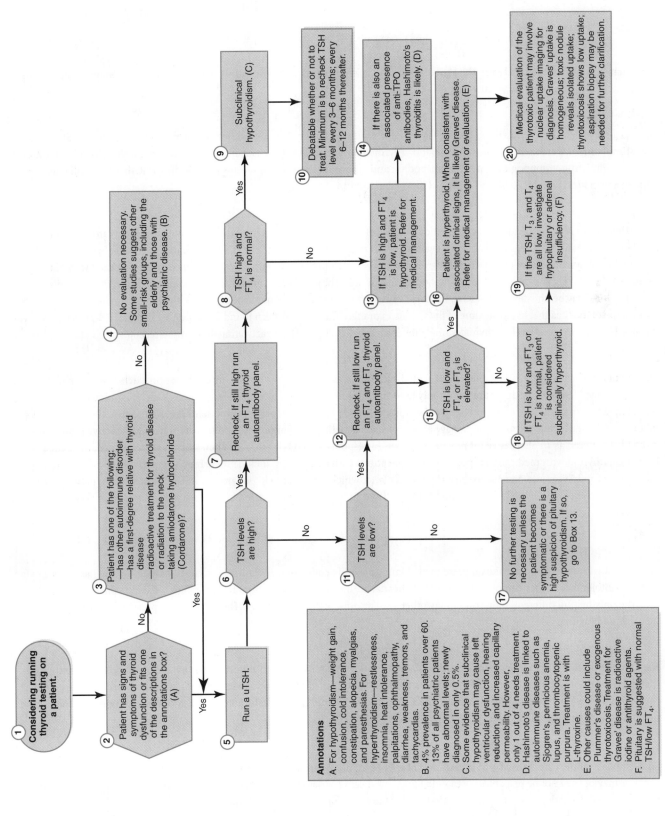

Figure 50–1 Thyroid Lab Evaluation—Algorithm

Selected Thyroid Disorders

Graves' Disease

Classic Presentation

A woman (8:1 ratio to men) between the ages of 20 and 40 years presents with complaints of nervousness, weight loss, palpitations, fatigue, heat intolerance, or menstrual irregularities.

Cause

Graves' disease (also called Basedow's disease) is an autoimmune disorder. Autoantibodies are formed that bind to the TSH receptors, stimulating hyperactivity of the thyroid gland. Thyroid autoantibodies that cause increased secretion of thyroid hormone are thyroid-stimulating immunoglobulin (TSI) antibodies, and activating thyrotropin receptor antibodies (TRAbs). A familial tendency with an association with HLA-B8 and HLA-DR3 has been found.

Evaluation

Hyperthyroidism is usually evident on examination because of the hypermetabolic state and ophthalmopathy. Tachycardia and atrial fibrillation are possible findings and should be evaluated with an electrocardiogram (ECG).[13, 14] A fine resting tremor, hyperreflexia, fine hair, and moist, warm skin are often found. The eyes may appear protuberant (exophthalmos) and this may be associated with other eye signs, including lid lag and diplopia due to lymphocytic infiltration. The eye changes are not an indication of the severity of the disease.[15] Exophthalmos may be unilateral or bilateral. Pretibial "myxedema" is found in about 3% of patients with Graves' disease. This is an infiltrate on top of the tibia that has the texture of the skin of an orange. The classic pattern found on lab testing includes a decreased TSH with elevated FT_4 with elevated levels of thyroid-stimulating immunoglobulin (TSI), and activating thyrotropin receptor antibodies (TRAbs).

Management

Treatment involves symptomatic management with β-blockers and the use of drugs that inhibit function, such as methimazole or propylthiouracil.[16] The latter drugs are commonly used in children and pregnant women. Alternatives include radioactive iodine treatment and surgery. Radioactive iodine treatment is contraindicated in pregnancy. Opponents feel that radioactive iodine will predispose the individual to cancer or damage an individual's genetic pool. Surgery is used less often than radioactive iodine and is more likely offered as an alternative for pregnant women unresponsive to medication.[17] When surgery is performed, the patient must be made euthyroid with medication if possible. Complications with surgery can include recurrent laryngeal nerve damage, leading to vocal cord paralysis, and damage to the parathyroid gland, which may lead to hypoparathyroidism. Post surgery, patients may eventually become hypothyroid requiring prescription of synthetic thyroid medication.

Hashimoto's Disease

Classic Presentation

The patient with overt hypothyroidism presents with multiple body complaints including weakness, fatigue, arthralgias, constipation, and cold intolerance. Other complaints may include headache, menstrual dysfunction, thinning hair, dry skin, and mental difficulties. The only helpful differentiation from many other similar presentations is a goiter. The patient may present first with a goiter and no other complaints.

Cause

Hashimoto's disease is an autoimmune disorder characterized by lymphocytic infiltration of the thyroid. Antibodies to the thyroid that decrease thyroid production with Hashimoto's include those against thyroglobulin called anti-TG antibodies and those against thyroperioxidase called anti-thyroperoxidase, also called anti-TPO antibodies. Hashimoto's disease is more common in women and demonstrates a familial relationship.

Evaluation

Signs may be subtle. Check for loss of lateral third of eyebrows, bradycardia, an enlarged tongue, and decreased deep tendon reflexes. A goiter may or may not be palpable due to individual and disease variation. The classic pattern found on lab testing for Hashimoto's is an increased TSH, decreased FT_4 and elevated levels of anti-TG and/or anti-TPO antibodies.

Management

Levothyroxine replacement therapy is used for primary hypothyroidism. Reevaluation is performed at six- to eight-week intervals until the TSH levels have normalized. After normalization of TSH, the level should be checked every six to twelve months.

Subacute Thyroiditis (De Quervain's Thyroiditis)

Classic Presentation

The patient is more likely Caucasian or Chinese and presents with a complaint of anterior neck pain that followed a viral prodrome (myalgia, low-grade fever, sore throat, and tiredness), often in the summer or fall. Associated symptoms may be palpitations, diaphoresis, and tachycardia.

Cause

Apparently viral in origin, subacute thyroiditis is an acute, self-limited inflammatory disorder of the thyroid. There appears to be an autoimmune abnormality and an association with HLA-Bw35 in Caucasian and Chinese patients. Women are more commonly affected (range from 3:1 to 6:1), with an onset between ages 30 and 50 years.[18]

Evaluation

Palpation usually reveals a very tender, nodular goiter, but a goiter is not always found. Thyroid function tests indicate hyperthyroidism; however, a coupled finding of a reduced radioactive iodine uptake is diagnostic. A normal thyroglobulin level generally rules out primary hyperthyroidism.

Management

Referral for medical management is necessary, although many patients are treated with aspirin in the initial stages. Occasionally, patients with dysphagia due to an enlarged gland need prednisone (20% experience rebound swelling when drug is withdrawn).[19] β-blockers are occasionally used for the hypermetabolic symptoms. Antithyroid drugs are useless; the disorder has nothing to do with synthesis of thyroid hormone, only release of existing preformed hormones. Recovery is common in three to six weeks; however, 30% of patients develop hypothyroidism due to follicular cell destruction. Ninety percent of these patients recover in four to six weeks. Ten percent are permanently hypothyroid.[20]

Silent Thyroiditis

Classic Presentation

A women who is four to eight weeks postpartum presents with complaints of nervousness and palpitations.

Cause

Antithyroid antibodies are found in 50% to 80% of patients, suggesting an autoimmune process. Although this entity may occur in men and women, the most common form is found in women (4:1). Thyroiditis may occur sporadically in either gender, but postpartum presentation is common in women. Hormonal shifts postpartum may act as a trigger. The postpartum and sporadic types account for between 5% and 20% of all hyperthyroidism. Six percent of patients may have persistent hypothyroidism.[21]

Evaluation

Thyroid palpation will reveal a nontender goiter in almost 50% of patients. Other findings are secondary to an initial hyperthyroidism for a few weeks, which may be followed by a 4- to 16-week period of hypothyroidism in 40% of patients. There is a low radioactive uptake in this disorder, distinguishing it from true hyperthyroidism.

Management

Generally reassurance is all that is needed. However, in some patients, referral may be necessary for medical management of transient symptoms, including β-blockers. There is no place for antithyroid medication in the treatment of silent thyroiditis.

Acute Thyroiditis

Classic Presentation

Patients present with an abrupt onset of intense anterior neck pain with associated signs of fever and chills; it occurs more often in women.

Cause

Sometimes referred to as suppurative thyroiditis, this rare disorder is usually due to *Staphylococcus aureus, Streptococcus pyrogens,* or pneumonia, although parasites and fungi are possible causes. Infection is hematogenous, lymphatic, or through a persistent thyroglossal duct. Fifty percent of patients have a history of thyroid disease.

Evaluation

Acute thyroiditis is usually apparent because of the abrupt onset and a tender thyroid. Laboratory results indicate normal thyroid function, an elevated white blood cell count with a shift to the left, and a normal radioactive iodine uptake.

Management

Refer for medical management of underlying infection.

Riedel's Thyroiditis

Classic Presentation

A middle-aged or elderly woman presents with a slowly enlarging, hard anterior neck mass that is not tender.

Cause

This extremely rare condition is due to replacement of thyroid tissue with dense fibrous tissue.

Evaluation

Palpation reveals a very hard thyroid gland. Laboratory tests usually reveal a normally functioning gland. In some patients, complete replacement of thyroid tissue will result in hypothyroidism evident on laboratory tests.

Management

Generally, the patient is monitored for progression to hypothyroidism, at which time thyroid replacement therapy is necessary. Surgical treatment is reserved for those with compressive complaints due to thyroid enlargement.

Thyroid Cancer

Classic Presentation

A patient with a past history of irradiation of the head or neck presents with a painless swelling in the region of the thyroid.

Cause

Papillary carcinoma or mixed papillary/follicular cancer accounts for 70% of all thyroid cancers, yet it is the least aggressive. Follicular cancer accounts for about 15% of cancers and is responsible for more metastases. Thyrotoxicosis rarely occurs with thyroid cancer.

Evaluation

Palpation of the thyroid will reveal a hard nodule in an enlarged gland and in some cases, palpable lymph nodes. Fine-needle biopsy is most useful in distinguishing benign (70% of time) from malignant (5%) tumors.[22] Thyroid function tests are usually normal. Occasionally, calcitonin levels are elevated. Radioiodine uptake testing usually demonstrates malignancies as "cold" lesions representing nonfunctioning tissue. Fine-needle aspiration is the test of choice. Metastatic lesions may be visible on radiographs or bone scans.

Management

Refer to oncologist.

APPENDIX 50–1

References

1. Surks MI, Chopra IJ, Mariash CN, Nicoloff JT, Solomon DH. American Thyroid Association guidelines for use of laboratory tests in thyroid disorders. *JAMA.* 1990;263:1529–1532.

2. U.S. Preventive Services Task Force. Screening for thyroid disease. In: *Guide to Clinical Preventive Services.* Baltimore: Williams & Wilkins; 1996:209.

3. Ladenson PW. Diagnosis of hypothyroidism. In: Braverman LE, Unger RD, eds. *Werner and Ingbar's The Thyroid: A Fundamental and Clinical Text.* 6th ed. Philadelphia: JB Lippincott; 1991:1092–1098.

4. Berlowitz I, Ramot Y, Rosenberg T, et al. Prevalence of thyroid disorders among the elderly in Israel. *Isr J Med Sci.* 1990;26:496–498.

5. Sobel R. Screening for thyroid disease (editorial). *Isr J Med Sci.* 1990;26:516–517.

6. Helfand M, Crapo LM. Screening for thyroid disease. *Ann Intern Med.* 1990;112:840–849.

7. DeGroot LJ, Mayor G. Admission screening by thyroid function tests in an acute general care teaching hospital. *Am J Med.* 1992;93:558–564.

8. Enns M, Ross C, Clark P. Thyroid screening tests in psychiatric inpatients. *Gen Hosp Psychiatry.* 1992;14:334–349.

9. Siminoski K. Does this patient have a goiter? *JAMA.* 1995;273:813–817.

10. Kilpatrick R, Milne JS, Rushbrooke M, Wilson ESB. A survey of thyroid enlargement in two general practices in Great Britain. *Br Med J.* 1963;1:29–34.

11. Dingle PR, Ferguson A, Horn DB, Tubmen J, Hall R. The incidence of thyroglobulin antibodies and thyroid enlargement in a general practice in northeast England. *Clin Exp Immunol.* 1966;1:277–284.

12. Brody MB, Reichard RA. Thyroid screening: how to interpret and apply results. *Postgrad Med.* 1995;98:54–66.

13. Woeber KA. Thyrotoxicosis and the heart. *N Engl J Med.* 1992;327:94.

14. Sawin CT, Geller A, Wolf PA, et al. Low serum thyrotropin concentration as a risk factor for atrial fibrillation in older persons. *N Engl J Med.* 1994;331:1249–1252.

15. Barrie WE. Graves' ophthalmopathy. *West J Med.* 1993;158:591.

16. Singer PA, Cooper DS, Levy EG, et al. Treatment guidelines for patients with hyperthyroidism and hypothyroidism. *JAMA.* 1995;273:808–812.

17. Patwardham NA, Moroni M, Rao S, et al. Surgery still has a role in Graves' hyperthyroidism. *Surgery.* 1993;114:1108–1113.

18. Sakiyama R. Thyroiditis: a clinical review. *Am Fam Physician.* 1993;48:615–621.

19. Singer PA. Thyroiditis: acute, subacute, and chronic. *Med Clin North Am.* 1991;75:61–77.

20. DeGroot LJ, Larsen PR, Refetoff S, et al. Acute and sub-acute thyroiditis. In: Braverman LE, Utiger RD, eds. *The Thyroid and Its Diseases.* 5th ed. New York: John Wiley & Sons; 1984: 717–727.

21. Schubert MF, Kountz DS. Thyroiditis: a disease with many faces. *Postgrad Med.* 1995;98:101–112.

22. Gharib H, Goellner JR. Fine needle aspiration biopsy of the thyroid: an appraisal. *Ann Intern Med.* 1993:118:282.

Hyperlipidemia

Context

The leading cause of death in the United States is coronary artery (heart) disease (CAD or CHD).[1] It is estimated that by the year 2020 cardiovascular disease will be the leading cause of death and disability.[2] Although there are many contributing factors to the development of coronary heart disease (CHD), a recent study emphasized that 80% to 90% of individuals with CHD have the four "conventional" risk factors.[3] These are cigarette smoking, hypertension, diabetes, and hyperlipidemia. The focus must be on lifestyle changes, including smoking cessation and the control of the other three factors that are interrelated. The second leading cause of death by disease is cancer; the third is diabetes.[4] There is evidence to suggest that some cancers are linked to high-fat diets. Adult-onset diabetes is strongly linked to diet. It would seem that the philosophy of prevention held by the chiropractic profession would dictate that part of a patient's care must involve intervention in areas such as these that do not require (and may prevent) the use of drugs or surgery and may prevent morbidity and mortality. Realistically, changes in diet and smoking habits are some of the most difficult to effect. Yet, the chiropractor is ideally positioned to provide either a direct or indirect comprehensive "wellness" program for his or her patients. Promotion of healthful eating and exercise should be a cornerstone in the management of all patients, regardless of current CHD status.

There are at least 10 meta-analysis studies of randomized trials that have attempted to address the effectiveness of cholesterol reduction and its effect on CHD.[5–7] It appears that for each 1% decrease in serum cholesterol, there is a 2% to 3% reduction in risk for CHD. This occurred in trials using drugs or diet. There is some controversy regarding the use of drugs in patients without CHD regarding cost, and an interesting increase in noncoronary mortality.[8] However, most agree that symptomatic men unresponsive to diet will benefit from drug intervention if it is monitored and reduced when appropriate. The reduction of serum cholesterol and decrease in CHD risk is not as clear in women. Women statistically have their onset of CHD approximately 10 years later than men, beginning at age 45 years. This delay is probably related to the protective effects of estrogen.[9] However, 49% of all CHD-related deaths in the United States are women.[1]

General Strategy

- Do not screen all individuals. Men aged 35 years and over, women aged 45 years and older, those with CHD or more than two risk factors, and children with a familial predisposition should be screened. Further testing is based on baseline results.
- Determine an individual's risk factors for CHD, including age, gender, physical activity/inactivity, smoking, obesity, hypertension, and diabetes.
- Order a lipid panel that includes total cholesterol, high-density lipoprotein cholesterol (HDLc), low-density lipoprotein cholesterol (LDLc), and triglycerides if the patient is at risk for CHD or has known CHD.
- Combine findings from the lipid panel with risk factors and make treatment/referral decisions.
- Order lipoprotein electrophoresis if patients have an isolated elevation of triglycerides that is suggestive of a familial disorder.
- Remember that for those patients without CHD or less than two risk factors, diet and exercise are the main approach; for those with CHD or two or

more risk factors, a trial of diet therapy is usually attempted for three to six months; when not responsive, drug therapy may be indicated.

Relevant Physiology

Cholesterol is not in and of itself bad. It is, in fact, essential to the body for the production of bile and the construction of cell membranes, myelin, and steroid hormones. The liver produces half the body's cholesterol; the remainder is acquired through the diet.[10] There are two main fats carried in the blood: cholesterol and triglycerides. They are packaged with proteins (apoproteins) into lipoproteins. The lipoproteins are classified based on density. The higher the triglyceride content, the less dense they are. The three main lipoproteins are HDLs, LDLs, and very-low-density lipoproteins (VLDLs). Therefore, LDLs contain about 75% lipid and 25% protein, whereas HDLs contain about an equal ratio. The general sequence of interaction is that VLDLs produced in the liver transport triglycerides to cells. When the VLDLs have lost a sufficient amount of triglyceride, they become LDL particles. LDL then provides cholesterol to the cells. Any excess of LDL is metabolized in the liver, providing cholesterol for bile. LDLs that are oxidized are potentially more harmful because of the direct effects on the arterial wall, and possibly through antibodies developed against the oxidized LDLs.[11] HDLs are produced in the liver and assist in transfer of apoproteins among the other lipoproteins. It is well known that HDLs may be protective through a mechanism referred to as reverse cholesterol transport—carrying excess cholesterol to other lipoproteins or to the liver.[12]

Hyperlipidemia is a term used to describe an increase in either plasma cholesterol or plasma triglycerides. These may occur in combination or in pure forms. Generally there are three main causes: (1) dietary, (2) genetic, and (3) secondary to other diseases or drugs. One distinction is that the dietary forms are generally milder than the genetic forms. In effect, hyperlipidemia is the same as hyperlipoproteinemia because there is always a problem with one of the steps in lipoprotein metabolism. For example, there may be a problem with the production, lipolysis, removal, or conversion of VLDL. The diagnosis is usually made when a lipid electrophoresis reveals an abnormally high fraction or combination of fractions of the lipoprotein pool.

One cause of high LDLc is familial hypercholesterolemia.[13] It is believed to be due to a defect in the LDL receptor gene, resulting in a reduced ability to process LDLc particles. This results in an LDLc level that is approximately twice that of normal. Many patients have an additional contribution to high LDLc from high dietary intake. These patients have an increased risk of developing CHD in their 30s and 40s. They are more likely to need drug therapy, especially if their LDLc levels remain above 190 mg/dL. Patients with a rare homozygous (two abnormal genes) form have absent surface receptors for LDLc and have extremely high levels of LDLc, with atherosclerosis development in childhood.

Another condition is called mixed hyperlipidemia, metabolic syndrome X, or familial hyperlipidemia (although these are not always synonymous). Most patients show a central obesity, hyperinsulinemia, hypertension, elevated triglycerides, low HDLc, and elevation of small LDL subfractions. Because these patients are prone toward diabetes and hypertension, they should be evaluated and monitored for these conditions. Patients with mixed hyperlipidemia respond favorably to even small decreases in weight. One ironic complication is that if total fat is reduced below 30% of total calories, there may be a compensatory increase in carbohydrate intake that may then stimulate the production of very-low-density lipoprotein cholesterol (VLDLc).

Triglycerides are more subject to changes in food consumption prior to laboratory investigation. An isolated increase in triglyceride levels is often due to a patient's not fasting or perhaps drinking coffee with cream prior to giving the laboratory sample. There are a number of lipid disorders that result in isolated triglyceride elevation. Usually the triglyceride levels are 1,000 mg/dL or above while the LDLc levels are often low or normal. Although there appears to be a genetic component, poor diet and lack of exercise seem to make the disorder more obvious. These patients can have a predisposition to pancreatitis, especially if they drink alcohol. Therefore, questioning regarding abdominal pain and counseling against excessive alcohol ingestion are warranted. Exercise and weight loss are the main treatment approaches. If unsuccessful, referral for medical management is necessary. There is disagreement as to the risk for patients with an isolated triglyceride elevation without a concomitant LDLc elevation.

Evaluation

History

The history is important in determining the level of concern with any individual cholesterol level. There are specific risk factors for CHD that significantly affect management decisions. Nonmodifiable, but significant, factors include age (45 years or older in men; 55 years or older in women), male gender, premature menopause (without estrogen replacement therapy), and a family history of premature CHD (myocardial infarction or sudden death before age 55 years in father or other male first-degree relative or before age 65 years in mother or other female first-degree relative). The modifiable risk factors include cigarette smoking (more than 10 per day), obesity (more than 130% of ideal total body weight), hypertension, physical inactivity, an HDLc level below 35 mg/dL, and diabetes mellitus. It is interesting to note that with the exception of smoking, the other risk factors are often interdependent. In other words, a patient who is inactive is more likely to become obese. Being obese is a predisposition for adult-onset diabetes, which is associated with hypertension. The other modifiable factor is diet. Although diet cannot always lower cholesterol levels, a low-fat diet is often instrumental in controlling obesity, diabetes, and hypertension.[14] Therefore, a careful diet history is important in determining the level of daily fat intake and its possible relationship to high levels of cholesterol and LDLc.

Laboratory Evaluation

There is some basic agreement as to who should be screened for high blood cholesterol. Men between the ages of 35 and 65 years and women between the ages of 45 and 65 years should be screened with either a fasting or nonfasting specimen to obtain a baseline reading.[15] The recommendation for how often these individuals should be screened varies. The strictest guidelines are from the National Cholesterol Education Program (NCEP) Adult Treatment Panel II, which recommends screening of nonfasting total cholesterol and HDLc every five years in all asymptomatic individuals aged 20 years and older.[16] These recommendations are similar to those of the American Academy of Family Physicians and the American College of Obstetricians and Gynecologists.[17,18] Most groups recommend selective screening of children and adolescents based on risk factors.[19,20] Children with a parental history of hypercholesterolemia should be screened with a nonfasting test for total cholesterol. Those with a family history of premature CHD should be screened with a fasting lipid profile. Children with multiple risk factors such as obesity and smoking should be considered for a screening lab test. Most groups agree that screening of individuals over the age of 75 years is not warranted.[21]

Total cholesterol is the sum of HDL-C, LDL-C, and very-low-density lipoprotein cholesterol (VLDL-C). Although total cholesterol and HDL-C and triglycerides are relatively easy and inexpensive to measure, LDL-C and VLDL-C are not.[22] To resolve this issue and provide a practical approach clinically, a formula was developed by Friedewald in the 1970s. Using this formula, VLDL-C can be estimated based on a ratio to the total level of triglycerides. This ratio of triglycerides to VLDL-C (TG:VLDL-C) levels is on average 5:1. Using this observation, the Friedewald formula was created to estimate the LDL-C: This formula is LDL-C = (TC) − (HDL-C) − (triglycerides / 5) in mg/dL. Several attempts have been made, even as late as 2013, to better this estimate given some known concerns, primarily that the formula is not accurate when triglycerides are high. If the triglyceride levels are above 400 mg/dL, the formula is inaccurate and requires a more costly direct LDL-C measurement be utilized. In addition, the TG:VLDL-C ratio is not constant across the range of triglyceride levels and also varies based on the total cholesterol levels. Newer formulas are complicated and may not add to the clinical value of this estimation. Many argue that given that higher levels of both LDL-C and VLDL-C are the concern regarding atherosclerosis it may be better to continue to use the approach that has been used for years, which simply divides the total cholesterol into the "good" (HDL-C) and the "bad" (non–HDL-C). In other words, treatment approaches as measures could be based on non–HDL-C instead of those for LDL-C.

Interpretation of laboratory results is not a simple process of using a high cut-off value; for example, all levels above 200 mg/dL are bad. The relationship of cholesterol to risk is multivariable, including modifiable and nonmodifiable factors as discussed above. It is also important to refer to a cholesterol result as fitting into a range as opposed to a specific value. The reason for this caution is that cholesterol levels vary with many "outside" influences such as minor illness, stress, posture, and season.[23] This variation may be as much as 4% to 11% for an individual. In addition, laboratory values may not reflect a "true" cholesterol. Laboratory error and variation in equipment or operation of the equipment may affect readings. Finger-stick methods are biased toward a high range averaging between 4% and 7% more than a venipuncture specimen.[24] New desktop machines have been introduced that produce reliable readings; however, some machines do not meet required standards. Given the possible influences on a specific reading, the variation in an individual can be as high as 14%. It is important to note that reliability for HDLc is less than that for total cholesterol, with an average variation as much as 10% from a reference standard. Triglycerides are even less reliable. Therefore, a single measure is insufficient if high, and rechecking with a second sample is often suggested. If the two measurements (performed on different days) differ by more than 16%, a third sample is recommended.

Generally, if a patient's total cholesterol is 240 mg/dL or above or the level is between 200 and 239 mg/dL with known CHD or two risk factors, a lipid panel (cholesterol LDLc, HDLc, and triglycerides) should be performed. Based on the LDLc levels, decisions regarding diet or medication can be made. For patients with an isolated low level of HDLc (cholesterol, LDLc, and triglycerides are normal), it is important to rule out secondary causes. Investigation for possible thyroid, liver, or renal dysfunction should be included. Other possible causes are medications and acute illness.

Additional testing beyond a standard lipid panel is warranted when a primary (familial) hyperlipoproteinemia is suspected. The suspicion is based on either extremely elevated, isolated levels of triglycerides, or cholesterol, or LDLc, or a history of unresponsiveness to dietary changes. For these patients, a lipoprotein electrophoresis will help distinguish among the five types and their subtypes. Refer to **Table 51–1** for a description of these familial disorders, their associated risk for CHD, and general treatment recommendations.

New biomarkers that are linked to the pathogenesis of atherosclerosis progression may be used to help determine further cardiovascular risk in some patients.[25] Some possible future testing approaches follow:

- Markers of lipoprotein and lipid metabolism such as lipoprotein (a) or apolipoprotein B
- Measures of vitamin B_{12} metabolism such as vitamin B_{12} levels (possible inverse relationship to homocysteine)
- Homocysteine levels
- C-reactive protein levels (increased in patients prone toward coronary events)
- Infectious agents such as Chlamydia, cytomegalovirus, *Helicobacter pylori,* and herpes simplex have been tied to increased risk of CHD through involvement in atherosclerotic plaque development[26]
- Increased levels of fibrinogen, fibrinogen beta mutation, plasmin-alpha-antiplasmin complex, plasminogen activator inhibitor I, tissue-type

plasminogen activator, and D-dimer may identify high-risk individuals for coronary events
- Increased levels of markers for endothelial function and cell adhesion
- Angiotensin
- Levels of vitamins C and E (antioxidants) and vitamin D
- Markers of oxidative stress such as serum 7 beta-hydroxycholesterol, F2-isoprostanes, and nitric oxide synthase polymorphisms

A recent study indicated that although C-reactive protein, lipoprotein (a), fibrinogen, and homocysteine are clear indicators of risk for atherosclerotic disease, how to use them in routine screening has yet to be determined.[27]

Although a number of lipid measures for prediction of coronary heart disease (CHD) are available, it has been unclear as to their value when matched to standard measures. A study published by Inglesson et al.[28] in 2007 indicates that measurement of apoB/apoA-1 ratio provided no more sensitivity in prediction of CHD than the traditional lipid ratio of total cholesterol/HDLc.

Management

Using only total cholesterol measurements to make management decisions may lead to unwarranted concern or confidence. As discussed above, high-normal levels may be the result of lab error or variation. Approximately 20% of men with confirmed CHD have a cholesterol level below 200 mg/dL with an HDLc below 35 mg/dL. It is clear that women with high cholesterol levels, especially those who appear healthy, should not be assumed to be at risk unless confirmed with an associated low HDLc. Men who have a low cholesterol level but either are symptomatic for CHD or have significant risk factors should be tested for a low HDLc. In the past, a simple ratio was used between total cholesterol and HDLc, but this may be misleading. For example, two individuals may have a ratio of 5:1. In one individual the total cholesterol is 240 mg/dL with an HDLc of 48 mg/dL; the other individual has a total cholesterol of 150 mg/dL with an HDLc of 30 mg d/L. The second individual may be at more of a risk than the first based on the low HDLc, especially when other risk factors are added.

Published in 2013 was a new ACC/AHA Guideline on the Treatment of Blood Cholesterol to Reduce Atherosclerotic Cardiovascular Risk in Adults: A Report of the American College of Cardiology/American Heart

Table 51–1 Characteristics of the Primary Hyperlipoproteinemias

Type	Name	Clinical Presentation	Risk of Coronary Heart Disease	Plasma Cholesterol Level	Plasma Triglyceride Level	Genetic Form	Secondary Causes	Treatment
I	Exogenous hypertriglyceridemia Familial hyperglyceridemia Familial chylomicronemia Fat-induced hyperlipidemia Hyperchylomicronemia	Pancreatitis Eruptive xanthomas Hepatosplenomegaly Lipemia retinalis	Risk not increased	Normal or slightly increased	Very greatly increased	Autosomal recessive, rare	Systemic lupus erythematosus; dysgammaglobulinemia; insulinopenic diabetes mellitus	Dietary: low intake of fat; no alcohol
II	Familial hypercholesterolemia Familial hyperbetalipoproteinemia Familial hypercholesterolemic Xanthomatosis	Accelerated atherosclerosis Xanthelasma Tendon and tuberous xanthomas Juvenile corneal arcus	Very strong risk, especially for coronary atherosclerosis	Greatly increased	Normal Slightly increased	Autosomal dominant; common	Excess dietary cholesterol; hypothyroidism; nephrosis; multiple myeloma; porphyria; obstructive liver disease	Dietary: low-cholesterol, low-fat diet Drugs: cholestyramine, colestipol, niacin, probucol Possible surgery
III	Broad beta disease Familial dysbetalipoproteinemia Floating betalipoproteinemia	Accelerated atherosclerosis of coronary and peripheral vessels Planar xanthomas Tuberoeruptive and tendon xanthomas	Very strong risk for atherosclerosis, especially in peripheral and coronary arteries	Greatly increased	Greatly increased	Mode of inheritance unclear; uncommon but not rare	Dysgammaglobulinemia; hypothyroidism	Dietary: reduction to ideal weight; maintenance of low-cholesterol, balanced diet Drugs: niacin, clofibrate
IV	Endogenous hypertriglyceridemia Familial hyperprebetalipoproteinemia Carbohydrate-induced Hyperlipoproteinemia	Possible accelerated atherosclerosis Glucose intolerance Hyperuricemia	Possible risk, especially for coronary atherosclerosis	Normal or slightly increased	Greatly increased	Common, often sporadic when familial; genetically heterogeneous	Excess alcohol consumption; oral contraceptives; diabetes mellitus; glycogen storage disease; pregnancy; nephrotic syndrome; stress	Dietary: weight reduction; no alcohol Drugs: niacin, gemfibrozil

(continues)

Table 51–1 Characteristics of the Primary Hyperlipoproteinemias (continued)

Type	Name	Clinical Presentation	Risk of Coronary Heart Disease	Plasma Cholesterol Level	Plasma Triglyceride Level	Genetic Form	Secondary Causes	Treatment
V	Mixed hypertriglyceridemia Combined exogenous and endogenous hypertriglyceridemia Mixed hyperlipidemia	Pancreatitis Eruptive xanthomas Hepatosplenomegaly Sensory neuropathy Lipemia retinalis Hyperuricemia Glucose intolerance	Risk of atherosclerosis not clearly increased	Normal or slightly increased	Very greatly increased	Uncommon but not rare; genetically heterogeneous	Alcoholism; insulin-dependent diabetes mellitus; nephrosis; dysgammaglobulinemia	Dietary: weight reduction; no alcohol Drugs: niacin, gemfibrozil

Modified with permission from D.S. Fredrickson and R.I. Levy, Familial Hyperlipoproteinemia, in *The Metabolic Basis of Inherited Disease*, 5th ed., J.B. Stanbury, J.B. Wyngaarden, and D.S. Fredrickson, eds., © 1983, The McGraw-Hill Companies, Inc.

Association Task Force on Practice Guidelines[29] and an online calculator to determine risk. Immediately criticism arose regarding the implications of adopting this new approach. In particular, the calculator appears to overestimate the risk to the point where individuals using the prior estimation of risk are now double the risk using the new calculator. It appears that this might be an attempt to increase the use of statin drugs. It is conjectured that because the calculator data were collected more than a decade ago, at a time when more people smoked and had strokes and heart attacks earlier in life, that the data do not reflect the current status of the general population. It has been estimated that the calculator may overpredict risk by as much as 75% to 150%, depending on the population.

The guidelines recommend an expanded group of individuals in whom statins should be used and for that group they believe the benefits outweigh the risks. This includes patients with:

- clinically evident atherosclerotic cardiovascular disease
- primary low-density lipoprotein (LDL) cholesterol levels of at least 190 mg per deciliter
- type 1 or type 2 diabetes and an LDL cholesterol level of 70 mg per deciliter or higher, or
- a 10-year risk of atherosclerotic cardiovascular disease of at least 7.5%, according to the new cohort equations, and an LDL cholesterol level of at least 70 mg per deciliter.

The implications for how physicians would change their prescribing behaviors based on these new guidelines include:

- Have patients use a new risk calculator that will target many more individuals for the need for statins.
- Decrease the use of indirect biomarkers of risk such as C-reactive protein or calcium scores.
- Increase the use of statins and avoidance of non-statin LDL cholesterol–lowering agents in statin-tolerant patients.
- Eliminate the need for routine checks of LDL cholesterol levels in patients receiving statin therapy, because target levels are no longer considered important.
- In patients older than 75 years of age who have no clinical atherosclerotic cardiovascular disease, become more conservative with the use of statins.

Generally, level of risk is known to increase by approximately 3% for each 1% increase in total cholesterol for middle-aged men. Based on the Framingham study, the level of risk is determined by adding point values for each risk factor and using a conversion table to determine the percentage of risk. These simple calculations may be helpful in defining risk for the patient and illustrate how significant each additional risk factor becomes. In practical application, the level of concern for two patients with a cholesterol level of 240 mg/dL is obviously different. If the patient is a middle-aged man with any risk factors, monitoring levels while applying intervention with diet or medication is warranted, whereas a woman with the same cholesterol level and a high HDLc would warrant less concern. However, recent evidence suggests that it is not always true that higher HDLc levels are protective. Researchers have found that based on genetic mechanisms that raise plasma HDL cholesterol for these individuals, higher levels do not seem to lower risk of myocardial infarction.[30]

Given the controversy over the newer guidelines, it is important to remember the recommendations from the National Cholesterol Education Program, which publishes an "at-a-glance" quick reference to the Adult Treatment Panel (ATP) III Guidelines.[31] They created an evidence-based, sequential, step-by-step approach to the management of patients with hyperlipidemia, which still appears relevant until the newer guidelines can be further evaluated. More than in the past, lifestyle and dietary approaches are emphasized as initial management in most patient scenarios except those with serious risk factors. There are clear indicators of when medical therapy should be pursued. A summary of these steps follows, and **Figure 51–1** shows an algorithmic representation of the guidelines. A website access address is provided at the end of this chapter.

LDL Cholesterol: Primary Target for Therapy
<100: Optimal
100–129: Near optimal/above optimal
130–159: Borderline high
160–189: High
≥190: Very high

Total Cholesterol
<200: Desirable
200–239: Borderline high
240: High

HDL Cholesterol
<40: Low
≥60: High

- Step 1: Determine the patient's lipoprotein levels utilizing a complete lipoprotein profile test after a 9- to 12-hour fast.
- Step 2: Identify risk factors for coronary heart disease (CHD) event (CHD risk equivalent) evident by the presence of clinical atherosclerotic disease. These include clinical CHD, symptomatic carotid artery disease, peripheral arterial disease, or abdominal aortic aneurysm. Diabetes is considered a CHD risk equivalent.
- Step 3: Determine any major risk factors (other than LDL), including cigarette smoking, hypertension (BP ≥140/90 mmHG or on antihypertensive medication), low HDL cholesterol (<40 mg/dL), family history of premature CHD (CHD in first-degree male relative <55 years; CHD in first-degree female relative <65 years), and men ≥45 years old or females ≥55 years old. Note that HDL cholesterol >60 mm/dL is a "negative" risk factor, allowing the subtraction of one of the other risk factors from the total count.
- Step 4: If there are 2 + risk factors (other than LDL) without CHD or CHD risk equivalents, assess the 10-year (short-term) CHD risk using the Framingham tables. There are three levels of 10-year risk: (1) >20% CHD risk equivalent, (2) 10% to 20%, and (3) <10%.
- Step 5: Determine the patient's risk category. This includes establishing the LDL goal of therapy, determining the need for therapeutic lifestyle changes (TLC), and determining the need for referral for drug consideration. Following is a summary:
  1. *For CHD or CHD risk equivalents:* The LDL goal is <100 mg/dL and the LDL level to initiate TLC is ≥100 mg/dL; drug therapy is considered if ≥130 mg/dL.
  2. *For 2+ risk factors (10-year risk <20%):* The LDL goal is 130 mg/dL, at which point TLC is initiated; drug therapy is considered at ≥130 mg/dL if the 10-year risk is 10% to 20% and if the 10-year risk is 10% drug therapy begins at ≥160 mg/dL.
  3. *For 0 to 1 risk factors:* The LDL goal is <160 mg/dL, at which point TLC are initiated; drug therapy is considered if LDL is ≥190 mg/dL. (For 160–190 mg/dL, drugs are considered optional.)
- Step 6: Initiate therapeutic lifestyle changes (TLC) if the LDL is above the goal level. These include dietary recommendations: saturated fats should equal <7% of calories, cholesterol <200 mg/day, possible use of viscous (soluble) fiber 10–25 g/day and plant stanols/sterols (2g/day) in attempting to reduce LDL, weight management, and increased physical activity.
- Step 7: Consider referring for drug therapy if the LDL exceeds recommended levels (see **Table 51–2** for list of medications and proposed effects).[5]
- Step 8: Identify whether the patient has metabolic syndrome and treat if present after three months of TLC. Risk factors include abdominal obesity indicated by a waist circumference of >102 cm (>40 in.) in males and 88 cm (>35 in.) in females, elevated triglycerides ≥150 mg d/L, HDL cholesterol <40 mg/dL in males and <50 mg/dL in females, blood pressure ≥130/85 mmHg, and a fasting glucose 110 mg/dL. Treatment includes weight management and increased physical activity to treat the underlying causes. Treatment for lipid and nonlipid risk factors is initiated if TLC were ineffective. Hypertension should be managed; aspirin is considered for CHD patients to reduce prothrombotic state; and referral made, if necessary, to decrease triglyceride levels or increase HDL if conservative approaches are not effective.
- Step 9: Treat elevated triglyceride levels. See the algorithmic representation of this step plan for management.

Classification of Serum Triglycerides (mg/dL)
150 = normal
150–199 = borderline high
200–499 = high
≥500 = very high

The primary treatment aim is still to reach LDL goal. Weight management and increased physical activity are emphasized. If triglycerides are ≥200 mg/dL after the LDL goal is reached, a secondary goal is set for non-HDL cholesterol (total cholesterol minus HDL) 30 mg/dL higher than LDL goal.

- *For CHD or CHD risk equivalents:* The LDL goal is <100 mg/dL and the non-HDL goal is <130 mg/dL.
- *For 2+ risk factors (10-year risk <20%):* The LDL goal is 130 mg/dL and the non-HDL goal is <160 mg/dL.
- *For 0–1 risk factors:* The LDL goal is <160 mg/dL and the non-HDL goal is <190.

Table 51–2 Nutritional Support for Hyperlipidemia

Substance	How Does it Work?	Dosage	Special Instructions	Contraindications for Possible Side Effects
Gugulipid	Increases liver's metabolism of LDL; increases uptake of LDLc from the blood; may prevent the formation of atherosclerosis.	25 mg (most extracts contain 5%–10% guggulsterones) 3 times/day.	Best taken with meals. Should be taken with pyridoxal 5 phosphate (included in recommended supplement).	Do not combine with Imitrex or other SSRI or MAOI antidepressants. Taking more than recommended dose may lead to serotonin syndrome. Should not be taken with history of liver disease or inflammatory bowel disease or diarrhea is found. Safety unknown for pregnant or lactating women.
Omega-3s (EPA & DHA)	Lowers triglyceride levels.	3,000 mg/day (add EPA & DHA content to determine omega-3 content).	Omega-3s may raise LCLc levels; taking 900 mg/day of garlic may neutralize this effect.	Cod liver oil is less expensive; however, it contains large amounts of vitamins A and D, which may cause side effects.
Flaxseed oil	Another form of omega-3 but does not lower triglyceride levels; may lower total cholesterol; increases HDL.	1–2 tablespoons daily.	Keep refrigerated; away from light; do not heat.	None at recommended dosage.
Inositol Hexaniacinate (Flush Free Niacin)	Lowers LDLc; fibrinogen (blood protein that causes clot formation); raises HDL level.	650 mg 3 times/day.	Best taken with meals.	Although safest form of niacin, it should be used with caution with diabetics and preexisting liver disease.
Chromium	Reduces LDLc and raises HDLc.	200 mcg/day	None.	At very high levels (>1,000 mcg/day) severe liver or kidney disease is possible. For those using brewer's yeast, some people have allergies.
Pantethine	Inhibits cholesterol production and increases utilization of fats as energy source.	250–300 mg 3 times/day.	Best taken with meals.	Diarrhea with increased dosage. Megadoses (over 6 g/daily) may increase calcium oxalate stone formation in susceptible individuals.
Vitamin E	Protects LDL from oxidation; may increase HDLc.	400–800 IU/day.	None.	Side effects for vitamin E are rare.
Vitamin C	Reduces total cholesterol; protects LDL from oxidation; may increase HDL levels.	350–1,000 mg 3 times/day Ascorbyl palmitate.	Best taken with meals.	Diarrhea with increased dosage. Megadoses (over 6 g/daily) may increase calcium oxalate stone formation in susceptible individuals.
B Complex (B$_6$, B$_{12}$, and folic acid)	Lowers homocysteine levels.	Per bottle recommendations.	Best taken with meals.	None
Carnitine	May lower triglyceride levels.	1–3 g/day	L-isomer not DL mixture is more safe and effective.	DL-carnitine has caused weakness in some kidney patients on dialysis. L-carnitine at 1.6 g/day for 1 year has not caused side effects.
Wild yam	May lower triglyceride levels.	2–3 ml of tincture 3–4 times/day.	None	None at recommended dose.

Note: The following have not been approved by the Food and Drug Administration for the treatment of this disorder.
Other substances that may benefit a patient with dyslipidemia include soy protein, chondroitin sulfate, beta-sitosterol, octacosanol, and royal jelly.
Key: SSRI, selective serotonin reuptake inhibitor; MAOI, monoamine oxidase inhibitor; EPA, eicosapentaenoic acid; DHA, docosahexaenoic acid; DL, dextro/levo (right/left).

If the triglycerides are 200–499 mg/dL after the LDL goal is reached, consider referral for drug therapy to reach the non-HDL goal. If triglycerides are ≥ 500 mg/dL, it is important to lower the triglycerides first to prevent pancreatitis. This includes recommendation for a very low-fat diet (< 15% of calories from fat), weight management and physical activity, and nicotinic acid (or referral for fibrate). Only after triglycerides are lower than 500 mg/dL should the emphasis switch to lowering LDL.

For patients with isolated low levels of HDLc, non-pharmacologic means should be used first including weight loss, exercise, cessation of smoking, and use of nutritional support.[32,33] Moderate alcohol consumption (two drinks/day for males; one drink/day for females) has also been demonstrated to increase HDLc levels; however, the negative effects probably outweigh the benefits of recommending this to patients.

Grundy et al.[34] published an update of the National Cholesterol Education Group Adult Treatment Panel III Guidelines based on published trials since their implementation. Following are some recommended modifications:

- High-risk patients—the recommended LDLc goal is <100 mg/dL; however, when the risk is very high an LDL of <70 mg/dL is a reasonable clinical option even for patients with a baseline LDLc of <100 mg/dL. If the high-risk patient has high triglycerides or low HDLc, combining a fibrate or nicotinic acid with an LDL-lowering drug should be considered.
- Moderately high-risk persons (2+ risk factors and 10-year risk of 10% to 20%)—the LDLc recommended goal is <130 mg/dL but a goal of <100 mg/dL is a therapeutic option even if baseline LDLc is <100 mg/dL.
- For both high-risk and moderate-risk persons— goal of therapy is at least a 30% to 40% reduction in LDLc levels and regardless of LDLc level, all of these patients must address therapeutic lifestyle changes.

Recent recommendations by the American College of Cardiology and American Heart Association focus on two general categories including advice to adults wishing to lower LDLc and advice to adults wishing to lower blood pressure (BP).[35] A synopsis of these recommendations for both groups is based on diet and exercise as follows:

- Consume a diet with emphasis on vegetables, fruits, and whole grains including low-fat dairy products, poultry, fish, legumes and nontropical vegetable oils and nuts; decrease sugars and meats. This can be accomplished without a plan or using the DASH diet, the USDA food pattern or the AHA diet. Reduce percent of calories from saturated fats and trans fat.
- For BP lowering they add the advice to lower sodium intake consuming no more than 2,400 mg of sodium/day.
- For both groups, it is recommended to exercise aerobically three to four times per week, 40 minutes per session involving moderate to vigorous activity.

There are a number of named dietary approaches. The NCEP two-step program is a staged approach to this reduction.[36] The step-one diet is to reduce dietary fat to less than 30% of total calories (saturated fat less than 10% of total calories). If after a three-month trial the step-one diet is unsuccessful, the step-two diet is implemented. This diet restricts saturated fats to 7% of total calories and dietary cholesterol to 200 mg/day. It begins with a focus on healthful choices. A list of foods that are high in fat and a substitute for that food allows for an educated participation by the patient rather than a strict diet menu. The goal of the step-one diet is to reduce the total serum cholesterol by 30 to 40 mg/dL. Reduction from the step-two diet is targeted at an additional 15% of total calories. Reduction in LDLc is based on the baseline measure. Generally, if the level is above 160 mg/dL, a goal is simply to achieve levels below this. For those between 140 and 159 mg/dL, the goal is to reach 130 mg/dL if there are two risk factors or to reach 100 mg/dL if the patient has CHD. Failure to achieve these goals after six months of using the step-one and step-two diet plans may indicate an individual who is noncompliant or unresponsive to diet therapy (e.g., familial hyperlipidemia). Referral for drug management may be appropriate.

Another recommended approach is the Ornish program.[37] Ornish demonstrated that a low-fat diet can reverse some CHD and help prevent development of CHD. His program is divided into a reversal diet and a prevention diet. The reversal diet is for those who have CHD, and restricts fat to less than 10% of total calories; protein, 15% to 20% of total calories; and carbohydrates (complex), 70% to 75% of total calories.[38] Cholesterol is limited to 5 mg/day. The prevention diet is less strict, but it is still more conservative than the NCEP guidelines. Ornish recommends the prevention diet for those with cholesterol levels above 150 mg/dL or if the total cholesterol to HDLc ratio is greater than 3. With the prevention diet, fat is still restricted to no more than 20% of total calories. Ornish also recommends other lifestyle changes, such as avoidance of caffeine and other stimulants and inclusion of exercise and meditation. Some studies indicate that modest dietary fat reduction is as beneficial as more aggressive approaches. A recent study[39] comparing four fat-restriction diets demonstrated that all were effective. The range of restriction in the four diets was 30%, 26%, 22%, and 18% of energy from fat.

There are several specifics regarding dietary recommendations for lowering cholesterol. A Mediterranean diet (MeDi) has been shown to decrease cardiovascular risk factors including blood pressure, C-reactive protein, and lipid profile. One study[40] indicated that a MeDi with a focus on nuts (specifically walnuts) did better than a typical MeDi in decreasing both cholesterol and triglycerides. In fact, contrary to intuition given the fat content of nuts, there is strong and increasing evidence that at least among subjects with higher LDL-C levels, nut consumption improves blood lipid levels in a dose-related manner.[41]

Studies have shown that dietary fiber, specifically barley bran flour and oil, and whole grain consumption in general all assist in decreasing cholesterol and perhaps CHD risk.[42–44] One study[45] indicated no additional benefit for children taking psyllium fiber who already follow a low-fat, low-saturated-fat, low-cholesterol diet. A new product line of foods marketed under the name Benecol is available. This product uses plant sterol mixtures (campestanol/sitostanol) to decrease serum cholesterol through increased absorption and decreased synthesis.[46] There are some concerns that the use of plant sterols will lower serum vitamins D and E, retinol, and alpha- and beta-carotenes. Recent evidence[47] suggests that only the carotenes were decreased.

There is increasing evidence[48,49] that the original excitement regarding the lipid-lowering effects of garlic may have been premature. Several large studies[50,51] using various types of garlic supplementation including garlic powder and garlic oil indicated no significant effect at lowering plasma lipids or lipoproteins. A study by Gardner et al.[52] tested several standard approaches to garlic use in attempting to lower cholesterol. Their study indicated that regardless of the type of administration there was no significant decrease in LDLc or plasma lipid concentrations in patients with moderate hyperlipidemia after a six-month trial and follow-up. This conflicts with earlier reports.

Gugulipid has been recommended for many years as a potentially effective herbal treatment for hypercholesterolemia. Some studies have indicated that this may occur because guggulsterones (the bioactive components) are antagonists for farnesoid X receptor and bile acid receptor, two hormone receptors that contribute to bile acid and cholesterol regulatory function. A recent study done through a randomized controlled trial concluded that, although there is evidence for a bioactivity model for the effects of gugulipid, there was no improvement in serum cholesterol over a two-month period.[53] Some concerns from this study were the potential for raising LDL cholesterol and a dermatologic hypersensitivity reaction in some patients.

Other nutritional factors that may be of benefit include diets high in or supplemented with vitamin E and omega-3 fatty acids. Vitamin E supplementation at 200 to 400 IU/day may be beneficial (Table 51–2).[54] The benefit is derived mainly from prevention of free-radical damage that may lead to atherosclerosis. There appears to be no additional benefit for using tocotrienols versus the standard alpha-tocopherol form.[55] Other antioxidants include vitamin C and bioflavinoids.[56] For omega-3 fatty acids, 8 mg of eicosapentaenoic acid (EPA) and docosahexaenoic acid (DHA) have been demonstrated to have a protective effect.[57] This protective effect is believed to be due to several actions. First, it is believed that omega-3 fatty acids prevent oxidation of LDL. Second, they may protect against CHD by reducing clot formation and coronary artery spasm through a reduction in production of thromboxane and an increase in prostacyclin and tissue plasminogen activator production. Foods high in omega-3s are fish (salmon, herring, mackerel, sardines, anchovies, albacore tune, and black cod), whole grains, beans, seaweed, and soybean. Adler and Holub[58] suggested that omega-3s may increase LDLc levels and that adding garlic (900 mg/day) to the diet may mitigate this effect, lowering cholesterol, LDLc, and triglycerides. Chromium supplementation (600 mcg/day) increases serum HDLc in men taking beta-blockers.[59]

Exercise has increasingly been demonstrated to be effective in reducing cardiovascular risk. A recent study by Johnson et al.[60] indicates that a modest amount of moderate intensity exercise even without dietary changes improves metabolic syndrome, supporting the recommendation of 30 minutes of moderate intensity exercise every day for adults. It appears that there is a dose-dependent effect in that a high amount of exercise had greater benefits regardless of whether it was moderate intensity or vigorous intensity. Specifically, a study by Slentz et al.[61] indicates that significant increases in LDLc occur with inactivity while a modest amount of exercise prevents this increase. Moderate intensity results in a sustained reduction in VLDL, whereas a high-intensity group had significant improvements in HDLc maintained at 15 days after exercise has stopped.

In one study,[62] subjects who performed an individualized exercise program for six months showed a 58.3% decrease in mononuclear cell production of atherogenic cytokines and a 35% decrease in serum levels of C-reactive protein. It has also been shown that exercise increases HDLc levels.[63,64] This effect may be less dramatic in women.[65] It is still unclear how much of the effect on HDLc is due to the exercise itself and how much is attributable to the related weight loss. A recent study[66] indicated that moderate-intensity exercise is just as effective as high-intensity exercise at improving HDLc levels. There is evidence[67] that a program of resistance training for 45 to 50 minutes a day, three times per week, may yield an average 10% reduction in total cholesterol, increased HDLc levels, and decreased LDLc levels. An enormous data pool indicates that exercise has effects on weight reduction, risk and degree of diabetes, and hypertension, among other benefits. The debate that is still being resolved is the degree of exercise needed to achieve these results. A recent study evaluated the level of exercise that tended to predict risk for death from CVD by comparing men with no evidence of CVD and following them for 11 years.[68] This study indicates that those classifying their leisure exercise as heavy or vigorous had an associated reduced risk for death from CVD.

Medications

There are several classifications of drugs used to lower lipids.

- 3-hydroxy-3-methylglutaryl coenzyme A (HMG CoA) reductase inhibitors ("statins" such as lovastatin)—inhibits the conversion of HMG CoA to mevalonic acid, which is needed for cholesterol production; this leads to an increase in LDLc receptors, lowering LDLc levels
- bile acid–binding resins (cholestyramine [Questran] and colestipol [Colestid])—combines with bile acids and salts and then is excreted in feces; removal of bile acids causes conversion of cholesterol to bile acids, which reduces blood levels of cholesterol
- nicotinic acid (niacin)—decreases hepatic production of LDLc and increases levels of HDLc (significantly lower doses are needed to increase HDLc)
- fibric acid derivatives (gemfibrozil [Lopid])—decreases triglycerides, raises HDLc, does not have much effect on LDLc
- probucol (Lorelco)—may inhibit the absorption of cholesterol and decrease LDLc levels
- estrogen replacement therapy—estrogen raises HDLc levels, lowers LDLc; however, may increase triglyceride levels; progestogens typically lower HDLc levels

The use of these drugs is somewhat controversial given that there are, as with most drugs, contraindications to their use, side effects, and cost considerations. In general, in patients with isolated LDLc elevations, bile acid-binding resins or statins are used first. For those with mixed hyperlipidemia, nicotinic acid (if tolerated) is the first drug used; if not effective, gemfibrozil or one of the statins is used. For isolated triglyceride elevation, niacin is used. However, niacin can unmask or increase the risk of developing diabetes. **Table 51–3** is a summary of commonly used medications in the management of hyperlipidemia.

Comanagement with a team including the chiropractor, dietitian, and medical doctor is recommended when a patient is noncompliant or does not seem to respond to individual provider recommendations with diet and exercise.

Algorithm

An algorithm for hypercholesterolemia management is presented in **Figure 51–1**.

Table 51–3 Hyperlipidemia Medications

Drug Class	Examples	General Mechanism	Interactions/Side Effects
HMG CoA reductase inhibitors (statins)	**Atorvastatin** Lipitor	A statin: a HMG CoA reductase inhibitor. This blocks the enzyme that controls production of cholesterol in the liver. Therefore, used in the treatment of hyperlipidemia. Lowers both total cholesterol and LDL cholesterol while increasing HDL cholesterol. Atorvastatin is different from other statins in that it reduces triglycerides. These effects may retard or reverse coronary artery disease.	GI upset, headache, myalgia, weakness, rhabdomyolysis, ocular and liver toxicity. Should have liver enzymes monitored.
	Lovastatin Mevacor	A statin: a HMG CoA reductase inhibitor. This blocks the enzyme that controls production of cholesterol in the liver. Therefore, used in the treatment of hyperlipidemia. Lowers both total cholesterol and LDL cholesterol while increasing HDL cholesterol.	May cause GI upset, headache, myalgia, weakness, rhabdomyolysis, ocular and liver toxicity. Should have liver enzymes monitored.
	Pravastatin Pravachol	A statin: a HMG CoA reductase inhibitor. This blocks the enzyme that controls production of cholesterol in the liver. Therefore, used in the treatment of hyperlipidemia. Lowers both total cholesterol and LDL cholesterol while increasing HDL cholesterol.	GI upset, headache, myalgia, weakness, rhabdomyolysis, ocular and liver toxicity. Should have liver enzymes monitored.
	Simvastatin Zocor	A statin: a HMG CoA reductase inhibitor. This blocks the enzyme that controls production of cholesterol in the liver. Therefore, used in the treatment of hyperlipidemia. Lowers both total cholesterol and LDL cholesterol while increasing HDL cholesterol.	GI upset, headache, myalgia, weakness, rhabdomyolysis, ocular and liver toxicity. Should have liver enzymes monitored.
Statins combined with other medications	**Amlodipine/ atorvastatin** Caduet	A combination antihypertensive (selective calcium channel blocker) medication with a statin (5 reductase inhibitor) used as an adjunct to diet in the treatment of primary hypertension.	Back pain, myalgia, constipation, diarrhea, flatulence, palpitations, tachycardia, facial edema, postural hypotension, headache, sexual dysfunction
	Ezetimibe and simvastatin Vytorin	Used for patients with primary (heterozygous familial and nonfamilial) hypercholesterolemia or mixed hyperlipidemia. Ezetimibe is a selective inhibitor of intestinal cholesterol and phytosterol absorption combined with simvastatin an HMG CoA reductase inhibitor.	Urticaria, arthralgia, myalgias, angioedema, anaphylaxis, elevated liver transaminases, hepatitis, pancreatitis, cholelithiasis, thrombocytopenia, GI signs/symptoms, such as nausea, abdominal pain, constipation, diarrhea, etc. rare cause of rhabdomyolysis/ myopathy.
	Ezetimibe Zetia Ezetrol	Used alone or in combination with statins (HMG CoA reductase inhibitors) for the treatment of primary hypercholesterolemia. At the lining of the small intestine, inhibits absorption of cholesterol but does not inhibit cholesterol synthesis in the liver.	Fatigue, arthralgia, myalgia, dizziness, headache, abdominal pain, angioedema, rhabdomyolysis (monitor liver enzymes when used with a statin)
Bile acid–binding resins	**Cholestyramine** Questran Lo-CHOLEST Prevalite	By combining with bile acids in exchange for chloride ions, an insoluble complex is formed which is excreted in the feces. Used in the management of hypercholesterolemia with reductions in both total cholesterol and LDL cholesterol.	May cause constipation, weight loss or gain, deficiencies in vitamins A, D, and K, and decreased erythrocyte folate levels, nausea, vomiting and other GI disturbances.

(continues)

Table 51–3 Hyperlipidemia Medications(continued)

Drug Class	Examples	General Mechanism	Interactions/Side Effects
	Colestipol Colestid Lestid Cholestabyl	By combining with bile acids in exchange for chloride ions, an insoluble complex is formed which is excreted in the feces. Used in the management of hypercholesterolemia with reductions in both total cholesterol and LDL cholesterol.	May cause constipation, weight loss or gain, deficiencies in vitamins A, D, and K, and decreased erythrocyte folate levels, nausea, vomiting and other GI disturbances.
Fibric acid derivatives	**Gemfibrozil** Lopid	Through blocking lipolysis of stored triglycerides and inhibiting uptake by the liver of fatty acids, there is a reduction in VLDL, LDL, total cholesterol, and triglycerides synthesis and an increase in VDL. Used in the management of patients with high triglyceride levels including familial hypercholesterolemia (type IIa and IIb).	May cause GI upset, headache, dizziness, musculoskeletal pain, rash, or hypokalemia.
Nicotinic acid	**Niacin** Nicobid Nicolar Novo-Niacin	Vitamin B_3 is used in the management of hypercholesterolemia. It has vasodilation effects on vascular smooth muscle and inhibits hepatic synthesis of VLDL, cholesterol and triglycerides, and LDL. May also be used in the treatment of pellagra.	May cause a generalized flushing sensation of warmth, transient, headache, tingling in the extremities, increased sebaceous gland activity, hyperuricemia, hyperglycemia, abnormalities of liver function, and jaundice.
Other	**Probucol** Lorelco	May inhibit the absorption of cholesterol and decrease LDLc levels	

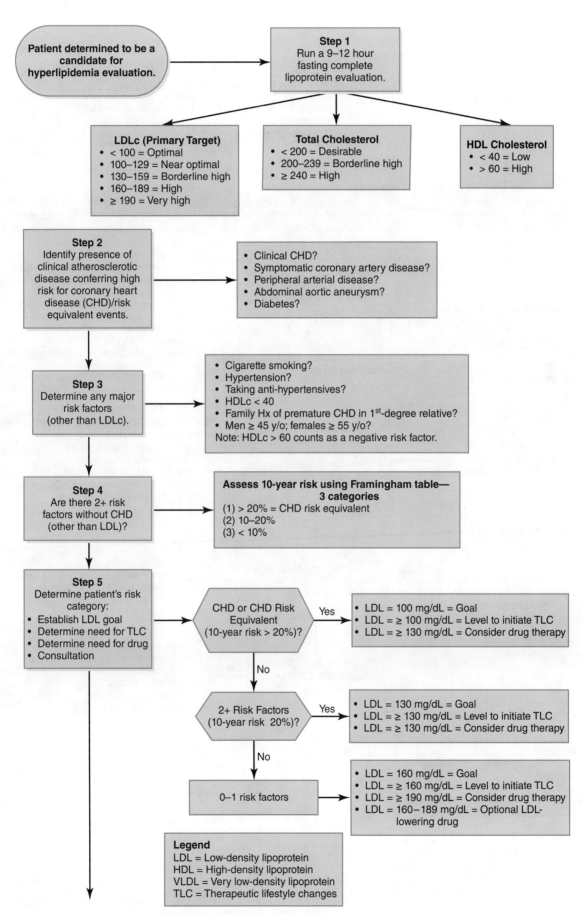

Figure 51–1 NCEP Hyperlipidemia Management—Algorithm

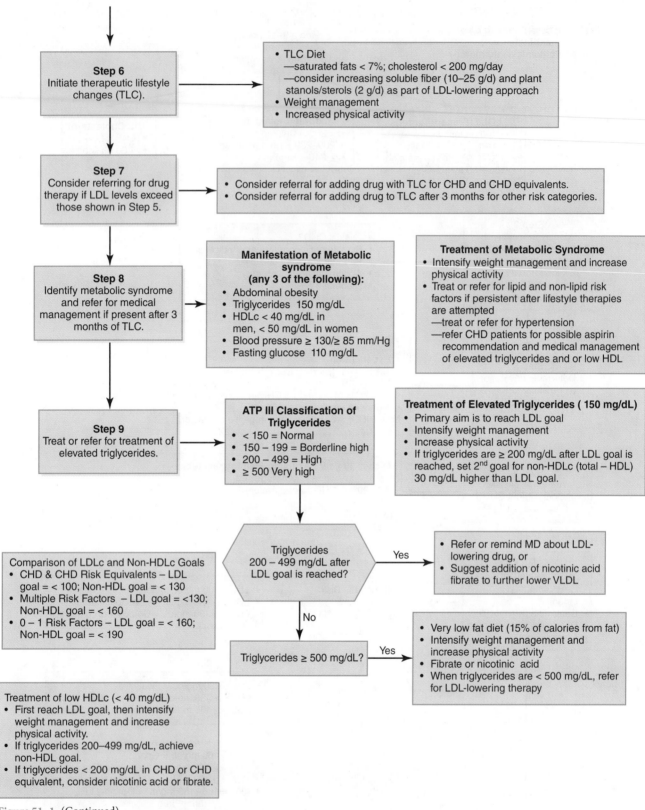

Figure 51–1 (Continued)

APPENDIX 51–1

Web Resource

National Cholesterol Education Group
http://cvdrisk.nhlbi.nih.gov/ncep_slds/menu.htm

APPENDIX 51–2

References

1. National Center for Health Statistics. Annual summary of births, marriages, divorces, and deaths: United States; 1993. *Monthly Vital Statistics Rep.* 1994;42(13).

2. Murray CJ, Lopez AD. Mortality by cause for eight regions of the world: Global Burden of Disease Study. *Lancet.* 1997;349:1269–1276.

3. Khot UN, Khot MB, Bajzer CT. Prevalence of conventional risk factors in patients with coronary heart disease. *JAMA.* 2003;290:898–904.

4. La Vecchia C. Cancers associated with high-fat diets. *Monogr Natl Cancer Inst.* 1992;12:79–85.

5. Law MR, Waid NJ, Thompson SC. By how much and how quickly does reduction in serum cholesterol lower risk of ischemic heart disease? *Br Med J.* 1994;308:367–373.

6. Law MR, Thompson SC, Waid NJ. Assessing possible hazards of reducing serum cholesterol. *Br Med J.* 1994;344:1833–1839.

7. Gordon DJ. Cholesterol lowering and total mortality. In: Rifkind BM, et al., eds. *Lowering Cholesterol in High-Risk Individuals and Populations.* New York: Marcel Dekker; 1995:333–348.

8. Heady JA, Morris JN, Oliver MF. WHO clofibrate/cholesterol trial: clarifications. *Lancet.* 1992;340:1405–1406.

9. Bush TL, Fried LE, Barrett-Connor E. Cholesterol, lipoproteins, and coronary heart disease in women. *Clin Chem.* 1988;34:B60–B70.

10. Mayes PA. Cholesterol synthesis, transport, and excretion. In: Murray RK, Granner DK, Mayes PA, Rodwell VW, eds. *Harper's Biochemistry.* 23rd ed. Norwalk, CT: Appleton & Lange; 1993.

11. Lipscomb TA. Antibodies to oxidized LDL in atherosclerosis. *Lancet.* 1992;339:899.

12. Franceschini G, Maderna P, Sirtori CR. Reverse cholesterol transport: physiology and pharmacology. *Atherosclerosis.* 1991;88:99–107.

13. Fredrickson DS, Levy R. Familial hyperlipoproteinemia. In: Stanbury JB, Wyngarden JB, Fredrickson DS, eds. *The Metabolic Basis of Inherited Disease.* 5th ed. New York: McGraw-Hill; 1982.

14. Vanltallie TB. Health implications of overweight and obesity in the United States. *Ann Intern Med.* 1985;103:983–988.

15. U.S. Preventive Services Task Force. *Guide to Clinical Preventive Services.* 2nd ed. Baltimore: Williams & Wilkins; 1996:15–38.

16. NCEP Adult Treatment Panel II. Summary of the Second Report of the National Cholesterol Education Program Expert Panel on detection, evaluation, and treatment of high blood cholesterol in adults. *JAMA.* 1993;269:3015.

17. American Academy of Family Physicians. *Age Charts for Periodic Health Examination.* Kansas City, MO: American Academy of Family Physicians; 1994. Reprint no. 510.

18. American College of Obstetricians and Gynecologists. *The Obstetrician–Gynecologist in Primary Preventive Health Care: A Report of the ACOG Task Force on Primary and Preventive Health Care.* Washington, DC: ACOG; 1993.

19. American Medical Association. *Guidelines for Adolescent Preventive Services (GAPS): Recommendations and Rationale.* Chicago: AMA; 1994.

20. National Cholesterol Education Program. *Report of the Expert Panel on Blood Cholesterol Levels in Children and Adolescents.* Bethesda, MD: National Institutes of Health, National Heart, Lung, and Blood Institute; 1991. NIH publication 91–2732.

21. American College of Physicians. Serum cholesterol, high-density lipoprotein cholesterol, and triglyceride screening tests for the prevention of coronary heart disease in adults. *Ann Intern Med.* 1996;124:327.

22. Gaziano JM, Gaziano TA. What's new with measuring cholesterol? *JAMA.* 2013;310(19):2043–2044.

23. Copper GR, Meyers GL, Smith SJ, et al. Blood lipid measurements: variations and practical utility. *JAMA.* 1992;267:1652–1660.

24. Greenland P, Bowley NL, Meikljohn P, et al. Blood cholesterol concentration: fingerstick plasma vs. venous serum sampling. *Clin Chem.* 1990;36:628–630.

25. Pahor M, Elam MB, Garrison RJ. Emerging noninvasive biochemical measures to predict cardiovascular risk. *Arch Intern Med.* 1999;159:237–245.

26. De Luis DA, Garcia Avello A, Lasuncion MA, et al. Improvement in lipid and haemostasis patterns after

Helicobacter pylori infection eradication in type I diabetic patients. *Clin Nutr.* 1999;18:227–231.

27. Hackam DG, Anand SS. Emerging risk factors for atherosclerotic vascular disease: a critical review of the evidence. *JAMA.* 2003;290:932–940.

28. Ingelsson E, Schaefer EJ, Contois JH, et al. Clinical utility of different lipid measures for prediction of coronary heart disease in men and women. *JAMA.* 2007;298(7):776–785.

29. Goff DC, Jr., Lloyd-Jones DM, Bennett G, et al. 2013 ACC/AHA Guideline on the Assessment of Cardiovascular Risk: A Report of the American College of Cardiology/American Heart Association Task Force on Practice Guidelines. *Circulation.* 2013:127(16);1730-1753

30. Voight BF, Peloso GM, Orho-Melander M, et al. Plasma HDL cholesterol and risk of myocardial infarction: a Mendelian randomisation study. *Lancet.* 2012;380(9841):572–580.

31. NCEP Expert Panel. Detection, evaluation and treatment of high blood cholesterol in adults (adult treatment panel III): executive summary. NIH Publication No. 01-3670, May, 2001.

32. Crique MH, Wallace RB, Heiss G, et al. Cigarette smoking and plasma high-density lipoprotein cholesterol: the Lipid Research Clinics Program Prevalence Study. *Circulation.* 1990;62(suppl 4):70–76.

33. Stampfer MJ, Golditz GA, Willet WC, et al. A prospective study of moderate alcohol consumption and the risk of coronary disease and stroke in women. *N Engl J Med.* 1988;319:267–273.

34. Grundy SM, Cleeman JI, Merz CN, et al. Implications of recent clinical trials for the National Cholesterol Education Program Adult Treatment Panel III guidelines. *Circulation.* 2004;110(2):227–239.

35. Eckel RH, Jakicic JM, Ard JD, et al. 2013 AHA/ACC guideline on lifestyle management to reduce cardiovascular risk: a report of the American College of Cardiology/American Heart Association Task Force on practice guidelines. *Circulation.* Nov. 12, 2013. (ePub ahead of print).

36. National Cholesterol Education Program. Report of the National Cholesterol Education Program expert panel on detection, evaluation, and treatment of high blood cholesterol in adults. *Arch Intern Med.* 1988;148:360–369.

37. Ornish DM, Scherwitz LW, Brown SE, et al. Adherence to lifestyle changes and reversal of coronary atherosclerosis. *Circulation.* 1989;80:11–57.

38. Ornish DM. *Dr. Dean Ornish's Program for Reversing Heart Disease.* New York: Ivy Books; 1990.

39. Knopp RH, Walden CE, Retzloff BM, et al. Long-term cholesterol-lowering effects of 4 fat-restricted diets in hypercholesterolemic and combined hyperlipidemic men: the dietary alternatives study. *JAMA.* 1997;278:1509–1515.

40. Estruch R, Martinez-Gonzalez MA, Corella D, et al. Effects of a Mediterranean-style diet on cardiovascular risk factors: a randomized trial. *Ann Intern Med.* 2006;145(1):1–11.

41. Sabate J, Oda K, Ros E. Nut consumption and blood lipid levels: a pooled analysis of 25 intervention trials. *Arch Intern Med.* 2010;170(9):821–827.

42. Lapton JR, Robinson MC, Morin JL. Cholesterol-lowering effect of barley bran flour and oil. *J Am Diet Assoc.* 1994;94:65–70.

43. Stampler LS, Hu FB, Giovannucci E, et al. Whole-grain consumption and risk of coronary heart disease: results from the Nurses' Health Study. *Am J Clin Nutr.* 1999;70:412–419.

44. Wolk A, Manson JE, Stampfer MJ, et al. Long-term intake of dietary fiber and decreased risk of coronary heart disease among women. *JAMA.* 1999;28:1998–2004.

45. Dennison BA, Levine DM. Randomized, double-blind, placebo-controlled, two-period crossover clinical trial of psyllium fiber in children with hypercholesterolemia. *J Pediatr.* 1993;123:24–29.

46. Gylling H, Miettinen TA. Cholesterol reduction by different plant sterol mixtures and with variable fat intake. *Metabolism.* 1999;48:575–580.

47. Gylling H, Puska P, Vartiainen E, Miettinen TA. Retinol, vitamin D, carotenes, and alpha-tocopherol in serum of a moderately hypercholesterolemic population consuming sitostanol ester margarine. *Atherosclerosis.* 1999;145:279–285.

48. Jain AK, Vargas R, Gotzkowsky S, McMahon FG. Can garlic reduce levels of serum lipids? A controlled clinical study. *Am J Med.* 1993;94:632–635.

49. Simmons LA, Balasubramaniam S, von Konigsmark M, et al. On the effect of garlic on plasma lipids and lipoproteins in mild hypercholesterolemia. *Atherosclerosis.* 1998;113:219–225.

50. Berthold HK, Sadhop T, von Bergmann K. Effect of a garlic oil preparation on serum lipoproteins and cholesterol metabolism: a randomized controlled trial. *JAMA.* 1998;279:1900–1902.

51. Silagy C, Neil A. Garlic as a lipid lowering agent: a meta-analysis. *J R Coll Physicians Lond.* 1994;28:39–45.

52. Gardner CD, Lawson LD, Block E, et al. Effect of raw garlic vs commercial garlic supplements on plasma lipid concentrations in adults with moderate hypercholesterolemia: a randomized clinical trial. *Arch Intern Med.* 2007;167(4):346–353.

53. Szapary PO, Wolfe ML, Bloedon LAT, et al. Guggulipid for the treatment of hypercholesterolemia: a randomized controlled trial. *JAMA.* 2003;290:765–772.

54. Byers T. Vitamin E supplements and coronary heart disease. *Nutr Rev.* 1993;51:333–345.

55. Mensink RP, von Houwellingen AC, Kromhout D, Hornstra G. A vitamin E concentrate rich in tocotrienols had no effect on serum lipids, lipoproteins, or platelet function in men with mildly elevated serum lipid concentrations. *Am J Clin Nutr.* 1999;69:213–219.

56. Simon J. Vitamin C and cardiovascular disease: a review. *J Am Coll Nutr.* 1992;11:107.

57. Leaf A, Weber PC. Cardiovascular effects of omega-3 fatty acids: an update. *N Engl J Med.* 1988;318:549–557.

58. Adler AJ, Holub BJ. Effect of garlic and fish-oil supplementation on serum lipid and lipoprotein concentrations in hypercholesterolemic men. *Am J Clin Nutr.* 1997;65:445–450.

59. Roebeck JR, Jr, Hila KM, Chambless LE, Fletcher RH. Effect of chromium supplementation on serum high-density lipoprotein cholesterol levels in men taking beta blockers. A randomized, controlled trial. *Ann Intern Med.* 1991;115:917–924.

60. Johnson JL, Slentz CA, Houmard JA, et al. Exercise training amount and intensity effects on metabolic syndrome (from Studies of a Targeted Risk Reduction Intervention through Defined Exercise). *Am J Cardiol.* 2007;100(12):1759–1766.

61. Slentz CA, Houmard JA, Johnson JL, et al. Inactivity, exercise training and detraining, and plasma lipoproteins. STRRIDE: a randomized, controlled study of exercise intensity and amount. *J Appl Physiol.* 2007;103(2):432–442.

62. Smith JK, Dykes R, Douglas JE, et al. Long-term exercise and atherogenic activity of blood mononuclear cells in persons at risk of developing ischemic heart disease. *JAMA.* 1999;281:1722–1727.

63. Milani RV, Lavei GJ. Prevalence and effects of non-pharmacologic treatment of isolated low-HDL cholesterol in patients with coronary artery disease. *J Cardiopulm Rehabil.* 1995;15:439–444.

64. Sagiv M, Goldbourt U. Influence of physical work on high density lipoprotein cholesterol: implications for the risk of coronary heart disease. *Int J Sports Med.* 1994;15:261–266.

65. Hiu FB, Stumpfer MJ, Manson SE, et al. Dietary fat intake and the risk of coronary heart disease in women. *N Engl J Med.* 1997;337:1491–1499.

66. Spate-Douglas T, Keyser RE. Exercise intensity: its effect on the high-density-lipoprotein profile. *Arch Phys Med Rehabil.* 1999;80:691–695.

67. Prabhakaran B, Dowling EA, Branch JD, et al. Effect of 14 weeks of resistance training on lipid profile and body fat percentage in premenopausal women. *Br J Sports Med.* 1999;33:178–185.

68. Yu S, Yarnell JW, Sweetnam PM, et al. What level of physical activity protects against premature cardiovascular death? The Caerphilly Study. *Heart.* 2003;89:502–506.

Anemia

Context

Although the *Job Analysis on Chiropractic* report from the National Board of Chiropractic Examiners[1] indicates that few chiropractors order laboratory studies on their patients, all chiropractic colleges teach students that laboratory studies are a diagnostic tool to be used when appropriate. This discrepancy probably occurs for several reasons. One is that students often feel that they have not had enough exposure in the college setting to feel comfortable ordering labs. There is often the concern of reimbursement. This is easily defended (as for any procedure) with an explanation of why the test was ordered. Also, the vast majority of patients are probably being seen by a medical doctor (MD); it is often the assumption of the chiropractor that the MD will order any appropriate laboratory work and, in fact, the chiropractor refers the patient to the MD for the lab work and follow-up. Yet there is a significant group of patients who request and/or need laboratory work for screening of certain values such as cholesterol/triglyceride levels, urinalysis with symptoms of a urinary tract infection, and a cross-check of possible causes with complaints of fatigue. These are easy tests to order and generally easy to interpret. It is important to remember that the patient population seen by chiropractors is ambulatory—not hospitalized; therefore, the types of disorders seen are already restricted. From a cost-effectiveness perspective, it may be less expensive for the patient within the context of the smaller chiropractic setting.

There is often an assumption that all patients with anemia will present as pale, fatigued, clay-eating individuals. It is far more common for a patient to be unaware of an underlying anemia. The absence of pallor and other physical signs of anemia as a diagnostic rationale for ruling out anemia has a false-negative value of between

45% and 55%.[2] If fatigue is present, it is initially felt only with exertion. If the patient is not in a position to exert himself or herself, anemia may remain silent. It is also crucial to regard anemia as a sign of disease rather than as a disease in itself. In other words, the doctor is only half finished with the evaluation process when anemia is discovered on laboratory testing. The next step in the process is to determine why. Anemia, in general, is due to one of three processes: (1) decreased production, (2) increased breakdown, and (3) blood loss. With each there is a limited number of common causes, and significant associated laboratory findings usually aid in the diagnosis. (See **Table 52–1** for less common anemias.)

General Strategy

History

- Determine whether there are any clear historical clues of anemia such as blood loss, dietary deficiencies, ethnic or familial predispositions, pregnancy or alcoholism, or past history of anemia; obtain a thorough drug history.
- Determine whether there are any secondary clues such as tiredness with exertion, gastrointestinal (GI) pains (GI bleeding source), heavy menstrual flow, pallor, pica (dirt/clay eating, ice eating, or starch eating), or bone pain (sternal pain in particular).

Examination

- Examine the patient for signs of tachycardia, systolic flow murmurs, a loud S1 and S2, a widened pulse pressure, a venous hum, and pale conjunctivae.

- If screening for a specific anemia, order an anemia panel that best demonstrates that anemia; if screening the patient generally, order a complete blood cell (CBC) count, blood chemistry, and urinalysis.
- Interpret the lab with a focus on the size (combined findings of mean corpuscular volume [MCV] and a morphologic description such as microcytosis or macrocytosis) and shape of the red blood cells (RBCs), the RBC distribution width (RDW), and a search for signs of hemolysis (increased bilirubin, lactate dehydrogenase [LDH], and/or potassium), or blood loss (increase in reticulocytosis).
- Combine the laboratory and historical findings to determine a working diagnosis.

Management

- Iron-deficiency anemia (IDA) requires a further determination of a bleeding source (and more rarely a dietary source); if not an occult process, use iron supplementation for two weeks; a recheck for response is necessary.
- Thalassemia minor is usually asymptomatic and not in need of intervention except to counsel parents who both have the same thalassemia (trait or minor) about risk for their children and also prenatal counseling.
- A patient with macrocytic anemia due to pernicious anemia is referred for cyanocobalamin (vitamin B_{12}) injections or other approaches;

Table 52–1 Some Less Common Anemias

Type	Findings	Management
Heredity Spherocytosis	An autosomal dominant disease with variable presentation. An abnormality of spetrin, an important protein used in the structure of the RBC membrane results in a spheroid cell rather than the normal bioconcave cell. As a result, the cell is destroyed earlier than normal RBCs, leading to a chronic hemolytic anemia. Findings include: • Reticulocytosis • Spherocytes on peripheral blood smear • Microcytosis with an increased MCHC • Hematocrit may be normal • May have an increase in indirect bilirubin (common with hemolytic anemias) • Negative Comb's test	Patients are supplemented with folic acid (1 mg/d). Splenectomy is usually performed to decrease the degree of hemolysis (does not correct the disorder).
Glucose-6-Phosphate Dehydrogenase Deficiency	An X-linked recessive disorder affecting approximately 10–15% of American black males. The defect in this enzyme leads to episodic hemolytic anemia to oxidative disruption of the RBC. Many drugs can exacerbate this anemia, such as sulfonamines, quinine, and quinidine, among others. The blood is normal when there is no hemolytic event. During hemolytic events, lab findings may include: • Reticulocytosis • Increased indirect bilirubin • May have "bite" cells (looks like a bite was taken out of cell) • Heinz bodiesan enzyme assay may reveal a low level of G6PD	No treatment. Avoid drugs known to increase hemolytic events.
Sickle Cell	An autosomial recessive disorder causing a single DNA base change of valine for glutamine in the sixth position of the b chain. This leads to hemoglobin S formation and "sickle-shaped" cells. The hemoglobin S gene is found in 8% of American blacks. One out of 400 American blacks will have sickle cell anemia. Onset is within the first year of life. Clinical presentation includes jaundice, pigment gallstones, splenomegaly, and poorly healing ulcers of the lower tibia. Hemolytic "crises" occur when viral infection or folate deficiency is present. Vaso-occlusive crisis may occur after infection, dehydration, hypoxia, or spontaneously. This leads to hours/days of extremely painful bone or organ pain with associated low-grade fever. Patients are at risk for delayed puberty, infections of bone, stroke, and infarction. Prenatal diagnosis is available. Laboratory findings include: • Hemtrocrit is 20–30% • Sickle cells compose 5–50% of RBCs	No treatment or cure for the disease. Patients remain on folic acid supplementation. Exchange transfusion is used, especially during painful crises.

Table 52–1 Some Less Common Anemias (continued)

Type	Findings	Management
	• Reticulocytosis (10–25%) • Nucleated RBCs • Howell Jolly bodies and target cells • WBC count is elevated and thrombocytosis may occur • Indirect bilirubin is high • Abnormal electrophoresis pattern indicating hemoglobin S	
Autoimmune Hemolytic	An acquired hemolytic anemia that is idiopathic in half of cases. Causes include systemic lupus erythematosis, chronic lymphocytic leukemia, and some lymphomas. IgG autoantibody if directed against mainly the Rb system. IgG antibodies coat the RBC, which is turned into a spherocyte to spleen macrophages. Must be differentiated from drug-induced hemolytic anemia. The onset of the anemia is acute, with the patient presenting with fatigue, jaundice, and splenomegaly. Laboratory findings include: • Hematocrit may be <10% • Reticulocytosis • Spherocytes on peripheral smear • Indirect bilirubin is increased • May have nucleated RBCs • May have coexisting immune thrombocytopenia (Evan's syndrome) • Direct Comb's test is positive; indirect may/may not be positive	Patients are treated initially with prednisone. Immunosuppressive agents may be used. Splenectomy is considered in some cases. High-dose intravenous immunoglobulin is also used.
Cold Agglutinin Disease	An acquired hemolytic anemia with the IgM autoantibody attaching to 1 antigen on RBCs. Most cases are idiopathic. Some are associated with Waldenstrom's macroglobulinenemia. Cold agglutinin disease may also occur after mycoplasma pneumonae or infectious mononucleosis. Symptoms may occur on exposure to cold with findings of mottled skin or numbness in fingers and toes. Lab findings include: • Reticulocytosis • Spherocytosis • Comb's test positive for complement only • A micro-Comb's test may be used • A bedside cold-agglutinin test demonstrates small clumps of blood on an iced glass slide	Treatment is primarily symptomatic with avoidance of exposure to cold.
Aplastic	Aplastic anemia is due to damage to the hematopoietic stem cell in the bone marrow. As a result, all components are affected including RBCs, WBCs, and platelets. Causes include radiation therapy, chemotherapy, SLE, toxins, drug induced (mainly RA and anti-epileptic medications), posthepatitis, pregnancy, and paroxysmal nocturnal hemoglobinuria. Anemia symptoms include fatigue and weakness; neutropenia predisposes the individual to infections; bleeding tendencies result from the decrease in platelets. Splenomegaly, hepatomegaly, pallor, and lymphadenopathy may be present. Lab findings include: • Pancytopenia without changes in RBC morphology • Bone marrow aspirate and biopsy appear hypocellular with small amounts of normal hematopoietic progenitors	High-dose immunosuppressants are most often used. Bone marrow transplant may be necessary.
Sideroblastic	A group of refractory disorders that may be either hereditary or acquired (e.g., drug-induced) or idiopathic (myelocytoplastic syndromes). Erythroid hyperplasia of bone marrow is the characteristic that unites these disorders. Iron utilization is impaired. • Hypochromic, microcytic RBCs (although macrocytes may prevail, making the MCV normal or high) • Often there is basophilic stippling • Serum iron and ferritin levels are normal or high • The serum total iron-binding capacity is normal or low with a high percent saturation • Free erythrocyte porphyrin levels may be high • Bone marrow evaluation reveals increased iron and ringed sideroblasts	Dependent on cause, erythropeitin may be used. Transfusion is usually avoided.

temporary deficiencies not associated with a loss of intrinsic factor may be managed nutritionally.

- Folic acid deficiencies are usually dietary and respond to supplementation; a trial of 100 mg for 10 days and a check for a reactive reticulocytosis may help distinguish between vitamin B_{12} and folate deficiency. A cross-check for indicators of a B_{12} deficiency is necessary given these do not respond to folic acid supplementation and the consequences of long-term B_{12} deficiency include irreversible neurological dysfunction.

Relevant Physiology

Anemia is an indication of an underlying disorder, not a disease itself. Anemia indicates a decreased ability of oxygen-carrying capacity and will usually result in attempts by the body to compensate. These compensations may be an increase in heart rate and/or an increase in RBC production. Anemia has been described several ways. However, anemia usually involves a decrease in hematocrit, hemoglobin, or RBCs. All of these are not necessarily decreased when anemia is present. In adult women a hemoglobin of less than 12 g/dL is considered anemia; in men, less than 13.5 g/dL is considered anemia. Hematocrit values indicating anemia are less than 36% in adult women and less than 39% in adult men. These values, which were established by the World Health Organization (WHO), are guidelines, not absolutes.[3]

Decreased Production

Although a decrease in production is idiopathic 50% of the time, there are some common identifiable reasons. Many of these aplastic anemias are pancytopenic, meaning there is a concomitant decrease in white blood cells (WBCs) and platelets. Chemotherapeutic agents and other drugs are often the cause. A distinction between blood loss and decreased production is determined through the reticulocyte count. The reticulocyte count (or index) is a reflection of new RBC production in response to a loss of blood. This does not occur with aplastic disorders.[4]

Increased Breakdown

Breakdown of RBCs is either intravascular or extravascular (within the cells of the reticuloendothelial system

[RES]). Intravascular hemolysis is rare in the ambulatory patient, usually due to a transfusion reaction, extensive burns, aortic valve prosthesis, or acute glucose-6-dehydrogenase deficiency. Intravascular hemolysis leaves a trail of clues. With RBC breakdown there is an increase in the released constituents such as bilirubin (indirect), LDH, and potassium. These same findings may occur if there was mishandling of the blood sample with consequent hemolysis but to a lesser degree. Urine hemosiderin may be found several days after intravascular hemolysis has occurred. Extravascular hemolysis, not occurring within the vascular system but within the cells of the RES, leaves few clues. However, most causes can be determined by an abnormality in the hemoglobin or shape of the RBC. Other causes are autoimmune. These are determined by the Coombs' test. A history of transfusion or pregnancy is often found.

Blood Loss

When blood is lost, a historical report of a bleeding source is not always obvious. Abortions, childbirth, stab wounds, and surgeries are obvious causes, but the majority of patients in an ambulatory setting have less obvious causes. The most common cause is heavy menstrual flow in women. Occult sites of bleeding are often GI. GI bleeding may be frank, as with hemorrhoids; however, higher GI bleeding is often not evident in the stool without guaiac testing. Associated GI symptoms such as upper GI pain associated with meals or lower GI pain with a change in bowel habits may be the only clues.

Laboratory Evaluation

The distinction among the various major types of anemia begins with an evaluation of size. This is done two ways: (1) indices, mainly the MCV, and (2) RBC morphology. These two values often coincide. For example, small cells are morphologically described as microcytic and are usually associated with a decreased MCV. Conversely, large cells are referred to as macrocytes and are accompanied by an increased MCV.

Microcytic Anemia

Microcytic anemia is mainly due to IDA and thalassemia minor. Anemia of chronic disease may present as normocytic or microcytic. IDA has some characteristic associated findings that often will clinch the diagnosis. RDW is the coefficient of variation of RBCs. This is determined by dividing the standard deviation of the erythrocyte volume distribution by the MCV. The result is then multiplied by 100 and expressed as a percentage. RDW is either normal or increased. An RDW increase often precedes changes in the MCV because the MCV is sensitive to large RBC population changes only. The sensitivity of RDW in diagnosing IDA is between 87% and 100%.[5] The RDW is normal with thalassemia minor (except in rare cases of severe anemia).

Serum ferritin is highly specific for IDA (99% to 100%). Therefore, IDA is diagnosed by finding a microcytic anemia with a combination of a decrease in RBCs and an increase in RDW that is confirmed by a concomitant decrease in serum ferritin. Other supportive findings are a decreased hemoglobin, an increased total iron-binding capacity (TIBC), and a decreased transferrin percent saturation.

Patients with thalassemia minor are usually asymptomatic. Although the anemia is microcytic and sometimes hypochromic, the serum ferritin is usually normal or slightly elevated, distinguishing it from IDA. More important, an elevated RBC count is virtually diagnostic, being 75% sensitive and 97% specific for thalassemia syndromes. RDW is normal. Further confirmation may be necessary with hemoglobin electrophoresis.

Anemia of chronic disease (ACD) may present in a pure form or associated with IDA. ACD is microcytic in only 25% of cases.[6] When microcytic, the MCV rarely is below 78 fL. When ACD is pure, the distinction between IDA is clearer. A decrease in TIBC, an increase in ferritin, and often an increase in the erythrocyte sedimentation rate (ESR) are found with pure ACD. Serum ferritin is often increased because it is an acute-phase reactant; it is increased in inflammatory diseases. Total serum iron is low in both ACD and IDA. IDA and ACD may coexist for various reasons. One possibility is that patients with rheumatoid arthritis, for example, may be taking medications that cause GI bleeding and an associated IDA. The serum ferritin will then be low or borderline.

Macrocytic Anemia

The most common causes of macrocytic anemia are vitamin B_{12} deficiency, folate deficiency, alcoholism, hypothyroidism, and liver disease. A distinction is made between megaloblastic and nonmegaloblastic anemia. This requires a bone marrow aspirate. This is rarely

needed, however, because of the sensitivity and specificity of other laboratory values, coupled with the history. When the MCV is greater than 130 fL the probability is 100% for vitamin B_{12} or folate deficiency (megaloblastic).[7] Levels below 95 fL equal a 0.1% probability. Antimetabolite or antifolate drugs may also cause a megaloblastic anemia. A mild elevation in the range of 100 to 110 fL is suggestive of other causes, such as alcoholism, liver disease, or hypothyroidism. Further laboratory testing for liver enzymes and ultrasensitive thyrotropin (TSH) will differentiate these possibilities.

Some lab values are elevated in both vitamin B_{12} and folate deficiencies, such as RDW. Also, RBC folate concentrations are low and serum homocysteine levels are elevated with both vitamin B_{12} and folate deficiencies.

A differentiation between vitamin B_{12} deficiency and folate deficiency is important because of the potential neurologic consequences of vitamin B_{12} deficiency. In other words, folate supplementation will not correct the neurologic abnormalities of vitamin B_{12} deficiency. Also, vitamin B_{12} deficiency is less often a "nutritional" deficiency (only 2% of all cases) and more often either a malabsorption consequence or due to a lack of intrinsic factor. Pernicious anemia is differentiated from dietary B_{12} deficiency by testing for anti-intrinsic antibody titers. The Schilling test is rarely used but is an option.

Serum levels of vitamin B_{12} and folate may be measured. In addition, serum methylmalonic acid (MMA) and total homocysteine levels are high in patients with vitamin B_{12} deficiency (95% sensitive).[8, 9] Folate deficiency will usually raise the homocysteine level only and not MMA. RBC folate is less valuable in distinguishing between the two anemias because it is often found to be low in both vitamin B_{12} and folate deficiency. RBC folate is better used as an indicator of tissue stores.

A therapeutic trial may be acceptable as an initial attempt to differentiate between vitamin B_{12} and folate deficiency; however, most authors warn against this approach due to the possibility of misinterpretation and the result of neurologic deficits in patients who actually have pernicious anemia. The approach involves oral folate at 100 mg/day for 10 days. The patient's reticulocyte response is then measured. If the underlying cause of macrocytic anemia is folate deficiency, there will be an increase in reticulocytes; however, there will be no increase in patients with a vitamin B_{12} deficiency. Although likely to differentiate between folate and vitamin B_{12} deficiency, there are many factors that influence test results and the inadvertent misdiagnosis in a patient with pernicious anemia as the cause of B_{12} deficiency may result in irreversible neurologic damage.

Management

Dietary management of anemias through supplementation must be preceded by a thorough diagnostic search that provides sufficiently convincing information that there is not an underlying cause that needs comanagement or referral. For example, IDA may be a dietary issue in pregnant women, infants, and adolescent or adult athletes. Dietary supplementation (or an iron-enriched formula for infants) is appropriate. However, in the case of occult GI bleeding, heavy menstrual flow, and urinary loss, referral for determination of underlying pathology is needed prior to institution of dietary correction. ACD also requires at the minimum a consultation with the physician treating the primary disorder. Vitamin B_{12} deficiency that is due to a strictly vegetarian diet is responsive to a change in diet or supplementation; patients with pernicious anemia should be referred for lifelong treatment with injectable or intranasal vitamin B_{12}. There is some evidence from Swedish studies, however, that daily supplementation of 1,000 mg (2,000 mg twice daily for the first month) is sufficient to cover the variable absorption rate in some individuals. There are no toxic effects known.[10] The main reasons given for not using this approach are compliance and cost. The cost currently is not a consideration.

Some basic recommendations for dietary supplementation, when appropriate, follow.[11]

Iron-Deficiency Anemia

- For adults, ferrous sulfate (or ferrous forms of lactate, fumarate, gluconate, glycine sulfate, or glutamate), 200 mg to 325 mg two to three times per day, is given for 6 to 12 months after hemoglobin levels are normal (the dose is dependent on patient tolerance).
- Side effects such as constipation may be decreased by starting with a lower dosage and slowly increasing gradually over several days or by taking the supplement in three divided doses.

Dietary recommendations include the following:

- Avoid substances that may affect iron absorption, including tea, coffee, milk or dairy products, calcium, and some medications at least for one hour before and after ingestion of iron supplementation.
- Include a source of vitamin C at every meal.
- Include foods rich in iron, such as dried beans and peas, poultry, seafood, and red meat.
- Increase dietary fiber moderately to offset the possible side effect of constipation associated with iron supplements.

Folate Deficiency

- Oral folic acid at 1 to 5 mg/day for two to three weeks is necessary to replenish tissues.
- Maintain levels with 50 to 100 mg/day.
- Remember that orange juice, asparagus, beef liver, wheat germ, red beans, and peanut butter are high in folic acid.

Vitamin B_{12} Deficiency Anemia— Pernicious Anemia

- Very large doses are necessary to attain a high enough level that 1% to 3% of vitamin B_{12} that does not require intrinsic factor equals therapeutic levels; doses at 1,000 mg/day are necessary.
- Increase sublingual B_{12}.

Vitamin B_{12} Deficiency Anemia—Nutritional

- Supplementation with B_{12} is best achieved through a B-complex formula to avoid imbalances.
- Dietary sources include liver, beef, pork, eggs, and milk and milk products.

Algorithm

An algorithm for microcytic anemia is presented in **Figure 52–1**.

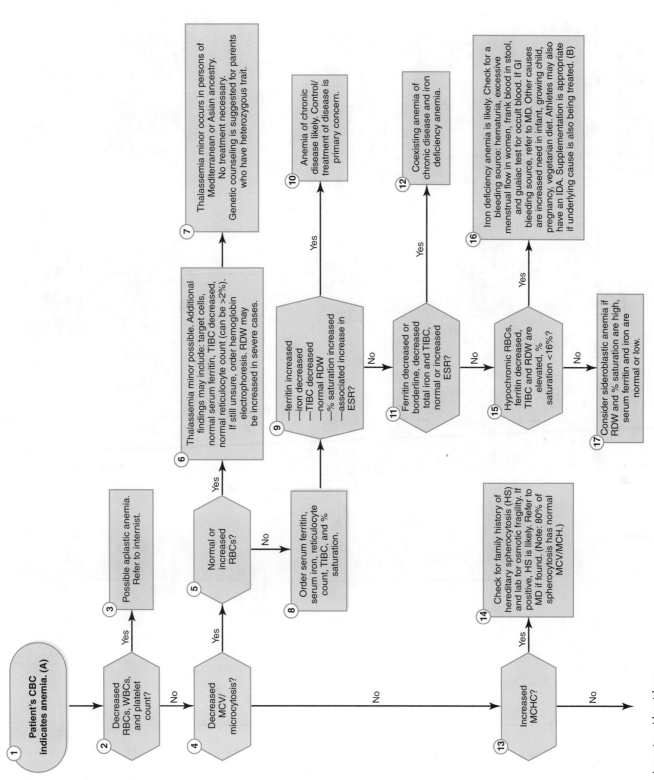

Figure 52–1 Anemia—Algorithm

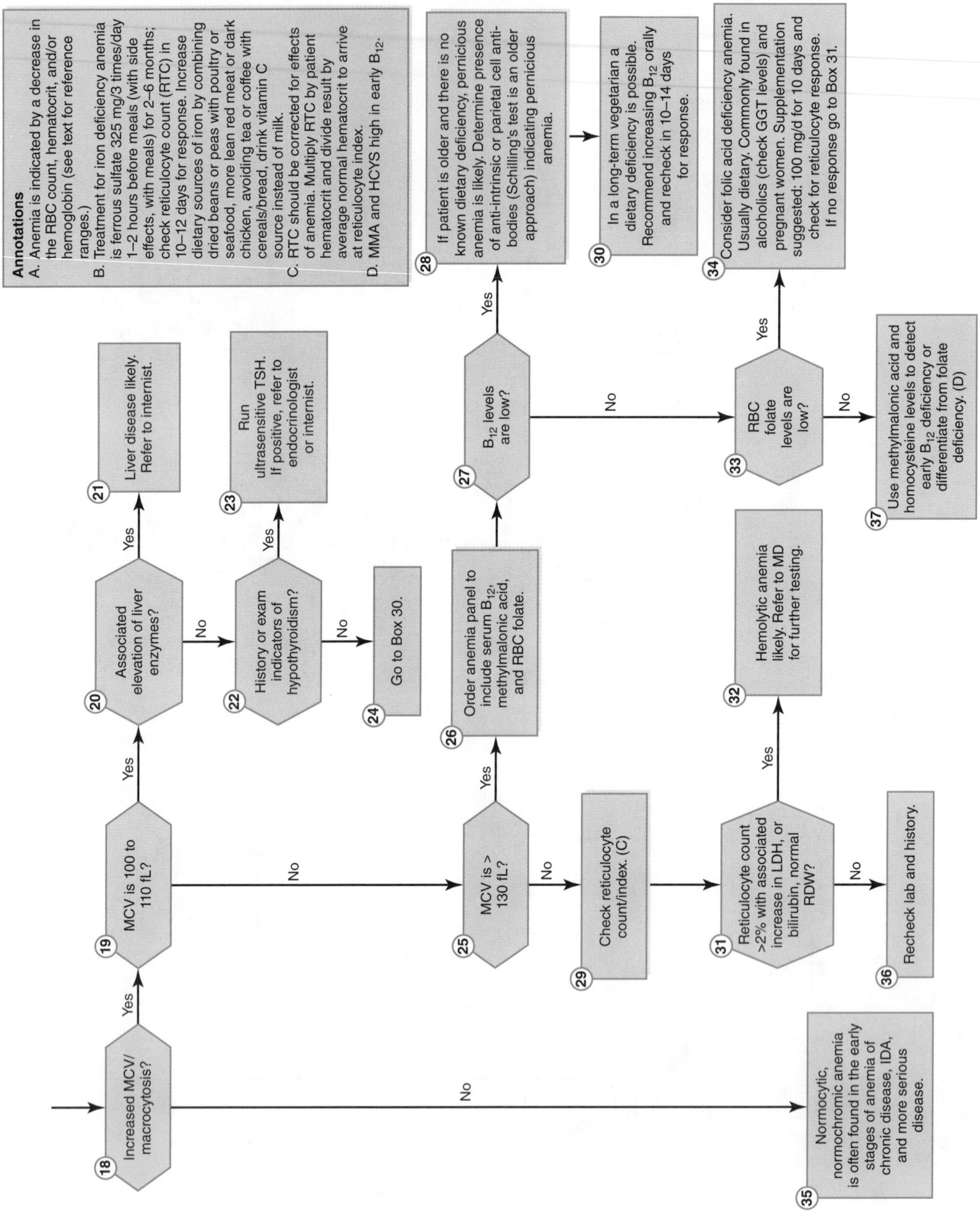

18 Increased MCV/ macrocytosis?
Yes
No
19 MCV is 100 to 110 fL?
Yes
No
20 Associated elevation of liver enzymes?
Yes
No
21 Liver disease likely. Refer to internist.
22 History or exam indicators of hypothyroidism?
Yes
No
23 Run ultrasensitive TSH. If positive, refer to endocrinologist or internist.
24 Go to Box 30.
25 MCV is > 130 fL?
Yes
No
26 Order anemia panel to include serum B_{12}, methylmalonic acid, and RBC folate.
27 B_{12} levels are low?
Yes
No
28 If patient is older and there is no known dietary deficiency, pernicious anemia is likely. Determine presence of anti-intrinsic or parietal cell antibodies (Schilling's test is an older approach) indicating pernicious anemia.
29 Check reticulocyte count/index. (C)
30 In a long-term vegetarian a dietary deficiency is possible. Recommend increasing B_{12} orally and recheck in 10–14 days for response.
31 Reticulocyte count >2% with associated increase in LDH, or bilirubin, normal RDW?
Yes
No
32 Hemolytic anemia likely. Refer to MD for further testing.
33 RBC folate levels are low?
Yes
No
34 Consider folic acid deficiency anemia. Usually dietary. Commonly found in alcoholics (check GGT levels) and pregnant women. Supplementation suggested: 100 mg/d for 10 days and check for reticulocyte response. If no response go to Box 31.
35 Normocytic, normochromic anemia is often found in the early stages of anemia of chronic disease, IDA, and more serious disease.
36 Recheck lab and history.
37 Use methylmalonic acid and homocysteine levels to detect early B_{12} deficiency or differentiate from folate deficiency. (D)
Annotations
A. Anemia is indicated by a decrease in the RBC count, hematocrit, and/or hemoglobin (see text for reference ranges.)
B. Treatment for iron deficiency anemia is ferrous sulfate 325 mg/3 times/day 1–2 hours before meals (with side effects, with meals) for 2–6 months; check reticulocyte count (RTC) in 10–12 days for response. Increase dietary sources of iron by combining dried beans or peas with poultry or seafood, more lean red meat or dark chicken, avoiding tea or coffee with cereals/bread, drink vitamin C source instead of milk.
C. RTC should be corrected for effects of anemia. Multiply RTC by patient hematocrit and divide result by average normal hematocrit to arrive at reticulocyte index.
D. MMA and HCYS high in early B_{12}.

Figure 52–1 (Continued)

Selected Anemias

MICROCYTIC AND NORMOCYTIC ANEMIAS

Iron-Deficiency Anemia

Classic Presentation

Most patients are initially asymptomatic. When symptomatic, the patient may present with symptoms related to a decreased oxygen-carrying capacity of the blood, such as fatigue (mainly on exertion), orthopnea, headaches, dizziness, learning disability/decreased attention span (in children), syncope/presyncope, or angina (if predisposed with coronary artery disease).

Cause

IDA is the most common hematologic disorder, affecting as many as 30% of the world's population. However, in the United States, it affects 0.2% to 2% of adult males and 2% to 10% (one study[12] indicated up to 20%) of adult females.[13] The likelihood of IDA development is increased in certain patient populations: pregnant women (increased demand), 60%; heavily menstruating women, 80%; and individuals with pica symptoms, 90%. Other groups at risk include infants (especially those infants fed unfortified cow's milk and/or those who substitute with juices) to age 4 years, adolescents who exercise heavily, long-distance runners (malabsorption, megaloblastic anemia), and patients with chronic diseases (i.e., rheumatoid arthritis, cancer).[14]

Anemia is not the first sign of iron deficiency. There are generally five stages: (1) depletion of storage iron, (2) decreased serum iron, (3) anemia with normal cells, (4) microcytosis, then hypochromia, and (5) symptoms and signs of IDA. The main cause of IDA is blood loss. When IDA is diagnosed, a search for a bleeding source is a requisite prior to treatment. However, a factor for individuals without blood loss is nutritional demand for and availability of iron at varying stages of life.

Evaluation

In the early stage of iron deficiency, there are no signs or symptoms. When a patient has reached the later stages, patients with chronic IDA often will have an unusual craving 50% of the time, referred to as pica (craving for ice, clay/dirt, or starch); pagophagia (ice eating) is most common.[15] Chronic, severe IDA may have signs, including spoon-shaped nails (koilonychia), brittle nails, skin cracking at the corners of the mouth (angular stomatitis), a smooth tongue (atrophic glossitis), or blue sclerae.[16] Remember that these signs and symptoms are the last clinical indicator of IDA. Laboratory evaluation can detect anemia prior to the development of these indicators. The classic laboratory presentation is a decrease in RBCs and hemoglobin, microcytosis, and a decreased MCV with an increase in the RDW. Specific indicators include a decrease in serum ferritin (<10 ng/mL), an increase in total TIBC, and a decrease in transferrin saturation (<16%). Other indicators are due to blood loss, such as increase of blood or RBCs in the urine, or a positive guaiac test for occult blood. If IDA is discovered, a thorough search for a source of blood loss must be made. The most common will be heavy menstruation, GI loss from ulcer or cancer, and urinary/renal pathology.

Management

The first decision to make before treatment is whether IDA is caused by nutritional need due to increased demand or due to blood loss. Blood loss from heavy menstruation should be comanaged with a gynecologist to determine whether there is an underlying hormonal imbalance. If occult blood is found, referral for medical evaluation should occur. Nutritional causes may be managed with dietary supplementation. Between 200 and 325 mg of ferrous sulfate two to three times per day for 10 to 14 days should be prescribed (higher doses may be necessary in some individuals).[17] Calcium supplementation may interfere with iron absorption, and therefore should be staggered. At about two weeks, the reticulocyte count is checked to determine a response (increase). The hemoglobin concentration should increase to normal in six to eight weeks. If responsive, continue for a total of six months. If not, consider another cause. Remember to counsel and possibly screen high-risk individuals (or their parents). In a recent preliminary study,[18] individuals who had IDA had no finding other than infection by *Helicobacter pylori*. These same patients did not respond well to iron supplementation. Eradication of the infection led to a cure of the anemia. At one-year post-treatment, 90% of patients were free of anemia. The authors note that many of the patients were women who were told that the anemia was due to menstrual blood loss.

Thalassemia Minor

Classic Presentation

The patient is usually asymptomatic.

Cause

Thalassemia (TS) is the second most common anemia in humans and the most common genetic disorder. The thalassemias are characterized by a reduction in globin chains that results in reduced hemoglobin synthesis. There are different types with varying degrees of severity. α-Thalassemia trait and β-thalassemia minor (heterozygous) are by far the most common. α-TS is more common in individuals from Asia/China and in blacks. β-TS is more common in persons of Italian or Greek ancestry and less common in blacks and Asians/Chinese. Thalassemia major is quite rare in the United States, representing less than 1,000 cases. These patients are homozygous and develop severe life-threatening problems within the first year of life.

Evaluation

An elevated RBC count with a low MCV is 75% sensitive and 95% specific for thalassemia syndromes. This combination distinguishes TS from IDA in most cases. Other findings may include microcytosis, target cells (basophilic stippling with β-TS), a normal serum ferritin, TIBC normal or decreased, and a reticulocyte count that is normal or slightly elevated. It is important to recognize that a patient suspected of having IDA yet is unresponsive to iron supplementation may have an underlying TS.

Management

Patients with α-TS trait or β-TS minor need no treatment. It is important to note that both parents who are heterozygous for a specific TS (i.e., both parents have TS minor or both parents have α-TS trait) are at risk of producing a homozygous (TS major) child. Given the severity and poor prognosis for a TS child, genetic counseling should be suggested and the option of prenatal diagnosis should be discussed with those already pregnant.

Anemia of Chronic Disease

Classic Presentation

Patients with ACD usually have rheumatoid arthritis (RA), cancer, chronic infection or inflammation, or liver disease.

Cause

The cause is unknown. Several theories have been proposed: (1) impairment of protein synthesis (decrease in transferrin, albumin, and erythropoietin), (2) activation of macrophages or reticuloendothelial (RE) cells, and (3) an impaired ability to recirculate iron from phagocytosed RBCs. Iron deficiency often coexists with ACD. A distinction is made between ACD and that caused by chronic renal failure; however, the mechanisms may overlap.

The iron deficiency seen with ACD is thought to be due to several mechanisms centered around the release of inflammatory cytokines that result in a disruption of iron homeostasis, impaired erythropoiesis, and RBC destruction. The inflammatory cytokines cause an increased uptake and decreased release of iron from the reticuloendothelial system creating a deficiency for heme biosynthesis. This is reflected in the often-found decrease in total iron on a general lab screen. The same mediators increase the release of hepcidin from hepatocytes. Hepcidin is a major negative iron regulator decreasing iron absorption from the duodenum. Erythropoiesis is downregulated by inflammatory cytokines due to a decrease in erythropoietin (EPO) precursors, and cells that produce these precursors go through apoptosis. The net result is a decrease in EPO production leading to a decrease in RBC production. Finally, RBC destruction is facilitated by the inflammatory cytokines by increasing phagocytosis of RBCs and increasing free radical destruction of RBCs.

Evaluation

Coexisting indications or diagnosis of an underlying chronic disease help in the diagnosis. Laboratory diagnosis is sometimes confusing because values are similar for ACD and IDA. This is often due to the fact that they coexist (especially in patients with RA). ACD is usually normochromic and normocytic (75% of the time). Twenty-five percent of the time ACD is microcytic with an associated decrease in the MCV. Classically, the hematocrit is rarely below 25% and there is a decreased TIBC. While serum iron may be decreased, RDW is usually normal unless there is coexisting iron depletion that would lead to an elevated RDW. The likelihood of ACD is strong when there is a normal or increased serum ferritin and a decreased TIBC.

Management

Usually treatment of the underlying disease is mainly what is necessary. If there is an associated IDA, iron supplementation may be beneficial. In severe cases, transfusion or erythropoietin injection may be necessary.

MACROCYTIC ANEMIAS

Vitamin B$_{12}$ Deficiency

Classic Presentation

In the early stages, most patients are asymptomatic. In later stages, the patient may complain of general weakness, shortness of breath, numbness and tingling, difficulty walking, or a swollen tongue.

Cause

Vitamin B$_{12}$ (cyanocobalamin) is a water-soluble vitamin that requires a glycoprotein, intrinsic factor for absorption in the terminal ileum. Vitamin B$_{12}$ stores in the liver are usually sufficient for three to five years. Vitamin B$_{12}$ is a coenzyme in DNA synthesis and is important for myelin production. It is found in dairy products and meats. A nutritional cause due to lack of ingestion of appropriate foods is an uncommon cause occurring in only about 2% of cases. Even vegetarians can obtain necessary amounts through the consumption of legumes. With pernicious anemia (PA) and atrophic gastritis, intrinsic factor is unavailable, making vitamin B$_{12}$ unabsorbable (except for 1% to 3%). PA is due to an autoimmune response against the parietal cells and intrinsic factor, leading to atrophic gastritis. Although the classic presentation of a gray-haired, middle-aged, northern European has been the standard description of a person with PA, PA is found in all ethnic groups; it is found more often in older patients[19] and young (<40 years old) black women.[20]

Malabsorption of vitamin B$_{12}$ may be due to lack of intrinsic factor due to atrophic gastritis, an *H. pylori* infection which impairs release of B$_{12}$ from protein, malabsorption syndromes including Crohn's disease, medications that decrease acidity and also impair the release of B$_{12}$ from protein such as proton pump inhibitors, H2 antagonists, and antacids, and pancreatic insufficiency that decreases proteases necessary to cleave the B$_{12}$-R factor complex. Other less common causes of vitamin B$_{12}$ deficiency include malabsorption from blind loop syndrome, fish tapeworm, and certain drugs. Nutritional deficiency is most common in chronic alcoholics and vegetarians. Vitamin B$_{12}$ deficiency in vegetarians is not inevitable if they eat a balanced diet. It would take three to five years of a diet free of dairy products and meat before clinical signs would become evident.

Evaluation

Differentiation between vitamin B$_{12}$ and other causes of macrocytic anemia is necessary. A history of alcoholism, nutritional deficiency, or gastric surgery may be helpful. About 20% of individuals with cobalamin deficiency have no anemia and no macrocytosis. Laboratory diagnosis is based on several classic findings: an MCV greater than 130 fL is 100% sensitive for vitamin B$_{12}$ and folic deficiency. Further distinction is that vitamin B$_{12}$ deficiency is usually associated with a low serum vitamin B$_{12}$, and a high serum or urine methylmalonic acid (MMA; 95% sensitive).[21] Total homocysteine levels are also elevated. MMA is not elevated with folic acid deficiency. Currently the standard for PA is to test for anti-intrinsic antibodies. The Schilling test is rarely used but is an option.

It is possible to take these values and create a couplet of findings that help negotiate the differential for macrocytic anemia. Using MMA and homocysteine levels, if both are normal, B$_{12}$ deficiency is ruled out. If both are positive, B$_{12}$ deficiency is ruled in (sensitivity 94%; specificity 99%). If MMA is normal and homocysteine is elevated, folate deficiency is likely.

Coexisting IDA and PA occurs 20% to 25% of the time.[22] This or coexisting thalassemia may result in a normal MCV.

Management

Folic acid replacement will correct the anemia of vitamin B$_{12}$ deficiency; however, there will usually be no reticulocyte count increase in response to folic acid supplementation. Vitamin B$_{12}$ deficiency due to PA requires injections (daily injections for one week, weekly injections for one month, monthly injections for life). When correction of the anemia has been achieved based on a normal laboratory investigation, intranasal cyanocobalamin (Nascobal) may then be used. Initial dose is one spray in one nostril once per week. Monitoring will determine effectiveness or need to return to intramuscular injection. Oral supplementation requires very large dosages (1,000 mg/day) and strict patient compliance (1% to 3% is absorbed without intrinsic factor).[10] Early treatment of PA may prevent or reverse neurologic manifestations. PA patients with neurologic findings less than three months before treatment may have these findings reversed. This may take between 6 and 18 months. Hematologic response is indicated by an increased reticulocyte count in 10 days and correction within six weeks. Patients generally feel physically better almost immediately. It is recommended that because of a higher predisposition to gastric carcinoma, PA patients should be examined with endoscopy every five years.

Folate Deficiency

Classic Presentation

Early folate (folic acid) deficiency is asymptomatic. The patient is often either an alcoholic or a pregnant woman who complains of generalized fatigue.

Cause

Folate is a water-soluble vitamin needed for DNA synthesis and erythropoiesis. Folate stores last for three to six months. It is found in most fruits and vegetables (especially citrus fruits and green leafy vegetables). There are numerous causes of deficiency. Inadequate intake is found in infants, adolescents, the elderly, and chronic alcoholics. Increased need is found in pregnant women. Malabsorption syndromes and drugs such as oral contraceptives, methotrexate, and phenytoin interfere with absorption. Smoking appears to be a risk factor with folate deficiency. Overcooking foods and a lack of vitamin C may also contribute to a deficiency.[23] It is important to note that low folate levels may be associated with an increased risk of colorectal and cervical cancer.[24] There may also be a relationship to chronic fatigue.[25] Low folate levels during pregnancy may result in neural tube defects in the fetus.

Evaluation

Folate deficiency is difficult to differentiate from early vitamin B_{12} deficiency. There are initially no neurologic findings with either. Eventually vitamin B_{12} deficiency might develop neurologic manifestations. Laboratory evaluation is helpful. Shared findings include an MCV >130 fL, macrocytosis, and decreased hemoglobin. Specific findings include low levels of serum and RBC folate. Although RBC folate is the better test, it may not indicate folate deficiency for several months. Some authors suggest a trial of oral folate at 100 mg/day for 10 days followed by a check for a reticulocyte count increase helps to differentiate between vitamin B_{12} deficiency and folate deficiency. At this level of supplementation there will not be a response with vitamin B_{12} deficiency.[26] However, most authors warn against this approach due to the potential of misdiagnosis and subsequent development of irreversible neurologic deficits with patients having pernicious anemia.

Management

When dietary deficiency or increased demand is the cause, supplementation at 1 to 2 mg/day for two to three weeks is needed. Daily supplementation of between 50 and 100 mg is needed. This can be achieved through a diet rich in orange juice, asparagus, red beans, peanut butter, and beef liver. The reticulocyte response occurs within 10 days. Unresponsiveness suggests other causes.

APPENDIX 52–1

References

1. National Board of Chiropractic Examiners. *Job Analysis of Chiropractic.* Greeley, CO: National Board of Chiropractic Examiners; 2005.
2. Nardonne DA, Roth KM, Mazur DJ, McAfee JH. Usefulness of physical examination in detecting the presence or absence of anemia. *Arch Intern Med.* 1990;150:201.
3. Djulbegovic B. Anemia: diagnosis. In: *Reasoning and Decision Making in Hematology.* New York: Churchill Livingstone; 1992:13–17.
4. Crosby WH. Reticulocyte counts. *Arch Intern Med.* 1981;147:1747.
5. Witte DL, Kraemer DF, Johnson GF, et al. Prediction of bone marrow findings from tests performed on peripheral blood. *Am J Clin Pathol.* 1986;85:202.
6. Schilling RF. Anemia of chronic disease: a misnomer. *Ann Intern Med.* 1991;115:572.
7. Scates S, Glaspy J. The macrocytic anemias. *Lab Med.* 1990;21:736.
8. Green R. Metabolic assays in cobalamin and folate deficiency. *Baillieres Clin Haematol.* 1995;8:533–566.
9. Stabler SP, Lindenbaum J, Allen RH. The use of homocysteine and other metabolites in the specific diagnosis of vitamin B_{12} deficiency. *J Nutr.* 1996;126:126–127.
10. Berlin H, Berlin R, Brante G. Oral treatment of pernicious anemia with high doses of vitamin B_{12} without intrinsic factor. *Acta Med Scand.* 1968;184:247–258.
11. Branson RA, Bowers LJ. Nutritional anemia: iron, cobalamin, or folate deficiency? *Top Clin Chiro.* 1995;2(4):33–42.
12. Scrinshaw NS. Iron deficiency. *Sci Am.* 1991;265:46–52.
13. Djulbegovic B. Iron deficiency anemia. In: *Reasoning and Decision Making in Hematology.* New York: Churchill Livingstone; 1992:21–24.
14. Williams SR. *Nutrition and Diet Therapy.* 7th ed. St. Louis, MO: Mosby-Year Book; 1993.
15. Hamilton HK. *Professional Guide to Diseases.* 2nd ed. Springhouse, PA: Springhouse Corp; 1987.
16. Robbins SL. *Robbins Pathologic Basis of Disease.* 4th ed. Philadelphia: WB Saunders; 1989.
17. Brigden ML. Iron deficiency anemia. *Postgrad Med.* 1993;93:181–192.
18. Annibale B, Marignani M, Monarca B, et al. Reversal of iron deficiency anemia after *Helicobacter pylori* eradication in patients with asymptomatic gastritis. *Ann Intern Med.* 1999;131:668–672.
19. Pippard JD. Megaloblastic anemia: geography and diagnosis. *Lancet.* 1994;344:6–7.
20. Carmel R, Johnson CS. Racial patterns in pernicious anemia: early age at onset and increased frequency of intrinsic-factor antibody in black women. *N Engl J Med.* 1978;298:647.

21. Pruthi RK, Tefferi A. Pernicious anemia revisited. *Mayo Clin Proc.* 1994;69:144–150.

22. Chanarin I. Pernicious anemia. *Br Med J.* 1992;304:1584–1585.

23. Bailey LB. Folate status assessment. *J Nutr.* 1990;120:1508–1511.

24. Butterworth CE, Jr, Hutch KD, Macaloso M, et al. Folate deficiency and cervical dysplasia. *JAMA.* 1992;267:528–533.

25. Jacobson W, Saich T, Borysiewicz LK, et al. Serum folate and chronic fatigue syndrome. *Neurology.* 1993;43:2645–2647.

26. Speicher CE. Hematological diseases. In: *The Right Test: A Physician's Guide to Laboratory Medicine.* 2nd ed. Philadelphia: WB Saunders; 1993:208.

Special Patient Groups

The Pediatric/Adolescent Patient

Context

A survey[1] of patients in Canada evaluated the use of complementary and alternative medicine (CAM) for the pediatric population. The range of use was between 42% to 71% representing wide regional differences. The most common CAM practitioners used were massage therapists and chiropractic physicians.

Data are limited regarding how much of a chiropractor's patient base is pediatric and adolescent. Preliminary studies, primarily done in countries outside the United States, indicate that pediatric visits account for between 4.6% and 10% of daily visits, and adolescent visits account for approximately 15% of daily visits.[2] With adolescents, back pain accounted for about 33% of visits. Neck and headache pain accounted for approximately 40% of visits. Probably unrepresentative of a field practice, a college clinic demonstrated that 33% of pediatric/adolescent patients presented for a general physical examination.

Interestingly, a Canadian study of pediatric visits to alternative care practitioners indicated that the majority of patients presented with nonmusculoskeletal complaints such as respiratory and eyes, ears, nose, and throat (EENT)-related symptoms.[3] In 2012, a review[4] noted that the reason for visits broken down by percentage equaled for skeletal (57.0%), neurologic (23.7%), gastrointestinal (12.4%), infection (3.5%), genitourinary (1.5%), immune (1.4%), and for miscellaneous conditions (0.5%). A review[5] of the literature in 2012 regarding chiropractic management of pediatric complaints revealed there were six clinical trials investigating the effectiveness of spinal manipulative therapy (SMT) for colic, two each for asthma and enuresis, and one each on hip extension, otitis media, suboptimal breastfeeding, autism, idiopathic scoliosis, and jet lag. The authors note that in their review none of the studies evaluated effectiveness of SMT on spinal pain.

Authors of a 2010 review[6] of pediatric care by chiropractors concluded that there is a paradox within the chiropractic profession (similar to the medical profession's use of medication) that although the main reason for pediatric patients (or their parents) to seek a chiropractor is for spinal pain, there are no studies other than case studies for this predominant complaint.

An individual chiropractor's involvement in pediatric/adolescent care is dictated by the chiropractor's pediatric/adolescent focus, expertise, and his or her involvement in school examinations, scoliosis screenings, and sports preparticipation examinations.

Generally, the pediatric/adolescent patient presents a complex and dynamic challenge based on constantly changing "normals" and milestones of development. Specific issues include:

- musculoskeletal and neurologic development
- prevention of injury issues (e.g., sports, motor vehicle collision, and abuse)
- social/psychologic challenges (e.g., attention-deficit disorder, hyperactivity, depression, eating disorders)

In addition to evaluating the young patient with a specific complaint or complaints, monitoring of normal development and screening for disorders and risk factors specific to a particular age range are responsibilities of the managing doctor. Counseling may be particularly important in the prevention of addictive behaviors (e.g., smoking, alcoholism, gambling), nutrition and exercise, sexually transmitted disorders, and birth control. Regarding unusual patient presentations, a review by Miller et al. evaluated the literature regarding child medication errors over a five-year period. The reviewers estimate that between 5% and 27% of medication errors occur during ordering, which includes prescribing, dispensing, and administering. The majority of these (72% to 75%) occur with administering the medication. Other "errors" include the use of medications designed and tested on adults but not on children. Most of these errors are hospital-based.[7]

Specific challenges arise when eliciting historical information with limitations presented by the inability of the infant or child to verbalize a complaint or the issue of privacy in an adolescent patient. Overreactive responses to physical examination procedures introduce a challenge to interpretation of orthopaedic and palpation positives. Radiologic challenges occur due to the overlap between normal variants and areas of complaint and age-related, and therefore changing, normal radiographic anatomy.

The following discussion is intended as an overview of an extremely broad specialty, focusing on some age-related complaints that are nonmusculoskeletal, but primarily on complaints and concerns of the musculoskeletal system.

General Strategy

- Consider the purpose and requirements for evaluation in three common scenarios:
  1. The periodic health examination—intended to check for milestones in development, screen for risk factors for a specific age group, and counsel on health-related topics for that age group
  2. The sports preparticipation examination—intended to screen for developmental markers related to the type of sport, screen for risk factors for injury, and determine deficiencies in performance to aid in exercise/training prescription
  3. The child or parent concerned about pain, dysfunction, or cosmetic appearance
- Address vaccination issues.
- Be vigilant with regard to ominous signs suggestive of cancer or tumor.
- Be vigilant with regard to child abuse and have a referral source for suspected cases.
- Be aware of normal variants of growth centers and bony development in children, always considering a bilateral radiographic evaluation if involving an extremity.
- Consider injuries or conditions that are more common or exclusive to the child/adolescent such

as developmental asymmetry, epiphyseal and apophyseal injury, and different types of fracture patterns.
- Refer for second opinion in the following settings:
  1. signs of abuse
  2. orthopaedic problems that have a tendency to progress without surgical management
  3. ear infections associated with high fever and chills
  4. suspicion or identification of fracture (with the exception of a torus fracture), osteomyelitis, septic synovitis, or tumor/cancer
- When adjusting the pediatric spine, consider anatomic and developmental issues, modifying the degree of force and positioning of the child.[8]

The Periodic Health Examination

For the asymptomatic patient, many agencies, including the U.S. Preventive Services Task Force (USPSTF), have developed strategies focusing on age-related concerns.[9] The examination components include screening, counseling, and immunization recommendations. General evaluation recommendations include:

- Measure vitals including height, weight, and blood pressure.
- Determine if normal growth and neurologic development are occurring. These signposts are particularly important in the first few years of life (see **Table 53–1**).
- Be vigilant regarding signs of physical or sexual abuse.
- Screen for vision between the ages of 3 and 4 years.
- Screen for lead toxicity and hypercholesterolism in high-risk groups.
- Focus counseling on the risk areas based on age; however, always counsel on a healthy diet and adequate exercise.

A 2007 study by Hansen et al.[10] indicates that there is an underdiagnosis of hypertension in children and adolescents. In a group of 507 children and adolescents, 3.6% had hypertension. Only 26% of those with HTN had an entry in their medical records, while only 11% with prehypertension had an entry in their medical records. Factors related to an increased associated risk were older age, increase in 1% height-for-age percentile, obesity, and frequency of degree of prior abnormal BP readings.

Many conditions due to inborn errors are evident at birth or as the child develops. A short list of some of

Table 53–1 Developmental Milestones

Age	Observational Activities	Activities Reported by Patients	Language Capabilities
1–2 months	Holds head up Raises head prone 45° Turns head and eyes to sound Acknowledges faces Follows objects through visual fields Drops objects (toys) Is alert in response to voices	Smiles responsively and spontaneously Recognizes parents	Engages in vocalizations (coo)
3–5 months	Smiles, laughs, giggles Holds head high and raises body with hands while in a prone position Reaches for and brings objects to mouth Makes "raspberry" sound Sits with support (head steady) Holds rattle briefly	Anticipates food on sight Rolls from front to back Turns from back to side Excited upon recognizing familiar people	Squeals Babbles, initial vowels Guttural sounds ("ah," "go") Consonants: m, p, b Vowels: o, u
6–8 months	Initiates "bye bye" Reaches Sits alone for a short time Some weight-bearing Passes object from hand to hand in midline First scoops up a pellet then grasps it using thumb opposition	Rolls front to back and back to front Is indifferent to the word "no"	Babbles/initiates speech sounds Syllables: da, ba, ka
9–11 months	Sits alone Pulls to stand Stands alone Creeps Initiates pat-a-cake and peek-a-boo Uses thumb and index finger to pick up pellet	Feeds self finger foods Walks supported by furniture Follows one-step verbal commands (e.g., "Come here," "give it to me")	MaMa/DaDa nonspecifically Approximates names: babba/bottle
12 months	Walks with support or independently Pincer grasp Gives toys upon request Brings two blocks together; tries to build tower Releases objects into cup after demonstration	Points to desired objects Looks for hidden objects	MaMa/DaDa specific Jargon begins (own language) 2–3 words understandable
18 months	Throws ball Climbs/descends stairs with aid Turns pages Uses a spoon Identifies body parts Seats self in chairs Scribbles spontaneously Builds tower of 3–4 blocks	Feeds self Carries and hugs doll Understands a 2-step command	Says 10–15 words Consonants: t, d, w, h, n 2-word phrases understandable
24 months	Kicks ball Holds cup securely Points to named objects or pictures Jumps off floor with both feet Stands on one foot alone	Verbalizes toilet needs Mimics domestic activities Pulls on simple garments	3-word phrases understandable (contains subject, verb, and object) Use of pronouns: mine, me, you, I

(continues)

Table 53–1 Developmental Milestones (continued)

Age	Observational Activities	Activities Reported by Patients	Language Capabilities
	Builds tower of 6–7 blocks		Vowels uttered correctly
	Climbs/descends stairs unaided		Approximately 100-word vocabulary
	Turns pages of a book singly		
30 months	Refers to self as I	Helps put things away	Counts 3 objects correctly
	Copies a crude circle		Repeats 3 numbers or a sentence of 6 syllables
	Walks backwards		Carries on a conversation
	Begins to hop on one leg		Uses prepositions
	Holds crayon in fist		
36 months	Shares playthings	Dresses with supervision	Some degree of hesitancy and uncertainty common
	Copies a circle	Rides tricycle using pedals	Intelligible 4-word phrases
	Holds crayon with fingers	While looking at picture book, able to answer: "What . . . doing?"	Approximately 900 words
	Initiates a vertical line		
	Builds a tower using 9–10 blocks		
	Gives first and last name		
3–4 years	Walks on heels	Takes off shoes and jacket	Intelligible 5-word phrases
	Climbs/descends stairs with alternating feet	Feeds self at mealtime	Answers questions using plurals, personal pronoun, and verbs (What do you want to do that is fun?)
	Responds to command to place objects in, on, or under table		
	Draws a circle when asked to draw a person (man, boy, girl)		
	Knows own sex		
	Finger opposition		
	Begins to button and unbutton		
	General knowledge: Full name, age, address (2 out of 3)		
4–5 years	May stand on one leg for at least 10 seconds	Dressing and undressing without supervision	Intelligible 6-word phrases
	Runs and turns without losing balance	Buttons clothes and laces shoes but does not tie	Names 4 colors
	Tiptoes	Self-care with toilet needs (may need help wiping)	Repeats sentence of 10 syllables
	Tells a simple story	Plays outside for at least 30 minutes	Approximately 1,540 words
	Knows the days of the week		
	Draws a person		
	Counts to 4 by rote		
	Begins understanding rules (right and wrong)		
	Cuts and pastes		
	Gives appropriate answers to: "What must you do if you are sleepy? Hungry? Cold?" etc.		
5–6 years	Skips	Goes to school unattended or meets school bus	Intelligible 6–7 word sentences
	Catches a ball	Helps with simple chores at home (taking out the garbage)	Approximately 2,560 words
	Copies a + that is already drawn	Good motor capability, but little aware of dangers	
	Tells own age		
	Knows right and left		
	Draws a recognizable person with at least 8 details		
	Understands the concept of 10 (is able to count out 10 objects)		
	Describes favorite television program or video in some detail		

Reproduced from *Nelson Essentials of Pediatrics*, R.E. Behrman and R. Klingman, pp. 80–82, © 1990, with permission from Elsevier.

these conditions is given in Tables 53–1 and **53–2**. These lists are not comprehensive; rather, they are a reminder that hereditary disease must be considered when neurologic development is abnormal, or when unusual signs or symptoms develop.

Focused Concerns (Not Covered in Other Areas of This Text)

Sudden Infant Death Syndrome

Sudden infant death syndrome (SIDS) is death in an infant younger than 1 year old that cannot be explained after complete autopsy, death scene investigation, or review of the family history. SIDS is the leading cause of death between 1 month and 1 year of age. In the United States the incidence is about 1.5 per 1,000 live births.[11] Although rare in the first month of life, there is a peak incidence in months two through four. Although there are no clear explanations as to the pathophysiology, there are identifiable risk factors including maternal smoking, prematurity, and perhaps bottle-feeding as compared with breastfeeding. The most successful modifiable risk factor, though, is the prone sleeping position.[12] SIDS rates decrease dramatically when parents are educated to the safer sleeping position of side-lying or supine.[13]

Table 53–2 Chromosomal Abnormalities with Examples of Each

Type with Example	Overview
Structural WGAR syndrome (Deletion of short arm of chromosome 11) Retinoblastoma (Deletion of long arm of chromosome 13)	Stands for congenital Wilms' tumor of the kidney, anindia (lack of iris), general malformations, and mental retardation. This condition results in tumor due to loss of a Wilms' tumor suppressor gene.
Numerical Trisomy 21 (Down's syndrome)	1 in 800 births. Common combinations of characteristics in varying degrees of severity, including mental retardation, wide face, low-bridged nose, closely set slanted eyes with epicanthus (medial fold of the upper lid), macroglossia (large tongue), short limbs, simian crease across palms, clinodactyly (fifth finger shorter and crooked), heart defects, gastro defects (atresia and stenosis), infertility in males and most females, possible mild anemia, and predisposition to leukemia. Down's syndrome affects longevity mainly due to cardiac problems; average age of death is 55 years. Prenatal diagnosis for Down's syndrome includes chorionic villus biopsy or amniocentesis.
Sex chromosome Turner's syndrome	Monosomy X (45 XO) occurs in 1 in 3,000 births. Abnormal segregation of sex chromosome during meiosis in female or male gonads. Characteristics include short stature, increased valgus angle at the elbows, webbed neck, barrel chest, and sometimes heart defects and coarctation of the aorta. Normal female genital organs except ovaries transform into "streak" gonads. Females do not develop secondary sexual characteristics and are generally infertile. Hormonal replacement may help body image but not the infertility.
Klinefelter's syndrome	Trisomy of sex chromosomes (47 XXY) occurs in 1 in 700 births. Abnormal segregation of sex chromosome during meiosis in female or male gonads. Phenotypically male and infertile. Puberty does not develop. Patients typically have a small penis, scant pubic hair; generally tall and effeminate with possible gynecomastia (enlargement of breast tissue).
Single gene disorders **Autosomal dominant** (over 1,000 disorders total)	Trait is apparent in heterozygotes with a 50% chance of passing on the gene to offspring with expression in every generation. Unaffected offspring of a symptomatic carrier do not transmit gene.
Marfan's syndrome	Occurs in 1 in 10,000 births. Dysfunction of the gene that codes for fibrillin, a connective tissue protein involved in the structure of many organs. Features include a tall, slender stature with elongated head (dolichocephalic) and prominent frontal bosselation, scoliosis and kyphosis, aortic aneurysm and other dissecting predisposition, valvular insufficiency, subluxation of the lens in the eyes, retinal detachment, cataracts, and sometimes blindness. Must be distinguished from anorexia nervosa, and in tall athletes diagnosis may affect participation.

(continues)

Table 53–2 Chromosomal Abnormalities with Examples of Each (continued)

Type with Example	Overview
Achondroplastic dwarfism	A type of osteochondrodysplasia dwarfism (many other types). Short limbs, bulky forehead, saddle nose, lumbar lordosis, and bowlegs. Parents are not affected by dwarfism in 90% of cases. Spinal stenosis is common as is basilar impression and stenosis of the foramen magnum. This may lead to apnea and sudden death.
Osteogenesis imperfecta	There are two main types, and some subdivisions, of this disorder that is characterized by abnormal maturation of collagen due to an ATPase enzyme deficiency. The clinical features include osteoporosis with resulting fragility of the skeleton, blue sclerae (90% of individuals), abnormal dentition (dentinogenesis imperfecta), and premature otosclerosi. Fractures, bowing of the extremities, dislocations, kyphoscoliosis, basilar impression, ligamentous laxity, and deafness are all found. The tarda form usually allows a normal life expectancy.
Polycystic kidney disease	Occurs in 1 in 400 to 1 in 1,000 births. The abnormal gene is (in most cases) located on the short arm of chromosome 16 (sometimes 4). In addition to kidney cysts development, cysts may be found in the liver (most common), pancreas and spleen (less common), and CNS arachnoid. Individuals are more prone to cerebral aneurysms. Diagnosis is made by a positive family history of polycystic kidney disease and three or more cysts in both kidneys detected on renal ultrasound or abdominal CT. Medication treatment for associated hypertension. If end-range kidney disease occurs, dialysis or renal transplantation is considered.
Spherocytosis	The membrane defect is found in the protein spectrin (there are two structural proteins for the red blood cell: spectrin and actin). The result is a round cell instead of a biconcave disk, making the cell vulnerable to lysis in the spleen. As a result, the individual will develop splenomegaly. The diagnosis is based on a positive family history, general signs of anemia, and a finding of spherocytes and increased reticulocytes on peripheral blood smear. Treatment includes splenectomy and daily dose of folic acid.
Huntington's disease	A trinucleotide repeat problem located on the short arm of chromosome 4. Occurs in 33.1–35.4 out of 100,000 births. Initially small oculomotor dysfunction and choreiform movement problems that progressively worsen. Usually the onset is in ages 30 to 40 years; however, may occur at any age. Progression to full neuropsychiatric instability (insanity) with associated neuronal loss in the caudate nucleus.
Neurofibromatosis	May also occur as a new mutation and not autosomal dominant. Of two types, characteristics include peripheral nerve tumors (neurofibromas) and pigmented skin lesions (café au lait spots).
Familial hypercholesterolemia	Occurs in 1 in 500 births. One of several familial hyperlipidemias. Involves the receptor for low-density lipoprotein (LDL). Gene for the receptor is mutated, which results in dysfunctional cholesterol removal. Deposition of lipids occurs, resulting in accelerated atherosclerosis, xanthomas (made up phagocytized cholesterol in macrophages that deposit in skin, especially around eyes). Requires low-fat diet and medical management.
Autosomal recessive	Only homozygotes have the gene effect, with both parents of the homozygote as asymptomatic carriers of the trait. The children of the homozygote are not symptomatic but 50% carry the gene for the trait. In siblings of the affected zygote, 25% are symptomatic homozygotes, 50% are asymptomatic carriers for the trait, and 25% are unaffected and do not carry the gene.
Cystic fibrosis	Occurs in 1 in 2,500 births in U.S. with an estimated 1 in 25 individuals being asymptomatic carriers. Seen primarily in Caucasians. Results in a more viscid glandular secretion (mucoviscidosis) from all exocrine glands, leading to obstruction, in particular in the pancreas, bronchi, and intestines. This is due to a defect in the gene for the protein that is involved in the chloride transport channel in the cell membrane. Fetal effects can include meconium peritonitis and meconium ileus. The primary concern is accumulation of viscid mucus makes breathing difficult and allows for the development of bronchiectasis and the development of life-threatening infection (the usual cause of death). Testing of sweat indicates increased salt content (pilocarpine test). Management includes antibiotic therapy for prevention of fulminant infection coupled with daily clearing of airways and some dietary manipulation.

Table 53–2 Chromosomal Abnormalities with Examples of Each *(continued)*

Type with Example	Overview
Sickle cell	Sickle cell disease is a hemolytic anemia occurring primarily in blacks (0.3% of blacks in the U.S.) characterized by abnormally shaped red blood cells (sickled) due to homozygous inheritance of hemoglobin S. Hepatosplenomegaly is common. Growth retardation with associated radiographic findings are salient features. Individuals are prone to infections. Upon exposure to acute infection (often viral) an aplastic crisis occurs due to a decrease in erythropoiesis. This results in bone infarcts and vascular occlusions causing severe pain in the hands, feet, and lower legs. Abdominal pain also occurs due to the vascular occlusion. Life expectancy is greater than 50 years old. Death is usually due to infection, pulmonary emboli, and renal failure.
Thalassemia	A group of hereditary disorders that involve decreased synthesis of globin chains (alpha or beta). The result may either be the trait for alpha or beta (heterozygous) or the full-blown beta thalassemia major (homozygous). The result is a microcytosis out of proportion to the degree of anemia. Individuals with the traits are mildly anemic and generally require no treatment, but should be given a recommendation for genetic counseling. Those with the beta trait have Mediterranean (e.g., Greek or Italian) or Chinese ancestry. Those with the alpha trait are either from southeast Asia or China; less commonly black. Those with full-blown beta thalassemia major usually require bone marrow transplantation with a relatively high degree of success in selected individuals (80%).
Tay-Sachs (hexosaminidase A deficiency or gangliosidosis GM2)	Found in Ashkenazi Jews, this gangliosidosis results in accumulation of sphingolipids in the brain. There is an early onset, with progressive retardation leading to death at ages 3 to 4 years. Indicators are progressive paralysis associated with dementia and cherry-red retinal spots seen ophthalmologically. Prenatal screening is available.
Niemann-Pick	There are three types (A, B, and C) of this lysosomal accumulation disorder. Types A and B involve defective sphingomyelinase activity leading to accumulation of sphingomyelin in the reticuloendothelial cells. Type C allows lysosomal accumulation of unesterified cholesterol. Prenatal diagnosis may be done through amniocentesis or chorionic villus sampling. Diagnosis in the infant or child is prompted due to hepatosplenomegaly. Treatment is supportive and nonspecific.
Hurler's	A mucopolysaccharidosis, involves primarily the skeletal system and central nervous system leading to body deformity (gargoylism), neurological dysfunction, and mental retardation. Urinary excretion finding of dermatan sulfate and heparin sulfate. Death occurs usually before age 10 years.
Hunter's	A mucopolysaccharidosis, with iduronate-2 sulfinate similar to but milder than Hurler's. No corneal clouding. Associated skeletal dysplasia, mental deficiency, and hepatosplenomegaly. Death at early age is still common before age 15 years.
Albinism	The enzyme tyrosinase defective affecting tyrosine and leading to an absence of pigment in the skin, hair, and eyes. Management involves protection from actinic radiation for skin and eyes.
Phenylketonuria (PKU)	This is an enzyme defect disorder that involves a deficiency of the enzyme that metabolizes phenylalanine into tyrosine (phenylalanine hydroxylase [PAH]). The result is an accumulation of dietary phenylalanine in the blood and body tissues and a shift in breakdown leading to the formation of phenyl pyruvic acid and other phenylketones excreted in the urine (reason for the term PKU). This disorder is screened for at birth in the U.S. If undetected, leads to pigmentation problems due to deficient melanin production and, more importantly, impairs nervous system development leading to slow, progressive mental retardation. If detected, a specific diet is prescribed.
X-linked recessive	Gene defect evident primarily in males, transmitted via asymptomatic mother (unaffected brothers do not carry the gene; sisters of affected males are asymptomatic). Sons of a female carrying the gene have a 50% chance of being affected; however, affected males do not pass on gene to sons but all daughters are asymptomatic carriers.
Hemophilia	Leads to bleeding disorder due a defect in gene (inherited or through mutation) that codes for coagulation factors VIII (hemophilia A; most common) or IX (hemophilia B; less common). Hemophilia A can exist anywhere from a mild to a severe form. Hemophilia B is always severe. Internal bleeding into joints (hemarthrosis) is common, which leads to deformity; cerebral hemorrhage is rarer than in the past. Genes for each hemophilia are available as recombinant clotting factors.

(continues)

Table 53–2 Chromosomal Abnormalities with Examples of Each (continued)

Type with Example	Overview
Muscular dystrophy	Several types: Most common are Duchenne (1 in 3,300 males) and Becker's (1 in 20,000 males) muscular dystrophy DBMD. Affects primarily males. Gene located to the midportion of the short arm of X chromosome for coding of dystrophin. Dystrophin is needed as a structural protein for the integrity of cell form. With Duchenne there is severe muscle wasting. Gower's sign may be evident, indicating proximal muscle wasting. Most confined to wheelchairs and die in teens. Becker's is less severe.
Fragile X syndrome	A trinucleotide repeat disorder (cytosine, guanine, and guanine [CGG triplet repeat]) in the chromosomal area Xq27. Eighty percent of males have mental retardation. It is the most common form of hereditary mental retardation (deficiency) in males. Even children of normal mental function carriers of Fragile X may be mentally retarded.

Infantile Colic

Infantile colic is a relatively common condition that usually occurs within the first weeks after birth. The incidence reported is quite variable (8% to 40%) due to the existence of several definitions of what infantile colic is and the reliance on parental interpretation of these definitions.[14] Probably the most accepted criteria are crying for three hours a day for more than three days a week for a minimum of three weeks.[15] Given that newborns have a tendency to cry with a reported average of about 2.75 hours/day, it is not surprising that the reported incidence can be so high.[16] The stress on the parents of infants with colic may lead to abuse (i.e., shaken infant syndrome) or feelings of guilt by the parents due to a feeling of being unable to meet the needs of their new child. Although the cause would seem to be gastrointestinal based on the reports of increased flatulence and association with onset after feeding, there is little evidence to support this theory. Radiologic studies have not shown any more air in the intestines of infants with colic compared with infants who do not have colic.[17] Other investigations of intestinal origin including measure of intestinal hormones, fecal analysis, and occult blood analysis have not shown abnormal findings.[14] Studies regarding mode of delivery (e.g., breech versus normal, those with epidurals, those with oxytocin) have not demonstrated any clear connection. One plausible theory is that due to an immature nervous system the infant is neurolabile with an overreaction to normal negative (e.g., hunger, gas, fatigue) or positive (e.g., music, voices, handling) stimuli.

The medical management of colic is primarily with dimethicone (Simethicone, Mylicon). However, it appears to be no better than placebo.[18] The new trend of physicians prescribing proton-pump inhibitors for colic should be discouraged due the potential effect on absorption of important minerals and a reduction in immune response. Studies[19,20] from Denmark seem to indicate that chiropractic manipulation is effective at improving or resolving infantile colic. The most recent study[21] compared manipulation to dimethicone as a treatment strategy. Generally, improvement in the manipulation group was a 2½-hour reduction in crying time compared with a one-hour reduction in the dimethicone group at one week.

Abuse and Neglect

Childhood abuse is divided into physical abuse, mental abuse, and sexual abuse. Given the common musculoskeletal focus of most chiropractors and given that 50% to 70% of physical abuse results in skeletal trauma, it is likely that the chiropractor will see signs of abuse.[22] The most commonly injured area is the face. More than half of abused children are in the age range of birth to 4 years. In one large, hospital-based study,[23] the percentage of childhood maltreatment cases relating to physical abuse was 41%, sexual abuse 35.4%, and neglect 23.6%. A recent study[24] indicates that approximately 20% of all head injuries seen at a metropolitan children's hospital were due to abuse. Given that even a suspicion of childhood abuse is a reportable event in some jurisdictions, it is a difficult task to weigh what may be circumstantial evidence against what may appear to be reasonable explanations in deciding whether to report. For chiropractors, it may be appropriate to refer for second opinion, voicing concerns to the medical physician.

There are some potential risk factors that, when taken together with physical evidence, suggest the possibility of abuse. Factors may include an early or unwanted pregnancy, foster care, poverty and/or unemployment, history of family psychologic problems (including a parent's childhood experience of separation or abuse), and postpartum depression. The infant/child who is premature, colicky, hyperactive, handicapped, sick, or biologically unrelated to the abuser is at higher risk.

Suspicion of abuse is supported by multiple bruises of areas not usually exposed to trauma (such as the back or trunk area); fractures of the skull, face, or spine; or pattern-shaped burns. Interestingly, children may report the abuse, but more commonly will lie to protect themselves. The child may demonstrate fear of the parent/caregiver or may even demonstrate a closeness to the abuser fostered by the need to be loved and not abused. One of the most serious injuries is the "shaken infant" or "shaken impact" syndrome where the caregiver violently shakes the infant, usually holding onto the shoulders while the head and neck are whipped back and forth.[25] Without evidence of outside trauma, intracranial injury including subarachnoid hemorrhage, subdural hematoma, and cerebral edema may occur. Shaken infant syndrome is suspected when any of the following are present:[26]

- There is a decreasing level of consciousness or lethargy, orbital or lid ecchymosis, retinal hemorrhages, disconjugate eye movement, bulging fontanelle, or focal or generalized motor weakness.
- There is an uncertain or illogical explanation offered by the caregiver. Common caregiver reports are no causative event, a minor fall, a seizure, or respiratory arrest.
- A new onset of seizures is reported associated with retinal hemorrhages and intrathecal hemorrhages seen on computed tomography (CT) scan or magnetic resonance imaging (MRI).

Radiographic clues to physical abuse include:[27]

- Evidence of multiple fractures that have healed or are in a healing stage without appropriate orthotic support.
- Multiple or bilateral skull fractures; linear fractures of the parietal bone may be due to an unintentional fall off of a bed but are rare.
- Fractures that are shaft or metaphyseal suggest abuse; supracondylar fractures of the humerus would typically indicate a fall with hyperextension and are not suspicious.
- Femoral fractures in children under 1 year of age are suspicious given the child is not yet

Table 53–3 Dysplasias	
Dysplasias	**Diagnostic Features and Considerations**
Achondroplasia	This is the most common cause of dwarfism. Although it may be transmitted as a single-gene abnormality, most new cases are due to new mutation. There is an abnormality in endochondral ossification with intramembranous bone formation normal. This short-limb dwarfism is recognized at birth as an enlarged head, frontal bossing, a low nasal bridge, and generalized hypotonia. Head and motor control milestones are delayed. All patients have foramen magnum stenosis that is associated with an increased incidence of sleep apnea and sudden infant death syndrome. Forty-four percent of neurologically intact achondroplasts demonstrate abnormal somatosensory evoked potential. Cervicomedullary compression is common enough to warrant extreme concern with cervical adjusting. A thoracolumbar kyphosis is seen at birth. There are two forms, with the fixed type caused by a triangular-shaped vertebral body with anterior wedging (seen on lateral radiograph). The more common flexible type extends over several levels. It appears that it many resolve over time. If persistent past age 3 years, a brace is recommended. Those with a kyphosis > 40° should have surgery.
	Spinal stenosis due to a congenitally small canal is common, with more than half of achondroplasts developing symptoms.
	Symptoms generally appear in the 20s or 30s. There are mixed results with surgical decompression. It is particularly worse in those with a thoracolumbar kyphosis. Extreme care should be taken when adjusting the spine. Hyperlordosis is common in the lumbar spine due to a heavy, larger head, lax ligaments, and vertebral malformation. Flexion deformities of the hip are also common.
Pseudoachondroplasia	This short-limbed dwarfism is an autosomal dominant disorder characterized by normal facies, joint laxity, and abnormalities in epiphyseal and metaphyseal development. There is abnormal proteoglycan accumulation in the chondrocyte rough endoplasmic reticulum. The disorder is not apparent at birth, with the first findings appearing within the first years of life. The spinal abnormalities that are of concern are atlantoaxial instability, a thoracic kyphosis (with anterior vertebral body wedging), and scoliosis. Hip deformities are also more common with achondroplasts.

(continues)

Table 53–3 Dysplasias (continued)

Dysplasias	Diagnostic Features and Considerations
Osteogenesis imperfecta	A large number of inherited connective tissue disorders are classified under osteogenesis imperfecta. The most common features are small, triangular faces, fragile bones with associated multiple and recurrent fractures, abnormal teeth, deafness, and blue sclera and tympanic membranes. Defects in or the quantity of type I collagen accounts for most of these findings. In addition to the frequency of nontraumatic fractures, the other orthopaedic/neurologic concerns are basilar impression and scoliosis. Scoliosis is common and progresses most in patients with a biconcave type of thoracic vertebrae. Compression fractures also factor into the development of kyphosis and scoliosis. Treatment for scoliosis is generally ineffective. Spinal or extremity adjusting should not be performed on these patients due to the brittleness of their bone.
Spondyloepiphyseal dysplasia	This form of dwarfism is a short-trunk type with involvement of the vertebrae and long bone epiphysis. An autosomal-dominant condition, it is usually seen at birth with a clinical appearance of a flat face with wide-set eyes, short neck, cleft palate, retinal detachment, barrel-chest, and shortening of the limbs with hip flexor contractures. A later form seen first in adolescence is the X-linked form only appearing in males. The first signs are osteoarthritis in a major joint and delay in the appearance of ossification centers. The major concerns are atlantoaxial instability seen in 40% of patients, often due to os odontoideum or odontoid hypoplasia. As a result, cervical myelopathy may develop, signaled by regression of motor milestones, respiratory problems, or simply fatigue. Kyphoscoliosis is not uncommon due to flattening of the vertebral bodies and other abnormalities in development. Radiographs for atlantoaxial instability are a requirement in making decisions regarding spinal adjusting.
Diastrophic dysplasia	This is a short-limb dwarfism, autosomal-recessive disorder associated with severe clubfeet, "hitchhiker thumb," cleft palate, and eventually in most patients, a cauliflower ear. Spinal concerns center around a cervical spine kyphosis associated with spina bifida and anterior wedging of apical vertebrae. Spontaneous resolution occurs in many cases by age 5 years; however, some cases may progress to spinal cord compression and death. Atlantoaxial instability is not a common feature. Kyphoscoliosis commonly develops with walking. The most rapid progression is between ages 8 and 12 years. Early bracing is recommended.
Ehlers-Danlos syndrome	A group of related disorders characterized by abnormal collagen production and structure. Although there are ten types listed, they generally have three common clinical manifestations: (1) hypermobile joints, (2) fragile blood vessels, and (3) various cutaneous abnormalities including hyperelasticity. Other areas that may be affected are the eyes (may have blue sclerae), bronchopulmonary (higher incidence of bronchiectasis and spontaneous pneumothorax), cardiovascular (tetralogy of Fallot, aortic and other aneurysms), gastrointestinal (spontaneous rupture or hemorrhage of the bowel), among others. Clinically the patient often is tall and exhibits a gait of hyperextension at the hips and genu recurvatum (hyperextended knees). Redundant skin folds around the eyes, hyperelastic skin, and joint hypermobility are evident upon examination. Radiographically, small "spherules" of subcutaneous fat may be seen (mainly pretibial and at forearms). Musculoskeletally, these patients are more prone to dislocations and early degenerative changes.
Marfan's syndrome	An autosomal dominant disorder of connective tissue, Marfan's is a condition associated with abnormal collagen organization with defects in cross-links leading to problems in three distinct organ systems (1) musculoskeletal, (2) ocular, and (3) cardiac. The condition is not all that rare, with a prevalence of about 1 in 10,000. Patients are often tall with long legs and hypermobile joints. The major musculoskeletal concerns are an enlarged concavity of the superior and inferior endplates of spinal vertebrae with widening of the spinal canal and dural ectasia. There is thinning of the cortex, dilation of the neural foramina, and dura protrusion outside the canal. There is some concern for both atlantoaxial instability and basilar invagination found in one-third to one-half of patients. Although spondylolisthesis is not seen more often than in general population, slippage is twice as common. Scoliosis is seen in three-fourths of patients with a single thoracic, thoracolumbar, and double major curve most common. Hyperkyphosis is also common. Scoliosis progression is more common, and therefore early bracing is recommended. Surgery is more likely with these patients. Ocular concerns are ectopia lentis (subluxation of the lens). Other orthopaedic concerns are pectus carinatum/excavatum and ligament laxity. Acetabular protrusion is seen in half of patients, and a higher incidence of slipped capital femoral epiphysis is also seen. Dissecting aortic aneurysm, valvular insufficiency, and mitral valve prolapse are all concerns for these patients, and a cardiovascular evaluation should be performed frequently.

Table 53–3 Dysplasias (continued)	
Dysplasias	**Diagnostic Features and Considerations**
Morquio's syndrome	Although not technically a dysplastic disorder, Morquio's syndrome represents one of several lysosomal storage diseases characterized by specific enzyme deficiencies resulting in accumulation of mucopolysaccharide glycos-aminoglycan (GAGS) in different tissue, resulting in disease. Clinically the patient is of short stature. Normal at birth, there is progression to short-trunk dwarfism, corneal opacities, hearing loss, and generalized laxity. Of particular concern is atlantoaxial instability (due to odontoid abnormalities) and the abnormal shape of thoracolumbar vertebrae. They are typically flame-shaped with flattening and an anterior projecting central tongue. Also, an increase in soft tissue anterior to the spinal cord may cause neurologic injury.

weight-bearing in most cases; the most common fractures in abuse cases are subtrochanteric and distal metaphyseal chip fractures.

- Chip fracture or bucket-handle fracture indicates an injury caused by sudden twisting of a limb; metaphyseal ligaments are stretched to the point of fracturing and avulsing bone at their insertion point at either one or both metaphyseal corners; a specific distinction between acute injury versus healing fractures is localized radiolucent extension of the growth plate into the metaphysis indicating hypertrophic cartilage extension found more often with past abuse.
- Rib fractures in young children are rare and should raise the suspicion of abuse, especially if associated with head trauma.

Sexual abuse should be suspected when there is vaginal bleeding in a child, persistent vaginal discharge, infection in the genital area and associated recurrent urinary tract infections, and genital/anal trauma with questionable explanation.[28] Pregnancy in adolescents should also be investigated for possible abuse. Behaviors suggesting abuse are sexual knowledge or behavior inappropriate for age, inappropriate sexual activities or game-playing with adults, fear of having diaper changed or being bathed, or sudden avoidance of being left with familiar adults or in familiar places. Later signs are depression, suicidal behavior, "night terrors," drug and alcohol abuse, and prostitution or promiscuity.

Neglect may be subtle. It is a generalized term including not only abandonment/desertion, but also medical, environmental, nutritional, safety, and emotional neglect. Signs of malnutrition, fatigue, poor hygiene, or inadequate clothing may indicate neglect. Emotional growth may be severely impacted by neglect. This may lead to problems in school performance or relationships with peers. Suspicion of neglect should be referred to the appropriate social services or welfare department.

Lead Toxicity

Although the prevalence of elevated blood lead levels has decreased dramatically over the last 20 years, it is still as high as 17% of preschool children in the United States (> 15 μg/dL).[29] More than 3 million children under age 6 years had blood lead levels greater than 10 μg/dL based on a 1990 estimate. It is recommended that all children at risk of exposure be screened for blood lead levels at age 12 months or in all children in communities where high environmental lead exposure is likely. Risks include minority race/ethnicity, central city living environment, low income and educational level, and living in the northeast United States. Sources include lead-based paint in pre-1950 housing, lead-soldered pipes, and lead dust from areas of heavy traffic and industry. Suspicion of lead intoxication should be raised and tested when there are indicators of either developmental delay, learning disabilities, convulsions, autism and other behavioral disorders, speech and hearing problems, or recurrent abdominal pain or vomiting. The effect on development and on central nervous system (CNS) function is due to the incomplete development of the blood–brain barrier before age 3 years, which allows accumulation of lead in the CNS.

The American Academy of Pediatrics recommends that intervention occur for children with blood lead levels greater than 10 μg/dL:[30]

- investigate and eliminate lead sources, including removal of lead-based paint
- use cold tap water, let water run for one to two minutes to rinse out pipes
- wash and clean toys frequently
- change shoes and clothing before returning home from work if there is potential lead exposure
- do not store food in inverted bread bags (printed with colored ink)

Children deficient in calcium, iron, zinc, and ascorbate more readily absorb lead. For those with levels 25 to

45 µg/dL, more aggressive attention to environmental exposure should be made and monitored. Levels above 45 µg/dL require chelation therapy; however, there is no indication that this can reverse any existing neurotoxicity.

Attention Deficit-Hyperactivity Disorder

Although there is little debate about the existence of attention deficit-hyperactivity disorder (ADHD), there are grave concerns about the overlap between normal childhood activity (especially in boys) and the diagnostic criteria for ADHD resulting in misdiagnoses and subsequent inappropriate prescription of medication. Although the incidence is reported to be between 3% and 5%, in one report, the proportion of children taking medication for ADHD is as high as 10% in second through fifth grades and 20% in fifth graders.[31]

The hallmarks of ADHD are a decrease in attention span, hyperactivity, and poor impulse control that spans across developmental norms and situations (e.g., occurs both at home and school). The signs of ADHD generally occur before age 7 years. The *Diagnostic and Statistical Manual of Mental Disorders,* fifth edition (DSM-V)[32] currently divides ADHD into three categories: (1) predominantly inattentive, (2) predominantly hyperactive/impulsive, and (3) a combination of both. The categories use the following signs/symptoms as indicators of ADHD, if six or more are present:

- Inattentive
  1. Has difficulty following instructions
  2. Has difficulty keeping attention on work or play activities at home and at school
  3. Loses things needed for activities at school and at home
  4. Appears not to listen
  5. Does not pay close attention to details
  6. Seems disorganized
  7. Has trouble with tasks that require planning ahead
  8. Forgets things
  9. Is easily distracted
- Hyperactive/Impulsive
  1. Fidgety
  2. Runs or climbs inappropriately
  3. Cannot play quietly
  4. Blurts out answers
  5. Interrupts people
  6. Cannot stay in seat
  7. Talks too much
  8. Is always on the go
  9. Has trouble waiting turn

It would strike most parents that these are common in most children, in particular boys. The concern is that given the easy out of medication, parents and schools encourage and steer the diagnosis to obtain what many feel is a medical form of behavioral therapy. With such a broad criteria overlap with "normal" behavior, it is not surprising that numerous suspected causes have been identified. These include inheritability, family environment, culture, lead poisoning, fetal anoxia, maternal smoking or use of alcohol, and many others. In those who do truly have ADHD there appears to be a processing dysfunction in the motor cortex that results in inappropriate motor response to stimulus.[33] The inattentive type may be due to parietal lobe dysfunction with an impairment in stimulus detection. In addition, specific defects have been found including reduced blood flow to the basal ganglia, small right hemispheres, and dopamine transporter density imbalance. Because ADHD is associated with comorbid conditions such as dyslexia and other learning disabilities, the diagnostic waters are muddied by potential overlap findings in patients with other conditions.

The primary medical approach to ADHD is methylphenidate (Ritalin) and amphetamine /dextroamphetamine (Adderall). Common side effects are a decrease in appetite, increased pulse and blood pressure, nervousness, mood lability, and sleep disturbance. Some of these side effects may be mediated by how and when the drug is administered. The biggest concern is the potential of growth retardation. **Table 53–4** summarizes the medical management of ADHD. Although recommended management opportunities include behavioral therapy, cognitive therapy, family counseling, and collaborative management with a team composed of the parents, physician, and school personnel, many rely on the medication to control the condition. Parental recommendations include:

- Present an organized schedule for the child.
- Set up house rules.
- Make sure directions are understood.
- Be consistent and positive.
- Help with homework and praise effort, not grades.
- Talk to school and child's teachers.

There are no chiropractic studies on ADHD at this time. However, it would seem prudent to aid in the

Table 53–4 ADHD Medications

Generic Drug	Examples	General Mechanism	Interactions/Side Effects
Methylphenidate	Concerta	A central nervous system stimulant used in the management of attention deficit-hyperactivity disorder (ADHD).	Slowing of growth height, seizures (in patients with Hx of seizures), blurred vision, GI blockage, heart racing, headache, stomach ache, decreased appetite, dizziness, nervousness, difficulty sleeping, anaphylaxis
Atomoxetine	Strattera	Strattera is a selective norepinephrine reuptake inhibitor used for the treatment of attention deficit-hyperactivity disorder (ADHD).	Decreased appetite, sleeping problems, constipation, dry mouth, nausea, allergic reactions, dizziness, tiredness, mood swings, are the most common reported side effects.
Methylphenidate	Ritalin	Causes the release of norepinephrine, dopamine, and serotonin from storage vesicles resulting in CNS stimulation. This causes an increase in performance, coordination, and energy. There is a decrease in appetite with an increase in blood pressure. Used for narcolepsy and attention deficit disorder.	May cause restlessness, insomnia, dizziness, anorexia, psychic disturbances, and arrhythmias
Pemoline	Cylert	Causes the release of norepinephrine, dopamine, and serotonin from storage vesicles resulting in CNS stimulation. This causes an increase in performance, coordination, and energy. There is a decrease in appetite with an increase in blood pressure. Used for attention deficit-hyperactivity disorder.	May cause restlessness, insomnia, dizziness, anorexia, psychic disturbances, and arrhythmias
Amphetamine and dextroamphetamine	Adderall	A combination of amphetamine and dextroamphetamine used for the management of ADHD; also used for narcolepsy.	High potential for abuse. Weight loss, dry mouth, nausea, dizziness, headache, diarrhea, nervousness, irregular or rapid heart rate, increased blood pressure, and allergic reactions

parental need to obtain a valid diagnosis without reliance only on meeting symptom criteria. This would include an evaluation of diet, exercise, home environment, and the child's self-appreciation. For an accurate diagnosis, a referral to a specialist, preferably a psychologist who specializes in ADHD, is needed. The psychologist specialist is trained in the administration and interpretation of neurocognitive tests and is less likely to rely on the drug solution to ADHD.

Childhood Cancer

Unfortunately, childhood cancer is a major cause of death in U.S. children. For children ages 1 to 14 years, cancer is second only to accidents as a cause of childhood mortality.[34] Although the survival rate has increased dramatically for some cancers, many types are still resistant to treatment or are clinically evident too late in the course of the illness to apply effective treatment. It is crucial that the chiropractor be vigilant in watching for red flags in a child's presentation that suggest cancer. Some of these red flag indicators follow:[35]

- unexplained weight loss
- bone pain that is resistant to analgesics or accompanied by recurrent or relapsing fever
- sternal tenderness, with recurrent nosebleeds

- lymphadenopathy that is persistent for more than 3 weeks and lymph nodes that are hard, rubbery, fixed, and nontender
- occult or frank blood in the urine or stool
- abdominal masses
- recurrent or severe (unbearable) headache associated with nausea and vomiting or persistent headache

It is important to remember that childhood cancer presents differently than adult cancer. By the time of diagnosis, approximately 80% of pediatric cancers are in their advanced stage. Pediatric cancers more commonly involve white blood cells (leukemias), brain, bone, lymphatic system (Hodgkin's and non-Hodgkin's), muscle, kidney, and the nervous system. A summary of the most common pediatric cancers is given in **Tables 53–5** and **53–6**.

Other Specific Concerns

Some of the following conditions or concerns are discussed in this chapter, but please consult the related chapters listed:

- Scoliosis/kyphosis—Chapters 4 and 5
- Headache—Chapter 17
- Dizziness—Chapter 18
- Seizures—Chapter 19
- Depression—Chapter 20
- Fatigue—Chapter 21
- Fever—Chapter 22
- Skin disorders—Chapter 27
- Weight loss—Chapter 28
- Obesity—Chapter 29
- Enuresis—Chapter 35

Table 53–5 Cancers and Tumors More Common in Childhood and Adolescence

Tumor	Diagnostic Features and Considerations	Management Considerations
Leukemias	Leukemias are the most common malignancy in children, with an age of onset of between 2 and 10 years (peak onset at age 4 years). There is a slightly increased incidence in boys, whites, and in siblings of children with leukemia. Signs and symptoms include hepatosplenomegaly (60% of patients), fatigue, bone pain (commonly in the pelvis, vertebral bodies, and legs), easily bruised, and other signs of vascular fragility such as petechiae or purpura, fever, lymphadenopathy, and, in boys, testicular enlargement. Laboratory testing includes a complete blood cell (CBC) count, which usually shows at least one cell type deficiency. A white blood count (WBC) above 50,000 is a strong indicator of leukemia. Radiographic findings may include diffuse osteopenia, radiolucent metaphyseal bands, new periosteal formation, and signs of osteosclerosis and bone destruction. Chest x-rays may reveal a mediastinal mass. Bone marrow aspiration and biopsy are needed for a definitive diagnosis.	Acute lymphoblastic leukemia (ALL) is the most common. Acute myelogenous leukemia (AML) has the poorest cure rate. Various drug regimens and chemotherapy are the treatments of choice, with localized radiation treatment when necessary. Bone marrow transplantation is reserved for unresponsive cases. Prognosis is best for children diagnosed between ages 3 and 7 years, with a more favorable outcome for patients with a total WBC count of 25,000 or less and no central nervous system (CNS) involvement at the time of diagnosis. The overall cure rate for ALL is 75%, with initial remission seen in 75%. Generally, girls have a more favorable prognosis than boys.
Brain tumors	25% to 30% of all childhood cancers are found in the CNS. The age of onset is generally between ages 5 and 10 years. Signs and symptoms include headaches, nausea and vomiting, seizures, cranial nerve dysfunction, or cerebellar signs such as dysarthria and ataxia; precocious or delayed puberty or a personality change may also occur. Referral for computed tomography (CT) and magnetic resonance imaging (MRI) is required for the differential diagnosis.	One-half of pediatric brain tumors occur above the tentorium and the other half in the posterior fossa. The most common type of brain tumor in children is astrocytomas. The ten-year survival rate with surgical excision is approximately 80%; however, central astrocytomas carry a less than 25% two-year survival rate. Most brain tumors are treated with a combination of surgery, radiation, and chemotherapy.

Table 53–5 Cancers and Tumors More Common in Childhood and Adolescence (continued)

Tumor	Diagnostic Features and Considerations	Management Considerations
Hodgkin's	Hodgkin's is a malignancy of the lymphatic system. 60% of Hodgkin's lymphoma occurs in children 10 to 16 years old. Signs and symptoms include fatigue, fever, chronic cough, night sweats, weight loss, painless cervical or supraclavicular lymphadenopathy, pruritus, and pain worse with alcohol ingestion. Radiographically, it is important to x-ray the chest in a search for a mediastinal mass (seen in 50% of patients). Further evaluation is based on staging defined by the Ann Arbor classification system. CT scans, lymphangiography, bone marrow aspirate, and biopsies are all used to determine spread of the disease. The presence of malignant Reed-Sternberg cells is pathognomonic for Hodgkin's. The CBC is often normal with a possibly increased erythrocyte sedimentation rate (ESR).	Those patients with early stages at time of treatment have an 85% to 90% five-year survival rate, while those with more advanced disease (stages III and IV) have a 50% to 80% five-year survival rate. Radiation therapy and chemotherapy are used in treatment.
Non-Hodgkin's	Mainly occurs in children ages 15 years or older. Accounts for only 7% to 13% of all childhood malignancies. Symptoms and signs include fever, chills, night sweats, loss of appetite, chronic cough, abdominal pain, headaches, hepatosplenomegaly, and lymphadenopathy, among others. Medullary destruction or pathologic fracture may be seen radiographically. The diagnosis is based on biopsy and subsequent typing of the cells. CT, bone scan, abdominal ultrasound, and bone marrow are also used.	Chemotherapy is the standard treatment with 90% survival rate if only localized disease is found. Poorer prognosis is expected with advanced disease, in particular to the CNS or bone.
Neuroblastoma	Neuroblastoma is the most common solid neoplasm outside the CNS, accounting for 7% to 10% of all pediatric malignancies. They occur at an early age with 50% occurring before age 2 years and 90% before age 5 years. Signs and symptoms are fever, weight loss, failure to thrive, neurologic signs, bone and abdominal pain, swelling around the eyes, and bowel and bladder dysfunction. Radiographically, widened skull sutures with "sunburst" spiculations and diffuse, multiple, osteolytic lesions are seen. CT and MRI are needed to detect spread and extent of lesions. Bone scans are used for peripheral sites.	Chemotherapy is the standard treatment, with 90% survival rate if only localized disease is found. Poorer prognosis is expected with advanced disease, in particular to the CNS or bone.
Wilms' tumors (Nephroblastoma)	Wilms' tumor is an embryonal tumor of the kidney seen mainly in children under age 5 years. A palpable abdominal mass, fever, anorexia, and abdominal pain are commonly seen. When hematuria is present, invasion of the collecting system has occurred. Hypertension may also occur. Abdominal ultrasound and CT are used to diagnose. Chest x-rays are needed to evaluate pulmonary metastasis.	Combined approaches of surgery, radiation, and chemotherapy are used. The Wilms' tumor study group has established criteria for staging and prognosis.
Neurofibromatosis (NF)	NF is an autosomal dominant disorder classified as type 1 or peripheral NF (von Recklinghausen's disease) and type 2 or central NF (characterized by bilateral acoustic neuromas) seen usually in the over 20-year-old patient. One-third of type 1 patients are asymptomatic, yet carry physical characteristics that allow clinical diagnosis by cosmetic or neurologic signs. Café-au-lait spots (brown spots) are seen as freckle-like macules in the flexor creases of the elbows and knees (found in 90% of patients at birth or in infancy). Various cutaneous tumors, subcutaneous nodules representing Schwann cell tumors (plexiform neuromas), are seen less often initially; more often after puberty. Varying types of skeletal involvement may occur including vertebral scalloping, scoliosis, and the absence of the greater wing of the sphenoid bone. Neurofibromas of the nerve roots grow in the intervertebral foramina (iVFs) (dumbbell tumors) and may grow intra- or extraspinally resulting in related dysfunction or pain. Optic gliomas and acoustic neuromas are common, with related loss of function.	Surgery and radiation therapy are the treatments of choice. When neurofibromas are removed, loss of function of the involved nerve is common. Genetic counseling is recommended.

Table 53–6 Bone Tumors More Common in Childhood and Adolescence

Tumor	Diagnostic Features and Considerations	Management Considerations
Benign tumors		
Fibrocortical defects	Fibrous lesions of bone that have a cortical location and are small and well delaminated with sclerotic margins. There are no symptoms; therefore, these are found incidentally on x-ray.	Resolve over 1–2 years.
Nonossifying fibroma	A larger version of the fibrocortical defect. Metaphyseal and large. Concern is the possibility of pathologic fracture.	If the lesion is large or fractures, curettage and bone grafting are used.
Fibrous dysplasia	Neoplastic fibrosis replaces bone, weakening it and predisposing it to pathologic fracture. Two types are monostotic or polyostotic. In the proximal femur, it may result in the "shepherd's crook" deformity.	The weakened area is strengthened with intramedullary rods that are left in indefinitely.
Osteochondroma	Endochondral ossification under a cartilage cap results in pedunculated or sessile lesions that often grow to the extent that they protrude enough to be seen. The multiple form is common and is an inherited, autosomal-dominant condition. Standard radiography of the area reveals the characteristic lesion; therefore, biopsy is not needed. Osteochondromas may become symptomatic if there is direct trauma or they grow large enough to protrude against pain-sensitive structures.	Only symptomatic lesions need excision. Rarely there is transformation to a chondrosarcoma; prophylactic removal is not recommended. When transformation does occur, it is usually in the adult and around the pelvic area.
Enchondroma	These tumors calcify in bone and are often multiple, occurring in the fingers and long bones. Radiographically, speckled calcification can be seen within the lesion.	Usually do not require surgical excision.
Chondroblastoma	Rare tumor of the epiphysis. Aggressive and recurrent, these lesions may be confused with infection or arthritis.	Curettage and bone grafting are needed.
Osteoid osteoma	These are highly vascular, bone-producing tumors. They often appear in the spine and result in a characteristic patient presentation of night pain relieved by aspirin. There is often an acute-angle scoliosis if found in the spine. Radiographically, there is a small radiolucent nidus surrounded by sclerosis.	Excision is necessary.
Unicameral bone cysts	These solitary bone cysts are more commonly found in the proximal humerus and femur. They are metaphyseal and have well-defined margins. They are usually symptomatically silent until there is a pathologic fracture.	If found before fracture, treatment involves steroid injection.
Malignant tumors		
Osteogenic sarcoma	Most common malignant tumor occurring in the second decade, often around the knee. Patient complains of night pain. A mass is sometimes palpable. Radiographs demonstrate osteolytic or osteogenic lesions of the metaphysis. Bone scans, computed tomography, and magnetic resonance imaging (MRI) are useful in determining other sites and the extent of the lesion.	Surgical elimination through resection or amputation is followed by chemotherapy. Limb salvage may be possible with allograph or metallic implant, yet creates a higher risk for the patient. The five-year survival rate is about 75% with aggressive treatment.
Ewing's sarcoma	The second most common malignant tumor of childhood. This round-cell tumor is often diaphyseal and osteolytic, creating large soft tissue masses. The child is febrile with an increased erythrocyte sedimentation rate. Bone scan and MRI help differentiate the cause and reveal the extent of involvement; biopsy confirms the diagnosis.	Chemotherapy and resection result in a five-year survival rate of 50%–60%.

- Otitis media—Chapter 44
- Specific joint complaints—See chapter specific to joint

For the special-abled child, please refer to a brief overview presented in **Table 53–7**. Check the index for conditions or problems not described in detail in this chapter.

Sports-Related Issues in the Young Patient

Sports-related injuries in children and adolescents are relatively common. Chiropractors should be aware of specific aspects of the young athlete's anatomic and

Table 53–7 Selected Special Needs Children

Disorder	Diagnostic Features and Considerations
Autism spectrum disorder (includes autism, Asperger's, childhood disintegrative disorder, and pervasive developmental disorder)	A syndrome characterized by deficits in social communication, and restricted repetitive behaviors and activities (RRBs). Social communication disorder is diagnosed if RRBs are absent. Autism usually manifests itself within the first year, often misinterpreted as deafness or mental retardation. The diagnosis is fairly clear by age 3 years. Abnormal behaviors include aloofness (detached, not making eye contact, not answering questions, avoiding physical contact), attachment to sameness (resists changes in environment or routine, develops rituals, repetitive behaviors), and speech/language problems (ranges from muteness to other idiosyncratic behavior such as echolalia [repeating words spoken by others], and pronoun reversal ["you" instead of "I"]). Other manifestations are with play, spinning objects or repetitive activity often demonstrating hyperactivity. Many autistic children demonstrate bursts of violent behavior. Some children will demonstrate remarkable skills in music or mathematics (savant). The cause is unknown, although the brainstem is shorter than normal and structures are closer together, especially at the lower medulla, with the appearance that a band of tissue is missing. A subgroup of patients has enlarged ventricles visible on computed tomography or hypoplasia of the cerebellar vermis on magnetic resonance imaging. Other isolated cases have been associated with congenital rubella and other infections. Behavioral therapy has mixed results dependent on the technique and the uniqueness of the child. Many "fringe" approaches are suggested including certain forms of music therapy, diets, and other approaches. The use of sign language has also been advocated as an alternate means of initial communication. None seems consistent in the results obtained. Speech therapy is recommended based on the severity of the child's case. Some children need medication to control violent or aggressive behavior. Some children have to wear protective headgear to protect against banging their head during repetitive or violent outbursts. In dealing with treatment of these children it is important to be almost ritualistic in the sameness from treatment to treatment, with an emphasis on avoiding disturbances such as loud noises. If the child is being treated chiropractically, distraction during adjusting is necessary.
Cerebral palsy syndromes	A group of nonprogressive motor disorders that affect approximately 2 out of every 1,000 children in the United States, that results in involuntary movement. The etiology is unclear and may range from in utero problems to perinatal and neonatal factors. Birth trauma, asphyxia (15% of cases), abnormal birth position, prematurity, and central nervous system trauma or systemic disease have been identified as causes. There are four types: (1) spastic, (2) athetoid or dyskinetic, (3) ataxic, and (4) mixed. Seventy percent to 80% are the spastic type characterized by stiffness, weakness, muscle hypertonicity, and a tendency toward contractures; a "scissors" gait; toe-walking; and increased deep tendon reflexes (DTRs). Milder forms may affect lingual/palatal movement resulting in speech disorders. With basal ganglia involvement, the athetoid/dyskinetic type (20% of cases) occurs. Either slow writhing movements of the extremities (athetoid) or the proximal muscle groups of the trunk (dystonic), or abrupt jerking type movements (choreiform) are found. Dysarthria is quite common and often severe. Due to the large variation in presentation, it would be difficult to outline all the options for patients with cerebral palsy. The goal is to develop as much independence as possible. This is accomplished mainly through physical therapy training, bracing, occupational therapy, orthopaedic surgery, and speech therapy. When possible, children who are not severely affected should attend school and develop social interaction skills.
Down's syndrome	Down's syndrome is due to an abnormality of chromosome 21 (trisomy 21). It occurs rather frequently; 1 out of every 800 births. This varies based on maternal age, with a much higher incidence in mothers over 40 years (1/40 births). The need for prenatal screening is necessary for mothers who would consider abortion. Characteristics of Down's children are low-set ears, almond-shaped eyes with persistent epicanthus, short physical size, mental retardation, shallow palate, Simian crease in palms, short fifth digit, Brushfield spots on the iris (peripheral spots that disappear during year 1), and heart defects. Like many disorders, there are varying degrees of expression. The biggest concern for the chiropractor is the common finding of atlantoaxial instability. Although it has been a requirement to screen all Down's children with flexion/extension views prior to participation in the Special Olympics, recent changes have not required this screening procedure. It is important to note that in addition to cardiac abnormalities, thyroid dysfunction is also common in these children.

physiologic uniqueness and how they affect participation in sports activities. As always, prevention is the major goal in working with athletes; when injured, the goals are proper diagnosis and rehabilitation. An overview of the more common concerns with children and adolescents follows.

Statistics

- Seven million individuals are involved in high school sports.[36]
- Twenty million individuals between the ages of 8 and 16 years are involved in non-school community athletic programs.
- Another 20 million participate in unstructured, relatively unsupervised recreation.[37]
- Fifty percent of all boys and 25% of all girls present as patients due to involvement in competitive sports.
- Approximately 79% of middle and junior high schools have sports programs.

Motivational Factors

Generally, all children initially participate in an activity for the purpose of fun. Other considerations are to (1) attain self-confidence, (2) avoid boredom, (3) socialize, and (4) further life goals. Health is not usually a motivational factor for children.

Characteristics of Young Athletes

- Physical growth affects exercise as well as the reverse; exercise may affect physical growth. Only one of the three growth spurts in life occurs while major physical activity is possible: puberty. The first is in utero during the fourth month. The second bridges on possible athletic interest: between 48 and 60 months. Minimum amounts of exercise may stimulate growth, while excessive exercise may retard growth.
- Exploration. Children and adolescents are interested in investigating new experiences. Sports may provide this experience for them.
- Maturation. At puberty there is an increase in strength, agility, and endurance that allows the individual to participate at a higher level than previously attainable.
- Body proportion changes. There is a gain of 15% of adult height and an increase in skeletal mass of 48% during puberty.

- Body composition. The male body fat decreases 11% on average through adolescence. Females increase body fat on average 25% during this same period. Prepubescent males and females are equal in body fat composition.[38] Exercise habits carry over into adulthood. The percentage of body fat of adults who exercised as adolescents is lower.

Predisposing Factors to Injury in the Skeletally Immature Athlete

Children's response to injury is often different from an adult's given the same mechanism and severity. Some of the factors involved include:

- *Weakness of epiphyseal and apophyseal areas.* A child is more likely to injure these areas than the surrounding or attaching ligaments or tendons; the reverse is true for adults.
- *Differential growth rate between bone and muscle.* Soft tissue lengthening lags behind skeletal growth. Therefore, during growth spurts a relative tightness occurs around the joint. This tightness may predispose the individual to overuse injury.
- *Malalignment of the pelvis, hip, and lower extremity.* Conditions affecting version (i.e., angle of alignment) of the hips and lower extremity are common. Differences in leg length due to growth alterations are also common.
- *Imbalance of muscle strength.* The most common example is a ratio of quadriceps to hamstring strength of 2:1 versus the adult ratio of 3:2.
- *Ligament laxity.* This finding is more common in females; although it allows flexibility, there is a predisposition to certain types of injuries such as patellar dislocation or subluxation.

Specific Concerns with the Young Athlete

Thermoregulatory Capacity

Children have less thermoregulatory capacity than adults.[39] This is more apparent in extremes of heat and cold. There are three factors:

1. larger surface area per kilogram of body weight
2. lower cardiac output at a given oxygen uptake level
3. lower sweating rate

Fractures

Generally there are four important differences between children and adults when considering fractures:[40]

1. A long bone fracture may heal in 3 weeks in a neonate; 6 weeks in a 7-year-old; 8 to 10 weeks in an adolescent; and up to 12 weeks in an adult.
2. In a child, a "sprain" is more likely to be a skeletal injury because bones (growth centers in particular) are weaker than ligaments.
3. Bone is more resilient than in the adult. Therefore, a full fracture in an adult would more likely be a "greenstick" fracture in a child.
4. Skeletal injury in children is usually at the growth plate, and therefore may have consequences regarding bone growth (although this sequela is uncommon).

Epiphyseal Injury

Growth plate fractures are generally classified according to the Salter-Harris system (see **Figure 53–1**).

- Type I—The type I injury is due to a shearing force applied to the junction of the epiphysis and metaphysis. It usually occurs during early childhood or infancy (occasionally due to a difficult labor). The perichondrium on one side remains intact as does the blood supply. Reduction is rarely necessary, and resolution is usually uneventful.
- Type II—These injuries are also due to a shearing force; however, in addition to separating the epiphysis from the metaphysis, there is a triangular avulsion of the metaphysis. This usually occurs falling on an outstretched hand or other similar injury between the ages of 6 and 12 years. The growth spurt period is when the physis is weakest. Again, the perichondrium on one side is intact as is the blood supply. Occasionally reduction is necessary; however, healing is uneventful.
- Type III—The forces here are directed both transversely and longitudinally across the physis and epiphysis, resulting in epiphyseal separation. The type of mechanism involves

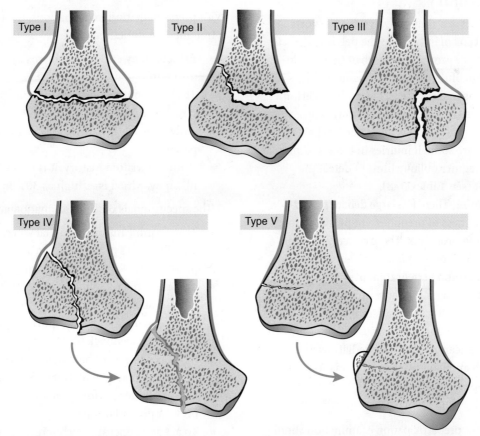

Figure 53–1 Salter-Harris type fractures. Type I: split of the growth plate. Type II: split of the growth plate with fracture producing triangular metaphyseal fragment. Type III: vertical fracture through the epiphysis that enters the epiphyseal plate. Type IV: fracture extending across the epiphysis, epiphyseal plate, and metaphysis. Type V: compression of a portion of the epiphyseal plate.

a lateral or rotational component. Prompt restoration is necessary to prevent the major complication: a bone bridge. The bone bridge is due to intermingling of separate vascular systems forming parallel to the plane of the physis. This effectively arrests cell growth in the physis. Open reduction is usually required.

- Type IV—The fracture extends the full thickness of both the epiphysis and physis and additionally splits off a portion of the metaphysis. Again, a bone bridge may form. In the upper extremity this may occur with a fall on an outstretched hand. Reduction, often with pin fixation, is frequently necessary.
- Type V—This is the rarest of growth plate fractures. It is a crushing injury that can severely affect bone growth. Unfortunately, it is not always easy to detect radiographically. A common scenario is a fall from a great height, crushing the distal radius. Again, it may be misdiagnosed as a sprain. Radiographically it may not be readily apparent, and the growth retardation may not be evident for months.

Apophyseal Injury

Apophyseal injuries are almost always due to sports activity.[41] They occur mainly about the pelvis and occur in the adolescent age group. This is when there is closure but not fusion of the apophyseal ossific nucleus. Common locations include the ischium, the anterior superior iliac spine (ASIS) or anterior inferior iliac spine (AIIS), the iliac crest, and the lesser trochanter. Oftentimes these are sudden injuries in track and field. They frequently require oblique films to detect the avulsed fragment (see **Table 53–8**).

Strength Training There is a large debate regarding the appropriateness of prepubescent participation in strength training programs. These concerns center on the tendency toward strains, tendinitis, epiphysitis, avulsions, fractures, and vertebral injuries. Most of these injuries are avoidable with proper training, supervision, and progression. It has been demonstrated that prepubescent children do increase muscle strength with training. The American Academy of Pediatrics, the National Strength and Conditioning Association, and the American Orthopedic Society of Sports Medicine have made the following eight recommendations:[42]

1. A mandatory preparticipation examination should be performed
2. Emotional maturity to accept coaching and instruction should be required

3. Adequate supervision should be provided by coaches who are knowledgeable in the area of children's weight training
4. Strength training should be a part of a more comprehensive program
5. Training should be preceded by a warm-up and followed by a cool-down
6. Training should emphasize full range of motion concentric contractions
7. Competition is prohibited
8. No maximum lift should ever be attempted

The prescribed program should be as follows:

1. Exercise sessions should be limited to two to three times per week, 20- to 30-minute periods.
2. No resistance should be applied until proper form is demonstrated.
   - 6 to 15 repetitions
   - 1 to 3 sets per exercise
3. Weight should be increased in 1- to 3-lb increments after the child is able to do 15 reps with good form.

Preparticipation Screening

With preparticipation examinations, the medical history is fraught with difficulties:

- Athletes may exclude problems they feel might disqualify them.
- They may not recognize the significance of positives in their past histories.
- Only 39% of athletes' histories agreed with their parents'.[43]
- With the written history, it is important to consider illiteracy, which is as high as 30% in some areas.

The specific goals of the examination are:

- To determine information that will exclude or modify an individual's performance in a particular sport and possibly refer for further medical evaluation.
- To determine the musculoskeletal status of an individual compared with the documented requirements for a given sport.
- To provide feedback to the individual about his or her general level of health, and, more specifically, point out areas in which the individual needs to focus to better perform the sport or activity and prevent potential injury.
- To act as a general health screen that is reproducible, establishing a baseline assessment for future comparison.
- To meet state or insurance requirements.

Table 53–8 Disorders of the Skeletally Immature Patient—The Extremities

Regional Disorder	Diagnostic Features and Considerations	Management Considerations
SHOULDER GIRDLE		
Os Acrominale (Bipartite Acromion) *Before Age 22*	Found in 2% to 8% of individuals (62% of the time bilateral). There are two secondary centers of ossification that enlarge and merge during the adolescent growth period. A third may appear during adolescence that may either represent an ossification center or possibly an avulsed fragment. An incomplete fusion of these centers may be due to a direct blow or repetitive overhead activity resulting in symptoms of rotator cuff irritation and inflammation. It is proposed that when the deltoid contracts it pulls the ununited fragment and any associated spur into the rotator cuff causing tearing. Most often seen on an axillary or Stryker radiographic view.	Limited activity and a balanced, progressive strengthening program are generally all that are needed. Rarely a persistent, symptomatic, nonunion requires surgical intervention such as open reduction and screw fixation.
Acromial Apophysitis *Before Age 19*	Similar to os acrominale; however, the ossification center is not abnormal, yet irritated. Pain is felt at the lateral acromion, due to repetitive traction by the deltoid attachment to the distal acromion.	Rest from or modification of the inciting activity, protection (i.e., padding) if involved in contact sports will usually resolve the problem over time. Generally, self-resolving; however, may progress to nonunion.
Coracoid "Apophysitis" *Before Age 21*	The cause is stress due to repetitive upper extremity activity (e.g., baseball pitchers, swimmers, tennis players). Pull of the lower center at the base of the coracoid is most common. This is the anchor site for the pectoralis minor. Tenderness on palpation of the coracoid (compare to opposite side) and a widened physeal line at the base on radiographic examination are the keys to the diagnosis.	Modification of the inciting activity and time will suffice for most cases. The condition is self-limiting and rarely causes functional long-term problems.
Little League Shoulder	Usually seen in young baseball pitchers or sometimes catchers, due to repetitive torque stress placed on the proximal humeral epiphyses (type I Salter-Harris injury). Widening of the epiphyseal plate may be evident on anteroposterior and lateral radiographs. It is also important to consider fracture through a unicameral bone cyst in the differential.	Healing is usually complete with 4–6 weeks of rest. Prevention is accomplished by following rules set by the Little League Association to limit the time of non-relief pitching.
Sprengel's Deformity	Failure of migration of the mesenchyme during fetal growth results in a congenital elevation of the scapula. Seventy percent of cases are unilateral.	Mild elevation that is not cosmetically obvious may be left untreated (except for stretching). More severe deformity must be corrected surgically, usually involving soft tissue release and possible excision of the superior/medial scapula and/or osteotomy of the clavicle.
Clavicular Fracture	The most common skeletal injury during delivery is a clavicular fracture. Risk increases with the size of the infant. The left side is fractured more often than the right. The clavicle is the fourth most common children's fracture (8% to 16%). Middle-third fracture is most common in children. Falls and blows to the clavicle are the most common injury seen in sports and abuse. Radiographs demonstrate the location and extent of injury.	Birth fractures rarely need treatment except to avoid picking the child up by the arms (use waist). Rapid healing occurs. In older children, a figure-of-eight brace is generally all that is needed. Although there may be an initial large deformity, this almost always resolves with time in children. Healing occurs in a few weeks.

(continues)

Table 53-8 Disorders of the Skeletally Immature Patient—The Extremities (continued)

Regional Disorder	Diagnostic Features and Considerations	Management Considerations
ELBOW		
Little League Elbow	A complex of changes seen in the Little League pitcher. Due to distraction forces medially and compressive forces laterally during late cocking phase of pitching and posterior traction and compressive forces at radial-capitellar joint with the quick pronation seen with follow-through. Elbow pain that may localize may be combined with flexion contracture or an increased valgus carrying angle. Radiographically, medial epicondyle hypertrophy or fragmentation, trochlear or olecranon fragmentation, and widening of medial epicondyle and humeral metaphysis space may be seen alone or in combination. These may represent, to some degree, normal variants in response to increased forces at the elbow. However, if symptomatic, the patient should be treated. Osteochondritis dissecans may also be seen as part of this complex.	Management simply involves limiting the activity to allow healing. Strict adherence to the Little League rules for pitching will be helpful. Generally, if caught early the prognosis is good; however, occurrence or persistence in the later stages of adolescence warrants a surgical consult due to the risk of the formation of loose osteocartilagenous fragments that will lead to early degeneration.
Osteochondritis Dissecans *Ages 13–16*	Avascular necrosis (local subchondral infarction) of the capitellum or radial head is due to vascular insufficiency and compressive trauma seen most often in Little League baseball pitchers; however, it may occur in gymnasts, basketball players, or any active adolescent. Patient presents with lateral elbow pain. Radiographs should include radial-capitellar view.	Restriction of inciting activity coupled with rest for a number of weeks to months may be successful in some cases. Loose-body formation, failure to heal, or persistent symptoms often require surgical debridement, excision of loose bodies, and occasionally drilling or curettage to vascularize the area to assist healing.
Panner's Disease *Ages 4–12*	An osteochondrosis of the capitellum distinguished from osteochondritis dissecans by some authors because of the younger occurrence (still primarily male) and that the entire physis is involved (more similar to Legge-Calvé-Perthes) with sequential change of sclerosis, fissuring, fragmentation, collapse, and remodeling. Enlargement of the radial head may occur. Patient presents with lateral elbow pain.	Healing occurs over a 2-year period. Temporary immobilization and avoidance of rapid forearm pronation/supination and activities that increase lateral compressive forces (valgus) may help prevent the complication of loose fragments. A brace to prevent flexion contractures is also used. Loose-body formation, failure to heal, or persistent symptoms often require surgical debridement, excision of loose bodies, and occasionally drilling or curettage to vascularize the area to assist healing.
Medial Epicondyle Fracture/ Separation	Due either to repetitive forces of distraction and/or rotation or may be due to an acute injury, such as falling on an outstretched hand, or any valgus loading force. The patient complains of medial elbow pain and possible swelling. Standard radiographs will demonstrate the degree of displacement; stress views may help determine stability of physis.	Displacement less than 5 mm may be managed with a long arm cast for 3 weeks. Radiographs while in the cast will help detect any further displacement that can occur due to the pull of the flexor/pronator group of muscles. Displacement greater than 5 mm requires orthopaedic consult with a surgical attempt at fixation with pins likely.
Olecranon Apophysitis	Repetitive activities that require forceful contraction of the triceps, such as the acceleration phase of throwing, may result in a triceps tendinitis or olecranon apophysitis. The patient complains of posterior elbow pain with resisted extension or occasionally with passive overpressure on extension. Radiographs are not generally helpful, although the late consequence may be hypertrophy or spurring of the olecranon with eventual impingement or loose-body formation (usually seen in the adult).	Primarily an overuse phenomenon; therefore, rest and modification of the activity (i.e., reduction in numbers of throws) coupled with ice and stretching are usually sufficient. Chronic apophysitis may rarely progress to avulsion of the olecranon apophysis.

Table 53–8 Disorders of the Skeletally Immature Patient—The Extremities (continued)

Regional Disorder	Diagnostic Features and Considerations	Management Considerations
Radial Head Subluxation (Nursemaid's Elbow) *Younger than Age 7*	Subluxation (medical) of the radial head may occur in the young child due to a traction force that pulls the radial head through the annular ligament and then traps the ligament between the radial head and capitellum. Common descriptions include swinging the child by the arms or sudden tugging or lifting by the arms. The child has sudden pain in the lateral elbow and holds the arm against the side unable to use it (pseudoparalysis).	Reduction may be accomplished with one thumb placed on the radial head while the other hand applies gentle traction through the wrist. This is followed by a quick, gentle supination of the forearm while pressing on the radial head. A click is usually felt when reduction occurs. Ability to move the arm is usually immediate.
Supracondylar Fractures	Hyperextension of the elbow, often seen with falling on an outstretched arm, may result in a supracondylar fracture, whereas in the adult, a dislocation would more likely occur. Displacement of the distal humerus may be palpable. Radiographs will demonstrate the relative posterior displacement of the distal humerus and a positive fat pad sign on the lateral view. Oblique views may be necessary. Neurovascular complication is not uncommon and may result in Volkmann's ischemic contracture and deformity.	Expert orthopaedic attention must be given immediately to avoid Volkmann's contracture. Generally, reduction and percutaneous pinning fixation are used. Malunion will result in a "gunstock" deformity.
WRIST/HAND		
Distal Radial Epiphyseal Injury	Injury to the distal radial (or ulnar) epiphyses may occur due to a fall on an outstretched hand or a twisting injury with the wrist weight bearing. Repetitive changes may occur due to the compressive maneuvers of gymnasts and weight lifters. Radiographs will help differentiate between physeal injury and soft tissue injury through demonstration of characteristic patterns for Salter I–IV fracture.	If the injury is severe, an effect on bone growth may occur. Long-term management should include follow-up radiographs to determine if growth is occurring normally.
Kienbock's	An avascular necrosis of the lunate is usually symptomatically silent without obvious traumatic onset. Hypermobility or an ulna minus (shortened ulna) may contribute to the development of Kienbock's. Even when the patient presents with wrist pain, radiographic changes may not yet be evident. When evident, there is an apparent increased density (i.e., appears brighter) of the bone compared with the other carpals.	If caught early, avoidance of repetitive, compressive activities may help. Recent studies indicate that conservative, nonsurgical care has a good outcome. Surgical options involve osteotomy of the radius and arthrodesis of the carpals.
Torus and Greenstick Fractures	With torus, or buckling, fractures the child usually reports falling on an outstretched hand. The wrist may be swollen and painful. The lateral radiograph may better demonstrate the buckling. The cortical bulge is usually 2 to 4 cm from the growth plate and may take 2 to 4 weeks to become visible. Greenstick fractures are usually due to a longitudinal force. A bowing deformity will be evident and an incomplete break may be seen radiographically. The child will have a definite problem with pronation/supination.	Torus fractures do not usually displace and simply require immobilization for 2–4 weeks. Greenstick fractures are manipulated by an orthopaedist to reduce bowing deformity. They heal in 4 to 6 weeks.
HIP/PELVIS		
Developmental (Congenital) Hip Dysplasia (DHD)	DHD is a generic term that encompasses a wide variety of anatomic abnormalities that are predispositions for dislocation or instability in the infant/child and degenerative arthritis in the adult (especially females). A shallow acetabulum, inverted acetabular labrum, enlarged	0 to 6 months—If caught early, fixation of the hips in a Pavlik brace (position of flexion/abduction) for a minimum of 6 weeks. Other approaches such as the use of double-diapers should be discouraged. The intent is to allow

(continues)

Table 53–8 Disorders of the Skeletally Immature Patient—The Extremities (continued)

Regional Disorder	Diagnostic Features and Considerations	Management Considerations
	ligamentum teres or an iliopsoas tendon interposed between the femoral head and acetabulum are common features. There is a genetic tendency (10% family history). Breech delivery, neonatal positioning in adduction and/or extension, and neonatal hormonal contributions to ligament laxity all are factors. Examination should be performed at birth and rechecked throughout the first year. Tests include Ortolani's sign (abduction/external rotation of femur produces a "clunk" with reduction), Barlow test (flex/abduct with long axis traction or posterior pressure of femoral head creates "clunk"), and Galeazzi's test (comparing level of knees with infant prone, hips and knees flexed). Ultrasound may be a useful tool for diagnosis (operator dependent); however, radiographic interpretation may be difficult. Radiographic findings are usually found later with a disruption of Shenton's line, femoral head in superior lateral quadrant, and a Skinner angle greater than 35° in newborn, 27° in pre-walking stage, and 25° at 1 year.	sufficient growth in the hip to establish stability and to avoid the consequences of early degenerative changes or avascular necrosis. 6 to 18 months—Traction to stretch out any hip contractures prior to manipulation under anesthesia is followed by spica casting. 18 to 36 months—Surgery is generally necessary with a pelvic osteotomy to correct the acetabular dysplasia. 36 months or older—Open reduction, femoral shortening and/or pelvic osteotomy is often necessary to correct deformity.
Transient Synovitis	A transient synovitis of the hip is a relatively common occurrence in children. The cause is unknown; however, over half of children have had a recent previous upper respiratory infection. Trauma and allergic etiologies are also possible. It is difficult or impossible to place weight on the affected hip and the hip is held in abduction. The key is to distinguish between septic and nonseptic synovitis. The erythrocyte sedimentation rate (ESR) is normal, and the hip radiograph is negative for bony pathology with transient synovitis. With septic synovitis, there is often a fever, elevated ESR, and joint aspiration may demonstrate leukocytosis with a positive culture. Bone scans are generally not helpful.	Rest and non-weight-bearing will allow resolution within a few days to a week. Persistence or worsening suggests a septic etiology and requires referral for joint aspiration. Recurrent cases may indicate a tendency toward Perthes' disease (2% to 3% of cases). Residual effects of transient synovitis may include a mild coxa magna or widening of the femoral neck.
Slipped Capital Femoral Epiphyses (SCFE) *Between Ages 8 and 15*	Progressive or sudden posterior/inferior slippage of femoral epiphysis; 10% to 25% (as high as 41%) bilateral; classified as acute or chronic; acute slippage is a type I physeal fracture occurring in 5% to 10% of children with SCFE (some authors feel that there is a distinction between SCFE and a transphyseal fracture where a single traumatic event is more likely); chronic SCFE designated as symptoms having been present for more than 3 weeks; two types of "typical" patients seem evident: (1) tall, rapidly growing children, and (2) a Frolich-type young male (obese); more common in blacks; pain is usually in the hip but may be referred to thigh or knee; patient may have a limp and inability to bear weight; on physical examination when hip is taken passively into flexion it tends to externally rotate; internal rotation is often limited, although any attempt at hip range of motion may be extremely painful with acute slippage; lateral radiograph is necessary to view slippage; slippage is graded I–III; grade I involves less than 33% displacement, grade II 33% to 50% slippage, and grade III is greater than 50% slippage; computed tomography (CT) may be necessary to demonstrate accurately the degree of slippage.	Never attempt to manipulate back into place due to the high risk of subsequent avascular necrosis. Medical management involves a short period of traction followed by internal rotation to achieve reduction. Good results with operative positioning have been found in 50% of cases without formal manipulation. Percutaneous fixation with cannulated screws is a common approach to management. Newer approaches include bone graft epiphysiodesis. For chronic slips no attempts at closed reduction should be made (i.e., avascular necrosis complication). Percutaneous pinning in situ is usually recommended.

Table 53–8 Disorders of the Skeletally Immature Patient—The Extremities (continued)

Regional Disorder	Diagnostic Features and Considerations	Management Considerations
Legge-Calvé-Perthes *Between Ages 4 and 9* *(80% of time)*	Avascular necrosis of femoral head with associated subchondral fracture; four to five times more common in males; only 17% of patients report an associated traumatic onset; symptoms may be minimal with only a chronic limp and mild pain aggravated by activity during previous several months; pain is often referred to the knee; limited abduction and internal rotation secondary to muscle spasm may be seen; the Trendelenberg test may be positive; leg length inequality and thigh atrophy may be present; radiographs are often initial tool to identify characteristic staging signs such as a crescent sign, fragmentation of the epiphysis, reossification of femoral head shape (flattened), and residual deformity in the later stage.	Bed rest with skin traction are often helpful. Approaches to femoral containment in acetabulum include prescription of an abduction orthosis, femoral osteotomy, and innominate osteotomy. Few asymptomatic hips with normal initial radiographs are at risk for pain or radiographic abnormalities. When the uninvolved hip does become involved, the process is slow and surgical intervention is rarely indicated.
Apophysitis **(General Comments)**	Usually the result of trauma, specifically sports activities that involve sudden contraction of muscles causing avulsion at tendon insertions. Sixty percent to 90% involve males. The apophysis is weakest at the time of its appearance. Occurrence is primarily in the adolescent population. Sudden pain and limitation of activity usually accompany the injury. When there is no obvious single traumatic event, radiographs may be difficult to interpret due to variation in the appearance of secondary ossification centers and also may be confused with osteosarcoma, Ewing's sarcoma, or osteomyelitis. Refer films to chiropractic or medical radiologist.	Controversy exists regarding treatment of avulsion. 1. Nonsurgical management—Studies indicate excellent results. Five-stage rehabilitation program consists of an initial period of rest for up to 7 days using ice and analgesics; positioning of the leg to decrease tension of involved muscle group. Week 2 begins when acute pain is decreased and consists of protected walking, isometrics, and limited stretching. Week 3 includes a progressive resistance exercise program, and week 4 increases resistance when 50% of anticipated strength is achieved. Sports-specific training usually begins in weeks 5–6. The only concern is bony exostosis formation, which occurs rarely and occasionally requires surgical excision. 2. Surgical management—Still recommended by some orthopaedics, especially for displaced avulsions of the ischial tuberosity; open reduction and internal fixation are recommended with displacement of more than 2 cm of the avulsed fragment.
ASIS Apophysis *Appears between* *Ages 13 and 15* *Fuses between* *Ages 18 and 25*	Caused by sudden contraction of the sartorius with hyperextension of hip with knee in flexion; mainly occurs in sprinters (middle of run), hurdlers, noncontact football players, or runners (running accounts for 75% of injuries). Patient may report a snap at the time of injury; pain at ASIS with passive hip extension or active hip flexion. Avulsed fragment may be palpable. Patient demonstrates antalgia forward and lateral to same side; oblique radiographs of area may be needed to view fragment.	Nonsurgical management is recommended with an emphasis on an initial period of rest, ice, analgesics, and crutch ambulation; follow above general recommendations for apophyseal injury. Average time of return to normal activity is 6 to 10 weeks. Surgical management is recommended only with severe displacement.

(continues)

Table 53–8 Disorders of the Skeletally Immature Patient—The Extremities (continued)

Regional Disorder	Diagnostic Features and Considerations	Management Considerations
AIIS Apophysis *Appears between Ages 13 and 15* *Fuses between Ages 16 and 18*	Due to rare injury of rectus femors overcontraction; mechanism same as ASIS injury (sprinter-type injury) and may also occur in soccer/football with kicking; antalgic gait with pain increased by active hip flexion. Radiographs should include obliques; caution in misinterpreting an os acetabuli (normal variant) as an avulsion (contralateral comparison films may help).	Nonsurgical management recommended; follow general recommendations above; average return to full activity is 6 to 8 weeks.
Lesser Trochanter Apophysis *Appears between Ages 8 and 12* *Fuses between Ages 16 and 17*	Avulsion occurs with forceful contraction of the iliopsoas against resistance (sprinters, jumpers, kickers); may occur in running or football. Antalgic gait on same side; anterior hip pain with radiation occasionally into groin; leg may be held in slight adduction/internal rotation; resisted hip flexion, passive extension, and internal rotation increase pain; positive Ludloff's sign—inability to actively flex hip while seated. Radiographs should include slight external rotation to clearly see lesser trochanter.	Nonsurgical management recommended; follow general recommendations above; average return to full activity is 10–12 weeks.
Greater Trochanter Apophysis *Appears around Age 4* *Fuses between Ages 16 and 18*	Due to excessive, sudden contraction of the hip abductors (e.g., cutting); sudden pain at greater trochanter with leg held in slight flexion/abduction; trochanteric fragment may be palpable. Patient is unable to perform a single-leg stance on affected side; Trendelenberg's may be positive; active abduction or passive adduction of hip will increase pain. Radiographs usually demonstrate a fragment displaced proximally, posteriorly, and medially; on rare occasions a small accessory ossification may be confused with avulsion and a comparison view assists in the differentiation.	Surgical management recommended if fragment is displaced more than 1 cm. Nonsurgical management for all other cases following recommendations above for general apophyseal rehabilitation. In addition, a hip abduction orthosis with a thigh cuff may assist in the early phases of healing.
Iliac Crest Apophysis *Appears between Ages 12 and 15* *Fuses between Ages 18 and 25*	Excessive muscle pull from either abdominal obliques, tensor fascia lata, or gluteus medius anteriorly and latissimus dorsi and gluteus maximus posteriorly. There are three forms (1) acute contact—fall or blow to crest (hip pointer), (2) acute noncontact—due to sudden change in direction, and (3) overuse—often due to torsional strains. Pain and tenderness worse with resisted abduction of hip, contraction of abdominal muscles, or lateral bending of the torso; caution when viewing radiographs due to common occurrence of normal variants simulating pathology.	Nonsurgical management recommended for most cases; follow general recommendations above; average return to full activity is 4–6 weeks. Surgical management recommended if fragment is displaced more than 3 cm.
Ischial Tuberosity Apophysis *Appears between Ages 14 and 16* *Fuses between Ages 18 and 25*	Classified as acute separation (apophyseolysis), chronic apophyseolysis with slow separation, and osteochondrosis (avasular necrosis or Kremser's disease); mechanism in acute injury is forceful eccentric contraction of hamstrings with knee in extension and hip in flexion found primarily with runners and also broad jumpers, hurdlers, and gymnasts/cheerleaders (performing splits). Patient is antalgic; pain is reproduced with passive stretching or active contraction of hamstrings or hip adductors; tenderness at ischial tuberosity or sacrotuberous ligament. Defect or gap may be palpable; diagnosis confirmed with radiographs. Displacement is usually distal and lateral.	Concern with nonsurgical management is fibrous nonunion (up to 68%). If nonunion does occur, excision of fibrous nonunion and reattachment of hamstrings are usually successful. Nonsurgical management is still recommended for most cases. Open reduction and internal fixation is recommended with displacement of more than 2 cm.

Table 53–8 Disorders of the Skeletally Immature Patient—The Extremities (continued)

Regional Disorder	Diagnostic Features and Considerations	Management Considerations
Adductor Avulsion of Symphysis Pubis	Usually a sprinting injury with onset of sudden groin pain; resisted adduction or passive abduction increase pain. Radiographs are difficult to interpret; no avulsed fragments are seen.	Usually conservative treatment is sufficient. Figure-of-eight wrap for assisted walking is beneficial followed by mild stretching and strengthening for several weeks.
KNEE		
Blount's Disease (Tibia Vara)	Disruption of growth at the medial proximal tibial growth plate leads to a varus deformity. There is a higher incidence in children who are black, obese, and who have a familial history or live in certain geographic areas. The cause is unknown but may be due to stress or trauma. There is an infantile and juvenile form. Initial radiographs may be negative. Increased uptake on bone scan is diagnostic. There is an associated medial tibial torsion in many cases.	There are six stages. In the first two stages braces are used during play and at night. If there is progression to later stages osteotomy is recommended (especially before the age of 4).
Posttraumatic Genu Valgum	Although rare, overgrowth may occur as a result of proximal tibial metaphysis fractures. The deformity may be due to soft tissue caught in between the fracture segments or malunion.	Prevention is possible with correct positioning in casting the leg for these fractures. If the deformity develops, osteotomy or hemi-epiphysiodesis may be used dependent on the degree.
Osgood-Schlatter's *Age 11–15*	An apophysitis at the tibial tubercle commonly seen in running/jumping sports, in hockey with boys and gymnastics and figure skating for girls. Pain and swelling over the tibial tuberosity are relatively diagnostic. Radiographs may be misleading due to normal variant of tibial tuberosity fragmentation and should generally be used either to rule out tumor (if suspected) and full avulsion (seen generally in patients complaining of pain with activity and rest; <1% of all patients).	Activity modification (reduction of intensity or frequency), icing, stretching, and strengthening are the mainstay of management. Focus is on hamstring, quadriceps, iliotibial band, and Achilles stretching and eccentrically strengthening the quadriceps. An Osgood-Schlatter brace may provide some limited symptom relief. The condition generally resolves in 6 to 9 months in most cases.
Sinding-Larson-Johannsen Syndrome *Ages 10–14*	An apophysitis of the inferior pole of the patella, this condition is seen primarily in males. The causes are similar to Osgood-Schlatter's including running and jumping, but also climbing stairs or kneeling may be aggravating. Radiographic appearance is of an irregular calcification at the inferior pole of the patella. Occasionally, this process affects the proximal pole of the patella.	Same as Osgood-Schlatter's.
Bipartite/Tripartite Patellae	Secondary centers of ossification may produce a bipartite or tripartite patella. These centers are connected to the patella by fibrous or cartilagenous tissue (not visible on radiographs). Symptoms are produced with direct trauma to the patella or pull from tight quadriceps (common during growth spurts). The most common location is the superior/lateral patella. Radiographs clearly demonstrate the center; however, bilateral views may be necessary to differentiate from a fracture when direct trauma to the patella has occurred (bipartite patellae are often bilateral).	Rest from any inciting activity and quadriceps stretching are usually sufficient for symptom resolution. On occasion, the pain is resistant to conservative care due to an associated chondromalacia of the affected region. In rare cases, surgical excision or a lateral retinacular release is recommended.

(continues)

Table 53–8 Disorders of the Skeletally Immature Patient—The Extremities (continued)

Regional Disorder	Diagnostic Features and Considerations	Management Considerations
Tibial Eminence Fracture	Tibial spine fractures are more common in children. Causes include avulsion from anterior cruciate ligament (ACL) injury or direct trauma from a fall or direct blow to the area (common in bicycle injuries). ACL-related injuries are due to the fact that the incompletely ossified eminences are weaker than the attached ACL. Tunnel and oblique radiographs will demonstrate the fracture in most cases.	Dependent on the degree of fracture, management may range from closed reduction and cast immobilization to surgical fixation. Although this injury is not usually associated with other damage, it is not uncommon to have some indications of ACL instability after healing has occurred.
Discoid Meniscus	Usually found laterally, this abnormally shaped meniscus has abnormal attachments that allow too much mobility. The patient complains of the knee giving way, or snapping, or sometimes locking and pain. Full extension may not be possible passively, and joint line tenderness laterally may be found. Magnetic resonance imaging (MRI) is usually necessary for the diagnosis.	Meniscectomy should be avoided. Meniscoplasty may help in reshaping the meniscus or a partial meniscectomy may be performed.
Plica	A redundant synovial fold may persist. The most common is a medial shelf plica. Symptoms often appear during the growth spurt when bone grows, yet the plica does not. This tethering may cause erosion pain at the femoral condyle and/or snapping with knee flexion. Also direct trauma may cause irritation. A CT or MRI is necessary for confirmation.	Management may be conservative with rest, ice, and anti-inflammatories. If persistent, surgical release is effective.
Epiphyseal Injury	When a twisting, hyperextension, or valgus injury occurs at the knee, epiphyseal injury is more likely than soft tissue injury in a young patient. Valgus testing will reveal opening that must be confirmed with a stress fluoroscopic study demonstrating epiphyseal opening (usually a Salter type II fracture).	Closed reduction is sufficient for Salter I and II injuries. Open reduction may be necessary for Salter III and IV. Long-term follow-up includes monitoring for any growth disturbances.
Osteochondritis Dissecans (OCD)	OCD is partial or incomplete separation of a distal femoral osteochondral fragment. The cause is unknown but is likely the result of trauma, ischemia, aberrant ossification, or a hereditary epiphyseal abnormality. The juvenile/adolescent form is probably the result of a combination of these factors. Symptoms usually appear in adolescence and may be bilateral in 20% to 30% of individuals. The most common site is the lateral area of the medial, distal femoral condyle. If the fragment is still attached, symptoms are usually of vague knee pain with swelling occurring in some cases. If the fragment dislodges or hinges into the joint, mechanical symptoms such as locking may then occur. Physical examination may reveal tenderness at the condyle with palpation of the area (knee is flexed 90° or more to access area). Wilson's test may be positive. Radiographs must include a tunnel view. Other imaging tools may be necessary to confirm the configuration and extent of the lesion.	If the fragment is intact, the management goal is to support healing. This includes rest and restriction from activity (to the extreme of cast immobilization if necessary). Sequential radiographs must be taken. If the patient is still symptomatic and/or there is no evidence of healing after 3 to 6 months of conservative care, surgical management may be considered. Surgery includes drilling to allow increased vascularization and healing or the use of fixation devices if the fragment is unstable and likely to separate off the condyle. The adult form of this condition has a higher rate of nonunion and need for surgical intervention.

Table 53–8 Disorders of the Skeletally Immature Patient—The Extremities (continued)

Regional Disorder	Diagnostic Features and Considerations	Management Considerations
Patellar Dislocation *Most Common: Ages 9 and 15*	Occurrence is 1 in 1,000 children. Associated osteochondral fracture is approximately 50%. This associated fracture may occur on relocation as the patella hits the lateral femoral condyle. Injury may include hyperextension or twisting injury with femur rotating medially or, less commonly, a direct blow to the medial patella. In unreduced dislocations, the deformity is usually obvious but may be obscured by a swelling (due to tearing of retinacular vessels or osteochondral fracture). If reduced, tenderness is found on the medial patella due to tearing of the retinaculum and other soft tissue.	Management of unreduced dislocation includes a gentle attempt at relocation. If not possible, transport to the emergency department is suggested due to the high rate of osteochondral and lateral femoral condyle fracture seen with aggressive relocation. For first-time dislocators without osteochondral involvement, 3 to 6 weeks of immobilization with knee extension and a lateral compression pad are sufficient. The chance of recurrent dislocation is one in six. If biomechanical predispositions can be determined such as patella alta, an attempt at conservative accommodation may be helpful. Surgical stabilization for recurrent dislocators is recommended.
ANKLE/FOOT		
Snowboarder's Fracture	Although not exclusive to the snowboarder, fracture of the lateral process of the talus is three times more common in snowboarders than in the general population. An "ankle sprain" with a complaint of anterolateral ankle pain, especially if the pain is persistent after a reasonable period of time, should raise the suspicion of this fracture. Although often missed on radiograph, a mortise view with internal rotation might catch the fracture; found just distal to the lateral malleous. Lateral radiographs at 0° dorsiflexion and 10° to 20° inversion may demonstrate the fragment. If still suspected but not seen on radiographs, a CT scan should be ordered.	Generally it is accepted that nondisplaced fractures can be managed with a short-leg, non-weight-bearing cast for about 4 weeks followed by 2 weeks of walking. Minimally displaced fragments will probably also do well with this treatment. With more displacement there is some disagreement as to whether the above protocol is sufficient or whether surgery is indicated.
Freiberg's *Ages 14–18*	Avascular necrosis of the head of either the second or third metatarsal. This condition is more common in females. Metatarsal pain in an adolescent would warrant a differentiation between stress fracture and Freiberg's. However, symptoms may appear 6 months prior to radiographic changes. Changes include a sequence of irregular articular surfaces progressing to sclerosing, fragmentation, and remodeling. Bone scans are occasionally used in the differential; however, uptake varies based on the staging of disease.	If caught early, rest, an orthotic designed to relieve metatarsal head stress, and a sole orthotic to reduce motion of the joint may be successful. If not, a short-leg walking cast may be necessary. Advanced changes with fragmentation or overgrowth may require surgical excision and debridement.
Kohler's *Ages 3–6*	There is still some debate as to whether this represents an avascular necrosis of the tarsal navicular or whether it is a normal variant (may be found bilaterally and unassociated with symptoms). This condition is more common in males. Therefore, patients who are symptomatic should have comparative films taken and the findings correlated to clinical symptoms. A navicular subluxation should be considered.	This condition usually resolves over 3 to 9 months. Arch supports may provide some symptom relief. Adjusting of a navicular subluxation may also prove effective in relieving symptoms.

(continues)

Table 53–8 Disorders of the Skeletally Immature Patient—The Extremities (continued)

Regional Disorder	Diagnostic Features and Considerations	Management Considerations
Sever's Phenomenon *Ages 11–12*	Irregularity of the secondary ossification center of the calcaneous is often misinterpreted as a cause of adolescent heel pain. The following scenario occurs and should be managed as an insertional tendinitis. Presentation is more frequent in boys. Pain at the heel exacerbated by running activities. Predispositions may include repetitive microtrauma, tight gastroc-soleus, weak ankle dorsiflexors, fast growth spurt, and biomechanical abnormalities including genu varum, or subtalar and forefoot varus. Rarely is there swelling. Tenderness with compression on the medial and lateral calcaneus is suggestive. Radiographs are of little help because of the normal variant of increased density seen at the apophysis.	A self-resolving condition in most cases. Management is conservative with temporary reduction or elimination of inciting activities and stretching of the plantarflexors and strengthening of the dorsiflexors. Orthotics may help compensate for some associated biomechanical predispositions.
Tarsal Coalition	Connections or fusion between tarsal bones with bone, cartilage, or fibrous tissue causing loss of inversion and eversion movement. Often familial, these may be unilateral or bilateral. Pain, flatfoot, and peroneal spasm may be seen. The most common at the calcaneonavicular joint is best seen on an oblique radiograph of the foot. The next most common is the talocalcaneal joint. This type is less visible on radiographs (occasionally seen on a Harris view); best seen on CT scan.	A short-leg walking cast for 4 weeks may provide relief from pain. When symptoms recur quickly after removing cast, surgical resection is used.
Accessory Tarsal Bones	Irritation or disruption of the connection (syndesmosis) between primary and secondary centers of ossification (accessory bones) may be the cause of pain in children and adolescents. There are about 21 accessory bones in the feet; therefore, pain may be localized to many different sites dependent on the involved syndesmosis. Common sites are at the navicular and below the medial or lateral malleolus. It is equally important not to mistake an avulsion fracture for an accessory ossicle. This is most common at the base of the fifth metatarsal, where an inversion injury may occur (through contraction of the peroneus brevis tendon) causing an avulsion fracture.	Short-leg walking cast immobilization may be sufficient for 2 weeks. If unresponsive, surgical excision may be required.
Iselin's	Considered a traction apophysitis of the base of the fifth metatarsal, this condition is considered either rare or nonexistent by some authors. The consideration is whether there is actually a fracture versus an apophysitis. Lateral pain at the site of irritation is increased with running, cutting, or jumping. Resisted eversion may also increase pain. Radiographically, the apophyseal space may be enlarged and the apophysis irregular.	Management is conservative with relative rest and avoidance of any symptom-producing activities for a period of a few weeks to 2 months. Rehabilitation may include stretching of the evertors and plantarflexors and strengthening of the invertors and dorsiflexors. In rare cases, a period of soft-cast immobilization may be needed.

The preparticipation evaluation is not intended as a substitute for a full physical. A portion of the examination is intended as a health screen to discover any serious disorders. The primary focus is musculoskeletal. However, for many school-aged children, the sports physical may be the only direct health evaluation access these children will have.[44]

A protocol for administration of the examination follows:

- Meet with the contact individual at an institution or sporting organization to determine specific needs. The variables to be discussed include:

   1. Which group of individuals is being examined (specific sport or general exam)?

2. Where will the examination be performed?

3. Which type of examination format will better suit the institution based on the numbers of individuals being examined, the facilities for the examination, and the intent of the examination?

- Send letters explaining to parents the intent of the examination, who is performing the examination, and where parents can call to ask questions. This letter would include an informed consent section to be signed by the parent.
- Perform the examination.
- Provide parents and students an evaluation summary with a copy sent to the coach and placed in the student's file. The information would include:
  1. Vitals and anthropometric measurements (blood pressure, temperature, pulse/respiration rate, height, weight, eyesight and hearing screening)
  2. Flexibility, strength, and endurance results with a sex- and age-matched comparison column
  3. A summary and recommendation section explaining areas that are below normal and how they may be improved

Dependent on the type of examination, the components of the preparticipation evaluation may vary. The constant component would be completing a general health questionnaire. The focus of the questionnaire is to screen for known problems such as disease, organ dysfunction (or absence), prior injuries, allergies, current medications, and familial tendencies. Focus is placed on two common tendencies; one is rare (but catastrophic), the other is common (but often undetected). The primary focus for detection of serious disorders is sudden death often due to undetected cardiac abnormalities such as hypertrophic cardiomyopathy. The history may be helpful, including a family history of cardiac disease causing death in a young, close relative and a personal history of syncope or heat intolerance. A screen for Marfan's syndrome is typically performed with a family history and physical examination. The second condition is exercise-induced bronchospasm. This condition may occur in as many as 15% of adolescents. Clues are exertional dyspnea or a complaint of wheezing during or after exercise.

The typical components of the examination include the following:

- Evaluation of vitals

- Evaluation of anthropometric measurements such as height, weight, body type, body fat composition, and general range of motion
- Medical evaluation including:
  1. vision evaluation
  2. auscultation of heart and lungs
  3. palpation of abdomen
  4. determination of Tanner staging (direct or indirect) to estimate physiologic maturity (optional)

The Tanner age classification system is as follows:

- Male Tanner staging[45]
  1. Stage 1: preadolescent with small testes, scrotum, and penis (same as proportions in childhood); no pubic hair
  2. Stage 2: scrotum and testes enlarge with some reddening of the scrotal area; sparse growth of pubic hair
  3. Stage 3: growth of penis in length and some breadth in addition to continued growth of testes/scrotum; pubic hair is darker, coarser, and curlier
  4. Stage 4: penis has enlarged with development of the glans; adult pubic hair but has not covered full area as in adult
  5. Stage 5: genitals and pubic hair are adult in size and shape
- Female Tanner staging of pubic hair development[46]
  1. Stage 1: preadolescent; no pubic hair
  2. Stage 2: sparse growth of long, downy hair, straight or curled mainly around labia
  3. Stage 3: hair is darker, denser, and coarser, spreading to junction of pubes
  4. Stage 4: hair is adult in type but not spread as far, not extending to medial thigh
  5. Stage 5: hair is adult in type and fully spread to medial thighs

More specific examination would include testing (**Table 53–9**) for:

- Strength: using sit-ups or push-ups, the squat, or one maximum-lift bench press (dependent on facilities and type of examination)
- Power: using the vertical jump or medicine ball toss
- Anaerobic endurance: using jumping jacks, 20-yard dash, shuttle run, or hexagon drill
- Aerobic endurance: using either step test or timed mile run

Table 53–9 Summary of Preparticipation Examination

Station	Tests	Equipment
Check-in	• Medical history	• Questionnaire and pens
	• Blood pressure	• BP cuff and stethoscope
	• Pulse	• Watch
	• Height	• Scale
	• Weight	• Scale
	• Vision	• Eye chart
	• Urinalysis (optional)	• Urine cups and dip sticks
	• Body fat measurement	• Calipers
Flexibility	• Sit and reach	• Sit and reach box
	• Goniometric joint measurement	• Goniometers
Strength	• Sit-ups	• Watch and mat
	• Push-ups, or	• Mat
	• Squats	• Squat bench and weights
Power	• Vertical jump	• Jump flags or chalk/tape measure
	• Medicine ball throw	• Medicine ball and tape measure
Anaerobic endurance	• Jumping jacks in 1 minute, or	• Watch
	• 20-yard dash, or	• Tape and tape measure
	• Shuttle run, or	• Five tennis balls, stopwatch, tape
	• Hexagon drill, or	• Tape, stopwatch
	• Sit-ups in 1 minute	• Watch, mat
Aerobic endurance	• Step test, or	• Metronome, step box
	• Mile run, timed	• Stopwatch
General medical evaluation	• Medical exam	• Standard medical bag equipment
	• Orthopaedic/neurological exam	
Check-out	• Records review and summary	• History forms from entry station
		• All other forms from previous stations

• Flexibility: sit -and -reach test and goniometric measurement

These may be general examinations or examinations focused on target areas based on the specific sport or sports in which the individual will participate. Statistically, there are common biomechanical requirements for specific sports and common injury patterns for that sport.[47] The intent of the preparticipation examination is to focus on these requirements and give suggestions to prevent injury.

The age of the athlete will also influence the focus of concern.[48] Children between ages 6 and 10 years are more involved in spontaneous play, becoming increasingly involved in organized sports. The focus of the examination in this group is on scoliosis, congenital anomalies, visual problems, and mesenchymal disorders such as Marfan's syndrome. In the young athlete, generally between the ages of 11 and 15 years, the focus shifts to more complex areas such as psychosocial influences. Particular attention is given to questioning regarding sexual activity, drug and alcohol use, and a determination of physical maturity with regard to risk of injury in contact sports. The most appropriate time for a preparticipation physical is six weeks prior to the season. This usually gives adequate time to further investigate any areas of concern or follow a prescribed program of stretching or strengthening.

The seven most important physical examination factors are:

1. *Are there any major medical restrictions or contraindications to a specific sport activity?* (major eyesight, hearing, cardiorespiratory, renal, or hematologic concerns)

2. *Any past injuries that tend to be recurrent?* (shoulder and patellar dislocations/subluxations, etc.)

3. *What are the major areas of imbalance musculoskeletally?*

4. *What is the level of maturation?* (The Tanner criteria determine skeletal maturity indirectly through the maturity of secondary sexual characteristics such as pubic hair growth or breast development. Stages are 1 through 5; musculoskeletal injuries occur more often during the peak height velocity phase of growth, which corresponds to Tanner 3 or 4. Also, mismatched Tanner-staged individuals are more likely to create a scenario where injury will occur to the lower Tanner individual such as matching a Tanner 1 with a Tanner 4, particularly in a contact sport.)

5. *What is the individual's motivation regarding participation?*

6. *Is there a family history of sudden death in relatives under the age of 50 years?* (hypertrophic obstructive cardiomyopathy)

7. *Are there any allergies to insect bites?*

Table 53–10 contains specific questions by organ or system.

Nine areas of special concern follow:[49]

1. *Viral infections.* Most viral infections are worsened by physical activity. They may adversely affect performance in the following situations:
   ○ Pharyngeal inflammation may decrease upper airway capacity.
   ○ Inner ear infections may affect balance and equilibrium.
   ○ Viral disease can occasionally lead to myocarditis.
   ○ Infectious mononucleosis may result in splenomegaly, which may predispose the spleen to blunt trauma.
   ○ Herpetic skin lesions can be transmitted between players.

2. *Hematologic disorders.* Hematologic disorders are not screened for in all individuals; however, in those complaining of fatigue:
   ○ Be careful to test for suspected anemia or abnormalities of the red blood cells (RBCs).
   ○ Sickle cell crisis can be precipitated by dehydration, lactic acidosis, or hypoxia.
   ○ False physiologic anemia is associated with increased volume expansion.

3. *Asthma.* Up to 17% of youngsters have exercise-induced bronchospasm.[50]
   ○ Dry, cold weather is usually worse.
   ○ Prolonged intense activity is worse.

4. *Renal disorders.* If the patient has a unilateral kidney, he or she is predisposed to serious renal problems with dehydration.

5. *Cardiovascular disease.* Key cardiovascular concerns on the physical examination include the following:
   ○ Heart rate over 120 beats per minute or any inappropriate tachycardia
   ○ Arrhythmias
   ○ Midsystolic clicks
   ○ Murmurs that are grade 3 or 4. (Most innocent murmurs should diminish with Valsalva. The murmur associated with hypertrophic cardiomyopathy increases with sitting and standing and with exercise. Individuals who have structural heart disease or a significant conduction defect [e.g., abnormal auscultation, chest radiograph, electrocardiogram, or echocardiogram] or those who are symptomatic [i.e., have syncope, near syncope, chest pain, pallor, or other related symptoms] require consultation with a cardiologist for recommendations/restrictions with regard to sports participation.[51])
   ○ Hypertension (HTN). Resting blood pressures (includes range of systolic/range of diastolic):[52]
      □ age 6 to 9 years: 122–129/70–85 mm Hg is considered significant HTN; >129/>85 mm Hg is considered severe
      □ age 10 to 12 years: 126–133/82–89 mm Hg is considered significant HTN; >133/>89 mm Hg is considered severe
      □ age 13 to 15 years: 136–143/86–91 mm Hg is considered significant HTN; >143/>91 mm Hg is considered severe
      □ age 16 to 18 years: 142–149/92–97 mm Hg is considered significant HTN; >149/>97 mm Hg is considered severe
      □ over 18 years is considered an adult (see Chapter 24)

   If there is no target organ damage or heart disease, significant hypertension should not limit sports activities; however, the individual should be monitored frequently and given advice regarding exercise and diet. Those with severe hypertension should be restricted from competitive sports and highly isometric activities and referred for evaluation by a specialist. All young people with HTN should be given advice regarding avoidance of

Table 53–10 Screening Questions for Specific Organs or Systems

Questions	Concern/Disorder
Pulmonary	
Do you experience long periods of coughing?	Asthma (including cough-variant asthma and exercise induced)
Do you experience coughing after exercise or sports?	
Do you experience shortness of breath or wheezing during or after exercise?	
Cardiovascular	
Have you ever passed out with exercise or sports or felt like you would?	Arrhythmias and structural abnormalities
Do you ever get dizzy with exercise or sports?	Vertigo versus cardiopulmonary
Have you ever experienced chest pain with exercise or sports?	Angina
Do you fatigue earlier than you feel is normal when exercising or playing?	General cardiopulmonary
Do you have hypertension?	Hypertension
Do any of your immediate family members have heart problems or hypertension?	
Has anyone in your immediate family (including uncles) died suddenly of a heart problem before the age of 50 years?	Hypertrophic cardiomyopathy
Neurologic	
Have you ever been knocked out or lost consciousness?	Concussion, risk of second-impact syndrome
Have you ever had a head injury?	
Have you ever had a seizure?	Epilepsy
Have you ever had what is called a "burner" or a "stinger"?	Narrow spinal canal or instability
Have you ever not been able to move a limb after an accident?	
Do you ever have headaches when you exercise?	Aneurysm, tumor, AVM versus dehydration or primary headache
Musculoskeletal	
Have you ever broken a bone or bones?	Past fracture history
Have you ever dislocated or "put a joint out"?	Instability of shoulder, knee, ankle, etc.
Have you ever sprained or torn a ligament?	
Have you ever strained a muscle or tendon that took a long time to recover?	Predisposed area
Do any of your joints swell?	Spondylolisthesis, Scheuermann's, scoliosis, etc.
Have you ever been told you have a condition of your spine?	
Urogenital	
Do you ever experience burning when you urinate?	Urinary tract infection
Have you ever noticed any discharge or skin lesions around your genitals?	Sexually transmitted disease
Have you ever noticed any blood in your urine?	Kidney, bladder, or urethra
Have you ever been diagnosed with any kidney, bladder, or other genitourinary conditions?	Congenital or acquired kidney problems
Have you ever been told that you had blood, protein, or sugar in your urine?	Kidney disorders or diabetes

exogenous androgens, growth hormone, drugs (in particular cocaine), asthma medications, alcohol, and tobacco.

- Discrepancy between femoral and brachial pulse (coarctation of the aorta)
- Other conditions that have cardiovascular risk potential and should be looked for on the history and physical include:
  □ hypertrophic cardiomyopathy (HC)
  □ mitral valve prolapse syndrome
  □ Marfan's syndrome
  □ congenital heart disease
- Other concerns include:[51]
  □ Some forms of congenital heart disease are contraindications for sports participation including some conduction deficits.
  □ Certain medication or drug abuse may cause dysrhythmias such as antidepressants, asthma inhalants, and cocaine.
  □ Patients with anorexia nervosa may develop a prolonged QTc interval or have significant bradycardia.
  □ If there is an obvious immediate family history of cardiovascular disease it might be prudent to test the child for cholesterol/high-density lipoprotein (HDL).
  □ Most children with high blood pressure are "hyperadrenergic" and in fact benefit from exercise. Still it would be best to avoid purely anaerobic activities such as weight lifting. Also prolonged isometric exercise should be avoided.

6. *Epilepsy.* Physical and mental activities seem to be deterrents to seizure activity. Many school systems make little distinction between epileptic and nonepileptic children in their athletic programs. Concerns regarding risk for seizure should include:[53]
- fatigue
- sleep deprivation
- hypothermia, hyperthermia, and hypoxia due to high altitude
- dehydration
- skipped meals and hypoglycemia
- excessive alcohol intake and ingestion of "street drugs"
- hyperventilation with activity is not a concern; it is different from voluntary or forced hyperventilation, which may precipitate petit mal spells

Epilepsy is not a contraindication to sports participation although caution should be used with climbing, horseback riding, diving, and swimming in general. Buddy participation is recommended. With gymnastics the biggest concern is a fall, due to a seizure, from a height that may lead to serious injury. Those with uncontrolled seizures should avoid water, heights, and speed.

7. *Diabetes.* Regularly exercising diabetics are better controlled than sedentary diabetics. Special focus should include:
- Anticipate a reduction in insulin requirements.
- Food may be necessary before, during, and after exercise to avoid hypoglycemia.
- Exercise should be avoided before bedtime to avoid hypoglycemia during sleep.
- Changes in insulin and diet need to be established by trial and error, realizing that a reduction is often necessary on days of strenuous exercise.
- Active children are better controlled with two doses of insulin a day (before breakfast and dinner).
- There is an increased release of insulin from the injection site that can be decreased by:
  □ twice-a-day, meal-related dose
  □ injection in the abdomen instead of the arms or legs
- A portable snack is necessary.
- In long-duration diabetes with severe micro-angiopathic complications, exercise should be limited because:
  □ Decreased splanchnic blood flow during strenuous exercise may lead to renal cortical ischemia.
  □ The exercised-induced increase in blood pressure may stress the vasculature in the eye leading to hemorrhage.
  □ Increased transglomerular passage of albumin (exercise induced) may lead to nephropathy.
- Children must be taught to give prompt attention to abrasions and lacerations and burning or freezing of the feet; they should trim their toenails properly and not wear tight shoes or socks.
- Dehydration can complicate diabetes.

8. *Chronic fatigue.* Fatigue is common with illness, lack of sleep, and poor diet. Chronic fatigue lasting

weeks or longer should be investigated. Some of the possibilities include:

- infection
- anemia
- burnout
- depression
- overtraining
- ergolytic drugs
- endocrine dysfunction
- respiratory and cardiovascular dysfunction

9. *Other concerns.*
   - Document unequal or unreactive pupils prior to sports participation to serve as a comparison should head trauma occur.
   - Look for necrotic or perforated nasal septum, which indicates drug (i.e., cocaine) abuse.

The decision to disqualify or modify an individual's participation in a particular sport is based on the American Academy of Pediatrics guidelines.[54] The format of this decision matrix is to classify sports into:

- contact/collision (e.g., boxing, hockey, lacrosse, martial arts, soccer, wrestling, football)
- limited contact/impact (e.g., baseball, basketball, bicycling, diving, high jump, pole vault, gymnastics, volleyball, skiing)
- noncontact; divided into:
   1. strenuous (e.g., aerobic dancing, crew, fencing, running, swimming, tennis, track, discus, javelin, shot put, weight lifting)
   2. moderately strenuous (e.g., badminton, curling, table tennis)
   3. nonstrenuous (e.g., archery, golf, riflery)

A full list of conditions or disorders is then matched with these categories with a recommendation regarding participation. Absence of a paired organ would, for example, exclude an athlete from a contact sport if the organ was a kidney, whereas it would require an eye guard if it was an eye (or functional loss of 20/400). An acute illness with a fever greater than 38.3°C (101°F), a pulse greater than 100, or severe or uncontrolled hypertension may prevent participation in all sporting activities until the illness resolves or is treated. If a parent (or coach) has a concern about the recommendation, he or she should seek a second opinion with the student's personal physician.

There are no standard legal guidelines in most states. However, based on a screening for serious problems and those problems that may increase the chance of

injury for a specific sports profile, recommendations should be made. Generally, there are four levels of recommendations:

1. *unrestricted and unconditional.* This level of approval includes all sports regardless of level of exertion or degree of contact/collision.
2. *approval with restrictions, or pass with conditions or reservations.* This level of approval allows recommendations with regard to referral for medical evaluation of suspected conditions, restrictions with regard to the level of activity or type of activity (i.e., contact/collision), recommendations for strengthening/stretching, or requirements for protective gear not usually required in a sport.
3. *fail with reservations or conditions.* This designation allows restriction from participation in some sports; however, it may allow participation in others (e.g., collision vs no collision). It would also allow medical consultation to determine whether the failure can be reversed by meeting certain criteria (e.g., diabetic patient is under control, asthmatic is properly medicated).
4. *fail.* No participation in any sport under any conditions.

Obviously, some of the concerns and restrictions may be transient when the underlying concern is self-resolving or treatable. Exclusion from sports based on the preparticipation physical is extremely rare. Studies have shown a rate between 0.3% and 1.3%.[55]

A Region-Based Approach to Complaints and Concerns of Patient/Parent

The young patient has the potential of presenting with complaints that reflect an underlying disorder seen at any age or disorders that are age-specific. The following section discusses the differential approach to the young patient based on regional concerns. These concerns generally will fall into two categories: (1) pain, and (2) deformity or asymmetry.

Each section approaches the patient based on region and type of complaint or concern and differentiates based on type of onset—traumatic versus nontraumatic, overuse, and insidious. Although most of the conditions are covered in more detail in other areas of this text, a brief overview is presented here with reference to the appropriate chapter. For those conditions that are not covered in other areas of this text, a more detailed description is given. Accompanying tables summarize the salient differential features of disorders that are region-related (see Table 53–8).

The approach to musculoskeletal complaints in the young patient must include a focus on specific developmental issues (see **Table 53–11**).

Table 53–11 Selected Disorders and Anomalies of the Spine	
Regional Disorder or Anomaly	**Diagnostic Features and Considerations**
Arnold-Chiari	These malformations are characterized by elongation of the brainstem and/or protrusion of the cerebellar tonsils below the foramen magnum. Type I cases usually present later in life with mild hydrocephalus and possible syringomyelia. Headache and cervical spine pain may be the only symptoms. An atypical scoliosis pattern may develop with a left-sided thoracic, right-sided lumbar curve. Type II cases are more severe and appear during infancy with breathing and feeding problems most common. Hydrocephalus is more evident. Other concerns are dorsal kinking of the medulla and spinal problems such as spina bifida and meningomyelocele. Posterior fossa and upper cervical decompression along with shunting if a syrinx is present are the standard approach.
Syringomyelia	A congenital or developmental dilation of the central canal of the spinal cord. When acquired it may be secondary to trauma or an intramedullary tumor. Often associated with Arnold-Chiari malformation and an atypical double major scoliosis (left thoracic/right lumbar). Symptoms and signs include loss of pain and temperature sense in a shawl-like distribution over the upper trunk and arms. This may lead to painless injury visible superficially at the skin. Atrophy and areflexia may be present. Magnetic resonance imaging will demonstrate the level and extent of the syrinx and whether there is associated Arnold-Chiari malformation. Treatment is to shunt fluid into the peritoneum and decompress the area such as with laminectomy of the cervical spine.
Klippel-Feil syndrome	A spectrum of disorders characterized by various congenital osseous abnormalities of the cervical spine. Primarily the upper cervical spine is affected with blocked vertebrae, occipitalization of C1 and platybasia, and odontoid abnormalities. Classically, the patient has a short neck, low posterior hairline, and limitations of lateral bending and rotation of the cervical spine. However, these occur in only about half of patients. Congenital scoliosis, Sprengel's deformity, hearing problems, and congenital heart disease occur in half of patients. It is also possible that renal agenesis or other renal abnormalities may be present. Patients may be asymptomatic or complain of neck pain. Radiographs should include the cervical, thoracic, and lumbar spines and audiologic testing is recommended. If there is instability of the upper cervical spine or platybasia, neurologic evaluation is necessary and caution with sports and obviously cervical adjusting is recommended. It is recommended that yearly neurologic examination and flexion/extension views of the cervical spine be performed in high-risk patients. In others, these exams should occur every 3 years.
Juvenile rheumatoid arthritis (RA)	Onset of RA in childhood occurs at two times, between the ages of 2 and 5 years and again at ages 9 to 12 years. There is a 2:1 ratio of male to female. Unlike the adult form, systemic signs are common including high fever, rash, uveitis, and possible pericarditis. When an acute attack occurs it is referred to as Still's disease. Unfortunately, rheumatoid factor is usually negative, and the acute onset of symptoms seems flu-like except for the fever pattern of spiking once or twice daily to 39.4°C (103°F) or 40°C (104°F) combined with a migratory maculopapular rash that is generally nonpruritic. The diagnosis is more assured with at least 6 weeks of joint swelling in a characteristic joint such as the knee, ankle, or wrist, although other causes such as Lyme disease must be considered. Concerns include the involvement of type II or pauciarticular RA where involvement of the SI joint or lumbar/thoracic vertebrae is typical. This may represent a precursor to ankylosing spondylitis. The polyarticular type involves joints symmetrically with the hip, knee, ankle, elbow, and small joints most commonly affected. The temporomandibular joint is also affected. There is always a concern of atlantoaxial instability. Flexion/extension views of the cervical spine are required prior to adjusting.

(continues)

Table 53–11 Selected Disorders and Anomalies of the Spine (continued)

Regional Disorder or Anomaly	Diagnostic Features and Considerations
Odontoid anomalies **Agenesis/hypoplasia** **Os odontoideum** **Os terminale**	These anomalies are more frequent with disorders such as Klippel-Feil, Down's, and Morquio's. The odontoid process may be absent (agenesis) or hypoplastic. Instability may be present, requiring flexion/extension views and orthopaedic/neurologic consult if found. Os odontoideum is possibly due to traumatic interruption of growth and may represent an ununited fracture or nonunion of the dens at the neurocentral synchondrosis. Although the transverse ligament is usually intact, it is important to check for spinal cord signs and to radiographically evaluate for instability. Os terminale is failure of the tip of the dens to completely ossify. Ossification generally should occur by age 12 years. There seems to be little clinical relevance to this finding.
Congenital torticollis (wryneck)	May be apparent at birth or within a few weeks. Usually due to fibrous contracture and/or hematoma of the sternocleidomastoid (SCM). A mass may be palpable. May be associated with congenital hip dysplasia or spinal developmental disorders. It must be differentiated from other causes usually evident radiographically. This condition usually self-resolves. Mild stretching may aid in resolution.

Spine

- Congenital anomalies may represent, in some cases, a source of a patient's complaint or a caution flag for modification of adjusting procedures.
- Rheumatoid, hyperelasticity conditions (e.g., Marfan's syndrome, Ehlers-Danlos syndrome) or abnormal chromosome conditions (e.g., Down's syndrome, Turner's syndrome) may cause laxity, in particular in the cervical spine.
- Developmental disorders of vertebrae may be the cause of blocked motion (e.g., blocked vertebrae, Klippel-Feil syndrome) or curvature of the spine (e.g., hemivertebrae, unilateral bar vertebrae, butterfly vertebrae).
- Developmental disorders may cause spinal cord or nerve compression (e.g., spinal cord/brainstem—Arnold-Chiara syndrome, syringomyelia [not technically compression], spondylolisthesis).

Extremities

- Muscle/tendon tightness occurs during growth spurts due to disproportionately more bone growth, which may predispose the young athlete to overuse injury.
- With trauma, the "weak" points are tendon and ligament attachment to bone (e.g., apophyseal injury) and epiphyseal injury. Given the same mechanism of injury in a child compared with an adult, the child will likely injure the ligament/ tendon attachment and growth plate, whereas the adult will likely sustain a soft tissue injury such as a mid-substance ligament tear.
- Secondary centers of ossification (e.g., bipartite patellae) and accessory bones (e.g., os talotibiale) may be misdiagnosed radiographically as the cause of an extremity complaint if the doctor is unaware of these normal variants and age-related issues; trauma or repetitive stresses to these anomalies may cause irritation and pain.
- Fractures heal more quickly in young patients than in adults.
- Developmental changes in the angulation of the lower extremity are age-related and may not represent pathology, especially when bilateral; most resolve over time.
- Asymmetric angulation of the hip, knee, or foot/ ankle often represents a disturbance in growth (e.g., Blount's disease), lack of differentiation (e.g., tarsal coalition), or hereditary predisposition.
- Certain tumors are more likely in the young versus the older patient (see Tables 53–5 and 53–6).

Neck

In addition to the information presented here, the reader is referred to Chapter 2.

Pain

Neck pain is a relatively uncommon complaint as an isolated regional presentation. Acute onset of pain with trauma warrants radiographic evaluation first. Nontraumatic acute pain should be cross-checked against systemic and neurologic signs. Neck pain with extreme limitation in motion and associated fever should be evaluated with Kernig's and Brudzinski's tests to determine if meningeal irritation causes a flexion reaction in the extremities. If present, it is often due to septic meningitis. Referral for medical management is required. Neck pain associated with cranial nerve dysfunction or signs of upper motor neuron lesion should result in referral to a neurologist. Lateral flexion injuries often result in a "burner" or "stinger" seen commonly in sports. Radiographic evaluation of these patients is recommended to both determine the approximate size of the spinal canal and determine if any instability is present. If instability or a very small canal is present, it is prudent to consider restrictions in sports (e.g., football) where head and neck trauma is common.

Deformity

- *Torticollis.* Parental concern over a fixed head tilt in their infant or child is not uncommon. In infancy, the most common cause of torticollis (wryneck) is a contracture of the sternocleidomastoid (SCM) muscle, presumably due to a breech delivery or other birth trauma resulting in a hematoma or fibrous mass in the SCM. Plagiocephaly, which is common with this type of torticollis, is visually seen as a flattening of the malar prominence and occiput opposite the side of head tilt. Ninety percent of these cases resolve spontaneously. There is debate as to whether gentle stretching accelerates this resolution.[56] If unresolved, it is recommended that if surgery to release the SCM is considered, it should be delayed for at least one to two years. Also, it is important to refer for an ultrasound or radiograph of the pelvis (after the child is 10 weeks old) to determine whether there is an associated hip dysplasia. In the differential list of possibilities, it is important to rule out other possible causes including infection and spinal cord tumor prior to diagnosing the benign form. In older children, torticollis may be acute following no specific event, minimal trauma, or a respiratory infection. The muscle spasm may be secondary to lymphadenitis or subluxation. Spontaneous resolution is generally in a day or two. Adjusting the cervical spine may

decrease any associated pain and may resolve the problem earlier although there are no studies comparing natural history and treatment results. Chronic torticollis in an older child is often due to contracture in both heads of the SCM muscle. If due to muscle spasm, gentle stretching and adjusting the cervical spine may be of benefit. Failure to respond likely indicates the rare, fixed type requiring surgical release.

- *Short Neck.* It is unusual to have a parental complaint of the appearance of a short neck in their child without accompanying concerns. When a short neck is the only concern, evaluation for Klippel-Feil syndrome should be performed. In addition to a radiographic confirmation indicated by blocked vertebrae, occipitalization of C1, and associated odontoid anomalies, a referral to a pediatric specialist with recommendation for evaluation of renal structure with diagnostic ultrasound should be part of the overall management strategy.

Thoracic Region

The reader should also see Chapters 4 and 5.

Pain

Midback pain is a common complaint with children and adolescents. Most pain described as diffuse and aching is generally a postural problem. A stooped forward posture and wearing of heavy backpacks are common causes. When associated with a stooped posture, a search for Scheuermann's disease should be included. An acute pain that is rather localized is found with infection, tumor (usually osteoid osteoma), or trauma.

Scoliosis Scoliosis is discussed in detail in Chapter 5. Painful scoliosis is rare in children and would dictate a radiographic search for processes such as osteoid osteoma or infection. The general approach to scoliosis is to determine if the scoliosis is present using Adam's test and lateral bending to determine if the curve corrects (functional) or does not (structural). Those patients with curves that do not improve on forward bending should be measured for rotational deformity using a scoliometer. Congenital causes include neurologic deficit disorders and congenital disorders that affect the growth of vertebrae including hemivertebrae, unilateral bar vertebrae, and butterfly vertebrae. These underdevelopments or failure of segmentation (becoming separate) may occur with a portion of or the entire segment. Radiographic discrimination is usually evident on standard radiographs; however, CT differentiation may be required. Dependent on the level, number, and degree of compensation, the prognosis varies (see Chapter 5 for recommendations regarding management and referral). Radiographic evaluation of all scolioses involves a determination of the degree of severity measured by the Cobb angle (although this is a one-dimensional view of a three-dimensional problem). Generally, the initial radiographs include a full-spine evaluation.

"Stooped Posture" A hunched or stooped posture is often evident in the adolescent. Generally this represents a postural syndrome with varying degrees of psychologic causes including self-confidence seen most often in shy or tall individuals, or with females during breast development. The primary differential goal is to determine whether the hyperkyphosis is structural or functional. The difference clinically is to observe whether correction occurs on forward bending in the standing position or with hyperextension in the prone position. Failure to correct with hyperextension or an accentuation of the kyphosis on forward bending is indicative of a structural cause and necessitates a radiographic evaluation. The most common cause of structural kyphosis is Scheuermann's disease. The incidence is estimated at between 1% and 8%.[57] Although approximately 50% of adolescents will have pain initially, by the time of skeletal maturity this number has decreased to 25%. A modified Cobb angle is taken off the lateral thoracic radiograph to determine severity. Generally, most cases less than 60° do not progress, and extension exercises of the trunk combined with hamstring stretching seem to be the standard (yet unsubstantiated) approach.[58] For a kyphosis greater than 60°, a Milwaukee brace has been recommended with apparently good initial correction (10° to 20°); however, many studies are flawed and the success rates may be overestimated due to lack of follow-up to determine which curves regress when the brace is removed.[57] For severe curves (>80°), surgical correction has been successfully performed. It is important to note, though, that this is an expensive procedure that carries some formidable risks.

Straight Back Occasionally, there is a concern by the parent of a flattened appearance to the midback. This may present as a secondary effect to a severe spondylolisthesis. More often this is due to a condition referred to as "straight back syndrome" (sometimes referred to as cobbler's chest). With the thoracic kyphosis diminished,

the anterior-to-posterior diameter of the chest is also decreased. Pectus excavatum is also seen with this disorder. With a narrowed chest dimension, mediastinal structures are compressed. On a posteroanterior (PA) chest view, the heart appears "pancake" shaped with a shift to the left and prominent upper left border. There may also be downward angulation of the anterior ribs. On a lateral thoracic view, the straightly stacked thoracic vertebrae are visible with no apparent structural abnormality. Patients with this condition often have a functional murmur often due to mitral valve prolapse (MVP) syndrome. Sixty-seven percent of individuals have echocardiographic (definitive test) evidence of MVP syndrome (see Chapter 39). Straight back syndrome may be inherited as an autosomal-dominant condition.[59]

Low Back/Pelvis

The reader should also see Chapter 6.

Pain

It appears that although as many as 36% of adolescents will have had low back pain by age 15 years, only about 2% will seek treatment.[60] A 25-year prospective study followed 14-year-old adolescents to age 39 years and found that those with low back pain at age 14 years were significantly more likely to have low back pain as an adult.[61] Although 36% of individuals had findings of radiographic abnormalities, these changes were not related to an increased risk of low back pain as an adult. In fact, one study[62] indicated that about 26% of asymptomatic individuals at age 18 years had signs of degenerated discs and 16% had signs of disc protrusion. Radiographic findings and evidence of disc protrusion are higher in symptomatic individuals, yet do not seem to be a reliable diagnostic indicator of cause given the high incidence in the asymptomatic population.[63]

Although the most frequent causes of persistent low back pain are either postural, sprain/strain, or spondylolisthesis, less frequent, but certainly more serious, causes can include tumor and infection. In children it is more common to develop an infective discitis than in adults. This infection is often self-resolving. In fact, the diagnosis is often made late in the course due to nonspecific clinical indicators. With infants, children, and adolescents, a fever may be present, yet the child may simply complain of a stiff back and try to remain relatively still. With infants or children, they may be reluctant to bear weight and walk due to the jarring effect on the spine. Adolescents are more likely to report a poorly localized pain. Radiographically, findings may be delayed. These findings may include narrowing of the disc space to the point of fusion. End-plate irregularities are common. If discovered at an earlier stage, antibiotic treatment (usually for staphylococcal infection) is recommended in an attempt to prevent these residual destructive changes. Spondylolysis occurs in approximately 6% of the population.[64] It may be due to repetitive microtrauma such as hyperextension. Spondylolysis is more common in female gymnasts, college football linemen, weight lifters, and rowers. Spondylolisthesis in adolescents is generally the dysplastic or isthmic type. Oblique lumbar radiographs will demonstrate a pars defect. Standing lumbosacral, lateral radiographs will indicate the degree of slippage. Generally, slippage is categorized based on grades of slippage 1 through 4 of 25%, 50%, 75%, or 100%, respectively. Single-photon emission tomography (SPECT) is often used to distinguish athletic patients who require an antilordotic brace and rest from those patients who do not have an "active" lesion.[65] Spondylolisthesis (also see Chapter 9) is not a common sequela to spondylolysis. There are several factors that may increase risk of slippage including the growth spurt, being female, and trauma. Recommendations for management are as follows:[66]

- For slippage up to 25% in asymptomatic children, observe radiographically every six months up to age 15 years and then annually up to age 18 years. This schedule is sufficient to catch any significant slippage. Slippage after adolescence is rare.
- For slippage between 26% and 50% in asymptomatic individuals, the above approach is reasonable with the addition of caution and perhaps the recommendation to avoid contact sports and hyperextension sports (such as gymnastics) if possible.
- For symptomatic cases less than 50% slippage, follow up with radiographs as indicated above, perform spinal and pelvic adjusting, recommend strengthening exercises for the abdominals and stretching of the paraspinals and hamstrings, and consider bracing. Lumbopelvic manipulation is considered safe in the up-to-25%-slip group. Modification of adjusting procedures may be required including anterior drop maneuvers for those with slips greater than 25%.

- For slippage greater than 50% in a growing child or in patients who have persistent pain with lesser slippage, surgery should be considered. In situ posterolateral fusion is the recommended surgery for those cases of intractable pain and slips under 50%. Past 50%, anterior and posterior fusion with cast immobilization and instrumentation are sometimes required.

Hyperlordosis

A hyperlordotic posture may:

- Be visually confused with prominent buttocks.
- Occur as a result of pathology in the lumbosacral area such as spondylolisthesis.
- Be due to a hip flexion contracture.
- Be compensatory to a hyperkyphosis in the thoracic region.

The diagnostic approach is to determine if the hyperlordosis decreases with forward bending. If persistent with forward bending, a fixed deformity seems likely. If a hip flexion contracture is the cause, the hyperlordosis will decrease when the child is sitting. Also, determine if a flexion contracture exists by performing the Thomas test (see Chapter 11). Radiographic evaluation will determine if there is a structural cause. In most cases this would be represented by some degree of spondylolisthesis. Myofascial stretching of hip flexors, strengthening of the abdominals, stretching of the paraspinal muscles, and possibly adjusting of the anterior superior (AS) iliums will be effective only if the hyperkyphosis is functional. Fixed deformities usually indicate a cause that requires surgical correction.

Shoulder/Acromioclavicular Joint

The reader should also see Chapter 7.

Pain

Nontraumatic pain at the shoulder is an unusual complaint by children. Adolescents may complain of pain secondary to overuse as the level and intensity of sports involvement increase. Due to the relative looseness of the shoulder capsule, it is not uncommon to have overstrain of the rotator cuff muscles acting as secondary stabilizers. Caution should be recommended with overstretching in sports such as swimming. Also, some children can spontaneously dislocate their shoulders posteriorly and may feel this "party trick" is benign. It is important to discourage this activity due to chronic and permanent stretching of the shoulder capsule. Persistent or acute-onset pain in the shoulder due to throwing activities warrants a radiographic evaluation to determine involvement of the proximal epiphysis of the humerus or, in acute scenarios, the possibility of pathologic fracture through a tumor or bone defect (i.e., unicameral bone cyst). Also, persistence of various secondary growth centers may cause pain due to sprain of the fibrous connections, avulsions of these centers, or secondary impingement of other structures. Persistent pain at the shoulder unrelated to activity and present at night warrants a radiographic evaluation for possible tumor.

Traumatic pain at the shoulder may be the result of falls or blows. The differential list is similar to that in adults, yet fracture is more common in the growing child, in particular, mid and distal clavicular fractures in place of acromioclavicular (AC) separation.

Deformity and Masses

Deformity at the shoulder may be localized or generalized. Generalized deformity having to do with carriage and shape or size is often either congenital or associated with nerve damage. Examples of congenital deformity may include Sprengel's deformity (congenital elevation of the scapula), varying degrees of underdevelopment of the limb, or absence of muscle (i.e., Poland's syndrome—unilateral absence of the pectoralis muscle). Upper brachial plexus damage may result in Erb's palsy with adduction, internal rotation, and pronation of the arm (waiter's tip) deformity. Lower brachial plexus damage may result in Klumpke's palsy with hand paralysis and hyperextension of the metacarpophalangeal joints and wrist flexion (no sensory loss). Localized masses may be due to osteochondromas (see Table 53–8) or at the clavicle due to pseudarthrosis.

Elbow/Forearm

The reader should also see Chapter 8.

Pain

Nontraumatic pain at the elbow is also an unusual presentation. Nontraumatic osteochondroses such as Panner's disease of the capitellum may spontaneously occur in later childhood and must be considered (see Table 53–10). Overuse in sports is the most common scenario,

especially with baseball and gymnastics. Constant medial stress or lateral compression at the elbow may result in varying degrees of soft tissue and bony consequences. Generically called Little League elbow, this spectrum of changes may affect either epiphyseal or apophyseal centers about the elbow (see Table 53–10). Evaluation for traumatic causes of pain unassociated with obvious deformity is based on mechanism and location of pain. A medically subluxated radial head causes lateral elbow pain following a traction stress such as being lifted by the arms or dragged by the arm. Falls onto an outstretched hand may result in a variety of fractures or dislocations that may not be visually apparent (see Table 9–1).

Deformity and Masses Deformity may be congenital with the same possibilities as outlined in the shoulder section. In addition, an increased carrying angle, hyperextension angle, or flexion contracture may be the sequelae to a fracture or dislocation (i.e., supracondylar fractures may result in all of the above). Hyperextension may also be the result of a connective tissue disorder; however, this hypermobility will be evident at the wrists and knees also. Caution must be used in jumping to the conclusion of a connective tissue problem due to the normal hypermobility of many young people's joints. It is clear that there is a statistically significant increase in the number of distal forearm fractures in both children and adolescents.[67] There is still some debate regarding the primary reasons for this: one being a changing pattern of physical activity and the other being decreased bone density due to a decrease in calcium intake. The theory is that there is a transient increase in cortical porosity due to increased bone turnover, possibly resulting from an increase in calcium demand during longitudinal bone growth spurts.

Deformity secondary to trauma is almost always an indicator of fracture and/or dislocation. It is important to consider supracondylar fractures when a deformity following hyperextension occurs. Supracondylar fractures are more often the cause of residual deformity at the elbow and forearm due to neurovascular involvement such as Volkmann's contracture of the forearm.

Wrist/Hand

The reader should also see Chapters 9 and 10.

Pain

Nontraumatic pain in the hand or wrist is unusual. A forgotten fall on an outstretched hand may eventually reveal the source of the problem. Traumatic causes include occult fracture without deformity (i.e., torus fracture) and dislocation. It is always prudent to check the proximal radius and ulna for associated fracture/dislocation. Soft tissue concerns from overuse are uncommon with the exception of gymnasts. Various types of capsular and osseous reactions may occur in the gymnast due to the repetitive compressive and distractive forces applied to the wrist. Epiphyseal damage should always be considered with a single traumatic event such as a fall on an outstretched hand or a history of repetitive trauma from weight-bearing forces such as handstands. Varying degrees of carpal dissociation must be considered with single-event traumas (see Chapter 9).

Deformity and Masses Congenital deformity may result from brachial plexus damage (as mentioned under the shoulder section), developmental defects such as syndactyly (abnormal connections between digits), polydactyly (extra digits), bent fingers (camptodactyly, clinodactyly, or delta phalanx), macrodactyly (i.e., overgrowth of digits), radial club hand (absence of radius or associated musculature), or Madelung's deformity (radial epiphyseal defect). Various chromosomal and metabolic disorders may result in a variety of changes in the shape of the hand or its creases. Traumatic considerations include the deformity or mass associated with fracture, healing from a fracture, or results of an unattended dislocation or fracture of a finger. Rotation deformities of the fingers (evident with flexion of fingers to the palm) are often the residual of a failure to address a metacarpal fracture. A bony mass subsequent to wrist trauma may indicate lunate dislocation and associated scapulolunate dissociation. Small painful nodules at the dorsum of the wrist often represent ganglion cysts that are the result of repetitive microtrauma. Deformity may rarely be associated with tumors such as enchondromas.

General Lower Extremity Overview

Torsion

Developmental twisting of the tibia or femur is referred to as *torsion*. *Version* indicates forward or backward projection of a bony landmark from the coronal plane. Specifically, *tibial version* is the angular difference between the axis of the knee and transmalleolar axis. *Femoral version* is the angular difference between the transcervical and transcondylar axes. *Anteversion* is associated with internal femoral torsion, and *retroversion* is associated with external femoral torsion. The consequence of version is often compensatory, involving a toeing in or out or

bowing in or out of the knee. It is important to note that version often represents developmental change that is normal (**Figure 53–2**). For example, femoral anteversion is normal in the adult progressing from about 30° at birth to about 10° as an adult. Lateral tibial torsion progresses from about 5° at birth to an average of about 15° as an adult. There are also familial tendencies to increases in torsion, and it is suggested that evaluating the parents is an important diagnostic and prognostic tool. When there is concern, the following approach will help in identifying serious causes of abnormal torsion:

- Screen for possible congenital or early acquired disorders such as cerebral palsy, hip dysplasia, achondroplasia, etc.
- Check the foot for abnormalities that commonly self-resolve such as metatarsus adductus (inward curved forefoot), pes planus, etc.
- Check hip range of motion and follow with Craig's test for a check of anteversion/retroversion of the femur.
- Check internal/external (medial/lateral) tibial torsion by first noting the position of the feet in a seated position (outward rotation of the dependent ankle may suggest lateral tibial torsion; a turned-in ankle may represent internal tibial torsion) and measuring the angle at the malleoli (usually the lateral malleolus is 15° [range of 13° to 18° in adults, less in children] behind the medial malleolus using the coronal plane as the reference point; greater than 30° may indicate external tibial torsion; less than 15° may represent internal tibial torsion).
- Observe the walking child and estimate the angle between a straight line of progression and the angle of the feet to that angle (foot progression angle). Greater than 15° in-toeing indicates a more severe problem and should be referred for orthopaedic consult, especially if unilateral.

Many orthopaedic appliances can be prescribed to correct version. It is important to note that most bilateral and some unilateral problems correct over time with no intervention. There are numerous studies showing no long-term difference in outcome with most patients.[68,69]

Leg Length Inequality

Leg length inequality may be clinically silent, evident as a limp, or suggested by scoliosis. The key in evaluation is to consider significant causes that might require medical intervention versus functional causes that either

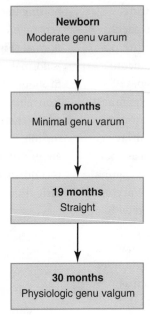

Figure 53–2 Physiologic evolution of lower limb alignment at various ages in infancy and childhood.

self-resolve or may be managed conservatively through treatment or orthotics. Evaluation should always include an observation of gait. Orthopaedic tests to determine a possible anatomic short or long leg include:

- Ali's test is performed with the patient supine and the legs and hips flexed. A long tibia is evident by a higher patella. A longer femur is evident laterally by a tibial tuberosity forward of the opposite leg. It is important to consider that the abnormal leg may be the long leg or the short leg. With hemihypertrophy it is important to consider an association with Wilms' tumor warranting an abdominal ultrasound evaluation. Also a lengthening occurs in the active phase of osteomyelitis of the femur. The majority of growth in the lower extremity occurs at the distal end of the femur.
- Tape measure assessment of true and anatomic leg length is performed using the medial malleoli and ASIS as the fixed points and the umbilicus as the functional comparison mark. A discrepancy evident with ASIS to malleoli comparison is indicative of an anatomic deficiency that warrants a radiographic evaluation.
- Orthodiagrams (orthoroentgenograms) are radiographs that include three exposures using a full spine film. Divided into thirds, the top third includes the femoral heads, the middle third the knees, and the bottom third the ankle joint.

Differences can then be determined and a site of inequality determined. For infants who can neither stand nor be immobile, a teleroentgenogram is used as a screen for radiographic apparent causes such as hip dysplasia. Large discrepancies should be referred for orthopaedic consult.

General orthopaedic rules of management are:[70]

- Calculation of projected height is made using one of several methods including the arithmetic, growth remaining, or straight-line graph method.
- Discrepancy at maturation may also be used in estimating corrective procedures.
- If the projected difference is large or would adversely affect total height, various procedures are considered including epiphysiodesis, bone shortening, or limb lengthening. The choice is based on whether the abnormal leg is short or long and the bone age of the individual coupled with growth spurt occurrence or projection.

Hip/Groin

The reader should also see Chapter 11.

Limp

The limping child may potentially have a problem anywhere from the pelvis to the foot. The type of limp and the history should first indicate whether it is due to pain or compensatory for a biomechanical deficiency. Painful limping is then pursued based on which is the painful joint. Pain at the hip may represent a myriad of problems that are to some degree age-specific. Considerations include stress fracture (history of repetitive weight-bearing activity), Legg-Calvé-Perthes disease, slipped capital epiphysis, transient synovitis, and infection, among others. Radiographic discrimination is often possible and must include lateral views. One recent study[71] indicated that the primary diagnosis in the emergency department was "irritable hip"/transient synovitis. Only 2% represented Legg-Calvé-Perthes disease. In another study,[72] predictors for the possibility of septic (versus aseptic [transient] synovitis) were identified:

- fever/chills
- inability to bear weight
- an elevated erythrocyte sedimentation rate (ESR)
- leukocytosis (>12,000 cells/mm^3)

Patients with three or four predictors were good candidates for aspiration; those with two predictors had an intermediate risk and may be candidates; those with no predictors were considered low-risk and not in need of aspiration. Biomechanical compensation may be due to an angulation abnormality of the femoral head/neck, femoral torsion problem, or muscle weakness pattern.

Deformity

Femoral anteversion (medial torsion) is a common cause of in-toeing in children older than 3 years. This inward twisting of the femur usually resolves between the ages of 10 and 12 years. Children with excessive anteversion may exhibit an "eggbeater" pattern when running with legs flailing outward during the swing phase. During resolution, signs and symptoms of patellofemoral tracking problems may be found due to a possible increase in the quadriceps (Q) angle increasing medial stress to the knee and lateral tracking of the patella. Femoral anteversion or retroversion is evaluated using Craig's test (see Chapter 11).

Knee

The reader should also see Chapter 12.

Pain

In children, pain at the knee may represent a referral phenomenon from the hip. Always evaluate possible hip pathology as a source. Nontraumatic pain at the knee should always raise the suspicion of infection or tumor

especially if accompanied by systemic or "red flag" indicators such as fever, swelling, or night pain. Other causes of nontraumatic pain, but associated more often with snapping or clunking at the knee, are a plica (see **Table 53–10** and Chapter 12) and discoid lateral meniscus, respectively.

Overuse pain is first approached by location. It is not uncommon to have pain and swelling at the tibial tuberosity (Osgood-Schlatter disease) or lower patella (Sinding-Larsen) indicating an apophysitis (especially with a history of running or jumping). Pain at the proximal or middle tibia warrants an investigation into possible stress fracture (especially with runners). With children, pain at the medial joint line more often indicates a medial collateral ligament sprain rather than a meniscal lesion.

Traumatic causes of knee pain are similar to the adult with the following age-specific, radiographic-evident exceptions:

- patella: bipartite patella irritation
- medial knee: epiphyseal injury (especially with any valgus or rotational mechanism of injury)
- anterior knee: tibial spine fractures and tibial plateau avulsions (anterior cruciate ligament [ACL] injury in children)

Rarely, pathologic fracture may occur through a large fibrocortical defect or undetected tumor secondary to trauma.

Deformity and Masses

- *Tibial Bowing:* Lateral bowing is a normal variant in infants and often resolves spontaneously. Anterior bowing may be associated with fibular hemimelia (absence) and requires radiographic confirmation. Posteromedial bowing is often associated with calcaneal deformity and often resolves with a residual of midlimb shortening. Anterolateral bowing is serious and requires orthopaedic referral. It may progress to fracture with a complication of pseudarthrosis of the tibia with nonunion. If attempts at union fail, amputation is unfortunately necessary.[73] Parental concern over a knock-kneed or bow-legged appearance in their child is common. General rules of thumb include:
  1. There are familial tendencies toward a more knock-kneed or bow-legged appearance. Always check the parents.

2. There are developmental changes that emphasize different angulations with different ages. For example, when learning to walk through the second year, a bow-legged appearance is normal (especially if bilateral). During the third and fourth years, a knock-kneed appearance is often a normal developmental variation with a wide range of severity (see Figure 53–2).

3. Bilateral appearance suggests a physiologic cause that resolves the vast majority of time, whereas unilateral deformity raises the suspicion of a pathologic cause. A full lower extremity evaluation should occur including an evaluation of femoral torsion, tibial torsion, foot deformity, and leg length differences. Radiographic evaluation should include weight-bearing views.

4. Local deformity is often physiologic, whereas, when generalized throughout the lower limb, it suggests a more serious cause and warrants an investigation of metabolic problems. The evaluation, in addition to a full physical examination, should include a laboratory evaluation of calcium, phosphorus, creatine, alkaline phosphatase, and hematocrit.

- *Genu Varus* (bow-legged): The fetal position in utero often involves flexion of the lower extremity with internal rotation of the knee and foot. Contractures of the medial capsule of the knee (especially the posterior oblique fibers) may persist, causing a restriction that is compensated by external rotation of the femur when walking. If persistent past 6 months of walking, stretching at each diaper change may help. This involves gradually stretching the tibia into external rotation with the knee flexed to 90°. Rarely, a varus deformity is due to either Blount's disease (see **Table 53–10**) or epiphyseal damage secondary to trauma. This would, of course, be unilateral in most cases.

- *Genu Valgus* (knock-kneed): It is a physiologic condition in most cases, seen primarily in children age 3 to 8 years, especially when seen bilaterally. Unilateral valgus appearance warrants a weight-bearing radiographic search for rare causes including posttraumatic genu valgum secondary to overgrowth following proximal tibial metaphyseal fracture. Also, malunion or soft tissue interposition may be the cause.

- *Genu Recurvatum:* Hyperextension at the knees is often a normal variant, especially in females. However, connective tissue disorders such as Marfan's or Ehlers-Danlos syndrome (see **Table 53–10**) may cause hyperelasticity manifested as hyperextension at the knees. A check of elbows and wrists may suggest a further search is necessary. Hyperextension predisposes the individual to patellar malalignment and subluxation/dislocation.

Bulging or masses at the joint line may represent meniscal cysts (seen more commonly in adults). These cysts usually represent an outward sign of meniscal damage. Anterior swelling at the tibial tuberosity is usually Osgood-Schlatter disease. Localized masses at the medial proximal tibia or at the patella usually represent localized bursitis. A posterior-medial mass is usually a popliteal (Baker's) cyst. This represents a lesion of the synovial sheath in children and is not as commonly associated with intra-articular disorders as in the adult (e.g., rheumatoid arthritis or infection). In children, these popliteal cysts are smooth, fixed, and transilluminate. They usually resolve over a year or two and, unless large or painful, do not require excision. A posterior-medial mass above the joint line may represent a fascial herniation of the semimembranosus muscle. This is apparent with contraction. Osteochondromas may be large enough to be seen at the knee (see Table 53–8). Differentiation is made radiographically. Ganglion cysts around the knee are also possible.

Lower Leg

The reader should also see Chapter 13.

Growing Pains

Although the exact cause of "growing pains" is unknown, it is recognized as a diagnostic entity. Growing pains

- are characterized by intermittent, bilateral pain, usually in the lower legs
- occur at night and are severe enough to awaken the child
- usually are asymptomatic during the day with no swelling, tenderness, or stiffness reported
- are associated with complaints of headache and stomach ache

The incidence is approximately 15% in children between the ages of 6 and 19 years, with a bimodal distribution peaking first at ages 3 through 9 years and again at adolescence.[74] Although it might be assumed that these pains would be associated with growth spurts or gains in the child's weight, there are no clear direct indicators of a relationship between height, weight, or rate of growth. Although the list of differential diagnostic causes is quite long and often contains serious conditions, the process of elimination is begun with a careful history. Bilateral pain unrelated to activity level and unassociated with systemic indicators such as fever or fatigue is likely benign and often represents "growing pains." Unilateral pain that is associated with systemic signs or associated with activity warrants a careful palpatory examination followed by a radiographic search for infection, tumor, or other potential causes. A screening lab test including a complete blood cell (CBC) and ESR will usually screen out serious causes. If radiographic and laboratory screens are negative, growing pains are not likely due to a serious cause.

Deformity

- *Internal tibial torsion:* An inward twisting of the tibia results in compensatory changes in walking. Although visually the patella faces forward, the foot is turned inward. It is apparent clinically by noting the lateral malleolus is in line or anterior to the medial malleolus. Spontaneous resolution is common. Prior to resolution, malalignment at the knee may result in patellofemoral tracking signs/ symptoms.
- *External tibial torsion:* Visually the patella faces forward; however, the foot is turned outward. When the angle between the malleoli is measured, it is greater than 25°. External (lateral) tibial torsion may be progressive due to the natural developmental increase in lateral rotation. Combined with femoral anteversion, there may be an associated knee pain due to patellofemoral tracking abnormalities.

Ankle/Foot

The reader should also see Chapter 14.

Pain

Although pain in the foot or ankle may be the result of sprain, strain, or other forms of trauma, there are some age-related considerations to add to the list of possibilities. These include the following:

- Osteochondritis. Pain secondary to avascular necrosis may occur in the navicular (Kohler's disease) or metatarsal head (Freiberg's disease). Both conditions are rarely treated surgically. Radiographic demonstration of increased radiopacity or increased uptake on bone scan may be found. Symptomatic treatment with orthotic support and protection of the involved bone is usually the only treatment needed.
- Syndesmosis sprains or fractures. Persistence of accessory ossicles (secondary centers of ossification that remain ununited) may cause pain in children or adolescents. Sprain or total disruption of the fibrous or cartilaginous connection between the two fragments may occur. It is important, though, not to assign a diagnosis simply based on the finding of an accessory ossicle. Pain localized to the site combined with an appropriate mechanism of injury is needed to raise the suspicion of syndesmosis sprain or rupture. Rest, immobilization, and support will assist in healing. One of the most common accessory bones in the foot is an accessory navicular found in about 2% of the population as a nonunion into adulthood. Late childhood or adolescence is a common time for this to become symptomatic. Immobilization with a soft cast for a limited period of time usually allows healing. Another common location is inferior to the lateral malleolus, which must not be confused with an avulsion fracture secondary to an ankle sprain.

Deformity

- *Flatfoot:* Although a common parental concern, flatfeet are often either part of normal development or, if persistent, an inherited tendency. This type of flatfoot is referred to as physiologic and accounts for 99% of cases.[75] From a developmental perspective, flatfoot is normal prior to the development of a bony support (i.e., sustentaculum tali) and with inherent pediatric ligament laxity. Even if persistent, flatfoot does not necessarily lead to symptoms, and in fact may be somewhat protective for stress fractures. A stiff flatfoot is found in only 1% of cases. Generally, when the foot is non-weight-bearing, an arch will appear in the flexible (physiologic flatfoot) whereas no arch will appear with the stiff (pathologic) form. A check of Achilles flexibility and a radiographic evaluation will help distinguish the pathologic form causes (the difference between soft tissue contracture and bony developmental problems). Specifically, when no arch appears (without weight-bearing), a search for causes includes a distinction based on the following possibilities:

1. Flexible flatfoot (FF) with tight Achilles tendon—contracture of the heel cord may be associated with a hypermobile FF causing obligatory heel valgus

2. Calcaneovalgus deformity—caused by a calcaneus that is in dorsiflexion due to intrauterine crowding (*Note:* associated with hip dysplasia); resolves spontaneously

3. Vertical talus—congenital deformity where the talus is in a vertical orientation (seen on a lateral radiograph); causes not only FF but also convexity of the sole

4. Tarsal coalition—connections between tarsal bones decreasing inversion and eversion; often familial; symptoms often appear during adolescence; either radiographs or CT scans are needed dependent on whether the connection is bony or fibrous

5. Neurogenic FF—common with spastic cerebral palsy, poliomyelitis, or myelodysplasia

- *High Arch (Cavus Foot):* Like FF, a high-arched foot is most often a physiologic variation of normal. When not, it is most often associated with neurologic disease that results in muscular tightening including Charcot-Marie-Tooth, spinal dysraphism, or muscular dystrophy. A search using radiographs, electromyography (EMG), and nerve conduction studies or creatine phosphokinase (CPK) evaluation will help differentiate among these possibilities.

- *Toe Walking (Equinus Gait):* Some children may have a tendency to toe walk constantly. Although this may represent "hysterical" manifestations, often it represents a muscular/soft tissue contracture or neurologic disorder. Children with cerebral palsy, muscular dystrophy, and uncorrected clubfeet may have this deformity. Gastrocnemius contracture is probably the most common cause. It is differentiated by a plantar-flexed foot that improves with the knee flexed (i.e., dorsiflexion of the foot increases significantly with knee flexion). Another rarer possibility is an accessory soleus. Both conditions usually require surgical lengthening and are not likely to respond to traditional stretching or physical therapy.

- *Toe-in (Pigeon-toed):* Often this is a compensatory position when first learning to walk. Medial (internal) torsion of the tibia is the most common cause in children under age 3 years. It resolves in most cases over time. In children over age 3, femoral anteversion (medial femoral torsion) is the most common cause. Spontaneous resolution is seen usually by age 10 years.[76] Metatarsus adductus is a deformity due to intrauterine positioning resulting in an inward turning of the forefoot with a normal hindfoot. It can be unilateral or bilateral and spontaneously resolves in almost all cases over a year or two.

- *Toe-out:* Three causes of toe-out walking should be considered: (1) talipes equinovarus (clubfoot; **Figure 53–3**), (2) calcaneovalgus foot, and (3) pes planus (flatfeet).

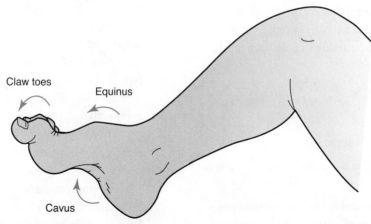

Figure 53–3 Components of talipes equinovarus.

Clubfoot is either congenital or teratologic (associated with spina bifida and other spinal deformities requiring surgical correction), or it can be postural (due to intrauterine position), which resolves after birth.

Calcaneovalgus is due to intrauterine positioning of extreme dorsiflexion of the ankle to the tibia, which resolves after birth. For pes planus, see the discussion above or Chapter 14.

Some Childhood Diseases*

Measles (Rubeola)

Classic Presentation

The patient presents with a history of a high fever 39.4°C to 40.5°C (103°F to 105°F), runny nose, sore throat, and cough several days before the appearance of a bright red rash. The rash began on the face and behind the ears and then spread to the trunk and extremities.

Cause

Infection is by paramyxovirus acquired through inhalation of droplets. Measles is most communicable before the rash appears and is essentially noncommunicable when the rash disappears. The incubation period is 10 to 14 days. Worldwide, 1 million children per year die of measles.

Evaluation

Prior to the onset of the rash, the patient may have a pathognomonic finding of tiny white spots on the mucous membranes in the mouth; they are called Koplik's spots. The spots are still present when the rash appears. Laboratory testing is usually not necessary. A serum hemagglutination inhibition antibody level that is found to be four times normal is diagnostic for measles. Standard laboratory tests demonstrate leukopenia and possible proteinuria.

Management

Treat measles symptomatically.

German Measles (Rubella)

Classic Presentation

The patient may report having had a mild fever or malaise up to a week prior to the appearance of a light rash that appeared on the face first and then spread to the trunk and extremities. The rash faded (or is fading) quickly over one day per site.

Cause

Rubella is caused by inhalation of droplets of togavirus. The incubation period is between two and three weeks. Communicability occurs one week before the rash and continues for up to two weeks.

Evaluation

There is a characteristic cervical and postauricular lymphadenopathy in most patients. The rash does not appear in all cases and, without its appearance, the diagnosis is difficult to make unless there is a history of exposure. Laboratory testing with rubella virus hemagglutination inhibition and fluorescent antibody tests is usually not necessary except in the case of pregnancy. A pregnant female infected with rubella during the first trimester carries the risk of conveying congenital rubella 80% of the time.[36]

Management

Treat rubella symptomatically.

Varicella (Chickenpox)

Classic Presentation

The patient presents with a history of mild malaise, anorexia, mild headache, and fever followed in 24 hours by the appearance of a pruritic, vesicular rash that began first on the trunk (and oropharynx), spread to the face, and spread less to the extremities. New vesicles are appearing as the older ones are crusting (over one to five days).

Cause

Chickenpox is a highly contagious infection with human herpes virus 3 (the same organism for herpes zoster [shingles]). Infection is through either inhalation of infective particles or direct contact with lesions. The incubation period is 10 to 20 days.

Evaluation

The rash is usually diagnostic. Laboratory evaluation could include a Tzanck test of vesicle scrapings for confirmation, although it is rarely necessary.

Management

The patient should be isolated because of the contagious nature of the vesicles. Topical calamine lotion or over-the-counter antihistamines may help with the itching. It is important to keep the skin clean and to avoid scratching in order to prevent scarring. Children should not be given aspirin because of the possibility of acquiring Reye's syndrome.

The use of a herpes zoster (shingles) vaccine has been recently evaluated. The decrease in incidence appears to be about 50%.[37,38] This is particularly important for seniors who may develop a painful and disabling condition given that herpes zoster is far more common in older age groups.[39,40]

Mumps

Classic Presentation

The patient presents with painful, swollen parotid glands. Mild malaise or fever may be present.

Cause

Paramyxovirus is the cause of mumps. Inhalation of infective droplets is the mechanism. The salivary glands become inflamed. Complications such as orchitis, pancreatitis, and meningitis are more likely to occur when the patient is older. The incubation period is two to three weeks.

Evaluation

The presentation of parotid gland swelling is usually quite clear, often beginning with one gland first and in one to three days the other. A headache and stiff neck suggest meningeal involvement. Abdominal pain with nausea and vomiting suggests pancreatitis. Testicular pain suggests orchitis. Lymphocytosis and an elevated serum amylase (with or without pancreatitis) are often found. The organism may be tested in saliva; if present, there is a sharp increase in complement-fixing antibodies.

Management

Isolate the patient while the glands are swollen. If the patient has a fever, require bed rest because of the strong possibility of aseptic meningitis. Watch for complications.

Fifth Disease (Erythema Infectiosum)

Classic Presentation

A child presents with a facial rash ("slapped cheek" appearance), but no fever. The rash is spreading to the trunk and limbs.

Cause

There are generally five causes of rashes in children: rubella, measles, scarlet fever, Filatov-Dukes disease (a mild form of scarlet fever), and erythema infectiosum (Fifth disease). Fifth disease is caused by human parvovirus B19. It is spread via the respiratory route. The incubation period is 4 to 14 days. The rash is maculopapular.

Evaluation

No evaluation is necessary unless accompanied by a high fever. Refer to pediatrician if a high fever is present.

Management

No treatment is necessary. The typical course is a fading and intensifying of the rash from hour to hour. Fading often takes a few weeks. There are no limitations to activity for the child; however, exercise, sunlight, heat, or fever may exacerbate the rash.

APPENDIX 53–1

Web Resources

Pediatrics

National Institute of Child Health and Human Development
(800) 370-2943
www.nichd.nih.gov
Nemours Foundation's Center for Children's Health Media
www.kidshealth.org
Centers for Disease Control and Prevention
http://www.cdc.gov
National Institute of Allergy and Infectious Diseases
http://www.niaid.nih.gov/factsheets/cold.htm
http://www.niaid.nih.gov/factsheets/antimicro.htm
American Academy of Pediatrics
http://www.aap.org

Burns

U.S. Consumer Product Safety Commission
(800) 638-CPSC (2772)
http://www.cpsc.gov
American Burn Association
(312) 642-9260
http://www.ameriburn.org

Child Abuse and Head Injury

Centers for Disease Control and Prevention National Center for Injury Prevention and Control
http://www.cdc.gov/ncipc/factsheets/tbi.htm
American Academy of Pediatrics
http://www.aap.org
Childhelp USA Child Abuse Hotline
(800) 422-4453
http://www.childhelpusa.org
American Academy of Child & Adolescent Psychiatry
(202) 966-7300
http://www.aacap.org

Mental Retardation

American Association on Intellectual and Developmental Disabilities
(800) 424-3688
http://www.aamr.org
National Dissemination Center for Children with Disabilities
(800) 695-0285
http://www.nichcy.org
The Arc
(301) 565-3842
http://www.thearc.org

Government Response to Public Concerns

www.cdc.gov
www.aap.org
www.vaccinesafety.edu

APPENDIX 53–2

References

1. Adams D, Dagenais S, Clifford T, et al. Complementary and alternative medicine use by pediatric specialty outpatients. *Pediatrics.* 2013;131(2):225–232.
2. Ebrall PS. A descriptive report of the case-mix within Australian chiropractic practice: 1992. *Chiro J Aust.* 1993;23:92–97.
3. Spigelblatt L, Laine-Ammara G, Pless B, Guyver A. The use of alternative medicine by children. *Pediatrics.* 1994;94:811–814.
4. Marchand AM. Chiropractic care of children from birth to adolescence and classification of reported conditions: an internet cross-sectional survey of 956 European chiropractors. *J Manipulative Physiol Ther.* 2012;35(5):372–380.
5. Gleberzon BJ, Arts J, Mei A, McManus EL. The use of spinal manipulative therapy for pediatric health conditions: a systematic review of the literature. *J Can Chiropr Assoc.* 2012;56(2):128–141.
6. Hestbaek L, Stochkendahl MJ. The evidence base for chiropractic treatment of musculoskeletal conditions in children and adolescents: The emperor's new suit? *Chiropr Osteopat.* 2010;18:15.
7. Sharek PJ, Classen D. The incidence of adverse events and medical error in pediatrics. *Pediatr Clin North Am.* 2006;53(6):1067–1077.

8. Plaugher G, Alcantara J. Adjusting the pediatric spine. *Top Clin Chiro*. 1997;4(4):59–69.

9. U.S. Preventive Services Task Force. *Guide to Clinical Preventive Services*. 2nd ed. Baltimore: Williams & Wilkins; 1996.

10. Hansen ML, Gunn PW, Kaelber DC. Underdiagnosis of hypertension in children and adolescents. *JAMA*. 2007;298(8):874–879.

11. Willinger M, Hoffman HJ, Harford RB. Infant sleep position and risk for sudden death syndrome: report of meeting held January 13 and 14, 1994. National Institutes of Health, Bethesda, MD. *Pediatrics*. 1994;93:814–819.

12. Gibson E, Cullen JA, Spencer S, et al. Infant sleep position following new AAP guidelines. *Pediatrics*. 1995;96:69–72.

13. Kattwinkel J, Brooks J, Meyerberg D. American Academy of Pediatrics task force on infant position- ing and sudden infant death syndrome (SIDS) in the United States: joint commentary from the American Academy of Pediatrics and selected agencies of the federal government. *Pediatrics*. 1994;93(5):820.

14. Talmage DM, Resnick D. Infantile colic: identification and management. *Top Clin Chiro*. 1997;4(4):25–29.

15. Wessel MA, Cobb K, Jackson EB, et al. Paroxysmal fussing in infancy: sometimes called colic. *Pediatrics*. 1954;14:421–434.

16. Brazelton TB. Crying in infancy. *Pediatrics*. 1987;29:579–588.

17. Klug BH. Behandling af spaedbarnskolik: en kritisk komentar. *Manedsskr Prakt Lagegern*. 1991;22(3):275–276.

18. Metcalf TJ, Irons TG, Shee LD, Young PC. Simethicone in the treatment of infant colic: a randomized, placebo-controlled, multicenter trial. *Pediatrics*. 1994;94(1):29–34.

19. Klougart N, Nilsson N, Jacobsen J. Infantile colic treated by chiropractors: a prospective study of 316 cases. *J Manipulative Physiol Ther*. 1989;12:281–288.

20. Nilsson N. Infantile colic and chiropractic. *Eur J Chiro*. 1985;33:264–265.

21. Wiberg JMM, Nordsteen J, Nilsson N. The short- term effect of spinal manipulation in the treatment of infantile colic: a randomized controlled clinical trial with a blinded observer. *J Manipulative Physiol Ther*. 1999;22:517–522.

22. Deltoff M. Non-accidental pediatric trauma: radio- graphic findings in the abused child. *J Can Chiro Assoc*. 1994;38:98–105.

23. DeFonesca JA, Feigal RJ, tan Bensel RW. Dental aspects of 1248 cases of child mistreatment on file at a major county hospital. *Pediatr Dent*. 1992;14:152–157.

24. Reece RM, Serge R. Childhood head injuries: accidental or inflicted. *Arch Pediatr Adolesc Med*. 2000;154:15–22.

25. Coody D, Brown M, Montgomery D, et al. Shaken baby syndrome: identification and prevention for the nurse practitioner. *J Pediatr Health Care*. 1994;8:50–56.

26. DiScala C, Serge R, Guohua L, Reece RM. Child abuse and unintentional injuries. *Arch Pediatr Adolesc Med*. 2000;154:16–22.

27. Merten DF, Carpenter BL. Radiologic imaging of inflicted injury in the child abuse syndrome. *Pediatr Clin North Am*. 1990;37:815–837.

28. Ebrall FS, Davies NJ. Non-accidental injury and child mistreatment. In: Arnig C, Plaugher G, eds. *Pediatric Chiropractic*. Baltimore: Williams & Wilkins; 1998:14–23.

29. Brody DJ, Pirkle JL, Kramer RA, et al. Blood lead levels in the US population. Phase I of the Third National Health and Nutrition Examination Survey (NHANES III 1988–1991). *JAMA*. 1994;272: 277–284.

30. American Academy of Pediatrics Committee on Drugs. Treatment guidelines for lead exposure in children. *Pediatrics*. 1995;96:155–160.

31. LeFever GB, Dawson KV, Morrow AL. The extent of drug therapy for attention deficit-hyperactivity dis- order among children in public schools. *Am J Public Health*. 1999;89:1359–1364.

32. American Psychiatric Association. *Diagnostic and Statistical Manual of Mental Disorders*. 4th ed. Washington, DC: APA; 1994.

33. Barkley RA. Behavioral inhibition, sustained atten- tion, and executive functions: constructing a unified theory of ADHD. *Psychol Bull*. 1997;121:65–71.

34. Kennedy LB, Miller BA, Ries LA, et al. Increased incidence of cancer in infants in the United States: 1980–1998. *Cancer*. 1998;4:1396–1400.

35. Barnes T. Understanding childhood cancer: keys for the chiropractor. *Top Clin Chiro*. 1999;6(1):25–36.

36. Smith NJ. Children and parents: growth, develop- ment, and sports. In: Straus RH, ed. *Sports Medicine*. Philadelphia: WB Saunders; 1984:207–217.

37. Thornburg HD, Clark DC. Middle school/junior high school research needs questionnaire. National Middle School Association Symposium, 1980.

38. Goldberg B. Pediatric sports medicine. In: Scott WN, Nisomon B, Nicholas J, eds. *Principles of Sports Medicine*. Baltimore: Williams & Wilkins; 1984:403–426.

39. Bar-Or O. *Pediatric Sports Medicine for the Practitioner*. New York: Springer-Verlag; 1983.

40. Pappas AM, Cummings NM. Sports injuries in the skeletally immature. In: Pappas AM, ed. *Upper Extremity Injuries in the Athlete*. New York: Churchill Livingstone; 1995:117.

41. Paletta GA, Jr, Andrish JT. Injuries about the hip and pelvis in the young athlete. *Clin Sports Med.* 1995;14:591.

42. Duda M. Prepubescent strength training gains support. *Phys Sportsmed.* 1986;14:157–161.

43. Risser WL, Hoffman HM, Bellah G. Frequency of preparticipation sports examinations in secondary school athletes. Are the university interscholastic legal guidelines appropriate? *Tex Med.* 1985;81:35–39.

44. Smith DM. The preparticipation physical examination. *Sports Med Arthroscopy Rev.* 1995;3:84–94.

45. Tanner JM, Whitehouse RH, Marshall WA, et al. *Assessment of Skeletal Maturity and Prediction of Adult Height*. London: Academic Press; 1975.

46. Marshall WA, Tanner JM. Variations in patterns of pubertal changes in girls. *Arch Dis Child.* 1969; 44:291–303.

47. Kibler WB. *The Sports Preparticipation Fitness Examination*. Champaign, IL: Human Kinetics Books; 1990.

48. McKeag DB. Preparticipation screening of the potential athlete. *Clin Sports Med.* 1989;8:373–397.

49. Small E, Bar-Or O. The young athlete with chronic disease. *Clin Sports Med.* 1995;14:709.

50. Lacroix VJ. Exercise-induced asthma. *Physician Sports Med.* 1999;17(12):163–172.

51. Committee on Sports Medicine and Fitness. Cardiac dysrhythmias and sports (RE9525). *Pediatrics.* 1995;95:786–788.

52. Committee on Sports Medicine and Fitness. Athletic participation by children and adolescents who have systemic hypertension (RE9715). *Pediatrics.* 1997;99:637–638.

53. Steven JI, Varrato J. Physical activity and epilepsy: what are the rules? *Physician Sports Med.* 1999;27:3.

54. Swander H, ed. *Preparticipation Physical Evaluation*. Kansas City, MO: American Academy of Family Physicians, American Academy of Pediatrics, American Medical Society for Sports Medicine, American Orthopedic Society for Sports Medicine, and American Osteopathic Academy of Sports Medicine; 1992.

55. Shaffer TE. The adolescent athlete. *Pediatr Clin North Am.* 1983;28:4.

56. Canale ST, Griffin DW, Hubbard CN. Congenital muscular torticollis: a long-term follow-up study. *J Bone Joint Surg Am.* 1982;64:810–816.

57. Wenger DR, Frick SL. Scheuermann kyphosis. *Spine.* 1999;24:2630–2639.

58. Lowe TG. Scheuermann's disease. *Orthop Clin North Am.* 1999;30:475–485.

59. Davies MK, Mackintosh P, Cayton RM, et al. The straight back syndrome. *Quebec J Med.* 1980;49:443–450.

60. Olsen TL, Anderson RL, Dearwater SR, et al. The epidemiology of low back pain in the adolescent population. *Am J Public Health.* 1992;82:608–609.

61. Harreby M, Neergaard K, Hesselsoe G, Kjer J. Are radiographic changes in the thoracic and lumbar spine of adolescents risk factors for low back pain in adults? *Spine.* 1995;20:2298–2302.

62. Salminen JJ, Erkintalo M, Laine ML, Pentti J. Low back pain in the young. *Spine.* 1995;20:2101–2108.

63. Tertti MO, Salminen JJ, Paajamen HE, et al. Low back pain and disc degeneration in children: a control MR imaging study. *Radiology.* 1991;180:503–507.

64. Fredrickson A, Baker K, McHolick W, et al. The natural history of spondylolysis and spondylolisthesis. *J Bone Joint Surg Am.* 1984;66:699–707.

65. Rosen PR, Micheli LJ, Treves S. Early scintigraphic diagnosis of bone stress and fractures in athletic adolescents. *Pediatrics.* 1982;70:11–15.

66. Lonstein JE. Spondylolisthesis in children: cause, natural history, and management. *Spine.* 1999;24:2640–2648.

67. Khosla S, Melton LJ, Dekutoski MB. Incidence of childhood distal forearm fracture over 30 years: a population-based study. *JAMA.* 2003;290:1479–1485.

68. Svenningsen S, Terjessen T, Auffem M, Borg V. Hip rotation and intoeing gait. *Clin Orthop.* 1990;251:177–181.

69. Staheli LT, Corgett M, Wyss C, et al. Lower extremity rotational problems in children. Normal values to guide management. *J Bone Joint Surg Am.* 1985;67:39–47.

70. Paley D. Modern techniques in limb lengthening: section I symposium. *Clin Orthop.* 1990;250:152–159.

71. Fischer SU, Beattie BR. The limping child: epidemiology assessment and outcome. *J Bone Joint Surg Br.* 1999;81:1029–1034.

72. Kocher MS, Zurakowski D, Kasser JR. Differentiating between septic arthritis and transient synovitis of the hip in children: an evidence-based clinical prediction algorithm. *J Bone Joint Surg Am.* 1999;81: 1662–1670.

73. Crossett LS, Beaty JH, Betz RR, et al. Congenital pseudarthrosis of the tibia: long-term follow-up study. *Clin Orthop.* 1989;245:16–18.

74. Bowyer SL, Hollister R. Limb pain in childhood. *Pediatr Clin North Am.* 1984;31:1053–1081.

75. Staheli LT, Chow DE, Corbett M. The longitudinal arch: a survey of eight hundred and eighty-two feet in normal children and adults. *J Bone Joint Surg Am.* 1987;69:426–428.

76. Bleck EE. Developmental orthopaedics III: toddlers. *Dev Med Child Neurol.* 1982;24:533–555.

The Geriatric Patient

Context

Studies suggest that the senior or geriatric patient (over age 65 years) represents approximately 12% to 17% of most chiropractic practices.[1-3] This percentage will likely increase given the projection that in the United States between the years 1989 and 2030 the population over age 65 years will double (12.5% to 22% of the total population).[4] Although currently accounting for only about 12.5% of the population, geriatric patients account for 21% of patient visits and purchase almost one-third of prescription medications.[5] The over-85 age group represents approximately 3 million individuals in the United States and is the fastest growing segment of the population. Currently, the average age of death is about 75 years. This may increase to 80 years by the year 2020. A 2007 survey by Wolinsky et al.[6] indicates that utilization by older adults in the United States for chiropractic care is only 4.6% on an annual average. Over a four-year period the percentage who had one or more visits to a chiropractor was 10.3%. Demographically, Caucasians, patients reporting pain, those who could afford care, and those who were close in vicinity to the chiropractor and who had transportation, were more likely to see a chiropractor. What this represents to the physician is a unique patient population with specific needs that must be addressed. Logically the majority of problems in the senior patient are represented by signs and symptoms that reflect the accumulation of lifelong environmental impact combined with decreased function of most organ systems. Ironically, signs and symptoms may be minimal or often minimized by the patient and may misdirect the doctor to the wrong organ system. Also, atypical presentations of common disorders are more likely in the senior.

The ultimate goal with the senior patient is to prevent or delay functional decline and restore and/or maintain function to allow as much independent living as possible.

It is clear that the ability for the senior to remain independent has a significant effect on his or her perceived quality of life.[7] Generally, independent living is more satisfying and less expensive than institutionalized living.

There are some myths with regard to senior citizen function and capacity. Following are some statistical corrections of these assumptions:[8]

- Only 5% of individuals over the age of 65 years live in nursing homes.
- Eighty-five percent of individuals between the ages of 65 and 69 years experience no difficulty in self-care activities or walking (66% of individuals between ages 80 and 84 years).[9]
- One-third of individuals over the age of 80 years have no difficulty walking a quarter of a mile, lifting 10 lb, or climbing 10 steps without resting.

The senior patient is often viewed with some degree of ambivalence. Often signs and symptoms are attributed to the normal aging process. It is logical that normal aging does result in some decreases in function; however, the distinction between this process and other disease processes is not always readily evident. Being cognizant of the effects of normal aging may facilitate a more focused examination allowing modification of the examiner's interpretation of "normal." Unfortunately, working off of the assumption that all decreases in function are age-related may delay intervention or allow a misdiagnosis that seriously restricts a patient's lifestyle; in turn, this may compound his or her problems.

One solution to this overgeneralization is not to look at all seniors as the same. Shepard[10] suggests dividing the elderly population into the following functional categories:

- Young-old: Patients who have maintained a level of fitness that allows participation in recreational and daily activity requirements.

- Middle-old: Patients who are independent with daily activities; however, they need assistance with more demanding tasks.
- Old-old: Disabled patients who require nursing care.

These three categories often correspond to the age categories of 65 to 75 years, 75 to 85 years, and older than 85 years, respectively. Generally, classifying a person as being a senior is based largely on social and political events that take place when a person reaches the age of 65 years.[11]

Second, it is important to understand those changes expected with aging and those that are the result of disuse or misuse (modifiable aspects). With this anticipation, the patient may also be educated as to what is normal and what is pathologic and perhaps become a more responsible partner in his or her healthcare. An educated patient and doctor may decrease the number of unnecessary visits and therefore increase the doctor's concern when a senior does have a complaint.

In the primary care setting, the 10 most common chronic conditions in the elderly, in decreasing order of occurrence, are as follows:[12]

1. Osteoarthritis
2. Hypertension
3. Hearing impairment
4. Heart disease
5. Orthopaedic deformity or impairment
6. Chronic sinusitis
7. Visual impairment
8. Diabetes
9. Varicose veins
10. Abdominal hernia

It is striking that four out of the five top conditions are treatable and in some cases preventable. The disability represented by many of these conditions may be minimized with appropriate strategies that allow for acceptable function. Heart disease, cancer, and stroke account for 75% of deaths in the senior population.[8] Campbell et al.,[13] performing a systematic review, evaluated the effects of various dosages of aspirin to determine the most desirable dose that would have the fewest gastrointestinal (GI) complications. Long-term use of dosages greater than 75 to 81 mg/D were found not to be any more effective, but did increase the risk of GI bleeding. It is important, however, to note some oddities with regard to mortality. One is that the suicide rate in the elderly

is five times the national average.[7] Second, the death rate from complications associated with a hip fracture is approximately 15%. Particular attention must be paid to the most common conditions seen in the elderly (see **Table 54–1**).

There are obviously numerous possible causes of morbidity and mortality in the senior. Most are addressed under the chapter associated with the related symptom or complaint. The focus of this chapter will be appropriate evaluation and screening of the senior patient, the most common diseases/disorders in this population, and the underlying physiologic and social causes of morbidity.

The doctor must always consider the following in evaluating the senior patient:

- Seniors often present atypically for a specific disease/disorder, usually due to symptoms in the most vulnerable organs rather than the organ of involvement (e.g., goiter, tremor, or exophthalmos are less common signs of hyperthyroidism as compared with atrial fibrillation, signs of heart failure, confusion, or weakness, because the "weakest link" in the older patient is more often the brain and cardiovascular system).
- An abrupt onset of symptoms or signs will usually represent a disease rather than "normal aging."
- Seniors are more likely to develop drug side effects and at lower doses.
- Seniors often suffer the effects of multi-pharmaceutical prescription.
- Seniors often develop symptoms at an earlier stage of disease due to a decreased physiologic reserve.
- Seniors have less reserve to deal with infections such as pneumonia or simple viral infections.
- Seniors are particularly vulnerable to the effects of inactivity, creating a downward spiral of disability and risk of injury mainly through falls and the continued inactivity during recovery from fractures.
- A substantial percentage of seniors are prone to depression and alcoholism.
- Seniors, in particular those being cared for, are often victims of verbal or physical abuse and/or neglect.
- Seniors who are "successful" at aging are more active physically, are involved socially, and adapt to their disabilities.

Table 54–1 Most Common Conditions Seen in the Elderly

Musculoskeletal	Cardiovascular/Renal
• Arthritis (osteoarthritis, rheumatoid arthritis, DISH [diffuse, idiopathic, skeletal hyperostosis], crystalline arthritides such as gout and pseudogout) • Osteoporosis (in particular in the postmenopausal female) and associated fractures • Paget's disease • Fat pad syndrome (common cause of heel pain)	• Congestive heart failure • Coronary artery disease and associated angina or myocardial infarction • Hypertension • Stroke • Abdominal aneurysm • Temporal arteritis • Chronic renal failure • Incontinence (stress incontinence and detrusor instability)

Neurologic and Neuropsychiatric	Female/Male Reproductive
• Alzheimer's • Parkinson's • Multi-infarct dementia • Depression • Normal pressure hydrocephalus	• Breast cancer • Ovarian cancer • Prostate cancer

Eyes, Ears, Nose, and Throat	Gastrointestinal
• Vision loss (includes cataract, glaucoma, age-related macular degeneration, amaurosis fugax, temporal arteritis, vitreoretinal traction) • Hearing loss (with focus on presbycusis) • Tinnitus • Chronic sinusitis	• Hiatal hernia and reflux • Constipation • Diverticulitis • Colorectal cancer

Endocrine	
• Diabetes • Hyperparathyroidism	

General Strategy

Evaluation

For all geriatric patients, perform a full baseline evaluation to include:

- a focused history
- an examination
- evaluation of mental function
- evaluation of socioeconomic health
- nutritional status
- risks to health including a screening for risk of falling, a thorough drug history, history of last examination for screening of senior-related disorders (e.g., colorectal cancer, breast cancer, prostate cancer, diabetes, hearing, glaucoma, cataracts)
- a nonfasting total blood cholesterol, urinalysis (dipstick for hematuria, bacteriuria, and proteinuria), mammography (up to age 75 years), and thyroid function tests (in older females) in asymptomatic seniors[14]
- an electrocardiogram, fecal occult blood, sigmoidoscopy or colonoscopy, fasting plasma glucose or glucose tolerance test, Pap smear (females), and tuberculin skin testing in high-risk seniors

The general strategy for the symptomatic patient includes:

- Consider the most common conditions seen in the elderly.

- Consider atypical presentations of common conditions.
- Consider that the symptoms may be the result of a drug or interactions of drugs.
- Screen for cancer if complaints include weight loss, night pain, unresponsiveness to previous care, or history of cancer.
- Perform a more comprehensive evaluation than in a younger patient, taking into account that symptoms or signs are more often the consequence of deterioration or dysfunction of the brain, cardiovascular, lower urinary tract, or musculoskeletal systems.

Management

For all geriatric patients:

- Establish a regular routine of an annual physical examination and focused examinations based on risk factors and national guideline recommendations. Give advice with regard to the general benefits of exercise and nutrition including the potential of prolonging functional capacities.
- Provide information with regard to reducing risk of disease.
- Provide information with regard to reducing the risk of falling.
- Provide the patient contacts for a support network of individuals or agencies including mobility, social contact, and care, including referral sources to other healthcare services.

For patients with diagnosed or suspected conditions:

- Refer patients who are suspected of having drug-related symptoms or signs to their prescribing physician.
- Refer patients with suspected cancer or serious visceral condition for further evaluation by a specialist.
- Comanage patients with hypertension, obesity, and non-insulin-dependent diabetes to aid in the support network for patient compliance with diet and exercise prescriptions.
- Manage musculoskeletal complaints with an emphasis on stability, pain reduction, and maintenance of as much joint mobility as possible.
- Modify adjusting procedures based on the patient's underlying health status and bone and joint integrity (see **Table 54–2**).

Relevant Anatomy and Physiology

Theories of Aging

There are many theories of aging; however, they can be organized into two main groups: (1) genetically determined, and (2) accumulated damage to key cellular processes. It seems clear that there are certain cultures in which age is independent of environment and must therefore have a strong genetic component. This has also been demonstrated with simple organisms; however, the degree to which this affects humans is unknown.

Change in technique approach or modification to most of the above presentations includes:

- Specific recommendations include:
  1. Flat hand contact for anterior thoracic maneuvers begun in supine position (versus seated to supine) or light-force techniques for osteoporotic patients
  2. Avoidance of excessive rotational techniques for neck and low back
  3. Avoidance of extreme spinal flexion positions with osteoporotic patients
  4. Allow the headpiece (i.e., elevated to position the head/neck in flexion) to provide support for patient's head/neck to allow for more relaxation
  5. With extremity adjusting, always provide some degree of distraction prior to thrusting and avoid thrusting into a full flexion or extension position
- Light-force technique options may be considered such as:
  1. Logan basic
  2. Distraction techniques (e.g., Cox traction)
  3. Pelvic blocking (e.g., Sacro-occipital technique [SOT])
  4. Instrumented adjusting (e.g., Activator)
- Soft-tissue approaches

There are generally two theories put forth regarding accumulated damage with aging. The first of these focuses on the damage caused by oxidative metabolism with the production of superoxide and hydroxyl free radicals (also hydrogen peroxide). The transcription of genes encoded for protective enzymes (e.g., superoxide dismutase, catalase) decreases with age. This has led to the recommendation by some nutritionists to supplement these enzymes.

Table 54–2 Yellow Flag Indicators of Caution with Possible Modification of Manipulative/Adjustive Procedures

Caution Disorder of Indicator	History or Exam Indicator(s)	Concern
Osteoporosis	• Suspicion due to age or posture • Radiographic confirmation	• Fracture
Scoliosis	• Adam's • Radiographic confirmation	• Which segments to adjust • Proper positioning of patient • Block vertebra
Spinal stenosis	• Patient presentation • Radiographic confirmation	• Risk of exacerbating symptoms • Proper positioning of patient
Spinal instability	• Past or current history of rheumatoid condition or trauma • Radiographic confirmation	• Spinal cord irritation
Diagnosis of disc herniation or sequestration	• Patient presentation • Physical examination indicators of nerve root or spinal cord involvement • MRI confirmation	• Exacerbation of symptoms
Previous surgery	• Patient report • Scars	• Instability • Damage to surgical stabilization
Use of corticosteroids or Cushing's disease	• Patient presentation • Past diagnosis • Current history of medications • Radiographic indicators	• Fracture
Use of anticoagulant medication	• Patient report	• Bleeding (e.g., subarachnoid bleeding)
Psychiatric disorder	• Indicators from history or questionnaire • Past diagnosis	• Abreactive response to manipulation
Previous adverse reaction to a specific therapy or therapeutic trial	• Past history from patient description	• Repeating adverse reaction
Acute pain presentation	• Patient presentation	• Increase in symptoms

The glycation theory postulates that glucose reactions with certain proteins and nucleic acids generate glycoadducts called advanced glycosylation end-products (AGEs). Through either cross-linkage or other modifications, molecules are altered, reducing certain key physiologic functions. Prevention of AGE formation has been demonstrated to retard the aging process in animals.

It is unclear whether the above indicators of increased damage or insufficient repair are the cause or the result of aging. Many of the theories regarding the mechanisms of aging have not been supported by the literature.[15] These theories include:

- somatic mutation theory—aging results from cumulative spontaneous mutations

- error catastrophe theory—aging is due to errors in protein synthesis
- intrinsic mutagenesis theory—aging results from DNA "rearrangements"

Age-Related Physiologic Changes

At the molecular level, aging does result in the following:

- protein deamidation, oxidation, cross-linking, and glycation increase
- DNA cross-linking
- single-strand breakage
- decrease in DNA methylation

- decrease in DNA telomeric sequences (length of telomeres)

On the macro level, there are age-related organ and system changes that must be considered when evaluating a patient's complaint or apparent dysfunction. **Table 54–3** illustrates some of these changes and the possible clinical consequence.

Evaluation

General Examination Approach

Comprehensive Geriatric Assessment

The approach to geriatric assessment is to gain a comprehensive appreciation of the total patient in order

Table 54–3 Consequences of "Normal" Aging

Structure	Changes	Clinical Consequences
Spine		
Intervertebral disk	Dry, fibrocartilaginous, islands of hyaline cartilage, little or no proteoglycans; after age 40 years virtually no nucleus pulposus	Disk herniation not likely in the elderly
Uncinate processes	Become flat, and project bone laterally and posterolaterally	Prevent disk herniation
Dural root sleeves	Become fibrotic and rigid	More prone to stretch injury
Spinal canal	Hypertrophied ligamentum flavum and osteophytes compromise canal space	Cord compression more likely than in younger patients
Zygapophyseal joints	Menisci have tendency to proliferate as a fibrous pannus	Joints less mobile
Cardiovascular		
Blood vessels	Some degree of atherosclerosis and thickening, which create aortic stiffening	Increase in blood pressure
Heart	Ventricular thickening in response to increased peripheral resistance, leading to LVH Decrease in pacemaker cells Decreased response to sympathetic, specifically beta-adrenergic, stimulation	Decrease in stroke volume
Baroreceptors	Decreased sensitivity	Decreased response to pressure changes
Respiratory		
Chest wall	Stiffening	Increases work of breathing
Lungs	Decrease in elastic tissue, destruction of alveolar septa, loss of capillaries, and calcification of bronchi	Reduction in various measures of air flow with an increase in residual volume
Gastrointestinal		
Esophagus	Diminished peristalsis amplitude and decreased lower sphincter tone	Slower transit time to stomach Reflux and hiatal hernia
Stomach	Decrease in acid production and hyposecretion of intrinsic factor	Digestion less effective B_{12} deficiency more common
Small intestine	Absorption functions decreased; in particular calcium	Decrease in vitamins B_{12}, C, and D

Table 54–3 Consequences of "Normal" Aging (continued)

Structure	Changes	Clinical Consequences
Liver	Slower biotransformation of lipid-soluble drugs Decrease in albumin production	Relative increase in drug bioavailability Serum concentrations of albumin decreased (liver function tests are normal)
Pancreas	Usually unimpaired	
Colon	Transit time is usually normal	Constipation is not necessarily a result of aging unless associated with diabetes or other disorders
Genitourinary		
Kidney	Shrinkage with loss of almost half of the glomeruli	Decreased excretion function (significant with drugs)
Bladder	Bladder capacity, bladder and urethral elasticity are reduced (combined with decrease in CNS inhibition)	Nocturia and frank incontinence increase with age
Endocrine		
Female	Ovarian secretion of estrogens and progestins ends	Atrophic changes in uterus, vagina, and mammary glands
Male	Increased prostatic binding of dihydrotestosterone	Prostatic hypertrophy
Blood sugar	Decreased peripheral response to insulin (pancreatic function of insulin secretion is usually normal)	Fasting blood sugar increases 5 mg/dL per decade after age 50 years (do not confuse with diabetes)
Thyroid	Thyroid function should not decline with age; however, the thyroid may migrate down toward manubrium	Thyroid function tests are normal. Palpate lower in elderly for thyroid.
Musculoskeletal		
Bone	After age 40 years, bone mass decreases by 5%–10% per decade (faster in women until seventh decade)	Osteopenia more likely, leading to susceptibility to compression fractures of the spine and hip fractures
Muscle	Decrease in muscle mass (increase in fat)	Gradually declining strength; may be more susceptible to injury
Nervous System		
Brain	Shrinkage of cerebral sulci and enlargement of gyri with fibrosis of meninges; 20%–25% loss of cerebral and cerebellar neurons; lipofuscin accumulates Decrease in stage 4 sleep Decrease in dopaminergic synthesis	More susceptible to subdural hematoma with minor head trauma
Peripheral nerves	Slower transmission; velocity decreases by 10%	Reaction time and adaptive responses to posture
Eyes/ears	Decreased accommodation and increased lens opacity Decrease in high-frequency perception	May need more light and possibly cataract surgery May have difficulty hearing in noisy rooms

Key: LVH, left ventricular hypertrophy; CNS, central nervous system.

to establish a baseline for comparison and to avoid or prevent potential risks for disease, misdiagnosis, and functional decline.[16] The intention is to provide the best care and advice to an older patient in the hope of extending the quality and sometimes quantity of life. A comprehensive database is also useful in communication with the patient's other healthcare providers.

History Strategies

In addition to eliciting a history of chief complaint in those presenting with complaints, it is important to include a screening history of current drug history, dietary history, history of falling, history of incontinence, and questioning or questionnaires evaluating possible depression, anxiety, and mental functioning. It is also important to include a history of significant medical events such as surgeries, illnesses, accidents, and any diagnosed conditions. *Significant* may be defined as a condition or event that resulted in an appreciable loss of time at work, hospitalization, or being bedridden. Family history questions are less crucial given that many hereditary or family-related disorders would have appeared at an earlier age. Those factors that have significance to the elderly include a family history of cancer (in particular colon cancer and breast cancer), Alzheimer's, Huntington's chorea, osteoporosis, and hypertension. Questioning regarding mental function is addressed later.

Examination Strategies

All seniors should have baseline vitals taken on the first visit, and more frequently than younger patients on subsequent visits. Establishing a baseline is particularly important for height and weight. For patients who have not had a physical within the previous year or for patients who do not have a medical physician, it is requisite to perform a comprehensive evaluation of the whole person with particular focus on senior-related concerns. **Table 54–4** outlines the various portions of a comprehensive senior examination and the specific concern or focus of each.

Physical Examination Focus

Vitals

It is particularly important to check vital signs frequently with older patients. The role of the initial measurements is to establish a baseline from which to make future comparisons. This is especially important when trying to determine if there has been significant weight loss (i.e., possible cancer, depression, or metabolic dysfunction) or significant height loss (i.e., osteoporotic vertebral compression fractures). The senior response to infection and inflammation may be blunted. It is important to establish the patient's baseline temperature on a well visit for

Table 54–4 Important Aspects of the Physical Examination of Older Patients

Area	Pathology Screen	Examination
Eyes	Acuity (far/near vision)	Snellen eye chart, normal print
	Macular degeneration	Grid matrix
		Peripheral fields by confrontation
	Cataracts	Lens opacification
	Glaucoma	Funduscopic (increased cupping)
Head	Temporal arteritis	Palpate temporal arteries for tenderness, nodularity, and pulsations, scalp tenderness and nodules
Ears	Hearing	Hand-held audioscope
		Free-field voice testing at 0.6 m (e.g., "What is your first name?" is a simple question even for the individual with cognitive impairments)
		Weber, Rinne tests
		Hearing Handicap Inventory for the Elderly
Mouth	Gingivitis	Inspect for erythematous, edematous gingiva, bleeding gums, loose teeth, exposure of the root surfaces of the teeth
	Dentures	Check fit, food debris, bacterial plaque
	Oral cancers	Inspect for persistent erythroplasia

Table 54–4 Important Aspects of the Physical Examination of Older Patients (continued)

Area	Pathology Screen	Examination
Neck	Decreased mobility	Range of motion, observe dizziness
	Thyroid disease	Palpate thyroid for nodules or enlargement
	Jugular venous pulse	Check on right side of neck
	Carotid artery stenosis	Bruits
Thorax	Chronic obstructive pulmonary disease	Chest expansion
	Lung disease	Auscultation
Cardiovascular	Orthostatic hypotension	Measure blood pressure supine and upright (a drop of 20 mm Hg or more systolic and 10 mm Hg or more diastolic)
Breasts	Breast cancer	Annual clinical breast examination
Back	Vertebral compression fracture	Spinous percussion
	Osteoporosis	Kyphosis
Abdomen	Osteoporosis	Skin bunched into folds from collapse of multiple vertebra
	Urinary retention	Percussion of suprapubic area
	Aortic aneurysm	Lateral or anteroposterior pulsatile mass, bruit
	Constipation	Palpable mass
Prostate	Cancer	Palpable, hard nodule
	Benign prostatic hypertrophy	Enlarged, smooth soft prostate
Gynecologic	Stress incontinence	Pad test (have patient cover urethral area with a small pad and cough forcefully three times in the standing position to check for leakage of urine)
Extremities	Decreased mobility	Range of motion
	Arterial insufficiency	Peripheral pulses, temperature, ulcers
	Diabetic foot	Ulcers, fungal infections
	Falls	Check for proper footwear
Skin	Hydration status	Check skin turgor
	Senile purpura	Dorsum of hand and forearm
	Actinic keratosis	Sun-exposed areas of skin
	Physical abuse	Unexplained bruising
	Melanoma	Lesion larger than 6 mm across, deep black areas, irregular borders and shape
Neurologic	Balance	Push gently with eyes open, then closed
	Range of motion	Seated: Place hands behind head and back, touch toes (if normal, has adequate range of motion to allow normal grooming and dressing)
	Gait and mobility	Ask patient to sit and then rise from armless chair, ask patient to walk across room, turn 180°, and return to chair
	Gait	Normal older female: Waddling, narrow-based, decreased arm swing
		Normal older male: Wider-based, smaller-stepped, decreased arm swing
	Parkinsonism	Short steps, shuffling feet, stooped trunk, decreased arm swing, festination, tendency to fall backward
	Pernicious anemia	Sensory ataxic gait (wide based)
	Motor tone	Check for spasticity, lead pipe stiffness, paratonia
	Tremor	Check for Parkinson's disease, cerebellar dysfunction, hyperthyroidism, or essential tremor
	Vibratory sense	Normal decrease (especially in lower extremities)
	Primitive reflexes	Normal release (snout, glabella, palmomental)

future comparison. Generally, a rise above 1.33°C (2.4°F) is a significant rise and should be investigated.

Blood pressure (BP) measurements are important for two reasons: (1) to determine if the patient has hypertension, and (2) to determine if the patient has orthostatic hypotension (common side effect of medications and secondary to diabetes). Blood pressure and pulse are measured with the patient seated and standing. Systolic pressure often increases with age. In the patient age 65 years or older a BP of 160/90 mm Hg constitutes the beginning level of mild hypertension. An isolated systolic BP over 160 mm Hg without an associated proportionate increase in the diastolic pressure warrants a referral for medical management. A pseudohypertension may be present due to stiff arteries. Osler's maneuver attempts to distinguish this type from true hypertension.[17] While taking the pulse, the artery proximal to the pulse is occluded with a finger or BP cuff. If the distal pulse remains unchanged, there may be sufficient stiffness in the arteries to falsely raise the BP measurement.

Orthostatic hypotension is common in the senior and may account for complaints of lightheadedness or falling when rising from a lying or seated position. If the pulse increases less than 10 beats per minute or the blood pressure drops from a lying to a seated position, a baroreceptor reflex dysfunction may be the cause. Generally, if the systolic BP drops 15 mm Hg or the diastolic BP decreases 10 mm Hg after moving from a lying to seated or seated to standing position, the patient has orthostatic hypotension. The most fruitful line of questioning is about medication. Common causes are antihypertensive medications. Also, diabetes may blunt the reflex splanchnic vasoconstrictive response that should occur on rising.

Respiratory rate for the older patient is within the range of 12 to 20 breaths per minute. If the rate is above this normal range, investigate the possibility of a lower respiratory tract infection.

Eyesight and Hearing

Approximately 8% of U.S. seniors are significantly visually impaired.[18] In addition to using either a Snellen eye chart or a handheld Jaeger chart, the Activities of Daily Vision Scale helps determine functional capacity of those with vision loss.[14] Visual impairment places the individual at risk of falls and others at risk due to motor vehicle accidents. Several disorders are more common in the senior including age-related macular degeneration, glaucoma, cataracts, vitreoretinal traction, and amaurosis fugax (see Chapter 42).

Significant hearing loss is claimed by only 30% of older individuals; however, when tested with audiometric evaluation, 60% of individuals over the age of 70 years have a deficit. Routine screening should be part of all initial geriatric assessments given the psychosocial impact and commonality of this problem in the elderly. A handheld audioscope is a useful screening tool for detecting significant hearing loss, particularly in the frequency range for speech. The most common age-related problem in seniors is presbycusis (see Chapter 45). It is believed that this dysfunction involves the loss of high-frequency hearing first due to degeneration of the hair cells in the organ of Corti.

Functional Assessment

Although many disorders of the elderly are not reversible, many individuals can adapt and function enough to retain their independence. A functional assessment is as important, if not more important, than a diagnosis in determining a patient's ability to function independently. Assessments are based on questions or questionnaires that focus on self-assessment. The basic intention is to determine a patient's ability to care for himself or herself.

Activities of Daily Living

The assessment of self-care functions is often divided into three categories: (1) basic activities of daily living (ADLs), (2) intermediate ADLs, and (3) advanced ADLs. The basic ADLs include:

- bathing
- dressing/grooming
- self-feeding
- toileting
- maintaining continence (bowel/bladder)
- mobility level
- transferring (within the home)

The activities assessed have a somewhat hierarchical order. For example, if bathing is possible many of the following functions are available: continence, dressing, feeding, completing one's toilet, and transfer.

Intermediate ADLs include:

- using the telephone
- preparing meals
- performing work around the house
- doing laundry
- shopping

- transportation
- self-medication
- managing money

Advanced ADLs include:

- strenuous physical activity (e.g., hiking, bicycling, running, walking briskly)
- heavy work around the house
- number of times one can walk 1 mile or more without rest
- number of times one can walk a quarter of a mile or more without rest

The ADL score is an important indicator of health outcome compared with basing the prediction of outcome on a diagnosis.[19]

Ancillary Testing

As with all patients, it is imperative that the following questions be posed prior to ordering what often is expensive, and occasionally uncomfortable, testing:

- What is the likelihood that the test will introduce information that appears to be related, yet has no proven relationship to the patient's complaint or dysfunction?
- What is the cost of the test and the ability of the patient to cover that cost?
- What is the availability of the test?
- Does the confirmation of a disorder by use of the test alter the treatment plan or prognosis for the patient?

Radiographic Evaluation

Many bone- and joint-related disorders are manifested by characteristic radiographic changes. The value in radiographs is therefore quite high in the differential diagnosis of musculoskeletal pain. However, the correlation between these findings, clinical symptoms, and patient function is not as directly related as might be assumed. Studies have indicated that radiographic indications of spinal degeneration, in either the cervical or lumbar spine, do not correlate with an increased incidence of pain or dysfunction.[20] Bone scans may be a useful tool for the evaluation of primary cancer or metastasis. Refer to Chapter 1 for a comparison of magnetic resonance imaging (MRI) to computed tomography (CT) in the evaluation of musculoskeletal disorders.

Laboratory Values

Clear data on the geriatric reference ranges for many tests are lacking. Each laboratory makes an attempt at adjusting the reference range based on gender and age; however, the ranges vary from lab to lab. The following information may help guide the ordering and interpretation of laboratory findings on the older patient:

- Erythrocyte sedimentation rate (ESR) increases with age at a rate of 0.22 mm/hour/year beginning at age 20 years. Also, this test is easily affected by handling variations leading to increased values. Generally, unless values are above 50 mm/hour it is unlikely that any significant disorder is present. Levels above 80 mm/hour do correlate with the finding of neoplasm, rheumatic disease, or infection.[21]
- The definition of anemia by the World Health Organization (WHO) is a hemoglobin concentration below 7.5 mmol/L (120 g/L) in women and below 8.3 mmol/L (130 g/L) in men. Values below this level correlate well in establishing a concern in the elderly with an increased mortality risk (e.g., infection, malignant neoplasms, and respiratory disease) two times that of individuals with normal hemoglobin concentrations. Therefore, a low hemoglobin concentration indicates significant disease in the older patient. Eighty percent of anemic women and 92% of anemic men have normocytic anemia.[22]
- The level of antinuclear antibodies (ANA) is somewhat age-dependent, with a rise of 16% of normal older individuals having a positive ANA evaluation.
- Rheumatoid factor (RF) increases with age to 15% to 25% of healthy individuals testing positive in the age group over 70 years.
- Serum albumin level may decrease with kidney disease, especially in patients with rheumatoid arthritis (RA) or systemic lupus erythematosus (SLE); however, malnutrition, which is common in the elderly, may also be a cause. A screening for malnutrition is to check for decreased serum albumin (4 g/dL or less) and/or a decreased cholesterol level (160 mg/dL or less).
- Caution must be used in interpreting a finding of a monoclonal protein in the serum or urine. As many as 10% to 23% of patients between the ages of 75 and 84 years tested positive for a monoclonal

protein.[23] In one study,[24] 55% had a monoclonal gammopathy of unknown origin, 18% had multiple myeloma, and 12% had amyloidosis. The distinction between multiple myeloma and that of monoclonal gammopathy of undetermined significance (MGUS) is that those with MGUS have immunoglobulin G (IgG) monoclonal protein less than 3.5 g/dL or IgA less than 2 g/dL with Bence-Jones protein (<1 g/24 hour) and less than 10% plasma cells in the bone marrow. There are no bony lesions, anemia, hypercalcemia, or renal insufficiency with MGUS. Still, about 30% of MGUS patients develop a malignant process in the future. Stability of the monoclonal protein levels over time is more predictive of a benign outcome.

Focused Concerns

Mental Health

Mental Health Status Evaluation

The most common mental health problems seen in older patients are dementia, depression, and delirium. Each condition may mimic the other. The consequences of mistaking one condition for the other is that management is often entirely different. For example, if a patient is incorrectly diagnosed as having dementia, or more specifically Alzheimer's disease (AD), when in fact the patient is severely depressed, effective treatment may be withheld and major decisions regarding institutionalized living versus independent living may be made with an unfortunate outcome for the patient.

Age-related memory loss is distinct from other causes. It has been demonstrated that with age-related memory decline, there is no decline in language, visuo-spatial skills, or abstract reasoning.[25] Also, the decline with age-related memory loss is specific to the acquisition and early retrieval of new information, and not memory retention. Anatomically, this correlates with the hippocampal formation. Dementia is defined as the development of multiple cognitive deficits, not memory deficits alone. The severity must be enough to impair occupational or social functioning and must be shown to decline compared with previous functioning. The two main causes of dementia are Alzheimer's disease and multi-infarct dementia (MID). Characteristically, the clinical presentation is distinct. MID is characterized by

a more abrupt onset of focal neurologic signs that have a stepwise deterioration. Associated factors are hypertension and other signs of cardiovascular or atherosclerotic disease. Common motor problems that more often dominate MID are dysarthria, dysphasia, pseudobulbar paralysis, seizures, and gait disturbances, with pathologic reflexes sometimes evident.

The differential diagnosis for dementia should also include a multitude of other causes as illustrated by the mnemonic DEMENTIA:[26]

- **D**rugs
- **E**motional illness including depression
- **M**etabolic/endocrine disorders
- **E**yes/ear/environment
- **N**utritional/neurologic
- **T**umors/trauma
- **I**nfection
- **A**lcoholism/anemia/atherosclerosis

The work-up (in addition to evaluation of mental function as discussed below) includes a neurologic and cardiovascular evaluation. Neurologic deficits are unusual with early and intermediate AD. Laboratory testing must include vitamin B_{12} and thyroid function. Additional tests may include folate, blood urea nitrogen (BUN) and creatinine, hematocrit and hemoglobin, alanine transaminase, glucose, electrolytes, venereal disease research laboratories (VDRL), and calcium. An electrocardiogram and electroencephalogram should be ordered if seizures are present. In the search for structural central nervous system (CNS) causes, an MRI or CT may be necessary.

Delirium is more often an acute, reversible brain dysfunction associated with many disorders. The onset is usually abrupt and associated with illness, drugs, or acute metabolic imbalances. The symptoms often fluctuate frequently (even within minutes); they are often worse late in the day (sundowning). Clouding of consciousness, confusion, irritability, inappropriate behavior, delusions, and hallucinations are all characteristic of delirium. The distinguishing tests are the same as for dementia; however, the urgency for an early diagnosis is important due to the reversibility of delirium in many cases.

In the portal of entry of the primary care setting, various tools and questionnaires are available to screen individuals at risk. In the distinction among delirium, depression, and dementia, it is helpful to use screening tools prior to laboratory testing or neuropsychologic testing. A test designed to screen for the five most common mental/behavioral disorders is the PRIME-MD (Primary Care Evaluation of Mental Disorders).[27] These disorders include depression, anxiety, alcohol abuse, somatoform disorders, and eating disorders. The first versions were administered by the doctor and took approximately 8 to 10 minutes. The most recent version is the self-administered PRIME-MD Patient Health Questionnaire (PHQ).[28] This tool has been shown to be diagnostically valid and efficient.

The most commonly used test when patients appear to have a memory or other cognitive dysfunction is the Mini-Mental Status Exam (MMSE). This cognitive screening examination assesses orientation, language, attention, concentration, mental flexibility (i.e., working memory), short-term memory, and constructional praxis (see **Exhibit 54–1**). The MMSE does not test abstract thinking or judgment, and it is more sensitive to left-hemisphere dysfunction than right. A score range of 0 to 30 is possible.

Exhibit 54–1 The Annotated Mini-Mental State Examination (AMMSE)

NAME OF SUBJECT _____   Age _____

NAME OF EXAMINER _____   Years of School Completed _____

Approach the patient with respect and encouragement.   Date of Examination _____

Ask: Do you have any trouble with your memory?   ☐ Yes   ☐ No

May I ask you some questions about your memory?   ☐ Yes   ☐ No

SCORE ITEM

5 (   ) TIME ORIENTATION

Ask:

What is the year _____(1),   season _____ (1),

month of the year _____(1),   date _____ (1),

day of the week _____(1)?

5 (   ) PLACE ORIENTATION

Ask:

Where are we now? What is the state _____ (1), city _____ (1),

part of the city _____ (1), building _____ (1),

floor of the building _____ (1)?

3 (   ) REGISTRATION OF THREE WORDS

Say: Listen carefully. I am going to say three words. You say them back after I stop. Ready? Here they are . . . PONY (wait 1 second), QUARTER (wait 1 second), ORANGE (wait 1 second). What were those words?

_____ (1)

_____ (1)

_____ (1)

Give 1 point for each correct answer, then repeat them until the patient learns all three.

(continues)

Exhibit 54–1 **(continued)**

5 ( ) SERIAL 7s AS A TEST OF ATTENTION AND CALCULATION

Ask: Subtract 7 from 100 and continue to subtract 7 from each subsequent remainder until I tell you to stop.

What is 100 take away 7? _____ (1)

Say:

Keep going. _____ (1), _____ (1),

_____ (1), _____ (1).

3 ( ) RECALL OF THREE WORDS

Ask:

What were those three words I asked you to remember?

Give one point for each correct answer. _____ (1),

_____ (1), _____(1).

2 ( ) NAMING

Ask:

What is this? (show pencil) _____ (1). What is this? (show watch) _____ (1).

1 ( ) REPETITION

Say:

Now I am going to ask you to repeat what I say. Ready? No ifs, ands, or buts.

Now you say that. _____ (1)

3 ( ) COMPREHENSION

Say:

Listen carefully because I am going to ask you to do something:

Take this paper in your left hand (1), fold it in half (1), and put it on the floor (1).

1 ( ) READING

Say:

Please read the following and do what it says, but do not say it aloud. (1)

Close your eyes

1 ( ) WRITING

Say:

Please write a sentence. If patient does not respond, say: Write about the weather. (1)

_____

_____

1 ( ) DRAWING

Say: Please copy this design

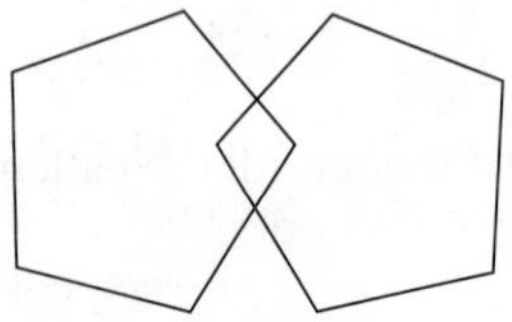

Exhibit 54–1 **(continued)**

TOTAL SCORE _____ Assess level of consciousness along a continuum

	Alert	Drowsy	Stupor	Coma

	YES	NO
Cooperative:	☐	☐
Depressed:	☐	☐
Anxious:	☐	☐
Poor Vision:	☐	☐
Poor Hearing:	☐	☐
Native Language: _____		
Deterioration from previous level of functioning:	☐	☐
Family History of Dementia:	☐	☐
Head Trauma:	☐	☐
Stroke:	☐	☐
Alcohol Abuse:	☐	☐
Thyroid Disease:	☐	☐

FUNCTION BY PROXY

Please record date when patient was last able to perform the following tasks. Ask caregiver if patient independently handles:

	YES	NO	DATE
Money/Bills:	☐	☐	_____
Medication:	☐	☐	_____
Transportation:	☐	☐	_____
Telephone:	☐	☐	_____

Information from "Mini-Mental State." A Practical Method for Grading the Cognitive State of Patients for the Clinician, *Journal of Psychiatric Research*, 12(3):189–198, 1975, © 1975, 1998 MiniMental LLC.

If a score of 24 is used as a cutoff point for normal, the MMSE has a sensitivity of 87% to 90% and a specificity of 80% to 82%.[29] Adjusted for education level, a score of 17 or less is abnormal in those with eight or fewer years of education. For all others, a score below 24 would direct a search for the types of questions missed. Alzheimer's patients often fail the memory portion. Another quick screening assessment for nonverbal ability is the Draw-a-Clock test. Alzheimer's patients do poorly on this task. The patient is asked to draw a clock with all the hour numbers on it. They are then asked to place hands on the clock to read 11:15.

Alzheimer's Disease

AD is the most common cause of dementia in the United States and accounts for approximately 65% to 75% of all cases.[30] There are more than 4 million Americans affected by AD. Women with AD live longer than men with AD and as a result, represent twice as many cases. The combined cost of direct management and lost productivity is currently at least $100 billion annually.[31] AD is characterized pathologically by the accumulation of senile plaques in the cerebral cortex and subcortical gray matter. These plaques contain β-amyloid and neurofibrillary tangles made up of tau protein. The cause of AD is not entirely understood. However, the elevation of amyloid-peptide prior to the development of significant tau pathology suggests an initiating role in mediating pathologic progression, especially in the frontal cortex.[32] The enzyme responsible for the accumulation of amyloid appears to have been uncovered. It appears that β-secretase splitting of the Alzheimer amyloid precursor protein is by the transmembrane aspartic protease (BACE) enzyme.[33] Future therapeutic strategies will be focused on inhibition of endogenous BACE messenger-RNA and other related approaches. There are some common features of neurodegenerative disorders. One feature is that overstimulation of the N-methyl-D-aspartate (NMDA) receptor by glutamate leads to neuronal damage in a phenomenon termed *excitotoxicity*. It is believed that such excitotoxicity leads to neuronal calcium overload. An approved drug, memantine, is an uncompetitive NMDA-receptor antagonist (antiglutamatergic) that may be effective in reducing clinical deterioration in moderate to severe AD.[34]

There are many risk factors, but, most define only subgroups at risk. For example, the early-onset form of AD is associated with an autosomal-dominant transmission with gene mutations on chromosomes 21, 14, and 1. However, this accounts for only 2% of all cases of AD. Associated with the more common, late-onset AD is the presence of the *APOEε4* allele on chromosome 19.[35] The presence of a single allele increases the risk of AD twoto fourfold, whereas the presence of the double *ε4* allele increases the risk four- to eightfold. Those patients with the *APOE ε4* allele in combination with atherosclerosis, peripheral vascular disease, or diabetes mellitus are at substantially higher risk of cognitive decline.[36] However, it is not currently recommended to use genotyping as a predictive test in asymptomatic individuals because having the *APOEε4* allele does not consistently predict AD, and not having it does not protect an individual from acquiring AD. Other factors being investigated are:

- Hyperhomocysteinemia. Patients in the upper third of serum homocysteine have at least a twofold increase in risk of developing AD (independent of all other known risk factors).[37] Also, an inverse relationship exists between serum folate and vitamin B_{12} levels and risk of AD. It is unknown whether decreased levels are functionally related to hyperhomocysteinemia.
- In a recent study, serum total cholesterol levels were not associated with an increased risk for AD.[38]

- A recent study indicates that depression is a possible risk factor for AD.[39] Depression, in addition to contributing to a higher risk of suicide attempt, also appears to be a risk factor for coronary heart disease.[40] Associated is the growing evidence that low Vitamin D levels are associated with the risk for AD.
- The effects of estrogen on prevention of dementia have been well documented, including neurotrophic effects, reductions in β-amyloid accumulation, augmentation of neurotransmitters, and some oxidative damage control.[41, 42] Estrogen receptors are found in areas of the brain related to memory and learning, including the hippocampus and amygdala. Yet recent studies have failed to demonstrate a significant effect in large populations of postmenopausal females. In fact, a randomized controlled study indicated there was no beneficial effect for estrogen therapy in women with known Alzheimer's.[43] Combined therapy with estrogen and progestin appears to increase the risk to some extent. A Women's Health Initiative project evaluating estrogen/progestin therapy and stroke provided data that indicated an increased risk of ischemic (but not hemorrhagic) stroke in generally healthy postmenopausal women.[44] A memory study portion of the Women's Health Initiative concluded that estrogen/progestin combination therapy did not improve cognitive function in postmenopausal women 65 years or older, and in fact may cause a small increased risk of clinically meaningful cognitive decline.[45] A part of the same study indicated increased risk for probable dementia.[46]
- Smoking. Although smoking has been found to increase the risk for AD, quitting smoking may cause a slight reduction in risk for AD.[47]
- Hippocampal atrophy. Hippocampal atrophy based on premorbid MRI-based volume measurement may be predictive for conversion to AD in patients with mild cognitive impairment.[48]
- Cerebrospinal fluid (CSF). CSF levels of β-amyloid appear to be decreased in patients with AD as compared with normal individuals.[49]

Factors that may be protective for AD include higher education, nonsteroid anti-inflammatory drugs (NSAIDs), vitamins D and E, and high monounsaturated fatty acid intake.[50,51]

The diagnosis of AD is both one of exclusion and inclusion. Although a definitive diagnosis cannot be made without autopsy or biopsy of the brain, there are clinical distinguishing features described in the *Diagnostic and Statistical Manual of Mental Disorders,* fifth edition (DSM-V).[52]

- The development of multiple cognitive impairments that impact significantly on the occupational or social functioning of the patient. This decline is significant when compared with previous levels of functioning. The decline is not associated with any other known cause of dementia or delirium.
- Memory impairment and one or more of the following: aphasia, apraxia, agnosia, or disturbance in executive functioning (i.e., planning, organizing, sequencing).

Other distinguishing factors are:

- A slower onset than a vascular cause of dementia or delirium
- Late onset of motor dysfunction
- Classic behavioral problems including:
  1. sundowning (late-day agitation)
  2. wandering
  3. sleep disturbances

The differential diagnosis is discussed above under dementia.

Management of AD is complex, involving not just the patient but also the caregiver. Early diagnosis and a correct diagnosis are important for future planning regarding living environment, supervision and care, and estate planning. The caregiver now has access to centers and groups offering training, support, and counseling. The AD patient cannot be cured; however, the process may be slowed or the cognitive and behavioral problems may be managed medically. For the cognitive impairment associated with AD, the primary medications are cholinesterase inhibitors such as tacrine (Cognex) and donepezil (Aricept). These drugs inhibit degradation of acetylcholine at the synaptic cleft. Cholinesterase inhibitors appear to provide modest benefit on neuropsychiatric and functional outcomes for mild to moderate Alzheimer's disease.[53] Memantine, is an uncompetitive NMDA-receptor antagonist (antiglutamatergic) and has been shown to be effective in reducing clinical deterioration in moderate to severe AD.[34] **Table 54–5** is a list of common medications used in the management of AD. Disease-altering strategies include the use of *ginkgo biloba* extract, vitamin E, monounsaturated fatty acids, NSAIDs, and estrogen (see **Table 54–6**).[54,55] A recent randomized, double-blind, placebo-controlled study[56] did not demonstrate any effect of slowing AD in women

Table 54–5 Alzheimer's Medications

Drug Class	Examples	General Mechanism	Interactions/Side Effects
Cholinesterase inhibitors	**Donepezil HCL** Aricept	A cholinesterase inhibitor used in the management of mild to moderate Alzheimer's disease. Works in the cerebral cortex blocking degradation of acetylcholine.	May cause headache, fatigue, insomnia, nausea, diarrhea, vomiting, cramps, anorexia, or muscle cramps.
	Tacrine Cognex	A cholinesterase inhibitor used in the management of mild to moderate Alzheimer's disease. Works in the cerebral cortex blocking degradation of acetylcholine.	May cause headache, fatigue, insomnia, nausea, diarrhea, vomiting, cramps, anorexia, or muscle cramps
	Rivastigmine tartrate Exelon	A cholinesterase inhibitor used in the management of mild to moderate Alzheimer's disease. Works in the cerebral cortex blocking degradation of acetylcholine.	May cause headache, fatigue, insomnia, nausea, diarrhea, vomiting, cramps, anorexia, or muscle cramps
NMDA-receptor antagonist	**Memantine** Axura Namenda	Memantine is an uncompetitive NMDA-receptor antagonist (antiglutamatergic) and has been shown to be effective in reducing clinical deterioration in moderate to severe Alzheimer's.	May cause emotional agitation, confusion, stomach upset, and nervousness.
Butyrophenone derivative	**Haloperidol** Haldol Peridol	A butyrophenone derivative similar to phenothiazines but with more extrapyramidal effects and less hypotensive and sedative effects. Used for psychotic disorders, tics, Tourette's syndrome, management of agitated states with Alzheimer's, and severe behavioral problems with children.	May cause extrapyramidal effects such as Parkinsonian symptoms, tardive dyskinesias, neuroleptic malignant syndrome. Agranulocytosis, laryngospasm, hyponatremia, hyperglycemia, and EEG changes.

Table 54–6 Nutritional Support for Dementia

Substance	How Might It Work?	Dosage	Special Instructions	Contraindications for Possible Side Effects
Gingko (*ginkgo biloba*)	Has antioxidant properties and platelet-inhibiting activity; may be neuroprotective and may improve circulation.	120–240 mg twice daily	None	Gastrointestinal upset and transient headache may occur in first few days of use. Interactions with anticoagulants may occur. Pregnancy and lactation are not contraindications.
Ginseng (Panax ginseng)	An adaptogen that enhances the immune system and acts also as an energizer and mood elevator (especially in the elderly).	0.5 to 1 g in two divided doses (capsules commonly contain 250 mg of the root/capsule); can also be taken as a tea with 3 g (1 teaspoon) ginseng steeped in 1 cup boiling water for 5–10 minutes.	Take in the morning and evening on an empty stomach. Limit the use to 3 months at a time.	Massive overdosages may result in ginseng abuse syndrome with sleeplessness, hypertonia, and edema.
Vitamin E	Antioxidant used to prevent progression of Alzheimer's disease.	2,000 IU/day	None	None at recommended dosage.
Acetyl-L-carnitine	Contributes to the production of acetylcholine.	1 g taken three times daily	None	Rare reports of skin rash, increased appetite, and body odor.
Coenzyme Q10	Assists in mitochondrial function.	Minimum dose usually 90–150 mg/day	Take with iron and B_6 (according to study demonstrating effect).	Congestive heart failure patients should not abruptly discontinue use.

Note: The following have not been approved by the Food and Drug Administration for the treatment of this disorder.

who took estrogen replacement therapy (ERT) for one year. It appears that ERT may not slow the progression, but more research is needed to determine if it has a protective effect if started early enough. Novel approaches are being developed for the treatment of AD. One approach is based on the observation that mice minus one-third of the cells needed for cognitive function were able to regain cognitive function when their brains were infused with nerve growth factor (NGF).[57] Apparently, this research implies that function of the remaining cells can be enhanced enough to make up for the loss of other cells.

A promising study was published in 2008 that indicates that a novel approach to Alzheimer's may be effective. Reger et al.[58] found that intranasal insulin improved cognition and actually modulated beta-amyloid in patients with early AD. This follows on the heels of an earlier publication that indicated that insulin increased levels of cerebrospinal fluid norepinephrine in normal patients, which correlated with better

cognition.[59] Dimebon (dimebolin) is an antihistamine showing promise.

Two reports of note involve the Mediterranean diet (MeDi) and a decrease in risk for Alzheimer's, as well as a decrease in mortality with Alzheimer's.[60, 61] A MeDi is high in vegetables, fruits, legumes, and cereals, high in unsaturated fatty acids (primarily olive oil), low in saturated fatty acids, a moderately high intake of fish, meat, and poultry, a moderate amount of wine (usually with meals), and a low intake of dairy products. Interestingly, according to one recent study,[62] a low-carbohydrate diet may not be preventive as some suggest.

Depression

Although when compared with younger patients, older patients are affected less often (7% to 10% of community dwellers) by obvious depression, atypical presentations are more common in the elderly.[63] Most specifically is the misdiagnosis of dementia (i.e., memory loss), when in fact depression is the cause (i.e., pseudodementia). Also, older patients may suffer from the depression associated with chronic disease, cancer, and prescribed medications. Some drugs that can cause depressive symptoms include antibiotics, anticonvulsants, antihypertensives, antineoplastic agents, antiparkinsonian agents, corticosteroids, digitalis, and hormones. Depression is covered more extensively in Chapter 20; however, for the older patient two screening tools may be useful: the Beck Depression Inventory (BDI) and the Geriatric Depression Scale (GDS).[64] These questionnaires can identify almost 90% of patients with depression. The longer version of the GDS takes approximately 10 to 15 minutes to fill out, whereas the shorter 15-item version (GDS15) takes only a few minutes and is recommended by some groups as the screening tool of choice (see **Exhibit 54–2**).[65] The BDI

Exhibit 54–2 Geriatric Depression Scale

	Yes/No Key
Are you basically satisfied with your life?	no
Have you dropped many of your activities and interests?	yes
Do you feel that your life is empty?	yes
Do you often get bored?	yes
Are you hopeful about the future?	no
Are you bothered by thoughts you can't get out of your head?	yes
Are you in good spirits most of the time?	no
Are you afraid that something bad is going to happen to you?	yes
Do you feel happy most of the time?	no
Do you often feel helpless?	yes
Do you often get restless and fidgety?	yes
Do you prefer to stay at home rather than go out and do new things?	yes
Do you frequently worry about the future?	yes
Do you feel you have more problems with memory than most people?	yes
Do you think it is wonderful to be alive now?	no
Do you often feel downhearted and blue?	yes
Is it hard for you to get started on new projects?	yes
Do you feel full of energy?	no
Do you feel that your situation is hopeless?	yes
Do you think that most people are better off than you are?	yes
Do you frequently get upset over little things?	yes
Do you frequently feel like crying?	yes
Do you have trouble concentrating?	yes
Do you enjoy getting up in the morning?	no
Do you prefer to avoid social gatherings?	yes
Is it easy for you to make a decision?	no
Is your mind as clear as it used to be?	no
Total score (number of answers matching key)	
Score 0–10 = No depression	
Score 11–14 = Mild depression	
Score >15 = Moderate to severe depression	

is short and takes only 5 to 10 minutes to complete; it is considered reliable and valid for screening.

Drugs

The elderly account for about 30% of prescription drug purchases and 40% of nonprescription drug purchases. Over a five-year period, 90% of the elderly are taking at least one medication, with the average noninstitutionalized patient often taking three to four medications.[66] The risks from drug usage increase exponentially with each additional drug. Forty percent of the elderly must take one drug each day to perform ADLs.[67] In addition to the high percentage of the elderly taking medication, the issues of polypharmacy and age-related changes affecting dosage are of particular concern. The taking of several medications at a time is common for several reasons:

- Many medical physicians rely on medications to achieve treatment goals because it is less time-consuming than nondrug management and gives greater immediate patient satisfaction.
- The patient seeks care from several medical physicians forgetting or purposefully omitting information regarding other prescribed (self or doctor) medications.
- The patient takes a friend's or family member's medication because he or she feels that his or her symptoms are the same.

It is also important to consider drug interaction with over-the-counter medications and herbal/supplemental products. Some common adverse reactions and associated medications are listed in **Table 54–7**. Be particularly vigilant in investigating drug interactions or cause when patients present with signs or symptoms of cognitive impairment, gastrointestinal bleeding, syncope and falls, arrhythmias, and extrapyramidal effects.

The physiologic factors related to drug absorption and concentration in the older patient are:

- Absorption. Decreases in splanchnic blood flow and hypochlorhydria may decrease absorption of some medications and also herbal/ supplement products. Interference in absorption includes:
  1. the effects of cholesterol-binding medications (e.g., cholestyramine or colestipol) on drugs such as digoxin, warfarin, and thyroxin
  2. the binding of tetracycline by dairy products, antacids, and iron
  3. the effects on gastrointestinal motility by anticholinergics, antidepressants, and narcotics
- Distribution. Many drugs bind to albumin. As part of normal aging and particularly with renal or liver disease, the amount of albumin decreases. The effect is that for drugs that usually bind to albumin, there is a greater amount of free, active drug available. Total body water and lean body mass decrease while body fat increases in the elderly. Therefore, drugs that are hydrophilic have higher concentrations. This is true of ethanol, digoxin, and cimetidine, among others. Lipophilic

Table 54–7 Common Adverse Drug Reactions in Older Persons

Adverse Reaction	Example	Common Causes
Sedation	Drowsiness and sleepiness	Sedative-hypnotics, narcotic analgesics, antipsychotics
Confusion	Disorientation, delirium	Antidepressants, narcotic analgesics, anticholinergic drugs
Depression	Intense sadness and apathy	Barbiturates, antipsychotics, alcohol, antihypertensive agents
Orthostatic hypotension	Dizziness or syncope when assuming an upright position	Antihypertensives, antianginal agents
Fatigue and weakness	Strength loss and inability to perform normal activities	Muscle relaxants, diuretics
Dizziness	Loss of balance and falling	Sedatives, antipsychotics, narcotic analgesics, antihistamines
Anticholinergic effects	Confusion, nervousness, drowsiness, dry mouth, constipation, urinary retention	Antihistamines, antidepressants, certain antipsychotics
Extrapyramidal symptoms	Tardive dyskinesia, pseudoparkinsonism, dystonias	Antipsychotic medications

Reproduced from K. A. McCarthy, Management Considerations in the Geriatric Patient, *Topics in Clinical Chiropractic*, Vol. 3, No. 2, p. 69, © 1996, Aspen Publishers, Inc.

drugs will have a higher concentration in the elderly including steroids and benzodiazepines.

- Hepatic and Renal Effects. Due to decreases in hepatic blood flow, there may be an increased half-life of medications that are processed through the liver for elimination. These include imipramine, amitriptyline, long-acting benzodiazepines, and theophylline. Decreases in renal blood flow are about 1% per year after age 50 years accompanied by decreases in creatinine clearance. This may result in proportionately more drug availability over any given period of time due to slowed elimination.

It is imperative for the chiropractor to obtain a full list of prescribed and nonprescribed medications, herbs, and supplements. Often the patient is more open about the total list knowing that chiropractors do not prescribe medication. Of particular concern for the chiropractor is that chronic or excessive use of analgesics is more likely to have serious renal and gastric effects in the older patient as compared with a younger patient. Also sedatives or CNS depressants carry with them a higher degree of sedation and risk of extrapyramidal effects. The complexities of interaction are beyond the training of the chiropractor; however, if the patient presents with suspicious complaints and a drug interaction, overdose, or underdose is the possible cause, a written or verbal referral to the primary prescribing physician is in the patient's best interest.

Falls

A longitudinal study by Baloh et al.[68] evaluated vestibular, visual, auditory, and somatosensory decline in normal older people. Although there were declines, they did not seem to contribute to changes in gait and balance. Highly correlated were white matter hypersensitivities on magnetic resonance imaging. Researchers in another study[69] found that certain reflexes were diminished such as the visual-vestibular-ocular reflex and the vestibulo-ocular reflex and likely accounted for some of the changes in gait seen in older individuals. In a review by Ganz et al.[70] the only indicators for risk of falling were a history of a fall within the past year and abnormalities found on assessment of gait and balance. Orthostatic hypotension, impaired cognition, visual impairment, medication variables, or decreased levels of activities of daily living were not predictive. Although falls are considered an almost natural result of growing

older, the impact is far greater than often assumed. With the exclusion of nontraumatic causes of death, falls are the leading cause of death due to trauma, primarily from head injury and complications associated with hip fracture.[71] A fall may be the decision point for nursing care or extended-care residency. In addition to the obvious pain, the associated loss of mobility leads to dependence and often results in depression and other secondary consequences. The increased risks of injury from falling arise from poorer reaction time, osteoporosis, and, if the head is involved, more intracranial space, which allows more shear to the dura and blood vessels. As many as one-third of patients over the age of 65 years report one or more falls per year. This rate dramatically increases over the age of 85 years. Women fall more often than men, with estimates as high as twice the rate of men. The major causes of falling include (in order): accidents, gait disturbance, dizziness/vertigo, drop attacks (no loss of consciousness), confusion, postural hypotension, visual disturbance, and syncope.[72] The reasons for these causes include primarily age-related changes in posture and proprioception and the effects of medication(s).[73] In the elderly, postural changes exhibit an extrapyramidal pattern of more flexion, a gait that involves shorter stride length and slower walking with increased muscle tone (stiffness). Increased sway is commonly the first sign of gait imbalance in the senior. Decreases in proprioception may be the result of normal aging; however, they are accelerated or augmented by dysfunction in the upper cervical spine and the result of diseases such as diabetes. Balance is coordinated through vestibular, visual, and proprioceptive interaction. Loss of one of these functions is more easily compensated for than loss or decrease of two. With poorer vision and/or proprioceptive loss or decrease, the patient is at substantial risk of loss of balance.

The first step in the differential is to attempt to determine whether an "accident" or a spontaneous fall occurred. Often these overlap and are hard to differentiate. The acronym SPLAT (**S**ymptoms associated with the fall, **P**rior falls, **L**ocation of the fall, **A**ctivity at the time of the fall, and **T**ime of day the fall occurs) may help.[74] For example, if the fall occurred after rising quickly from a seated or lying position and was associated with presyncope or syncope, orthostatic hypotension would be suspected. The most common causes considered would be medications (e.g., antihypertensives) or the autonomic reflex blunting effect of diabetes. If the patient stated that the fall occurred at night in a dimly lit area, proprioceptive dysfunction would be considered. If the patient stated that the fall occurred upon standing without ambulating, a cardiac or CNS cause would be suggested. A screening test that may be used is the Get Up and Go Test (GUGT). The patient is directed to stand up from a seated position, walk 3 meters (10 feet), turn, walk back, and sit down. The doctor observes and times the task to determine problems with rising, maintaining balance, and maintaining coordination. It is imperative to check for proprioceptive loss in the distal extremities, measure visual acuity, test for cerebellar dysfunction (in particular, Romberg's test), and measure blood pressure lying and standing (to detect orthostatic hypotension). Laboratory investigation should include a general screen to determine problems with anemia and glucose metabolism. Further investigation may include evaluation of vitamin B_{12} deficiency, thyroid disorders, or other specific concerns. In the patient with a suspected arrhythmia, a resting electrocardiogram (ECG) may be used as a screen; however, Holter monitoring is probably necessary in most cases due to the low sensitivity of a resting ECG.

Management approaches include:

- Referral to prescribing physician if medication is the suspected cause
- Referral for change in eyewear prescription, if necessary
- Lower extremity strengthening exercises
- Recommendation for t'ai chi classes; t'ai chi has been shown to improve balance in seniors[75]
- A home-site investigation of potential risks and suggestions on modifying or otherwise altering living environment to decrease risks (see **Table 54–8**)
- Assisted devices such as walkers or canes may be necessary for some patients

Urinary Incontinence

Incontinence is an involuntary loss of urine that is not an inevitable result of aging. Statistics vary based on living environment, time frame, and definition; however, estimates are that urinary incontinence affects approximately 30% to 50% of older adults.[76] The prevalence specifically in community-dwelling individuals older than age 65 years is approximately 15% to 30%. Women are twice as likely to be affected. Only about one-third of incontinent adults seek management. Those who do are patients with severe incontinence and those with better access to healthcare. Interestingly, the management strategies of men differ from those of women.[77] Men are more likely to limit fluids and traveling, and in fact are more likely to see a physician about incontinence. Women more frequently wear pads or perform exercises for their incontinence. In part, these differences reflect some differences in the types of incontinence seen based on gender. Men are more likely to have detrusor instability (i.e., involuntary contractions of the bladder) that increases with age. Also, enlargement of the prostate lengthens the urethra and moves the bladder neck more superiorly. Stress incontinence (due to urethral hypermobility in women) is uncommon in men, although radical prostatectomy may increase stress on the external urethral sphincter. Childbirth, aging, and hormonal influences may result in descent of the bladder neck or affect innervation to the bladder in women. Generally, the most frequent causes of urinary incontinence (UI) in women are stress incontinence and urge incontinence, whereas in men overflow incontinence and urge incontinence are more common. The cause of overflow incontinence in men is due to anatomic blockage of the bladder outlet, usually due to benign prostate hypertrophy, prostate cancer, or urethral stricture. For both men and women, incontinence associated with low back and/or leg pain warrants an investigation of cauda equina syndrome.

Table 54–8 Home Safety Evaluation and Recommendations

Area	Recommendations
General home environment	Floors/Rugs—Secure carpet edge, especially on stairs; remove throw rugs; keep areas clear of clutter, especially cords and wires; do not wax floors
	Other—Make sure there is adequate lighting especially at night; make sure that chairs are not too low and that the phone is accessible from floor
Bathroom	Install handrails for toilet and shower; use rubber bath mat; raise toilet seat if necessary
Outdoors	Make sure sidewalk and driveway are free of cracks; install handrails at areas with stairs; ensure adequate lighting; keep shrubbery trimmed

Focused questioning topics for UI include:

- frequency and amount of voiding
- situational aspects related to onset of UI (mechanical stimulation of voiding from coughing, laughing, sneezing, or jumping is likely stress incontinence, whereas UI without mechanical stimulation is more often due to detrusor instability)
- any associated signs/symptoms of urinary tract infection
- bowel movements, in particular constipation (a distended distal colon with stool may affect bladder function through a pressure effect)
- diagnosed conditions that may be the cause of voiding difficulty (e.g., congestive heart failure, diabetes, prostate or pelvic surgery for various conditions) or the medications used for the condition may exacerbate voiding problems
- drug history (some medications may cause retention and lead to overflow incontinence [e.g., α-agonists and stimulants such as ephedrine found in nasal decongestants] while others may act as diuretics [e.g., prescription and herbal diuretics, alcohol, and caffeine])
- previous diagnosis and/or management of UI
- patient's desired goals of management

The evaluation may be limited for the chiropractor given that a rectal examination for both sexes and a pelvic examination for women are necessary for a complete evaluation. If these examinations are not part of the practitioner's skills, a referral for these evaluations is requisite. In addition to a urogenital examination, the following should be included in the work-up of UI:[78]

- Palpation for suprapubic tenderness, lower abdominal masses, and bladder distention
- Neurologic testing of the perianal area and lower extremity may be warranted when complaints of pain or numbness are reported
- The cough test (a screening test for stress incontinence) to determine if there is loss of urine with coughing
- Maintenance of a frequency-voiding record by the patient
- Urinalysis to determine if glucosuria, blood, or infection may indicate an underlying pathologic cause

- Referral for more extensive testing includes an estimation of post-void residual, uroflowmetry, and pressure flow studies

Based on the type of UI, treatment options vary. Refer to Chapter 34 for a more extensive discussion of the options. Generally, if stress incontinence is the cause, Kegel exercises are beneficial. If detrusor instability is the cause, bladder training, habit training, pelvic muscle exercises, and biofeedback are important nonsurgical, drugless approaches. Drug therapy involves antimuscarinic medications including oxybutynin and tolterodine.

Male-Specific Concerns

A number of male-specific problems can occur in the senior patient. These include benign prostatic hypertrophy, prostate cancer, erectile dysfunction, and low testosterone. Prostate problems are discussed in the Selected Causes section of Chapter 34, Urinary Incontinence/Dysfunctional Voiding.

Erectile Dysfunction

The inability to acquire or sustain an erection for sexual intercourse is most often due to a secondary disorder, the most common cause being diabetes. Other medical conditions or the medications used to treat these conditions are also possible causes. Risk factors, in fact, include several of these disorders including diabetes, cardiovascular disease, metabolic syndrome, and smoking. Those patients with prior prostate surgery for prostatectomy are also at risk. Age is also a risk with the prevalence being quite high, with reports as high as 52% for males 40 to 70 years old; most of these cases are from ages 50 to 70 years.

Erection occurs with parasympathetic control of the central release of nitric oxide, which increases production of cAMP. This leads to a relaxation of the cavernous smooth muscle allowing an increase in penis blood flow. There are sinusoids in the cavernous muscle that fill with blood and compress the veins decreasing outflow. There are basically three general mechanisms that can interfere with this sequence. One is psychological including acute stress or chronic depression, vascular blockage, and the final possible contributor is neurological. The diagnostic work-up should then include a screen for pulses, reflexes, signs/symptoms (and lab) for diabetes, and psychological questioning.

Treatment of underlying disease such as diabetes is the first approach. For those with continuing problems, medications that act to increase blood flow to the penis are a form enzyme blocker for phosphodiesterase type 5 (PDE-5). Familiar drugs are Viagra, Cialis, and Levitra. Common side effects are flushing, headache, orthostatic hypotension, and for those taking Levitra, low back pain. It is important to avoid grapefruit and limit alcohol intake when taking any of these drugs. Failing this approach, some patients are directed to intraurethral and intracavernosal injectables such as Alprostadil (prostaglandin E1). **Table 54–9** is a list of these drugs and their potential side effects.

Low T Syndrome

Low testosterone is defined as levels <300 ng/dL. Symptoms in addition to low sexual drive include decreases in muscle mass and strength, and fatigue. Clearly, these low levels may also be related in part to aging, and certainly are related to other disorders that may be risk factors such as obesity, diabetes, and COPD. Causes may include undescended testicles, mumps infection (orchidis), Cushing's syndrome, hemochromatosis, TB, HIV/AIDS, and testicular trauma. Luteinizing hormone released from the pituitary stimulates the release of testosterone from the testes. Treatment is with testosterone gels such as AndroGel or Testim. Those taking these medications are cautioned not to transfer the gel to females or children, which may result in increased testosterone and its effects. Other approaches include a patch (Androderm or Testoderm), and injection with Delatestryl or Depo-Testosterone.

Nutrition

With the elderly, loss of weight is often more of a concern than weight gain. Chronic diseases can be tied to increases in weight, in particular diabetes, however. The focus here will be on the more immediate issue of weight loss. Weight loss is a multifactorial problem based primarily on feeding and appetite issues related to an underlying disease or disorder or secondarily due to psychosocial influences including accessibility to food sources, financial resources, nutritional knowledge, and social aspects of eating (i.e., not wanting to prepare a meal for self only). A line of questioning that centers around a typical daily meal schedule and content is the best approach to investigating a senior's nutritional status. If concerns surface, focus on common causes:

- Lack of appetite. Investigate medication use and underlying diseases and disorders. If necessary, follow up with appropriate laboratory investigation. The most common causes of lack of appetite in the elderly are depression and medication use.
- Difficulty with eating. Investigate dental problems including ill-fitting dentures and difficulties with swallowing or digesting food.

Table 54–9 Erectile Dysfunction Medications			
Drug Class	**Examples**	**General Mechanism**	**Interactions/Side Effects**
Tadalafil	Cialis	Used in the treatment of erectile dysfunction, it is a selective cyclic guanosine monophosphate (cGMP) inhibitor (specific phosphodiesterase type 5 [PDE5])	Headache, dizziness, abdominal pain, rash, chest pain, myalgias, spontaneous or long-lasting erections; caution if patient is taking alpha-blockers or nitrates
Vardenafil	Levitra	A phosophodiesterase-5 inhibitor. Used for erectile dysfunction. Causes a vasodilation effect in the corpus cavernosus of the penis through effect with nitric oxide.	May cause facial edema, postural hypotension, palpitations, headache (and other "cerebral signs/symptoms"), MI, angina, dermatitis, photosensitivity, and gout. For some, may experience a slight bluish tinge to vision.
Sildenafil citrate	Viagra	Used for erectile dysfunction. Causes a vasodilation effect in the corpus cavernosus of the penis through effect with nitric oxide.	May cause facial edema, postural hypotension, palpitations, headache (and other "cerebral signs/symptoms"), MI, angina, dermatitis, photosensitivity, and gout.
Vardenafil HCL	Levitra	Used in the management of erectile dysfunction in men. It acts as an enzyme blocker for phosphodiesterase type 5 (PDE-5), which results in increased blood flow to the penis.	Headache, indigestion, flushing, stuffy nose, and dizziness.

- Difficulty with preparing food. Evaluate for disorders that affect the use of the hands or the ability to ambulate around the kitchen.
- Difficulty obtaining food. Investigate transportation availability, affordability of groceries, and whether patient knows of resources such as home-delivery services including Meals-on-Wheels and other resources.
- Nutritional knowledge. Investigate the senior's general knowledge of appropriate nutritional balance in diet, ability to read labels, and attitude toward maintaining a healthy diet and lifestyle.

More sophisticated approaches include the Nutrition Screening Initiative (NSI), a tiered approach to nutritional screening in the elderly.[79] The first-line screen is basically a checklist filled out by the patient, and two screening tests. These two screening tests are based on information obtained by the social service or other healthcare professional. Physical examination screens should include a check for weight loss, an estimation of percentage body fat, and a check for oral problems with a focus on dentition. Laboratory screening can include an evaluation for decreases in serum albumin (4 g/dL or less) or cholesterol (160 mg/dL or less).

Attention to underlying disorders and appropriate management is the primary focus. This may require referral or comanagement. Assisting with issues regarding food accessibility should include a list of phone numbers of resource centers or individuals who can provide continuity in a schedule of regular meals and quality of those meals. Education of the senior patient of proper food intake through choice and preparation may be part of the services provided by the chiropractor or referred to focused sources such as a dietitian or other expert source.

Physical/Verbal Abuse or Neglect

Elder abuse or neglect is often undetected and may represent the most underreported type of domestic violence.[80] The National Center on Elder Abuse estimates that in 1996 there were over 1 million individuals over the age of 65 years who were mistreated.[81] Although there are laws in all states to protect the elderly from mistreatment, the specific criteria and penalties vary enormously. However, most states do require that all healthcare professionals report incidents of actual and suspected abuse. Types of mistreatment are numerous and include physical abuse, sexual abuse, emotional abuse, caregiver neglect, and material. When seniors have depression, dementia, falls, fractures, decubitus ulcers, or loss of

Table 54–10 Indicators of Possible Elder Abuse

General Indicator	Specific Indicator
Elderly patient environment	Social isolation, primarily dependent on others, shared living environment, incontinence, dementia, or behavioral problems
Caregiver elements	Stress, substance abuse, mental or physical illness, dependence on elder for housing or finance, history of violence, unwillingness to leave elder alone with doctor, implausible explanation of physical injury
Physical findings in elderly patient	Depression, anxiety, dehydration, undernourished, weight loss, medical issues that go unresolved, bruises in unusual areas, patterned bruises, abrasions or burns, decubitus ulcers, clothing that is unclean or inappropriate for weather

weight, mistreatment must be considered. Screening with questions regarding who takes care of the individual or attempting to determine if the patient is afraid of his or her spouse or caretaker may initiate the dialogue. Frank questions about whether someone has struck or hurt the patient in any way must be approached delicately. About one-third of elderly patients who are mistreated deny abuse when questioned specifically. More alarming, physicians report as few as 2% of all cases.[82]

The signs of mistreatment may be more clear when physical abuse has taken place. Emotional abuse or neglect is more difficult to detect. **Table 54–10** provides a list of risk factors and physical findings that suggest abuse.[83] **Table 54–11** suggests various avenues of management. Generally, the approach is to provide social

Table 54–11 Strategies for Managing Elder Abuse/Neglect

Management Aspect	Specific Suggestions
Prevent social isolation	Provide resource contacts for home health services, adult day-care or connection to senior center, meal-delivery services, and churches
Support for caregiver	Establish possible relief support for caregiver, connect to support groups to help deal with psychologic stresses, simplify activities by using central resource for medication and medical services
Determine home needs	Determine safety; provide resources for obtaining any special medical equipment; assess patient for activities of daily living performance; and determine need for caregiver or a higher level of care at a group home, assisted living, or skilled nursing facility

support to reduce isolation, decrease caregiver stress, manage any medical issues, and evaluate the living environment to determine the need for a higher level of care.

Specific Management Issues

Modification of Adjusting Procedures

There are a number of concerns to be considered when adjusting or manipulating the senior patient. The susceptibility of the elderly to injury varies; however, the primary issues are:

- Generally decreased flexibility and elasticity of soft tissue may predispose the elderly patient to a sprain-strain effect from treatment. Also, the senior patient, in an effort to assist with the doctor's positioning, often has difficulty relaxing in the end-range position for adjusting. This makes the adjustment more difficult and increases the possibility of overstretch.
- Generally seniors are more osteoporotic, which increases the risk of vertebral compression fractures and rib fractures with specific positions and high-force approaches.
- Generally, the senior patient has more degenerative joint disease, which may include osteophyte formation into the neural foramina or spinal canal increasing the risk of nerve irritation.
- Generally, in the senior, early degenerative changes and/or lack of appropriate muscle tone and reaction result in functional instability.

Table 54–3 summarizes the specific focus for the senior patient including physical examination/history indicators, concerns, and modification options.

Exercise Prescription

The ability to function, maintaining mobility and independence, is among the most important goals for the senior patient. It affects quality and, indirectly, quantity of life. The benefits of exercise are far-reaching and exponential. Individuals who exercise regularly have a better chance at preventing, slowing, or accommodating to the effects of many chronic diseases including congestive heart disease, coronary artery disease, diabetes, osteoarthritis, and intermittent vascular claudication, among others.[84] A regular exercise program combined with an appropriate diet is important for avoiding obesity and

its consequences. Exercising has been shown to improve balance and decrease the chance of falling in the elderly. With exercise, joint reaction time is decreased and muscle mass is increased, which provides some protection from falls. A sedentary life due to lack of motivation or the consequence of chronic or progressive disease will often cause a downward spiral in function. Some of the most important concepts for older patients to understand are:

- Prolonged rest decreases and prolongs recovery.
- Moderate exercise does not increase the chance or progression of arthritis.
- Seniors can benefit from exercise in strength, flexibility, balance, and endurance.
- Osteoarthritis pain often responds to toning exercises even though existing degenerative changes (seen on radiograph) remain.

The primary concerns with exercise and the older patient include:

- Isometric exercises should not be performed at a maximum or held for longer than a few seconds due to the vascular effect of increased blood pressure.
- Sudden changes in posture may result in presyncope or syncope due to a blunted reflex vascular response causing a postural hypotension (e.g., drug effect from antihypertensives or from diabetes).
- A safe aerobic exercise goal must be established for the older patient based on the patient's response to cardiopulmonary and endurance testing to determine cardiovascular response and avoid a cardiac event.
- Spinal flexion exercises place more stress on the vertebral body and have been shown to increase the risk of compression fracture.

Preparticipation Evaluation

The preparticipation evaluation attempts to determine any known limitations, contraindications, or motivational issues with regard to an exercise program and to establish a baseline recommendation. Historical information on known chronic diseases including hypertension, chronic obstructive disease, coronary and cardiac disease, and orthopaedic limitations are important for determining exercise testing restrictions and future recommendations. Also needed is a list of medications, type of activities the individual is interested in, and availability of a facility or equipment (if appropriate).

Prior to exercise testing it is important to note the following absolute and relative contraindications:

- Absolute contraindications to office exercise testing
    1. recent ECG changes or acute myocardial infarction
    2. unstable angina, third-degree heart block, or acute congestive heart failure
- Relative contraindications to office exercise testing
    1. uncontrolled hypertension
    2. cardiomyopathies, valvular heart disease, and complex ventricular ectopic arrhythmias
    3. uncontrolled metabolic diseases such as diabetes; thyroid or adrenal disorders

General Cardiovascular Fitness

The office evaluation can be performed in approximately 20 minutes. The American College of Sports Medicine (ACSM) recommends cardiac treadmill stress-testing prior to engaging in vigorous exercise (i.e., > 60% of maximal oxygen uptake) for men over age 40 years, women over age 50 years, and all individuals who have cardiac risk factors with or without symptoms.[85] Because treadmill tests are generally unavailable in-office for the chiropractor, referral for off-site testing or an in-office alternative testing approach is acceptable. Most physicians use the Kasch pulse recovery test to assess the patient's functional and aerobic capabilities.[86]

General Musculoskeletal Evaluation

Although more formalized evaluation with equipment and testing protocols may be available, a general in-office approach may include:

- Strength—A general measure of upper body strength can be estimated using a dynamometer for grip strength and push-ups or modified push-ups for proximal muscle (i.e., shoulder/elbow) strength; lower body strength may be estimated by watching a patient perform the sit-and-rise test. The patient leans back against a wall or door and slides down the surface bending the knees (no more than 90°) and then rises. The ability of the patient to perform and repeat this test is a good general screen for lower body strength.
- Balance—Balance can be assessed using Romberg's test or observing the patient rise from a seated position, walk 10 steps, turn, return, and sit.
- Flexibility—Low back and hamstring flexibility are often measured using the sit-and-reach test.

Range-of-motion testing for other joints may aid in evaluating flexibility.

Other Areas

- Body mass index (BMI)—BMI is a value used to determine, in particular, a threshold for obesity. It is determined by dividing body weight in kilograms by height in meters squared. A BMI over 25 indicates obesity. Skin-fold measurement may be used to estimate body-fat content.
- Bone density—In particular for the senior woman, bone-density estimation using x-ray absorptiometry may be useful in determining risk and/or degree of osteoporosis.
- Lipid profile—It is important to determine a baseline measure of lipids to measure the effect of exercise on these values.

Exercise prescription must take into account the limitations and needs established above. A summary of general recommendations is given in **Table 54–12**. In determining the frequency, duration, and intensity of exercises, a target heart range of 120–145 beats per minute or muscle fatigue in 8 to 12 repetitions is often used. More specifically, an exercise target heart rate (ETHR) is determined by measuring the resting heart rate (RHR); determining the maximum heart rate (MHR) through exercise tolerance testing or through an estimate by subtracting the patient's age from 220; and estimating the exercise target heart rate using the following formula:

$$ETHR = P \times (MHR - RHR) + RHR$$

where P equals the percentage of MHR desired; for seniors P is between 60% and 80%.

Many seniors can surpass these cautionary limitations. Generally, two indicators are used for aerobic activities:

1. Metabolic equivalents (METs): 3.5 mL of O_2 per kg of body weight per minute. Estimated METs for common activities include:
    - bowling or playing music: 2–4 METs
    - pleasure cycling, social dancing, walking while golfing carrying a bag, stair climbing, swimming, tennis, skiing downhill: 3–9 METs
    - running, cross-country skiing, aerobic dancing: 6–12 METs
2. Borg Scale of Perceived Exertion:[87] A scale from 0 to 20 based primarily on the individual's ability to

Table 54–12 General Exercise Recommendations for the Older Patient

Element	Recommendations
Cardiovascular/Pulmonary Capacity	Perform a minimum of 30 minutes of physical activity, preferably aerobic, most days of the week.
Strength	• Perform 1–3 sets of 8–12 repetitions 2–3 times per week with emphasis on both upper and lower body exercises. • If osteoporotic, begin with aquatic or bicycling, progress to walking, and gradually introduce weight training while weight bearing. • Include balance training and emphasis on strong lower body strength to prevent falls.
Flexibility	• Perform 6–10 general body stretches before and after activity; use prolonged stretch while continuing to breathe; do not hold breath creating a prolonged isometric contraction. • Emphasize the combination of lower body strength and flexibility to maintain mobility.
Weight	• For men: 12% to 20% fat; lean body mass between 125 and 150 lbs. • For women: 20% to 30% fat; lean body mass between 90 and 110 lbs. • Emphasize the combination of diet and exercise in maintaining proper weight. • Diet should include plenty of fruits/vegetables, and patient should be educated in reading labels in order to make proper choices.

talk while exercising and with his or her perceived muscle fatigue with exercise.

- ○ 7 = very, very light exertion
- ○ 9 = very light
- ○ 11 = light
- ○ 13 = moderate
- ○ 15 = heavy
- ○ 17 = very heavy
- ○ 19 = very, very heavy

3. Light is considered about 30% to 49% maximum oxygen uptake, while heavy is about 85% maximum oxygen uptake.

Osteoarthritis

A recent literature review of athletes and osteoarthritis (OA) reveals some interesting findings:[88]

- Runners older than 60 years running three hours per week for 12 years showed no greater prevalence of OA when matched to nonrunning controls (they did demonstrate a 40% greater bone density of vertebral bodies).
- Radiographic evidence of OA in a group of middle-aged runners was associated with genu varum, a history of a prior major joint injury, and more years of long distance running.
- Those with knee ligament or meniscal injury demonstrated a higher risk of developing degenerative changes earlier.

- Other factors that may be considered in some athletes are joint incongruity or joint dysplasia, muscle weakness, neurologic deficits, and increased weight.
- The ability to repair articular damage decreases with age; therefore, the healing response is less efficient as one ages.

What is clear clinically and substantiated in some literature reports is that moderate activity is beneficial to joints. It is also clear that, radiographic findings not withstanding, patients improve symptomatically with toning exercises for the involved joint or joints. For weight-bearing joints, it is often helpful to begin with non-weight-bearing simulations of weight-bearing activities. For example, pool (aquatic) training is a valuable initial exercise prescription for those with lower extremity OA. Muscles must function against the resistance of water; however, the load applied is decreased due to the buoyancy of the water. Also there is no direct impact loading of body weight as would occur with walking, jogging, or running. Bicycle riding is also a great alternative, allowing passive and active range of motion with minimal loading of the joint. This accomplishes both goals of decreasing impact loads to the knee and toning of muscles around the knee joint. With walking, a lateral heel wedge is often beneficial for relieving the pain of an osteoarthritic knee. As the medial meniscus degenerates, patients with OA develop a varus deformity or a closing down on the inside of the knee. A lateral heel wedge biomechanically shifts weight, opening up the medial joint area.

Nutritional management includes both glucosamine and chondroitin sulfate. Glucosamine seems to stimulate regeneration of articular cartilage and prevent its breakdown. Chondroitin draws fluid into cartilage, which helps to draw in nutrients. Recommended doses vary based on the size of the individual, but, in general are 1,500 mg of glucosamine sulfate and 1,200 mg of chondroitin sulfate. These daily doses should be divided into two to four doses and taken with food.

APPENDIX 54–1

Web Resources

Alzheimer's Disease

Alzheimer's Association
(800) 272-3900
http://www.alz.org
Alzheimer's Disease Education and Referral Center
(800) 438-4380
http://www.nia.nih.gov/alzheimers
Administration on Aging (Department of Health and Human Services)
(202) 619-7501
http://www.aoa.gov

Stroke

National Institute of Neurological Disorders and Stroke/National Institutes of Health
(800) 352-9424
http://www.ninds.nih.gov

APPENDIX 54–2

References

1. Association Research Group. *American Chiropractic Association 1992 Annual Physician Survey and Statistical Study.* Arlington, VA: American Chiropractic Association; 1992.
2. Coulter ID. The chiropractic patient. A social profile. *J Can Chiro Assoc.* 1985;29:25–28.
3. National Center for Health Statistics. Public Use Tape Documentation Part I, National Health Interview Survey 1989 [machine-readable data file and documentation]. Hyattsville, MD: National Center for Health Statistics; 1990.
4. Shock MW, ed. Normal human aging. In: *The Baltimore Longitudinal Study of Aging.* Washington, DC: Government Printing Office; 1984.
5. U.S. Dept of Health and Human Services. *Vital and Health Statistics: Health Data on Older Americans: United States, 1992.* Series 3: Analytic and Epidemiology Studies. Hyattsville, MD: US Dept of Health and Human Services, Public Health Service, Centers for Disease Control and Prevention, National Center for Health Statistics; 1993.
6. Wolinsky FD, Liu L, Miller TR, et al. The use of chiropractors by older adults in the United States. *Chiropr Osteopat.* 2007;15:12.
7. Fleming KC, Evans JM, Weber DC, Chulka DS. Practical functional assessment of elderly persons: a primary care approach. *Mayo Clin Proc.* 1995;70:890–910.
8. Chappell NS. Aging and social care. In: Binstock RH, George LK, eds. *Handbook of Aging and the Social Sciences.* 3rd ed. San Diego, CA: Academic Press; 1990.
9. National Center for Health Statistics. Current estimates from the National Health Interview Survey, 1988. In: *Vital Health Statistics.* Series 10, No. 173. Washington, DC: Public Health Service; 1989. DHHS publication 89-1501.
10. Shepard RJ. Physical training for the elderly. *Clin Sports Med.* 1986;5:515–533.
11. Andres R, Bierman EL, Hazard WR. *Principles of Geriatrics Medicine.* New York: McGraw-Hill; 1985.
12. American Medical Association. White paper on elderly health: report of the Council on Scientific Affairs. *Arch Intern Med.* 1990;150:2459–2462.
13. Campbell CL, Smyth S, Montalescot G, Steinhubl SR. Aspirin dose for the prevention of cardiovascular disease: a systematic review. *JAMA.* 2007;297(18):2018–2024.
14. Beck JC, Freedman ML, Warshaw GA. Geriatric assessment: focus on function. *Patient Care.* Feb. 1994:10–32.
15. Resnick NM. Geriatric medicine. In: Fauci AS, Braunwald E, Isselbacher KJ, et al., eds. *Harrison's Textbook of Medicine.* New York: McGraw-Hill; 1998:37–46.
16. Pereles LRM, Boyle NGH. Comprehensive geriatric assessment in the office. *Can Fam Physician.* 1991;37:2187–2194.
17. Fields FD. Special considerations in the physical exam of older patients. *Geriatrics.* 1991;46:39–44.
18. Ochs M. Selecting routine outpatient tests for older patients. *Geriatrics.* 1991;303:130–135.

19. Miller DK, Kaiser FE. Assessment of the older woman. *Clin Geriatr Med.* 1992;9:1–11.

20. Peterson CK, Bolton JE, Wood AG. A cross-sectional study correlating lumbar spine degeneration with disability and pain. *Spine.* 2000;25:218–223.

21. Duthie EH, Abbasi AA. Laboratory testing: current recommendations for older adults. *Geriatrics.* 1991;46:41–50.

22. Izaks GJ, Westendorp RGJ, Knook DL. The definition of anemia in older persons. *JAMA.* 1999;281:1714–1717.

23. Brigden ML. The search for meaning in monoclonal protein: is it multiple myeloma or monoclonal gammopathy of undetermined significance? *Postgrad Med.* 1999;106(2):135–142.

24. Aguzzi F, Bergani MR, Gasparro C, et al. Occurrence of monoclonal components in general practice: clinical implications. *Eur J Haematol.* 1992;48(4):192–195.

25. Small SA, Stern Y, Tang M, Mayeux R. Selective decline in memory function among healthy elderly. *Neurology.* 1999;52:1392–1396.

26. Ham RJ, Sloane PD, eds. *Primary Care Geriatrics: A Case-Based Approach.* 2nd ed. St. Louis: Mosby-Year Book; 1992.

27. Spitzer RL, Williams JRW, Kroenke K, et al. Utility of a new procedure for diagnosing mental disorders in primary care: the PRIME-MD-1000 study. *JAMA.* 1994;272:1749–1756.

28. Spitzer RL, Kroenke K, Williams JRW, et al. Validation and utility of a self-report version of PRIME-MD: the PHQ primary care study. *JAMA.* 1999;282:1737–1744.

29. Folstein MF, Folstein SE, McHugh PR. "MiniMental State": a practical method for grading the cognitive state of patients for the clinician. *J Psychiatric Res.* 1975;12(3):189–198.

30. Bachman DL, Wolf PA, Linn RT, et al. Incidence of dementia and probable Alzheimer's disease in a general population: the Framingham Study. *Neurology.* 1993;43:515–519.

31. Ernst RL, Hay JW. The US economic and social costs of Alzheimer's disease revisited. *Am J Public Health.* 1994;84:1261–1264.

32. Näaslund J, Haroutunian V, Mohs R, et al. Correlation between elevated amyloid-peptide in the brain and cognitive decline. *JAMA.* 2000;283:1571–1577.

33. Vassar R, Bennett BD, Babu-Khan S, et al. β Secretase cleavage of Alzheimer amyloid precursor protein by the transmembrane aspartic protease BACE. *Science.* 1999;286:735–741.

34. Reisberg B, Doody R, Stoffler A, et al. Memantine in moderate-to-severe Alzheimer's disease. *N Engl J Med.* 2003;348:1333–1341.

35. Stritmatter WJ, Roses AD. Apolipoprotein E and Alzheimer's disease. *Annu Rev Neurosci.* 1996;19:53–67.

36. Haan MN, Shemanski L, Jagust WJ, et al. The role of *APOE ε4* in modulating effects of other risk factors for cognitive decline in elderly persons. *JAMA.* 1999;282:40–46.

37. Clare R, Smith AD, Jobst KA, et al. Folate, vitamin B12, and serum total homocysteine levels in confirmed Alzheimer disease. *Arch Neurol.* 1998;55:1449–1455.

38. Tan ZS, Seshadri S, Beiser A, et al. Plasma total cholesterol level as a risk factor for Alzheimer's disease: The Framingham Study. *Arch Intern Med.* 2003;163:1053–1057.

39. Green RC, Cupples LA, Kurz A, et al. Depression as a risk factor for Alzheimer's disease: The MIRAGE Study. *Arch Neurology.* 2003;60;753–759.

40. Ferketick AK, Schwartzbaum JA, Frid DJ, Moeschberger ML. Depression as an antecedent to heart disease among women and men in the NHANES I study. National Health and Nutrition Examination Survey. *Archives of Internal Medicine.* 2000;160(9):1251–1258.

41. Xu H, Gouras GK, Greenfield JP, et al. Estrogen reduces neuronal generation of Alzheimer beta-amyloid peptides. *Nat Med.* 1998;4:447–451.

42. Gruber CJ, Tschugguel W, Schineeberger C, Huber JC. Production and actions of estrogens. *N Engl J Med.* 2002;346:340–352.

43. Mulnard RA, Cotman CW, Kawas C, et al. Estrogen replacement therapy for treatment of mild to moderate Alzheimer's disease: a randomized controlled trial. Alzheimer's Disease Cooperative Study. *JAMA.* 2000;284:2597–2602.

44. Wassertheil-Smoller S, Hendrix SL, Limacher ML, et al. Effect of estrogen plus progestin on stroke in postmenopausal women. The Women's Health Initiative: a randomized trial. *JAMA.* 2003;289:2673–2684.

45. Rapp SR, Espeland MA, Shumaker SA, et al. Effect of estrogen plus progestin on global cognitive function in postmenopausal women. The Women's Health Initiative Memory Study: a randomized controlled trial. *JAMA.* 2003;289:2663–2672.

46. Shumaker SA, Legault C, Rapp SR, et al. Estrogen plus progestin and incidence of dementia and mild

cognitive impairment in postmenopausal women. The Women's Health Initiative Memory Study: a randomized controlled trial. *JAMA.* 2003;289:2651–2662.

47. Merchant C, Tang MX, Albert S, et al. The influence of smoking on the risk of Alzheimer's disease. *Neurology.* 1999;52:1408–1411.

48. Jack CR, Petersen RC, Xu YC, et al. Prediction of AD with MRI-based hippocampal volume in mild cognitive impairment. *Neurology.* 1999;52:1397–1401.

49. Andreasen N, Hesse C, Davidson P, et al. Cerebrospinal fluid β amyloid in Alzheimer disease: differences between early- and late-onset Alzheimer disease and stability during the course of the disease. *Arch Neurol.* 1999;56:673–680.

50. Richards SS, Hendrie HC. Diagnosis, management, and treatment of Alzheimer disease: a guide for the internist. *Arch Intern Med.* 1999;159:789–798.

51. Solfrizzi V, Panza F, Torres F, et al. High monounsaturated fatty acid intake protects against age-related cognitive decline. *Neurology.* 1999;52:1563–1571.

52. American Psychiatric Association. *Diagnostic and Statistical Manual of Mental Disorders.* 4th ed. Washington, DC: APA; 1994.

53. Trinh NH, Hoblyn J, Mohanty S, Yaffe K. Efficacy of cholinesterase inhibitors in the treatment of neuropsychiatric symptoms and functional impairment in Alzheimer's disease: a meta-analysis. *JAMA.* 2003;289:210–216.

54. Le Bars PL, Katz MM, Berman N, et al. A placebo-controlled, double-blind, randomized trial of an extract of *Ginkgo biloba* for dementia. North American Egb Study Group. *JAMA.* 1997;278:1327–1332.

55. Sano M, Ernesto C, Thomas RG. A controlled trial of selegiline, alpha-tocopherol, or both as treatment for Alzheimer's disease. *N Engl J Med.* 1997;336:1216–1222.

56. Mulnard RA, Cotman CW, Kawas C, et al. Estrogen replacement therapy for treatment of mild to moderate Alzheimer disease: a randomized controlled trial. *JAMA.* 2000;283:1007–1015.

57. Wagner JP, Black IB, Di-Cicco-Bloom E. Stimulation of neonatal and adult brain neurogenesis by subcutaneous injection of basic fibroblast growth factor. *J Neurosci.* 1999;19(4):6006–6016.

58. Reger MA, Watson GS, Green PS, et al. Intranasal insulin improves cognition and modulates beta-amyloid in early AD. *Neurology.* 2008;70(6):440–448.

59. Watson GS, Bernhardt T, Reger MA, et al. Insulin effects on CSF norepinephrine and cognition in Alzheimer's disease. *Neurobiol Aging.* 2006;27(1):38–41.

60. Luchsinger JA, Noble JM, Scarmeas N. Diet and Alzheimer's disease. *Curr Neurol Neurosci Rep.* 2007;7(5):366–372.

61. Scarmeas N, Luchsinger JA, Mayeux R, Stern Y. Mediterranean diet and Alzheimer disease mortality. *Neurology.* 2007;69(11):1084–1093.

62. Luchsinger JA, Tang MX, Mayeux R. Glycemic load and risk of Alzheimer's disease. *J Nutr Health Aging.* 2007;11(3):238–241.

63. Welsh-Bohmer KA, Morgenlander JC. Determining the cause of memory loss in the elderly: front in-office screening to neuropsychological referral. *Postgrad Med.* 1999;106(5):99–128.

64. Ochs M. Selecting routine outpatient tests for older patients. *Geriatrics.* 1991;46:39–50.

65. Yesavage JA, Brink TL, Rose TL, et al. Development and validation of a geriatric screening scale: a preliminary report. *J Psychiatr Res.* 1983;17(1):37–49.

66. Jones-Grizzle AJ, Craugalis JR. Demographics. In: Bressler R, Katz MD, eds. *Geriatric Pharmacology.* New York: Mc-Graw-Hill; 1993.

67. Cadieux RJ. Drug interactions in the elderly: how multiple drug use increases risk exponentially. *Postgrad Med.* 1989;86:179–186.

68. Baloh RW, Ying SH, Jacobson KM. A longitudinal study of gait and balance dysfunction in normal older people. *Arch Neurol.* 2003;60(6):835–839.

69. Kerber KA, Ishiyama GP, Baloh RW. A longitudinal study of oculomotor function in normal older people. *Neurobiol Aging.* 2006;27(9):1346–1353.

70. Ganz DA, Bao Y, Shekelle PG, Rubenstein LZ. Will my patient fall? *JAMA.* 2007;297(1):77–86.

71. Bowers LJ. Clinical assessment of geriatric patients: unique challenges. *Top Clin Chiro.* 1996;3(2):10–22.

72. Robbins AS. Prediction of falls among elderly people: results of two population-based studies. *Arch Intern Med.* 1989;149:1625–1631.

73. Tinneti ME, Speechley M, Gintern SF. Risk factors for falls among elderly persons living in the community. *N Engl J Med.* 1988;319:1701–1705.

74. Fields SD. History taking in the elderly: obtaining useful information. *Geriatrics.* 1991;46:26–35.

75. Hain TC, Fuller L, Weil L, Kotsias J. Effects of t'ai chi on balance. *Arch Otolaryngol Head Neck Surg.* 1999;125:1191–1195.

76. Herzog AR, Fultz NH. Prevalence and incidence of urinary incontinence in community-dwelling populations. *J Am Geriatr Soc.* 1990;38:273–281.

77. Hunskaar S, Sandvik H. One hundred and fifty men with urinary incontinence. III. Psychosocial consequences. *Scand J Prim Health Care.* 1993;11:193–196.

78. Johnson TM II, Ouslander JG. Urinary incontinence in the older man. *Med Clin North Am.* 1999;83:1247–1267.

79. *Report on Nutrition Screening I: Toward a Common View.* Washington, DC: Nutrition Screening Initiative; 1992.

80. O'Brien ME. Elder abuse: how to spot it—how to help. *N C Med J.* 1994;55:409–411.

81. Executive summary. In: Tatara T, Kuzmeskus LB, eds. *Summaries of the Statistical Data on Elder Abuse in Domestic Settings for FY 95 and FY 96.* Washington, DC: National Center on Elder Abuse; 1997:vii–ix.

82. Rosenblatt DE, Cho KH, Durance PW. Reporting mistreatment of older adults: the role of physicians. *J Am Geriatr Soc.* 1996;44(1):65–70.

83. Kruger RM, Moon CH. Can you spot the signs of elder mistreatment? *Postgrad Med.* 1999;106(2):169–183.

84. Petrella RJ. Exercise for older patients with chronic disease. *Phys Sports Med.* 1999;27(11):79–104.

85. Mahler DA. *American College of Sports Medicine: Guidelines for Exercise Testing and Prescription.* 5th ed. Baltimore: Williams & Wilkins; 1995:1–37.

86. Kasch FW, Philips WH, Ross WD, et al. A comparison of maximal oxygen uptake by treadmill and step-test procedures. *J Appl Physiol.* 1966;21(4):1387–1388.

87. Borg GA. Psychosocial bases of perceived exertion. *Med Sci Sports Exerc.* 1982;14(5):377–381.

88. Buckwalter JA, Lane NE. Athletics and osteoarthritis. *Am J Sports Med.* 1997;25:873–881.

The Female Patient

Context

The female patient presents a unique challenge to the chiropractor. Many of the distinctions between male and female presentations are based on hormonal differences manifested often as gynecologic dysfunction or pathology. The inclusion of gynecologic differentials often requires that physical examination skills include breast and pelvic evaluation. For many chiropractors, examination skills and expertise are limited in these areas and would therefore affect the course and scope of evaluation. For example, in the evaluation of abdominal or pelvic pain, a pelvic examination is requisite in evaluating gynecologic causes. If the chiropractor is not experienced in pelvic examination, referral to the patient's obstetrician/gynecologist is necessary to complete a comprehensive search for cause. However, for many complaints, a clinical impression may still be gained through appropriate questioning resulting in either a limited trial of treatment or a referral for further testing or management.

Until recently, women were considered a subcohort of men; therefore, separate research studies for women were not performed. Also, women were excluded due to concerns regarding the effects of pregnancy or hormonal changes on the results of treatment studies. Most research efforts were directed at men with the assumption that the results could be extrapolated to women. Several major historical changes have updated the focus and strategic approach to research:

- In 1983, the U.S. Public Health Task Force on Women's Health Issues was established.
- In 1990, the National Institutes of Health (NIH) established the Office of Research on Women's Health.
- In 1991, the Women's Health Initiative (WHI) (a large prevention-based study) was developed.

One of the largest prospective studies, the Nurses' Health Study, evaluated women for 20 years (and continues to follow patients).[1] Interesting findings include the following:

- A strong relation between weight gain, heart disease, and mortality
- A lack of relation between calcium and osteoporotic fractures
- A positive relation between postmenopausal hormone use and the risk of breast cancer

Through ongoing research, several important differences have surfaced regarding women's health compared with men's health:[2]

- Women live longer than men.
- Women (primarily through what is believed to be an estrogen-protective effect) develop cardiac disease 10 years later than men, on average.
- Women may present atypically for heart disease; in particular, cardiac ischemia (i.e., dizziness, headache, or backache instead of chest discomfort).
- Women have a higher incidence of certain types of sports injuries; in particular, at the knee (e.g., anterior cruciate ligament).
- Women may have different nutritional needs than men.
- In addition to gender-specific disorders, women have a higher incidence of certain disorders including migraine headache, depression, specific immune-mediated diseases (e.g., rheumatoid arthritis, systemic lupus erythematosus, multiple sclerosis, Graves' disease, and thyroiditis), cholelithiasis, eating disorders, urinary incontinence, obesity, progressive scoliosis, osteoporosis, and osteoporotic-related fractures, among others.

Among women ages 24 to 34 years in the United States, the leading causes of death are accidents, homicide, and suicide. From ages 45 to 54 years, the leading causes of death are ischemic heart disease (IHD) and lung cancer. In women ages 65 to 74 years, the leading causes of death in order are IHD, lung cancer, cerebrovascular disease, and breast cancer.[3] IHD is, by far, the leading cause of death overall with a mortality rate five to six times higher than that of lung or breast cancer.

The top ten cancers in women (listed in order) are:

1. Breast
2. Lung
3. Colorectal
4. Uterine/Cervical
5. Urinary tract
6. Lymphoma
7. Melanoma
8. Thyroid
9. Ovarian
10. Leukemia

A Creighton School of Medicine study stated that vitamin D could cut the risk of any cancer by 60%.[4] A regimen of 15 minutes of sun exposure two to three times a week or 1,000 IUs of vitamin D with 1,400 to 1,500 mg of calcium per day was shown to be effective in reducing cancer risk. Vitamin D3 versus D2 is the recommended version.

The focus of this chapter is on issues specific to women. Many disorders are just as likely to be seen in either gender, and these conditions are covered in other areas of this text. Also, some female-related conditions are discussed under the related symptom-based chapter (e.g., the chapter on abdominal pain includes pelvic inflammatory disease, ectopic pregnancy, and dysmenorrhea). For those issues that are related to menstruation or not covered in detail in other areas of this text, a more detailed approach and description are given.

General Strategy

Evaluation

For female patients there are generalized guidelines for evaluation based on age and potential risks. While recommendations vary, a general summary follows:

- Screen for a family history of cancer, heart disease or hypertension, osteoporosis, depression, rheumatic diseases, headache, obesity, and diabetes.

- Perform or refer for the following screening examinations based on age-related concerns:
  1. blood pressure: every 2 years (if normal)[5]
  2. clinical breast examination: every 3 years for ages 20 to 39 years, then annually thereafter[6]
  3. mammography: every 1 to 2 years for women ages 40 to 49 years, annually for women ages 50 to 69 years (controversy exists regarding the benefits of screening annually after age 69 years)[7,8]
  4. pelvic examination: every year
  5. Papanicolaou (Pap) smear testing: beginning at age 18 years or when a woman becomes sexually active, every year until three satisfactory results, then future testing is based on doctor's discretion (usually every 3 years thereafter); Pap smears can be discontinued in women after age 65 years[9]
  6. eye examination: once between puberty and age 40 years, then every 2 to 4 years through age 64 years, then annually after age 65 years; high-risk groups for screening of glaucoma include African American women over age 40 years and Caucasian women over age 50 years[10]
  7. fasting plasma glucose: every 3 years if at high risk such as obesity or family history
  8. cholesterol (total and high-density lipoprotein [HDL]): every 5 years (if normal)[11]
  9. fecal occult blood: every year after age 50 years[12]
  10. colorectal cancer testing (sigmoidoscopy, colonoscopy, barium enema, digital rectal exam): every 5 to 10 years based on familial risk
  11. skin self-exam: monthly and every 3 years by a physician and annually for over age 40 years[13]
  12. thyroid stimulating hormone: every 3 to 5 years in patients over age 65 years[14]
  13. bone mineral density testing: use for screening purposes in high-risk females
- Evaluate the patient's nutritional status with a focus on common deficiencies such as:
  1. inadequate calcium or vitamin D in all women
  2. iron deficiency, B12 and folate deficiency, and gestational diabetes in the pregnant patient
  3. iron deficiency, calcium/vitamin D/phosphorous deficiency in athletic females
  4. calcium/vitamin D/phosphorous and iron deficiency in the elderly female
- Evaluate patient's weight and make recommendations regarding appropriate diet and exercise for weight loss when appropriate.

The general strategy for the symptomatic patient includes:

- Consider the most common conditions that are seen in females.
- Consider the atypical (compared with males) presentation for cardiac disease (e.g., dizziness, headache, backache).
- Be vigilant for detection of signs and symptoms related to possible abuse.

For the athletic patient, the general strategy is as follows:

- Screen for regional weakness; in particular, the upper extremity.
- Screen for indicators of generalized joint instability, paying particular attention to the knee and shoulder.
- Screen for patellar tracking abnormalities.
- Watch for indicators of the female athlete triad: disordered eating, amenorrhea, and osteoporosis.
- Make recommendations with regard to specific nutritional demands for the female athlete (i.e., iron and calcium).
- Watch for signs of stress fractures, especially of the tibia and proximal femur.

For the pregnant patient, the strategy includes the following:

- Reinforce the need for regular prenatal check-ups with the patient's chosen specialist.
- Support prenatal recommendations regarding supplementation of folate and possibly iron, avoidance of alcohol and smoking, control of diabetes, adequate weight gain during pregnancy, and safe exercise.
- Monitor patient's blood pressure.
- Be alert to hyperthyroidism, postpartum blues and depression, and endometritis (uterine infection following birth [more common after caesarean section] or abortion) in the postpartum patient.

For the postmenopausal patient, the strategy is as follows:

- Pay particular attention for signs of osteoporosis.
- Watch and screen for indicators of diminishing cognitive function.
- Watch and screen for signs of breast cancer.
- Watch and screen for signs of colon cancer.
- Pay attention to psychosocial needs of women living alone.

Management

For all female patients, management consists of the following:

- Stress the importance of monthly breast and skin self-exams.
- Ensure that the patient has an established routine of periodic health check-ups and counseling/education to address age-related concerns for females.
- Give advice with regard to the general benefits of exercise, nutrition, and smoking cessation in relation to prevention of obesity, heart disease, and diabetes.
- Provide information with regard to reducing the risk of osteoporosis.
- Modify adjusting procedures based on differences in anatomy and with pregnancy.

For patients with diagnosed or suspected conditions, management consists of the following:

- Refer patients with suspected gynecologic pathology.
- Manage musculoskeletal complaints with an emphasis on stability, pain reduction, and maintenance of as much joint mobility as possible.

Female Hormonal and Reproductive Physiology

The balance of reproductive hormones with endocrine and target organ interaction is a complex but essential coordination necessary for sexual development, puberty, and menarche. Ovulation and menstruation do not occur or are abnormal if the required level and balance of hormones and endocrine function are not correctly timed. Estrogen and progesterone have stimulating effects on reproductive target organs such as the breasts, uterus, and vagina. Through negative and positive feedback loops with the central nervous system (CNS)-hypothalamic-pituitary axes, estrogen and progesterone join with the gonadotropins, luteinizing hormone (LH), and follicle-stimulating hormone (FSH), in providing the correct balance for ovulation, pregnancy, or menstruation.

LH and FSH, although elevated at birth, are at low levels until puberty. Adrenal androgens dehydroepiandrosterone (DHEA) and DHEA sulfate (DHEAS) seem to initiate the development of pubic and axillary hair growth due to gradual increases seen during the few years preceding puberty.

The menstrual cycle is divided into different phases based on whether the uterine changes are the prime focus or whether endocrine changes are the primary focus. With uterine changes as the focus, there are three phases (see **Figure 55–1**):

1. Menstrual phase: shedding of endometrium with vaginal bleeding; first week of cycle

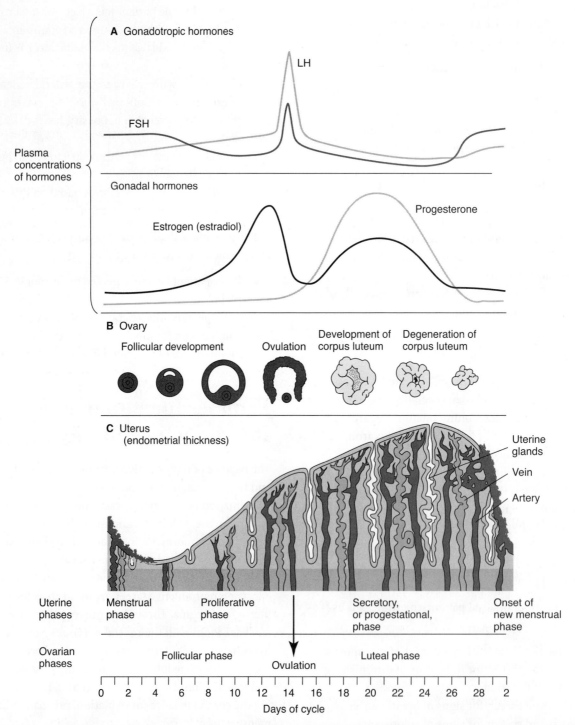

Figure 55–1 Physiologic events of the normal menstrual cycle. During days 1 to 14, the egg follicle in the ovary grows to maturity. The abrupt rise in luteinizing hormone (LH) as ovarian estrogen production increases during the first 2 weeks of the cycle triggers ovulation. The corpus luteum then develops and functions until it disintegrates at cycle's end if the egg is not fertilized. These events are reflected indirectly by visible and palpable changes in cervical mucus.

2. Proliferative phase: estrogen release from ovaries stimulates proliferation of endometrium; second week of cycle

3. Secretory phase: progesterone release from ovarian follicle stimulates endometrial secretion in preparation for implantation of the embryo; final two weeks of cycle

When the focus is on endocrine changes, the phases are described as follows:

1. Follicular (preovulatory) phase: first day of menses to the day before the LH surge

2. Ovulatory phase: release of the ovum from the Graafian follicle (i.e., ovulation) due to LH surge occurring approximately 16 to 32 hours after the surge

3. Luteal (postovulatory) phase: cells of the follicle reorganize to form the corpus luteum, which secretes increasing amounts of progesterone peaking at about six to eight days after the LH surge

The sequential hormonal events of the cycle proceed as follows:

- Low levels of estrogen and progesterone released from the ovaries cause the secretion of releasing factors from the hypothalamus. These releasing factors cause the anterior pituitary to release FSH and LH. The FSH increase stimulates primordial follicles, with one follicle becoming dominant.

- This dominant follicle matures and secretes estrogen causing proliferation of the endometrial lining of the uterus and the breast's glandular and ductal tissue. With increasing estrogen levels, FSH decreases while LH increases dramatically. The LH increase is referred to as the LH surge.

- This LH surge is necessary for the follicle to release an egg (i.e., ovulation). Ovulation then occurs at around the 14th day of a 28-day menstrual cycle. The corpus luteum inside the ruptured follicle develops and secretes progesterone. Due to the thermogenic effect of progesterone, basal body temperature rises about 0.5°C (0.9°F) and remains elevated until menstruation begins. Progesterone prevents further development of the endometrium and stimulates differentiation into a secretory epithelium in preparation for implantation of the embryo. Progesterone also has an inhibitory effect on LH secretion.

- If conception does not occur by day 23, low levels of LH cause the degeneration of the corpus luteum. Levels of progesterone and estrogen then drop.

- If fertilization does occur, the fertilized ovum travels from the fallopian tube to the uterus for implantation. The trophoblastic cells of the outer layer of the embryo (precursors of the placenta) secrete human chorionic gonadotropin (hCG). Serum level of hCG is the primary laboratory indicator of pregnancy.

During adolescence, ovulation does not occur initially. Gonadotropin levels must reach a level high enough to stimulate development of ovarian follicles, which in turn produce estrogen, which in turn leads to the necessary LH surge leading to ovulation. This LH surge may not occur until as late as five years postmenarche. Approximately 75% of abnormal bleeding in the adolescent is due to immaturity of this system.[15]

Dysfunctional bleeding occurs in the perimenopausal (before menopause) woman because of the decreased sensitivity of the ovary to FSH and LH. The resulting decrease in estrogen prevents the LH surge necessary for ovulation. However, similar to the adolescent, there is still enough estrogen being produced to stimulate endometrial growth. Without the balance of progesterone (that would normally be produced by the corpus luteum), the endometrium becomes extremely vascular and friable, leading to intermittent sloughing. This type of bleeding is often referred to as estrogen withdrawal bleeding. Estrogen breakthrough bleeding may be due to (1) constant low levels of estrogen, causing portions of the endometrium to degenerate (often seen with low-dose oral contraceptive use) and (2) high levels of estrogen, which allow the endometrium to become hyperplastic and outgrow its blood supply, leading to degeneration and often profuse bleeding. Another type of hormonal imbalance bleeding is progesterone withdrawal and breakthrough bleeding. This is usually the result of exogenous administration of progesterone.

Focused Issues

Menstrual-Related Concerns

Amenorrhea

Amenorrhea is generally classified into primary, if menarche has not occurred by age 16 years, and secondary, when menses have ceased for at least three months. Amenorrhea is normal before menarche, during pregnancy and early lactation, and after menopause.

Pathologic causes of primary amenorrhea include both anatomic abnormalities such as cervical stenosis or imperforate hymen, or vaginal or uterine aplasia. These conditions are rare and will generally be evident prior to the age of menarche. Hormonal imbalances or dysfunction of the hypothalamic-pituitary-gonadal-uterine axis and endocrine dysfunction are the most common causes of amenorrhea. There are many influences on hypothalamic function including modifiable factors such as weight loss (including anorexia nervosa), emotional stress, and excessive exercise. Rarer causes include tumors, Prader-Willi syndrome, or Kallmann syndrome. Metabolic abnormalities include adrenal and thyroid dysfunction, medications (e.g., antipsychotics and antidepressants), androgenic tumors, obesity, and polycystic ovary syndrome.

Investigation for amenorrhea should occur with the following presentations:

- No signs of puberty by age 13 years, or menarche has not occurred by age 16 years, or five or more years have passed since puberty without menarche
- Women who have had menses, however, are amenorrheic for three or more months or who have fewer than nine menses per year

For the girl who has not achieved menarche, it is important to have anatomic abnormalities ruled out. Second, an evaluation of normal secondary sexual characteristics development using a Tanner scale (see Chapter 53) is useful. Abnormalities in this development suggest hormonal imbalances due either to congenital problems or possible tumor.

The most common source of amenorrhea other than pregnancy is lifestyle excess and its effect on hypothalamic dysfunction. Questioning with regard to diet, dieting, weight loss, excessive stress, and excessive exercise often reveals a potential underlying cause.

The congenital or developmental abnormalities that may cause amenorrhea are complex and should be referred to a specialist; however, indicators that may necessitate the referral include:

- signs of androgen imbalance indicated by virilization (masculinization), hirsutism, a deep voice, balding, increased muscle mass, clitoromegaly, or galactorrhea
- abnormal development of the breasts or genitalia or abnormalities in the growth of pubic hair or its distribution
- internal obstruction to menstrual outflow would be difficult to ascertain; however, it may be

represented by a bulging vagina or pelvic mass (accumulation of menstrual blood or distention of uterus)

Laboratory investigation for amenorrhea is complex; however, it is based on a sequential approach:

- A basal measure of thyroid stimulating hormone (TSH), FSH, and prolactin may be helpful; when prolactin is increased, it needs to be remeasured due to increases found with stress, sleep, or food stimuli. When prolactin is increased with normal thyroid, a prolactin-secreting tumor is possible. When prolactin is normal with an increased TSH, hypothyroidism is the cause (although increased prolactin may occur). Increased FSH suggests ovarian failure.
- If the above tests are normal, and there are signs of hirsutism or other androgen effects, total serum testosterone and DHEAS tests should be ordered. Testosterone greater than 200 ng/dL indicates an androgen-producing tumor. If the levels are twice as high, an adrenal neoplasm is likely.
- Other testing may include a check for Cushing's syndrome (check for cortisol excess) or a measure of LH to help distinguish between polycystic ovary disease versus hypothalamic or pituitary dysfunction. With polycystic ovary disease there are increases in LH, whereas LH and FSH are generally normal or decreased with hypothalamic or pituitary disease. If pituitary disease is suspected, a radiograph of the sella turcica is warranted. If positive for possible tumor, magnetic resonance imaging (MRI) or computed tomography (CT) scan to determine the extent is then necessary.

Management of amenorrhea is obviously based on the suspected underlying mechanism. **Table 55–1** lists some medications used to manipulate the hormonal status of females including use for birth control and dysfunctional bleeding. For those found to have polycystic ovary disease, there is no known treatment, although hormonal manipulation may be possible if pregnancy is desired. For those with possible structural abnormalities or hormonal imbalance (including neoplasm induced), referral for appropriate therapy is required. Those who have no known structural or hormonal imbalance may benefit from modification of exercise, stress, and diet. This would be most common in the high-level female athlete.

Table 55-1 Medications Affecting Hormonal Status of Women

Drug Class	Examples	General Mechanism	Interactions/Side Effects
Estrogen (conjugated) and esterified	C.E.S. Premarin Cenestin Progens Estratab Menest Menrium Neo-Estrone Kestrone	A short-acting estrogen used in the treatment of atrophic vaginitis, postmenopausal symptoms, postmenopausal osteoporosis, and abnormal bleeding, and palliative treatment of both breast and prostate carcinoma.	May cause libido changes, depression, nausea, mastodynia, hypertension, and thromboembolic disorders.
Estrogen-progestin combinations	*Monophasic* Alesse Demulen Desogen Levlite Levora Loestrin Necon Nordene Ogestrel Others *Biphasic* Jenest Kariva Mircette Others *Triphasic* Ortho-Cept Triphasil Trivora Others	In addition to oral medications listed to the left, there are transdermal (Ortho Evra), intravaginal (Nuva Ring), and postcoital contraceptives (Plan B, Preven). Monophasic has the estrogen and progestin amounts remain the same. Biphasic has the estrogen remain the same with progestin initially less in first half of cycle, and increased in second. Triphasic has the progestin vary and the estrogen remains the same or varies. Prevents ovulation and creates a hostile environment for sperm.	May cause early or midcycle breakthrough bleeding, nausea, gallstones, thrombotic disorders such as thrombophlebitis, decreased glucose tolerance pyridoxine deficiency, vaginal candidiasis, weight gain, paresthesias, hypertension, and chloasma.
Progesterone	Crinone gel Gesterol Progestaject Progestasert Prometrium	Transforms endometrium from proliferative to secretory state and has pituitary gonadotropin secretion suppression as another effect. Not used as much due to newer medications. Can be used for secondary amenorrhea, dysfunctional uterine bleeding, and premenstrual syndrome.	May cause breakthrough bleeding, many GI symptoms, migraine headache, weight change, dizziness, and possible thromboembolic disorders.
Danazol	Cyclamen Danocrine	A synthetic androgen derivative from testosterone used in the management of endometriosis and fibrocystic breast disease. Causes a reduction in FSH and LH leading to anovulation and amenorrhea.	May cause hypersensitivity reaction, weight gain, hair loss, deepening of voice, breast reduction, hot flashes, hirsutism, irregular menstrual periods/amenorrhea, dizziness, tremor, and rarely hepatic damage. May increase LDL cholesterol.
Tamoxifen	Nolvadex Nolvadex-D Tamofen	Competes with estradiol and estrogen receptors causing a strong anti-estrogen effect. Used in the palliative treatment of advanced breast cancer in postmenopausal women and adjunctively with surgery for women with breast cancer and positive lymph nodes.	May cause hot flashes, thrombosis, leucopenia, thrombocytopenia, with nausea and vomiting occurring in about 25% of patients.

Premenstrual Syndrome

Premenstrual syndrome (premenstrual tension) is a hormone-mediated, varied response to fluctuating levels of progesterone and estrogen. The timing of the onset of symptoms is characteristically 7 to 10 days prior to menses (luteal phase) and improves within hours to days following the onset of menses (although dysmenorrhea may then appear). Symptoms vary in severity and frequency from woman to woman but generally represent the consequences of emotional lability (e.g., mood swings, anxiety, depression) and hormonal effects on neuroendocrine function including headaches, food cravings, fluid retention, breast tenderness or fullness, and back pain. When premenstrual syndrome (PMS) is chronic and severe, a psychologic disorder may be the primary source; it is referred to as premenstrual dysphoric disorder (PDD).

The theories proposed to explain why PMS symptoms occur and why they vary from woman to woman include the following:

- Some women may metabolize progesterone differently with the result of less allopregnanolone (enhances gamma-aminobutyric-acid [GABA]) resulting in a pregnenolone increase that decreases GABA effects.
- Serotonin levels decrease.
- There is estrogen excess or progesterone deficiency (through stimulation of the renin-angiotensin system, increased levels of aldosterone lead to fluid retention).
- Thyroid dysfunction exists. (Hypothyroid state may lead to increased levels of prolactin, which has been associated with increased PMS in some studies.)
- There are nutritional imbalances in B_6 and magnesium, altered blood sugar levels, and prostaglandin imbalance (see **Table 55–2**).
- Psychological factors exist.

Recommendations for conservative management include:

- Exercise. Although no specific exercise appears to have benefit, exercise may help decrease the frequency or intensity of PMS symptoms.[16]
- Smoking cessation
- Diet. Recommendations for diet modifications include:

  1. Eat small, regular meals.
  2. Follow a low-fat or vegetarian diet; limit red meats, dairy products, foods with a high sugar content, and fried foods.
  3. Increase carbohydrate consumption with a temporary reduction in protein.
  4. Limit or eliminate caffeine and alcohol.
  5. Increase dietary fiber and water (increase to six to eight glasses/day for natural diuresis).

- Spinal manipulation. Most studies have tested the treatment effect for dysmenorrhea; however, some studies[17, 18] have indicated manipulation has a positive effect on PMS.

Medical therapeutic approaches include:

- Serotonin reuptake inhibitors (e.g., fluoxetine and nefazodone)
- Hormones (e.g., oral contraceptives, Danazol [testosterone derivative], and Lupron [a gonadotropin-releasing hormone agonist])
- Benzodiazepines (e.g., alprazolam [Xanax] taken during the luteal phase)

Dysmenorrhea

Dysmenorrhea is classified as either primary or secondary. Primary dysmenorrhea is common and is considered a functional problem without an underlying pathologic cause. Secondary dysmenorrhea is due to a pathologic etiology that, in most cases, represents endometriosis. Other causes include a tight cervix, endometrial polyps, or pelvic inflammatory disease.

Primary dysmenorrhea usually begins in adolescence and diminishes with age and/or after pregnancy. There is a wide range of severity among women, yet a given woman generally has a baseline of discomfort that is consistent with each period. The patient is at least one to two years postmenarchal with increasing pain associated with menses. The pain is felt in the lower abdomen and pelvis, sometimes radiating to the back or inner thighs. The pain may begin before or with menses, peaking after 24 hours. Discomfort continues, on average, approximately two days after the onset. Some possible structural factors include a narrow cervical os or malposition of the uterus. Functional relationships have been found with lack of exercise and with anxiety.

Pain is mediated via prostaglandins. The cause is a combination of vasoconstriction and myometrial contraction leading to uterine ischemia. Increased discomfort may be caused by fluid retention (estrogen causes salt retention). No examination usually is necessary unless the pain is "new" or suddenly increased. Then a pelvic examination is warranted. With primary

Table 55–2 Nutritional Support for Premenstrual Syndrome

Substance	How Does it Work?	Dosage	Special Instructions	Contraindications and Possible Side Effects
Primrose oil	Source of omega-6 fatty acids (in particular, gamma linolenic acid [GLA]), which act as precursors to synthesis of prostaglandin E_1 (anti-inflammatory prostaglandin).	1,000 to 2,000 mg/day (researchers have used as high as 3,000 to 6,000 mg/day, which provides 270–540 mg of GLA).	None.	None at recommended dosage.
Flaxseed and borage oil	Source of omega-3 fatty acids, which are precursors to synthesis of anti-inflammatory prostaglandins.	1–2 tablespoons flaxseed daily.	Keep refrigerated; keep away from light; do not heat.	None at recommended dosage.
Vitamin B$_6$	Cofactor in the production of dopamine.	50 to 500 mg/day.	None.	Dosages above 600 mg/day have been associated with peripheral neuropathy.
Vitamin E	Possible reduction in breast pain.	100 to 400 IU/day.	None.	None at recommended dosage.
Magnesium	Cofactor in the production of dopamine.	400 to 1,000 mg/day.	None.	High dosage may cause diarrhea.
Valerian (*Valeriana officinalis*)	Unknown; however, used for anxiety and as a sleep aid.	2 to 3 g taken 1–3 times/day.	Valerian smells bad even when encapsulated. The active ingredients are unstable, therefore, should use only fresh valerian.	Should not be taken during pregnancy or with drugs used to treat anxiety or as sleep enhancers.
St. John's wort (*Hypericum performatum*)	Works synergistically with 5-HTP; also anti-inflammatory and analgesic properties.	(0.3% hypericin content) 300 mg. 3 times/day (as high as 600 mg 3 times/day for some patients).	If taken with 5-HTP, reduce 5-HTP dose to 100 mg/day.	Possible mild stomach irritation; may cause photosensitivity of skin in fair-skinned individuals; rarely allergy, tiredness, weight gain, headache, or restlessness.

Note: The above substances have not been approved by the Food and Drug Administration for the treatment of this disorder.
Key: HTP, hydroxytryptophan.

dysmenorrhea there are no obvious pathologic findings, but the examination may be more uncomfortable during menses.

Management of primary dysmenorrhea draws from a variety of therapeutic interventions. Some examples of conservative approaches include:

- Exercise. Studies indicate that exercise may decrease the frequency or intensity of pain with dysmenorrhea.[19]

- Nutritional and herbal supplementation. Magnesium, calcium, omega-3 polyunsaturated fatty acids, and vitamin B$_{12}$ are recommended (see **Table 55–3**).

- Spinal manipulation. Studies[20, 21] indicate a possible benefit with the use of spinal manipulative therapy. A recent study[22] failed to determine the superiority of a low-force mimicking maneuver versus a high-velocity, short-lever, low-amplitude, high-force manipulation approach.

Table 55–3 Nutritional Support for Dysmenorrhea

Substance	How Might It Work?	Dosage	Special Instructions	Contraindications and Possible Side Effects
Niacin	Relieves menstrual cramping.	200 mg/day throughout menstrual cycle and 100 mg/day every 2–3 hours while having menstrual cramping (may be combined with 300 mg of vitamin C and 60 mg of rutin/day to increase effectiveness).	Generally not effective unless taken 7–10 days prior to menstrual flow.	A flushing effect, headache, and stomachache may occur with high doses of niacin. Also high doses should not be taken if the patient has gout, diabetes, liver damage, or eye damage.
Calcium	Maintains normal muscle tone.	1,000 mg/day throughout the month; during cramping, 250–500 mg every 4 hours for a total of 2,000 mg/day.	Some sources of calcium such as bonemeal, oyster shell, dolomite, and amino acid chelates may contain lead.	Calcium supplementation should not be used in individuals with sarcoidosis, hyperparathyroidism, chronic kidney disease, or milk-alkali syndrome.
Magnesium and vitamin B$_6$	Possible decrease in menstrual cramping.	400 mg/day throughout the cycle; 100 mg/2 hours as needed during menses.	None.	High doses of magnesium may cause diarrhea.
Omega-3s (*EPA & DHA*)	Source of omega-3 fatty acids increases anti-inflammatory prostaglandins.	1,000 mg of EPA and 700 mg of DHA daily for at least 2 months.	None.	Long-term use of fish oils at more than 3–4 g/day may cause problems due to elevated blood sugar, cholesterol, or glucose levels. Side effects may then include nose bleeds or gastrointestinal upset.
Cramp bark (*Viburnum opulus*) Black Haw (*V. prunifolium*)	A spasmolytic effect on the uterus.	Extract is a tea combination with Black Haw Bark, camomile flowers, and peppermint leaves.	None.	None.
Black cohosh	Has a weak estrogen-like effect to help reduce hot flashes. May decrease levels of luteinizing hormone.	Highly concentrated extract at 40 mg 2 times/day in a 40%–60% alcoholic extract.	Because long-term studies have not been conducted, it is recommended to limit to 6 months of usage.	Not to be used in pregnant or lactating women. Women on ERT should consult prescribing doctor. High doses may cause abdominal pain, nausea, headaches, and dizziness.
Blue cohosh (*Caulophyllum thalictroides*)	Mild estrogenic, spasmolytic effect.	0.3–1 g of drug or 0.5–1 mL of liquid extract.	None.	Should not be used during the first 3 months of pregnancy due to estrogenic effects.

Note: The above substances have not been approved by the Food and Drug Administration for the treatment of this disorder.

Key: EPA, eicosapentaenoic acid; DHA, docosahexaenoic acid; ERT, estrogen replacement therapy.

- Stimulation of sacral and low-back reflex points. Stimulation via acupressure, electrical stimulation,[23] or acupuncture may provide relief.[24]

Secondary dysmenorrhea is usually due to endometriosis or other pelvic pathology. A pelvic examination followed by special imaging may help identify the site, extent, and type of lesion (also see Chapter 31 and **Table 55–5**).

Menopause

Natural menopause represents an age-related ovarian failure. Progressive decline in pituitary gonadotropins (FSH and LH levels) results in shorter menstrual cycles with fewer ovulations and a decrease in progesterone. This progressively leads to failure of the follicle to respond due to low levels of hormones and correspondingly results in less estrogen production. As a feedback loop, this is followed by increased levels of LH and FSH in response to decreased estrogen. Most of the circulating estrogen in postmenopausal women is due to conversion of androgens to estrogens in primarily fat cells and the skin. During this transitional phase, referred to as the climacteric or perimenopausal period, the frequency of bleeding eventually is less often and irregular; however, prior to this, there is often a phase of increased bleeding that is irregular and unassociated with ovulation. This type of anovulatory bleeding is the most common cause of "abnormal" bleeding in the perimenopausal female. Menopause may also be induced through surgery, medication (usually chemotherapy), radiation, or trauma to the ovarian blood supply.

When menses have not occurred for one year, the female has reached menopause. This occurs on average at age 50 or 51 years in the United States. Any vaginal bleeding that does occur in a female who apparently has reached menopause or has not had any vaginal bleeding for six months should be further evaluated. Premature menopause is defined as occurring before age 40 years and is of unknown origin. There have been associations to smoking, nutritional deficiencies, or high-altitude living.

Clinical manifestations of menopause include:[25]

- Decreased circulating levels of estrogen appear to affect the CNS via the hypothalamus. As a result, 95% of perimenopausal and menopausal women experience "hot flashes" manifested as flushing and sweating episodes. These episodes are sudden in onset, last several minutes, and are felt as a sensation of face and neck hotness that extends to the anterior chest. The skin temperature may increase as much as 5°C and may result in wetting of clothing through excess perspiration. Physiologic responses that also occur include an increase in heart rate perceived sometimes as palpitations. There may be associated symptoms of headache, dizziness, and nausea during the episodes. It is important to distinguish these occurrences from thyroid storm (i.e., sudden increases in thyroid hormone). Approximately 80% of women experience these episodes for more than one year, with as many as 20% of women having symptoms for more than five years. Sleep is also affected. Many women have night sweats and also have difficulty falling asleep (prolonged sleep latency phase) and often awaken early without being able to fall back to sleep. It is important to distinguish this type of sleep disturbance from a similar problem seen in endogenous depression. Given a growing concern regarding estrogen replacement therapy, a search for alternatives in the management of hot flashes has begun. A randomized controlled trial demonstrated that a selective serotonin reuptake inhibitor (SSRI) (paroxetine controlled-release [CR]) was effective in treating menopausal hot flashes.[26] SSRIs are usually used in the treatment of depression. There also appears to be an increased risk for Alzheimer's disease in postmenopausal women not taking estrogen replacement therapy.
- Estrogen deficiency leads to a decrease in bone mass accelerating the osteoporosis process.
- Estrogen deficiency leads to an increased risk of cardiovascular disease and death including coronary artery disease and stroke. Increases in low-density lipoprotein (LDL) levels and decreased levels of HDL are seen.
- Tissue that is estrogen-sensitive will undergo atrophy. Common manifestations are:
  1. vaginal atrophy resulting in vaginal itching, burning, and painful sexual intercourse
  2. decrease in collagen content of the uterus, bladder, and rectum resulting in prolapse of these structures and/or an increased incidence of recurrent urinary tract infections and rectal or urinary incontinence

3. decrease in collagen also results in thinning of skin and decreased elasticity
4. thinning of scalp hair with an increase in facial hair

Based on the severity of the clinical manifestations and the perceived effect on quality of life and risk for death, estrogen replacement therapy (ERT) should be considered. It is known that exogenous estrogen replacement can decrease flushes and sweating, vaginal and other related atrophy, and skin/hair changes when taken for a period of one to five years. Longer use (10 years and beyond) has a significant effect on decreasing risk for osteoporosis and cardiovascular disease (decreased by 50%). There still remains much controversy regarding the risks versus benefits of oral contraceptive use and hormonal replacement therapy. A recent review summarizes what is known at this time about oral contraceptives:[27]

Benefits

- Ovarian cancer is reduced by at least half.
- Endometrial cancer is reduced (presumably due to progestin-mediated suppression of estrogen-induced proliferation of endometrial cells).
- Acne is substantially reduced.
- The severity of dysfunctional uterine bleeding may be reduced, thereby reducing associated anemia.

Risks

- The relative risk for myocardial infarction has been estimated at between 1.4 to 5 and 2 to 5. Differences may be due to the factor of either smoking and/or undiagnosed hypertension.
- Venous thromboembolism increases by a factor of 3 to 4 for women using low-estrogen oral contraceptives. New studies of combination oral contraceptives using low-dose estrogen with third-generation progestins indicated an increased risk. The risk of thromboembolism is much higher for women who have thrombophilia (deficiency in protein C or protein S or having the factor V Leiden or prothrombin G20210A mutation).
- There appears to be no increased risk for hemorrhagic stroke among women who are not hypertensive and no increased risk for hepatocellular carcinoma.

One significant change over the last few years is the caution given to the use of HRT in the treatment of postmenopausal complaints or as a cardiovascular protector. The Women's Health Initiative Randomized Trial, a randomized, double-blind, placebo trial of more than 16,000 postmenopausal women over five years suggests that combined estrogen plus progestin may increase the risk of ovarian cancer.[28] Endometrial cancers rates were similar to placebo. A second part of the study evaluated combined therapy (estrogen and progestin) in preventing the risk of fracture through an increase in bone mineral density. The researchers concluded that there was an increase in BMD and a decreased risk of fracture; however, when weighed against the risk of other diseases, there was no net benefit.[29]

A Women's Health Initiative project evaluating estrogen/progestin therapy and stroke provided data that support an increased risk of ischemic stroke in generally healthy postmenopausal women.[30] A memory study portion of the Women's Health Initiative concluded that estrogen/progestin combination therapy did not improve cognitive function in postmenopausal women 65 years or older and in fact may cause a small increased risk of clinically meaningful cognitive decline.[31] A part of the same study indicated increased risk for probable dementia.[32]

Nutritional recommendations are given in **Table 55–4**. Recent interest is in the use of phytoestrogens (plant estrogens derived from soy or clover) to prevent or reduce hot flashes. The isoflavones in the extracts may have additional benefits related to cholesterol levels and bone loss. Soy-derived isoflavones have been recommended for the treatment of hot flashes in menopausal women. A recent randomized, double-blind, placebo-controlled trial found that daily administration of 72 mg of soy-derived isoflavones was no more effective than placebo in reducing hot flashes.[33]

Vaginal Bleeding

Vaginal bleeding is usually due to uterine bleeding. The causes of vaginal bleeding are limited and are usually the result of trauma or atrophic vaginitis found in elderly women. Uterine bleeding should be correlated with the woman's menstrual history in an attempt to place her in a stage of menstrual development. Uterine bleeding may occur (1) when no ovarian function is occurring as in premenarcheal and postmenopausal stages, (2) when

Table 55-4 Nutritional Support for Menopause

Substance	How Might It Work?	Dosage	Special Instructions	Contraindications and Possible Side Effects
Vitamin E	Unknown.	800-1,000 IU/day	Take for 3 months to determine effectiveness.	Generally safe at recommended dose.
Vitamin C	May reduce symptoms of hot flashes.	1,200 mg of vitamin C and 1,200 mg of bioflavonoid hesperidin.	None.	Bioflavonoid Some individuals are sensitive to vitamin C and may have diarrhea; high levels of vitamin C may deplete the body of copper.
Black cohosh	Has a weak estrogen-like effect to help reduce hot flashes. May decrease levels of luteinizing hormone.	Highly concentrated extract at 40 mg 2 times/day in a 40%–60% alcoholic extract.	Because long-term studies have not been conducted, it is recommended to limit to 6 months of usage.	Not to be used in pregnant or lactating women. Women on ERT should consult prescribing doctor. High doses may cause abdominal pain, nausea, headaches, and dizziness.
Dong Quai	Adaptogenic effect on female hormonal system.	Powdered root as herbal extract, capsules or tablets, or tea at 3–4 g/day.	None.	Not recommended in pregnant or lactating women. May cause sensitivity to ultraviolet light (decrease exposure to sunlight).

Note: Other possibly helpful substances include the phytoestrogens (plant estrogens derived from soy or clover) for management of hot flashes.

Note: The above substances have not been approved by the Food and Drug Administration for the treatment of this disorder.

normal ovulation occurs, (3) anovulatory (more common in the first years following menarche or perimenopausal years), and (4) during pregnancy. Chronologically, a woman's reproductive system's development may be divided into the following five stages:[34]

1. premenarchal
2. menarche
3. the reproductive years
4. perimenopausal
5. postmenopausal

This categorization is useful in considering the most likely causes in each stage of development. Bleeding in stages 1 and 5 is abnormal and warrants investigation. In premenarchal years, the most common cause is direct trauma and/or sexual abuse. In postmenopausal years, any bleeding that appears to be uterine should be suspected to be cancerous in origin. Irregular bleeding during menarche and perimenopausal stages is often the natural consequence of fluctuations in hormonal balance. However, one-fifth of abnormal bleeding during menarche is due to a bleeding diathesis. During the reproductive years, the major concerns are that there may be excessive bleeding and that there may be bleeding during pregnancy. Also, it is important to recognize the classic presentation of cervical cancer, which includes painful intercourse, postcoital bleeding, and foul smelling vaginal discharge. Alterations in the degree and timing of bleeding related to the menstrual cycle are defined by specific terms as follows:

- polymenorrhea—more frequent than every 20 days
- oligomenorrhea—less often than every 42 days
- menorrhagia—bleeding lasting longer than 8 days
- metrorrhagia—bleeding between periods

The time limits listed above are generalizations and may vary with other text definitions by a few days.

The major differential pivot point is whether bleeding is ovulatory or anovulatory. Ovulatory bleeding is cyclic and is associated with dysmenorrhea and some premenstrual symptoms. In general, the cause of abnormal ovulatory bleeding is usually a pelvic lesion such as endometriosis, fibroids, an intrauterine device (IUD), pelvic inflammatory disease (PID), or pelvic tumors (see **Table 55–5**). Anovulatory bleeding is irregular and usually painless; it is often heavy. Endocrine dysfunction or contraceptive use is often the cause. Anovulation often is due to lack of production of LH during the midcycle. The type of bleeding may suggest an underlying cause. If bleeding is bright red with associated clots,

Table 55-5 Tumors and Cancer in Females

Disorder	Diagnostic Features and Considerations	Management Considerations
Endometriosis	Endometriosis is a condition characterized by uterine tissue (glands and stroma) located outside the uterus. Most commonly the tissue is found on the serosa of the ovaries or the peritoneum, although endometriosis may be found almost anywhere in the pelvic cavity and sometimes beyond. The etiology is believed to be from regurgitation during normal menstruation with the tissue traveling retrograde through the fallopian tubes instead of out the vagina. Endometriosis is found in an estimated 15% to 20% of women of reproductive age (the highest rates in infertile women); primarily in the age group 25–29. Classically, there is a triad of dysmenorrhea that has worsened coupled with dyspareunia (painful intercourse), and infertility. The pelvic pain is associated more with the depth of infiltration versus the extent of the disease. A pelvic examination may reveal involvement of the uterosacral ligaments, the cul-de-sac, with a fixed retroversion of the uterus, or tenderness only. Diagnostic ultrasound or magnetic resonance imaging (MRI) may be used to detect the extent of lesions; however, laparoscopy is needed for a definitive diagnosis. Colonoscopy is recommended if there is associated rectal bleeding.	Although painful, endometriosis is a benign, self-limited disorder; it does not progress to cancer. There are two general approaches dependent on whether pregnancy is still desired. Medical approaches may attempt to decrease estrogen influence through creating a pseudopregnancy using contraceptive pill approach, androgens (danazol), or gonadotropin-releasing hormone. Surgery may be used to remove lesions to correct infertility. For those not wishing to have children and having extensive disease, surgery involves a total hysterectomy with bilateral salpingo-oophorectomy.
Uterine Myomas (Leiomyomas, Fibromyomas, Fibroids)	Uterine fibroids are the most common uterine tumor occurring in about 25% of all white women and 50% of all black women. These myometrial tumors develop only in women having reached menarche; however, not after menopause. They are often multiple and are estrogen sensitive. Signs and symptoms are dependent on the location. Small tumors are often asymptomatic. Larger tumors that are subserosal tend to cause signs/symptoms due to compression of the bladder or rectum such as urinary urgency or constipation. Those that are submucosal cause menstrual irregularities or bleeding. Infertility may also be due to fibroids. A pelvic examination is the initial evaluation tool followed by diagnostic ultrasound, computed tomography (CT), or MRI for confirmation. Occasionally, calcified uterine fibroids are seen radiographically on an anteroposterior (AP) lumbopelvic film.	Asymptomatic fibroids are not treated. Symptomatic lesions may be medically manipulated using various hormonal approaches to manage the abnormal bleeding or use of either gonadotropin-releasing hormone agonists or danazol (an andronergic agonist) to decrease the size of the fibroids. These drugs carry with them common side effects (in particular, danazol has a virilization effect). Surgery is used for those symptomatic women who have large masses or for those who are infertile (secondary to the fibroids). Surgical options include myomectomy (shelling-out the lesion) for those women wishing to still conceive or hysterectomy for those who do not.
Meigs' Syndrome	Meigs' syndrome involves the development of ascites and right hydrothorax (pleural effusion) secondary to a large, benign fibroma. It is theorized that the fibroma has an inadequate lymphatic drainage. Meigs' syndrome occurs primarily in middle-aged women.	Surgical removal.
Cervical Cancer	Cervical cancer is the third most common gynecologic cancer. It is often considered a sexually transmitted disease due to the association with risk factors such as early-age first time intercourse, multiple sexual partners, venereal disease, and infection with human papillomavirus (HPV). However, smoking is also associated with a higher risk. The average age of onset is about 50 years; however, cervical cancer may occur in younger women. Early cancer is asymptomatic. The first signs are usually painful intercourse, postcoital bleeding, or a foul smelling discharge. As the cancer progresses, other signs or symptoms may develop. Screening for cervical cancer is important given the initial asymptomatic phase. Papanicolaou (Pap) smears are the initial screening test. Although the false negative rate can be as high as 40% dependent on lab, it is extremely important that Pap smears be a routine part of a women's check-up; in particular, those at high risk. If abnormal cells are found, further investigation proceeds systematically with colposcopy-directed biopsy. If equivocal,	Based on the staging of the disease, various forms of therapy are available. Preinvasive disease may require only conization biopsy. To prevent spread to lymphatics, radiation therapy may be required and, in fact, is used often in advanced disease. More radical surgery such as hysterectomy is reserved for more advanced disease. Bilateral pelvic lymph node dissection and removal of all adjacent ligaments may be required. The 5-year survival rate is quite high for early-stage disease (80% to 90%); however, for late-stage disease, the 5-year survival rate is dismal with the best possible rate at 15%. This reemphasizes the need for regular Pap smears in an effort to detect early-stage disease. A vaccine (Gardacil) against HPV is now available.

Table 55–5 Tumors and Cancer in Females (continued)

Disorder	Diagnostic Features and Considerations	Management Considerations
	a conization biopsy is required. A newer approach is to include an HPV DNA test (Digene Hybrid Capture test) with the Pap for women over age 30. The HPV DNA test is designed to detect certain specific groups of HPV more likely to cause cancer. If both the Pap and HPV test are normal, retesting is performed in 3 years.	
Ovarian Cysts	During the proliferative phase of the menstrual cycle, ovarian follicles enlarge and are transformed into Graafian follicles. Only one precedes to rupture at ovulation. The remaining follicles may continue to enlarge into fluid-filled folicular cysts or the ovulated follicle may fail to transform into a corpus albicans and fill with fluid becoming a corpus luteum cyst. When multiple cysts are found on both ovaries, the diagnosis is polycystic ovary syndrome. Affected females have complex hormonal dysfunction and are not able to ovulate even in an environment of high levels of gonadotropins. Sudden abdominal pain may occur with rupture, adnexal torsion, or hemorrhage.	For masses found on pelvic exam or with diagnostic ultrasound, a repeat evaluation in 4 to 6 weeks helps determine those cysts that will spontaneously resolve versus those that will persist or progress. Management varies dependent on size, number, and complications associated with cysts. Oral contraceptive treatment may reduce the size of cysts. Surgical excision may be necessary for symptomatic patients or those with other cyst complications.
Vaginal Cancer	Vaginal cancer is rare, occurring mainly in the 60–65 age group. Increased risk is found with a history of human papillomavirus infection, cervical or vulvar cancer, and diethylstilbesterol. Most vaginal cancers are squamous cell carcinomas. Spread of the tumor may be direct to local tissues, through inguinal or pelvic lymph nodes, or hematogenously. The most common finding is abnormal vaginal bleeding (usually postmenopausal) and sometimes a watery discharge. A punch biopsy is used for diagnosis. Screening for metastasis includes radiography.	Poorly differentiated lesions that have spread carry a poor prognosis of 15% to 20% 5-year survival. Small, differentiated lesions may carry a 5-year survival as high as 70%. Primary tumors are usually treated with radiation. Surgical procedures such as radical hysterectomy and vaginectomy with lymph node dissection may be needed for more advanced disease.
Fallopian Tube Cancer	Fallopian tube cancer is rare, occurring mainly in the 50–60 age group. There are no well-defined risk factors. Most patients have vague pelvic or abdominal complaints. Some have a triad of pelvic pain, watery discharge, and adnexal mass.	Diagnosis is via surgical exploration and, if found, surgical removal and postoperative radiation therapy are standard.
Ovarian Cancer	Ovarian cancer is made up of a number of different groups that include benign and malignant lesions. The categorization of these lesions is based on basically four main cell types: (1) surface epithelium (germinal), (2) germ, (3) sex cord stromal, and (4) nonspecific. Benign lesions are more common than malignant. However, ovarian cancer causes more deaths than all other gynecologic cancers. It ranks as the second most common gynecologic cancer, however, first as a cause of death by gynecologic cancer. Ovarian cancer is seen more often in industrialized countries, especially where high-fat dietary intake is found. Risk factors include multiparity, infertility, late child bearing, and late onset of menopause. A personal or family history of endometrial, breast, or colon cancer also increases risk. A small percentage of women who have the BRCA gene are at higher risk. Oral contraceptives are protective. Seventy-five percent of women have advanced disease at the time of diagnosis. Vague symptoms may include dyspepsia, a sense of bloating or gas pains, lack of appetite due to a sense of fullness with small amounts of food, or low back pain. Physical findings may include finding an abdominal mass on pelvic examination. Severe abdominal pain may occur with torsion of the mass. Germ cell or stromal tumors may create	Localized tumors are surgically removed. More advanced disease requires a combination of approaches including radical surgical procedures combined with chemotherapy. Response to chemotherapy is often monitored with CA 125 levels. The 5-year survival rate is variable from 5% to 40%. Use of BCP may be protective.

(continues)

Table 55–5 Tumors and Cancer in Females (continued)

Disorder	Diagnostic Features and Considerations	Management Considerations
	signs/symptoms secondary to the development of hyperthyroidism or androgen stimulation leading to feminization or virilization. Sonography may help; however, surgery may be needed for suspicious masses. Laboratory testing is nonspecific; however, beta-subunit-human chorionic gonadotropin, lactate dehydrogenase (LDH), alpha-fetoprotein, and the cancer antigen 125 (CA 125) should be evaluated.	
Endometrial Cancer	Endometrial cancer is most often found in postmenopausal women, peaking at ages 50 to 60. It is the most common gynecologic cancer in the United States and is more common in industrialized countries where there is a high dietary fat intake. Risk factors include obesity (3 to 10 times higher risk); and, where unopposed estrogen is common such as estrogen replacement therapy, polycystic ovary disease; and estrogen-producing tumors. Those with a history of breast or ovarian cancer or pelvic radiation therapy are at higher risk. Eighty percent of cases represent adenocarcinoma, with sarcomas accounting for only 5%. Sarcomas are generally more aggressive. Abnormal uterine bleeding is the most common initial complaint, occurring in 90% of women. Many are postmenopausal. In fact, one third of postmenopausal bleeding patients have endometrial cancer. Pap smears may show abnormal cells. However, endometrial tissue sampling is the definitive test (>90% accurate). Following a positive tissue sampling, investigation with laboratory, x-ray, and electrocardiogram is necessary to determine extra-uterine involvement.	Like most cancers, staging based on histologic differentiation is necessary. Prognosis is based on the staging, the patient's age (poorer prognosis with advancing age), and metastatic spread. For early-stage cancer, total hysterectomy, bilateral salpingo-oophorectomy, and peritoneal cytologic examination are used. For later stages, pelvic and para-aortic lymphadenectomy is often added. The 5-year survival rate is 70% to 95% for early stages and varies from 10% to 60% for late-stage disease.
Vulvar Cancer	Vulvar cancer is a geriatric cancer seen primarily in women over 70 years old. It is not common, accounting for only about 3% to 4% of all gynecologic cancers in the United States. Risk factors include having a premalignant lesion, human papillomavirus, or chronic vulvar pruritis. Those patients with cervix or vaginal cancer are also at higher risk. The most common presentation is a palpable, often visible, vulvar lesion with pruritis. Dermal punch biopsy is used for diagnosis.	The 5-year survival rate is based on staging, with as little as a 15% survival with widespread involvement to as high as 90% for local involvement. Treatment is radical excision and unilateral or bilateral inguinal and femoral lymph node dissection.

a nonmenstrual flow is suggested. Bleeding during pregnancy may be serious. Spotting is common in the first trimester; however, it may represent spontaneous abortion (50%), ectopic pregnancy, or a low-lying placenta. Past the 20th week of gestation, serious causes are likely, including placental abruption, placenta previa, marginal separation of the placenta, and vasa previa. Referral is indicated in all cases of vaginal bleeding during pregnancy.

The examination is limited to determination of endocrine causes or a bleeding tendency. An evaluation for thyroid dysfunction is prudent. Pelvic examination should be performed by chiropractors with training or referred to a medical physician in a search for a bleeding source such as a tumor. Laboratory evaluation may be helpful in determining whether the patient is anemic.

After performing a thorough history and brief examination, the patient should be given an explanation as to the different types of bleeding and what is specifically suggested in her case. Referral should be made, with a letter explaining the doctor's rationale or recommendations.

If a structural lesion is not found to be the source of bleeding, an attempt at controlling the bleeding and normalizing the cycle is made. The standard form of treatment is prescription of oral contraceptive pills (OCPs) or nonsteroid anti-inflammatory drugs (NSAIDs). Both OCPs and NSAIDs can reduce bleeding by up to 50% (NSAIDs usually are a little less effective).[35, 36] NSAIDs have a strong vasoconstrictive effect. A side benefit is possible reduction of any associated dysmenorrhea. A small number of women may have an increase in bleeding.

Vaginal Discharge

The first line of distinction with vaginal discharge is to determine if the discharge is physiologic or nonphysiologic. Physiologic discharge is not offensive in odor and is rarely associated with vulvar discomfort. Laboratory evaluation usually reveals few polymorphonuclear (PMN) leukocytes with predominantly Gram-positive bacillus found on culture or staining. Physiologic discharge is associated with ovulation, premenses, use of birth control pills, and sexual excitement. Nonphysiologic discharge often has an offensive odor with associated vulvar discomfort that may include local dermatologic involvement. Laboratory evaluation will generally indicate a high PMN count with specific findings on bacteriologic testing. Nonphysiologic categories include dermatologic, allergic, or toxic irritation from douches, vaginal sprays, perfumes, or contraceptive products (creams, jellies, foams, and suppositories), infection primarily from sexually transmitted diseases, neoplasms, and, on rarer occasions, anatomic problems such as a fistula or proctitis, or foreign body such as a tampon or intrauterine device.

Questioning regarding contraceptive and hygiene practices will often reveal the source of discharge with elimination, modification, or substitution as the primary solution. Infection should be suspected when there is an active sexual history, when discharge is accompanied by skin lesions, or when there is painful urination or intercourse. Generally, there are three primary causes of localized vaginitis, including:[37]

1. Bacterial vaginosis (anaerobes plus *Gardnerella*)— *Gardnerella* accounts for approximately 50% to 60% of vaginal infections. Clues include a mild to moderate gray/whitish discharge with mild itching. Laboratory testing includes a positive "whiff" test (a fishy odor is smelled when the discharge is mixed with 10% potassium hydroxide [KOH] on a clean slide). Examination of the slide microscopically may reveal vaginal epithelial cells covered with coccobacilli (clue cells). There are few PMNs. Treatment is usually with metronidazole (Flagyl).

2. Trichomoniasis *(Trichomonas vaginalis)*— Trichomoniasis accounts for approximately 15% to 20% of all vaginal infections. It is found most commonly when the pH of the vagina changes to a more alkaline environment (e.g., menstruation, abortion, post-delivery). This infection is generally sexually transmitted. One-fourth of patients are asymptomatic, one-fourth have pruritus, and one-half have both pruritus and discharge. The discharge is generally profuse and foul smelling, often being called "fishy" in odor. Diagnosis is made with a wet mount of vaginal secretions to identify the organism. A pelvic examination may reveal punctuate hemorrhages of the cervix ("strawberry cervix"). Treatment is with metronidazole (Flagyl).

3. Candidiasis *(Candida albicans)*—Candidiasis accounts for approximately 15% to 20% of all vaginal infections. Unlike the other infections, it is often a cause of extreme pruritus, especially at night. There are many predispositions including diabetes, contraceptive use, steroids (including corticosteroids), antibiotics, and late pregnancy. Sexual transmission is less common. Although the discharge is scanty, it has a cottage-cheese or curd-like appearance, often being thick and white. Marked pruritus leads to an erythematous, edematous, excoriated vulva. Diagnosis is via a KOH preparation or Gram stain. Treatment is often with over-the-counter medications such as clotrimazole or miconazole. If frequent and recurrent, prescribed treatment is usually with oral ketoconazole or fluconazole.

Gonorrhea and chlamydia are not direct infections of the vagina, but rather infect the endocervix. The discharge may lead one to think there is a local vaginal infection.

Infertility

Infertility is defined as a year of attempted conception without success and is clinically separate from recurrent spontaneous pregnancy loss. The time frame of one year is used because within one year 85% of couples attempting conception will be successful.[38] Approximately 6 million couples are affected in the United States. There are reasons for infertility evaluation prior to one year. This would be in patients older than age 35 years or those who have diagnosed or suspected pelvic pathology.

The evaluation for infertility involves the following procedures:

- Semen analysis.
- Assessment of ovulatory function (often used are urinary luteinizing hormone and midluteal phase serum progesterone level). Urinary ovulation prediction kits replace the basal body temperature

approach, and endometrial biopsy has been replaced by midluteal progesterone levels).

- Assessment of the uterus with a hysterosalpingogram (HSG) or sonohysterogram.
- Assessment of fallopian tube patency using either HSG or laparoscopy.
- Estimation of FSH on cycle day three in women 35 years or older or those with prior ovarian surgery. (Elevated FSH levels are associated with a poor ovarian response to hormonal stimulation.)

Management is dependent on cause and other factors. Two possible management approaches are in vitro fertilization (IVF) and intracytoplasmic sperm injection (ICSI). These are reserved for specific patients, and due to cost and complexity are still not commonly used. Also, IVF carries with it an increased risk of multiple births.

The primary identifiable causes of infertility include:

- Ovulation disorders (25% of cases) such as oligomenorrhea, amenorrhea, and hyperprolactinemia: Medical options include clomiphene citrate, gonadotropins, metformin, laparoscopic ovarian diathermy, and IVF.
- Tubal disease (20% of cases) such as obstruction from prior infection: Medical management includes tubal reparative surgery and IVF.
- Endometriosis (5% to 10% of cases): Treatment with danazol, GRH, or progestins does not seem to improve fertility; therefore, laser ablation of endometriosis is recommended.
- Male factors (20% to 25% of cases) such as oligospermia or azoospermia.
- Unexplained infertility (30% of cases): Medical options include clomiphene citrate, intrauterine insemination with or without gonadotropins, and IVF.

Some Specific Pregnancy-Related Concerns

Pregnancy is a natural process that in many cases is uncomplicated. Concerns ranging from decisions to screen for prenatal abnormalities, fetal development abnormalities, and other serious complications with pregnancy are beyond the scope of this overview. The primary focus of this discussion is on issues where the chiropractor can play a role in monitoring and

counseling and musculoskeletal issues associated with pregnancy.

The U.S. Preventive Services Task Force and other groups[5-14] have made specific recommendations for screening, follow-up visits, and counseling for the pregnant patient. The general purposes of screening include:

- To monitor for signs of hypertension and developing preeclampsia and eclampsia (see Chapter 24).
- To detect diabetes and monitor for gestational diabetes development.
- To screen for anemias.
- To screen for diseases that may affect the pregnancy or fetus such as rubella, hepatitis, chlamydia, and, in high-risk groups, HIV.
- To make recommendations regarding amniocentesis (generally recommended in women age 35 years or older) or laboratory testing of specific indicators of disorders such as Down's syndrome and spina bifida (e.g., serum alpha-fetoprotein).
- To counsel on issues such as alcohol, smoking, and other drug cessation; adequate nutrition (specifically folate supplementation) and calcium (for high-risk eclampsia patients); and avoidance of high-risk sexual behavior.
- To encourage breastfeeding, lap-shoulder seatbelt usage, infant safety, and car seats.

Postpartum concerns include the development of a hyperthyroid state and postpartum depression. Hyperthyroidism may develop in the first few weeks following delivery, and it should be suspected in any patient with increased blood pressure, palpitations, and anxiety (see Chapter 50). Postpartum blues are common in the first few weeks following delivery. It is due to fluctuating levels of estrogen and other hormones. Patients are often emotionally labile and appear irrational in their reaction or response to minor relationship issues. Postpartum blues will resolve over a number of weeks once hormonal levels have stabilized. Postpartum depression, however, occurs within the first few months up to one year following delivery. It is a poorly understood condition, but likely represents a version of endogenous depression often requiring medication due to the not uncommon result of infant abuse or neglect (see Chapter 20).

The American College of Sports Physicians (ACSM)[39] and the American College of Obstetricians and

Gynecologists (ACOG)[40] have made recommendations for exercise during pregnancy. Generally, women who already have an established exercise routine are advised to continue, with appropriate cautions and with close attention to any warning signs such as shortness of breath, dizziness, loss of balance, etc. For those women who have not established an exercise program prior to pregnancy, the ACSM guidelines recommend an intensity level where the heart rate is at or below 150 beats/minute, exercise of short duration (less than 20 minutes), and avoidance of ballistic movements. For the pregnant woman starting an exercise program, the ACOG recommends the following:

- Avoid dehydration and hypoglycemia by ensuring adequate caloric and fluid intake.
- Avoid extreme environmental conditions and dress appropriately to allow for heat dissipation.
- Avoid exercise in the supine position after the first trimester (decreased cardiac and venous return).
- Avoid vigorous exercise because of the preferential distribution of blood flow to the periphery and away from the uterus.
- Exercise regularly; intermittent exercise is not as effective or safe.

Absolute contraindications to exercise during pregnancy include ruptured membranes, premature labor, vaginal bleeding, suspected fetal distress, intrauterine growth retardation, preeclampsia, kidney disease, valvular or ischemic heart disease, multiple pregnancy, acute infection, or incompetent cervix.[41] Relative contraindications to exercise during pregnancy include hypertension; moderate to severe anemia; poorly controlled diabetes; excessive obesity; underweight; smoking; excessive alcohol intake; a history of premature delivery, preeclampsia, or significant pulmonary disease; twins after 24 weeks' gestation; and previous sedentary lifestyle. There are no apparent effects on length of labor with exercise; however, 85% of exercising women will have a normal spontaneous vaginal delivery as compared to only 50% to 55% for those women not exercising.[42, 43] Also, regular exercise appears to decrease musculoskeletal complaints. Even as little as 45 minutes of physical activity per week has an effect of decreasing lumbar pain in pregnancy.

Musculoskeletal concerns during pregnancy are primarily related to mechanical changes due to the growth and position of the fetus and hormonal changes that result in less ligament stability (i.e., relaxin). Following are some common problems and management issues:

- It is not uncommon for the pregnant female to develop a mechanical compensation to the anterior position and weight of the fetus and develop an increased thoracic kyphosis and anterior head positioning. These factors, plus the more direct effect of the weight of the breasts in some women, may contribute to mechanical strain to the cervical and thoracic areas. Development of myofascially related problems is common and warrants stretching of the anterior musculature (i.e., pectorals) and strengthening of the interscapular musculature (i.e., rhomboids and middle trapezius).
- With the anterior displacement of the gravity line that occurs with the frontal position of the fetus, anterior tilting of the pelvis with hip flexion results. This may place hyperextension forces to the knees, stretching the posterior capsule. It is important for the patient to consider this recurvatum position when standing and to shift weight as often as possible to avoid bilateral, chronic stretching. Maintaining good muscle tone about the knee through a standard knee exercise program may also help.
- A shift from the weight-bearing function of the calcaneus to the metatarsals occurs due to the shift in the center of gravity anteriorly. In addition, the extra weight incurred during pregnancy adds to the challenge of the foot ligamentous and fascial structures. Adjusting of the joints of the foot and ankle, and/or arch supports may be beneficial for these problems.
- Increasing anterior weight causes an increase in the lumbar lordosis. The hyperlordosis may contribute to the development of symptoms related to facet compression including some referral of pain into the lower extremity. Abdominal strengthening early in pregnancy and modified abdominal contractions during pregnancy may assist in providing more anterior support.
- Hip pain is common for the simple reason of increased weight bearing coupled with the later trimester effect of relaxin on the ligamentous support of the hip. Proactive approaches include a strengthening program for the hip musculature, in particular the abductors, and extra cushioning and support for the hips during sleep.

Low back pain is common in pregnant women.[44] There is some literature support[45] for the role of chiropractic treatment of the pregnant patient with low back pain. Adjusting of the pregnant female is safe if precautions are taken to protect against compression forces to the abdomen, consider positional effects of blood flow, and ensure comfort. Compression by the fetus and abdominal organ combination may block venous return and lead to a relative hypovolemic response due to position change to a seated or standing posture resulting in either presyncope or syncope.

Two excellent reviews of adjusting procedures for women and pregnant females include those by Bartol[46] and Esch and Zachman.[47] The primary modifications are to support the abdomen without causing compression, avoid excess compression to the breasts, and avoid prolonged recumbency in the supine position. Abdominal support and redistribution of forces off of the abdomen can be accomplished through the use of appropriately positioned pillows. Another excellent alternative for avoidance of abdominal compression is appropriately delivered knee-chest table adjusting. Alternatives to standard adjusting approaches include "softer" approaches such as Activator, massage, and reflex therapy. Certainly, in the last trimester and during labor, many practitioners focus on sacral mobility and reflex pain modulation through sacral reflex or acupressure/acupuncture points.

Breast Pain or Discharge

Breast pain (mastodynia) is usually due to local tissue involvement; however, it may represent referral or extension of pain from the chest wall, or it may emanate from cardiac or gastrointestinal origins. It is important to first make this distinction before proceeding to an evaluation of breast involvement. The breast is composed of epithelial-lined ducts organized into lobules surrounded by Cooper's ligaments. These ligaments extend throughout the breast and connect to both the skin and the chest wall. Most local pathology involves the ductal epithelium through hyperplasia, dysplasia, or neoplasm. The breast is sensitive to hormonal stimulation, in particular estrogen. As a result, the vast majority of "normal" breast discomfort is a result of this ebb and flow of estrogen related to menses. Discomfort is generally cyclic and bilateral. The associated pain, tenderness, and swelling are usually premenstrual in onset. The degree of discomfort may vary depending on pain threshold and the degree of fibrocystic changes. Fibrocystic "change" is manifested as multiple, well-defined nodules most seen in the upper outer quadrant and often bilateral. This fibrocystic involvement

is by far the most common cause of breast discomfort seen from ages 25 years through 60 years.[48] Management of fibrocystic disease includes some conservative options including caffeine (xanthine) restriction and vitamin E supplementation. Medical approaches are hormonal, involving androgens such as danazol or antiestrogens. Noncyclic breast pain in the premenopausal female or any breast pain in the postmenopausal female should be further investigated for possible fibrocystic disease, mastitis, or malignancy. This requires referral to a specialist.

Nipple discharge is a common concern. About 7% of patients with nipple discharge have carcinoma. There are some key factors that help distinguish benign physiologic causes versus those warranting concern. When there is bilateral nipple discharge that is seen only with nipple compression, never occurring spontaneously, and if the discharge is greenish or milky, there is rarely a concern. Usually this type of discharge is bilateral and is coming from multiple ducts. With this type of discharge there are several common causes:

- eczema or other dermatologic disease
- birth control pills, tranquilizers, rauwolfia alkaloids, or the patient is recently menopausal
- pregnancy, prolonged lactation, nonlactational galactorrhea, or elevated prolactin levels or other endocrine dysfunction

Serous or bloody discharge may occur with cystic mastitis, fibrocystic disease, Paget's disease of the breast (intradermal infiltration by ductal carcinoma), or Bowen's disease. This is more often represented by spontaneous discharge that is unilateral and arises from a single duct. When this scenario is present, further investigation by a specialist is requisite.

Breast Cancer

Breast cancer is a significant cause of mortality in women, second only to lung cancer as the leading cancer-related cause of death in women. Important statistics to consider when discussing breast cancer follow:[49]

- Women account for 99% of all cases of breast cancer.
- In 60% of all cases, the only identifiable risk factor is being female.
- Women 50 years and older account for 70% of all cases; the risk in women 80 to 85 years of age is 15 times higher than that for women 30 to 35 years old.

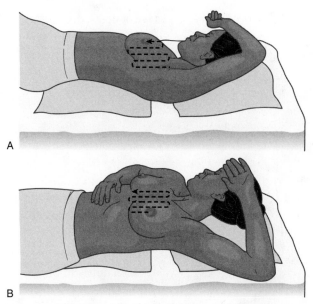

Figure 55-2 Position of patient and direction of palpation for the clinical breast examination. (A) The figure shows the lateral portion of the breast; (B) the medial portion of the breast. Arrows indicate vertical strip pattern of examination.

- Although those with genetic mutations in the BRCA1 gene (and less commonly the BRCA2 gene) have a significantly higher risk of developing breast cancer (50% to 80% over a lifetime), these women represent only 3% of all breast cancer cases.[50]
- An appropriate in-office breast examination can detect, at minimum, 50% of asymptomatic cancers.[51] (See **Figures 55-2** through **55-4**.)
- Twenty-one percent of women aged 40 years or older who are multiparous or had their first child after age 30 years account for 16% of new breast cancer cases each year.

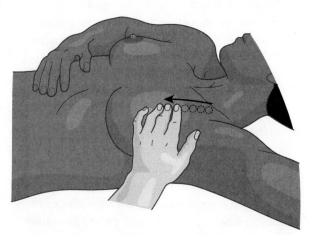

Figure 55-3 Palpation technique. Pads of the index, third, and fourth fingers (inset) make small circular motions, as if tracing the outer edge of a dime.

- One-third of women who develop breast cancer will succumb to it; therefore, the survival rate for breast cancer is approximately 60%.
- Most recurrences develop within two to six years following the initial diagnosis.
- Fifty percent of survivors will develop metastasis, with 40% to 60% of metastasis occurring in bone and 7% to 15% in soft tissue.

A large database regarding a woman's risk of developing breast cancer has been developed. Generally, there are those factors that have been strongly associated with breast cancer risk and those that may or may not play a role but are important to consider. Certainly significant risk factors are being female and increasing age (the most important). A list and a brief discussion of other major risk factors and a list of potential risk factors follow.[52]

Major Risk Factors

- Family history: Genetics contributes to about 5% of all breast cancers; however, it accounts for 25% of cases seen before age 30 years. Familial clustering is suspected when the patient has three or more affected first-degree or second-degree relatives on the same side of the family; or when fewer than three are affected, breast cancer is diagnosed before age 45 years, ovarian cancer has been diagnosed in one or more family members, a genetic mutation is detected in a family member, or the patient has an ethnic risk such as Ashkenazi Jews.
- Previous history of breast cancer: When there is a previous diagnosis; in particular, lobular carcinoma in situ (LCIS) or if the cancer was diagnosed before menopause, the risk of having another primary tumor is three to four times greater.
- Benign breast disease: Benign breast disease that necessitates a biopsy increases the likelihood of subsequent cancer, especially those with proliferative lesions or cellular atypia; in fact, 40% of those with proliferative disease and a family history of breast cancer in a first-degree relative develop carcinoma. Also, a history of biopsy before age 50 years is associated with a higher likelihood than a history of biopsy performed in older patients.
- Menstrual relationships: Menarche before 12 years of age or menopause after age 55 years allows for breast cells to be exposed to estrogen longer;

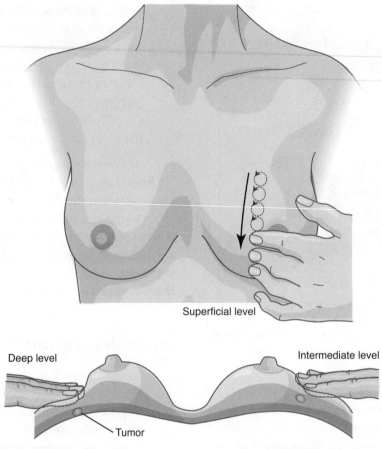

Superficial level

Deep level

Intermediate level

Tumor

Figure 55–4 Levels of pressure for palpation of breast tissue shown in a cross-sectional view of the right breast. The examiner should make three circles with the finger pads, increasing the level of pressure (superficial, intermediate, and deep) with each circle.

women who have reached menopause or have a hysterectomy before age 45 years have half the incidence of breast cancer compared to those reaching menopause after age 55 years. Early menarche, extremely lean body mass at age 10 years old, and taller adult height increase risk;[53] being multiparous or giving birth for the first time after age 30 years (risk doubles); pregnancy before age 20 years reduces the incidence of breast cancer.

- Hereditary/genetic factors: Mutation of the BRCA1 gene increases lifetime risk up to 85%; chance of acquiring a second primary breast cancer is 65% and risk of developing ovarian cancer is between 40% and 60%.[54] BRCA1 is located on chromosome arm 17q and is involved in encoding a tumor suppressor protein; BRCA2 (located on chromosome 13) is associated with similar risks for breast and ovarian cancer. Although the risk is extremely high for these patients, they account

for only a small percentage of all women with breast cancer.

- Hormonal replacement therapy (HRT): There is strong evidence that there is a causal relation between both endogenous estrogen levels and the use of postmenopausal estrogens and progestins and the incidence of breast cancer in postmenopausal women. Contraceptive use prior to menopause does not appear to be a significant risk.[55] A recent study[56] indicates that the assumed safer combination of estrogen/progestin actually carries more risk than estrogen alone. Some differences in data indicate that perhaps HRT promotes the growth of less aggressive, slower growing tumors. A recent study[26] indicated that HRT was associated with risk for invasive breast cancer when the woman had a more favorable histology. It is known that there are significant differences in prognosis between the two carcinomas. Eighty-five to ninety percent of carcinomas that metastasize are invasive tumors including infiltrating ductal and lobular carcinomas versus the less common medullary, papillary, tubular, and mucinous tumors that have a lower rate of metastasis.[57]

Potential Risk Factors

- Alcohol consumption: The relative risk of breast cancer increases slightly if one or two drinks (33 to 45 g) are ingested per day in the under-30-years age group; apparently this risk may be reduced with adequate folate intake (greater than 300 mg/day).[58]
- Smoking: Smoking is a risk factor in some women; in particular, those who have cytochrome P450 1A1 polymorphism.[59] However, the risk is relatively low.
- Fat intake: Although previous accusations of a high-fat intake as a cause of breast cancer have been discounted,[60] there may be a relationship between a high-fat diet and high linoleic acid.[61]
- Weight gain and obesity: Weight gain after age 18 years appears not to be associated with premenopausal breast cancer; however, it is positively associated with incidence after menopause, accounting for approximately 16% of all cases. When HRT is taken alone, it accounts for only approximately 5%; however, both weight gain and HRT taken together account for as much as one-third of postmenopausal breast cancers.[62] Estrogen levels in the postmenopausal female are not from ovarian production but result from androgen conversion to estrogen and the amount of adipose tissue. Estrone and estradiol are converted into estrogen via an enzyme found in adipose tissue, thereby increasing the level of active estrogen.
- Recently, attention has been focused on the contribution of low levels of vitamin D to many disorders; breast cancer included. A meta-analysis in 2013[63] determined that there was a dose-response. For every 10 ng/mL increase in serum 25(OH)D concentration, there was an associated 3.2 % reduction in breast cancer risk.

A potential positive factor is length of breastfeeding. A large epidemiological review of 47 studies in 30 countries indicates that the longer women breastfeed, the more they are protected from breast cancer.[64] The authors suggest that the shorter time that women breastfeed in

developed countries versus underdeveloped countries may in part explain the higher incidence.

Tools for evaluating a patient's risk are available through the National Cancer Institute at http://cancer-trials.nci.nih.gov. An interactive tool and an in-office program are available free of charge.

Types of Breast Cancer

Breast cancer is not a single entity. There are many different types, primarily categorized by invasiveness and location. Following is a brief description of each:

- *Noninvasive.* Noninvasive carcinomas account for approximately 10% of all breast cancers. They are considered as a group to be early-stage cancer or precancerous in most cases. There are two main types: (1) ductal carcinoma in situ (DCIS) arising from milk ducts, and (2) LCIS. DCIS is divided into comedo and noncomedo. Comedo is more aggressive, while noncomedo is slower growing over longer periods of time. DCIS is seen as clusters of microcalcification on mammogram. Nipple discharge or a palpable mass may be seen on exam. LCIS is more common in premenopausal women. LCIS is less often diagnosed from a clinical exam and more likely found on biopsy.
- *Invasive.* Ductal carcinoma accounts for 80% of all cases of breast cancer. There are many types including adenocarcinoma, tubular carcinoma, mucinous or colloid carcinoma, and medullary carcinoma. Each carries a different degree of risk. Invasive lobular carcinoma accounts for approximately 10% of cases.

Staging of breast tumors includes tumor, lymph node, metastasis (TNM) staging mainly used for research, and a clinical division using four stages. A zero stage is used for lesions found in situ that are noninvasive. Stage I is a lesion that is less than 2 cm and has no lymph node involvement. Stage II is an intermediary stage with small lesions with lymph node enlargement or larger lesions without lymph node enlargement. Stage III is more advanced, larger than 5 cm, with lymph node involvement. Stage IV indicates metastasis.

Signs and symptoms may be subtle and require vigilant attention to both observation and examination on a regular basis. Signs include:

- Detection of an abnormal lump on a monthly breast self-exam (BSE)

- A change in breast tissue size or shape
- Spontaneous bloody discharge from the nipple
- Skin changes including crusting, ulceration, or eczema
- Venous distention seen as an irregular pattern referred to as the "peau d'orange" or orange-peel appearance
- Any redness, warmth, or edema of the breast or axilla

Any abnormal breast examination findings (including breast exam and evaluation for axillary or supraclavicular lymphadenopathy) warrant a referral for mammography or a fine-needle aspiration (FNA). Biopsy can be performed as a core biopsy or surgical biopsy. If a surgical biopsy is performed, removal of the lesion and some surrounding normal tissue is the standard approach. A 2007 study by Lehman et al.[64] indicates that at the initial diagnosis of breast cancer, MRI evaluation of the contralateral breast can detect breast cancer missed on mammography or clinical examination.

Mammography remains a controversial topic, with disagreement on the application of the existing evidence.[66] A Cochrane review[67] in 2011 estimated that one in 2,000 women will have their life prolonged by 10 years of screening; however, another 10 women will be exposed to unnecessary treatment for breast cancer. With regard to mortality rates, they concluded that the evidence does not demonstrate a reduction in mortality. Also, most estimates are that about 30% of breast cancer is overdiagnosed (largely due to screening mammography).[68] This amounted to approximately 1.3 million in the United States over the last three decades; 70,000 women in 2008. Although the recommendation is for women to make an informed decision with their physician, such a decision is difficult when national groups for over 40 years have not entirely agreed. A brief history follows:[69]

- 1971—The Health Insurance Plan study reported that although breast cancer screening reduced mortality rates for women in the age range of 50 to 64 years, it did not for women in the age range of 40 to 49 years.
- 1997—The National Institutes of Health Consensus Development Conference summarized their findings by stating that no single recommendation can be made for all women regarding screening mammography yet in the same year. The American Cancer Society made the recommendation that all women in their 40s undergo annual mammography

and the National Cancer Institute recommended performing mammography every one to two years.
- 2002—The U.S. Preventive Services Task Force (USPSTF) reversed its recommendation and recommended mammography screening for women 40 years and older.
- 2009—The USPSTF made a recommendation against "routine" mammography among women aged 40 to 49 years with the advice that women make an informed decision with their physician. What is misinterpreted is that this is a recommendation for screening mammography. For patients at higher risk or with a palpable lump, it is still recommended to obtain a mammogram.

In a 25-year 2014 follow-up study of the Canadian National Breast Cancer Study, the conclusions by the researchers were that annual mammography in women ages 40 to 59 years did not reduce mortality from breast cancer beyond that for those screened by physical examination or usual care, and that over 22% of mammography-detected invasive breast cancer was overdiagnosed, meaning it eventually was determined not to be.[70]

It is likely that early detection has less benefit than previously assumed due to the fact that cancers detected often are curable at a later time due to advances in treatment, and that many tumors may recede on their own or grow so slowly that the woman dies of another cause.

Following is a summary of recommendations:

- Most groups agree that a recommendation can be made for biennial (every two years) screening mammography for women aged 50 to 74 years.
- Annual mammograms beginning at age 40 years—recommended by the American Cancer Society, the American College of Radiology, and the American Congress of Obstetricians and Gynecologists.
- Mammograms every one to two years for women ages 40 to 49 years—recommended by the National Cancer Institute.
- Individualized screening plans for women 40 to 49 years of age—recommended by the American College of Physicians.

Mammography ratings are based on the BI-RADS system (Breast Imaging Reporting and Data System) published by the American Radiology Society. It is a quality assurance approach using a scale of 6:

0 = incomplete
1 = negative

2 = benign

3 = probably benign

4 = suspicious abnormality

5 = suggestive of malignancy

6 = known biopsy-proven malignancy

Then by matching whether there is a palpable mass based on age, whether there is reproducible nipple discharge, or whether there is asymmetrical thickening, further testing is dictated using diagnostic ultrasound, needle biopsy, ductogram, or surgical excision.

Newer imaging approaches include:

- Scintimammography: uses an injected radioactive tracer called technetium sestamibi to attach to breast cancer cells and mark their presence.
- Tomosynthesis (3D mammography): is a variation of standard mammography that allows the construction of a 3D image generated by taking more images, requiring slightly more radiation. Studies are still needed to confirm the advantage of these images in a risk/benefit ratio analysis.

Although laboratory testing is possible, most tests are reserved for those with established breast cancer or those at high risk. Testing to determine a hereditary tendency or evaluating for BRCA1, BRCA2, or an altered tumor suppressor gene p53 is not used as screening except for those at high risk. Testing for those with breast cancer includes:

- An evaluation of estrogen receptors (those tumors that are positive are generally less aggressive)
- Detection of cancer cells in lymph nodes and blood vessels close to the tumor site
- Tumor grading (the lower the grade, and therefore the more differentiated, the less aggressive; the higher the grade, the more likely to metastasize)
- TRUQUANT BR RIA (test for serum levels of the antigen CA27–29; found in tumors that metastasize; high levels seen in tumors that recur)
- Oncotype Dx,[71,72] a diagnostic assay that analyzes a panel of 21 genes related to breast cancer to determine the risk of recurrence in women with newly diagnosed, early stage disease. Through the measurement of these genes it is possible to determine which women need chemotherapy beyond hormonal therapy. This approach may reduce the need for chemotherapy in as much as 23% of women with early stage breast cancer.

There are a number of treatment options dependent on type of lesion, risk factors, and the woman's preference.[73] General approaches include using selected estrogen response modifiers (SERMs) such as tamoxifen (Nolvadex, Soltamox) or raloxifene (Evista) for estrogen-receptor (ER) positive tumors. This approach is used for premenopausal women who have had their breast cancer removed or for those at high-risk as a preventive (50% effective in this group). Aromatase inhibitors are used for postmenopausal women with HER2/neu-positive results.

For those with stage I or II breast cancer, breast conserving surgery (BCS), which involves lumpectomy followed by radiotherapy, is the most common choice. For women who choose mastectomy over lumpectomy, a new study indicates that, instead of the standard five-week daily treatment, treatment may take only three weeks. Some doctors are even trying five days. Options also include chemotherapy and tamoxifen for prevention of recurrence. New findings indicate that women with breast cancer may survive longer with fewer numbers of recurrences by incorporating a strategy that combines the use of tamoxifen (a selective estrogen-receptor modulator) with a newer medication, letrozole (an estrogen synthetase [aromatase] inhibitor). Because tamoxifen is both an antagonist and a partial agonist of estrogen receptors, at some point the agonist action impairs any potential anticancer ability. As a result, after five years the beneficial effects are lost, and the guidelines are to discontinue use at that time. The result was recurrence. Researchers in a recent study placed women who had completed the five-year tamoxifen therapy on five years of letrozole.[74] The results indicate a significant degree of reduction in the frequency of recurrence. Although the increase in osteoporosis was higher in this group versus the placebo group, it was not substantial (5.8% versus 4.5% respectively). Herceptin (Trastuzumab) may reduce recurrence rates by as much as 50% in women who have HER2 protein-related breast cancer.[75] It is intended for those patients who have received one or more chemotherapy regimens for metastatic disease, or is used in combination with paclitaxel for those patients who have not received chemotherapy. Modified radical mastectomy is recommended for some patients, leaving the pectoral muscle intact and involving reconstruction with a saline implant or tissue flap. The survival rate for both procedures appears to be the same; however, those having BCS are more likely to have recurrence in the same breast. Tsangaris et al.[73] provide a more extensive discussion of treatment options with tamoxifen. Axillary node dissection is being recommended less often with local breast cancer due to the complications of nerve damage and arm edema. Lymphatic mapping with sentinel (main node involvement) lymphadenectomy is now recommended. For later-stage cancers, radical mastectomy is still the treatment option of choice. Radical mastectomy is also chosen as a prophylactic measure for women at extremely high risk of cancer based on hereditary likelihood and other risk factors.

Prevention may be possible to some degree; however, many of the risk factors are nonmodifiable. Some possible prevention strategies have less to do with preventing cancer and more to do with early detection and early treatment.

- Early detection is more likely with monthly breast examination, annual in-office breast examination, and mammography when there is a questionable finding or every one to two years in women over age 40 years.
- There are conflicting reports regarding the effect of physical activity and breast cancer risk. However, it does appear that higher levels of adult physical activity provide a modest degree of protection.[76]
- Dietary factors may have a bearing on survival of women with breast cancer. Interestingly, a recent study[77] indicated that there was no advantage to a low-fat diet after the diagnosis of breast carcinoma was made; however, there was an increased survival for women eating more protein, but not red meat. It has also been shown that a diet high in fruits and vegetables, specifically high in alpha-carotene, beta-carotene, lutein/zeaxanthin, total vitamin C, and total vitamin A, may reduce premenopausal breast cancer risk.[78]

Eating Disorders

Disordered eating is a common problem in females. The majority of problems occur with the female athlete or with women in occupations where a thin appearance is required (e.g., acting or modeling). The two primary disorders representing the extremes of disordered eating are anorexia nervosa (AN) and bulimia nervosa (BN). AN is a disorder associated with self-imposed weight loss due to a distorted body image and other psychologically related problems. The vast majority of individuals are young, affluent white females (85%). Eighty percent of AN patients develop the disorder within seven years after menarche if, in fact, menarche develops. The female is often a perfectionist, coming from a family and

environment of high expectations. The AN patient is sometimes identified as either restrictive dominant (i.e., avoiding eating) or binge-purge dominant (i.e., engaging in bulimic activities). The diagnosis of AN is based primarily on patient attitudes and self-perception with some indicators of malnourishment to support the diagnosis. Clinically AN criteria include the following[79]

- Weight is maintained at least 15% below that expected as normal based on height and gender.
- Intense fear of gaining weight even though obviously underweight
- Distorted sense of self
- Absence of at least three consecutive menstrual cycles (without any other known cause)

AN patients may have associated problems. In 50% of AN patients there is a tendency toward bulimic activities including compulsive exercise to lose weight, misuse of laxatives or diuretics, and purging activities such as vomiting. Due to nutritional deficiencies, some patients may have a hypo-functioning thyroid. Cardiovascular problems include bradycardia and hypotension manifested occasionally as orthostatic hypotension or syncope. Skin changes include facial lanugo, often giving a "furry" appearance, and also a yellowish discoloration (hypercarotenemia) of the skin. When bulimia is also present, additional findings may occur, as discussed below. Due to the associated amenorrhea, the diagnostic search will often include laboratory testing, as discussed under the amenorrhea section of this chapter. Treatment is aimed at dealing with the nutritional aspects and the psychologic impairment that maintains the disorder. Referral to an eating disorders clinic is requisite. Management is beyond the expertise of most general physicians.

Bulimia nervosa (BN) is characterized by a binge–purge cycle in an effort to avoid weight gain. Although BN is seen in about half of AN patients, it is also its own disorder, with many individuals being of normal weight or slightly above normal. Bingeing usually occurs when the individual is depressed, bored, or lonely. Binge meals are often the "forbidden" foods that are high in fat or carbohydrate. Many bulimics report being obese during childhood or adolescence; they diet as a first approach to weight loss. The most common bingeing activities include self-induced vomiting or laxative/diuretic abuse. This activity is so common it is seen in as many as 20% of college students, with about 4% reporting weekly binge/purge actions. Other BN patients use extreme amounts of exercise in an attempt to burn off anticipated weight gain. BN patients are more aware of their actions as being aberrant compared to the purely AN patient. The purging activities are easier to keep private and, given that extreme weight loss is not always seen, the disorder is silent to others. The only clues are indirect and reflect, in most instances, the secondary effects of self-induced vomiting. These signs include:

- Parotid or salivary gland swelling, giving a puffy-cheek appearance
- Bruising of knuckles from hitting incisors during self-induced finger vomiting
- Pharyngitis from reflux of gastric acid, detected as a chronic hoarseness that is unrelated to respiratory infection
- Dental erosions from gastric acid reflux
- Conjunctival hemorrhages from retching

Patients may have problems with esophageal irritation including Mallory-Weis syndrome and strictures. Cardiac and renal problems may occur secondary to problems with hypokalemic, hypochloremic metabolic alkalosis.

If a patient is suspected of having the disorder, subtle questioning should attempt to determine how often purging activities occur. If there appears to be enough evidence to warrant concern, referral to an eating disorders clinic is requisite.

Incontinence

Urinary incontinence (UI) is an involuntary loss of urine that is not an inevitable result of aging. Statistics vary based on living environment, time frame, and definition; however, estimates are that urinary incontinence affects approximately 30% to 50% of older adults.[80] The prevalence specifically in community-dwelling individuals older than age 65 years is approximately 15% to 30%. Women are twice as likely to be affected. Generally, the most frequent causes of UI in women are stress UI and urge incontinence. Focused questioning for UI addresses the following areas:

- Frequency and amount of voiding
- Situational questions regarding the onset of UI (mechanical stimulation of voiding from coughing, laughing, sneezing, or jumping is likely stress incontinence, whereas UI without mechanical stimulation is more often due to detrusor instability)

- Any associated signs/symptoms of urinary tract infection
- Bowel movements, in particular constipation (a distended distal colon with stool may affect bladder function through a pressure effect)
- Diagnosed conditions that may be the cause of voiding difficulty (e.g., congestive heart failure, diabetes, pelvic surgery for various conditions) or the medications used for the condition may exacerbate voiding problems
- Drug history (some medications may cause retention and lead to overflow incontinence [e.g., α-agonists and stimulants such as ephedrine found in nasal decongestants] while others may act as diuretics [e.g., prescription and herbal diuretics, alcohol, and caffeine])
- Previous diagnosis and/or management of UI
- Patient's desired goals of management

The evaluation may be limited for the chiropractor given that a rectal examination for both sexes, and a pelvic examination in women, is necessary for a complete evaluation. If these examinations are not part of the skills of the practitioner, referral for these evaluations is requisite. In addition to a urogenital examination, the following should be included in the work-up of UI:[81]

- Palpation for suprapubic tenderness, lower abdominal masses, and bladder distention
- Neurologic testing of the perianal area and lower extremity may be warranted when complaints of pain or numbness are reported
- The cough test (a screening test for stress incontinence in which the patient is asked to cough to determine if there is loss of urine)
- Maintenance of a frequency-voiding record by the patient
- Urinalysis to determine if glucosuria, blood, or infection may indicate an underlying pathologic cause
- Referral for more extensive testing includes an estimation of post-void residual, uroflowmetry, and pressure flow studies

Based on the type of UI, treatment options vary. Refer to Chapter 34 for a more extensive discussion of treatment options. Generally, if stress incontinence is the cause, Kegel exercises are beneficial. If detrusor instability is the cause, bladder training, habit training, pelvic muscle exercises, and biofeedback are important nonsurgical, drugless approaches. Pelvic floor electrical stimulation (PFES) has been used for half a century as a treatment approach to stress incontinence. PFES stimulates pudendal nerve afferents activating pudendal and hypogastric nerve efferents, resulting in contraction of smooth and striated periurethral muscles and the striated pelvic floor muscles. Researchers in a recent randomized controlled trial assigned women to an eight-week behavioral training program, behavioral training plus PFES, or gave women a self-help booklet.[82] There was significant improvement in those treated with behavioral training (69%) or behavioral training plus PFES (72%) but no significant difference between the two groups. Those using the self-help booklet also had improvement (52%). Drug therapy involves antimuscarinic medications including oxybutynin and tolterodine.

Physical Abuse

Partner abuse is unfortunately a common feature of many relationships. The statistics are staggering, with the minimum prevalence data indicating 30% to 35% of all couples having had at least one episode of violence.[83] Some estimates are as high as 50% to 60% of couples. Abuse during pregnancy is also troubling, with estimates between 17% and 45%. Other saddening statistics include the following:[84]

- Thirty percent of all female homicides are perpetrated by a husband, a boyfriend, or an ex-partner.
- Of all women who seek care in the emergency department, 21% are battered women.
- Around 4 million women are physically assaulted each year.

Unfortunately, once an anger reaction has crossed over the verbal boundary to violence, it is more likely to recur. Unbelievably, until the last few decades of the twentieth century, abuse by a woman's husband was considered a personal option and the woman was not protected under law.[85] It was not until 1971 that the first shelter for battered women was established in London.

There appear to be cycles of abuse behavior. Initially there is a tension-building phase that escalates into the violence phase. Ironically, often following the violence phase is a honeymoon phase where the abuser apologizes and promises to change and demonstrates renewed love interest. This often misleads the abused partner so that plans to leave are postponed in the hope of reconciliation. It is also not uncommon for the abuser to then

shift blame to the abused, minimize the occurrence, or even deny it ever happened. Despite the high prevalence of abuse, physicians rarely recognize the signs. This is in part due to the abused patient's attempt to hide these signs. The signs may be subtle or if obviously due to trauma may be explained away by the abused patient. Some physical signs that are suspicious include:

- Bruises are of different colors (old versus new abuse).
- Battering is more commonly in a central pattern at the head, neck, breast/chest, or abdomen, except for bilateral peripheral injuries (indication of defense attempts).
- Imprints of hands or shoes are on the skin (especially with rib fractures).
- Other types of suspicious injury include missing teeth, fractured mandible, choke marks on the neck, and scalp wounds including areas where hair has been pulled out.

Psychologically there are numerous possible consequences for the abused individual including chronic depression, sleep disorders, somatization disorders, anxiety disorders, and alcohol and drug abuse, among others.

In interviewing female patients, it is recommended that questions regarding abuse be asked in the past tense to prevent an avoidance response. If abuse is suspected, documentation is required. If a photo record of abuse is acceptable by the patient (indicated by a signed release form) it should be part of the patient record. In California, if abuse is even suspected, it is a requirement that a telephone or written report to the police be made. Many other states have similar requirements. In addition to reporting the suspected abuse and providing for appropriate care for injuries, it is equally important to provide resources for the abused patient including a shelter resource if it is determined that returning home is unsafe. All healthcare practitioners should have at hand contacts at centers for abused women. Social services and/or shelters will provide information regarding development of a safety plan. If the patient refuses help, the doctor must respect that the patient has the right to personal choice no matter how difficult it may seem. However, the doctor should be cautiously persistent if possible.

Osteoporosis

Although osteoporosis (loss of bone mass; see Chapter 30) is seen in both genders, the female-to-male ratio for vertebral osteoporosis and fracture is 6:1.[86] This is primarily due to the lack of estrogen stimulation seen in the postmenopausal female. Bone loss in early menopause is between 1% and 5% per year. This bone loss is relative to the premenopausal bone mass status of the female. Bone mass development occurs primarily before and up to the early twenties; therefore, any interruption or dysfunction in bone accumulation leaves the individual with less bone prior to menopause. Common factors are related to diet and exercise. Not enough calcium and too much or too little exercise are the primary risk factors in the adolescent group. The focus for the young female athlete is to determine menstrual status. Amenorrhea (as part of the female athletic triad) results in loss of estrogen stimulation for bone formation and, as a result, bone loss may equal that of early menopause.

It is important to screen all females, and in particular those with indicators of osteoporosis, on x-ray for known risk factors for osteoporosis including the following:[86]

- white or Asian background
- early menopause
- family history
- lean body habitus
- lack of exercise, or excessive exercise in the young
- glucocorticoids, phenytoin, aluminum antacids, lithium, loop diuretics, tetracycline, warfarin
- heavy alcohol consumption; smoking; low calcium intake or vitamin D deficiency; high phosphate, fiber, or sodium intake; more than four cups of coffee per day; carbonated drinks (several a day); and possibly a high-animal-protein diet (although a low-protein diet may also place the female at risk)
- high homocysteine levels

The resulting screen of the above factors will establish a baseline level of risk for osteoporosis or progression of osteoporosis. Given that osteoporosis is essentially a silent disease until fracture or deformity occurs, it is important to screen all females.

When osteoporosis is suspected, the primary initial evaluation tool is x-ray. Spinal x-rays may detect existing osteoporosis; however, only with bone loss between 30% and 50%. There are classic radiographic findings with osteoporosis; however, their appearance indicates advanced involvement. These findings include cortical thinning (pencil-thin cortex) and trabecular changes. Trabecular resorption may leave the remaining stress-surviving trabeculae more visible, in contrast to a background of radiolucency. Changes in the vertebral shape with osteoporosis include vertebra plana (pancake vertebra), wedged vertebra, and biconcave (fish, hourglass) vertebra.

More sensitive techniques include single- and dual-photon absorptiometry (SPA and DPA, respectively), quantitative computed tomography (QCT), dual-energy x-ray absorptiometry (DEXA), and possibly ultrasonography (US). Although DPA, QCT, and DEXA measure both types of bone, DEXA is now the measurement tool of choice. Laboratory evaluation is valuable only in the differential evaluation. Most bone-related lab levels, such as calcium, phosphorus, and alkaline phosphatase, are usually normal unless there has been a recent fracture.

Osteoporosis treatment includes both prevention strategies and treatment strategies for those with documented osteopenia or osteoporosis:

- For all women, establish a lifestyle habit of maintaining an adequate amount of calcium and vitamin D combined with an appropriate level of exercise; also recommendations for avoidance of known contributors to osteoporosis acceleration including smoking, alcohol, caffeine, carbonated drinks, etc.
- When a secondary cause of osteoporosis or a compression fracture is found or suspected (i.e., cancer, Paget's disease, hyperparathyroidism, or osteomalacia), medical consultation is necessary.
- If a compression fracture appears radiographically unstable, refer for medical consultation (see Chapter 6 for details).
- For all older women, establish a prevention program for falls including an environmental evaluation, exercise program, and nutritionally supportive regimen.
- For all osteoporotic patients, a comprehensive program is needed that includes patient education, appropriate exercise, and appropriate nutrition coupled with psychosocial support.

The amount of calcium intake is generally recommended to be 1,000 mg for premenopausal women and 1,500 mg for postmenopausal women. For the elderly or homebound patient it is important to consider the need for vitamin D supplementation. The recommended daily allowance is between 400 and 800 IU. A cup of milk will provide only 100 IU of vitamin D. This is a significant factor that is often overlooked (see Table 30–2).

Medical options for postmenopausal women include the following:

- ERT or HRT (hormonal replacement therapy)
- bisphosphonates such as alendronate (Fosamax)
- selective estrogen receptor modulators (SERMs) such as raloxifene
- calcitonin

Exercise prescription for the osteoporotic patient should meet two goals. First, it is important to stimulate bone production and prevent loss. Second, it is important to strengthen muscles to provide support and to provide proprioceptive training to prevent falls. The increases in bone mass seen with exercise are mild to modest, in the order of 1% to 3%. However, it must be kept in mind that simply preventing further bone loss is a major goal of an exercise prescription. The general rule of thumb for causing bone mass response is that the exercise must provide mechanical loading either through pull of muscle on bone or with weight bearing. Some important considerations follow:

- Walking does not seem to provide enough stimulation for increased bone mass; it must be combined with resistance exercise.[87]
- Non-weight-bearing exercises including swimming and cycling are relatively ineffective approaches.[88]
- Resistance exercise must exceed that provided by daily activities.[89]
- The effects of exercise are site-specific (e.g., running does not provide a stimulation for bone in the upper extremities).
- Impact activities that apply relatively large loads on bone quickly are the most osteogenic and are the most risky; therefore, a progression of exercise up to the level of these types of activities is the final goal.

The Female Athlete

A major milestone for females and sports occurred in 1972 with Title IX legislation.[90] This legislation mandated equal opportunity for females, providing for equity in sports programs at educational institutions and equal access to athletic competition and recreational exercise. It has led to an explosion of participation in many sports, including those previously male-dominated sports such as soccer, rugby, basketball, bodybuilding, bowling, and golf, among others. With this increased involvement, the number of injuries to females related to athletics has skyrocketed. There are many theories as to why this increase seems out of proportion to similar injury patterns in males. Some of the most obvious have to do with gender-specific training. Other factors relate to the anatomic and physiologic differences between males and females. These observations have spawned an interest in gender-specific research that increasingly demonstrates more similarities and fewer differences when body size and weight are factored in.

Prior to puberty, the differences between males and females are negligible. Due to the fact that girls reach puberty earlier than males, there is a small period in which females mature more quickly, have greater coordination, and in many cases are taller than their male counterparts. Prepubescent males and females are equal in body fat composition.[91] The male body fat decreases 11% on average through adolescence. Females increase body fat on average 25% during this same period. Postpuberty, there are some recognized differences between males and females:[92]

- The average female is 3 to 4 inches shorter than her male counterpart.
- Adult women have 8% to 10% more body fat than men on average. Percent body fat differs with each sport; endurance athletes average between 12% to 18%, white elite runners as low as 6% to 8%, and team sports (e.g., softball, volleyball, and swimming) 18% to 24%.
- Women have shorter limbs relative to body length when compared with men. This is most evident in the upper extremity where the humerus is shorter in women than in men. Women also have a more narrow shoulder width.
- The wider, shallower pelvis observed in women has been cited as a major cause of an increased quadriceps (Q) angle at the knee. The effect on the Q angle and its association with increased patellofemoral problems has not proven to be as major a concern as has been implied from earlier research.[93]
- Cardiopulmonary differences include the following: women have fewer red blood cells (RBCs), lower hematocrit and hemoglobin, smaller heart and stroke volume, smaller vital capacity and residual lung volume, and lower VO_2 max.
- As absolutes, the average female is two-thirds as strong as the average male; upper body strength is only 30% to 50% and lower extremity strength 70% that of the same size male. However, when

body mass and relative strength are considered, the female has about 55% of the male's upper body strength and is about equal in lower body strength.

- Statistically, there are no objectifiable differences between joint laxity compared with males, although clinically it has been observed that the knees and shoulders of females seem to be "looser."

Regarding the menstrual cycle, there appears to be no significant correlation between menstrual phase cycle and exercise performance.[94] However, injury rates appear to increase in athletes with premenstrual symptoms. Also, there has been some association suggested between estrogen and possible laxity of the anterior cruciate ligament.[95]

Specific concerns that should be addressed on preparticipation examinations and with all athletic females are as follows:[96]

- Shoulder laxity: Women who participate in upper body sports such as tennis, swimming, and volleyball should be instructed to focus on both strengthening the shoulder rotator cuff and serratus anterior and also trunk strengthening to decrease the stress to the shoulders. Given that women are generally weaker in upper body strength, focus on a generalized upper body-strengthening program will also be beneficial.
- Knee laxity: It has been observed that patellar instability is more common in females. This may be due in part to more of a tendency toward underdevelopment of the back surface of the patella and lateral condyle of the femur, decreased vastus medialis strength, tighter iliotibial band (ITB), or a high riding patella. This tendency, combined with a position of recurvatum (hyperextension) seen more commonly in females, may predispose toward either tracking problems, patellar subluxation, or patellar dislocation. Focus the patient on vastus medialis strengthening, ITB stretching, orthotics for pronation, and proprioceptive training. Anterior cruciate ligament (ACL) laxity or looseness is a concern for females, given a relatively high rate of injury when compared to males participating in similar sports. Although there are many theories, it appears that the main effective strategy for decreasing injury is training. It is clear that the vast majority (78% in one study) of ACL injuries are noncontact, often occurring when landing from a jump.[97] This is

even more true in sports such as basketball and volleyball. One study[98] divided these noncontact injuries into three types and documented the percentage of incidence. Together they accounted for most ACL injuries in the study and individually are essentially equal in occurrence (26% to 29%). The three types are:

1. planting and cutting
2. straight leg landing
3. one-step landing with the knee hyperextended

ACL injury rates were reduced among a group of women by almost 90% simply by modifying the plant-and-cut maneuver to a three-step stop with an emphasis on avoiding knee extension. Another study[99] indicated that the incidence of knee injury in female athletes is significantly reduced with a training program for jumping and landing. Noncontact ACL injury may be related to both genu recurvatum and hyperpronation. Intercondylar notch size is probably not a factor.[100]

- Stress fractures: Tibial and other stress fractures are more common in females who are amenorrheic and/or osteoporotic. Of particular concern is the "dreaded black line" seen radiographically at the tibia in dancers. Nonunion is particularly difficult with this fracture. Standard stress fractures should be managed with partial weight-bearing, aquatic and non-weight-bearing exercise, and an increase in calcium supplementation to 2 g/day for several weeks.
- Nutritional concerns: The primary nutritional concerns in the female athlete are iron deficiency and calcium insufficiency. Iron deficiency is seen in 20% to 25% of female athletes. The incidence is high in elite cross-country skiers, followed by female distance swimmers, then all collegiate athletes; the greatest deficiency is seen in adolescent female swimmers (47%).[101] These subsets of athletes should be screened as well as any athlete developing early fatigue, chest complaints, dizziness, or presyncope/syncope events. Vegetarian runners are more at risk than those consuming meat. Menstrual loss is the main cause; during menses loss of 1.2 to 2 mg of iron per day is common. This translates into a 1- to 2-mg drop in hemoglobin levels. Nonmenstruating women require 10 mg of iron per day, while menstruating women require at least 15 mg of iron per day. Calcium supplementation is discussed under the osteoporosis section.

- Pelvic floor laxity and incontinence: Either urethral sphincter insufficiency or loss of detrusor tone in combination with an increased intravesical pressure exceeding urethral pressure will result in incontinence. It is seen primarily in high-impact sports (high-impact aerobics, running, basketball, track and field, and volleyball) and in those activities associated with increased abdominal pressure (gymnastics, weight lifting, martial arts, and others). Management is discussed under the incontinence section in this chapter and in Chapter 34.

- Female athletic triad syndrome: The triad of disordered eating, amenorrhea, and osteoporosis is found in some female athletes; in particular, in the high-level amateur and professional. Each is discussed under its own section above. Females who are affected generally have low body fat, inadequate caloric intake, disordered eating, and/or are involved in a high-intensity exercise/sport. The amenorrhea (and subsequent development of estrogen-deficient osteoporosis) is believed to be a form of hypothalamic amenorrhea where decreased or abnormal secretion of gonadotropin-releasing hormone (GnRH) is due to either (1) adrenal activation inhibiting hypothalamic release of GnRH, or (2) increased caloric demand with inadequate caloric intake that leads to an "energy drain" that then may cause a relative hypothyroid state.

APPENDIX 55–1

Web Resources

Obstetrics and Other Female Issues

American Congress of Obstetricians and Gynecologists
(202) 863-2518
http://www.acog.org
National Women's Health Information Center
(800) 994-9662
www.nchealthywoman.org/
La Leche League
(847) 519-7730
http://www.lalecheleague.org/FAQ/mastitis.html
North American Menopause Society
(800) 774-5342
http://www.menopause.org

American Medical Women's Association
(703) 838-0500
http://www.amwa-doc.org

Postpartum Depression

"Postpartum Support International
http://www.postpartum.net

For Violence

American Bar Association
(202) 662-1744
http://www.abanet.org/domviol/home.html

Infertility

RESOLVE: The National Infertility Association
(888) 623-0744
http://www.resolve.org

Heart Disease

National Coalition for Women with Heart Disease
(202) 728-7199
http://www.womenheart.org

APPENDIX 55–2

References

1. Colditz GA, Manson JE, Hankinson SE. The Nurses' Health Study: a 20-year contribution to the understanding of health among women. *J Women's Health.* 1997;6(1):49–62.
2. Verbrugge LM, Wingard DL. Sex differentials in health and mortality. *Women Health.* 1987;12:103–108.
3. National Center for Health Statistics. *Vital Statistics of the United States, 1990.* Vol. II: Mortality, Part A. Washington, DC: Public Health Service; 1994:40–52. DHHS publication (PHS) 95–1101.
4. Lappe JM, Travers-Gustafson D, Davies KM, Recker RR, Heaney RP. Vitamin D and calcium supplementation reduces cancer risk: results of a randomized trial. *Am J Clin Nutr.* 2007;85(6):1586–1591.
5. U.S. Preventive Services Task Force. Screening for hypertension. In: *Guide to Clinical Preventive Services.* 2nd ed. Baltimore: Williams & Wilkins; 1996:39.

6. U.S. Preventive Services Task Force. Screening for breast cancer. In: *Guide to Clinical Preventive Services.* 2nd ed. Baltimore: Williams & Wilkins; 1996:73.

7. American Academy of Family Physicians. *Age-Charts for Periodic Health Examination.* Kansas City, MO: American Academy of Family Physicians; 1994. Reprint no. 510.

8. Canadian Task Force on the Periodic Health Examination. *Canadian Guide to Clinical Preventive Health Care.* Ottawa: Canada Communication Group; 1994:787–795.

9. U.S. Preventive Services Task Force. Screening for cervical cancer. In: *Guide to Clinical Preventive Services.* 2nd ed. Baltimore: Williams & Wilkins; 1996:105.

10. U.S. Preventive Services Task Force. Screening for glaucoma. In: *Guide to Clinical Preventive Services.* 2nd ed. Baltimore: Williams & Wilkins; 1996:383.

11. U.S. Preventive Services Task Force. Screening for high blood cholesterol and other lipid abnormalities. In: *Guide to Clinical Preventive Services.* 2nd ed. Baltimore: Williams & Wilkins; 1996:15.

12. U.S. Preventive Services Task Force. Screening for colorectal cancer. In: *Guide to Clinical Preventive Services.* 2nd ed. Baltimore: Williams & Wilkins; 1996:89.

13. American Cancer Society. *Cancer Facts and Figures— 1995.* Atlanta: American Cancer Society; 1995.

14. U.S. Preventive Services Task Force. Screening for thyroid disease. In: *Guide to Clinical Preventive Services.* 2nd ed. Baltimore: Williams & Wilkins; 1996:214.

15. Neinstein LS. Menstrual dysfunction in pathophysiologic states. *West J Med.* 1985;143:476–484.

16. Steege JF, Blumenthal JA. The effects of aerobic exercise on premenstrual symptoms in middle-aged women: a preliminary study. *J Psychosom Res.* 1993;37:127–133.

17. Oyelowo TA. Diagnosis and management of premenstrual syndrome in the chiropractic office. *Top Clin Chiro.* 1997;4:60–67.

18. Walsh MJ, Polus BI. A randomized, placebo-controlled clinical trial on the efficacy of chiropractic therapy on premenstrual syndrome. *J Manipulative Physiol Ther.* 1999;22:582–585.

19. Golomb LM, Solidum AA, Warren MP. Primary dysmenorrhea and physical activity. *Med Sci Sports Exerc.* 1998;30:906–909.

20. Liebl NA, Butler LM. A chiropractic approach to the treatment of dysmenorrhea. *J Manipulative Physiol Ther.* 1990;13:101–106.

21. Kokjohn K, Schmid DM, Triano JJ, Brennan PC. The effect of spinal manipulation on pain and prostaglandin levels in women with primary dysmenorrhea. *J Manipulative Physiol Ther.* 1992;15:279–285.

22. Hondras MA, Long CR, Brennan PC. Spinal manipulative therapy versus a low force mimic maneuver for women with primary dysmenorrhea: a randomized, observer-blinded, clinical trial. *Pain.* 1999;81:105–114.

23. Kaplan B, Rabinerson D, Lurie S, et al. Clinical evaluation of a new model of a transcutaneous electrical nerve stimulation device for the management of primary dysmenorrhea. *Gynecol Obstet Invest.* 1997;44:255–259.

24. Helms JM. Acupuncture for the management of primary dysmenorrhea. *Obstet Gynecol.* 1987;69:51–56.

25. Seler M, Danakas G. Menopause. In: Damakas G, Pietrontoni M, eds. *Practical Guide to the Care of the Gynecologic-Obstetric Patient.* St. Louis: Mosby; 1997.

26. Stearns V, Bebe K, Iyengar M, Dube E. Paroextine controlled release in the treatment of menopausal hot flashes: a randomized controlled trial. *JAMA.* 2003;289:2827–2837.

27. Petitti DB. Combination estrogen-progestin oral contraceptives. *N Engl J Med.* 2003;349;1443–1450.

28. Anderson GI, Judd HI, Kaumitz AM, et al. Effects of estrogen plus progestin on gynecologic cancers and associated diagnostic procedures. The Women's Health Initiative Randomized Trial. *JAMA.* 2003;290:1739–1748.

29. Cauley JA, Robbins J, Chen Z, et al. Effects of estrogen plus progestin on risk of fracture and bone mineral density: the Women's Health Initiative Randomized Trial. *JAMA.* 2003;290:1729–1738.

30. Wassertheil-Smoller S, Hendrix SL, Limacher ML, et al. Effect of estrogen plus progestin on stroke in postmenopausal women: the Women's Health Initiative: a randomized trial. *JAMA.* 2003;289:2673–2684.

31. Rapp SR, Espeland MA, Shumaker SA, et al. Effect of estrogen plus progestin on global cognitive function in postmenopausal women. The Women's Health Initiative Memory Study: a randomized controlled trial. *JAMA.* 2003;289:2663–2672.

32. Shumaker SA, Legault C, Rapp SR, et al. Estrogen plus progestin and incidence of dementia and mild cognitive impairment in postmenopausal women. The Women's Health Initiative Memory Study: a randomized controlled trial. *JAMA.* 2003;289:2651–2662.

33. Periotti M, Fabio E, Modena AR, et al. Effect of soy-derived isoflavones on hot flashes, endometrial

thickness, and the pulsatility index of the uterine and cerebral arteries. *Fertility and Sterility.* 2003;79:1112–1117.

34. Deprez DP. Abnormal vaginal bleeding. In: Greene HL, Fincher RME, Johnson WP, et al. eds. *Clinical Medicine.* 2nd ed. St. Louis, MO: Mosby-Year Book; 1996:821.

35. Nilsson L, Rybo G. Treatment of menorrhagia. *Am J Obstet Gynecol.* 1971;110:713–720.

36. van Eijkeren MA, Cristiaens GC, Scholten PC, et al. Menorrhagia: current drug treatment concepts. *Drugs.* 1992;43:201–209.

37. Kirchner JT, Emmert DH. Sexually transmitted diseases in women: *Chlamydia trachomatis* and herpes simplex infections. *Postgrad Med.* 2000;10(1):55–65.

38. Smith S, Pfeifer SM, Collins JA. Diagnosis and management of female infertility. *JAMA.* 2003;290:1767–1770.

39. Clapp JF. A clinical approach to exercise during pregnancy. *Clin Sports Med.* 1994;13:443–458.

40. American College of Obstetricians and Gynecologists. *Exercise during Pregnancy and the Postpartum Period.* Washington, DC: ACOG; 1994. ACOG technical bulletin 189.

41. American College of Sports Physicians. *ACSM's Handbook for the Team Physician.* Baltimore: Williams & Wilkins; 1996:435.

42. Sternfeld B, Quesenbery CP, Eskenazi B, Newman L. Exercise during pregnancy and pregnancy outcome. *Med Sci Sports Exerc.* 1995;27:634–640.

43. Horns PN, Ratcliffe LP, Leggett JC, Swanson MS. Pregnancy outcomes among active and sedentary primiparous women. *J Obstet Gynecol Neonatal Nurs.* 1996;25:49–54.

44. Fast A, Shapiro D, Ducommun EJ, et al. Low back pain in pregnancy. *Spine.* 1997;12:368–371.

45. Dialow DRP, Gadsby TA, Gadsby JB, et al. Back pain during pregnancy and labor. *J Manipulative Physiol Ther.* 1991;14:116–118.

46. Bartol KM. Considerations in adjusting women. *Top Clin Chiro.* 1997;4(3):1–10.

47. Esch S, Zachman Z. Adjustive procedures for pregnant chiropractic patients. *Chiro Tech.* 1991;3:66–71.

48. Donegan WI, Spratt JA. *Cancer of the Breast.* Philadelphia: WB Saunders; 1995.

49. Berestinasky-Sembrat L. Breast cancer: a current summary. *Top Clin Chiro.* 1999;6(1):9–17.

50. Whittemore AS, Gong G, Ibyre J. Prevalence and contribution of BRCA1 mutation in breast cancer and ovarian cancer. *Am J Hum Genet.* 1997;60:496–504.

51. Barton MB, Harris R, Fletcher SW. Does this patient have breast cancer? The screening clinical breast examination: should it be done? How? *JAMA.* 1999;282:1270–1280.

52. Vogel VG. Tools for evaluating a patient's 5-year and lifetime probabilities. *Postgrad Med.* 1999;105:49–60.

53. Berkey CS, Frazier AL, Gardner JD, Colditz GA. Adolescence and breast carcinoma risk. *Cancer.* 1999;85(11):2400–2409.

54. Schrag D, Kuntz KM, Garber JE, Weeks JC. Life expectancy gains from cancer prevention strategies for women with breast cancer and BRCA1 or BRCA2 mutations. *JAMA.* 2000;283:617–624.

55. Colditz GA. Hormones and breast cancer: evidence and implications for consideration of risks and benefits of hormone replacement therapy. *J Women's Health.* 1999;8(3):347–357.

56. Schairer C, Lubin J, Troisi R, et al. Menopausal estrogen and estrogen-progestin replacement therapy and breast cancer risk. *JAMA.* 2000;283:485–491.

57. Claus EB, Risch N, Thompson WD, Carter D. Relationship between breast histopathology and family history of breast cancer. *Cancer.* 1993;71:147–153.

58. Zhang S, Hunter DJ, Hankinson SE, et al. A prospective study of folate intake and the risk of breast cancer. *JAMA.* 1999;28:1632–1637.

59. Ishibe N, Hankinson SE, Colditz GA, et al. Cigarette smoking, cytochrome P450 1A1 polymorphisms, and breast cancer risk in the Nurses' Health Study. *Cancer Res.* 1998;58:667–671.

60. Holmes MD, Hunter DJ, Colditz GA, et al. Association of dietary intake of fat and fatty acids with risk of breast cancer. *JAMA.* 1999;281:914–920.

61. Rose D. Dietary fatty acids and cancer. *Am J Clin Nutr.* 1997;66(suppl):15815–15865.

62. Huang Z, Hankinson SE, Colditz GA, et al. Dual effects of weight and weight gain on breast cancer risk. *JAMA.* 1997;278:1407–1411.

63. Wang D, Velez de-la-Paz OI, Zhai JX, Liu DW. Serum 25-hydroxyvitamin D and breast cancer risk: a meta-analysis of prospective studies. *Tumour Biol.* 2013; 27.

64. Collaborative Group on Hormonal Factors in Breast Cancer. Breast cancer and breastfeeding: collaborative reanalysis of individual data from 47 epidemiological studies in 30 countries, including 50,302 women with breast cancer and 96,973 women without the disease. *Lancet.* 2002;360:187–195.

65. Lehman CD, Gatsonis C, Kuhl CK, et al. MRI evaluation of the contralateral breast in women

with recently diagnosed breast cancer. *N Engl J Med.* 2007;356(13):1295–1303.

66. Ransohoff DF, Harris RP. Lessons from the mammography screening controversy: can we improve the debate? *Ann Intern Med.* 1997;127(11):1029–1034.

67. Gotzsche PC, Jorgensen KJ. Screening for breast cancer with mammography. *Cochrane Database Syst Rev.* 2011;6:CD001877.

68. Bleyer A, Welch HG. Effect of three decades of screening mammography on breast-cancer incidence. *N Engl J Med.* 2012;367(21):1998–2005.

69. Woolf SH, Harris R. The harms of screening: new attention to an old concern. *JAMA.* 2012;307(6): 565–566.

70. Miller AB, Wall C, Baines CJ, Sun P, To T, Narod SA. Twenty five year follow-up for breast cancer incidence and mortality of the Canadian National Breast Screening Study: randomised screening trial. *BMJ.* 2014;348:366.

71. Paik S. Development and clinical utility of a 21-gene recurrence score prognostic assay in patients with early breast cancer treated with tamoxifen. *Oncologist.* 2007;12(6):631–635.

72. Paik S, Shak S, Tang G, et al. A multigene assay to predict recurrence of tamoxifen-treated, node-negative breast cancer. *N Engl J Med.* 2004;351(27):2817–2826.

73. Tsangaris T, Robert N, Love N. Update on treatment of early breast cancer: the trend toward less surgery, more systemic therapy. *Postgrad Med.* 1999;105:81–102.

74. Goss PE, Ingle JN, Martino S, et al. A randomized trial of letrozole in postmenopausal women after five years of tamoxifen therapy for early-stage breast cancer. *N Engl J Med.* 2003;349:1793–1802.

75. Kim SY, Kim HP, Kim YJ, et al. Trastuzumab inhibits the growth of human gastric cancer cell lines with HER2 amplification synergistically with cisplatin. *Int J Oncol.* 2008;32(1):89–95.

76. Willett RB, Hunter DJ, Manson JE, et al. A prospective study of recreational physical activity and breast cancer risk. *Arch Intern Med.* 1999;159:2290–2296.

77. Holmes MD, Stampfer MJ, Colditz GA, et al. Dietary factors and the survival of women with breast carcinoma. *Cancer.* 1999;86:826–835.

78. Zhang S, Hunter DJ, Forman MR, et al. Dietary carotenoids and vitamins A, C, and E and risk of breast cancer. *J Natl Cancer Inst.* 1999;91:547–556.

79. Drossman DA. The eating disorders. In: Bennett JC, Plum F, eds. *Cecil Textbook of Medicine.* 20th ed. Philadelphia: WB Saunders; 1996:1158–1160.

80. Herzog AR, Fultz NH. Prevalence and incidence of urinary incontinence in community-dwelling populations. *J Am Geriatr Soc.* 1990;38:273–281.

81. Johnson TM II, Ouslander JG. Urinary incontinence in the older man. *Med Clin North Am.* 1999;83:1247–1267.

82. Goode PS, Burgio KL, Leoher JL, et al. Effect of behavioral training with or without pelvic floor electrical stimulation on stress incontinence in women: a randomized controlled trial. *JAMA.* 2003;290:345–352.

83. Dickstein LJ. Spouse abuse and other domestic violence. *Psychiatr Clin North Am.* 1988;11(4):611–628.

84. American Medical Association. 4 million American women abused annually. *Hosp Health Netw.* Dec 1994:15.

85. Talmage DM. Partner abuse: recognition and intervention strategies. *Top Clin Chiro.* 1997;4(3):44–50.

86. Beck BR, Shoemaker R. Osteoporosis: understanding key risk factors and therapeutic options. *Phys Sports Med.* 2000;28(2):34–57.

87. Cavanaugh DJ, Cann CE. Brisk walking does not stop bone loss in postmenopausal women. *Bone.* 1988;9(4):201–204.

88. Taffle DR, Snow-Harter C, Connolly DA, et al. Differential effects of swimming versus weight-bearing activity on bone mineral status of eumenorrheic athletes. *J Bone Miner Res.* 1995;10(4):586–593.

89. Dalsky GP. The role of exercise in the prevention of osteoporosis. *Compr Ther.* 1989;15(9):30–37.

90. Agostini R. The athletic woman. *Clin Sports Med.* 1994;12:xi–xii.

91. Goldberg B. Pediatric sports medicine. In: Scott WN, Nisomon B, Nicholas J, eds. *Principles of Sports Medicine.* Baltimore: Williams & Wilkins; 1984:403–426.

92. Thein LA, Thein JM. The female athlete. *J Orthop Sports Phys Ther.* 1996;23(2):134–148.

93. Livingston LA. The quadriceps angle: a review of the literature. *J Orthop Sports Phys Ther.* 1998;28(2):105–109.

94. Morgenthal AP, Resnick DN. The female athlete: current concepts. *Top Clin Chiro.* 1997;4(3):11–20.

95. Liu SH, Al-Shaikh RA, Panossian V, et al. Estrogen affects the cellular metabolism of the anterior cruciate ligament: a potential explanation for female athletic injury. *Am J Sports Med.* 1997;25(5).

96. Morgenthal AP, Resnick DN. Health-related concerns unique to female athletes. *Top Clin Chiro.* 1997;4(3):51–59.

97. Noyes FR, Mooar PA, Mathews DS, et al. The symptomatic ACL-deficient knee. *J Bone Joint Surg Am.* 1983;65:154–174.

98. Griffis ND, Vequist SW, Yearout KM, et al. Injury prevention of the anterior cruciate ligament. In: *American Orthopaedic Society for Sports Medicine: Meeting Abstracts, Symposia, and Instructional Courses.* 15th annual meeting; June 19–22, 1989; Traverse City, Michigan.

99. Hewett TE, Lindenfeld TN, Ricobene JV, Noyes FR. The effect of neuromuscular training on the incidence of knee injury in female athletes: a prospective study. *Am J Sports Med.* 1999;27(6):699–706.

100. Teitz CC, Lind BK, Sacks BM. Symmetry of the femoral notch width index. *Am J Sports Med.* 1997; 25(5):483–491.

101. Risser WL, Risser JM. Iron deficiency in adolescents and young adults. *Phys Sports Med.* 1990; 18(12):87–101.

How to Incorporate Literature Evidence into Practice

This appendix will not satisfy the detail necessary for an understanding of statistics or even research design and so therefore will disappoint scientists and teachers of evidence-based methods. However, the intention is not to train clinicians on how to conduct research or to remind researchers how to construct or conduct research but rather is designed for the clinician as a foray into the world of the scientist to understand their methods and logic and how to begin to resolve the apparent disconnect between these two worlds.

The three components of evidence-informed practice must include not only the literature evidence, but also the practitioner's expertise and the patient's preferences. This is often biased toward a focus on the literature for scientists, and toward the practitioner's belief in his or her expertise for the field-doctor. The patient's preferences are perhaps biased toward the individual from whom he or she seeks help, but are also influenced by the information given by that practitioner. Because patient outcomes are somewhat unique to that context, evidence-informed knowledge and measurement must include both the literature evidence for a given topic and also the practice environment of each practitioner. Measurement in practice is not confined by the restraints of randomized controlled trials (RCTs) and other studies. Imposed by the practice context, using a less scientifically restrictive approach is allowable and preferable. This is because with no intention of extrapolation outside that practice, it reflects the context of that environment where future patients will be managed and where data are relevant. How then can one practice scientifically without being a scientist? Let's look at how a scientist views patients.

The Scientist Mindset

Here is the scientist's perspective:

- Attempt to systematically eliminate any bias in drawing conclusions and determine how much *chance* may play a part in the results.
- Address as many variations as possible through research design to include multiple patient populations, practice environments, and other variables to allow general application. At the same time, make patient groups homogenous so that comparison is appropriate (meaning comparing groups requires that both groups are similar in demographics and other elements regarding their condition, comorbidities, pain levels, acuteness, etc.).
- Scientists and researchers believe that clinical "expertise" is often the product of the classic representation of the "biased" environment. In other words, as a practitioner you see what you want to see and forget what does not support the perception of success.

To be sure, there are some flaws to most human observations. These can be generalized into two broad categories: (1) bias, and (2) misinterpretation of chance occurrence.

Bias

Bias has many forms, but the most common is having an expectation based on prior experience, or on trying to get a specific result. This applies both in practice and in research. Here are some examples:

- Bias can occur in the reader who believes a positive report from a research study because he/she wants to find support for his/her belief, and therefore discounts the results of studies that do not support his/her belief system.

- When bias enters into a study it is called an error. Bias can enter at all levels of a research study including the participants, examiners, staff, and reviewers. Bias in the selection of patients, bias in patient recall of events, bias based on preferences of patients, and so forth.

In practice, to be honest about our successes, we must first understand the caveats of human perception; our tendency toward a bias to believe in what we do. "Recall" bias is often focused on successes, so you remember those events that support your belief in the value of what you do; not in itself a bad thing, but not unbiased.

Consider the following:

- You may not count those patients who received benefit through referral to other healthcare providers.
- You may tend to selectively forget those patients who don't improve and attribute that result to their lack of compliance or attitude. Perhaps you do not count them as a non-responder because they never returned to convey that information.

Chance

The possibility that chance is the reason for an occurrence is more likely if it is seen rarely or by a single individual and less likely if it occurs frequently and is observed by many; for example your practice versus a large study, respectively. Chance occurrence is more common than we humans intuit. Researchers can measure this occurrence and calculate the probability that chance is the potential reason for a result. In general, the more individuals in a study and the more studies that support the same findings, the less likely it is that chance will play a role. Chance occurrence is reported in numbers such as *p* values and 95% confidence intervals (CI); more on that later.

Placebo and Nocebo

We are less concerned with placebo in our practices than in scientific studies because a positive placebo effect still results in a successful outcome; the patient's expectation and requirement of you are met. Scientifically we want to avoid placebo in order to determine the truth about an intervention's direct cause of an effect. In practice, this becomes less relevant but must nonetheless

be recognized and appreciated when tallying our successes. The ethical dilemma is this: Is a patient avoiding a known intervention that is safer, cheaper, or, of course, more effective? Nocebo is the reverse—a sham or inert substance or treatment that produces harm. New studies are indicating that some sham treatments result in adverse events.

The Clinician Mindset

The clinician's perspectives that may be contrary to the scientist's perspectives include the following:

- Do the best you can for the patient even if your choice of treatment does not match the literature.
- Each patient is unique and no amount of literature support for a given conclusion can cover all possible scenarios (i.e., patient variation; the real world).
- The major concern by clinicians—and an excuse for studies being ignored if they don't represent what the clinician wants to hear—is that the clinician may believe that the scientific perspective is the epitome of disconnect to the individual patient.

The danger is that the clinician will adopt a "desert island" approach where he or she stays isolated in practice without updated knowledge or comparison to others' experiences and opinions. This is defensible only when you have no choice; you use the best available tool to accomplish the task based on your experience. When you have access to a greater fund of knowledge, is it ethical to limit your scope of treatment, and become that person on the desert island?

Is what appears in studies enough to guide our clinical decisions? What are the potential limitations of applying strong literature conclusions that are scientifically sound? Good science is based on large groups of individuals where the potential for chance can be diminished statistically, yet these large groups are in fact averaged, so the group or that average may not represent the patient in front of you. Scientific studies cannot tell you how each patient will respond to you specifically, because of these unique elements:

- Your office space
- Your procedures
- Your demeanor
- Your patients' beliefs and attitudes
- Your techniques and expertise

Common questions and concerns clinicians voice about using only scientifically validated evidence from the literature or when adopting the scientific mentality are:

- If I question everything, what can I trust?
- If I question everything, how can I have confidence in what I do?
- If I don't try to stay up to date with techniques that promise high-tech advances, how can I provide the best care for my patients?
- Do I have to wait for evidence?

The solution is through the understanding that an evidence-informed practice allows, and demands that one generates, some of the evidence upon which one makes decisions. You become the clinician/scientist. The clinician/scientist mentality is simply a change in focus that requires that, whenever possible, one:

- Applies scientific principles to observations in practice (i.e., recognizes the potentials for biased observation)
- Applies literature recommendations (i.e., pilot studies) when possible even if this is not your customary management approach, to test out the literature
- Writes case reports
- Participates in research and research design

You may ask: What's in it for me?

- You can map out your patients by presentation and determine your effectiveness with each type.
- Your successes are marketable.
- Your weaknesses are remediable when you are part of a group that compares.

Before we illustrate some simple approaches to measurement, analysis, and change for your practice, let's review some basic scientific principles.

Evidence

Let's start with a world; a perfect world. In a perfect data-driven world, we would know all about all. We would have data on billions of individuals that would include all the demographic information, genetic information, disease/disorder information, and data on how all problems were managed and the success or failure of those methods. We therefore would know an individual's risk and the risk relationship to a multitude of environmental and genetic risk factors and triggers. We would even know the detail of what is the best diagnostic test and

most available test for a given context such as a country, region, or area. We would know the exact treatment method used to manage operationally defined disorders to the point of understanding what specific surgical, drug, or conservative treatment approach works in the majority of patients who are, in fact, the mirror-image of the patient in front of me; the whole person in front of me. Because this perfect data-driven world is not attainable, this appendix is about how to take only fragments of understanding and piece together an approach that is the best educated guess to what may work for our patient.

We could rely on our experience, but what if you are a novice with little experience or none in the specific area of concern for your patient? How would you approach this problem? You would look for what others know. You may ask colleagues, you may search the Internet using a broad search engine such as Google or Google Scholar. google. Even then, how much can you trust the information you find? Regardless of your choice of resource(s), you will still ask the same questions to know whether you are close to the truth:

- Does the information from a colleague, an article, or a blog reflect relevant information for my specific patient?
- On what is the opinion or conclusion based?
- What are the prejudices or biases of those resources?

Like any other search, we want information that is based on an attempt to look at what is fact and not based entirely on observation, opinion, or interpretation. That is where science comes in. That makes it sound like science is perfect. It is not. Scientific knowledge is always building on past observations, including misinterpretations or errors. That being said, the best we can do is to aggregate all available resources and weigh each one, and science should rank high on that list. How we attribute weight to that information is not a equal one-to-one proposition. And, how we value the information, how practical and usable it is, is not always a reflection of how scientifically rigorous the research has been.

It is relatively easy to rate the weight of information based on scientific rigor. For example, a randomized controlled study would certainly rate higher than one that is not, because that is the highest-order study for ruling out chance and bias if conducted properly. A prospective study, in general, is better than a retrospective study (more on this later). A case study of one to several patients is clearly not as strong scientifically as a larger study involving more participants. But regarding value, the weighting must be in the context of the patient in front of you and the confluence of the literature conclusions in an aggregate summary. Then each clue, whether historical or by clinical examination, must now be placed on a scale on the side of likely having the disorder in question versus not.

For example, a given historical clue may be placed on the side of having the disorder but only amount to the weight of a BB, whereas the value of an orthopaedic clue may have the weight of a bowling ball, or vice versa (**Figure A–1**). Or something may be intermediate, like the weight of a billiard ball. That being said, the value of the test may be different from the scientific rigor rating, especially if the study population matches the patient in front of you compared to studies where the population does not. Also, remember that risk factors are not diagnostic clues. They have value in rating risk, which is an association, but do not necessarily help in making a diagnosis.

The broadest and most important distinction of research studies is determining their intent. There are basically two types of research studies (**Figure A–2**):

1. Observational: A study can be designed to find an association or risk to a particular disease or disorder. These are observational studies without intervention.
2. Interventional: A study can be designed to determine the effect of an intervention on patients with a known disorder.

These studies can: (1) examine a patient group at one point in time, called a cross-sectional study; (2) follow a group of patients forward in time, called a prospective (or longitudinal) study; or (3) back through time, called a

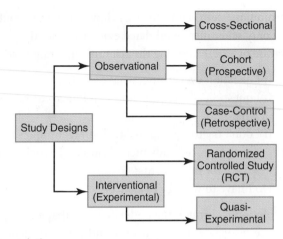

Figure A–2

retrospective study. We will begin by looking at interventional studies to determine how we approach the literature with regard to the effectiveness of an intervention.

Treatment Effects

How do you know if the treatment works, and if so, how well it works? To understand how the results of research can be utilized in practice, the clinician must be numerate. Numeracy is similar to literacy but instead of interpreting the meaning of words, it means to interpret the meaning of numbers. Note that this does not equate to doing the math and calculating the statistics, but it means that clinical application of the end result of the calculations is achievable and hopefully communicable.

What numbers mean depends on the interpreter. Of course it is human nature to convey our own bias and certainly use numbers in the most convincing light for what we mean to achieve. The variables are the study, the researchers who conduct the study, the patient, and the middle man—you, the doctor. Like it or not, the doctor becomes the inevitable translator of statistics for the patient. You need to be "bilingual": know the results for a group of patients (the study), and attempt to translate that information into results for your patient. You need to convey why you feel your care can help and also include reasonable options for the patient. Most would admit that second on the list for not reading a research article (the first being time) is that when you encounter the numbers, you just want to gloss over them and get to the conclusion, hoping that the researchers and editors of the publication have done their job and given you the bottom line. But you are rarely confident that you truly understand the meaning and relevance of the statistical terminology and numbers.

Not all evidence is equally weighted

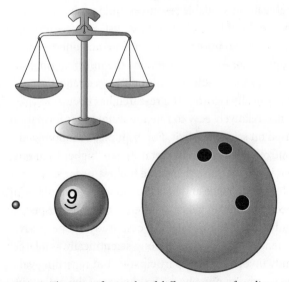

Figure A–1 The scientific weight of different types of studies.

If you don't see one of the following terms in the abstract of an article on an intervention or risk factor, you will have your first warning sign about the scientific validity of that study: Absolute Risk (AR), Relative Risk (RR) and Recurrence Rate Data (RRD), Number Needed to Treat (NNT), Odds Ratio (OR), Effect Size (ES), and mean differences. This is the vocabulary list of statistics, the words one needs for understanding the results found. It may sound daunting but the math used is almost always simple addition, subtraction, or division, which is now automated through online calculators, is easily accessed, and for the most part, mathematically related. By using examples and discussing results first, we will effortlessly learn the language used to express the results utilized in study papers. You should then be able to generally determine what a study is saying, despite the possibly confusing terminology, and determine whether it is worth reading, how important and valid the information is, and whether it is usable for your purposes.

Understand the patients' dilemma. They want to be in control of their health management choices, yet most are not trained in the language of statistics to make sense of that information if it is offered in terms such as *p* values, confidence intervals, and so on; in other words, they are not numerate. We need to assist patients in making decisions regarding their health. Although we are always sensitive to our patients' desires to be actively involved in their health management choices, we understand that they are relying on us to give them information in a manner that is usable. How we explain the benefits and risks of a given treatment, even to a colleague, is in need of edit and translation before explaining the same information to a patient.

Where do clinical questions about an interventions success come from? It may be a question based on lack of experience, but it just as often may reflect curiosity; an attempt to learn something new about something you already know. The question can also come from your patient. It probably will center on whether they will improve or if there is a risk to treatment. So what is the patient going to ask? What are the chances I will get better with this treatment and how long will it take? What are the chances of responding to a standard treatment such as medication, surgery, or no treatment?

Suppose a patient approached with a question about a report he or she heard on the news about a "miracle cure" for some disorder. Let's use an example. A news headline states that a new drug reduces cancer death by 33%. Thirty-three percent reduction of cancer, but compared to what, no treatment or another treatment

approach? In other words, 33% of these cancer patients will survive and 66% will not without treatment? Or does this mean the new treatment is compared to another existing treatment? What if the newer treatment is far more expensive and has more side effects? How this study was conducted would, like most studies, be based on two main goals of science: is there a difference between groups, and are there associations when evaluating risk?

Let's say that an oncologist needed to explain the study to one of his or her patients. Here is how it could be expressed.

- "You have one-third the risk of death with the newer treatment compared to the standard treatment."
- "The risk of death is about two-thirds that of those in the standard treatment group."

Or you could use a combination of the above two statements:

- "Your risk of death is reduced one-third with the newer treatment compared to standard treatment so that now you have only two-thirds the risk of someone using the standard treatment."

The first statement is called relative risk reduction (RRR), the next statement about having two-thirds the risk of someone on standard treatment is called relative risk or the risk ratio (RR), and it is just that, calculated by dividing the rates of death with the new treatment by those of the standard treatment. This indicates a comparison to another treatment, not comparison to natural history. What's missing? If the actual death rate for those on the standard treatment was only 5.7% and the death rate in the group with the newer treatment was only 3.8%, then we know the death rate using standard care for this cancer is not very high to begin with. The ratio between groups magnified the effect of the new treatment to 66%, which is a true comparison but as a ratio. The actual difference in death rates between the two groups is only 1.9%.

Let's discuss another set of hypothetical examples (**Figure A–3**). If the risk of death is 10% in the standard group compared to 6% in the new treatment group, the absolute difference is 4% AND this is also a 40% reduction in risk! If the risk of death is 1% in the standard treatment group and it is 0.6% in the new treatment group, it is still a 40% reduction AND this equals an added advantage of helping only 0.4% more people! So what makes the difference? The actual (not relative)

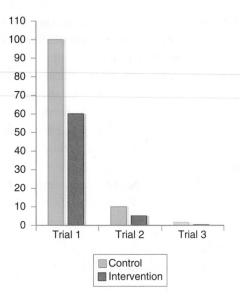

Figure A–3 40% RR in three different-sized groups.

outcome rate (event rate) difference is called the Absolute Risk Reduction (or Risk Difference). The relative risk and relative risk reduction calculations are blind to the actual numbers because they are only ratios between numbers. For example:

- 10 is 10% of 100
- 1 is 10% of 10 and
- 0.1 is 10% of 1

The ratio remains the same (10%) but clearly the actual numbers are magnitudes of difference lost when calculated as ratios. The problem is that RR and RRR create a magnification of effect often enlisted by researchers or pharmaceutical marketers attempting to sway the reader into thinking the effect of a newer treatment is greater than it really is greater than its actual clinical value would be. There are clearly some ethical considerations in the medication advertisements that illustrate attempts to exaggerate effects. It is disturbing to realize that to be considered effective, researchers have to show only that a new drug has a *statistically* significant difference (not due to chance) but not a clinically significant difference if compared to placebo.

Next, let's discuss some other terminology for events that occur with two treatment groups compared in a study. The term Exposed Group Event Rate (EER) is also called Treatment Event Rate (TER) and Intervention Event Rate (IER), and refers to the new treatment approach group. The term Control Group Occurrence (CGO), also called Control Event Rate (CER), refers to the comparison group. **Figure A–4** is a more detailed expression of how a two-by-two table is constructed and the resultant RRR, ARR, and NNT are mathematiclly derived. Although interesting and valuable, much of this is automated through online calculators so that you could take the results of studies and plug in the numbers without doing the math.

Let's review a study that uses these designations, comparing clopidogrel (Plavix) to aspirin for patients with risk of ischemic events. The ischemic events included

	+ Outcome	− Outcome
+ Intervention	A 10	B 50
− Intervention	C 26	D 34

CER = control group event rate   = c / (c+d) = 0.43 = 43%
EER = experimental group event rate = a / (a+b) = 0.17 = 17%

CER	EER	Relative risk reduction (RRR)	Absolute risk reduction (ARR)	Number needed to treat (NNT)
		$\dfrac{\text{CER−EER}}{\text{CER}}$		
		CER−EER / CER	CER−EER	1/ARR
43%	17%	60%	26%	4
		*95% CI ⇒	10.3% − 41.7%	2 − 10

*95% confidence interval (CI) on an NNT = 1/(limits on the CI of its ARR) =

$$\pm 1.96 \sqrt{\left[\frac{\text{CER} \times (1-\text{CER})}{\text{\#Control Pts}}\right] + \left[\frac{\text{EER} \times (1-\text{EER})}{\text{\#Exper Pts}}\right]} = \pm 1.96 \sqrt{\left[\frac{0.17 \times 0.83}{60}\right] + \left[\frac{0.43 \times 0.57}{60}\right]} = \pm 15.7\%$$

Figure A–4 Sample calculations—risk reduction.

These questions were adapted from the Oxford Centre for Evidence-Based Medicine and applied to physical therapist practice.

myocardial infarction, stroke, or vascular death. The control event group used aspirin. For them, the CER was 5.83% versus the EER for the clopidogrel group of 5.32%. The RRR = (5.83 − 5.32)/5.83, which equals 8.7% in favor of clopidogrel. The absolute risk is ARR =5.83 − 5.32, which equals only 0.51%!

The NNT is the inverse of the ARR (1/ARR) and represents the number of patients needed to be treated to avoid *one* adverse outcome (e.g., an ischemic event). In the previous example, the NNT is equal to 1/0.0051, which equals 196. Almost 200 patients would need to be treated with clopidogrel, *as compared to aspirin*, to avoid one adverse CV event. Does this make sense considering the high cost of the new drug?

Here is another study comparing endarterectomy versus aspirin for cervical artery stenosis. The CER was 26%, whereas for surgery the EER was 9%. Using standard calculations and statistics, RR = 35%; RRR = 65%; and ARR = 17%. The NNT = 5.9, meaning five to six patients need to be treated with surgery to prevent one stroke. The questions arise: Is it worth it? What are the costs and what are the risks of the treatment?

The use of statins is very popular for the reduction of cholesterol. What are the results, though, regarding reducing cardiovascular risk and death? Although Crestor (statin) sales were $4.5 billion ($3–$5/day for patients) with 80 million meeting the criteria, it was proposed the following criteria should also be included (effectively increasing eligible patients significantly):

- Patients over age 50 years if male; age 60 years if female
- One risk factor (smoking or hypertension)
- Elevated C-reactive protein (CRP) (> 6.5 mol)

The researcher (also the developer of the test C-reactive protein used as one of the indicators) claimed a reduction of 55% in myocardial infarction, 48% in stroke, and 45% in angioplasty. The real numbers for Crestor were that the CER in the placebo group was 0.37% (68/8901) and in the Crestor group the EER was 0.17% (31/8901). The RR = 54%; RRR = 46% (1 − RR), but the AR = 0.2% with an NNT = 500. So the author/researcher was correct but selective in the statistic he or she used, which appears to be an intentional decision to promote the use of statins.

When determining effectiveness, several questions need to be answered. The first is, did a statistical difference occur? This is determined, and is reported as the *p* value. The *p* value is a measure of how often something would happen beyond chance. In other words, is it statistically likely that the vast majority of the difference is NOT due to chance? The next question is, what is the magnitude of that difference? This is measured, and is reported as the 95% confidence interval (CI). The CI is the range of difference not just a point value representing an average.

Like CIs for diagnostic tests, a result of 1 means there is no value. Unlike CIs for diagnostic tests, CIs for intervention and/or risk must not include 0 or go below 0. In other words, if there is no difference between two treatment outcomes or risks, divided into each other the result is 1. If it is less than 1, the intervention being tested is less effective or the risk being evaluated turns out to be potentially protective and not a risk. CIs inform the clinician about the range within which the true treatment effect might lie. The greater precision (narrower range) results from larger sample sizes (i.e., assuming a larger number of events). It is calculated by finding the appropriate *z*-score, which is based on the degree of confidence. The CI is calculated as the standard deviation divided by the square root of the *n* and then multiplied by 1.96. The final step is to add and subtract it from the mean to determine the range.

The next question is, is it clinically relevant? This is determined by various means of measuring two issues: the *minimal clinically important difference* (MCID) and the *effect size* (**Table A–1**).

Table A–1 Minimal Clinically Important Difference (MCID)

Outcome Measure	Suggested MCID	Patient Population
Oswestry	4–6	Patients with LBP
Roland-Morris	2–5	Patients with LBP (1–2 with mild disability; 7–8 with high disability)
Neck Disability Index	7	Patients with cervical radiculopathy
VAS (100 points)	18	Patients with chronic LBP
Pain (11-point scale)	2–3	Patients with chronic pain

Table A–2 Effect Size Summary

Number	Difference between Treatment and Placebo
0.0	No difference
0.2	Small treatment effect
0.5	Moderate treatment effect
>0.8	Large treatment effect

The MCID is generally gauged by a comparison to a percentage or difference in points based on an outcome measure. This is by standard a 30% change; however, some researchers require a higher standard of up to 50% change. How is this change determined? This can be statistically determined in complicated formulas, but again, for the clinician, the quickest and most reliable way is by comparison to an outcome measure. These outcome measures are numerous but the most common for spinal conditions include the Roland-Morris Disability Questionnaire, the Oswestry, the Bournemouth Questionnaire, the Neck Disability Index, and the common measures of pain—the visual analog scale and the numerical rating scale. Some caution must be used when the baseline for these outcome measures does not indicate a high degree of disability or pain. As we have seen, a percentage change of let's say 50% may indicate only a change from a numerical rating scale (NRS) for pain of 2 to 1 (as compared to a more significant indicator of an NRS of 10 to 5). Therefore, the higher the severity indicated by the measure, the more reliable is the percentage change. The other determination is simply a point change relative to the outcome measure, as indicated in **Table A–2**. MCIDs can be used to simply look at the effect of treatment (intervention) in each group, or for a comparison between groups. When comparisons are made between groups, an effect size based on the mean differences between groups is more often utilized.

The effect size can be even trickier than the MCID. This statistic more often has to do with the difference between treatment groups. As a statistical calculation, the effect size is often described as a number with a point value of greater than 0.8 equal to a large treatment effect.

A summary approach is to compare several statistical values to see globally if there is an effect change that would likely be clinically valuable; i.e., valuable to your patient. **Table A–3** summarizes an approach using the NNT, EF, and OR in gauging the significance of a change. Remember that this is always an important comparison to what often is reported as a *statistically important change* or difference, which may have little or no value in practice.

Risk

When estimating risk, researchers are really looking for whether there is an association between an exposure and an event. Associations can be studied based on looking at risk factors such as smoking, hypertension, obesity, and so on. An association is not by definition the same as cause-and-effect, which requires more stringent study approaches including studying patients only forward in time rather than retrospectively. In studying risk, researchers attempt to compare the risk of an outcome in participants exposed to the risk factor compared to those non-exposed in observational (not interventional) studies (trials). For studies of risk factors versus interventions, there are two approaches, both observational (**Figures A–5**, **A–6**). One is the cohort or prospective study that follows people through time. The other is a case-control, retrospective study where researchers use a method that looks back in time to see if the patient with a specific disorder was exposed to a risk factor under investigation. The cohort study usually uses *relative risk* as a measure whereas the retrospective, case-control study must use an *odds ratio*.

Table A–3 Summary Comparison

Statistic	Good	Poor
NNT (Number Needed to Treat)	A single-digit number	A larger number; the higher number the more patients needing treatment to affect 1 patient
ES (Effect Size)	>0.8	<0.2
OR (Odds Ratio)	>2	1

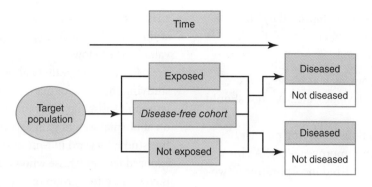

Figure A–5 The cohort study.

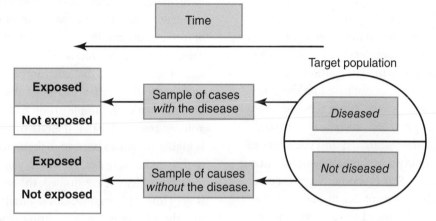

Figure A–6 The case control study.

So again with the prospective study you begin with disease-free subjects and see who develops the disease when exposed to a risk factor, whereas in a retrospective, case-control study, the individuals already have the disease, so you are looking back in their medical records to see how many of them were exposed to the risk factor. Here is a very important difference between these two approaches. In the cohort study, the item of interest is the *outcome* (**Table A–4**); who was exposed to the risk

factor develops the outcome, whereas in the case-control retrospective study, the item of interest is the *risk factor*, because we already know which individuals have the disease (**Table A–5**).

If you want to determine if the researchers or even peer-reviewers of a study missed an important factor on how the statistics were calculated based on the type of data, make sure you check for the following statistics. For the statistics used to determine the difference between

Table A–4 Cohort (Prospective)

		Condition/Health Problem		
		Present	**Absent**	**Risk**
Risk Factor	Exposed	a	b	a/a+b
	Not Exposed	c	d	c/c+d

Table A–5 Case-Control (Retrospective)

		Risk Factor		
		Exposed	**Not Exposed**	**Odds**
Condition	Case (those with)	a	c	a/c
	Those Without	b	d	b/d

groups (improved/not improved, improved by how much, prevents/does not prevent, etc.), the following questions and solutions are used:

- Are the data continuous such as blood pressure, ROM, temperature, lab values, etc.? A t-test should be utilized.
- Are the data dichotomous (meaning positive/negative, improved/not improved, etc.)? A chi-square test should be utilized incorporating a two-by-two table.

How do we determine the strength of these types of study results and conclusions? First, we need to look at a study's *p* value or confidence intervals. What does a *p* value indicate? It is the mathematical caution flag that indicates whether to proceed or not based on the study's accepted tolerance of whether the differences found are due to chance. A *p* value of 0.05, which is often used, basically indicates that the researchers and you are comfortable with the possibility that these values could occur 5% of the time by chance. Stated another way, you can be 95% sure that the findings are not due to chance. What about confidence intervals? They keep everyone honest by revealing the *range* of values in a study. The point values, such as relative risk, are a mean or average of all study participant outcomes. But clearly there is a range of findings in any sample of people including extremes. And just like the *p* value, a 95% confidence interval means that the true value is likely to be in that range 95% of the time and that conversely you can accept that 5% of the time it is not.

The confidence interval is one step closer to giving you a sense of the clinical significance of the findings. What is our clue that the range conflicts with the conclusion that there is a risk? If the ratio of the event being studied, the disease or the condition, is the same in both groups, numerically they will equal 1, meaning that if it occurred in 10 out of 100 patients in one group and the same in the other, dividing them into each other equals 1. If it is below 1, we must consider the possibility that this is not a risk factor, or at least in some patients it is not. And at the extreme it may be protective, especially if all the values were below 1.

So let's use a hypothetical example. What if you were studying the effect of diabetes during pregnancy on the fetus and subsequently wanted to determine the effect on abnormal weight gain as a child? This is a prospective study; forward in time and hopefully that cohort of exposed fetuses (those who had mothers with diabetes) is compared to a group of fetuses whose mothers did not have diabetes. In **Table A–6** we see how that would be constructed in a two-by-two table. Note that the outcome of interest, the condition, would be abnormal weight gain, and this is our focus. We then compare those fetuses exposed to a diabetic mother with those who were not to determine the risk of abnormal weight gain. Let's say that each sample group had 1,000 study subjects. You can see quickly that the rate of abnormal weight gain is higher in fetuses born to diabetic mothers compared to those who were not. However, you also see that the overall problem being studied, the abnormal weight gain, is very low. Although we can say that the absolute risk is low, the relative risk or risk ratio calculated by dividing the risk of those exposed by those who were not, is high at 10. Said another way, the children born to diabetic mothers have 10 times the risk of abnormal weight gain compared to those not born to diabetic mothers in our hypothetical study.

Now let's use a real study that illustrates a hybrid where patients were studied prospectively but then evaluated as a follow-up retrospectively for the relationship between cardiac risk factors and having a diagnosis of lumbar disc herniation.[1] Note that this is not a cause-and-effect study, but a study of associated risk. This is a key limitation of studies that look back in time. This is a 16-year follow-up study of nearly 3,000 nurses.[1] Multivariate analysis was used, meaning statistically an attempt to tease out overlap among factors is being incorporated so that there is some confidence that the factor's independent association to the outcome, in this

Table A–6 Cohort (Prospective) 1,000 Subjects in Each Group

		Condition/Health Problem		
		Present	Absent	Risk
Risk Factor	Exposed	30	970	0.03
	Not Exposed	3	997	0.003
Relative Risk (Risk Ratio) = 0.03/0.003 = 10				

Table A–7 Multivariate Analysis

Factor	Relative Risk	95% Confidence Interval
Diabetes	1.52	1.17–1.98
Hypertension	1.25	1.11–1.41
High Cholesterol	1.26	1.10–1.44
Smoking (age >45)	2.14	1.34–3.42
P value = 0.01 (for trend)		

Reproduced from Jhawar BS, Fuchs CS, Colditz GA, Stampfer MJ. Cardiovascular risk factors for physician-diagnosed lumbar disc herniation. *The Spine Journal*. 2006: 6;684–691.

case disc herniation, is estimated. Among the cardiovascular risk factors evaluated were diabetes, hypertension, high cholesterol, and smoking. **Table A–7** illustrates the relative risks and their association 95% confidence intervals for several of these CV risk factors. You can see the adjusted relative risk is above 1, which indicates an increased associated risk. None of the confidence intervals falls below 1, which means the range of values in this study population always indicates an increased risk. Also the *p* value is well within the 0.05 target. How can this be stated to a patient? As a diabetic there is an associated risk for disc herniation that is 52% higher than for people who don't have diabetes, or even though it might not seem obvious, having been or being hypertensive increases associated risk for disk herniation by 25%. This is stated as relative risk. As a side note, the proposed mechanism is an accelerated growth of atherosclerotic plaque to the arteries that supply the lumbar disc.

In a case-control study we are interested to see who with the disease was exposed to the risk factor. Looking back through medical records is a shorter, less expensive approach, but because patients cannot be randomized as in a cohort study, you can look only at an association and not a cause-and-effect relationship. You can see that what has changed with a case-control study is our focus of interest, which is the risk factor. That's because we already know who has the disease. What we don't know is who with that disease or disorder was exposed to the risk factor. That changes the two-by-two table. Because researchers are allowed to choose the number of patients to study in a retrospective study, we can only estimate risk through the odds ratio. This is the ratio of odds between those who have the disease/disorder and were exposed to the risk factor divided by those without the disease/disorder who were exposed to the risk factor. Plugging in numbers, let's see how this works. Let's say this is a hypothetical study of workers with carpal tunnel syndrome who use computers, the risk factor (**Table A–8**). You can see here the odds for those with carpal tunnel, the cases that were exposed to the risk factor of computer use, are 9, whereas the odds of those in the no carpal tunnel group exposed to computer use are only 0.82. The ratio equals 11. This could be stated as the associated risk between computer use and carpal tunnel syndrome in our hypothetical study is eleven times higher than those without carpal tunnel syndrome.

There is an important aspect regarding odds ratio interpretation. For the comparison of two groups, if they have equal odds, meaning the denominator and numerator are the same, numerically this will calculate to 1, which means there is no difference in associated risk. But remember if it is below 1 it may indicate either a decreased risk or protection.

Let's now use a real study of risk in a case-control study by Cassidy et al.[2] This is a measurement of association between visits to a chiropractor or a medical doctor's office prior to a VB stroke (**Table A–9**). We can see that the odds ratios are all above 1, which indicates some association for both visits to a chiropractor or MD's office and VB stroke. Note that the CIs are all above 1 and rather tight except visits to a PCP for patients under the age of 45 years. It is important to remember that as a retrospective study, all that can be established is an estimate of associated risk, not cause-and-effect.

Table A–8 Case-Control (Retrospective)

		Risk Factor		Odds
		Exposed	Not Exposed	
Condition	Case (those with)	90	10	9
	Those Without	45	55	0.82
Odds	Ratio = 9/0.82 = 11			

Table A–9 Odds Ratio- How Do I Interpret?

Parameter	Odds Ratio	95% CI
Visit to chiroprac-tor within 30 days	1.37	1.04–1.91
Visit to PCP – Pt. under 45 y/o	1.34	0.94–1.87
Visit to PCP – Pt. 45 y/o and older	1.52	1.39–1.67

Reproduced from Cassidy JD, Boyle E, Cote P, et al. Risk of vertebrobasilar stroke and chiropractic care: results of a population-based, case-control, and case-crossover study. *Spine.* 2008;33(4 Suppl):S176–183.

So let's review some summary take-home points about studies that evaluate risk.

- They can be forward in time, called a prospective, cohort study or backward in time, called a retrospective, case-control study.
- Although both may estimate odds ratios, case controls can only use odds ratios because the actual relative risk cannot be determined. This is because the samples of patients in each group are not necessarily equal. In case-control studies the researchers can choose the number of patients and who the controls are.
- If there is no difference between the groups being studied, the relative risk or odds ratio will equal 1. Always look for the corresponding CIs and see if the range goes below 1 or in studies of protective factors, rises above 1, in which case you will have some doubt about the significance of the difference between groups.
- Cause-and-effect may be implied in a prospective study, especially if it is an RCT. However, a case-control study can estimate an associated risk only through the odds ratio.

We have one final step in reaching a conclusion about the literature evidence for what we are investigating. We have been determining the value of studies related to interventions and risk. If we weigh these on our scale of determining yes or no for their value, case studies amount to only BBs (**Figure A–7**). If we have stronger studies, especially prospective studies that are blinded and randomized, we have the weight of billiard balls. What about the bowling ball? These are the systematic reviews (SRs) that include all relevant RCTs and other

Not all evidence is equally weighted

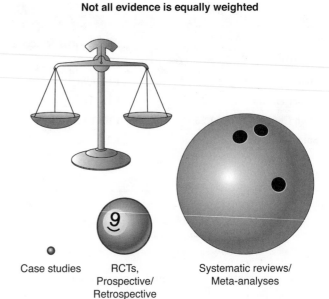

Case studies | RCTs, Prospective/Retrospective studies | Systematic reviews/Meta-analyses

Figure A–7 The scientific weight of different types of studies.

high-quality studies. And when these studies are homogenous (i.e., same group of patients, same measures) we have a potential for a meta-analysis (i.e., statistical comparisons). To be clear, reviews may also be narrative, not applying rigid rules of search and rating but expressing the summary opinion of an individual or groups. These are not systematic reviews.

With a high-quality SR, a group of researchers, using stringent inclusion/exclusion search criteria (similar to a study of patients but here it is studies), rates the quality and conclusions of all relevant studies. If they are homogenous, they can generate what are called *forest plots*. A forest plot is a very efficient way of visualizing all studies on the same page. Note in **Figure A–8**, we see a number of studies that are represented by dots and lines. The dots (diamonds or circles) represent the point estimate of the study. The line represents the CI. We can immediately gauge whether or not studies consistently reach the same results compared to each other. Additionally, we can see how many of the studies' CIs stay above the central line. That central line is our foul line. It is equal to 0 if there is a comparison of differences or mean difference among studies. When the comparison is a ratio such as relative risk, the center line is "1." If the CI line crosses that center line, the range of the CI becomes less trustworthy because it has a foot on either side of the result. In other words, in a study of risk, it would indicate there was some risk in some participants but less risk in others. So for example, if studying the risk of smoking on lung cancer,

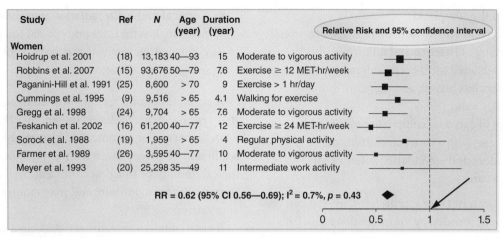

Figure A–8 Forest plot of risk.

it would imply both that there is risk in some participants but in some there was less risk (even the chance that this factor is protective).

So far we have examined how researchers study and report the results of treatment but how can we be confident that their research represents a strong, scientifically based study. We need to know there was a comparison between groups of similar patients with similar prognosis and that there was a control group or placebo group. A strong study will be designed to compare treatments or compare the treatment to natural history. We know that, in general, the larger the group of participants in the study, the more we can trust the results, especially if reflected in a tight CI. If the study is prospective (forward in time), it is stronger when randomized (meaning patients are randomly assigned to groups). It is even stronger if the patient is "blind" to which treatment he or she is receiving. When the treatment that the subjects are randomized to is also "blind" to those assigning randomization, those delivering the treatment, and those gathering outcome data, it is considered "double-blind."

When reviewing a study on risk related to either a treatment or risk related to no-treatment, we need to know that the same comparison groups of participants discussed above are incorporated. This could be done prospectively, which is the stronger study, or retrospectively (i.e., patients usually selected from past medical records), which is weaker scientifically and can only establish associations of risk. Finally, we know that a systematic review is the strongest scientific resource, where comparisons of high-level studies can be summarized and sometimes visualized in a forest plot.

How to Create an Evidence-Informed Practice: Your Practice

So how is it possible for a non-scientist clinician to establish a research approach that generates evidence about his or her practice? Let's review a template that is easy to incorporate by simply using the data you usually collect, adding some other items, entering this into a simple spreadsheet, and learning a few tricks to organize that data to provide meaningful information. You then become an evidence-informed chiropractor.

Evidence-informed knowledge and measurement must include the practice environment of each practitioner, given that patient outcomes are somewhat unique to that context. The data generated are relevant because they reflect the environment in which future patients will be managed.

What is important to measure? You should never measure anything you are not willing to use for change. Evaluating patients' responses based on their complaint and diagnosis matched with the management tools that were utilized is obviously the most important information that effects change. Capturing data can be as simple as entering it into a spreadsheet where it can be manipulated and sorted to produce reports based on your focus of interest. Comparative information should include the following:

- Demographic information including gender and age.
- Complaint information with regard to acute, subacute, or chronic complaints.

- Severity of the complaint.
- A measurement and documentation of a functional questionnaire at baseline and follow-up. This patient-completed form keeps judgment about effectiveness less biased, and therefore more scientifically valid.
- Frequency of care and compliance to that plan.
- Types of care, with a focus on the type of manipulation, and secondarily, columns for adjunctive care.

Figure A–9 illustrates one approach to this. You can see that the patient is coded by his or her diagnosis. This is extremely important for comparing results of care. Unfortunately, there is no standard. Even International Classification of Diseases (ICD) codes are not consistently used, and there is no code for all specific common problems. So either by using a coding system developed by the practitioner or by operationally defining some ICD codes, a distinction of patient groups allows better delineation of patient types. For example, a patient with a cervical spine complaint could have the following codes or distinctions further subcoded by the type (i.e., acute, subacute, or chronic):

- Cervical pain only with no radiation
- Cervical pain with radiation into the arm with no neurological findings

- Cervical pain with radiation into the arm with neurological findings and special imaging confirmation versus those that do not have special imaging confirmation

A separate column for each will allow sorting that may reveal differences based on whether the pain is acute, subacute, or chronic, and also might indicate a difference between those with or without neurological findings or imaging confirmation. Each may respond differently to care and may require different approaches.

If entered into a spreadsheet, making a copy allows manipulation of the data without disturbing the primary data sheet. Sorting can be by any column. For example, if you wanted to look at all patients with cervical pain and radiation with neurological findings and special imaging findings, you could group them together and look at their responses. In fact, you could average them into a point estimate. You could then visually, or through sorting, look for patterns with different responses based on the type of manipulation used or adjunctive care. **Figure A–10** illustrates how sorting by diagnosis allows the ability to average response rates for that diagnosis based on a pain scale or Oswestry score. Further sorting can illustrate if those who improved more had a specific chiropractic technique

File #	Age	Gender	Start Date	1st DIAGNOSIS	VAS 1st	VAS 2wk	VAS 4 wks	OSWESTRY 1	OSWESTRY 2 wks	OSWESTRY 4wks	TOTAL # Txs	LENGTH OF CARE (wks)	TECHNIQUE(S)	OTHER TREATMENT(S)
10922	45	M	03/09/12	722.1	7	3	4	82%	50%	42%	10	4	D	AC M ST
10923	23	M	03/10/12	847.2	3	1	0	30%	10%	0%	5	2	D C	E ST
10924	12	F	03/11/12	728.8	4	2	1	20%	22%	0%	6	2	D C	E
10925	56	F	03/12/12	722.1	5	1	0	38%	10%	0%	7	2	A	ST
10926	35	F	03/13/12	847.2	8	3	1	78%	48%	43%	12	4	T	AC M ST
10927	38	M	03/14/12	722.1	3	1	0	10%	3%	1%	4	1	A	D E
10928	22	F	03/15/12	728.8	5	1	0	34%	12%	0%	6	2	D	ST
10929	25	M	03/16/12	847.2	7	3	2	70%	30%	10%	10	4	D C	E
10930	28	M	03/17/12	846.0	5	3	2	29%	20%	4%	6	2	A	E
10931	57	F	03/18/12	847.2	6	3	0	56%	20%	0%	8	2	D C	ST
10932	53	M	03/19/12	722.1	7	5	2	44%	0%	0%	8	4	D	D
10933	43	M	03/20/12	724.3	6	3	1	64%	20%	0%	9	2	D C	E
10934	33	F	03/21/12	724.3	3	2	0	20%	11%	6%	5	1	D C	D
10935	22	F	03/22/12	722.1	8	4	4	64%	32%	38%	14	5	D A	AC M ST
10936	45	F	03/23/12	724.8	5	2	0	34%	10%	0%	7	2	T	D
10937	38	M	03/24/12	847.2	5	3	0	40%	20%	10%	8	3	D C	ST

MANIPULATIVE TECH	OTHER TREATMENTS
A = Activator	AC = Active Care
C = Cox	D = Decompression
D = Diversified	E = E-Stim
T = Thompson	M = Mechanical Traction
O = Other	ST = Soft Tissue
	U = Ultrasound
	O = Other

Figure A–9 Sample template for clinical practice data capture.

File #	Age	Gender	Start Date	1st DIAGNOSIS	VAS 1st	VAS 2wk	VAS 4 wks	OSWESTRY 1	OSWESTRY 2 wks	OSWESTRY 4wks	TOTAL # Trs	LENGTH OF CARE (wks)	TECHNIQUE(S)	OTHER TREATMENT(S)
10922	45	M	03/09/12	722.1	7	3	4	82%	50%	42%	10	4	D	AC M ST
10925	56	M	03/12/12	722.1	5	1	0	38%	10%	0%	7	2	A	D ST
10927	38	F	03/14/12	722.1	3	1	0	10%	3%	1%	4	1	A	D E
10932	53	F	03/19/12	722.1	7	5	2	44%	0%	0%	8	4	D	D
10935	22	F	03/22/12	722.1	8	4	4	64%	32%	38%	14	5	D A	AC M ST
				→	6	2.8	2	48%	19%	16%	9	3		
10933	43	F	03/20/12	724.3	6	3	1	64%	20%	0%	9	2	D C	E
10934	33	M	03/21/12	724.3	3	2	0	20%	11%	6%	5	1	D C	D
10936	45	F	03/23/12	724.8	5	2	0	34%	10%	0%	7	2	T	D
				→	5	2	0	39%	14%	2%	7	2		
10924	12	F	03/11/12	728.8	4	2	1	20%	22%	0%	6	2	D C	E
10928	22	F	03/15/12	728.8	5	1	0	34%	12%	0%	6	2	D	ST
				→	4.5	1.5	0.5	27%	17%	0%	6	2		
10930	28	M	03/17/12	846	5	3	2	29%	20%	4%	6	2	A	E
10923	23	F	03/10/12	847.2	3	1	0	30%	10%	0%	5	2	D C	E ST
10926	35	M	03/13/12	847.2	8	3	1	78%	48%	43%	12	4	T	AC M ST
10929	25	F	03/16/12	847.2	7	3	2	70%	30%	10%	10	4	D C	E
10931	57	F	03/18/12	847.2	6	3	0	56%	20%	0%	8	2	D C	ST
10937	38	M	03/24/12	847.2	5	3	0	40%	20%	10%	8	3	D C	ST
				→	5.8	2.6	0.6	55%	26%	13%	9	3		

MANIPULATIVE TECH	OTHER TREATMENTS
A = Activator	AC = Active Care
C = Cox	D = Decompression
D = Diversified	E = E-Stim
T = Thompson	M = Mechanical Traction
O = Other	ST = Soft Tissue
	U = Ultrasound
	O = Other

Figure A–10 Sorting of data by diagnosis.

or combination of adjunctive approaches that proved more successful. **Figures A–11** and **A–12** illustrate how by highlighting data and then creating a graph, one can visually look at responses to care effects.

As your database grows, patterns will emerge, and different responses based on specific patient types become more meaningful. The intention is to find your "best practices" and to see where there is need for improvement or change. These are the areas where conversations with other practitioners or literature searching become valuable. If other practitioners use the same approach to clinical measurement and data collection as you do and they demonstrate better responses in areas than you do,

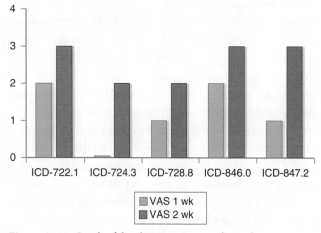

Figure A–12 Graph of data by pain response for each diagnostic group.

sharing the differences can influence change and hopefully improve your results. So the best-case scenario is to establish a working group of like-minded clinicians and meet to share sanitized information (data free of patient information that would violate HIPAA). A final step would be to aggregate that data into a publication that reflected not only the data, but changes made by practitioners who shared the information and the results of those changes.

Change this data to represent improvement

	VAS 1 wk	VAS 2 wk
ICD - 722.1	2	3
ICD - 724.3	0	2
ICD - 728.8	1	2
ICD - 846.0	2	3
ICD - 847.2	1	3

Figure A–11 Sorting of data by pain response for each diagnostic group.

Diagnostic Tests

Translating Terms and Numbers into Useable Information

Now let's switch to the other aspect of clinical practice, the tests we use to determine what is causing our patient's problem and the management approach we utilize. How do you know if the test you are using is of value? Although many diagnostic tests are taught and utilized, many have not passed the scientific rigor necessary to warrant their use. Let's look at the basic criteria by which a diagnostic test is tested, and from a scientific perspective how their value is determined. Although these can be discussed from a mathematical perspective, it is possible to use primarily a narrative explanation and when math is invoked, it will involve mainly simple addition, subtraction, and division. Ironically, we often approach a diagnostic test value like a simple math problem. For example, take a history indicator and a positive examination test finding, add them together (i.e., a + b) and you have the answer (i.e., c). The problem, as most clinicians intuitively know, is that the patient presentation is far too complex for this to work, except perhaps for the more classic presentations of a disorder. In fact, most of the time we can only get close to feeling entirely correct about our diagnosis based not only on the complexity of patient presentation, but the unlikelihood that we can narrow down the cause to a single pain-producing structure. And, as is the case many times, conditions can overlap, such as shoulder impingement and rotator cuff tendinitis. Diagnosis is more commonly the act of weighing the factors on the side of having the disorder versus those on the side arguing against having the disorder. What makes this complex is that all factors do not carry equal weight in value. As mentioned previously, the weighing of factors leading to a diagnosis must account for differences in value so that some amount to the weight of a BB, others a billiard ball, and others a bowling ball. All factors are not equal in determining whether an individual does or does not have a disorder.

When it is time to interpret and apply the statistics regarding whether a patient has or does not have a disorder, we face two obstacles: (1) gathering and analyzing the studies used to study a test, and (2) extrapolation to our patient.

Let's step back. Why do we do tests? It may seem obvious: to discover the cause of our patient's problem. But we soon realize there are a host of peripheral factors that determine whether we perform a test. These include what we are taught, what managed care, Medicare, or other outside agencies require, whether it costs money, and frankly some of the time, whether it protects us legally. But what really determines the value of a test for your patient? It begins with what is known about the statistical value of the test. We will focus on the true value of testing without the interference of outside influences, motivators, past prejudices, and tradition.

One initial purpose of a test is to rule out a serious concern; one that would cause one to refer the patient. Another is to determine if you can move onto treatment without further testing. For instructors, there is a different mindset. How do you determine which tests to teach? Is it the test list we were taught or the tests on a form that drive the instructor to want to prepare the student for either the real world or perhaps National Board testing? And why are those tests chosen by that group in the first place? How do we determine the value of the tests in relation to one another and how do we answer the student's question: should I combine tests into a cluster or is there one best test for this condition? There are any questions, but hopefully a few answers will satisfy most of them.

There are three main steps that determine the value of a test. The first is, are the test results valid? Secondly, what are the test results; and finally, if I use this test, will the results change anything in the management of my patient? For validity, we need to determine the type of patients used in the study. Are they representative of a spectrum of patients with the disorder from mild to severe, and are they representative of the types of patients I see? Is there a comparison to a gold standard? Is there, in fact, a gold standard? In other words, can this disorder be identified directly through visualization of the pathology through imaging, or of dysfunction through electrical testing or lab testing? Most importantly, is there an independent blinded comparison to that standard?

For studies that report results regarding the ability of diagnostic tests to find or exclude a disorder, a host of terms are used to describe values that seem mind-numbing in their scope and breadth. These include sensitivity, specificity, likelihood ratios, predictive values, and odds ratios, among others. It is a common clinician fear that if one does not understand the math behind the generation of these statistics, their use is not possible. Not true, as we will see.

For the value to my patient, we need to know if the test can be used in my office and whether the results apply to the types of patients I see to warrant extrapolation and application. Most importantly, will the result change my management? Finally, what are the costs and risks, if any, of the test?

With the evaluation of a test, we look for two values: Is the test reliable? Is it valid? The reliability of a test has two components. The examiners evaluating a particular test may or may not agree with the result. Each examiner, when comparing the current interpretation to his or her past interpretation of a test, may not agree with his or her original interpretation. This comparison is called intra-examiner reliability. The comparison of an examiner's results to other examiners' results is termed interexaminer reliability. If the test result is dichotomous (meaning one value or another, such as true or false) the statistic used is the *kappa coefficient*. If the test result is continuous (such as the values for blood pressure, temperature, or range of motion) the statistic *intra-class correlation coefficient* (ICC) is used. So the estimate of the chance that an examiner will find the same result on the same patient when tested a second time is termed intra-examiner reliability, and interexaminer reliability is the estimate of how often a different examiner testing the same patient would arrive at the same result as the first examiner.

Validity has to do with whether the test is measuring what it is supposed to measure. This is determined by its comparison to a gold standard. Validity is the degree of trust you should give to the result the test is giving you. Is it sensitive enough to find the disorder, and is the test specific, meaning is it unique enough that when positive, it identifies that disorder? If a test has not passed the requirements of reliability and validity, it likely will have no demonstrable value. It may surprise you that many tests never have been put to the task of meeting these requirements. Even after failing one or both, some tests are still widely used due to tradition and habit. In the past, a surefire guarantee of utilization of the test was a plausible mechanistic explanation of what the test was doing in relation to the pathology of the related condition, or by having someone naming the test after you. Great for writing test questions, useless for determining the value of the test on a patient.

As mentioned earlier, there are two ways of representing reliability, based on whether a test is simply positive or negative or whether there is a range of possible findings. Kappa is used for the dichotomous, or "one-or-the-other," type of test result. The other type of result is the ICC, when the test result is a range of values. What we can do is take the numbers for kappa and ICC and translate these, based on a range, into usable language so that when we see the results, we automatically know whether we can

Table A–10 Intrepreting Kappa

Value of Kappa	Strength of Agreement
<0.20	Poor
0.21–0.40	Fair
0.41–0.60	Moderate
0.61–0.80	Good
0.81–1.00	Very Good

trust that the test is interpreted similarly either among examiners or on repeated attempts by the same examiner. For example, a kappa of 0.21 to 0.40 is considered fair, and anything below 0.20 is considered poor (**Table A–10**). We should proceed with caution when considering adopting a test with such a rating. Lucky for us, the ICC produces similar number ranges and categories, making them relatively easy to remember and use (**Table A–11**).

So how is test performance measured—in other words, its ability to rule in or rule out a disorder? We tend to forget that there are really two contexts. One is the study itself—the tests in the study and the patients in that study. We then must find a way to translate the results of that study into a decision about the patient in front of you—the second context.

Test results that are dichotomous—positive or negative—are represented graphically in a two-by-two table. This deceptively simple-looking graphic serves as a source of frustration for many. The mathematical calculations and resulting terms are often confusing and tend to immediately turn off the clinician. Let's simplify these through some examples. In the example in **Figure A–13** we have true positives and negatives and false positives and negatives, meaning some test results have been compared to a gold standard and found to be either accurate in finding the disorder or not. When the test is positive and the disorder is not present, this is a false positive. When the test is negative but the disorder is present, the test is a false negative. How these are combined determines their value to us and to our patient. These values include sensitivity,

Table A–11 Intrepreting the ICC

Value of ICC	Strength of Agreement
<0.40	Poor
0.40–0.75	Fair to Good
>0.75	Excellent

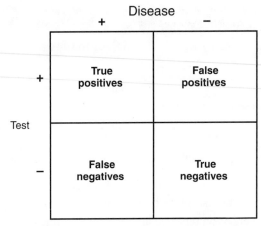

Figure A–13 Two-by-two table for diagnostic test results.

specificity, predictive values, and likelihood ratios. And it is important to know that these represent only the patients in the study. We will later find a way to take these values and help predict probability for the patient in front of us.

Sensitivity

By taking the true positives and false negatives, we account for all the patients with the disorder who were tested. Sensitivity is the proportion of the people with the disease or disorder who test positive (**Figure A–14**). Using an unrealistic scenario will allow us to use easily performed math. Let's say we have 100 patients who all have the disorder (**Figure A–15**). If the test is 84% sensitive, it means that it found 84 of the 100 patients with the disorder but missed 16.

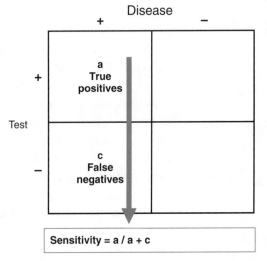

Sensitivity = a / a + c

Figure A–14 Sensitivity.

Proportion of people <u>with</u> the disease who have a positive test result.

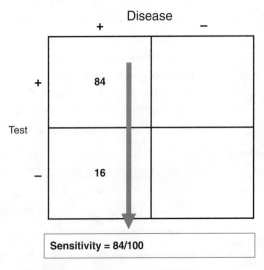

Sensitivity = 84/100

Figure A–15 Sensitivity.

Proportion of people <u>with</u> the disease who have a positive test result.

So, a test with 84% sensitivity....means that the test identifies 84 out of 100 people WITH the disease

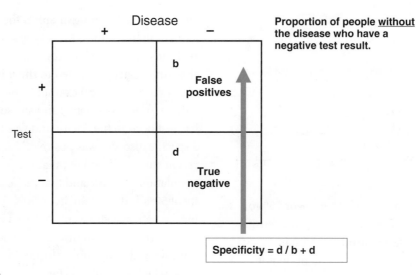

Figure A–16 Specificity.

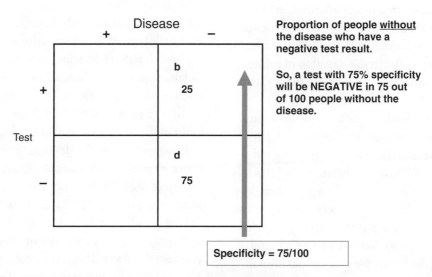

Figure A–17 Specificity.

Specificity

Specificity is a measure of the number of people without the disease who test negative. It combines the true negatives with the false positives to include all patients who do not have the disorder (**Figure A–16**). Again, using the same study where 100 patients have the disorder, a specificity of 76% would indicate that the test correctly identified 76 out of the 100 patients without the disorder but incorrectly implied that 24 had the disorder when they did not (**Figure A–17**). So how is this useful in determining the value of the test? It must first be understood that the sensitivity and specificity of a test are not affected by the prevalence of the disorder (**Figure A–18**).

Sensivity and Specificity are not *directly* affected by *prevalence*

- sensitivity
  131/143 = 92%
- specificity
  93/143 = 65%

		Condition		
		Present	Absent	
Test	Pos.	131	50	181
	Neg.	12	93	105
		143	143	286

Figure A–18 Sensivity and specificity are not directly affected by prevalence.

Table A–12 Sensitivity and Specificity

SnNout

A Highly SeNsitive Test , when Negative, points toward Ruling OUT the condition

SpPin

A Highly SPecific Test, when Positive, points toward Ruling IN the Disorder

In other words, it doesn't matter whether 5% or 75% of patients have the disorder. It will not change the sensitivity or specificity. We will soon introduce the statistics that do change with how many patients do or do not have the disorder.

How do we translate a statistic such as a test is 92% sensitive and 65% specific into useful information? We can use an acronym (**Table A–12**). Using *SnNout* for sensitivity, we remind ourselves that a highly sensitive test, when negative, tends to point in the direction of ruling out the condition/disorder. We can then use the acronym *SpPin* for specificity, reminding us that a highly specific test, when positive, tends to point in the direction of ruling in a condition/disorder. The degree to which each test should be weighted in ruling in or ruling out is clearly illustrated by the percentage value.

The next step is *predictive values*. These are affected by prevalence, so that the number of patients with the disorder does affect the values of positive and negative predictive values (**Figure A–19**). Now we can get a better sense of the value of the test in the study population of patients. Note that a positive predictive value is related to specificity, and a negative predictive value is related to sensitivity. This makes sense when we look at the meaning of SnNout for sensitivity and the negative predictive

- positive predictive value
  131/181 = 72%
- negative predictive value
  93/105 = 89%

		Condition		
		Present	Absent	
Value	Pos.	131	50	181
	Neg.	12	93	105
		143	143	286

Figure A–19 Predictive values are directly affected by prevalence.

value and the meaning of SpPin for specificity and positive predictive values. An easy way to remember this is that the *p* in positive relates to the *p* in specificity and the *n* in negative is related to the *n* in sensitivity.

Let's use a practical example. You get a call from a patient, friend, or relative and she sounds concerned. She has just been to the doctor and was told that her test for a specific disorder was positive. You look up the most recent study and find out that the prevalence in the study population was 30% and that the test used has a sensitivity of 50% and a specificity of 90%. We already know that for the patients who were studied a positive test was quite good at ruling in that disorder. But let's see if we can improve and have some information regarding our individual. Let's look at this (**Figure A–20**). We have a prevalence of 30%, a sensitivity of 50%, and a specificity of 90%. To keep the math simple, let's assume the study had 100 patients. In that study 30 patients had the disorder and 70 did not. With a sensitivity of 50%, the test will be positive in only 15 patients. Now, we are more interested in false positives for those without the disorder. You will see why in a moment. The false positive rate would be 10% given the specificity is 90%. With 70 patients without the disorder and a false positive rate of 10%, 7 patients were correctly identified as not having the disorder. Adding the 15 true positives and 7 false positives, we arrive at 22. The true positives divided by the total number of positives (15/22) is about 70%. The chance of having the disorder is 70% if your individual matches the demographics and prevalence of the patients in the study that tested the test. This is the positive predictive value. Now let's simply change one thing, the prevalence, and reduce it to 4% (**Figure A–21**). If the test is positive, now what is the chance the person has the disease? Now with a sample group of 100 patients, only 4 have the disease and 96 do not. With a sensitivity of 50% only 2 patients are identified correctly. Adding the true positive and false positives together we arrive at 11.6 who test positive, 2 of whom actually have the disorder. Dividing those patients who actually have the disorder by the number who tested positive (2/11.6) we arrive at a predictive value of only 17%. A lower prevalence seriously decreases the ability of the test to correctly detect the disorder even when sensitivity and specificity remain the same. Then back to your patient, friend, or relative with the positive test, the only way to truly know the predictive value for her test result is to match the results to the prevalence in the study population. In other words, if the patients in the study

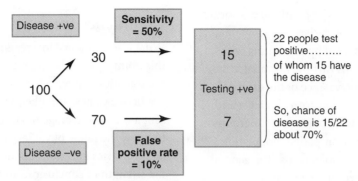

Figure A–20 Prevalence of 30%, sensitivity of 50%, specificity of 90%.

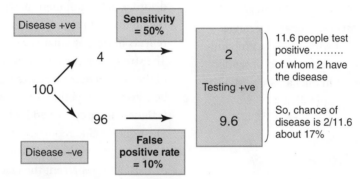

Figure A–21 Prevalence of 4%, sensitivity of 50%, specificity of 90%.

were referred to a specialty clinic but your patient is seen by a primary care physician, the prevalence would likely be higher in the study population than in the primary care setting. The predictive value of the test would not be guaranteed to be as high assuming the prevalence is lower in the primary care versus specialist context.

We still need more to determine the value for a patient not in the study—the one in front of us. We need to find the connecting statistic between the study and a real patient. We need the likelihood ratio. By taking the estimated prevalence of a disorder in our patient or patient population and combining it with the likelihood ratio, we can arrive at a post-test probability that our patient does or does not have the disorder. Likelihood ratios are

derived from values that include sensitivity and specificity. Although there are no actual positive and negative LRs, their values in ruling in or out a disorder have been categorized by that designation. A positive LR is sensitivity divided by 1 minus specificity and a negative LR is 1 minus sensitivity divided by specificity. You can see in **Table A–13** a representation of the value of ranges of likelihood ratios with regard to whether they affect the probability in a large, moderate, or small degree for both positive and negative LRs. Basically an LR of 10 would change the probability that a patient had a disorder in the realm of 45%. Conversely, a negative LR of 0.1 would change the probability 45% that the patient does not have the disorder. Also, an LR approaching 1 has no value in

Table A–13 Interpreting Likelihood Ratios				
% Change in INCREASE Probability	**+LR Power to RULE IN**	**Shift in Post-Test Probability**	**–LR Power to RULE OUT**	**% Change in DECREASED Probability**
10 = 45%	10	LARGE	<0.1	<0.1 = 45%
5 = 30%	5–10	MODERATE	0.1–0.2	0.2 = 30%
2 = 15%	2–5	SMALL	0.2–0.5	0.5 = 15%

discriminating between those with or without a disorder regardless of being positive or negative.

The value is further augmented by combining with a prediction of prevalence. This isn't the prevalence in the study but the predicted prevalence of the disorder in the general population, or if you are a specialist and that data are known, the prevalence for that subgroup of patients with this disorder in your patient population. Let's take a simple example of appendicitis. The general prevalence is 5%. This is called the pretest probability. By using a graphical tool called a nomogram (**Figure A–22**) we can draw a line starting at the pretest probability through the associated LR and the line will intersect on the far right in the post-test probability range (**Figure A–23**). Here we see that with a pretest probability of 5% and an LR of 3.4 for McBurney's point tenderness, a positive test would result in only a 20% post-test probability that the patient has appendicitis.

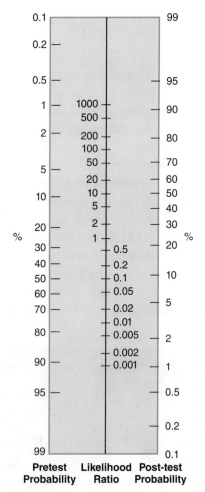

Figure A–22 Nomogram.

Confidence Intervals

What do confidence intervals add to the picture? Up to this point we have been discussing *point values*. These are the statistics that we referred to as sensitivity, specificity, predictive values, and likelihood ratios. But these represent a mean or average of all results of a study. We need to know the range of values, because when that range is large, it raises questions about the value of the data and the strength of conclusions that can be drawn from the data. The range is influenced by several factors, but one of the major ones is the number of occurrences of the disorder in the population, which is affected often by the number of participants in the study population. This reflects indirectly what is called the power of the study. The strength of the conclusions is highest when the range of the confidence interval is tight, meaning the numbers are close together. For example a CI of 7.8 to 12.9 is tight compared to a wider CI of let's say 7.8 to 128.8. The tighter value represents what is called more precision and strengthens the confidence that the point value can be trusted to represent the results. The wide range makes one question the size of the study population (meaning being too small) and number of occurrences. This indirectly affects the power of the conclusions.

What about the possibility that even though a single test performs only moderately with regard to sensitivity or specificity, its combination with other tests keeps it valuable as part of a cluster of exam findings? This is often the case with what are called clinical prediction rules (CPRs).

Clinical Prediction Rules

Clinical prediction rules (CPRs) represent a scientifically developed, validated, and tested set of factors that have been shown to assist clinically, in the hopes of saving time and expense, while benefitting the patient. CPRs are used to predict patients' diagnosis or prognosis but given the variation in patients and their presentations, clinical judgment must be part of the decision-making approach. CPRs are used for screening and diagnosis, prognosis, and interventions. Although designated as a rule, they really represent more of an algorithmic approach to a patient with the hope that prediction of the intended outcome is better than clinician best-guessing.

A number of screening CPRs have been developed to help guide the clinician in making decisions regarding the need for x-rays or imaging in the event of neck, knee,

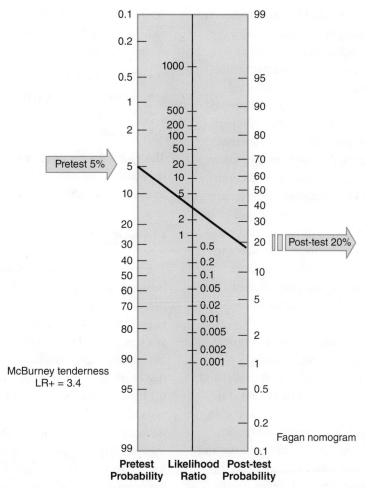

Figure A–23 Nomogram for appendicitis.

and ankle trauma; probably even more relevant for on-field sports practitioners where imaging access is limited. For prognosis it is important to recognize that patients, payers, and the doctor are interested in prediction of success. Many of the interventional CPRs were developed by physical therapists—at least those related to the types of patients seen by chiropractors. They are more prescriptive, and when involving manipulation must be viewed with some caution given the manipulation utilized in the study may not represent that done by chiropractors.

When would one consider using a CPR?

- When you encounter problems you do not see on a regular basis.
- When you wish to demonstrate the scientific basis for your treatment, plan perhaps in defense of a management plan to a payer or for patient confidence in what you are proposing
- When you wish to be cost-effective. Many CPRs were developed based on this primary motivation.

Let's review the process of CPR development. The first step is to begin with a search of the existing literature. Then it is important to analyze the data and put together a composite of validated predictors into a "rule" and conduct a derivation study. There are three progressive steps in the development of a CPR. These include:

1. Derivation—the study from which CPR factors are derived
2. Validation—when the CPR is tested in a different population of patients
3. Impact analysis—when the CPR is applied in multiple settings in the real world to see if it is accepted and utilized; in other words, if it is feasible and practical, and ultimately of value

To decide which factors out of many to pay attention to—the reliable indicators—researchers use a prospective cohort design with patients selected based on specific inclusion and exclusion criteria. Patients go through a standardized exam with a reference standard if a diagnostic

CPR is being developed and a specific treatment approach if an interventional CPR is being developed, or wait a specific period of time if it is intended to be prognostic.

For interventional studies, a validated outcome measure with strong psychometric properties is selected. This outcome measure should have been demonstrated to have discriminative value in confirming a "minimal detectable change," and possess a difference score that identifies a clinically important difference to the patient. For interventional CPRs, once the patients are dichotomized into successful versus unsuccessful, variables are compared with these two groups to determine univariate associations. Those with significant univariate associations are then combined into a multivariate analysis to determine the contribution of a group of predictors. Variables that become part of a group prediction of variables may not necessarily be the most significant individual predictor variables.

The process for diagnostic CPRs is to look at studies that measure validity (compare to a gold standard). Next, look at studies of reliability (intra- and interexaminer) and make sure the kappa values are used if data are not continuous; interclass coefficient if continuous. If acceptable, examine the statistical analysis that includes sensitivity, specificity, and positive and negative predictive values, and establish likelihood ratios. Next, based on experience or prevalence values, determine pretest probability. Finally, use the likelihood ratios to determine post-test probability.

At this point groups of tests (or historical features) can be applied to a group of patients to determine if combinations of tests yield high likelihood ratios for prediction. With this analysis, it can be determined if a number of positive (or negative) findings can provide more prediction than single tests.

One approach, not part of the CPR process, that is a "quick-and-dirty" approach, is using the positive finding of one test's post-probability as the new starting pretest probability. Another is to rank the test with regard to its value, not as a rule-in or rule-out test but in comparison to other tests for that disorder. This is accomplished using the Diagnostic Odds Ratio (DOR). Scientifically, far less sound but perhaps more useful for the busy clinician, the DORs allow the prioritization of several tests for the same condition. By calculating the DOR, the tests with overall better performance have higher numbers. The calculation is by simply dividing the +LR by the –LR. DORs do not, though, indicate the value of the test with regard to rule-out or rule-in; just its value compared to other tests. Sometimes this is close to the literature conclusion.

See in **Table A–14** the DORs for test findings for cervical radiculopathy. Now look at what the literature suggests.[3] A cluster including:

- Upper limb tension test
- Restricted cervical rotation <60°
- Distraction
- Spurling's

The +LR = 6.1 for three or more positives. History questions and standard neurological evaluation were not found to be sensitive.

Correlation

The strength of the linear relationship or associations between variables is statistically their *correlation*. A correlation coefficient is represented by *r*. Correlation coefficients range from –1 to +1. Graphically, this may be represented as a scatterplot (**Figure A–24**). As one decreases while the other increases, the coefficient is negative. Simple correlation coefficients are unit free. The closer a correlation is to 1 (–1 if looking for an inverse relationship) the more strongly associated the data. If a scatterplot is constructed, the closer the points are (tightly clustered), the stronger the relationship. Scatterplots demonstrate relationships by showing form, direction, and strength. The line through the data is a regression line or a "least-squares line" (calculated by minimizing the vertical distances between the data points; the sum of squared deviations) and the straight line that is fitted to the data: the average trend of the data points. It is tempting to imply causation when it is only association that is demonstrated. Correlation belongs to a large class of statistics called regression.

Table A–14 Diagnostic Odds Ratio Example for Cervical Radiculopathy

Test	+LR	–LR	DOR
Upper limb tension test	1.3	0.12	10.8
Decrease of C-spine ROM less than 60°	1.7	0.02	8.5
Cervical distraction	4.4	0.62	7.1
Spurling's	3.5	0.58	6.0
Decrease of C-spine ROM less than 55°	1.5	0.27	5.5
Weakness of any arm muscle	1.9	0.4	4.7

Reproduced from Wainner RS, Fritz JM, Irrgang JJ, Boninger ML, Delitto A, Allison S. Reliability and diagnostic accuracy of the clinical examination and patient self-report measures for cervical radiculopathy. *Spine*. 2003;28(1):52–62.

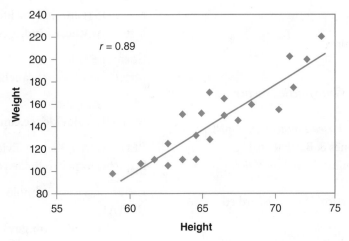

Figure A–24 Correlation scatterplot.

Regression describes the magnitude of change among variables. It is used to create therapeutic and diagnostic predictive models considering the role of several variables simultaneously (multivariate) and the weight each variable contributes to predicting the outcome of interest.

Several terms are used including "logistic regression," "discriminate function analysis," and "log-linear models."

Here is an example: To determine the need for densitometry, one is looking at a host of possible contributors to the prediction of low bone mineral density (BMD) indicating possible osteoporosis. One study[4] evaluated numerous items and arrived at six items—RA, history of previous fractures, older age, non-estrogen use, and low weight—that indicated low BMD. By assigning each a numerical weight based on the degree to which it contributed to prediction and summing the numeric weights, each variable that contributes to the predictive model is given its own coefficient.

Another Example

When several variables are used to predict a certain outcome (as in prognostic clinical prediction rule) multiple regression is used. For example, for prognostic indicators for sciatica, multiple regression analysis demonstrated that the following contributed to the recurrence or persistence of sciatica:[5]

- Driving more than 2 hours/day
- Carrying heavy loads at work
- High level of psychosomatic problems
- Sciatica symptoms the year before

Summary and Cautions

- Many CPRs serve as a starting point for what should be considered in looking at preventive, prognostic, or interventional approaches to patients but are not necessarily proven in larger impact studies.
- Most CPRs have only been taken through the derivation stage. Therefore, outside of the study population, one does not know if the CPR actually applies, given the variability of patient groups and the practice variables of doctors.
- For interventional CPRs, some do not compare to natural history when looking at the success of therapeutic interventions.
- For diagnostic testing, researchers gather together studies that look at:
  1. The diagnostic reliability and validity for the entity being considered.
  2. The variables that (through regression analysis) have been shown to help predict an outcome. These may be historical factors, diagnostic factors, or outcome measures.
- Then it is important to analyze the data and put together a composite of validated predictors into a "rule" and conduct a derivation study.

So if you are wondering if the data on diagnostic tests and clinical prediction rules have been gathered into combined resources, they have, and there are several opportunities to access this information. The best are the textbooks listed with other resources at the end of this appendix.

Resources

Textbooks

Haneline M. *Evidence-Based Chiropractic Practice.* Sudbury, Jones & Bartlett, 2007.

Jewell DV. *Guide to Evidence-Based Physical Therapist Practice.* 2nd ed. Sudbury, Jones & Bartlett, 2011.

Glynn PE, Weisbach PC. *Clinical Prediction Rules.* Sudbury, Jones & Bartlett, 2011.

McGee S. *Evidence-Based Physical Diagnosis.* 3rd ed. Philadelphia, Elsevier, 2012.

Cleland JA, Koppenhaver S. *Netter's Orthopedic Clinical Examination: An Evidence-Based Approach.* 2nd ed. Philadelphia, Saunders, 2011.

Tierney Jr. LM, Henderson MC. *The Patient History: An Evidence-Based Approach.* New York, Lange Medical Books/McGraw-Hill, 2005.

Evidence-Based Sites

Agency for Healthcare Research and Quality
http://www.ahrq.gov/

Cochrane Collaboration
http://www.cochrane.org/

Center for Evidence-Based Medicine
http://www.cebm.net/

Evidence-Based Medicine
http://ebm.bmjjournals.com/

Databases Search Sources

PubMed
http://www.ncbi.nlm.nih.gov/pubmed

CINAHL (Cumulative Index to Nursing and Allied Health Literature)
http://www.ebscohost.com/cinahl/

MANTIS (Chiropractic literature not on PubMed)
http://www.healthindex.com/

Cochrane Library
http://www.thecochranelibrary.com

Clinical Evidence
www.clinicalevidence.com

PEDro (Physiotherapy Evidence Database)
http://www.pedro.fhs.usyd.edu.au/

Health Services/Technology Assessment Text (HSTAT)
http://hstat.nlm.nih.gov/

References

1. Jhawar BS, Fuchs CS, Colditz GA, Stampfer MJ. Cardiovascular risk factors for physician-diagnosed lumbar disc herniation. *The Spine Journal.* 2006:6;684–691.

2. Cassidy JD, Boyle E, Cote P, et al. Risk of vertebrobasilar stroke and chiropractic care: results of a population-based, case-control, and case-crossover study. *Spine.* 2008;33(4 Suppl):S176–183.

3. Wainner RS, Fritz JM, Irrgang JJ, Boninger ML, Delitto A, Allison S. Reliability and diagnostic accuracy of the clinical examination and patient self-report measures for cervical radiculopathy. *Spine.* 2003;28(1):52–62.

4. Lydick E, Cook K, Turpin J, et al. Development and validation of a simple questionnaire to facilitate identification of women likely to have low bone density. *Am J Man Care.* 1998;4:37–48.

5. Fritz JM, Lindsay W, Matheson JW, et al. Is there a subgroup of patients with low back pain likely to benefit from mechanical traction? *Spine.* 2007;32:E793–E800.

Pharmacology for the Chiropractor: How Medications May Affect Patient Presentation and Management Outcomes

Although a heated debate may ensue when asked about the inclusion of medication prescription to the scope of practice of the chiropractor, it is often evident that a baseline of pharmacology knowledge is in fact realistic and necessary to fulfill the role of a portal-of-entry physician. Many patients are taking medications prior to entering the chiropractor's office. As a result, a basic knowledge of common prescribed and over-the-counter (OTC) medication is useful. Following are some important reasons:

- The patient often asks questions regarding the side effects of his/her medication.
- The patient may present with signs or symptoms directly related to a side effect of a medication or from lack of compliance in taking a prescribed medication.
- The medication taken by the patient is used for the condition or symptoms the chiropractor wishes to address.
- In a review of a patient's medical history, it is important to determine current and past medications. Even if the patient has forgotten why the medication was prescribed, a basic knowledge of commonly prescribed drugs will often offer a clue.
- Events may have changed in the patient's life that may influence the effect of medication. For example, certain foods, alcohol, fever, or illness may effectively increase or decrease the effects of the available drug.
- If laboratory studies are performed, drug interactions may have a significant effect on the results.

Here are just a few practical examples:

- A patient has a sense of difficulty breathing (sense of tightness) and multiple other complaints that range from musculoskeletal aches and pains to headaches. The patient is taking alprazolam (Xanax), which is often prescribed for anxiety, as an adjunct with antidepressants, or simply as a sleep inducer. Anxiety may have an effect on blood pressure, response to questions, and general well-being. Depression certainly may have an effect on patient complaints and their perceived response to care. Lack of sleep may have an effect on patient presentation as well.
- Another patient who takes lithium has a remarkable response one time to your care of midthoracic pain, yet another time is angry with you or simply nonresponsive. Knowing that lithium is used for manic depression may help in explaining the range of response if, in fact, the patient is not consistently taking his/her medication.
- A patient who has had chronic pain is taking large daily doses of naprosyn. The patient is complaining of constant heartburn and epigastric pain in addition to tinnitus. Understanding that naprosyn and similar medications are potentially ototoxic at high and prolonged use, and that these medications may lead to ulcers, and primarily gastric ulcers, may help to explain the patient's symptoms and direct the appropriate course of management.
- A patient is taking Lasix for congestive heart failure. He is starting to complain of some cramping and muscle weakness. When a lab is ordered, the patient's serum potassium level is very low. Knowing the Lasix is nonpotassium sparing helps in the explanation and results in an immediate referral to the prescribing physician with a suggestion that potassium supplementation is requisite.

- A patient with migraine headaches seemed to respond to chiropractic care, but when on vacation was in an area where she did not have a chiropractor available. The patient took sumatriptan prescribed by her physician. It helped, but now, three days later, her headache is back, and worse. Knowing that many medications prescribed for migraine may be the cause of a "rebound migraine" is helpful in making decisions about management and explains why this would occur.
- A patient is taking coumadin because of deep vein thrombosis discovered one month ago. You are considering adjusting the low back with a side-posture adjustment. Understanding that coumadin is an anticoagulant may have an effect on the degree of force used in the adjustment or whether another technique will be used during the time the patient is on the medication.
- A patient who was diagnosed with temporal arteritis is on a course of corticosteroids for six months. During that time the patient has midthoracic pain that seems fairly severe. Knowing that the patient is on corticosteroids would certainly warrant taking x-rays to determine whether a compression fracture was the cause, and may explain why if found. If not found, there would still be a caution against any position or exercise that would cause loaded flexion, including while adjusting, due to the osteopenic effect of long-term corticosteroid use.

Additionally, the patient is often taking many medications. With the senior patient, it is not uncommon to have obtained each medication from a different physician and each physician is unaware of the other's prescription. As a result, unforeseen interactions may occur. The chiropractor is in the advantageous position of being able to ascertain the complete picture of medications the patient is taking because the patient assumes the chiropractor is not involved in the regulation of these drugs.

The caveat for the chiropractor is that no advice regarding taking or withdrawing from, or increasing or decreasing dosage can be given without violating state scope-of-practice laws. However, when a problem is suspected or recognized, it is imperative that the chiropractor either sends the patient back to the prescribing physician with informative questions or contacts the prescribing physician to discuss the individual patient. It is extremely important to recognize that if a medication is stopped suddenly or the dose is decreased, a rebound effect or other reactions may occur that are potentially lethal. For example, sudden withdrawal of seizure medication may lead to status epilepticus (i.e., a seizure that continues and may lead to death).

It is important to understand that although a drug may have been developed for a specific system or condition, the same medication may be used as the primary or alternative drug for another condition. For example, although antihypertensive and antidepressant medications were designed for the associated condition, these medications are also used in the treatment of headache. Antihypertensive medications may also be used in the treatment of some cardiac disorders or reflex sympathetic conditions.

According to the IMS Institute for Healthcare Informatics, patients in the United States spent $307 billion in 2010 for prescription drugs; an increase of 2.4% over one year.[1] In 2011, 78% of all prescriptions were for generic drugs. The CDC's National Center for Health Statistics survey[2] reported the following (**Figures B–1** through **B–3**):

- The percentage of individuals taking five or more drugs increased from 6.3% to 10.7% from 1999 to 2008.
- Thirty-six percent of those age 60 years and older took five or more drugs over the preceding month.
- For those individuals 12 to 19 years of age, 30% took one drug over the previous month.
- For those age 60 years and older, 88.4% took one drug over the previous month.
- For those age 60 years and older, 90% of drugs are used to treat hypertension, high cholesterol, and heart disease—all modifiable through lifestyle changes.

The cost for the top ten drugs prescribed in the United States in 2010 was $48 billion.

The top grossing drugs and their primary use in the United States were:

1. Lipitor (atorvastatin)—high cholesterol
2. Nexium (esomeprazole) —gastroesophageal reflux disease (GERD)
3. Plavix (clopidogrel)—anticoagulant
4. Advair Diskus (gluticasone and salmeterol)—asthma/COPD
5. Abilify (aripiprazole)—schizophrenia, bipolar depression, clinical depression
6. Seroquel (quetiapine)—schizophrenia, bipolar depression (combined with an SSRI) clinical depression
7. Singulair (montelukast)—asthma/COPD
8. Crestor (rosuvastatin)—high cholesterol

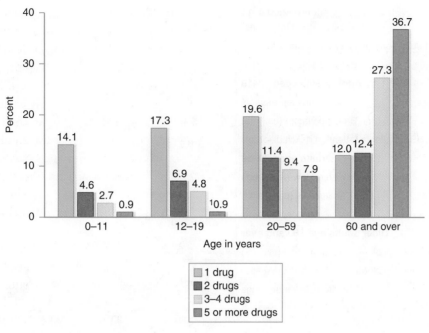

¹Estimate is unstable; the relative standard error is greater than 30%.

Figure B–1 Percentage of prescription drugs used in the past month, by age: United States, 2007–2008.

Reproduced from Gu Q, Dillon CF, Burt VL. Prescription drug use continues to increase: U.S. prescription drug data for 2007–2008. NCHS Data Brief. Sep 2010(42):1–8.

9. Actos (pioglitazone)—diabetes
10. Epogen (epoetin alfa)—anemia due to chronic renal failure

The most prescribed drugs in the United States were:

1. Vicodin (hydrocodone/acetaminophen)—analgesic
2. Zocor (Simvastatin)—hyperlipidemia
3. Prinivil and Zestril (Lisinopril)—hyperlipidemia

4. Synthroid (levothyroxine sodium)—thyroid
5. Norvasc (amlodipine besylate)—antihypertensive
6. Prilosec (omeprazole)—GERD
7. Zithromax (azithromycin)—antibiotic
8. Amoxicillin—antibiotic
9. Glucophage (metformin sodium)—diabetes
10. Hydrochlorothiazide—diuretic (antihypertensive/congestive heart failure)

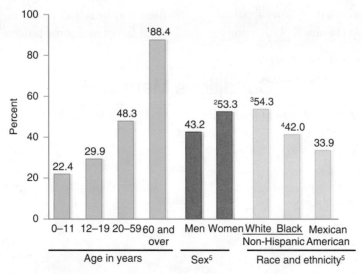

¹Significant linear trend over age.
²Significantly different from men.
³Significantly different from Non-Hispanic black and Mexican-American persons.
⁴Significantly different from Mexican-American persons.
⁵Age adjusted by direct method to the year 2000 projected U.S. population.

Figure B–2 Percentage of use of at least one prescription drug, by age, sex, and race and ethnicity: United States, 2007–2008.

Reproduced from Gu Q, Dillon CF, Burt VL. Prescription drug use continues to increase: U.S. prescription drug data for 2007–2008. NCHS Data Brief. Sep 2010(42):1–8.

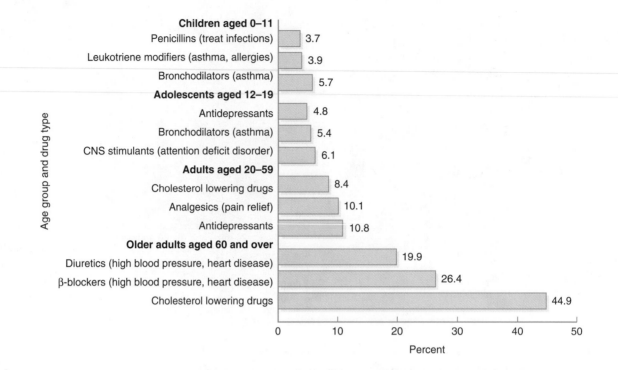

Figure B–3 Percentage of prescription drugs used most often, by drug type and age group: United States, 2007–2008.

Reproduced from Gu Q, Dillon CF, Burt VL. Prescription drug use continues to increase: U.S. prescription drug data for 2007–2008. NCHS Data Brief. Sep 2010(42):1–8.

11. Xanax (alprazolam)—anxiety
12. Lipitor (atorvastatin)—hyperlipidemia
13. Lasix (furosemide)—diuretic (antihypertensive/ congestive heart failure)
14. Ambien (zolpidem tartrate)—sleep induction
15. Lopressor (metoprolol tartrate)—hyperlipidemia

When matching these two lists, it becomes apparent that there is clearly an overlap (**Figure B–4**). Among the overlapping conditions, all are modifiable through lifestyle changes including diabetes, high cholesterol, GERD, hypertension, and chronic pain. To a lesser degree, asthma, depression, and rheumatoid conditions may be affected through lifestyle. Not generally modifiable through lifestyle changes after being diagnosed are thyroid disorders, chronic renal failure, and cancer, although there may be some opportunity for prevention for chronic renal failure and some cancers based on cause and type.

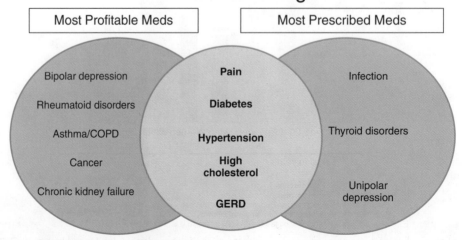

Figure B–4 Conditions managed.

It would be prudent for the chiropractic physician, although not prescribing, to have at least a general sense of these most commonly prescribed medications and their mechanisms of action to determine possible side effects related to a patient's clinical presentation. Following is a very brief overview of drug categories, mechanisms, examples within those categories, and possible side effects and concerns.

It is easy enough, with searchable databases, to find a specific medication, its mechanism of action, side effects, and concerns regarding timing and cross-reaction with other substances including foods and dietary supplements. However, prior to being specific, it is possible to have a general sense of these elements by simply understanding the general classification of a medication, its intended actions, and assuming the medication is taken and not specifically injected, understanding the systemic effects of that medication (which often translate into side effects or adverse reactions).

Our approach then will be to discuss some very basic biologic factors that relate to medication interactions including absorption, metabolism, and excretion, move to a broad-based discussion of some classifications of medication, and complete the discussion with an overview of commonly prescribed medications for specific diagnoses or patient complaints.

Some general principles of pharmacology allow a better understanding of prescribing practices. The primary concern is prescribing the optimal amount of medication to be effective but not toxic or wrought with side effects. This dosage varies for several important reasons:

- The amount of active drug in the body is determined by its metabolism in the liver and clearance from the kidneys. Obviously, liver or kidney disease may alter the available amount of drug in the system. Some special considerations include the infant and the elderly, for whom function of both organs is decreased compared to an average adult.
- The available amount of medication will vary with processes such as fever, other drugs, and metabolic conditions.
- Special concerns apply to particular groups, including pregnant females, the immunocompromised, the elderly, and infants. Some medications should not be used during pregnancy, and medication dosages for the other groups will vary based upon that group's specific factors.

A reminder that QID stands for four times/day; TID, three times/day; BID, two times/day; and QD is once a day. You can see how easily QID and QD could be confused and result in under- or overmedication.

Please refer to **Table B–1** for the basic terminology and definitions for medication usage. To find the location

Table B–1 Summary of Basics Regarding How Drugs Affect Patients

Principle	Definition
How Drugs Are Administered	
• Oral (PO)	The disadvantage of self-administration is that the drug must survive the acidity of the stomach and be capable of passing through the intestinal lining to reach the bloodstream. Drug absorption is thus related to whether the drug is taken with meals or without, and to some restrictions on type of foods.
• Sublingual	Absorbed quickly, directly into the bloodstream through the capillary bed of the tongue. Does not have to withstand the acidic environment of the stomach.
• Rectal	Rate of absorption is not reliable. Useful for infants and for patients who are unconscious or vomiting.
• Parenteral (outside GI tract)	Injection: Can be given intravenous (IV), intramuscular (IM), and subcutaneous (SubQ). IV has the advantage of rapid and continuous administration. Also good for unconscious patients and for delivery of insoluble drugs. IM has the advantage of passing through capillary walls in muscle. May be rapid absorption if aqueous, while oil-based preparations are absorbed slowly. SubQ is more easily self-administered and is delivered to the capillaries beneath the skin for fairly quick distribution.
Dosing	
• Safety Issues with Dosing	Drug safety is presented in animal studies as EC50 (Effective Concentration 50%)—the concentration of a drug that causes an effect in 50% of individuals; LD50 (Lethal Dose 50%)—the concentration that is lethal to 50% of subjects; the therapeutic index—determines safety through the ratio of dividing the LD50 by the ED50; and Margin of Safety—the margin between the therapeutic and lethal dose of the drug.

(continues)

Table B–1 Summary of Basics Regarding How Drugs Affect Patients (continued)

Principle	Definition
• Tolerance, Dependence, Withdrawal	Tolerance occurs when a larger dose is necessary to achieve a previous therapeutic effect. This can occur due to metabolic reasons (e.g., drug is metabolized more quickly), at the cellular level (there is a decrease in the number of drug receptors [i.e., downregulation]), or for behavioral reasons. Dependence is when the patient must have the drug to function at a normal level. Withdrawal refers to removing a drug from a dependent patient.
• Patient Profile	It is extremely important to consider weight, gender, age, and in females, whether the patient is pregnant or not. Newer considerations are genetic inheritance of mutations that render a drug more effective or less effective.
• Types	Some drugs are given at a higher initial dose, called a loading dose. This is followed by a maintenance dose that is lower.
• Abbreviations	Once a day—QD; twice a day—BID; three times a day—TID; four times a day—QID
Drug Absorption	Drug absorption is affected primarily by the formulation state (gel cap, pill, solution, etc.) and by the route of administration.
Drug Distribution	The factor that affects distribution is the membrane permeability. This includes some barriers such as the blood–brain barrier, blood–testes barrier, and the blood–placenta barrier. Another factor is whether the drug is lipophilic or not. Those that are passed through the gut wall easily tend to accumulate in fat. Other drugs may be bound and stored in other areas, such as bone. Calcium-binding drugs accumulate in bones and teeth.
Drug Metabolism	Drugs are metabolized primarily in the liver, and as a result are affected by liver disease and also may be toxic to the liver.
Drug Excretion and Clearance	Kidney function is important for the proper excretion and clearance of drugs. This is also a potential toxic factor for the kidneys. Proper kidney function is important for proper clearance. The older a patient is, the less effective this function becomes.
Drug Actions	Drugs bind to receptors and may act as agonists or antagonists that result in opening or closing channels (blockers), activated secondary messengers, inhibited normal cellular function (e.g., some antibiotics interfere with bacterial cell wall construction), or activated cellular function. Many of the newer drugs are enzyme inhibitors, such as cholinesterase inhibitors for Alzheimer's.
Drug Interactions	Drugs are generally described as interacting by addition, synergism, potentiation, or antagonism. Addition is the combined action of two drugs, equal to the combined response. Synergism results in a greater effect than a simple one, plus one additive response. Potentiation means that the drug has no inherent effect but enhances the effect of another drug. Antagonism is the opposite, whereby normally the drug has no effect but acts to inhibit the effect of another drug.

of a drug in Table B–1 by the product name, refer to **Table B–4**.

Food/Drug/Supplement Interactions

For chiropractors, it is particularly important to understand that recommendations in diet and advice regarding supplementation must be in the context of medications taken by a patient. There are several ways that this interaction can be affected:

- External effects based on how the drug is delivered (Type I interaction)

- Affect on absorption or transportation (Type II interaction)
- Distribution of the drug after absorption (Type III interaction)
- Excretion (Type IV interaction)

Our main concern with the latter three interactions is how they relate to timing with food/supplements, and the types of foods/supplements that interact with specific types of drugs. The effect may be less activity of the medication or more activity of the medication available for longer periods of time. Finally, medications can affect absorption or excretion of important vitamins and minerals leading to nutritional deficiencies and their consequences.

Absorption

Because most drugs are absorbed in the stomach and small intestine, any substances ingested at the same time may affect this process. A general rule, not always applicable, is that medications are often taken one hour before a meal or two hours after a meal. Otherwise, food may decrease absorption or delay the time needed for absorption. Following are some examples:[3]

- Soluble fiber, phytate, and oxalate found in some fruits, vegetables, whole grains, Metamucil, legumes, nuts, and cocoa may decrease the absorption of some medications.
- For patients taking coumadin/warfarin, foods that contain vitamin K may counteract the effects of the medication. These foods include dark green leafy vegetables, cabbage, avocado, liver, canola oil, soybean oil, and green tea. Also vitamin K, vitamin E, vitamin A, feverfew, garlic, ginger, ginkgo, inositol hexaphosphate, licorice, St. John's wort, turmeric, wheat grass, and fish oils may have the same effect, as does large amounts of alcohol ingestion (i.e., more than three drinks/day).
- Supplements containing fat-soluble vitamins (A, D, E, and K) and coenzyme Q10 need to be taken with 5 g of fat.

Metabolism

Foods, drugs, and supplements may interact in a way that increases or decreases the metabolism of specific drugs. One of the major principles upon which this interaction is based is called the cytochrome P450 system.

To understand why certain medications are different in their absorption, metabolism, and excretion, it is first important to understand, at least basically, the cytochrome P450 group of enzymes (also abbreviated as CYP). This large and diverse group is one of the major sets of enzymes involved in drug metabolism. Largely proteins, they are found on the inner membrane of mitochondria and in the endoplasmic reticulum of cells. There are a number of substrates that include lipids and steroidal hormones, drugs, and toxic materials that can cross-react due to shared similarities. There are many isoenzymes of the CYP system that are named according to a standard format that has CYP indicating the gene family, followed by the subfamily number, and finally the gene coding. So, for example, for CYP3A5, *CYP3*

indicates the gene family, *A* indicates the subfamily, and *5* indicates the gene coding. There are, in essence, eight primary isoenzymes of importance for the CYP system.

It is a system affected not only by drugs but also by herbs that can inhibit the CYP system or increase activity of the CYP system. Under the discussion of specific medications related to system or disorder, the specific cytochrome interactions affected are listed, but here is a brief list of some important specific examples:[3]

- Although St. John's wort is commonly utilized in Europe as an alternative to some antidepressants, it is known to increase CYP3A4 enzymes used to metabolize many drugs (speeds up clearance) and therefore should not be taken with other medications, specifically other antidepressants. Also, with a similar action to monoamine oxidase inhibitors, there is a risk for sudden increase in blood pressure when ingesting foods with high tyramine content. Some of the foods included in this list can be remembered by thinking of a pizza parlor, because they include aged cheeses, pepperoni, salami, sausage, draft beer, and red wine; other foods include bananas, chocolate, soy sauce, sauerkraut, avocado, and fava beans.
- Ingesting ¼ grapefruit or more per day slows down CYP3A4 enzymes. Known medications that are affected by grapefruit ingestion include NSAIDs, statins, some diabetes medications, antihypertensives, antibiotics, protease inhibitors, antihistamines, erectile dysfunction meds, and others.
- Certain medications slow the metabolism of caffeine, which may augment the effect of caffeine. These include Tagamet, Ciprofloxacin, and Luvox among others. Coffee may speed up the clearance of certain medications including theophylline, clozapine, estrogen, coumadin, and naproxen.
- As more individuals substitute meat with soy products it is important to note that soy interferes with tamoxifen and aromatase-inhibitor activity used for breast cancer therapy, and whole soy food interferes with thyroid medications.

Nutrient Depletion

The effect of medications on absorption and increased excretion of vitamins, minerals, and other nutrients is well known, with some specifics to be aware of:

- NSAIDs may interfere with the absorption of folate, iron, vitamins C and K, and melatonin.

- Antacids and proton-pump inhibitors (e.g., Nexium or Prilosec) may decrease the absorption of vitamins C, B_{12}, and D; calcium; iron; zinc; and folic acid. One major concern is osteoporosis.
- Some diabetes medications may interfere with vitamin B_{12}, folic acid, thiamin, magnesium, and CoQ_{10} metabolism.
- Some antihypertensives may interfere with the absorption of zinc, CoQ_{10}, vitamin B_{12}, copper, and melatonin.
- Statins used for the treatment of hyperlipidemias (e.g., Crestor, Lipitor) may interfere with the metabolism and availability of CoQ_{10}. Muscle soreness or achiness is a common complaint with the use of these medications.
- Selective serotonin reuptake inhibitors (SSRIs) (e.g., Prozac) may interfere with sodium and melatonin absorption.
- Nonpotassium-sparing diuretics used for hypertension and congestive heart failure may cause potassium deficiency (requiring potassium supplementation) and sodium deficiency.
- Certain antiepileptic medications may require the need for sodium supplementation.
- Antirheumatic medications such as methotrexate require the patient to take folate supplementation.

Before we discuss specific medications based on use, a shortcut to identifying some medications is that they often have identifying suffixes due to similar chemical configurations. For example:

- Most tricyclic antidepressants have the suffix *-iptiline.*
- Antibiotics that are chemically similar have the suffix *-cycline.*

- Leukotriene receptor antagonists used in the treatment of asthma end in *-lukast.*
- Cholesterol-lowering drugs that block the production of cholesterol are generically called "statins."
- Headache medications that are serotonin receptor agonists have the suffix *-triptin.*
- Drugs ending in *-mab* are monoclonal antibodies.
  1. Chimeric monoclonal antibodies end in *-ximab*, and those ending in *-zumab* are humanized monoclonal antibodies.

Pain Medications

Let's start with a review of one of the pathways for eventual inflammation (**Figure B–5**). Arachidonic acid and omega-6 fatty acids are converted to a group of metabolites called eicosanoids. One pathway is to convert arachidonic acid to prostanoids through the action of the cyclooxygenase enzyme called the COX enzyme. These prostanoids include the inflammatory prostaglandins, thromboxanes, and prostacyclins. Another conversion of arachidonic acid by the enzyme lipoxygenase or LOX enzyme, leads to the production of leukotrienes, which are responsible for some of the inflammatory reactions seen in asthma and other allergic reactions. A balance occurs through competition with the COX enzyme. This is between arachidonic acid and omega-3 fatty acids represented by DHA and EPA (**Figure B–6**). Anti-inflammatory omega-3s are found in most green vegetables, wild game, most grains, grass-fed meat, and EPA/DHA fish oil. Metabolites of EPA and DHA are a different series of thromboxanes and prostaglandins, which are either less inflammatory or noninflammatory compared to the prostaglandins associated with arachidonic acid

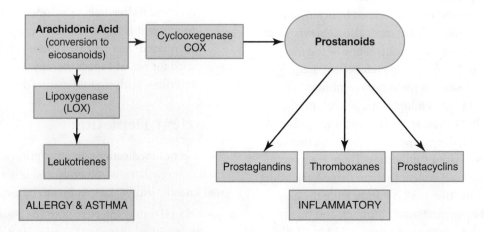

Figure B–5 One possibility.

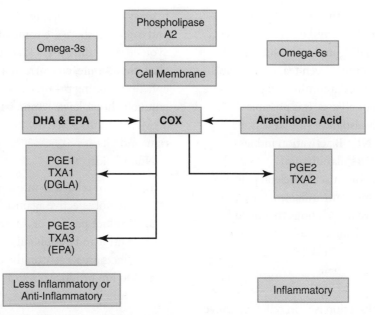

Figure B–6 Omega-3 and Omega-6 pathways.

metabolism. Medications generally affect or take advantage of these pathways through competition or blocking. For example, corticosteroids inhibit phospholipase A2, which inhibits arachidonic acid release from phospholipids in the cell membrane. Aspirin, NSAIDs and cyclooxygenase inhibitors block the COX enzyme that converts arachidonic acid to prostaglandin E2, thereby blocking or decreasing inflammation. Additionally, non-drug ingestibles such as turmeric, ginger, bioflavonoids, and boswellia have similar actions.

Many other components influence these processes with sometimes overlapping actions, so the following can only be a generalization for clinical purposes. One example is cell-signaling molecules, which stimulate genes to induce the expression of the COX enzyme. The expression of the coding gene for COX-2 for the production of prostaglandins is transcriptionally regulated by NFκ-B. It is in the cytoplasm and is bound to its inhibitor (**Figure B–7**). Free radicals release NFκ-B from the inhibitor, which then moves into the nucleus to activate

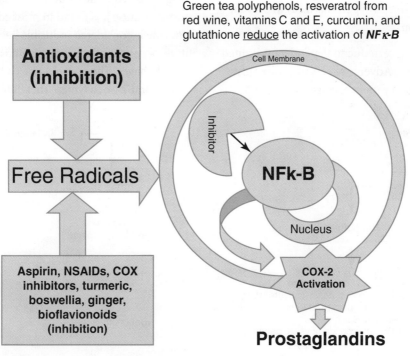

Figure B–7 NFk-B metabolism.

genes responsible for COX-2 activation and prostaglandin formation. Aspirin, NSAIDs, and corticosteroids inhibit binding of cell-signaling molecules such as NFκ-B, which reduces inflammation. Green tea, polyphenols, resveratrol, vitamins C and E, curcumin, and glutathione also reduce the activation of NFκ-B. It is possible that keratinoids and flavonoids also have similar actions. Without these inhibitors, NFκ-B activation induces COX-2 activation leading to inflammation.

Medications prescribed for musculoskeletal pain are not just analgesics but include anti-inflammatories, muscle relaxants, and adjunctive medications that include sedative, antidepression, and antiseizure medications.

Analgesics

Medications whose main function is pain relief are called analgesics. Analgesics are divided into opioids and nonopioids (**Figure B–8**). Opioids, previously referred to as narcotics, are derived from morphine and include morphine, oxycodone, methadone, and tramadol.[4] Their use is widespread either prescribed alone or in combination with other substances. Opioids bind to opioid receptors, mimicking endorphins with several receptors known including mu, kappa, and delta. There are basically three mechanisms for their actions, including:

1. Inhibiting neurotransmitter release through blockage of Ca2+
2. Inhibiting glutamate release
3. Opening K+ channels (hyperpolarized) to prevent pain transmission

Because abuse is a concern due to dependency, limited use of opioids is the rule. Adverse effects include confusion, nausea, vomiting, dry mouth, constipation, and urinary retention. Opioids are metabolized by CYP2D6 and therefore there are some inhibitors that should be avoided, including 5-HTP, adrenal extract, black tea, cat's claw, chamomile, chaparral, chromium, clove, DHEA, ephedra, evening primrose, fenugreek, ginger, ginkgo, gotukola, hops, kava, lemon balm, phenylalanine, sage, SAMe, St. John's wort, thyme, turmeric, tyrosine, valerian, and vitamin B_6.

Nonopioids:

1. Are not related to morphine
2. Are not effective against severe, sharp pain
3. Produce pain relief through actions on both the central and peripheral nervous systems (opioid's effects are largely on the CNS)
4. Do not produce physical dependency

Anti-Inflammatory Medications

Anti-inflammatory medications are divided into steroids and nonsteroids. Steroids include prednisone and methylprednisolone, hydrocortisone, and betamethasone (**Figure B–9**). Nonsteroid anti-inflammatory medications (NSAIDs) include salicylates (i.e., aspirin) and traditional NSAIDs; the nonselective COX inhibitors, and COX-2 inhibitors. The majority of patients given analgesics are given NSAIDs. Here we discuss their general mechanisms of action.

There are different isoenzymes of the COX enzyme (**Figure B–10**). The COX-1 enzyme is considered constitutive because it is found in most cells, whereas the COX-2 enzyme is considered inducible because it is mainly found in response to inflammation, and is found in activated macrophages. The nonselective COX inhibitors block both 1 and 2 isoenzymes. These include aspirin and

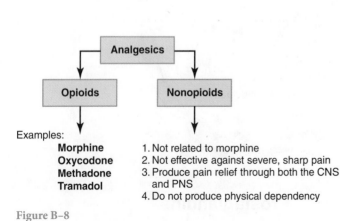

Examples:
Morphine
Oxycodone
Methadone
Tramadol
1. Not related to morphine
2. Not effective against severe, sharp pain
3. Produce pain relief through both the CNS and PNS
4. Do not produce physical dependency

Figure B–8

Figure B–9

Table B-2

Synthetic NSAIDs	Analgesic/Antipyretic Dosing	Anti-Inflammatory Dosing
Ibuprofen (Advil, Motrin, Nuprin)	200–400 mg every 6–8 hr	600 mg QID
Naproxen (Aleve, Midol)	200 mg every 6–8 hr	550 mg BID (or 275 mg every 6–8 hr)
Naproxen (Naprosyn, Anaprax, Naprolam)	200 mg every 6–8 hr	200–500 BID
Meloxicam (Mobic)	Not indicated for pain/fever	7.5–15 mg/day
Indomethacin (Indocin)	Not indicated for pain/fever	25–70 mg TID
Meclofenamate (Meclomen)	50–100 mg every 4–6 hr	200–400 mg/day

most NSAIDs. Selective COX inhibitors block the COX-2 enzyme. This is most often represented by celecoxib (Celebrex). Note that the functions of these enzymes are not always detrimental and are often essential for proper function, so their blockage carries with it adverse reactions. The most common problem is interference with the enzymes whose role is gastrointestinal protection particularly of the stomach lining, but also for renal blood flow and platelet aggregation. As a result, gastric irritation and bleeding may occur, and because of an increase in thromboxane with an inhibition of prostacyclin by COX-2 inhibition, there is an increase in thrombus formation. This may lead to an increase in heart attack and stroke. Additionally affected are the kidneys, with an increased risk of renal failure. Other concerns are that NSAIDs can deplete vitamin C, folate, iron, and zinc. Related to the gastrointestinal bleeding and anticoagulant effects,

it is important to avoid alcohol and to avoid supplements and products that have anticoagulant effects such as garlic, ginger, gingko, fish oils, and vitamin E, among others. NSAIDs are metabolized by CYP2C9 and therefore contraindicated are black tea, chamomile, chaparral, clove, ginger, milk thistle, St. John's wort, sage, thyme, and turmeric.

In **Table B–2** we see a list of common NSAIDs. Note that ibuprofen, represented by Advil, and Motrin and naproxen, represented by Aleve, are the most common OTC medications used for pain. They have analgesic, antipyretic, and anti-inflammatory effects, but the dosing for anti-inflammatory effects is higher.

Not all synthetic NSAIDs are used for their effects of reducing pain, fever, and inflammation. In fact, we can see that the only approved COX-2 inhibitor, Celebrex, is dosed only for its anti-inflammatory effects (**Table B–3**).

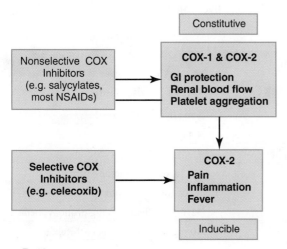

Figure B–10

Table B-3

Synthetic NSAIDs	Anti-Inflammatory Dosing
Oxaprosin (Daypro)	1200–1800 mg QD
Piroxicam (Feldene)	20 mg/day
Sulindac (Clioril)	200 mg BID: 400 mg/day
Selective COX-2 Inhibitor	
Celecoxib (Celebrex)	200 mg/day

Drugs such as Vicodin, Percodan, Percocet, Darvocet, and Darvon are combination drugs (**Table B–4**). They represent combinations of either aspirin or acetaminophen combined with either oxycodone, codeine, or hydrocodone. In other words, they are combinations of an NSAID or acetaminophen with an opioid. The concerns are the gastrointestinal and vascular effects of NSAIDs combined with the dependency and narcotic effects of the opioids. For chiropractors it is important to be aware of a commonly prescribed steroid for low back pain—the Medrol Dosepak. It is a card with twenty-one 4-mg pills. Patients start with six pills (24 mg) and take one less pill each day until finished. The pills are taken orally with a full glass of water before breakfast, after lunch, and after dinner.

Acetaminophen

Acetaminophen is an aniline analgesic. It blocks the COX prostaglandin H_2 synthase enzyme at its peroxidase rather than the cyclooxygenase catalytic site. Higher concentrations of peroxide in activated leukocytes and platelets block the effect of acetaminophen on inflammation and platelet thrombosis. Acetaminophen is able to inhibit prostaglandins in the CNS, reducing pain and fever. It is neither an anti-inflammatory nor an anti-thrombotic medication. It is metabolized by CYP2E; therefore certain supplements are contraindicated, including chaparral and dandelion.

Several concerns have been raised about chronic and/or large amounts of acetaminophen use. These center on three key issues:

- Exacerbation of asthma
- Elevation of liver enzymes
- Hearing loss

Another potential for confusion is that acetaminophen is labeled differently on different products, including but not limited to the following abbreviations and acronyms: AC, APAP, Acetaminoph, Acetamin, and Acetam.

Recently, there has been a concern about acetaminophen and asthma. Although this seems counterintuitive, the effect may possibly be through depletion of glutathione in bronchial mucosa, which could raise the risk of damage from oxidative stress. It appears that acetaminophen increases airway inflammation for those with asthma or for those predisposed to asthma, leading to an increase in severity and frequency of symptoms. Also, individuals may be more likely to develop asthma later in childhood if exposed to acetaminophen in utero or in the first year of life. Use of acetaminophen was associated with a 2.87-times increased risk of asthma.[5] Asthma symptoms related to acetaminophen exposure have been reported as high as 38% for 13- to 14-year-olds. Asthma prevalence in the United States showed a rapid increase in the 1980s when acetaminophen was being suggested for children in place of aspirin. There was a leveling off for that increase in the 1990s when acetaminophen use became the standard for fever management. This then seems a plausible explanation for an association with asthma increases given no other environmental changes occurred during that same period of time. Also, for 36 countries worldwide, the per-capita sales of acetaminophen are a predictor for the prevalence of childhood wheezing.

Another concern associated with acetaminophen, and a warning issued in 2011 by the FDA, is liver damage. There was a strong recommendation to limit the amount of acetaminophen to 325 milligrams per tablet or capsule. They also required a boxed warning on all prescription acetaminophen products highlighting the potential risk for severe liver injury.

Table B-4

Combined Analgesics	Nonopioid Medication	Other Medication
Vicodin or Panacet 5/500	500 mg acetaminophen	5 mg hydrocodone
Percodan	325 mg aspirin	4.4 oxycodone
Percocet	325, 500, 600 mg acetaminophen	2.5, 5, 7.5, 10 mg oxycodone
Tylenol with codeine	300 mg acetaminophen	15, 30, 60 mg codeine
Darvocet N (50 or 100)	325 or 650 mg acetaminophen	50 or 100 mg propoxyphene
Darvon Compound-65	389 mg aspirin	32.4 mg caffeine, 65 mg propoxyphene
Fiorinal	325 mg aspirin	40 mg caffeine, 50 mg barbituate

Cautions include:

- Taking more than the prescribed dose of an acetaminophen-containing product in a 24-hour period
- Taking more acetaminophen than the maximum daily dose of 4,000 milligrams (4 grams)
- Taking more than one acetaminophen-containing product at the same time
- Drinking alcohol while taking the drug

In one study,[6] a placebo-control group had no elevation of liver enzymes after two weeks as compared to a group that took 4 grams of Tylenol daily for two weeks. Of this group, 33% to 44% had elevations of ALT; >3 times the upper limit. Those with the highest elevations were 10 times the upper limit of normal. Elevations returned to normal after discontinuing the Tylenol.

In one study[7] evaluating almost 27,000 men for hearing loss related to analgesic use, researchers concluded that regular use of aspirin, NSAIDs, or acetaminophen increases the risk of hearing loss in men, with the highest risk group being those 50 years of age and younger. A similar association was found for women in a study[8] published in 2012; however, the researchers found no association with aspirin but with ibuprofen and acetaminophen. In all studies, the relationship is dose-dependent, with those chronically taking these medications more than twice per week. Specifically, men were classified into three groups: under 50 years of age, ages 50 to 59 years, and those 60 years of age or older. Compared to men not regularly taking aspirin, NSAIDs, or acetaminophen, the risk increase was on average about 33% for those 59 years of age or younger for all of these medications. There was a substantially increased risk compared to men who did not take acetaminophen regularly, so that those men who did had a comparative increased risk of 99%.

Disease-Modifying Antirheumatic Drugs (DMARDs)

A special class of medications used in the management of rheumatoid and rheumatoid-like inflammation is DMARDs. A broad classification for these diseases also includes the inflammatory bowel diseases (Crohn's and ulcerative colitis). There are two classifications, biologics and nonbiologics. The older nonbiologics include drugs such as methotrexate, cyclosporine, and sulfasalazine. The biologics work off different principles. Delivery is

either through self-injection subcutaneously (SQ) or through infusion therapy. Biologics are genetically engineered proteins used to address one of several aspects of immune regulation:

- Anti-TNF inhibitors—Cimzia, Enbrel, Humira, Remicade, and Simponi
- T cell inhibitors—Orencia
- IL-6 inhibitors—Actemra

Muscle Relaxants

Muscle relaxants used as adjuncts to musculoskeletal pain management are the most heterogeneous group of medications (**Figure B–11**). They include "antispasticity" medications used for the spasticity associated with upper motor neuron disease and the more common "antispasmodics," which are further divided into benzodiazepines (BZD) and nonbenzodiazepines. The original benzodiazepine was Librium. Marketed soon after was Valium. They are clearly known for their sedative effects. Benzodiazepines work primarily through augmenting the effects of the neurotransmitter gamma-aminobutyric acid (GABA). An alternative herb supplement is valerian root. Side effects for BZDs include rebound insomnia, nausea, and diarrhea. Special attention should be given to cross-reactions with Tagamet, alcohol, and other sedatives. Because BZDs are metabolized by CYP2C19, certain supplements are contraindicated and certain foods and teas need to be avoided such as black tea, chamomile, ginseng, chaparral, St. John's wort, thyme, turmeric, clove, ginger, gotukola, kava, milk thistle, and red yeast rice.

Like many medications in this category, there are many formulations and many delivery approaches, including orals and injectables. Because the effects on the CNS also include the limbic and reticular systems, they have effects related to sedation and sleep induction. Included

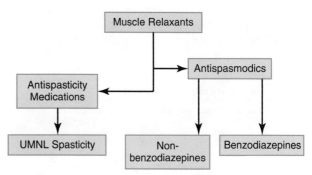

Figure B–11

Table B–5 Nonbenzodiazepine Muscle Relaxants

Generic Name	Brand Name
Carisoprodol	Soma
Cyclobenzaprine	Flexeril
Chlorzoxazone	Parafon-Forte
	Paraflex
	Strifon-Forte
Metaxalone	Skelaxin
Methocarbamol	Robaxin

in the BZDs are halcyon, Ativan, and Xanax, each with its own primary use such as decreasing anxiety, as a sedative, for pain, and antitremor and anticonvulsive effects. Some non-BZDS such as Lunesta, Sonata, and Ambien are best known for their sleep induction properties. Side effects may include dizziness, headache, dry mouth, and some GI disturbances. Metabolized by CYP3A4, interactions with certain supplements, foods, and teas should be monitored and potentially limited. Some are inhibitors and some are inducers. Inhibitors include black tea, cannabinoids, chamomile, Essiac herbal tea, ginger, ginseng, goldenseal, gotukola, grapefruit juice, kava, licorice, chaparral, clove, echinacea, milk thistle, peppermint oil, red yeast rice, sage, saw palmetto, St. John's wort, thyme, and turmeric. Inducers include chamomile, echinacea, garlic, goldenseal, hops, licorice, St. John's wort, and yucca.

Table B–5 lists some non-BZDs used to reduce muscle spasm for patients with back pain. Note that they do not relieve pain, but they either relieve muscle spasm or are sedating. There are common side effects including drowsiness, dizziness, and severe allergic reactions (**Table B–6**). They interact strongly with other sedatives and alcohol. Commonly prescribed are Norflex, Skelaxin, and Flexeril. Some, such as Flexeril, may cause urinary retention in males, and some may be habit-forming. Many are

metabolized by CYP1A2 and therefore may interact with some supplements, foods, and other substances including broccoli, cabbage, shiitake mushrooms, charbroiled meats, melatonin, chaparral, tobacco, herbal tea, and turmeric.

In summary, it is important for chiropractors to be aware of national guidelines and recommendations related to the medications prescribed for back pain.[9] Following are summaries of Clinical Practice Guidelines for NSAIDs and for muscle relaxants for chronic low back pain (LBP).

Summary for the Clinical Practice Guidelines (CPG) by Country for the Use of NSAIDs for Chronic LBP

- Europe, Italy, and the United States: CPG recommendations were that there was evidence for use (short-term).
- CPG recommendations in Belgium concluded there was no evidence for NSAID use or for aspirin.
- The U.S. CPG concluded there was insufficient evidence to estimate the effectiveness of aspirin.
- COX-2 inhibitors were recommended in the United Kingdom only if acetaminophen was not effective.

Summary for the Clinical Practice Guidelines (CPG) by Country for the Use of Muscle Relaxants for Chronic LBP

- Belgium in a 2006 review found only low-quality evidence to support the use of muscle relaxants in the management of chronic LBP; recommendation was that only short-term use be considered.
- European guidelines in 2004 found strong evidence for support of benzodiazepines for chronic LBP but conflicting results for nonbenzodiazepines.

Table B–6 Common Side Effects of Nonbenzodiazepine Muscle Relaxants

Concerns	Brand Name	Dosing
May be habit forming	Soma	350 mg/8 hr
May lead to urinary retention in males	Flexeril	10 mg/6 hr
Drowsiness, dizziness, and severe allergic reactions	Parafon-Forte Paraflex Strifon-Forte	500 mg/3–4 times/day
Drowsiness, dizziness, and severe allergic reactions	Skelaxin	800 mg/3–4 times/day
Drowsiness, dizziness, and severe allergic reactions	Robaxin	500 mg/2–3 tablets/QID

- For the U.S. guidelines in 2007, there was no evidence generally for the use of muscle relaxants but moderate benefit was found for benzodiazepines.

Medications with Neurological Effects

Medications used for local problems have systemic effects. This is no more true than for medications that affect the nervous system. The principles upon which these medications work are based first on a division between central nervous system (CNS) and peripheral nervous system (PNS) effects. Secondly, medications primarily have an effect on neurotransmitters and/or their receptors. Blocking or slowing transmission, inhibiting, blocking, or stimulating receptors, or preventing breakdown or reuptake of the neurotransmitter are the primary strategies of medications developed to affect the nervous system. As a reminder, the autonomic nervous system, which governs most visceral function, also serves functions related to stress, an increased demand for increased metabolism (such as exercise), and pain. Following are some primary drug mechanisms in relation to their nervous system effects.

Acetylcholine is the neurotransmitter for both the sympathetic and parasympathetic preganglionic neurons. For both, the receptors are nicotinic. For the postganglionic parasympathetic nervous system, receptors are muscarinic. For the sympathetic nervous system, the postganglionic (junctional) receptors are referred to as adrenergic because the neurotransmitter is norepinephrine. Acetylcholine is also the neurotransmitter for parasympathetic postganglionic neuron stimulation and sympathetic sweat gland stimulation. So the first obvious conclusion is that any effect on acetylcholine will have an effect on both divisions of the autonomic nervous system but clinically seem to have more effect on junctional or target tissue receptors post-synaptically. For example, the usual target organ effects of cholinergic parasympathetic activation are glandular secretion and peristaltic activity so that tears, mucus production, salivation, GI secretion, defecation, and urination are all facilitated by parasympathetic activity. Blocking these effects results in drying of secretions, constipation, and urinary retention. Parasympathetic activation also decreases heart rate and blood pressure. Receptors are divided into muscarinic and nicotinic. Muscarinic stimulation results primarily in cardiac and GI effects. Nicotinic receptor activation has effects on the heart and GI system, and nicotinic receptors in muscle are responsible for depolarization and subsequent muscle contraction.

Drugs affecting acetylcholine are called cholinergics. Cholinergics can be classified as cholinergic, anticholinergic, cholinesterase inhibitors, and nicotinic and muscarinic blockers and agonists.

- Cholinergics—used for glaucoma and urinary retention. Example, isoptocarpine. Side effects for cholinergics are nausea, vomiting, blurred vision, tremors, hypertension, and bronchial constriction.
- Anticholinergics—used for intestinal disorders such as irritable bowel syndrome, chronic obstructive pulmonary disease (COPD), and urinary incontinence. Examples are VESIcare and Detrol (urinary incontinence especially detrusor instability [unstable bladder]), and Spiriva (asthma and other COPD-reducing bronchoconstriction). Side effects include dry mouth, urinary retention, depression, flushing, fever, and constipation.
- Anticholinesterases—used in treatment of Alzheimer's disease, glaucoma, and as a local muscle relaxant. Examples include Aricept (Alzheimer's), Humorsol (glaucoma), and Botox (headaches due to local muscle entrapment and Dupuytren's). Side effects include nausea, diarrhea, confusion, and headache.
- Muscarinic receptor blockers or inhibitors—used in the treatment of asthma, tachycardias, and incontinence. Examples include Atrovent and Apovent (asthma), Ditropan (urinary incontinence), Artane and Cogentin (adjunctive for Parkinson's), Colofac, Duspatal, Duspatalin (irritable bowel syndrome), Benadryl (antihistamine), scopolamine (motion sickness), and atropine (anesthesia and bradycardia). Side effects include urinary retention and blurred vision.
- Nicotinic agonists—used in the treatment of smoking addiction. Examples include Nicorette, Nicoderm, and Chantix. Side effects include altered taste, heartburn, and nausea.
- Nicotinic inhibitors—used for hypertension. Example is Inversine. Side effects include dry mouth, constipation, hypotension, and incontinence.

There are supplements and herbs that are purported to have cholinergic and anticholinergic effects. Some examples include:

- Cholinergic supplements: Pulsatilla, American hellebore, and betel nut

- Anticholinergic supplements: Jimson weed, sage, Angel's trumpet, barberry, belladonna, and *Datura wrightii*
- Nicotinic receptor blockers: Jimson weed, scopolamine, and belladonna

Sympathetically focused medications target primarily respiratory and vascular issues such as COPD, hypertension, and congestive heart failure. The influences of the sympathetic nervous system are through junctional receptor types found pre- and postjunctional. Following is a breakdown with specific effects for each receptor.

Postjunctional Adrenoceptors

- *alpha-1 receptors* are largely responsible for constriction of small and large peripheral arteries, stimulation of the dilator papillae, constriction of many of the gastrointestinal tract sphincters, the bladder neck sphincter, and the vas deferens. So it is clear that blocking these receptors could help for several reasons: they decrease blood pressure through a decrease in peripheral resistance and prevent incontinence through bladder neck sphincter tightening, although this is more often a side effect of these medications inhibiting micturition.
- *beta-1 receptors* increase the pacemaker activity of the heart while at the same time increasing the force of contraction of the ventricles; additionally, if there is a sudden drop in blood pressure, activation of juxtaglomerular cells in the kidneys activates the rennin-angiotensin-aldosterone system. Blocking these receptors might be effective in decreasing blood pressure through decreasing cardiac force of contraction.
- *beta-2 receptors* are responsible for promoting smooth muscle relaxation for both blood vessels and bronchi, and they initiate glycogen breakdown. For asthmatics and those with constriction of bronchioles, promotion of smooth muscle may be effective, while their blockage for managing hypertension may allow bronchial constriction with difficulty in breathing as a side effect.

Prejunctional Adrenoceptors

- *alpha-2 receptors* (also called autoreceptors) are found on both sympathetic and parasympathetic

presynaptic synapses and when stimulated, inhibit the release of norepinephrine.
- *beta-2 receptors* facilitate the release of norepinephrine.

Nonadrenergic, noncholinergic (NANC) neurons include dopamine, vasoactive intestinal polypeptide, and nitric oxide. These substances modulate primarily the activity of parasympathetic cells.

Antidepressants

The basis upon which medical management has evolved follows the hypothesis development over several decades related primarily to the function of mainly three neurotransmitters: serotonin, norepinephrine, and dopamine. These neurotransmitters, also called the monoamines, are crucial to proper function related to, among others, emotion, sleep, appetite, sexuality, and reaction to stress. Medications increase one or more of these monoamines, decrease their breakdown (e.g., monoamine oxidase inhibitors), or normalize receptor sensitivity. Although the neurotransmitters are often increased within hours of ingestion, it may take weeks for the effects to be felt by the patient. This delay may be due to a hypothesized receptor sensitivity reaction. Upregulation may occur when decreased neurotransmitter is available leading to increased receptor sensitivity or an increased number of receptors. Medications may decrease this hypersensitivity or decrease the number of receptors through downregulation. This may take several weeks, partially explaining the delayed effects of antihypertensive medications. The permissive hypothesis restates the cause of depression through a proposed *imbalance* of neurotransmitters versus their actual levels. For example, low levels of serotonin may allow proportionately high levels of norepinephrine to cause mania.

Following are examples of drug categories and mechanisms of action.

- *Tricyclics* (e.g., amitriptyline [Elavil, Endep] and doxepin HCl [Adapin, Sinequan]) and heterocyclic antidepressants (e.g., trazodone HCl [Desyrel], nortriptyline [Aventyl], clomipramine [Anafranil]). Avoid alcohol, grapefruit juice, and St. John's wort. There is an increased risk for suicide. Tricyclics are metabolized by CYP2C19; therefore it is important to avoid black tea, chamomile, chaparral, clove, ginger, ginseng, gotukola, milk thistle, red yeast rice, thyme, and turmeric.

- *Selective serotonin reuptake inhibitors (SSRIs)* (e.g., fluoxetine HCl [Prozac], paroxetine HCl [Paxil], and sertraline HCl [Zoloft]). SSRIs are metabolized by either CYP2C9 or CYP2D6 and as a result, certain supplements and some foods are contraindicated:
  1. CYP2C9: black tea, chamomile, chaparral, clove, ginger, milk thistle, sage, St. John's wort, thyme, and turmeric
  2. CYP2D6: 5-HTP, tyrosine, adrenal extract, vitamin B$_6$, kava, black tea, cat's claw, chamomile, chaparral, chromium, clove, DHEA, ephedra, evening primrose, fenugreek, ginger, ginkgo, gotukola, hops, phenylalanine, sage, St. John's wort, SAMe, thyme, turmeric, and valerian root
- *Monoamine oxidase (MAO) inhibitors.* Inhibit the reuptake of dopamine, serotonin, and norepinephrine with the major affect on dopamine. With the older MAO inhibitors there is a caution regarding a sudden onset of hypertension. To prevent this, patients are instructed to avoid high tyramine foods such as aged cheeses, tap beer, licorice, soy sauce, miso, sauerkraut, homemade pizza, sausage, pepperoni, salami, fava beans, snow peas, tofu, soybeans, and meat substitutes, and to avoid tryptophan supplements and St. John's wort. There is also a recommendation to limit certain liquids including wine (2–4 oz/d), coffee and cola (<500 mg caffeine/d), and bottled beer (24 oz/d). Newer drugs such as Wellbutrin and Cymbalta are used in the treatment of depression, and Zyban has been approved as an aid for smoking cessation. Possible problems are seizures, hepatotoxicity, nausea, vomiting, headache, agitation, tremor, and anticholinergic effects. These drugs are generally CYP2D6 inhibitors and are metabolized by CYP2B6. As with many antidepressants, alcohol and St. John's wort should be avoided.

When stress reaction is managed medically, drugs such as Valium and Librium are also prescribed. These benzodiazepines inhibit the stimulation from the locus coeruleus to the amygdala, thereby decreasing norepinephrine release and subsequent sympathetic stimulation. These drugs are effective; however, due to their sedative and addictive properties they should be used with caution.

Lithium is still the standard for manic depression; however, patients with thyroid, kidney, or heart disorders should not take lithium. Other medications prescribed for manic depression include two anticonvulsants, carbamazepine (Tegretol) and valproate (Depakote), and lamotrigine (Lamictal) and gabapentin (Neurontin). However, the role of gabapentin was apparently misrepresented, and although effective for other disorders it has not been shown to be effective for depression.

Some possible side effects of these medications include:

- drowsiness and sedation—tricyclics
- insomnia and anxiety—SSRIs
- orthostatic hypotension and cardiac arrhythmia—tricyclic and heterocyclic agents
- weight gain—tricyclics, heterocyclics, and MAO inhibitors
- delirium—interactions between tricyclic and heterocyclic compounds and SSRIs may cause what has been coined "serotonin syndrome," which results in excess cerebral serotonin stimulation

Anti-Epileptic

With the understanding that seizure activity represents, in part, hyperexcitability, the mechanism of action for many of the medications prescribed for epilepsy becomes more evident. The development of effective medications is based on the premise that neurotransmitters that are primarily excitatory need to be diminished or blocked and those that are inhibitory need to be enhanced. Following are some common examples:

- Phenytoin (e.g., Dilantin) and carbamazepine (e.g., Tegretol) are part of a medication category termed glutamate antagonists. They block glutamate ionotropic receptors, rendering ion channels less permeable to sodium and/or calcium.
- Benzodiazepines and barbiturates used in the management of many disorders are used as therapy for seizures due to their glutamate inhibition by GABA through hyperpolarization.
- Sodium valproate is able to effectively block the conversion of GABA to glutamate by blocking the transaminase enzyme responsible for this conversion.
- Ethosuximide is a specific T-channel blocker affecting the excitability of thalamic relay neurons. This then blocks these neurons from entering a burst-firing mode.

Note that anti-epileptic medications are used for other disorders based on these neuronal inhibitory effects including prophylactic management of chronic headache and neuralgias such as trigeminal neuralgia and post-herpetic neuralgias.

The major concern with medical management of epilepsy is the chronic effect on psychomotor and cognitive function. Phenytoin and phenobarbital are of particular concern with long-term usage. A possible problem with anti-epileptic drugs is CNS toxicity, including sedation, dizziness, imbalance, diplopia, and nausea. Usually these are transient. Morbilliform rashes occur in 5% to 7% of patients. Common side effects for the three primary drugs include:

- Valproic acid (Depacon): tremor and weight gain
- Phenytoin (Dilantin): in young patients, gingival hyperplasia and hirsutism
- Carbamazepine (Carbatrol, Tegretol, Tegretol-XR) and oxcarbazepine (Trileptal): hyponatremia in patients who drink large amounts of fluids or are on diuretics

Psychomotor Stimulants

Psychomotor stimulants are utilized in the treatment of several disorders including narcolepsy and attention deficit hyperactivity disorder (ADHD). In the past, amphetamines have also been used as appetite suppressants. The substances stimulate the CNS by increasing norepinephrine (NE) and dopamine (D) activity in the brain. This is accomplished through several mechanisms including binding to NE and D receptors, stimulating the release of NE and D, and preventing the reuptake of NE and D. Examples include Adderall and Ritalin, used in the management of ADHD, and Dexedrine, used in the management of weight gain through appetite suppression. There is the risk of drug dependency with these medications. Some side effects include dry mouth, rapid heartbeat, hypertension, tremor, insomnia, and paranoia. It is recommended to avoid high-dose vitamin C and alcohol and to limit caffeine, high-acid foods (fruit juice), and antacids.

Anti-Infection Medications

Antibiotics are some of the most commonly prescribed medications. In addition, because they are introduced into the production of our food supply, they are ubiquitous. This allows organisms to develop resistance, which creates a never-ending battle to find the next generation of antibiotic. This has been a concern of the medical community and as a result, restrictions on the addition of antibiotics to the food supply of farm animals and the recommendations to avoid antibiotics as the first response to ear infections or persistent coughs are attempts at slowing down the ability of organisms to develop resistance. That being said, there are critical clinical scenarios where antibiotics and anti-infective agents are life-saving and necessary. A brief overview of organisms and their classifications is given in **Figures B-12** through **B-14**.

Bacteria are often categorized by their cell wall staining:

- Gram-positive organisms stain blue during gram staining because the cell wall is impenetrable, retaining the color of the dye. These are further divided into cocci and bacilli, and then further divided into aerobic and anaerobic. The most common aerobic bacteria are strep and staph. Mycobacteria such as tuberculosis (TB) and leprosy are unique in that they stain gram-positive weakly. They are often called "acid fast" because the stain remains even when washed with acid alcohol. These organisms are unique in their approach because they live inside mononuclear phagocytes, often for years, and are therefore intracellular parasites.
- Gram-negative organisms are negative to staining. They are unique in that they have an additional protection for their plasma membranes in the form of a rigid peptidoglycan wall covered by an outer membrane. Gram-negatives protect themselves against penicillin through the production of betalactamases, enzymes that destroy penicillin. Gram-negatives are also categorized as cocci and

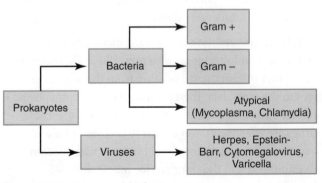

Figure B-12 Organism classification.

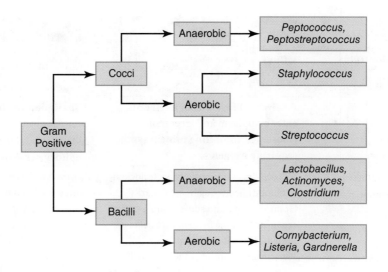

Figure B–13

bacilli, aerobic and anaerobic. Functionally, they are also categorized as:

1. Enterics (organisms infecting the GI tract)—*Escherichia*, *Shigella*, *Salmonella*, *Klebsiella*, *Enterobacter*, and others.
2. *Haemophilus influenza*
3. *Neisseria*
4. *Pseudomonas*

The following will give a cursory overview of the topic of how medications are designed to fight infection. **Table B–7** lists some commonly prescribed antibiotics, antiviral, and antifungal medications for quick reference. So how do anti-infection drugs work? There are several targets of effect.

The Cell Wall

The cell wall is one key feature for the categorization of organisms. If an organism does have a cell wall and is therefore less like human cells that, in fact, do not have cell walls, it is a prokaryote. These prokaryotes do not have a nucleus where DNA is housed. Prokaryotes include viruses and bacteria. These key differences allow for targeting of the organisms with agents that will in most cases do no harm to human cells, which are eukaryotes (i.e., have a nucleus with DNA but no cell wall). Eukaryotes include animals, plants, fungi, and parasites. Using the cell wall as the target, some antibiotics are designed to kill bacteria by inhibiting cell wall synthesis; these are termed bactericidal. Other agents are bacteriostatic, meaning that they inhibit bacterial proliferation and allow the host defense system to kill the organism. Common infections such as staph and strep rely on protection through glycoprotein cross-linking in their cell walls. Bactericidal agents affect the cross-linking necessary for the cell wall's integrity and include the penicillins and cephalosporins.

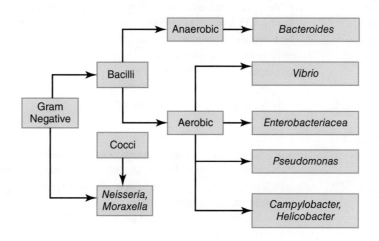

Figure B–14

Table B–7 Some Commonly Prescribed Antibiotic, Antiviral, and Antifungal Medications

Drug Class	Examples	General Mechanism/Used For	Interactions/Side Effects
Antibiotic			
Aminoglycosides		**Passively diffuse through cell wall, enter cytoplasm and irreversibly bind to ribosomes, inhibiting protein synthesis requiring oxygen**	**Usually administered parenterally due to poor GI absorption** **Side effects include damage to kidneys and auditory nerve (tinnitus) and hearing loss)**
Gentamycin	Garamycin Genoptic	A broad-spectrum usually bacteriocidal antibiotic effective against primarily Gram-negative and some Gram-positive organisms. Some include *Klebsiella, Proteus, E. Coli, Enterobacter, Pseudomonas*, among others. Usually reserved for serious infections when other less toxic antibiotics are ineffective.	Is ototoxic, hepatotoxic, and nephrotoxic with associated indications on lab testing. May cause a variety of hypersensitivity reactions, neuromuscular blockade, hypo-kalemia, and hypomagnesia with muscle cramps/weakness.
Streptomycin	Trobicin	A bacteriostatic antibiotic effective against numerous bacteria. Primarily used for *N. gonorrhoeae*.	Pain, swelling, tenderness at injection site. May cause dizziness, headache, and nausea. May elevate some liver enzymes or cause decrease in hematocrit or hemoglobin.
Penicillins		**Cross-linking of peptidoglycan strands by inhibiting transpeptidase enzymes**	**Most common type of drug allergy** **Nutrient interactions: avoid K supplements**
Penicillin (including G benza-thine, G potassium, G sodium, G procaine, and V/V potassium)	Bicillin Permapen Megacillin Pentids Pfizerpen Cryptocillin Benzylpenicillin Wycillin	An antibiotic in many different forms used for different infections. Penicillin G benzathine – mild to moderate infections, syphilis, and prophylaxis for rheumatic fever. Penicillin G potassium or sodium – moderate to severe infections, meningococcal meningitis. Penicillin G procaine – moderate to severe infections, pneumococcal pneumonia, uncomplicated gonorrhea, and syphilis. Penicillin V & V potassium – mild to moderate infections and endocarditis prophylaxis.	Anaphylaxis is common, hypersensitiv-ity symptoms, common GI disturbances, SLE-like syndrome, hypotension, rarely circulatory collapse, Loeffler's syndrome, thrombocytopenia, hemolytic anemia, and delayed skin rashes.
Ampicillin	Amcil Penbritin Omnipen Totacillin	Broad-spectrum antibiotic. Effective against Gram positives such as alpha- and beta-hemolytic streptococci, diplococci, pneumoniae, staphylococci, and *Listeria*. Also against some Gram-negatives such as *E. coli, N. Gonorrheae, Proteus, shigella, Salmonella*, mycoplasma, some viruses and fungi.	Possible anaphylaxis, diarrhea, pseudomem-branous colitis, and rash.
Amoxicillin	Amoxil Polymox Larotid Trimox	Penicillin-type antibiotic (bacterial cell-wall inhibitor). Inhibits mucoprotein synthesis of cell wall in rapidly reproducing cells. Used for infections of the middle ear, throat, bronchi, and lungs. Also for UTI, skin infections, and gonorrhea. Specific susceptible organisms include *H. influen-zae, N. gonorrhea, E. coli*, pneumococci, streptococci, some forms of *staphylococci*.	Similar to other penicillin medications; possibility of hypersensitivity with rash, anaphylaxis. Also possible are hemolytic anemia, eosinophilia, pseudomembranous colitis, pruritus, and urticaria.

Table B–7 Some Commonly Prescribed Antibiotic, Antiviral, and Antifungal Medications (continued)

Drug Class	Examples	General Mechanism/Used For	Interactions/Side Effects
Cephalosporins		**Same as penicillins: bind to and inhibit bacterial enzymes, causing defective cell wall formation and eventually bacterial death**	Nutrient interactions: depletes vitamin K; avoid alcohol, decrease sodium in diet while taking cephalosporins
Cephalexin	Keflex Keftabs	A semi-synthetic cephalosporin antibiotic (similar to penicillin; β-lactam binds penicillin binding proteins inhibiting crosslinking of bacterial cell wall). Susceptible bacteria are Gram-positive except for enterococci and methicillin resistant *Staph aureus* (MRSA), some Gram-negative; not anaerobes.	Hypersensitivity reactions (anaphylaxis, serum sickness), GI disturbances, rare neurologic problems (seizures), and hematologic abnormalities (cytopenias), and nephrotoxicity and hepatic enzyme increases.
Fluoroquinolones		**Same as penicillins: bind to and inhibit bacterial enzymes, causing defective cell wall formation and eventually bacterial death**	Nutrient interactions: divalent and trivalent minerals impair absorption (Zn, Mg, Ca, Fe, Al) – take 2 h prior or 6 h after drug; limit caffeine **Inhibits CYP1A2** **Contraindicated supplements: melatonin, chaparral, tobacco, herbal tea, broccoli, cabbage, charbroiled meats, shiitake mushrooms, turmeric**
Ciprofloxacin	Cipro	A synthetic quinolone that is bactericidal by inhibiting DNA-gyrase an enzyme required for bacterial DNA replication. Often used for urinary tract infections caused by *E. coli*. Also for *C. jejuni* and *Shigella*. Also used for bacterial conjunctivitis.	May cause nausea, vomiting, abdominal pain, cramps, and gas. May elevate liver enzymes and eosinophils. May cause tendon rupture, headache, vertigo, seizures, or rash. If used for conjunctivitis may precipitate buildup on cornea or crusting scales.
Macrolides and Ketolides		**Inhibit bacterial protein synthesis**	Nutrient interactions: avoid St. John's Wort and grapefruit, limit alcohol **Inhibits CYP3A4, CYP3A5 & CYP3A7** **Supplements affected: DHEA, eucalyptus oil, tea tree oil, yohimbine**
Erythromycin	Akne-Mycin Ery-Tab ApoErythroBase A/T/S/E-Mycin EryDerm Erythrocin Erythromid Illocyin Norvo-Rythro Robomycin Staticin T-Stat	A macrolide antibiotic effective primarily against Gram-positive. Effective against *Chlamydia trachomatis*. Also used for Pneumococcal and Mycoplasma pneumonia, *N. gonorrhea*, and *H. influenzae*. Main use is for ear, nose, and throat infections in those allergic to penicillin and cephalosporin.	Usual GI complaints, plus superinfection with yeast, nonsusceptible bacteria, and fungi. Also causes ototoxicity (reversible vertigo, hearing loss, and tinnitus), hypersensitivity reactions, and cholestatic hepatitis syndrome.

(continues)

Table B–7 Some Commonly Prescribed Antibiotic, Antiviral, and Antifungal Medications (continued)

Drug Class	Examples	General Mechanism/Used For	Interactions/Side Effects
Azithromycin	Zithromax	A macrolide antibiotic effective primarily against pyogenic streptococci, *S. pneumoniae*, *H. influenzae*, and *S. aureus*. Interferes with protein synthesis by binding to 50S ribosome of bacteria.	May cause headaches, dizziness, hepatotoxic effects such as mild elevation of liver enzymes, and usual GI complaints.
Nitromidazoles			
Metronidazole	Flagyl Metizol Metro-Gel Protostat Noritate	A synthetic agent that is effective against a wide variety of organisms including *Trichomonas vaginalis*, *Entamoeba histolytica*, and *Giardia lablia*. Also anti-bacterial anaerobic bacteria and some Gram-negatives. Used with other antibiotics (triple antibiotic regimen) for duodenal ulcers. Topical may be used for rosacea.	May cause a Candida infection (overgrowth), hypersensitivity, nausea and other GI symptoms, polyuria, dysuria, vertigo, headache, and a metallic or bitter taste. May decrease AST levels (interferes with chemical reaction).
Tetracyclines and Glycylcyclines		**Reversibly bind to ribosomes, inhibiting protein synthesis**	**Nutrient interactions: avoid St. John's wort; take Ca, Zn, Mg, Fe, or multivitamin at least 3 h before or 1 h after drug**
Tetracycline	Achromycin	A synthetic broad-spectrum antibiotic that is bacteristatic (inhibits protein synthesis by binding to 30s subunit blocking amino acid linked tRNA from binding to the A site of the ribosome). Susceptible bacteria include *M. pneumoniae*, *C. psittaci*, *C. trachomatis*, and *N. gonorrhea*. Used for respiratory infections, nongonococcal urethritis (ureaplasma), Rocky Mountain spotted fever, typhus, chancroid, anthrax, syphillis, cholera, brucellosis, chlamydia, acne, and Lyme disease. Doxycycline approved for malaria prophylaxis.	GI distress, reversible nephro- and hepatotoxicity, photosensitivity, and dental staining (not used in prepubertal children).
Doxycycline	Vibromycin	A synthetic broad-spectrum antibiotic that is bacteristatic (inhibits protein synthesis by binding to 30s subunit blocking amino acid linked tRNA from binding to the A site of the ribosome). Susceptible bacteria include *M. pneumoniae*, *C. psittaci*, *C. trachomatis*, and *N. gonorrhea*. Used for respiratory infections, nongonococcal urethritis (ureaplasma), Rocky Mountain spotted fever, typhus, chancroid, anthrax, symphillis, cholera, brucellosis, and acne.	May cause GI distress, reversible nephro- and hepatotoxicity, photosensitivity, and dental staining (not used in prepubertal children).
Folate Antagonists			
Trimethoprim-Sulfmethoxasole	**Bactrim** **Septra** **Co-Trimoxazole**	A combination drug that acts as a synthetic folate antagonist acting as an enzyme inhibitor preventing bacterial synthesis. Used with *Pneumocystis carini* pneumonitis, *Shigella* enteritis, and UTI caused by *Enterobacteriaceae*.	Possible toxic epidermal necrosis syndrome, pseudomembranous colitis, agranulocytosis, aplastic anemia (rare), and anorexia, nausea, and skin rash. May elevate liver enzymes and bilirubin.

Table B–7 Some Commonly Prescribed Antibiotic, Antiviral, and Antifungal Medications (continued)

Drug Class	Examples	General Mechanism/Used For	Interactions/Side Effects
Glycopeptides			
Vancomycin	Vancocin Vancoled	An antibiotic that interferes with cell membrane synthesis. Primarily for Gram-positive. Organisms include beta-hemolytic streptococci, staphylococci, pneumococci, enterococci, clostridia, and cornyeobacteria.	Is ototoxic, and nephrotoxic. May cause anaphylaxis, and hypersensitivity reactions, "red neck" syndrome with IV administration, thrombophlebitis, super-infections, and transient leucopenia and eosinophilia.
Antimycobacterials			
Isoniazid	INH Isotamine Laniazid Nydrazid Teebaconin	An anti-TB medication that interferes with the synthesis of bacterial proteins, lipids, and nucleic acids. Used also for high-risk individuals as a preventive. Additional use for tremors with multiple sclerosis.	May cause paresthesias, peripheral neuropathies, tinnitus, dizziness, hallucinations, increased liver enzymes, decrease in vitamin B absorption, RA and SLE-like syndromes, or possible agranulocytosis and aplastic anemia (rare).
Others			
Chloramphenicol	Chloromycetin Chlorofair Fenicol Novochloroscap	A broad-spectrum antibiotic that is primarily bacteriostatic (bacteriocidal to *H. influenzae*). Interferes with protein synthesis by binding to 50S ribosome of bacteria. Used when infection is serious and unaffected by other antibiotics. Examples include *Salmonella*, *Rickettsia*, *Chlamydia*, *Mycoplasma*, *Streptococcus pneumoniae* and *Neiserria* among others.	May cause hypersensitivity reactions, bone marrow suppression, neurotoxicity, angio-edema, pancytopenia, headache, confusion, stomatitis, glossitis, and the usual GI complaints.
Norfloxacin	Chibroxin Noroxin	A strong broad-spectrum antibiotic that alters DNA-gyrase inhibiting protein synthesis. Used primarily for UTIs and conjunctivitis. Effective against many organisms including *Klebsiella* and other pneumonias, *Salmonella*, *Shigella*, *Pseudomonas*, *S. aureus*, among others.	May cause joint pain, swelling, and erosions in weight-bearing joints. Usual GI complaints, headaches, dizziness, pruritus, elevated liver enzymes, and immunosuppressed swelling of ankle and hip with tendon tenderness and swelling of 3rd finger bilaterally after one month of continuous therapy.
Antiviral			
Valacyclovir	Valtrex	An antiviral medication that interferes with viral DNA synthesis. Due to increased GI absorption, plasma levels are higher than acyclovir. Used for the treatment of herpes zoster (shingles) and recurrent genital herpes.	Headache, weakness, fatigue, nausea, vomiting, dyspepsia, abdominal pain, renal damage, allergic reactions.
Acyclovir	Zovirax Acycloguanosine	Interferes with DNA synthesis for specific viruses including herpes simplex 1 and 2, varicella-roster, and cytomegalovirus. It does not eliminate the latent herpes virus.	May cause headache, nausea, vomiting, diarrhea, and rarely acute renal failure or thrombocytopenia purpura or hemolytic uremic syndrome.

(continues)

Table B–7 Some Commonly Prescribed Antibiotic, Antiviral, and Antifungal Medications (continued)

Drug Class	Examples	General Mechanism	Interactions/Side Effects
Amantadine	Symmetrel	A medication that is effective as an antiviral against influenza A (not B) and also an initial or adjunct therapy with anticholinergic drugs for Parkinson's. Antiparkinsonian effects may be due to effect of release of dopamine and other catecholamines.	May cause dizziness, lightheadedness, difficulty with memory, hallucinations, confusion, mood or other mental effects, nausea, vomiting, or dry mouth.
Hepatitis B Immune Globulin	H-BIG Hep-B-Gamma-gee HyperHep	Sterile human-based solution of IgG used to provide passive immunity for hepatitis B or post-exposure prophylaxis.	May cause a hypersensitivity reaction, muscle stiffness and aching, fever, dizziness, malaise, rash, or leg cramps.
Immunoglobulin	BayGam Gamimune Gammagard Gammar P Iveegam Sandoglobulin Venoglobulin	A sterile concentrated human globulin solution used both as prophylaxis or to modify the severity of a number of diseases including rubella, rubeola, varicella zoster, type A hepatitis, idiopathic thrombocytopenia purpura, among others.	Side effects related to site of injection. Also may cause hypersensitivity reactions, headache, GI symptoms, chest tightness, or wheezing.
Interferfon Alfa n-1, Alfacon-1, Alfa 2a, and Alfa 2b	Wellferon Infergen	A variety of medications used in the management of hepatitis C. Actions include suppression of cell proliferation and augmentation of lymphocyte natural killer cells.	Common to have side effects including headache, fever, chills, anxiety, nervousness, GI disturbances, alopecia, abnormal mood, emotional lability, and confusion. Possible lab effects on thrombocytes and granulocytes.
Antifungal			
Amphotericin B Amphotericin B Lipid Based	Amphocin Fungizone Amphotec Abelcet	An antifungal that binds to sterols in the fungus cell membrane. Produced from *Streptomyces nodosus*. Used intravenously to treat serious, life-threatening fungal infections such as aspergillosis, blastomycosis, coccidiomycosis, cryptococcosis, histoplasmosis, and others.	May cause fever, chills, anaphylaxis, cardiac arrest, nephrotoxicity, hypokalemia, hypomagnesemia, and super-infections.
Clotrimazole	Lotrimin Gyne-Lotrimin Canasten Mycelex	A broad-spectrum antifungal agent that alters the fungal wall permeability allowing loss of potassium and other important elements necessary for replication. Used for both dermal fungal infections and vaginal yeast infections.	May alter liver function tests and cause the usual GI disturbances, UTI symptoms, and pruritus.
Ketoconozole	Nizoral	Cell membrane function is disrupted by inhibiting sterol (ergosterol) synthesis in fungi. Used for serious systemic fungal infections such as Candida, coccidiomycoses, histoplasmosis, blastomycosis, and similar infections. Also used for superficial treatment of mycosis such as the "tineas."	May cause usual GI disturbances, anaphylaxis, gynecomastia, decreased libido, hair loss, acute hypoadrenalism, rarely hepatic necrosis, and may change multiple lab values such as decreases in cholesterol and triglycerides, and low serum testosterone.

Table B–7 Some Commonly Prescribed Antibiotic, Antiviral, and Antifungal Medications (continued)

Drug Class	Examples	General Mechanism	Interactions/Side Effects
Miconazole	Monostat (Derm, 3, 7) Femizole M-Zole Micatin Tetterine Fungoid Lotrimin Desenex	A broad-spectrum antifungal that inhibits absorption of essential material for cell reproduction, growth, and cell wall integrity. Used primarily for Candida, common dermatophytes, and tinea vesicolor. Used for a variety of body sites: vaginal Candida infection, athlete's foot (tinea pedis), and similar "tineas" caused by dermatophytes.	May cause burning at the site of application, skin reactions, or ulcerations.
Nystatin	Mycostatin Nadostine Nilstat Nyaderm Nystex	An antifungal antibiotic that binds to cell membrane and causes leakage of intracellular components. Used primarily for Candida infections.	May cause nausea, vomiting, epigastric pain, or diarrhea.
Terbinafine	Lamasil Lamasil Derma-Gel	Cell membrane function is disrupted by inhibiting sterol (ergosterol) synthesis in fungi. Used for superficial treatment of mycosis such as the "tineas."	May cause burning at the site of application, skin reactions, or ulcerations. Also, may cause headache, GI disturbance, liver function test abnormalities, taste abnormalities, and rarely liver failure or neutropenia.

Protein and DNA Synthesis

What if the organism does not have a cell wall such as some bacteria, fungi, and parasites? Then the approach is to affect DNA synthesis by disruption of the code or interference in protein synthesis. The DNA in a prokaryotic cell is coiled up in a region called the nucleoid not separated in a cell nucleus like animals, and consists of one long strand. Following are some examples:

- Fluoroquinolones, such as Cipro and Noroxin, introduce defective building blocks into DNA creation.
- Sulfonamides and acyclovir (used for many viral infections) inhibit enzymes or cofactors necessary for DNA synthesis. Sulfonamides are similar to paramino benzoic acid (PABA) and prevent the incorporation of PABA into folate necessary for its function. A commonly used sulfonamide combination is Septra (trimethoprim sulfamethoxazole), which is utilized against enteric Gram-negative infections such as *Shigella*, *Salmonella*, and *E. coli*, and for urinary tract infections.

- The antimetabolites disarm the synthesis of DNA, RNA, or proteins. Examples include tetrahydrofolate, which is able to donate a single carbon molecule affecting the synthesis of purines, pyrimidines, and some amino acids.
- Destroying the RNA code through the inhibition of RNA polymerase is another strategy used in the treatment of tuberculosis (TB). This is the mechanism of rifampin, one of two common drugs utilized in the treatment of TB.
- Drugs such as erythromycin, tetracycline, chloramphenicol, and the aminoglycosides all attack at the level of the ribosome (70s ribosome) preventing assembly of proteins from the mRNA.

The prescription of antibiotics is complex, involving the decision as to whether it is appropriate given the development of resistant organisms, the need to identify the organism and prescribe the appropriate medication, and the consideration of harm when the medication affects human cells. The patient must be reminded to adhere to the prescription regimen for antibiotics or risk failure and potential additional infection.

To understand the strategies utilized by prescribing physicians, it might be worth summarizing. Some general rules-of-thumb that prescribing physicians use in their decision making include:

- For Gram-positive organisms, most physicians rely on Nafcillin (IV) and dicloxacillin (PO) because they are not susceptible to penicillinases.
- For Gram-negative organisms, third-generation cephalosporins are effective. They can access the brain as well. Another approach is the combination of cephalosporins combined with penicillins, which augments the effectiveness of aminoglycosides.
- The combination of ampicillin and gentamycin ("amp and gent") is effective against the combination of Gram-positive and Gram-negative organisms.
- Amoxicillin is commonly prescribed for otitis media and many upper respiratory infections.
- Septra (trimethoprim-sulfamethoxazole [Bactrim/Septra]) is commonly prescribed for urinary tract infections.
- For anaerobic bacteria, metronidazole (Flagyl) and clindamycin are commonly employed.
- For infections of the brain, testes, joints, and eye, targeted therapy is necessary due to the inherent protection for these sites.
- Abscesses form a protective wall in many anaerobic infections and therefore must be drained and then treated.

Antiviral Medications

Antibiotics are for bacterial infections. Different agents are used for viruses because their structure and strategy of infection are different. Viruses are obligate intracellular parasites inserting themselves into cells and utilizing those cells to produce new viruses with the inserted viral DNA and RNA. There are commonly several viruses that are seen by medical physicians including:

- Herpes—including herpes simplex causing genital and oral involvement, and the varicella virus (chicken pox) leading to herpes zoster and latent infection of the dorsal root ganglion leading to skin lesions. These are often treated with acyclovir (Zovirax), which inhibits viral DNA polymerase.
- Influenza is of particular concern for the immunocompromised, the elderly, and some infants. Medications are either prophylactic or targeted to infection. Amantadine (Symmetrel) is

an example of a medication utilized to prevent the virus from infecting cells; prophylactic.

- Cytomegalovirus (CMV) is of particular concern in transplant patients, those with AIDS, and others who are immunocompromised. Ganciclovir (Cytovene) is used to prevent DNA synthesis through inhibition of DNA polymerase.
- HIV is a retrovirus. Its ability to mutate through substitutions of base-pair substitutions requires a different approach to treatment. Multiple medications are utilized. The drugs include nucleoside analogs, non-nucleoside reverse transcriptase inhibitors, and protease inhibitors given more as a "cocktail" of medications. Commonly used drugs are Retrovir, Videx, Viracept, and Norvir, among others.

Antifungal Medications

Fungi are either yeast or mold. Reproduction strategies and mechanisms are different for each. Yeast spreads through budding or spore formation, whereas mold spreads through extending hyphae; branching out. The most common yeast infection is Candida. Infection of the mouth is often referred to as thrush. This may be secondary to treatment of asthma with aerosol corticosteroids. Candida infections in women are common vaginally and are more common with the use of corticosteroids, antibiotic treatment, and diabetes. Treatment for oral Candida is usually with nystatin (Mycostatin), whereas vaginal infection is treated first with miconazole (Monistat). If the Candida infection is systemic, amphotericin B is incorporated; this is a very toxic medication.

Fungal infections are difficult to treat, with medications often being toxic. All may find their way to the lungs where granulomas develop. Although there are many different forms of fungal infection, following are some examples of common types:

- Histoplasmosis, blastomycosis, aspergillus, and San Joaquin Valley fever (coccidioidomycosis) are the most common fungal infections and usually present as pneumonia. Treatment is either with the older amphotericin B, or the newer fluconazole or itraconazole, both of which have the advantage of being taken orally versus the IV administration for amphotericin B.
- Cryptococcus is another fungal infection that may present as pneumonia, but more commonly

presents as meningitis. This requires medications that can cross the blood–brain barrier. Fluconazole is the most effective, followed by flucytosine. Fluconazole inhibits fungal cytochrome P-450 enzymes.

Antiparasitic Medications

Parasitic infections are more common in those who travel to foreign countries or, in some cases, are exposed to a crowded environment such as daycare centers. Parasites use the human as host and are difficult to treat. The standard treatment is with metronidazole (Flagyl), commonly used for the treatment of Giardia. Lindane is a medication used for the treatment of head lice. Malaria is even more complicated due to variations in regions and the growing resistance to antimalarial medications. Prophylactic treatment seems appropriate when traveling to endemic areas.

Cardiovascular Medications

Cardiovascular effects are needed to modulate a number of pathological processes or conditions including:

- Arrhythmias
- Cardiac ischemia
- Congestive and chronic heart failure
- Hypertension
- Atherosclerosis
- Anticoagulants

Some of the drugs overlap in their application such that management of hypertension, cardiac ischemia, and sometimes arrhythmias may be similar.

Antiarrhythmics

The mechanism of action is generally to block transmission through sodium and potassium blockade or through smooth muscle relaxation through calcium channel blockers or sympathetic blockers (i.e., beta blockers). Examples include:

- Sodium channel blockers—including Quinidine, Procanbid, and Lidocaine. Avoid Ca and K supplements and grapefruit, and maintain sodium. Metabolized by CYP2D6; therefore avoid substances as listed above.

- Beta blockers (B1)—Commonly used is Propranolol. Avoid alcohol, calcium, sodium, and licorice supplements. Also metabolized by CYP2D6.
- Potassium channel blockers—Example is Cordarone. Taken with food due to increased absorption with fat. Avoid St. John's wort and grapefruit. Metabolized by CYP3A4.
- Calcium channel blockers—Example is Cardizem. Avoid Ca supplements; decrease salt intake; limit caffeine; and high dose vitamin D (>2000 IU). Also metabolized by CYP3A4.

Some supplements with purported anti-arrhythmic activity include alpha-linolenic acid, cat's claw, coenzyme Q10, *Cordyceps*, fish oil, Indian snakeroot, lotus, and omega-3 fatty acids.

Anti-Anginal

The most common drugs used to manage an acute angina attack are vasodilators. Nitrates are the most common example, affecting both arteries and veins through conversion into nitric oxide (NO), a potent vasodilator due to smooth muscle relaxation. This is given sublingually during an attack or prophylactically using a dermal patch. A common side effect with sublingual administration is headache. Some herbals that may have anti-anginal properties include bilberry, feverfew, sweet Annie, horse chestnut, shark cartilage, and noni.

Antihypertensives

Medications reduce the pressure in the cardiovascular system by reducing the force of contraction of the heart, reducing the amount of fluid in the system, or reducing the tension in the arteries/veins. The following general classes of medications accomplish these actions:

- Diuretics (decrease fluid in system)
- Drugs that affect the sympathetic nervous system such as beta blockers and alpha adrenergic blockers (reduce force of contraction of the heart and/or tension in the vascular system)
- General vasodilators (often based on activation of nitric oxide)
- Calcium channel blockers (similar effect on heart and vasculature as sympathetic blockers)

- Angiotensin-converting enzyme (ACE) inhibitors (inhibit the renin-angiotensin-aldosterone cycle)
- Angiotensin receptor blockers

Each drug has its potential side effects. The most characteristic side effects are as follows:

- Diuretics—Thiazide diuretics include Diuril, Thalitone, and Lozol. Some diuretics will cause loss of potassium or magnesium and lead to some increase in low-density lipoprotein cholesterol.
- Beta blockers—These often have an effect of causing a decrease in energy or inducing general malaise.
- Calcium channel blockers—Some of the older types of calcium channel blockers have been associated with an increased risk for certain cancers.
- ACE inhibitors—Examples include Monopril, Lotensin, Capoten, and Captopril. Side effects include headache, dizziness, GI distress, and a chronic nonproductive cough. Other concerns are that ACE inhibitors may deplete iron and magnesium. Also patients should avoid potassium supplements and limit Na, Ca, and alcohol.

Some herbs that have purported antihypertensive effects include blue cohosh, cayenne, cola nut, ephedra, ginger, ginseng, grape seed, green tea, hawthorn, kola nut, *Verbena*, vervain, yerba mate, lavender, licorice, maté, and yohimbe.

It is important that the patient consult his or her physician prior to decreasing or increasing the dose of medication. Older patients may forget to take their medication (or with diuretics, potassium supplementation) or decide to stop taking medication because of the cost. It is important to ask questions regarding any change in medication, in particular with those patients who appeared to be under control, yet now have a high BP. For these patients, consider in the older patient renal stenosis as the cause.

Lipid-Lowering Drugs

There are several classifications of drugs used to lower lipids. The two major mechanisms are to block absorption and/or to block intrinsic production in the liver.

- 3-hydroxy-3-methylglutaryl coenzyme A (HMGCoA) reductase inhibitors ("statins" such as Lipitor, Crestor, Zocor, Mevacor, Pravachol)—

Inhibit the conversion of HMG-CoA to mevalonic acid, which is needed for cholesterol production. Also, statin use may lead to an increase in LDLc receptors, lowering LDLc levels. Avoid alcohol, red yeast rice, grapefruit, and St. John's wort. It is also important to limit soluble fiber at the time of ingestion of these drugs. They are metabolized by CYP3A4. Due to hepatotoxicity, statins require liver function testing every 6 to 12 weeks. A common complaint seen in the chiropractor's office is muscle achiness and sometimes weakness.

- Cholesterol absorption blockers—Ezetimibe (Zetia) is used alone or with statins (e.g., with Zocor it is marketed as Vytorin). It decreases cholesterol levels but has not been shown to improve cardiovascular risk compared to placebo. It prevents cholesterol absorption from the small intestine at the brush border. Another drug, probucol (Lorelco) may inhibit the absorption of cholesterol and decrease LDLc levels.
- Bile acid–binding resins (cholestyramine [Questran] and colestipol [Colestid])—These combine with bile acids and salts and then are excreted in feces; removal of bile acids causes conversion of cholesterol to bile acids, which reduces blood levels of cholesterol.
- Nicotinic acid (niacin)—Examples include Niaspan and Niacor. It is often combined with Lipitor. Nicotinic acid decreases hepatic production of LDLc and increases levels of HDLc (significantly lower doses are needed to increase HDLc) through inhibition of triglyceride lipase and induction of lipoprotein lipase. Common side effects are nausea, flushing (which can be avoided or decreased by taking aspirin 30 minutes prior to administration for first week), gout, jaundice, and liver damage (liver enzymes should be checked every three months). Nutrient interactions require a recommendation to avoid alcohol, hot liquids, and spicy foods.
- Fibric acid derivatives (gemfibrozil [Lopid])—Decrease triglycerides, raise HDLc, do not have much effect on LDLc.
- Estrogen replacement therapy—Estrogen raises HDLc levels, lowers LDLc; however, may increase triglyceride levels; progestogens typically lower HDLc levels.

The use of these drugs is somewhat controversial given that there are, as with most drugs, contraindications to their use, side effects, and cost considerations. In general, in patients with isolated LDLc elevations, bile acid–binding resins or statins are used first. For those with mixed hyperlipidemia, nicotinic acid (if tolerated) is the first drug used; if not effective, gemfibrozil or one of the statins is used. For isolated triglyceride elevation, niacin is used. However, niacin can unmask or increase the risk of developing diabetes.

Anticoagulants

For patients who have stroke or other thromboembolic events such as deep vein thrombosis, anticoagulants are often prescribed on a limited basis. As a prophylactic for patients at high risk, daily aspirin is recommended, although the value is less for those not at high risk. The most common prescribed drug is warfarin (Coumadin). Coumadin interferes with several clotting factors (II, VII, IX, X). Side effects may include nausea, diarrhea, hypotension, fatigue, headache, and alopecia. Patients should be constantly monitored for prothrombin time. Metabolized by CYP2C9, patients should avoid supplements containing vitamin K, vitamin E, vitamin A, CoQ_{10}, St. John's wort, turmeric, milk thistle, tea, anticoagulants (garlic, ginger, ginkgo, ginseng, saw palmetto, fish oils and avocado). More recently clopidogrel (Plavix) has begun to be used commonly as an anticoagulant.

Respiratory Drugs

Drugs used for management of the respiratory tract include the following categories:

- Infection (see below under anti-infection section)
- Allergic reactions
- Chronic obstructive pulmonary diseases (COPDs) including asthma, chronic bronchitis, and emphysema

Antihistamines

Antihistamines (H_1 blockers) such as Zyrtec, Dramamine, Benadryl, Claritin, and Sudafed all block the release of histamine from mast cells in response to IgE-mediated allergies. They bind to H_1 receptors on blood vessels, bronchiolar smooth muscle, and intestinal smooth muscle in an attempt to avoid itching, redness, and swelling, and inflammatory reactions in the bronchial tree (e.g., cromolyn sodium [Intal]). Benadryl inhibits CYP2D6.

Bronchodilators

For COPDs, beta-2 receptor stimulation or anticholinergic drugs that decrease parasympathetic activity both result in bronchodilation. Beta-2s such as Albuterol (Ventolin), Formoterol, and Terbutaline increase the synthesis of cAMP, which causes bronchodilation and prevents synthesis and secretion of inflammatory compounds from mast cells. Bronchodilators such as methylxanthines (a caffeine derivative) inhibit the enzyme that degrades cAMP. One example, theophylline (Theodur) is metabolized by CYP1A2 and may deplete B_6 and thiamine. Anticholinergics such as Spiriva are inhaled. These are not as effective as beta-2s. Combination drugs include Symbicort and Advair, which are a combination of a beta-2 agonist and anti-inflammatory.

Some substances with purported bronchodilator effects are alpha-linolenic acid, coffee, black tea, *Boswellia* (genus), *Tylophora* (genus), butterbur, choline, coleus, ephedra, fish oil, green tea, hawthorn, *Lactobacillus acidophilus*, lycopene, melatonin, omega-3 fatty acids, perilla, Pycnogenol, selenium, vitamin B_6, and vitamin C.

Anti-Inflammatory Drugs for COPD

Corticosteroids are utilized for those with severe COPDs. They inhibit activity of inflammatory cells, prevent the release of inflammatory compounds from mast cells, decrease the production of IgE, and reduce edema. They may be administered orally or through an inhaler (i.e., aerosol). Oral corticosteroids used for over seven weeks may result in severe adverse effects including osteoporosis, soft tissue damage, anemia, Cushing's disease, and so on. Aerosol corticosteroids are cleared on their first pass through the liver so do not carry as severe a restriction. However, used as an inhaler, they do carry the risk of causing oral candidiasis. This is decreased through the use of what is called a spacer added to the inhaler. Corticosteroids such as prednisone and hydrocortisone are metabolized by CYP3A4.

Lipoxygenase (LOX) inhibitors such as Zyflo prevent leukotriene formation, thus preventing bronchoconstriction and inflammation. It is metabolized by CYP1A2. Singulair is similar. Its main mechanism is to block leukotriene receptors, which then prevents the production of inflammatory cytokines. Singulair inhibits CYP2C8.

Gastrointestinal Drugs

Gastroesophageal Reflux Disease (GERD) and Peptic Ulcers

One concern in the upper GI is hyperchlorhydria. The result may be peptic ulcers that include the esophagus, stomach, or duodenum. The approach is either to decrease the production of hydrochloric acid, buffer its effects, or eradicate *H. pylori* as a source of hyperchlorhydria. As a normal process, acetylcholine (ACH) causes the release of enzymes, gastrin, histamine, and HCl. Specifically, gastrin releases histamine. Histamine then binds to H2-receptors on parietal cells, releasing HCl. Antacids or the newer OTC H₂ antagonists usually help for short-term relief. Alcohol and smoking also increase HCl production and limitation or cessation will help. Antacids such as Tums, Rolaids, Maalox, and Mylanta neutralize acid already released but may cause nutrient depletions for calcium, phosphorus, copper, iron, magnesium, potassium, and zinc. H2-receptor antagonists (antihistamines) such as Tagamet, Pepcid, Axid, and Zantac are now sold OTC and competitively inhibit histamine from binding to receptors, preventing acid secretion. They too should be used only for short-term relief. It should be noted that Tagamet inhibits CYP2C9, CYP2D6, and CYP3A4, thus impairing the metabolism of many drugs. Also, Zantac prevents warfarin (Coumadin) clearance and inhibits CYP2D6. An older less commonly used drug is Carafate (Sucralfate), which binds proteins building up a protective mucosal barrier.

The next step is to provide a neutralizing effect and also provide for ulcer healing. Proton pump inhibitors (PPIs) such as Nexium, Prevacid, and Prilosec inhibit the exchange of H+ and K+ ions in parietal cells, thus decreasing HCl secretion. Omeprazole (Prilosec) is the standard for treatment of GI reflux. However, long-term use may lead to problems with absorption of calcium and other important nutrients. The most serious side effect is osteoporosis and an increased risk of fracture.[10] Unfortunately, pediatricians are prescribing this medication for infants with colic, increasing the risk of decreased absorption and possible increased risk of infection.[11, 12] Prilosec prevents excretion of warfarin and diazepam, and inhibits the absorption of Plavix (an anticoagulant). Also, Prilosec induces CYP1A2 and inhibits CYP2C19.

Most importantly, gastroesophageal reflux should not be confused with the temporary reflux of infants. A concern that has warranted strong editorial warnings is that medical doctors are prescribing proton-pump inhibitors for infants with reflux. The critics of this approach feel that this practice is more for the parents than the infant and may harm the infant with regard to important nutritional absorption and potentially increase risk for infection.

For duodenal ulcers, the mainstay is not an attempt to irradiate an underlying *H. pylori* overgrowth infection. This "triple therapy" is a combination of omeprazole or lansoprazole (proton-pump inhibitor) with metronidazole (Flagyl) and amoxicillin (antibiotics). For gastric ulcers, discontinuing NSAIDs combined with a two- to three-month course of H₂ antagonists or sucralfate (a drug that acts locally as a mucous bandage) is usually effective.

Irritable Bowel Syndrome (IBS) Drugs

Generally, the two main problems with IBS are distention and pain, coupled with either or both diarrhea and constipation. The prescribing physician attempts to match the drug based on the predominance of either diarrhea or constipation related to specific serotonin receptors. For pain and diarrhea, selective serotonin (5-HT3) receptor antagonists (Alosetron) are utilized. These receptors are located throughout the myenteric plexus and have affect on distention perception, GI motility, and secretions. For patients with primarily constipation and pain, a serotonin 5-HT4 receptor agonist is used (Tegaserod). The 5-HT4 receptor, a serotonin receptor, normalizes intestinal contractions. In addition, this medication acts to raise the pain threshold for distention of the colon. Other medications specific to diarrhea or constipation may also be used.

Antidiarrhea Drugs

There are generally three types of medications available:

1. Antimotility drugs—Loperamide (Imodium) is the most common type and quite effective (codeine is an effective prescription drug).
2. Antisecretory drugs—Bismuth subsalicylate (Pepto-Bismol) reduces diarrhea through prostaglandin inhibition (aspirin has some effect).
3. Absorbents—Kaopectate (mainly clay and pectin from apples/citrus fruits) bulks up the stool.

The primary goal of management of the immunosuppressed or infants is to maintain proper glucose and electrolytes. Sports drinks are not appropriate because the fluid must be hypoosmolar. For infants, several OTC drinks are available, such as Pedialyte. A simple home concoction is a mixture of ½ tsp salt, 1 tsp baking soda, 8 tsp sugar, and 8 oz of orange juice diluted in water to produce 1 L of liquid.

Anticonstipation (Laxative) Drugs

Bulk-forming agents act similarly to fiber. When ingested these agents form emollients and gels when they mix with intestinal water, expanding their size. This distention increases peristaltic activity. One side effect with these agents is that they may contribute to gas production, causing distention and discomfort. Lubricants (i.e., mineral oils) are of limited value. Chronic use may impair fat-soluble vitamin absorption and lead also to a chronic perianal inflammatory response. Salts are used for their osmotic effects of drawing in fluid and increasing reflex colon contractions. They are usually the sulfate or phosphate salts of sodium and magnesium ions (saline cathartics). A similar action occurs with lactulose; however, lactulose has no effect on the small bowel. Another group of agents is referred to as surface-active agents. They act to decrease colonic absorption and increase secretion. Stimulation of adenylate cyclase and prostaglandin E, inhibition of sodium absorption, and alteration in mucosal permeability are all possible mechanisms of these agents. Castor oil is an example of a surface-acting agent.

Rectal enemas or suppositories are usually in the form of glycerin, bisacodyl, water (tap and saline), and soaps (usually castile). These should be reserved for the patient with impaction. Chronic use may lead to colitis.

Medications Used in the Management of the Female Patient

Contraceptives

Contraceptives are used to prevent pregnancy by inhibiting the release of follicle stimulating hormone (FSH) and luteinizing hormone (LH) necessary for ovulation. They are also used to regulate menstruation, especially for those with physiological vaginal bleeding. Either alone or in combination, estrogen and progesterone are the primary hormones utilized. Examples include some monophasics: Loestrin, Ortho-Novum, Yasmin, Yaz;

and triphasics such as Ortho Tri-Cyclen. Other options include an injection (Depo-Provera) or an intrauterine device (Mirena). Side effects are largely related to the sodium retention caused by estrogen, including edema, hypertension, weight gain, and depression. Diabetics may have restrictions due to an increase in insulin secretion that may occur with some of the drugs. Some nutritional concerns are depletion of many B vitamins including folate, vitamins B_6 and B_{12}, riboflavin, magnesium, and zinc.

Fertility Drugs

The opposite of contraceptives, fertility drugs are used to stimulate ovulation by effecting LH and FSH. The effect does not focus on the Graafian follicle but includes multiple follicles, which leads to a risk of multiple fetuses. Examples include Clomid, Follistim (peptide), and human chorionic gonadotropin (hCG). Side effects include those similar to dysmenorrhea including bloating, hot flashes, headache, pelvic pain, and breast pain. There may be an increase in ovarian cysts.

Medications for Osteoporosis

Although in the past, estrogen replacement therapy and calcitonin have been the mainstay for the prevention of further bone loss in postmenopausal females, three new therapies are now becoming first-line therapy:

- Selective estrogen receptor modulators (raloxifene)
- Bisphosphonates (alendronate and risedronate)
- Parathyroid hormone

Both raloxifene and the bisphosphonates comprise a group of medications classified as antiresorptive. These medications inhibit bone resorption but eventually reduce bone formation due to a decrease in overall bone turnover. A standard intermittent treatment program with parathyroid hormone is intended to increase bone formation; however, it also increases bone resorption. The net effect, however, is bone formation. It is clear that prolonged exposure to parathyroid hormone such as in hyperparathyroidism causes osteoporosis. Intermittent use through daily subcutaneous injections has an anabolic effect, particularly with trabecular bone. The effect on cortical bone may be an increase in cortical porosity, yet most of this occurs at the endocortical surface (partially at the Haversian canals), having little mechanical effect (i.e., no increased risk of fracture). A recent study confirmed the effect of increased trabecular bone content in parathyroid treated patients versus combination treatment with alendronate and parathyroid.[13] A separate study in men confirmed the same effect. Additional findings indicate that any initial benefit of combined therapy changes over time, so that those treated with parathyroid hormone had higher bone mineral density than with combination therapy.[14] In fact, it appears that alendronate may reduce the beneficial effects of parathyroid treatment. The positive effect of parathyroid hormone therapy on reducing the risk of fracture has been demonstrated in one study.[15] Although it appears that 5-reductase inhibitors (statins) have been demonstrated to increase bone formation in vitro and in vivo in some studies, a recent study indicated that this had no effect on fracture risk for postmenopausal females.[16]

Calcitonin appears to have two effects. In addition to increasing bone density, it may reduce pain significantly in some patients. The infrequent complaints of nausea and flushing are usually managed by beginning with a low dose given at bedtime. Newer approaches that are being investigated are fluoride and parathyroid hormone use.

Incontinence Medications

Parasympathetic activation is necessary for micturition. Medications for inhibiting this stimulation are directed mainly at the receptors, including muscarinic receptors, anticholinergics, or smooth muscle relaxants (antispasmodic). This is particularly true of drugs used in the management of detrusor instability or unstable bladder.

- Muscarinic receptor (antagonist) blockers—VESIcare, Ditropan, Detrol
- Anticholinergic, antispasmodic—Oxytrol

Medications Used in the Management of the Male Patient

Erectile Dysfunction

Frequently marketed in television advertising are medications to address erectile dysfunction (ED). However, prior to being prescribed these medications, it is important to understand that there are underlying treatable disorders that may lead to ED. The most common disorders are diabetes, atherosclerosis, surgery for prostate cancer, and a multitude of medications. When age is the primary factor, these medications may be of benefit. The primary mechanism of these medications is stimulation of central release of nitric oxide and selective inhibition of phosphodiesterase type 5, preventing metabolism of cGMP. Common examples include Viagra, Cialis, and Levitra. Side effects include hypotension and resulting orthostatic hypotension leading to a complaint of dizziness upon rising, headache, flushing, nasal congestion, rash, diarrhea, and photophobia. It is important to avoid grapefruit and limit alcohol intake.

Benign Prostatic Hypertrophy (BPH)

BPH is one of the most common disorders of older males. Compression of the urethra by the surrounding prostate results in symptoms related to difficulty starting a stream, frequent urination, and sometimes dysuria. Risk factors include the use of beta-blockers often used for hypertension. Higher physical activity seems to decrease risk. Lower androgen levels may also decrease risk as is seen in cirrhosis of the liver with chronic alcoholism. The most effective medications are alpha-adrenergic antagonists such as Flomax and Hytrin, which in part reduce smooth muscle tone in the prostate. Other commonly used drugs are 5-alpha reductase inhibitors, which block the conversion of testosterone to 5 alpha DHT (responsible for prostate hypertrophy). Examples are Proscar and Avodart.

Low Testosterone (Testosterone Deficiency)

Low testosterone is defined as levels < 300 ng/dL. Symptoms in addition to low sexual drive include decrease in muscle mass and strength, and fatigue. Clearly, these may also be related in part to aging, and certainly are related to other disorders that may be risk factors such as obesity, diabetes, and COPD. Causes may include undescended testicles, mumps infection (orchitis), Cushing syndrome, hemochromatosis, TB, HIV/AIDS, and testicular trauma. Luteinizing hormone released from the pituitary stimulates the release of testosterone from the testes. Treatment is with testosterone gels such as AndroGel and Testim. Patients who use these medications are cautioned not to transfer the gel to females or children, which may result in increased testosterone and its effects. Other approaches include a patch (Androderm and Testoderm) and injection with Delatestryl or Depo-Testosterone.

Hormonal Imbalance

Thyroid

There are primarily two main causes of thyroid dysfunction. For hyperthyroidism it is usually the auto-immune disorder Graves' disease and for hypothyroidism, the auto-immune disorder Hashimoto's disease. For hypothyroidism, Synthroid and Armour Thyroid are the primary synthetics utilized. When taking Synthroid separate by 4 hours from the ingestion of Ca, Fe, or Mg supplements, soy, walnuts, or high-fiber meals. For hyperthyroidism, primarily Graves' disease, treatment may be surgical, with radiation, or through medication. The primary drug used is Propylthiouracil. The intention is to destroy the function of the thyroid, leading to the eventual need of Synthroid or Armour Thyroid.

Diabetes

Diabetes is categorized as type-1 diabetes mellitus (DM) associated with pancreatic failure to produce insulin and the acquired, type-2 DM which starts as decreased insulin production and decreased sensitivity of insulin receptors. For type-1 DM, insulin is given by subcutaneous injection in the arms, abdomen, thighs, or buttocks using pen injections or pump delivery systems. There are many factors affecting insulin requirements and absorption when injected including colds, fever, infections, illness, surgery, stress, and exercise. Side effects are related mainly to hypoglycemia, but also include allergic reactions, and lipodystrophy at the injection site. Some contraindicated supplements include melatonin, chaparral, tobacco, herbal tea, broccoli, cabbage, charbroiled meats, shiitake mushrooms, and turmeric.

Medical management of type-2 diabetes includes the use of the following drugs prior to resorting to insulin:

- Sulfonylureas (e.g., glipizide [Glucotrol], glyburide [Glynase, Micronase, DiaBeta], glimepiride [Amaryl], chlorpropamide [Diabinese])—close energy-sensitive potassium channels on beta cells causing influx of calcium and subsequent release of insulin
- Biguanides (e.g., Glucophage [metformin])—hypoglycemic action is based on its effect of decreasing glucose production from the liver
- Thiazolidinones (e.g., Actos [pioglitazone], Avandia [rosiglitazone])—attach to nuclear receptors in cells to cause an increase in production of cellular proteins that facilitate glucose transport. Note Avandia has been taken off the market in Europe since fall of 2010 and restricted in the United States to patients who do not respond to other medications due to its associated increase in cardiovascular risk. Inhibits CYP2C8.
- Alphaglucosidase inhibitors (e.g., Acarbose [Precose], Miglitol [Glyset])—reduces the rate of digestion of carbohydrates by competitive inhibition of enzymes needed to digest carbohydrates
- Dipeptidyl peptidase 4 inhibitor (e.g., sitagliptin [Januvia])—increases incretin levels, which inhibit glucagon which allows increase in insulin secretion. Incretins are a group of proteins secreted by the GI tract along with glucose that enhance insulin secretion in the pancreas. These include glucagon-like peptide-1 (GLP-1) and gastric inhibitory peptide (GIP). GLP-1 also inhibits glucagon secretion and delays gastric emptying.
- GLP-1 receptor agonist injectables—Exenatide (Byetta) and Liraglutide (Victoza).
- SGLT2 inhibitors (e.g., canagliflozin [Invokana®], dapagliflozin [Farxiga®])—act by blocking the kidneys' reabsorption of glucose. The result is decreased plasma glucose due to loss in the urine. Soon to be released is a GLP-1 receptor agonist that is delivered intranasally not requiring injection.

Tables B–8 and **B–9** list common examples of medications based on generic and product name, and list common side effects. There are many handbooks with far

Table B–8 Some Common Medications (Listed by Generic Name)

Name	Examples	Mechanism/Use	Some Side Effects/Concerns
Abatacept	Orencia	A disease-modifying antirheumatic drug (DMARD) which inhibits T-cell proliferation and tumor necrosis factor alpha, gamma-interferon and interleukin-2, and decreases anticollagen antibody production. Used in the management of rheumatoid arthritis in patients who have an inadequate response to other MARDs. Used as monotherapy or in combination. Given as IV infusion.	May cause hypersensitivity reactions, headache, dizziness, hypertension, upper respiratory infection, malignancies, or urinary tract infections.

(continues)

Table B–8 Some Common Medications (Listed by Generic Name) (continued)

Name	Examples	Mechanism/Use	Some Side Effects/Concerns
Acyclovir	Zovirax Acycloguanosine	Interferes with DNA synthesis for specific viruses including herpes simplex 1 and 2, varicella-roster, and cytomegalovirus. It does not eliminate the latent herpes virus.	May cause headache, nausea, vomiting, diarrhea, and, rarely, acute renal failure, thrombocytopenia purpura, or hemolytic uremic syndrome.
Adalimumab	Humira	A disease-modifying antirheumatic drug (DMARD) used alone or with methotrexate for the treatment of rheumatoid arthritis and similar disorders. A human monoclonal antibody, it works by blocking tumor necrosis factor (TNF) alpha, a major protein involved in inflammation.	May cause a local injection response, rash, or increase the risk of serious infection such as tuberculosis, neurologic events, or malignancies. Very expensive.
Albuterol	Ventolin Proventil	Beta-2 agonist used in the treatment of asthma. Causes bronchodilation without secondary vascular and cardiac effects.	May cause anorexia, tachycardia, nausea, arrhythmias, tremor, hypertension, muscle cramps, convulsions, weakness, hallucinations, or postural hypotension.
Alendronate	Fosamax	Bisphosphonate; antiresorptive used in the treatment of osteoporosis and Paget's disease. These medications inhibit bone resorption but eventually reduce bone formation due to a decrease in overall bone turnover. A standard intermittent treatment program with parathyroid hormone is intended to increase bone formation; however, it also increases bone resorption. The net effect though is bone formation. It is clear that prolonged exposure to parathyroid hormone such as in hyperparathyroidism causes osteoporosis.	Hypocalcemia. GI effects include esophageal irritation/ulceration with abdominal pain, nausea, vomiting, diarrhea/constipation, arthralgias, myalgias, headache, and rash. Dairy products decrease absorption.
Allopurinol	Alloprin Lopurin Novopurinol Zyloprim	A xanthine oxidase inhibitor used in the treatment of gout. It decreases endogenous uric acid. Inhibiting xanthine oxidase prevents conversion of hypoxanthine to xanthine and then xanthine to uric acid. Not used for anti-inflammatory effect.	May cause nausea, vomiting, diarrhea, and abdominal pain. Concerns over possible hepatotoxicity, renal insufficiency, aplastic anemia, and thrombocytopenia. Check CBC and liver function tests.
Alosetron	Lotronex	Selective serotonin (5-HT3) receptor antagonist. These receptors are located throughout the myenteric plexus and affect distention perception, GI motility, and secretions. Used in the control of abdominal pain and diarrhea with irritable bowel syndrome in women.	May cause constipation, ischemic colitis, urinary frequency, muscle cramps, weakness, and anxiety.
Alprazolam	Xanax	A benzodiazepine sedative causing CNS depression. Suggested sites of action are the limbic, thalamus, and hypothalamus. Used in the treatment of anxiety, panic attacks, insomnia, and muscle spasms. Also used as adjunctive therapy with depression (associated anxiety).	May cause lethargy. Some concern over dependency/abuse and withdrawal problems.

Table B–8 Some Common Medications (Listed by Generic Name) (continued)

Name	Examples	Mechanism/Use	Some Side Effects/Concerns
Amantadine	Symmetrel	A medication that is effective as an antiviral against influenza A (not B) and also as an initial or adjunct therapy with anticholinergic drugs for Parkinson's. Anti-parkinsonian effects may be due to effect of release of dopamine and other catecholamines.	May cause dizziness, lightheadedness, difficulty with memory, hallucinations, confusion, mood or other mental effects, nausea, vomiting, or dry mouth.
Amiloride	Midamor	A potassium-sparing diuretic without direct effects on aldosterone used in the management of CHF, hypertension, or hepatic cirrhosis. Usually combined with a thiazide or loop diuretic.	May cause headache, diarrhea, nausea, aplastic anemia, rash, weakness, cramps, hyperkalemia, or hyponatremia.
Amitriptyline	Elavil Endep	Increases levels of serotonin and to a lesser degree norepinephrine through inhibition of reuptake at the presynaptic neuron in the brain. It is used for depression and associated insomnia, restlessness, and nervousness. Also used for fibromyalgia and chronic pain.	May cause drowsiness, sedation, dizziness, orthostatic hypotension, tachycardia, increased appetite, weight gain, urinary retention, or constipation.
Amlodipine/ Atorvastatin	Caduet	A combination antihypertensive (selective calcium channel blocker) medication with a statin (5 reductase inhibitor) used as an adjunct to diet in the treatment of primary hypertension.	May cause back pain, myalgia, constipation, diarrhea, flatulence, palpitations, tachycardia, facial edema, postural hypotension, headache, sexual dysfunction.
Amoxicillin	Amoxil Polymox Larotid Trimox	Penicillin-type antibiotic (bacterial cell-wall inhibitor). Inhibits mucoprotein synthesis of cell wall in rapidly reproducing cells. Used for infections of the middle ear, throat, bronchi, and lungs. Also for UTI, skin infections, and gonorrhea. Specific susceptible organisms include *H. influenzae*, *N. gonorrhea*, *E. coli*, pneumococci, streptococci, and some forms of staphylococci.	Similar to other penicillin medications, possibility of hypersensitivity with rash, anaphylaxis. Also possible are hemolytic anemia, eosinophilia, pseudomembranous colitis, pruritus, and urticaria.
Amphotericin B Amphotericin B Lipid Based	Amphocin Fungizone Amphotec Abelcet	An antifungal that binds to sterols in the fungus cell membrane. Produced from *Streptomyces nodosus*. Used intravenously to treat serious, life-threatening fungal infections such as aspergillosis, blastomycosis, coccidioidomycosis, cryptococcosis, histoplasmosis, and others.	May cause fever, chills, anaphylaxis, cardiac arrest, nephrotoxicity, hypokalemia, hypomagnesemia, and super-infections.
Ampicillin	Amcil Penbritin Omnipen Totacillin	Broad-spectrum antibiotic. Effective against Gram-positives such as alpha- and beta-hemolytic streptococci, diplococci, pneumoniae, staphylococci, and *Listeria*. Also against some Gram-negatives such as *E. coli*, *N. gonorrhea*, *Proteus*, shigella, *Salmonella*, mycoplasma, some viruses, and fungi.	Possible anaphylaxis, diarrhea, pseudomembranous colitis, and rash.
Aripiprazole	Abilify	A psychotropic drug used in the management of schizophrenia, bipolar disorder, and adjunctive therapy for major depressive disorder.	Not recommended for the elderly with dementia-related psychosis. May cause tardive dyskinesias, orthostatic hypotension, seizures, worsening of suicidal risk, neuroleptic malignant syndrome, hyperglycemia, diabetes, cognitive impairment, body temperature regulation interference, nausea, vomiting, constipation, headache, dizziness, anxiety, or insomnia.

(continues)

Table B–8 Some Common Medications (Listed by Generic Name) (continued)

Name	Examples	Mechanism/Use	Some Side Effects/Concerns
Aspirin (acetylsalicylic acid)	Alka-Seltzer A.S.A. Aspergum Bayer Cosprin Easprin Ecotrin Empirin Entrophen Novasen St. Joseph's Triaphen-10 ZORprin	Inhibits the formation of proinflammatory prostaglandins. Acts as an anti-inflammatory, antipyretic, and analgesic. Also has an antiplatelet effect. Used in the management of pain, fever, and prophylactically for its anticlotting action to prevent stroke (transient ischemic attack), recurrence of MI, and thrombus formation (such as deep vein thrombosis).	Some individuals are allergic to aspirin and may have a hypersensitivity reaction including an asthma-like response. Heartburn and stomach upset may be due to irritation leading to peptic ulcer formation. Anemia may be due to blood loss or hemolytic anemia. Ototoxic effects include tinnitus and hearing loss. High doses may impair renal function.
Atenolol	Tenormin	Beta-blocker: A β-adrenergic antagonist blocking primarily $\beta1$ receptors (less bronchoconstriction effect than $\beta2$ blockers), decreases heart rate and rennin release used in the treatment of hypertension.	CNS depressive effects with concerns for those with diabetes, heart block and heart failure, asthma, and emphysema.
Atomoxetine	Strattera	Strattera is a selective norepinephrine reuptake inhibitor used for the treatment of Attention Deficit Hyperactivity Disorder (ADHD).	Decreased appetite, sleeping problems, constipation, dry mouth, nausea, allergic reactions, dizziness, lethargy, mood swings.
Atorvastatin	Lipitor	A statin: An HMGCoA reductase inhibitor. This blocks the enzyme that controls production of cholesterol in the liver. Therefore used in the treatment of hyperlipidemia. Lowers both total cholesterol and LDL cholesterol while increasing HDL cholesterol. Atorvastatin is different from other statins in that it reduces triglycerides. These effects may retard or reverse coronary artery disease.	GI upset, headache, myalgia, weakness, rhabdomyolysis, ocular and liver toxicity. Should have liver enzymes monitored.
Azithromycin	Zithromax	A macrolide antibiotic primarily effective against pyogenic streptococci, *S. pneumoniae*, *H. influenzae*, and *S. aureus*. Interferes with protein synthesis by binding to 50S ribosome of bacteria.	May cause headache, dizziness, hepatotoxic effects such as mild elevation of liver enzymes, and usual GI complaints.
Bevacizumab	Avastin	A recombinant humanized monoclonal IgG1 antibody that binds to and inhibits vascular endothelial growth factor. In combination with other chemotherapy used in the treatment of non-small cell lung cancer and metastatic colorectal cancer. As an injectable into the eye, used for the treatment of the wet variety of age-related macular degeneration.	Intravenous use may cause GI perforation. May also cause delayed wound healing, hemoptysis, hypertensive crisis, nervous system and visual disturbances, neutropenia, nephrotic syndrome, or congestive heart failure.
Bisacodyl	Apo-Bisacodyl Bisacolax Deficol Dulcolax Fleet Laxit Theralax	Used in the management of constipation. It increases intestinal fluid volume through increasing epithelial permeability.	May cause mild cramping or nausea. May have mild electrolyte disturbances.

Table B–8 Some Common Medications (Listed by Generic Name) (continued)

Name	Examples	Mechanism/Use	Some Side Effects/Concerns
Bismuth	Pepto-Bismol	Hydrolyzed to salicylate that inhibits inflammatory prostaglandins. Used as an antidiarrheal both prophylactic and treatment. Also for temporary relief of indigestion.	May cause temporary darkening of stool, a metallic taste in the mouth, a bluish gum line, and possible bleeding tendencies.
Botulinum Toxin Type A	Botox	In addition to standard cosmetic uses, injectable Botox is used for patients with cervical dystonia, primary axillary hyperhidrosis, strabismus, or blepharospasm.	May cause anaphylaxis, dysphagia, cardiovascular adverse events such as arrhythmias, MI (some fatal), skin rash, or pruritus.
Bretylium tosylate	Bretylol Bretylate	An adrenergic blocker having an effect on ventricular fibrillation and also a peripheral vascular effect that initially leads to postural hypotension. Used specifically for re-entry arrhythmias.	May cause dizziness, headache, syncope, bradycardia, nausea, vomiting, and postural hypotension.
Bromocriptine	Parlodel	Reduces prolactin levels through a series of events, activation of dopaminergic receptors in the hypothalamus, which then releases prolactin inhibiting factor. Used for amenorrhea/galactorrhea or female infertility, but also used as adjunctive therapy to levodopa for Parkinson's.	May cause headache, agitation, nervousness, mania, orthostatic hypotension, Raynaud's, depression, acute MI, or shock.
Bupivacaine	Marcaine Sensorcaine	An anesthetic that acts as a sodium channel blocker resulting in effects primarily in the medulla and higher centers. Effects patient's reaction to pain, temperature, proprioception, and muscle tone. Used as a sympathetic and peripheral nerve block agent. Used for postoperative pain, trigeminal neuralgia, kidney (ureteral) stones, and accidental trauma pain.	May cause sedation, drowsiness, dizziness, headache, amnesia, insomnia, withdrawal symptoms, nausea, vomiting, or constipation.
Bupropion	Wellbutrin Zyban Wellbutrin SR	Inhibits the reuptake of dopamine, serotonin, and norepinephrine with the major effect on dopamine. Wellbutrin is used in the treatment of depression; Zyban has been approved as an aid for smoking cessation.	Possible problems with seizures, hepatotoxicity, nausea, vomiting, headache, agitation, tremor, and anticholinergic effects.
Captopril	Capoten	Angiotensin-converting enzyme (ACE) inhibitor used in the management of hypertension, congestive heart failure, diabetic nephropathy, left ventricular dysfunction, and post MI.	May cause hypersensitivity reactions, angioedema, persistent cough, orthostatic hypotension, altered taste sensation, or positive ANA titers.
Carbamazepine	Carbatrol Tegretol Tegretol-XR	Sodium potassium and calcium currents are reduced across neuronal membranes decreasing neuronal transmission. Has an antidiuretic effect. Used in the treatment of seizures and facial neuralgias, also sometimes schizophrenia.	CNS toxicity including sedation, dizziness, imbalance, and nausea/vomiting. Agranulocytosis or aplastic anemia. Also possible cause of birth defects.
Carbidopa	Sinemet Lodosyn	Prevents peripheral metabolism of levodopa, in effect making more available to the brain. Also prevents the inhibitory effects of pyridoxine (B_6) on levodopa. Used in the management of Parkinson's.	May cause visual disturbances, GI problems, confusion, involuntary movements, hallucinations, dyskinesia, hypotension, and depression with suicidal tendencies.

(continues)

Table B–8 Some Common Medications (Listed by Generic Name) (continued)

Name	Examples	Mechanism/Use	Some Side Effects/Concerns
Celecoxib	Celebrex	NSAID: Cyclooxygenase (COX) 2 inhibitor (does not inhibit COX-1) used primarily for arthritis (osteo and rheumatoid, and rheumatoid variants), acute pain, and menstrual cramps. Reduces fever. Also approved to prevent and reduce the size of polyps in patients with genetic disease.	May cause back pain, peripheral edema, GI problems, dizziness, headache, pharyngitis, and rash.
Cephalexin	Keflex, Keftabs	A semi-synthetic cephalosporin antibiotic (similar to penicillin; β-lactam binds penicillin-binding proteins inhibiting crosslinking of bacterial cell wall). Susceptible bacteria are Gram-positive except for enterococci and methicillin-resistant *Staph aureus* (MRSA), some Gram-negative; not anaerobes.	Hypersensitivity reactions (anaphylaxis, serum sickness), GI disturbances, rare neurologic problems (seizures), hematologic abnormalities (cytopenias), and nephrotoxicity and hepatic enzyme increases.
Chloramphenicol	Chloromycetin, Chlorofair, Fenicol, Novochloroscap	A broad-spectrum antibiotic that is primarily bacteriostatic (bactericidal to *H. influenzae*). Interferes with protein synthesis by binding to 50S ribosome of bacteria. Used when infection is serious and unaffected by other antibiotics. Examples include *Salmonella*, *Rickettsia*, *Chlamydia*, *Mycoplasma*, *Streptococcus pneumoniae*, and *Neisseria*, among others.	May cause hypersensitivity reactions, bone marrow suppression, neurotoxicity, angioedema, pancytopenia, headache, confusion, stomatitis, glossitis, and the usual GI complaints.
Chlordiazepoxide	Libritabs, Librium, Epoxide, Medilium, Novo Epoxide, Sereen	A benzodiazepine that affects sleep by suppression of REM and increasing stage 4 NREM with an increase in total sleep time. Has a mild anxiolytic effect. Used primarily for anxiety and tension and assisting sleep in these individuals.	May cause drowsiness, lethargy, depression, orthostatic hypotension, dry mouth, vertigo, syncope, photosensitivity, or urinary frequency.
Chlorothiazide	Diuril, Diachlor, SK-Chlorothiazide	A diuretic that acts at the distal convoluted tubules, inhibiting absorption of sodium, potassium, and chloride. Increases excretion of sodium, bicarbonate, and potassium. Used in the management of CHF, hepatic cirrhosis, and fluid retention from corticosteroid and estrogen therapy.	May cause hypokalemia (should supplement with potassium) with associated problems such as muscle cramps and cardiac arrhythmias, anaphylaxis, agranulocytosis (rare), hyperglycemia, or hyperuricemia.
Chlorpromazine	Chlorpromanine, Largactil, Ormazine, Promapar, Promaz, Somazina, Thorazine, Thor-Prom	A phenothiazine derivative that has alpha-adrenergic blocking effects, an antiemetic effect through depression on chemoreceptor trigger zone, and antipsychotic effects through actions (blocks post-synaptic dopamine receptors) in the hypothalamus and reticular formation. Used in the management of manic phase of manic depression, for psychotic disorders such as schizophrenia, and for severe nausea and vomiting. Also, sometimes used for behavioral disorders in attention deficit disorder in children.	A phenothiazine derivative that has alpha-adrenergic blocking effects, an antiemetic effect through depression on chemoreceptor trigger zone, and antipsychotic effects through actions (blocks post-synaptic dopamine receptors) in the hypothalamus and reticular formation. Used in the management of manic phase of manic depression, for psychotic disorders such as schizophrenia, and for severe nausea and vomiting. Also, sometimes used for behavioral disorders in attention deficit disorder in children.

Table B–8 Some Common Medications (Listed by Generic Name) (continued)

Name	Examples	Mechanism/Use	Some Side Effects/Concerns
Chlorzoxazone	Paraflex Parafon-Forte	Used as a muscle relaxant due to action of depression of nerve transmission. Has slight sedative action. Used in combination with other medications in the treatment of low back and neck pain associated with muscle spasm.	May cause drowsiness, dizziness, nausea, vomiting, constipation, rash, or jaundice.
Cholestyramine	Questran Lo-CHOLEST Prevalite	By combining with bile acids in exchange for chloride ions, an insoluble complex is formed that is excreted in the feces. Used in the management of hypercholesterolemia with reductions in both total cholesterol and LDL cholesterol.	May cause constipation; weight loss or gain; deficiencies in vitamins A, D, and K, and decreased erythrocyte folate levels; nausea; vomiting; and other GI disturbances.
Cimetidine	Novo-Cimetine Peptol Tagamet	An H2 (histamine) inhibitor blocking gastric acid secretion and raising pH of the stomach, decreasing pepsin secretion. Used as an OTC medication in the management of ulcers, GERD, and Zollinger-Ellison syndrome.	May cause the usual GI symptoms; increase pain in joints for patients with preexisting arthritis; rash; Stevens-Johnson syndrome; neutropenia; increase in uric acid, BUN, and creatinine; feminizing effects; and rarely, aplastic anemia or cardiac arrest.
Ciprofloxacin	Cipro	A synthetic quinolone that is bactericidal by inhibiting DNA-gyrase, an enzyme required for bacterial DNA replication. Often used for urinary tract infections caused by *E. coli*. Also for *C. jejuni* and shigella. Also used for bacterial conjunctivitis.	May cause nausea, vomiting, abdominal pain, cramps, and gas. May elevate liver enzymes and eosinophils. May cause tendon rupture, headache, vertigo, seizures, and rash. If used for conjunctivitis may cause precipitate buildup on cornea or crusting scales.
Cisplatin (cis-DDP or cis-PLATINUM II)	Carboplatin Oxaliplatin Platinol	A heavy metal medication (platinum) that cross-links in DNA or rapidly reproducing cells preventing DNA, RNA, and protein synthesis. Used as part of combination therapy (vinblastine and bleomycin) for patients with testicular cancer or ovarian cancer.	Anaphylactic reaction, nausea and vomiting, myelosuppression (25% to 30% of patients), hypomagnesemia, hepatio- and nephrotoxicity.
Citalopram	Celexa	A selective serotonin reuptake inhibitor (SSRI) (prevents reuptake at presynaptic neuron) making more serotonin available in the CNS. Used in the treatment of depression.	May cause fatigue, fever, arthralgia, myalgia, postural hypotension, anorexia, paresthesia, tremor, agitation, anxiety, migraine.
Clonazepam	Klonopin Rivotril	A benzodiazepine derivative that potentiates GABA and acts to inhibit seizure activity. Used alone or in combination with other medications for absence seizures, myoclonic seizures, Lennox-Gastaut, akinetic seizures, and restless leg syndrome.	May cause palpitations, dry mouth, anorexia, drowsiness, ataxia, sedation, respiratory distress, GI symptoms, diplopia, facial edema, hallucinations and other psychogenic problems.
Clonidine	Catapres	An α2 adrenergic agonist used as an anti-hypertensive. It decreases cardiac output, heart rate, and blood pressure.	Rash, drowsiness, headache, impaired ejaculation, dry mouth, and if stopped suddenly, rebound hypertension.

(continues)

Table B–8 Some Common Medications (Listed by Generic Name) (continued)

Name	Examples	Mechanism/Use	Some Side Effects/Concerns
Clopidogrel bisulfate	Plavix	Inhibits platelet aggregation by preventing ADP from binding to its platelet receptor. Used in combination with aspirin/NSAIDs to prevent stroke, MI, and vascular disease in patients who have had recent types of health events.	Should not be given to patients at risk for bleeding due to the increased bleeding time. Usual possible complaints of dizziness, headache, abdominal pain, chest pain/dyspnea, thrombocytopenia purpura, epistaxis, etc.
Clotrimazole	Lotrimin Gyne-Lotrimin Canesten Mycelex	A broad-spectrum antifungal agent that alters the fungal wall permeability allowing loss of potassium and other important elements necessary for replication. Used both for dermal fungal infections and vaginal yeast infections.	May alter liver function tests and cause the usual GI disturbances, UTI symptoms, and pruritus.
Codeine	Methylmorphine Paveral	An opiate derivative from morphine. Antihistamine effect stronger than morphine. Effective for pain relief and cough suppression.	May cause constipation, dizziness, urticaria, anaphylactic reaction, or urinary retention.
Colchicine	Novocolchine	Used as an anti-inflammatory agent in the treatment of gout. Sometimes used for sarcoid arthritis and pseudogout.	May cause nausea, vomiting, diarrhea, abdominal pain, steatorrhea, and pancreatitis. Also, a syndrome of muscle weakness may occur with accompanying elevation of serum creatine kinase.
Colestipol	Colestid Lestid Cholestabyl	By combining with bile acids in exchange for chloride ions, an insoluble complex is formed that is excreted in the feces. Used in the management of hypercholesterolemia with reductions in both total cholesterol and LDL cholesterol.	May cause constipation; weight loss or gain; deficiencies in vitamins A, D, and K, and decreased erythrocyte folate levels; nausea; vomiting; and other GI disturbances.
Cromolyn	Intal Disodium cromoglycate Fivent NasalCrom Gastrocrom Rynacrom Vistacrom	A prophylactic medication used in the management of asthma; specifically extrinsic or allergic-related asthma. Stabilizes sensitized mast cells preventing the release of histamine and SRS-A (slow-reacting substance of anaphylaxis). May also be used ophthalmologically for allergic ocular disorders.	Side effects mainly due to method of administration. Includes nasal stinging and burning, irritation of throat, nausea, rarely angioedema and bronchospasm.
Cyclizine HCL	Marezine Marzine	A specific antihistamine that depresses the labyrinth and vestibular/cerebellar pathways. Used in the management of vertigo, motion sickness, and nausea.	May cause dizziness, dry mouth, blurred vision, or fatigue.
Cyclobenzaprine	Cycloflex Flexeril	Similar in structure to tricyclic antidepressants, these medications are used as muscle relaxants acting primarily on the CNS specifically at the brainstem. Increases circulating norepinephrine by blocking reuptake effects and anticholinergic effects. Also has sedative effects and anticholinergic effects.	Drowsiness, dizziness, dry mouth, edema of the tongue, palpitations, chest pain, pruritus, and similar side effects of tricyclic antidepressants. Contraindicated for patients with heart problems.
Cyclosporine	Gengraf Neoral Sandimmune Restasis	An immunosuppressant used for organ transplant, RA, severe psoriasis, Sjogren's, and ulcerative colitis. Inhibits helper T cells. Also used for keratoconjunctivitis sicca to produce tears.	May cause hypertension, vomiting, tremor, hypermagnesemia, hyperkalemia, hyperuricemia, hyperglycemia, decreased sodium bicarbonate, pancytopenia, and nephrotoxicity. May cause sinusitis, sore throat, or tinnitus.

Table B–8 Some Common Medications (Listed by Generic Name) (continued)

Name	Examples	Mechanism/Use	Some Side Effects/Concerns
d-Amphetamine	Dexedrine	Causes the release of norepinephrine, dopamine, and serotonin from storage vesicles resulting in CNS stimulation, causing an increase in performance, coordination, and energy. There is a decrease in appetite with an increase in blood pressure. Used for narcolepsy and attention deficit disorder.	May cause restlessness, insomnia, dizziness, anorexia, psychic disturbances, and arrhythmias.
Danazol	Cyclamen Danocrine	A synthetic androgen derivative from testosterone used in the management of endometriosis and fibrocystic breast disease. Causes a reduction in FSH and LH leading to anovulation and amenorrhea.	May cause hypersensitivity reaction, weight gain, hair loss, deepening of voice, breast reduction, hot flashes, hirsutism, hot flashes, irregular menstrual periods/amenorrhea, dizziness, tremor, and rarely hepatic damage. May increase LDL cholesterol.
Dexamethasone	Decadron Aeroseb-Dex Decaderm Decaspray Dexasone Dexone Hexadrol Mymethasone Deronil Dalalone Alba-Dex	A long-acting adrenocorticoid with anti-inflammatory and immunosuppressant effects used in the treatment of adrenal insufficiency, cerebral edema, Addisonian shock, and short-term therapy for rheumatic disorders. Used as a diagnostic test for Cushing's. May also be used for antiemetic with cancer therapy.	Dependent on type of administration of medication. Can cause osteopenia, increased risk of compression fracture, posterior subcapsular cataract, hyperglycemia, impaired wound healing, ligament/tendon weakness, peptic ulcer, and skin changes.
Dextromethorphan	Balminil Benylin Delsym Mediquell Pertussin Romalar	Primarily a cough suppressant that acts on the cough center of the medulla.	May cause some drowsiness, constipation, or GI disturbances.
Diazepam	Apo-Diazepam Diastat Diazemuls Novo-Dipam Valium Vivol	Drug of choice for status epilepticus; also used as an anti-anxiety, sedative, or muscle relaxant. A long-acting benzodiazepine acting at the limbic, hypothalamic areas producing sedation.	May cause vertigo, dizziness, fatigue, laryngospasm, thorax or chest pain, incontinence or urinary retention, hiccups, hypotension, or cardiovascular collapse.
Digoxin	Lanoxin Lanoxicaps	A cardiac glycoside that increases the force and velocity of myocardial contraction. Also increases conduction velocity at AV node. Used in the management of congestive heart failure (CHF).	May cause fatigue, muscle weakness, facial neuralgia, visual disturbances, GI symptoms, paresthesias, hallucinations, arrhythmias, hypotension, and AV block.
Diphenoxylate and Atropine	Diphenatol Lofene Lomanate Lomotil Lomox Low-Quel Nor-Mil	A narcotic similar to meperidine is combined with atropine to possibly prevent deliberate overdose. Reduces GI motility by inhibiting receptors for peristalsis. Use in the management of diarrhea.	May cause hypersensitivity, swelling of gums, urinary retention, drowsiness, depression, lethargy, numbness, dry mouth, GI complaints, and palpitations or tachycardia.

(continues)

Table B–8 Some Common Medications (Listed by Generic Name) (continued)

Name	Examples	Mechanism/Use	Some Side Effects/Concerns
Diphenhydramine HCL	Allerdryl Banophen Belix Ben-Allergin Benadryl Benahist Benylin Diahist Nordryl Nytol with DPM Valdrene Many others	An H1 receptor antagonist used in the treatment of many varied conditions. Has significant anticholinergic effects and seems to prevent reuptake of dopamine. As a result, it is used for both allergic conditions, partial management of Parkinson's, as a non-narcotic cough suppressant, and as a sleep aid for those with intractable insomnia.	May cause dizziness, drowsiness, tachycardia, thickening of bronchial mucus with associated wheezing, anaphylaxis, dry mouth, and hypersensitivity.
Docusate	PMS Docusate Surfak Dialose Colace Regulax Therevac	Used as a stool softener. Through detergent action lowers surface tension allowing water and fats to penetrate stool.	May cause mild abdominal cramps, diarrhea, bitter taste, and throat irritation.
Donepezil HCL	Aricept	A cholinesterase inhibitor used in the management of mild to moderate Alzheimer's disease. Works in the cerebral cortex blocking degradation of acetylcholine.	May cause headache, fatigue, insomnia, nausea, diarrhea, vomiting, cramps, anorexia, or muscle cramps.
Doxepin	Adapin Sinequan Triadapin Zonalon	A tricyclic antidepressant that acts as a serotonin reuptake inhibitor and, to a lesser degree, norepinephrine. Used in the management of depression and anxiety.	May cause drowsiness, orthostatic hypotension, dry mouth, metallic taste, photophobia, urinary retention, or weight gain.
Doxycycline	Vibramycin	A synthetic broad-spectrum antibiotic that is bacteriostatic (inhibits protein synthesis by binding to 30s subunit blocking amino acid linked tRNA from binding to the A site of the ribosome). Susceptible bacteria include *M. pneumoniae, C. psittaci, C. trachomatis,* and *N. gonorrhea.* Used for respiratory infections, nongonococcal urethritis (ureaplasma), Rocky Mountain spotted fever, typhus, chancroid, anthrax, syphilis, cholera, brucellosis, and acne.	May cause GI distress, reversible nephro- and hepatotoxicity, photosensitivity, and dental staining (not used in prepubertal children).
Drospirenone and Estradiol	Yaz	A combination contraceptive pill that, in addition to preventing pregnancy, is used for the emotional symptoms manifested as premenstrual dysphoric disorder in a 24/4-day dosing.	May cause headache, nausea, breast pain, intermenstrual bleeding, decreased libido, upper respiratory infection, emotional lability, back pain, or urinary tract infection.
Duloxetine	Cymbalta	Used in the management of depression, it acts as a selective serotonin and norepinephrine reuptake inhibitor (SSNRI). Caution with narrow-angle glaucoma or patients taking MAOIs.	May cause fatigue, hot flashes, rashes, nausea, dry mouth, constipation, decreased appetite, decreased libido, insomnia, or tremors.

Table B–8 Some Common Medications (Listed by Generic Name) (continued)

Name	Examples	Mechanism/Use	Some Side Effects/Concerns
Dutasteride	Avodart	Blocks the conversion of testosterone to 5-alpha DHT (responsible for prostate hypertrophy). Inhibits both type 1 and 2 5-alpha reductase inhibitors.	May cause gynecomastia, ejaculation dysfunction, impotence, or decreased libido.
Edrophonium	Enlon Reversol Tensilon	An indirect cholinesterase inhibitor sometimes used as short-term management of myasthenia gravis and to reverse the effects of curariform muscle relaxants.	May cause muscle weakness, hypotension, convulsions, bronchospasm, or respiratory distress.
Enalapril	Vasotec	An ACE inhibitor. Blocks the conversion of rennin to angiotensin II thereby decreasing the release of aldosterone. This blocks the potent vasoconstriction effects of these substances resulting in a decrease in blood pressure without a compensation of increased heart rate or cardiac output.	May cause headache, dizziness, fatigue, postural hypotension, chronic cough, hoarseness, and rash. May increase potassium levels, BUN, or creatinine.
Epinephrine	Bronkaid Mist Epi E-Z Pen Epinephrine Primatene Mist Bromitin Mist Asthmahaler AsthmaNefrin Epitrate	Both synthetic and prepared from animal adrenal glands. Used in the treatment of asthma. Effects are to cause bronchial arterial constriction, bronchodilation (smooth muscle relaxation), and inhibit histamine release. Also used for anaphylactic shock, restoring sinus rhythm, open-angle glaucoma, and to reduce uterine contractions.	Causes sympathetic effects of nervousness, tremor, palpitations, tachycardia, anorexia, urinary retention, etc. Also may cause pulmonary edema, ventricular fibrillation, or MI.
Epoetin Alfa (Human Recombinant Erythropoietin)	Epogen Eprex Procrit	A glycoprotein that stimulates RBC production used to elevate the hematocrit for patients with anemia from secondary causes such as chronic kidney failure, AIDS, or malignancies.	May cause headache, nausea, diarrhea, iron deficiency, thrombocytosis, clotting of AV fistula, seizures, sweating, arthralgias, and bone pain.
Erythromycin	Akne-Mycin Ery-Tab Apo-Erythro Base A/T/S/E-Mycin Eryderm Erythromid Erythrosine Novo-Rythro Robimycin Staticin T-Stat	A macrolide antibiotic effective primarily against Gram-positive. Effective against *Chlamydia trachomatis*. Also used for pneumococcal and mycoplasma pneumonia, *N. gonorrhea*, and *H. influenzae*.	Usual GI complaints, plus superinfection with yeast, nonsusceptible bacteria, and fungi. Also causes ototoxicity (reversible vertigo, hearing loss, and tinnitus), hypersensitivity reactions, and cholestatic hepatitis syndrome.
Esomeprazole	Nexium	Similar to omeprazole (isomer of Prilosec). A proton pump inhibitor, it inhibits H+K+-ATPase (acid production from parietal cells of stomach). Used for erosive esophagitis, GERD, and in concert with antibiotics for *H. pylori* infection with duodenal ulcer management.	May cause headache, nausea, vomiting, constipation, abdominal pain, and dry mouth.

(continues)

Table B–8 Some Common Medications (Listed by Generic Name) (continued)

Name	Examples	Mechanism/Use	Some Side Effects/Concerns
Estrogen (conjugated) and Esterified	C.E.S. Premarin Cenestins Progens Estratab Menest Menrium Neo-Estrone Kestrone	A short-acting estrogen used in the treatment of atrophic vaginitis, postmenopausal symptoms, postmenopausal osteoporosis, abnormal bleeding, and palliative treatment of both breast and prostate carcinoma.	May cause libido changes, depression, nausea, mastodynia, hypertension, and thromboembolic disorders.
Estrogen-Progestin combinations	*Monophasic* Alesse Demulen Desogen Levlite Levora Loestrin Necon Nordene Ogestrel Others *Biphasic* Jenest Kariva Mircette Others *Triphasic* Ortho-Cept Triphasil Trivora Others	In addition to oral medications listed to the left, there are transdermal (ortho-Evra), intravaginal (Nuva-Ring), and postcoital (Plan B, Preven) contraceptives. Monophasic has the estrogen, and progestin amounts remain the same. Biphasic has the estrogen remain the same with progestin initially less in first half of cycle, and increased in second. Triphasic has the progestin vary and the estrogen remain the same or vary. Prevents ovulation and creates a hostile environment for sperm.	May cause early or midcycle breakthrough bleeding, nausea, gallstones, thrombotic disorders such as thrombophlebitis, decreased glucose tolerance, pyridoxine deficiency, vaginal candidiasis, weight gain, paresthesias, hypertension, and chloasma.
Eszopiclone	Lunesta	Used for the treatment of insomnia. It is a nonbenzodiazepine hypnotic; however, its main effects seem to relate more to GABA receptor complexes which may be coupled to benzodiazepine receptors. It shortens sleep latency and improves sleep maintenance.	May cause anxiety, confusion, depression, headache, tachycardia, pericardial infusion, left ventricular systolic dysfunction, dysmenorrhea, dry mouth, nausea, rash, or pruritus.
Etanercept	Enbrel	A recombinant DNA substance that binds to tissue necrosis factor (TNF)-alpha receptors. TNF is a cytokine that induces an inflammatory action through interleukins. Effective in the management of Crohn's disease and inflammatory arthritic disorders such as RA and psoriatic arthritis.	May cause the usual GI disturbances, headache, dizziness, fatigue, loss of hair, pruritus, and rarely may cause MI, serious infections, or pancytopenia.

Table B–8 Some Common Medications (Listed by Generic Name) (continued)

Name	Examples	Mechanism/Use	Some Side Effects/Concerns
Ethosuximide	Zarontin	A succinimide anticonvulsant used in the treatment of seizures. Specifically, absence seizure, myoclonic and akinetic epilepsy. Acts to depress the motor cortex and elevate CNS threshold for stimulation.	May cause drowsiness, hiccups, ataxia, dizziness, headaches, lethargy, sleep disturbances, myopia, nausea, vomiting, epigastric discomfort, eosinophilia, thrombocytopenia, positive direct Comb's test, hirsutism, pruritic skin rash, gingival hyperplasia, and weight loss.
Etidronate	Didronel	Bisphosphonate; antiresorptive used in the treatment of osteoporosis and Paget's disease. Decreases vascularity of bone with Paget's. These medications inhibit bone resorption but eventually reduce bone formation due to a decrease in overall bone turnover. A standard intermittent treatment program with parathyroid hormone is intended to increase bone formation; however, it also increases bone resorption. The net effect though is bone formation. It is clear that prolonged exposure to parathyroid hormone, such as in hyperparathyroidism, causes osteoporosis.	May cause hypocalcemia, hyperphosphatemia, or elevated serum phosphatase. GI effects include esophageal irritation/ulceration with abdominal pain, nausea, vomiting, diarrhea/constipation, arthralgias, myalgias, headache, and rash. Dairy products decrease absorption.
Ezetimibe and Simvastatin	Vytorin Zocor	Used for patients with primary (heterozygous familial and nonfamilial) hypercholesterolemia or mixed hyperlipidemia. Ezetimibe is a selective inhibitor of intestinal cholesterol and phytosterol absorption combined with simvastatin, an HMG-CoA reductase inhibitor.	May cause urticaria, arthralgia, myalgias, angioedema, anaphylaxis, elevated liver transaminases, hepatitis, pancreatitis, cholelithiasis, thrombocytopenia, GI signs or symptoms such as nausea, abdominal pain, constipation, diarrhea, etc. Also a rare cause of rhabdomyolysis or myopathy.
Ezetimibe	Zetia Ezetrol	Used alone or in combination with statins (HMG-CoA reductase inhibitors) for the treatment of primary hypercholesterolemia. At the lining of the small intestine, it inhibits absorption of cholesterol but does not inhibit cholesterol synthesis in the liver.	May cause fatigue, arthralgia, myalgia, dizziness, headache, abdominal pain, angioedema, or rhabdomyolysis. (Monitor liver enzymes when used with a statin.)
Famotidine	Pepcid	An H2 (histamine) inhibitor blocking gastric acid secretion, raises pH of the stomach, decreasing pepsin secretion. Used as an OTC medication in the management of ulcers, GERD, and Zollinger-Ellison syndrome.	May cause dizziness, headache, confusion, diarrhea, constipation, thrombocytopenia, rash, and may increase uric acid, BUN, and creatinine.
Fexofenadine	Allegra	An antihistamine (H1 receptor antagonist used for the management of seasonal allergic rhinitis and chronic urticaria).	May cause headache, nausea, fatigue, dyspepsia, or throat irritation.
Finasteride	Propecia Proscar	A 5-reductase inhibitor of the enzyme necessary for conversion of testosterone into DHT. Used in the management of benign prostatic hypertrophy and male pattern baldness.	May cause decreased libido, impotence, or decreased volume of ejaculation.

(continues)

Table B–8 Some Common Medications (Listed by Generic Name) (continued)

Name	Examples	Mechanism/Use	Some Side Effects/Concerns
Fluoxetine	Prozac	An SSRI making more serotonin available in the CNS. Used in the treatment of depression and obsessive-compulsive disorders.	About 15% of patients discontinue use due to nausea, anxiety, diarrhea, insomnia, or headache.
Flurazepam HCL	Apo-flurazepam Dalmane Durapam Novo-flupam	A benzodiazepine used for the management of sleep problems. Reduces stage 4 NREM sleep while increasing total sleep time. Sedative effects in CNS at limbic and subcortical levels.	May cause residual sedation effects, but also irritability, nervousness, nightmares, hyperactivity, euphoria or depression, and coma with overdose.
Fluticasone	Flonase Flovent Cutivate	A synthetic corticosteroid used for the management of nasal symptoms for allergic and nonallergic rhinitis.	May cause nosebleeds, nasal sores, nasal or oral fungal infections, glaucoma, or cataracts.
Fluticasone Propionate with Salmeterol	Advair	An inhaled medication for the treatment of asthma and chronic bronchitis. A combination of a long-acting beta-2 agonist (salmeterol) and oral corticosteroid. Not used for acute asthma attacks.	May increase the risk of asthma-related deaths. May cause dizziness, headache, palpitations, sinus tachycardia, respiratory arrest, or long-term steroid use effects.
Furosemide	Lasix Fumide Luramide Furomide	A sulfonamide "loop" diuretic that inhibits reabsorption of sodium and chloride at the loop of Henle and proximal and distal renal tubules. Used in the management of hypertension, fluid reduction for CHF, hepatic cirrhosis, and renal dysfunction.	May cause hypokalemia (supplement with potassium), GI complaints, circulatory collapse, or aplastic types of anemia.
Gabapentin	Neurontin	Related to gamma aminobutyric acid (GABA). Used as an adjunctive treatment of seizures; also used for herpes zoster.	May cause lethargy, ataxia, dizziness, or other CNS effects.
Gemfibrozil	Lopid	Through blocking lipolysis of stored triglycerides and inhibiting uptake by the liver of fatty acids, there is a reduction in VLDL, LDL, total cholesterol, and triglyceride synthesis and an increase in VDL. Used in the management of patients with high triglyceride levels including familial hypercholesterolemia	May cause GI upset, headache, dizziness, musculoskeletal pain, rash, or hypokalemia.
Gentamycin	Garamycin Genoptic	A broad-spectrum, usually bactericidal, antibiotic effective against primarily Gram-negative and some Gram-positive organisms. Some include *Klebsiella*, *Proteus*, *E. coli*, *Enterobacter*, *Pseudomonas*, among others. Usually reserved for serious infections when other less toxic antibiotics are ineffective.	Is ototoxic, hepatotoxic, and nephrotoxic with associated indications on lab testing. May cause a variety of hypersensitivity reactions, neuromuscular blockade, hypokalemia and hypomagnesaemia with muscle cramps/weakness.
Glipizide	Glucotrol Glucotrol XL	A sulfonylurea hypoglycemic agent used in the initial management of type 2 diabetes after dietary management without medication has failed. Has the effects of sensitizing functioning pancreatic beta cells to release insulin, and indirectly increasing the number and sensitivity of insulin receptors.	May cause hypoglycemia, heartburn, pruritus, nausea/ vomiting, hepatic porphyria, hypersensitivity, and visual disturbances.
Glyburide	DiaBeta Glynase Micronase Euglucon	A sulfonylurea hypoglycemic agent used in the initial management of type 2 diabetes after dietary management without medication has failed. Has an effect of sensitizing functioning pancreatic beta cells to release insulin.	May cause hypoglycemia, heartburn, pruritus, nausea, or vomiting.

Table B–8 Some Common Medications (Listed by Generic Name) (continued)

Name	Examples	Mechanism/Use	Some Side Effects/Concerns
Gold Sodium Thiomalate	Myochrysine	An injectable water-soluble gold compound used in the treatment of rheumatoid arthritis. Appears to have immunosuppressant and anti-inflammatory properties possibly through inhibition of inflammatory prostaglandins.	May cause photosensitivity, dizziness, syncope, proteinuria, stomatitis, GI symptoms, grey to blue discoloration of skin, hypersensitivity, and erythema dermatitis.
Haloperidol	Haldol Peridol	A butyrophenone derivative similar to phenothiazines but with more extrapyramidal effects and less hypotensive and sedative effects. Used for psychotic disorders, tics, Tourette's syndrome, management of agitated states with Alzheimer's, and severe behavioral problems with children.	May cause extrapyramidal effects such as Parkinsonian symptoms, tardive dyskinesias, or neuroleptic malignant syndrome, agranulocytosis, laryngospasm, hyponatremia, hyperglycemia, and EEG changes.
Heparin Dalteparin	Hepalean Heparin Hep-Lock Lipo-Hepin Liquaemin	Prepared from bovine lung tissue and porcine intestinal mucosa, this potent mucopolysaccharide anticoagulant enhances the inhibitory actions of antithrombin III. Used for the treatment of venous thrombosis and pulmonary embolism, prevention of thrombi/emboli following surgeries, and also used for the treatment of disseminated intravascular coagulation (DIC).	May cause spontaneous bleeding, transient thrombocytopenia, bronchospasm, anaphylaxis, osteoporosis, and hypoaldosteronism.
Hepatitis B Immune Globulin	H-BIG Hep-B-Gammagee HyperHEP	Sterile human-based solution of IgG used to provide passive immunity for hepatitis B or post-exposure prophylaxis.	May cause a hypersensitivity reaction, muscle stiffness and aching, fever, dizziness, malaise, rash, or leg cramps.
Hydrocodone/ Acetaminophen	Vicodin Vicodin ES Anexsia Lorcet Lorcet Plus Norco	Narcotic pain reliever and cough suppressant similar to codeine (CNS depression). The acetaminophen component is a non-narcotic pain reliever and fever reducer.	May cause dry mouth, nausea, vomiting, lightheadedness, dizziness, euphoria, dysphoria, some respiratory depression, and rash.
Hydromorphone Hydrochloride	Dilaudid Dilaudid-HP	Similar to morphine but with a much stronger analgesic effect. Used for mild to moderate pain and cough suppression.	May cause dry mouth, nausea, vomiting, lightheadedness, dizziness, euphoria, dysphoria, some respiratory depression, and rash.
Hydroxyzine	Vistaril Atarax Vistacon Vistaject	An antihistamine with anticholinergic and sedative properties. Tranquilizing effect mainly due to depression of hypothalamus and brainstem reticular formation. Primarily used to treat allergic reaction and to relieve nasal congestion and other symptoms.	May cause drowsiness, dizziness, headache, urticaria, dyspnea, wheezing, rash, or hypotension.
Ibandronate	Boniva	A nitrogen-containing bisphosphonate used in the management of osteoporosis. Bisphosphonates inhibit osteoclast-mediated bone resorption. Advantage over other similar medications is the once-per-month dosage. Requires adequate intake of calcium and vitamin D.	May cause upper GI problems such as esophagitis, dyspepsia, or esophageal or gastric ulcers.
Imipramine	Impril Tofranil	Used for endogenous and sometimes reactive depression. Works by blocking reuptake of norepinephrine and serotonin by presynaptic neurons (classified as a tricyclic antidepressant). Reduces REM sleep and increases stage 4 NREM sleep.	May cause upper GI problems such as esophagitis, dyspepsia, or esophageal or gastric ulcers.

(continues)

Table B–8 Some Common Medications (Listed by Generic Name) (continued)

Name	Examples	Mechanism/Use	Some Side Effects/Concerns
Immune Globulin	Baygam Gamimune Gammagard Gammar P Iveegam Sandoglobulin Venoglobulin	A sterile concentrated human globulin solution used either as prophylaxis or to modify the severity of a number of diseases, including rubella, rubeola, varicella zoster, type A hepatitis, idiopathic thrombocytopenia purpura, among others.	Side effects related to site of injection. Also may cause hypersensitivity reactions, headache, GI symptoms, chest tightness, or wheezing.
Indomethacin	Indameth Indocid Indocin Indocin SR	NSAID use to reduce pain and fever. May reduce activity of PMNs, development of cellular exudates, and vascular permeability when tissue is damaged.	Hypersensitivity possible with rash, dyspnea, asthma syndrome if patient is an aspirin-sensitive asthmatic, edema, or hypotension. Also, concern of GI bleeding and rarely, an aplastic anemia effect or renal function impairment.
Infliximab	Remicade	An IgG1-K monoclonal antibody that binds to TNF-alpha. TNF is a cytokine that induces an inflammatory action through interleukins. Effective in the management of Crohn's disease and inflammatory arthritic disorders such as RA and psoriatic arthritis.	May cause the usual GI disturbances, headache, dizziness, fatigue, etc., lupus-like syndrome, loss of hair, pruritus, and increased liver enzymes.
Insulin (many types)	NovoLog (RCA) Lantus (RCA) Humulin Novolin Iletin II Humalog (RCA)	These are recombinant human analogs (RCA) extracted from pork used in the treatment of diabetes. Effects are to lower blood sugar levels by increasing peripheral uptake in muscle and fat, and promoting conversion of glucose to glycogen (and inhibiting reverse).	Side effects related to hypoglycemia, profuse sweating, hunger, tremors, palpitations. Also, coma is possible.
Interferon Alfa n-1 Alfacon-1 Alfa 2a Alfa 2b	Wellferon Infergen	A variety of medications used in the management of hepatitis C. Actions include suppression of cell proliferation and augmentation of lymphocyte natural killer cells.	Common to have side effects including headache, fever, chills, anxiety, nervousness, GI disturbances, alopecia, abnormal mood, emotional lability, and confusion. Possible lab effects on thrombocytes and granulocytes.
Interferon Beta 1a and 1b	Avonex Rebif Betaseron	A recombinant DNA medication with effects that are antiviral, antitumor, antiproliferative, and immunomodulatory. Used in the management of relapsing multiple sclerosis.	Common to have side effects including headache, fever, chills, anxiety, nervousness, GI disturbances, alopecia, abnormal mood, emotional lability, and confusion. Possible lab effects on thrombocytes and granulocytes.
Isoniazid	INH Isotamine Laniazid Nydrazid Teebaconin	An anti-TB medication that interferes with the synthesis of bacterial proteins, lipids, and nucleic acids. Used also for high-risk individuals as a preventive. Additional use for tremors with multiple sclerosis.	May cause paresthesia, peripheral neuropathies, tinnitus, dizziness, hallucinations, increased liver enzymes, decrease in B vitamin absorption, RA and SLE-like syndromes, or possible agranulocytosis and aplastic anemia (rare).

Table B–8 Some Common Medications (Listed by Generic Name) (continued)

Name	Examples	Mechanism/Use	Some Side Effects/Concerns
Isoproterenol	Isuprel Dispose-a-Med	Used primarily as a bronchodilator with asthma. A β1 adrenergic agonist that causes increased expectoration, increased ciliary motility, and bronchodilation with increase in cardiac output and strength. Also used for cardiac stimulation with cardiac arrest, and various arrhythmias.	May cause anorexia, tumors, palpitations, tachycardia, flushing, or ventricular arrhythmias.
Kaolin-Pectin	Kaopectate Kaolin w/Pectin	Kaolin as an aluminum silicate may have adsorbent and demulcent actions. Pectin may help to consolidate stool. Used for mild to moderate diarrhea.	May cause mild constipation.
Ketoconazole	Nizoral	Cell membrane function is disrupted by inhibiting sterol (ergosterol) synthesis in fungi. Used for serious systemic fungal infections such as Candida, coccidiomycosis, histoplasmosis, blastomycosis, and similar infections. Also used for superficial treatment of mycosis such as the "tineas."	May cause usual GI disturbances, anaphylaxis, gynecomastia, decreased libido, hair loss, acute hypoadrenalism, rarely hepatic necrosis, and may change multiple lab values such as decreases in cholesterol and triglycerides, and low serum testosterone.
Labetalol	Trandate Normodyne	An antihypertensive that acts as an alpha-adrenergic blocker and nonselective beta blocker. Results are decreased peripheral resistance, decreased conduction at sinus node, AV node, and ventricular muscle. Often used with thiazide diuretics.	May cause postural hypotension, bronchospasm, dizziness, fatigue, malaise, tremors, and GI disturbance. May cause positive on ANA testing and SLE-like syndrome.
Lamotrigine	Lamictal	May have an affect on glutamate/aspartate release and help in stabilizing neurons. Used in the treatment of seizures; in particular, partial seizures.	May cause dizziness, headache, nausea, diplopia, blurred vision, ataxia, lethargy.
Levodopa (L-Dopa)	Dopar Larodopa	L-dopa is the metabolic precursor to dopamine. Its advantage is that it crosses the blood–brain barrier. Helps restore levels of dopamine in extrapyramidal areas of the brain. Used in the treatment of Parkinson's.	May cause choreiform and other involuntary movements, increase tremor and cause bradykinetic episodes (on-and-off phenomenon). Many other side effects occur including hallucinations, paranoid delusions, severe depression, and suicide tendencies. There are a host of other system effects that include possible dark sweat or urine and all the other common side effects of many medications.
Levothyroxine Sodium	Eltroxin Synthroid Levoxyl Levothroid Unithroid	A synthetic version of thyroxine (T4) used to treat hypothyroidism and to suppress thyroid hormone release with cancerous thyroid nodules.	May cause similar effects of hyperthyroidism related to increased metabolism including palpitations, hypertension, agitation, insomnia, heat intolerance, weight loss, leg cramps, arrhythmias, headache, and menstrual irregularities such as anovulatory bleeding.

(continues)

Table B–8 Some Common Medications (Listed by Generic Name) (continued)

Name	Examples	Mechanism/Use	Some Side Effects/Concerns
Lidocaine	Anestacon Dilocaine L-caine Lidopen Octocaine Nervocaine Xylocaine Xylocard	Acts as both a local anesthetic and also antiarrhythmic blocking automaticity of His-Purkinje system. Used both for rapid control of ventricular arrhythmias and also as an injectable local anesthetic.	May cause difficulty breathing, anaphylaxis, respiratory depression, numbness, paresthesias, confusion, disorientation, or cardiovascular collapse in rare cases.
Liothyronine (T3)	Cytomel Triostat	Replaces T3 in hypothyroid patients. Used in the 3 suppression test. Main use is for those patients who do not respond to levothyroxine (synthroid).	Overdose effects are signs/symptoms of hyperthyroidism.
Lisinopril	Zestril	An ACE inhibitor. Blocks the conversion of rennin to angiotensin II thereby decreasing the release of aldosterone. This blocks the potent vasoconstriction effects of these substances resulting in a decrease in blood pressure without a compensation of increased heart rate or cardiac output	May cause headache, dizziness, fatigue, postural hypotension, chronic cough, hoarseness, and rash. May increase potassium levels, BUN, or creatinine.
Lithium	Cibalith-S Lithonate Lithane Lithobid Eskalith	Competes with other ions and as a result accelerates catecholamine breakdown, inhibits the release of neurotransmitters, and decreases the sensitivity of post-synaptic receptors. Used in the treatment of acute mania and manic phase of mixed bipolar disorder.	May cause headache, lethargy, fatigue, recent memory loss, nausea, vomiting, abdominal pain, nephrogenic diabetes insipidus, fine hand tremors, muscle weakness, and reversible leukocytosis. Rare peripheral vascular collapse.
Loperamide	Imodium Maalox antidiarrheal Pepto Diarrhea Control	Synthetic piperidine derivative that inhibits GI peristaltic activity. OTC medication used in the treatment of acute diarrhea or chronic diarrhea associated with inflammatory bowel disease.	Toxic megacolon with overuse, may cause drowsiness, CNS depression, dizziness, bloating, constipation, or abdominal pain.
Loratadine	Claritin Claritin RediTab	An antihistamine used in the treatment of allergies, hives (urticaria), and other allergic inflammatory conditions. A long-acting selective peripheral H1 receptor blocker (prevents release of histamine).	May cause dry mouth, dizziness, fatigue, changes in salivation, flushing, hypotension, palpitations, tachycardia, arthralgias, myalgias, blurred vision, rash, and photosensitivity.
Lorazepam	Ativan	A benzodiazepine used for anti-anxiety. Acts to enhance the effects of GABA particularly in the thalamus, hypothalamus, and limbic areas. It is the most potent of the benzodiazepines, but has fewer interactions and is less toxic than most other benzodiazepines. Also used for insomnia and panic attacks.	Many side effects disappear with continued use including anterograde amnesia, weakness, dizziness, sedation, restlessness, hallucinations, hyper- or hypotension, blurred vision, or depressed hearing.
Lovastatin	Mevacor	A statin: An HMG CoA reductase inhibitor. This blocks the enzyme that controls production of cholesterol in the liver. Therefore used in the treatment of hyperlipidemia. Lowers both total cholesterol and LDL cholesterol while increasing HDL cholesterol.	May cause GI upset, headache, myalgia, weakness, rhabdomyolysis, ocular and liver toxicity. Should have liver enzymes monitored.

Table B–8 Some Common Medications (Listed by Generic Name) (continued)

Name	Examples	Mechanism/Use	Some Side Effects/Concerns
Mannitol	Rectisol Osmitrol	An osmotic diuretic causing increased excretion of sodium, potassium, and chloride. Used in the management of oliguric phase of acute renal failure, for ascites, increased intraocular or intracranial pressure, to help in the excretion of toxic substances, and pulmonary edema.	May cause fluid and electrolyte imbalance, in particular hyponatremia, headache, dizziness, hypotension, convulsions, and transient muscle rigidity.
Memantine	Axura Namenda	An uncompetitive NMDA-receptor antagonist (antiglutamatergic), memantine has been shown to be effective in reducing clinical deterioration in moderate to severe Alzheimer's.	May cause emotional agitation, confusion, stomach upset, and nervousness.
Meperidine	Demerol Pethadol Pethidine HCL	An opiate receptor agonist having the effects of analgesia, respiratory depression, and sedation.	May cause dizziness, sedation, nausea, constipation, allergic reaction, respiratory depression, convulsions, or cardiovascular collapse.
Metformin	Glucophage Glucophage XR	Biguanide hypoglycemic agent (not a sulfonylurease). Does not increase insulin production, but helps bind insulin to insulin receptors and potentate insulin activity. Used in the treatment of type 2 diabetes. Sometimes used in combination with a sulfonylurease.	May cause abdominal complaints of pain, nausea, or vomiting. May interfere with absorption of folic acid and B_{12} or amino acids. Patient may complain of a bitter or metallic taste. Caution for lactic acidosis.
Methimazole	Tapazole	Blocks transformation of inorganic iodine to organic iodine. Blocks conversion of T4 and T3. Often used to produce a euthyroid state prior to radiation or surgery. Long-term use may produce euthyroid state in half of patients.	May cause headache, vertigo, nausea, vomiting, hepatitis, myelosuppression, leukopenia, and rarely agranulocytosis. May elevate prothrombin time and liver enzymes.
Methotrexate	Rheumatrex Trexall	An antimetabolite that blocks the metabolism of fast-growing cells. Blocks folate reduction through inhibitory effect on dihydrofolate reductase. Used in the treatment of cancer and rheumatoid-like conditions such as psoriatic arthritis and RA. Cancers include acute lymphocytic leukemia; osteogenic sarcoma; Burkitt's lymphoma; non-Hodgkin's lymphoma; cancer of the brain, head, neck; and small-cell lung choriocarcinoma. Also used to induce miscarriage (e.g., ectopic pregnancy).	May cause bone marrow suppression, GI ulcers, nephrotoxicity, hepatotoxicity, nausea, diarrhea, or pulmonary infiltrates.
Methyldopa	Aldomet	An α2 adrenergic agonist used as an antihypertensive. It decreases cardiac output, heart rate, and blood pressure.	May cause dry mouth, possible postural hypotension, and sedation. May experience nightmares or psychic disturbances.
Methylphenidate	Ritalin Concerta	Causes the release of norepinephrine, dopamine, and serotonin from storage vesicles, resulting in CNS stimulation. This causes an increase in performance, coordination, and energy. There is a decrease in appetite with an increase in blood pressure. Used for narcolepsy and attention deficit disorder.	May cause restlessness, insomnia, dizziness, anorexia, psychic disturbances, and arrhythmias.

(continues)

Table B–8 Some Common Medications (Listed by Generic Name) (continued)

Name	Examples	Mechanism/Use	Some Side Effects/Concerns
Methysergide	Sansert	An ergot derivative, methysergide competes with serotonin receptors, decreasing the pro-inflammatory and vasoconstrictive effects of peripheral serotonin. Used in the treatment of migraine headaches.	May cause postural hypotension, nausea, vomiting, abdominal pain, heartburn, diarrhea, and the common side effects of most medications.
Metoprolol	Lopressor Toprol XL	Beta-blocker: A β adrenergic antagonist blocking primarily β1 receptors (less bronchoconstriction effect than β2 blockers), decreases heart rate and rennin release. Used in the treatment of hypertension.	CNS depressive effects with concerns for those with diabetes, heart block and heart failure, asthma, and emphysema.
Metaproterenol	Alupent	β2 agonist used in the treatment of asthma. Causes bronchodilation without secondary vascular and cardiac effects.	May cause anorexia, tachycardia, nausea, arrhythmias, tremor, hypertension, muscle cramps, convulsions, weakness, hallucinations, or postural hypotension.
Metronidazole	Flagyl Metizol Metro-Gel Protostat Noritate	A synthetic agent that is effective against a wide variety of organisms including *Trichomonas vaginalis*, *Entamoeba histolytica*, and Giardia. Antibacterial anaerobic bacteria, and some Gram-negatives. Used with other antibiotics (triple antibiotic regimen) for duodenal ulcers. Topical may be used for rosacea.	May cause a Candida infection (overgrowth), hypersensitivity, nausea and other GI symptoms, polyuria, dysuria, vertigo, headache, and a metallic or bitter taste. May decrease AST levels (interferes with chemical reaction).
Miconazole	Monistat (Derm, 3, 7) Femizole M-Zole Micatin Tetterine Fungoid Lotrimin Desenex	A broad-spectrum antifungal that inhibits absorption of essential material for cell reproduction, growth, and cell wall integrity. Used primarily for Candida, common dermatophytes, and tinea versicolor. Used for a variety of body sites: vaginal Candida infection, athlete's foot (tinea pedis), and similar "tineas" caused by dermatophytes.	May cause a Candida infection (overgrowth), hypersensitivity, nausea and other GI symptoms, polyuria, dysuria, vertigo, headache, and a metallic or bitter taste. May decrease AST levels (interferes with chemical reaction).
Milrinone	Primacor	A new type of drug that is an isotropic/vasodilator inhibitory against cyclic-AMP phosphodiesterase. Increases cardiac output while decreasing pulmonary wedge pressure. Used in the short-term management of CHF.	May cause arrhythmias such as PVCs, supraventricular and ventricular tachycardias, or hypotension.
Montelukast	Singulair	Used as prophylactic treatment of chronic asthma, exercise-induced bronchospasm, and allergic rhinitis. A leukotriene receptor antagonist.	May cause sinusitis, nausea, diarrhea, dyspepsia, otitis, viral infection, or laryngitis.
Nadolol	Corgard	Beta-blocker: Blocks both β1 and β2 adrenergic receptors, decreases heart rate and rennin release. Used in the treatment of hypertension. Also has bronchoconstriction effect due to β2 blockade.	May cause CNS depressive effects with concerns for those with diabetes, heart block and heart failure, asthma, and emphysema. Transient hypertension due to blockage of β2 receptors (which normally dilate large arteries).
Naproxen Naproxen sodium	Aleve Apo-naproxen Anaprox Naprosyn Naprolen	NSAID. Similar to ibuprofen, ketoprofen, etc. Inhibits inflammatory prostaglandin synthesis. Actions include analgesic, anti-inflammatory, and antipyretic. Inhibits platelet aggregation and prolongs bleeding time but does not affect clotting.	May cause headache, drowsiness, dizziness, anorexia, heartburn, nausea, GI bleeding, and rarely agranulocytosis.

Table B–8 Some Common Medications (Listed by Generic Name) (continued)

Name	Examples	Mechanism/Use	Some Side Effects/Concerns
Natalizumab	Antegren	A humanized monoclonal antibody used to treat multiple sclerosis and Crohn's disease. A receptor blocker that binds to alpha-4-beta-1 and alpha-4-beta-7 integrins, natalizumab prevents lymphocytes and eosinophils from moving from the bloodstream to outer tissue sites involved in inflammation. For multiple sclerosis it is used in combination with interferon beta 1-a.	Most common side effects are abdominal pain and headache.
Neostigmine Bromide and Methyl sulfate	Prostigmin	Prolongs effects of acetylcholine at cholinergic synapses (reversible cholinesterase inhibition) and has a direct stimulant action on voluntary muscle fibers and possibly on autonomic ganglia and CNS. Used in the treatment of myasthenia gravis.	Generalized cholinergic responses including constriction of bronchi and ureters with stimulation of salivary and sweat glands. May cause cramps, muscle facilitations, nausea, tight chest, generalized, weakness, hypotension, but increased BP.
Niacin (Nicotinic acid)	NiAc Nicobid Nicolar Novo-Niacin	Vitamin B_3 is used in the management of hypercholesterolemia. It has vasodilation effects on vascular smooth muscle and inhibits hepatic synthesis of VLDL, cholesterol and triglycerides, and LDL. May also be used in the treatment of pellagra.	May cause a generalized flushing, sensation of warmth, transient headache, tingling in the extremities, increased sebaceous gland activity, hyperuricemia, hyperglycemia, abnormalities of liver function, and jaundice.
Nifedipine	Adalat	A calcium channel blocker that causes smooth muscle relaxation of coronary and peripheral blood vessels decreasing peripheral resistance without affecting serum calcium levels. Used in the management of hypertension usually in combination with a diuretic and also vasospastic (Prinzmetal or variant) angina.	May cause dizziness, lightheadedness, postural hypotension, facial flushing, palpitations, peripheral edema, hepatotoxicity, sore throat, and various GI symptoms.
Norfloxacin	Chibroxin Noroxin	A strong broad-spectrum antibiotic that alters DNA-gyrase inhibiting protein synthesis. Used primarily for UTIs and conjunctivitis. Effective against many organisms including *Klebsiella* and other pneumonias, *Salmonella*, *Shigella*, *Pseudomonas*, *S. aureus*, among others.	May cause joint pain, swelling, and erosions in weight-bearing joints. Usual GI complaints, headaches, dizziness, pruritus, elevated liver enzymes, and immunosuppressed swelling of ankle and hip with tendon tenderness and swelling of third finger bilaterally after one month of continuous therapy.
Nortriptyline	Aventyl Pamelor	A tricyclic antidepressant that acts as a serotonin reuptake inhibitor and to a lesser degree norepinephrine. Used in the management of depression and anxiety.	May cause drowsiness, orthostatic hypotension, dry mouth, metallic taste, photophobia, urinary retention, or weight gain.
Nystatin	Mycostatin Nadostine Nilstat Nyaderm Nystex	An antifungal antibiotic that binds to cell membrane and causes leakage of intracellular components. Used primarily for Candida infections.	May cause nausea, vomiting, epigastric pain, or diarrhea.

(continues)

Table B–8 Some Common Medications (Listed by Generic Name) (continued)

Name	Examples	Mechanism/Use	Some Side Effects/Concerns
Omeprazole	Prilosec Losec	A proton pump inhibitor, it inhibits H+K+-ATPase (acid production from parietal cells of stomach). Used for erosive esophagitis, GERD, and in concert with antibiotics (usually metronidazole and amoxicillin) for *H. pylori* infection with duodenal ulcer management.	May cause headache, nausea, vomiting, constipation, abdominal pain, and dry mouth.
Orlistat	Xenical	An enzymatic blocker (gastrointestinal lipase) that inactivates pancreatic and gastric lipase reducing the absorption of fat. Used in the management of obesity.	May cause headache, dizziness, hypertension, oily discharges, and abdominal pain and cramping.
Oxybutynin Chloride	Ditropan Ditropan XL	A synthetic amine used for neurogenic bladder or detrusor instability (unstable bladder). Effects are antispasmodic through inhibition of muscarinic effect of acetylcholine on smooth muscle.	May cause drowsiness, blurred vision, dry mouth, constipation, urinary hesitation, dizziness, weakness, or skin rash.
Oxycodone	Roxicodone Percolone Oxycontin Oxyfast	Binds to stereospecific receptors in the CNS having the effects of a potent analgesic; ten times more potent than codeine. Used in the management of pain with fractures, bursitis, dislocations, post-surgery, and postpartum.	May cause sedation, constipation, respiratory depression, or hepatotoxicity.
Paroxetine	Paxil	An SSRI making more serotonin available in the CNS. Used in the treatment of depression and obsessive-compulsive disorders.	May cause nausea, vomiting, weakness, dizziness, agitation, insomnia, headaches, or abnormal ejaculation.
Pemoline	Cylert	Causes the release of norepinephrine, dopamine, and serotonin from storage vesicles resulting in CNS stimulation. This causes an increase in performance, coordination, and energy. There is a decrease in appetite with an increase in blood pressure. Used for attention deficit disorder.	May cause restlessness, insomnia, dizziness, anorexia, psychic disturbances, and arrhythmias.
Penicillamine	Cuprimine Depen	Forms a chelate with various metals such as zinc, copper, iron, lead, mercury, and perhaps other heavy metals. Used in the management of Wilson's disease (causes excretion of excess copper), management of RA (mechanism unknown), and prevention of cystinuria.	During initial use, patients with Wilson's disease may have a worsening of neuropathy. May cause excessive skin wrinkling, regular GI complaints, fever, arthralgia, SLE-like syndrome, thrombophlebitis, myasthenia gravis syndrome, optic neuritis, thrombocytopenia, skin reactions including rash and pruritus, pancreatitis, proteinuria, and hematuria.
Penicillin (including G Benzathine, G Potassium, G Sodium, G Procaine, and V/V Potassium)	Bicillin Permapen Megacillin Pentids Pfizerpen Cryptocillin Benzylpenicillin Wycillin	An antibiotic in many different forms used for different infections: Penicillin G benzathine—mild to moderate infections, syphilis, and prophylaxis for rheumatic fever. Penicillin G potassium or sodium—moderate to severe infections, meningococcal meningitis. Penicillin G procaine—moderate to severe infections, pneumococcal pneumonia, uncomplicated gonorrhea, and syphilis. Penicillin V & V potassium—mild to moderate infections and endocarditis prophylaxis.	Anaphylaxis is common, hypersensitivity symptoms, common GI disturbances, SLE-like syndrome, hypotension, rarely circulatory collapse, Loffler's syndrome, thrombocytopenia, hemolytic anemia, and delayed skin rashes.

Table B–8 Some Common Medications (Listed by Generic Name) (continued)

Name	Examples	Mechanism/Use	Some Side Effects/Concerns
Pentazocine	Talwin Talwin NX	A synthetic analgesic, narcotic, CNS depressant used in the management of moderate to severe pain and preoperative sedation.	Not to be used with head injury. Will cause drowsiness, lightheadedness, and sedation. May cause dizziness, nausea/vomiting, constipation, urinary retention, rash, respiratory depression, or shock.
Phenelzine	Nardil	A MAO inhibitor in the management of depression. Increases available levels of serotonin and norepinephrine. Also may affect the hepatic microsomal enzymes that metabolize drugs, prolonging the effects of these drugs.	May cause orthostatic hypotension, dry mouth, dizziness, constipation, anorexia, blurred vision, tremors, or muscle twitching. Caution for hypertensive crisis when ingesting foods containing tyramine.
Phenobarbital	Barbital Luminal Solfoton	A long-acting barbiturate used primarily for the management of epilepsy (grand mal). Inhibits the reticular activating system, causes CNS depression, and raises the threshold for stimulation of the cerebral cortex. Also used for pre- and postoperative sedation in pediatrics and pylorospasm in infants.	Causes CNS depression with possible extreme of coma and death. May cause usual GI symptoms, hyperkinesis, insomnia, nightmares, headaches, bradycardia, syncope, megaloblastic (macrocytic) anemia, agranulocytosis, thrombocytopenia, folic acid or vitamin D deficiency; if taken during pregnancy, birth defects (10%).
Phentermine	Adipex-P Fastin Ionamin Obenix Oby-Trim	Appetite suppressant similar to amphetamines, acting as a CNS stimulant. Used for a short period along with diet and exercise, and behavioral training for weight loss.	Most side effects are those of CNS stimulation including agitation, nervousness, tremor, hypertension, arrhythmias, etc. In addition, hypersensitivity reactions are possible and all of the common side effects reported for most drugs related to GI complaints and CNS effects, such as headache, dizziness, etc.
Phenytoin	Dilantin	Sodium, potassium, and calcium currents are reduced across neuronal membranes, decreasing neuronal transmission. Used in the treatment of epilepsy (except absence seizures).	CNS toxicity including sedation, dizziness, imbalance (ataxia), nausea, diplopia (nystagmus), also birth defects, hepatotoxicity, bone marrow suppression, and GI disturbances. Usually these are transient. Morbilliform rashes occur in 5% to 7% of patients. In young patients, gingival hyperplasia and hirsutism.
Physostigmine	Antilirium	An anticholinesterase inhibitor making more acetylcholine available at cholinergic sites. Used to reverse the overdose/toxic effects of tricyclic antidepressants, atropine, scopolamine, or diazepam.	May cause sweating, abdominal pain, diarrhea, nausea, salivation, weakness, convulsions, and rarely respiratory collapse.
Pilocarpine	Absorbocarpine Isopto carpine Minims pilocarpine Miocarpine Ocusert Pilocar	A tertiary amine that mimics acetylcholine causing miosis, spasm of accommodation, and decreased intraocular pressure. Used for both open-angle and closed-angle glaucoma.	May cause salivation, blurred vision, sweating, headache, dizziness, or in rare cases, retinal detachment.

(continues)

Table B–8 Some Common Medications (Listed by Generic Name) (continued)

Name	Examples	Mechanism/Use	Some Side Effects/Concerns
Pravastatin	Pravachol	A statin: An HMGCoA reductase inhibitor. Blocks the enzyme that controls production of cholesterol in the liver. Therefore, used in the treatment of hyperlipidemia. Lowers both total cholesterol and LDL cholesterol while increasing HDL cholesterol.	GI upset, headache, myalgia, weakness, rhabdomyolysis, ocular and liver toxicity. Should have liver enzymes monitored.
Prazosin	Minipress	Alpha blocker: α adrenergic antagonist causing dilation of arteries and veins used for the treatment of hypertension.	Postural hypotension, dry mouth, edema, congestion, headache, sexual dysfunction, and lethargy.
Prednisone	Dethasone Liquid Pred Prednisolone Pediapred Oral Liquid Medrol	Synthetic oral corticosteroid used to suppress immune system reaction including inflammation. These medications mimic actions of cortisol (hydrocortisone) produced by the adrenal gland. Used in the treatment of inflammatory arthritis, colitis such as Crohn's and ulcerative colitis, asthma, bronchitis, some skin rashes, and allergic or inflammatory conditions affecting the nose and eyes.	Long-term use may cause suppression of bone growth, osteopenia and resultant fractures, Cushing's syndrome (osteoporosis, skin atrophy, abnormal glucose tolerance, anemia, behavioral abnormalities, etc.). Increased risk of Candida (yeast) infection.
Pregabalin	Lyrica	Used in the management of neuropathic pain (diabetic peripheral neuropathy), postherpetic neuralgia, adjunctive therapy for partial seizures, and fibromyalgia.	May cause dizziness, sleepiness, edema, blurred vision, weight gain, or difficulty with concentration.
Probenecid	Benemid Benuryl Probalan	Used as an anti-arrhythmic, especially for atrial fibrillation and flutter. Decreases excitability of myocardium and increases refractory time with possible peripheral vasodilation effect.	May cause headache, GI complaints, hemolytic anemia, respiratory depression, and rarely hepatic necrosis.
Procainamide	Procan Procanbid Pronestyl	Used as an anti-arrhythmic, especially for atrial fibrillation and flutter. Decreases excitability of myocardium and increases refractory time with possible peripheral vasodilation effect.	May cause SLE-type syndrome, polyarthralgias, ventricular fibrillation, or agranulocytosis with prolonged use.
Procaine	Novocain	Used as a local anesthetic to block sensation and motor activity in local injection area. Blocks sodium into nerve cell. Also used for spinal anesthesia and nerve blocks.	There is a known hypersensitivity to procaine. May cause respiratory distress, anaphylactic reaction, arthralgias, tremors, convulsions, or headache.
Progesterone	Crinone Gel Gesterol Progestasert Prometrium Progestaject	A phenothiazine derivative that has alpha-adrenergic blocking effects, an antiemetic effect through depression on chemoreceptor trigger zone, and antipsychotic effects through actions (blocks postsynaptic dopamine receptors) in the hypothalamus and reticular formation. Used in the management of manic phase of manic depression, for psychotic disorders such as schizophrenia, and for severe nausea and vomiting. Also, sometimes used for behavioral disorders in attention deficit disorder in children.	May cause breakthrough bleeding, many GI symptoms, migraine headache, weight change, dizziness, and possible thromboembolic disorders.
Propranolol	Inderal	Beta-blocker: Blocks both β1 and β2 adrenergic receptors, decreasing heart rate and rennin release. Used in the treatment of hypertension. Also has bronchoconstriction effect due to β2 blockade.	CNS depressive effects with concerns for those with diabetes, heart block and heart failure, asthma, and emphysema. Transient hypertension due to blockage of β2 receptors (which normally dilate large arteries).

Table B–8 Some Common Medications (Listed by Generic Name) (continued)

Name	Examples	Mechanism/Use	Some Side Effects/Concerns
Propoxyphene	Darvon Novopropoxyn	Related to methadone; a strong opioid. Used for mild to moderate pain. Also used to manage narcotic withdrawal.	Caution that use with alcohol or high doses may cause death. Also, more commonly causes drowsiness, constipation, skin reactions, GI upset, and rarely circulatory collapse or coma.
Propylthiouracil (PTU)	Propyl-Thyracil	Blocks transformation of inorganic iodine to organic iodine. Often used to produce a euthyroid state prior to radiation or surgery. Long-term use may produce euthyroid state in half of patients.	May cause headache, vertigo, nausea, vomiting, hepatitis, myelosuppression, leukopenia, and rarely agranulocytosis. May elevate prothrombin time and liver enzymes.
Psyllium	Hydrocil Instant Karasil Konsyl Metamucil Modane bulk Per Diem Plain Reguloid Serutan Silybon V-Lax	A bulk-producing laxative made from colloid of psyllium seed. Promotes peristalsis. Used for constipation.	May cause eosinophilia, nausea, abdominal cramps, and GI tract strictures (using dry form).
Pyridostigmine	Mestinon	An indirect cholinesterase inhibitor sometimes used for short-term management of myasthenia gravis and to reverse the effects of curariform muscle relaxants.	May cause muscle weakness, hypotension, convulsions, bronchospasm, or respiratory distress.
Raloxifene	Evista	Selective estrogen receptor modulator; antiresorptive used in the treatment of osteoporosis. These medications inhibit bone resorption but eventually reduce bone formation due to a decrease in overall bone turnover. A standard intermittent treatment program with parathyroid hormone is intended to increase bone formation; however, it also increases bone resorption. The net effect though is bone formation. It is clear that prolonged exposure to parathyroid hormone such as in hyperparathyroidism causes osteoporosis. Raloxifene is believed to decrease total cholesterol and LDL cholesterol but does not raise HDL or lower triglycerides. Also, the selective estrogen receptor inhibition effect prevents tissue proliferation in the uterus and breasts.	May cause flu-like symptoms, also hot flashes, migraine headache, insomnia, depression, weight gain, vaginitis, breast pain, and vaginal bleeding.
Ranitidine	Zantac	An H2 (histamine) inhibitor blocking gastric acid secretion. Used as an OTC medication in the management of ulcers and GERD.	May cause usual GI symptoms, dizziness, depression, reversible leukocytosis, thrombocytopenia, and possible decreases in liver enzymes.
Reserpine	Serpalan Sk-Reserpine	Decreases binding of serotonin and synthesis of norepinephrine, and inhibits their reuptake. Decreases in these two neurotransmitters in the CNS. Primarily used in the treatment of hypertension. May also be used for the vasospastic feature of Raynaud's.	May cause drowsiness, sedation, lethargy, edema, bradycardia, nasal decongestion, hypersensitivity, menstrual irregularities, and other sexual effects. Also, orthostatic hypotension, and rarely respiratory distress.

(continues)

Table B–8 Some Common Medications (Listed by Generic Name) (continued)

Name	Examples	Mechanism/Use	Some Side Effects/Concerns
Risedronate	Actonel	Bisphosphonate; antiresorptive used in the treatment of osteoporosis and Paget's disease. These medications inhibit bone resorption but eventually reduce bone formation due to a decrease in overall bone turnover. A standard intermittent treatment program with parathyroid hormone is intended to increase bone formation; however, it also increases bone resorption. The net effect though is bone formation. It is clear that prolonged exposure to parathyroid hormone such as in hyperparathyroidism causes osteoporosis. Risedronate is believed to be more effective than other bisphosphonates at blocking bone dissolution.	Fewer GI side effects than other bisphosphonates.
Rivastigmine Tartrate	Exelon	A cholinesterase inhibitor used in the management of mild to moderate Alzheimer's disease. Works in the cerebral cortex, blocking degradation of acetylcholine.	May cause headache, fatigue, insomnia, nausea, diarrhea, vomiting, cramps, anorexia, or muscle cramps.
Rofecoxib	Vioxx	NSAID: cyclooxygenase (COX) 2 inhibitor (does not inhibit COX-1) used primarily for arthritis (osteo and rheumatoid, and rheumatoid variants), acute pain, and menstrual cramps. Reduces fever. Also approved to prevent and reduce the size of polyps in patients with genetic disease.	May cause flu-like symptoms, peripheral edema, GI problems, dizziness, headache, pharyngitis, and rash.
Ropinirole	Requip	Used in the treatment of Parkinson's and restless leg syndrome (Ekbom syndrome) through a mechanism that causes stimulation of postsynaptic dopamine D2-type receptors (for Parkinson's specifically within the caudate-putamen).	May cause increased sweating, dry mouth, flushing, fatigue, sleeping attacks, tachycardias, orthostatic hypotension, hyperkinesias, nausea, vomiting, or anorexia.
Rosiglitazone Maleate	Avandia	An oral medication used as adjunct therapy with diet and exercise for type 2 diabetes. It acts primarily by increasing insulin sensitivity but is not related to sulfonylureas, the biguanides, or the alphaglucosidase inhibitors.	Not to be used with nitrates. May cause hypoglycemic symptoms, edema, or exacerbation of congestive heart failure.
Salmeterol Xinafoate	Serevent	Similar to albuterol, it is a long-acting beta 2 receptor agonist. Effects include reduction of bronchospasm, increased motility of cilia, and decrease in inflammatory mediators such as histamine. Used in the treatment of asthma and hyperactive airway disease. Not used to treat acute bronchospasm.	May cause dizziness, headache, tremor, palpitations, and in rare cases, acute respiratory arrest.
Scopolamine	Hyoscine Murocoll Triptone	Resembles atropine producing CNS depression/sedation, and decreased secretions of salivary, sweat, and bronchial glands. Used as a preanesthetic.	Causes drowsiness, dry mouth and throat, constipation, dilated pupils, and decreased respiration.
Selegiline	Eldepryl	Increases dopaminergic activity, partial action due to MAO inhibition and inhibition of dopamine reuptake. Used as adjunctive treatment for Parkinson's.	May cause visual disturbances, GI symptoms, confusion, hallucinations, dyskinesia, and hypotension.
Senna (Sennosides)	Black Draught Gentlax Senexon Senokot Senolax	Dried leaf preparation that is converted to glycone, which causes an increase in peristalsis. Used for acute constipation.	May cause abdominal cramping, flatulence, diarrhea, weight loss, and associated loss of electrolytes.

Table B–8 Some Common Medications (Listed by Generic Name) (continued)

Name	Examples	Mechanism/Use	Some Side Effects/Concerns
Sertraline	Zoloft	An SSRI making more serotonin available in the CNS. Used in the treatment of depression and obsessive-compulsive disorders.	May cause nausea, diarrhea, dry mouth, dizziness, insomnia, fatigue, or impotence.
Sildenafil Citrate	Viagra	Used for erectile dysfunction. Causes a vasodilation effect in the corpus cavernosus of the penis through effect with nitric oxide. A phosphodiesterase-5 inhibitor.	May cause facial edema, postural hypotension, palpitations, headache (and other "cerebral signs/ symptoms"), MI, angina, dermatitis, photosensitivity, and gout.
Simvastatin	Zocor	A statin: An HMGCoA reductase inhibitor. This blocks the enzyme that controls production of cholesterol in the liver. Therefore, used in the treatment of hyperlipidemia. Lowers both total cholesterol and LDL cholesterol while increasing HDL cholesterol.	GI upset, headache, myalgia, weakness, rhabdomyolysis, ocular and liver toxicity. Should have liver enzymes monitored.
Solifenacin	VESIcare	A muscarinic receptor antagonist used in the management of overactive bladder (detrusor instability).	May cause dry mouth, constipation, or blurred vision.
Somatropin	Bio-tropin Genotropin Nutropin Humatrope Norditropin Serostim Saizen	A recombinant growth hormone used for growth hormone deficiencies, Turner's syndrome, and AIDS wasting syndrome.	May cause hypercalciuria, accelerated growth of intracranial tumors, hyperglycemia, gallstones, and myalgia.
Spironolactone	Aldactone Novospiroton	Blocks action of aldosterone by competing with receptor sites in distal renal tubules. Used as a diuretic without an effect of hyperglycemia or hyperuricemia. A potassium-sparing diuretic. Used in the management of CHF and other forms of edema, and adjunct therapy for hypertension.	May cause confusion, lethargy, rapid weight loss, gynecomastia, electrolyte imbalances, elevated BUN, gout, decreased glucose tolerance, or SLE.
Streptokinase (Tissue Plasminogen Activator: TPA is similar)	Kabikinase Streptase	Produced from beta-hemolytic streptococcus, this potent thrombolytic enzyme promotes conversion of plasminogen to plasmin. This process breaks apart clotting materials into a soluble form, clearing blocked areas in acute thrombotic or embolic situations. Used for acute treatment of deep vein thrombosis, pulmonary embolism, coronary artery thrombosis, etc.	Given that this is an antithrombotic agent, hypocoagulation exists, which may lead to bleeding at any body site. May also cause an allergic reaction, anaphylaxis, unstable blood pressure, ventricular arrhythmias, musculoskeletal pain, and flushing.
Streptomycin	Streptomycin	A bacteriostatic antibiotic effective against numerous bacteria, including Gram-positive, Gram-negative and acid-fast.	Pain, swelling, tenderness at injection site. May cause dizziness, labyrinth damage, headache, and nausea. May elevate some liver enzymes or cause decreases in hematocrit or hemoglobin.
Sucralfate	Carafate Sulcrate	Used as part of GI ulcer therapy due to effects of creating a protective mucosal "paste" and inhibits pepsin, decreases bile absorption, and blocks back diffusion of H_+ ions. Valuable for smokers treated for duodenal ulcers.	Very few side effects. May cause constipation.

(continues)

Table B–8 Some Common Medications (Listed by Generic Name) (continued)

Name	Examples	Mechanism/Use	Some Side Effects/Concerns
Sulfasalazine	Azulfidine Sulfasalazine Salazopyrin S.A.S.-500	A long-acting sulfonamide used in the management of *Clostridium* and *E. coli* infections, inflammatory bowel disease, and RA. Anti-inflammatory effect may be due to inhibition of prostaglandins, and may have antibacterial effect due to conversion to sulfapyridine and 5-ASA.	May cause nausea, vomiting, bloody diarrhea, anorexia, rash, and allergic reactions.
Sulfisoxazole	Gantrisin	A bacteriostatic antibiotic that interferes with p-amino benzoic acid (PABA) which interferes with folic acid biosynthesis necessary for bacterial growth. Used primarily for chronic UTIs, acute otitis media, resistant malarial infections, conjunctivitis and corneal infections, and topically for *H. vaginalis*.	A wide variety of potential side effects including headache, peripheral neuropathy, anaphylaxis, agranulocytosis, thrombocytopenia, Stevenson-Johnson syndrome, alopecia, goiter, depression, crystalluria, hematuria, and the usual GI complaints.
Sulindac	Clinoril	An indole prostaglandin inhibitor (similar to indomethacin) used similar to aspirin with fewer GI effects than aspirin. Primarily used for inflammatory arthritis such as RA, ankylosing spondylitis, acute attacks of gout, and acute bursitis of the shoulder.	May cause dizziness, headache, abdominal pain, prolonged bleeding time, aplastic anemia, anaphylaxis, and toxic epidermal necrosis syndrome.
Sumatriptan	Imitrex	A selective serotonin receptor agonist that causes vasoconstriction of cranial arteries. Used in the management of migraine headaches (with or without aura) and cluster headaches.	Depends on mode of delivery, but may cause angina, tingling, numbness, dizziness, lightheadedness, hypo- or hypertension, nausea, or vomiting. Also, a rebound migraine headache is common.
Tacrine	Cognex	A cholinesterase inhibitor used in the management of mild to moderate Alzheimer's disease. Works in the cerebral cortex, blocking degradation of acetylcholine.	May cause headache, fatigue, insomnia, nausea, diarrhea, vomiting, cramps, anorexia, or muscle cramps.
Tadalafil	Cialis	A phosophodiesterase-5 inhibitor. Used for erectile dysfunction. Causes a vasodilation effect in the corpus cavernosus of the penis through effect with nitric oxide.	May cause facial edema, postural hypotension, palpitations, headache (and other "cerebral sign/symptoms"), MI, angina, dermatitis, photosensitivity, and gout. For some, may experience a slight bluish tinge to vision.
Tamoxifen	Nolvadex Nolvadex-D Tamofen	Competes with estradiol and estrogen receptors causing a strong antiestrogen effect. Used in the palliative treatment of advanced breast cancer in postmenopausal women and adjunctively with surgery for women with breast cancer and positive lymph nodes.	May cause hot flashes, thrombosis, leucopenia, thrombocytopenia, with nausea and vomiting occurring in about 25% of patients.
Tamsulosin	Flomax	Used in the management of prostate hypertrophy, this is an antagonist to alpha 1A adrenoceptors in the prostate.	May cause orthostatic hypotension, priapism, allergic-type reactions, constipation, or vomiting.
Tegaserod	Zelnorm	A serotonin 5-HT4 receptor agonist used in the management of constipation-predominant irritable bowel syndrome. The 5-HT4 receptor, a serotonin receptor, normalizes intestinal contractions. In addition, this medication acts to increase the pain threshold for distention of the colon.	May cause headache, dizziness, migraine, abdominal pain, nausea, flatulence, or back pain.

Table B–8 Some Common Medications (Listed by Generic Name) (continued)

Name	Examples	Mechanism/Use	Some Side Effects/Concerns
Terazosin	Hydrin	An alpha 1-adrenergic blocker used in the management of hypertension in combination with a beta-adrenergic blocker and thiazide diuretic. Also used in the management of benign prostatic hypertrophy.	May cause weakness, dizziness, headache, weight gain, or syncope.
Terbinafine	Lamisil Lamisil DermGel	Cell membrane function is disrupted by inhibiting sterol (ergosterol) synthesis in fungi. Used for superficial treatment of mycosis such as the "tineas."	May cause burning at the site of application, skin reactions, or ulcerations. Also, may cause headache, GI disturbance, liver function test abnormalities, taste abnormalities, and rarely liver failure or neutropenia.
Teriparatide	Forteo	A parathyroid hormone agonist used in the management of postmenopausal osteoporosis.	May cause pain, transient increases in calcium levels, headaches, dizziness, arthralgias, myalgias, leg cramps, rash, or swelling.
Tetracycline	Achromycin	A synthetic broad-spectrum antibiotic that is bacteriostatic (inhibits protein synthesis by binding to 30s sub-unit, blocking amino acid-linked tRNA from binding to the A site of the ribosome). Susceptible bacteria include *M. pneumoniae*, *C. psittaci*, *C. trachomatis*, and *N. gonorrhea*. Used for respiratory infections, nongonococcal urethritis (ureaplasma), Rocky Mountain spotted fever, typhus, chancroid, anthrax, syphilis, cholera, brucellosis, chlamydia, acne, and Lyme disease. Doxycycline approved for malaria prophylaxis.	GI distress, reversible nephro- and hepatotoxicity, photosensitivity, and dental staining (not used in prepubertal children).
Theophylline	Bronkodyl Elixophyllin Pulmophylline Slo-Bid Slo-phyllin Somophyllin Theo-Dur Theospan Uni-Dur	A xanthine derivative that causes the relaxation of smooth muscle, stimulates the medullary respiratory center and the myocardium. Used primarily in the management of bronchospasm and prophylactic and acute attacks of asthma. Also may be used for edema associated with CHF.	May cause gastric upset, irritability, anorexia, abdominal pain, dizziness, headache, drug-induced seizures, palpitations, tachycardia, albuminuria, fever, dehydration, and rarely respiratory arrest.
Timolol	Blocadren	Beta-blocker: Blocks both β1 and β2 adrenergic receptors, decreasing heart rate and rennin release. Used in the treatment of hypertension. Also has bronchoconstriction effect due to β2 blockade.	CNS depressive effects with concerns for those with diabetes, heart block and heart failure, asthma, and emphysema. Transient hypertension due to blockage of β2 receptors (which normally dilate large arteries).
Tiotropium	Spiriva	A once-a-day inhaled anticholinergic specific for muscarinic receptors used in the management of bronchospasm associated with COPD.	May cause dry mouth, constipation, increased heart rate, blurred vision, glaucoma, or urinary difficulty.
Tolterodine	Detrol Detrol A	A synthetic amine used for neurogenic bladder or detrusor instability (unstable bladder). Effects are antispasmodic through inhibition of muscarinic effect of acetylcholine on smooth muscle.	May cause drowsiness, blurred vision, dry mouth, constipation, urinary hesitation, dizziness, weakness, or skin rash.

(continues)

Table B–8 Some Common Medications (Listed by Generic Name) (continued)

Name	Examples	Mechanism/Use	Some Side Effects/Concerns
Topiramate	Topamax	May affect GABA or kainate/AMPA receptors. Used in the treatment of partial seizures.	May cause ataxia, dizziness, and speech and psychomotor impairment.
Tramadol	Ultram	Tramadol and its main metabolite bind to μ-opioid receptors. Also reduces uptake of norepinephrine and serotonin. A pain reliever that is similar in action to narcotics with less of a risk for addiction or abuse.	May cause constipation, dizziness, nausea/vomiting, headache, and pruritus.
Tranylcypromine	Parnate	A MAO inhibitor used as a last-choice treatment for those unresponsive to other MAO in the management of depression.	May cause orthostatic hypotension, dry mouth, dizziness, anorexia, blurred vision, tremors, or muscle twitching. Caution for hypertensive crisis when ingesting foods containing tyramine.
Trastuzumab	Herceptin	Monoclonal antibody antineoplastic used in the treatment of metastatic breast cancer for tumors that overexpress HER2 proteins.	May cause anaphylaxis, pain, fever, abdominal pain, diarrhea, congestive heart failure, insomnia, dizziness, or headache.
Trazodone	Desyrel	Inhibits the reuptake of dopamine, serotonin, and norepinephrine with the major affect on serotonin. Used in the treatment of depression and also for aggressive disorders.	May cause a decrease in appetite, rash, hypertension, or shortness of breath.
Triamcinolone	Aristocort Atolone Kenacort Kenalog-E Aristospan Cenocort Triam-Forte Articulose Trilone Tristoject	A corticosteroid with anti-inflammatory and anti-rheumatic effects. Aerosol version commonly used in the management of asthma. A spacer is used with the inhaler to prevent possible Candida infection of the mouth. With the inhaled version the usual side effects associated with long-term glucocorticoid use are not seen, partially due to the clearance on first pass through the liver.	With injectable type may have Cushing's-like features, growth retardation, hyperglycemia, carbohydrate intolerance, nausea, vomiting, headache, euphoria, muscle weakness, osteoporosis, aseptic necrosis of bone, and delayed wound healing.
Triamterene	Dyrenium	Blocks action of aldosterone by competing with receptor sites in distal renal tubules. Used as a diuretic. It has direct effects on distal renal tubules to prevent excretion of potassium. Decreases glomerular filtration rate and increases BUN. Used in the management of CHF and other forms of edema, and adjunct therapy for hypertension.	May cause hyperkalemia and other electrolyte imbalances, anaphylaxis, some blood dyscrasias, GI disturbances, gout, rash, or hypotension.
Triazolam	Halcyon	A benzodiazepine derivative that has hypnotic effects through blocking of limbic and cortical arousal. Used for short-term management of sleep dysfunction.	May cause drowsiness, rebound insomnia, memory impairment and antegrade amnesia, GI symptoms, headache, or dizziness.
Trimethoprim-Sulfamethoxazole	Bactrim Septra Co-Trimoxazole	A combination drug that acts as a synthetic folate antagonist acting as an enzyme inhibitor preventing bacterial synthesis. Used with *Pneumocystis carinii* pneumonitis, *Shigella* enteritis, and UTI caused by Enterobacteriaceae.	Possible toxic epidermal necrosis syndrome, pseudomembranous colitis, agranulocytosis, aplastic anemia (rare), and anorexia, nausea, and skin rash. May elevate liver enzymes and bilirubin.

Table B–8 Some Common Medications (Listed by Generic Name) (continued)

Name	Examples	Mechanism/Use	Some Side Effects/Concerns
Valacyclovir	Valtrex	An antiviral medication that interferes with viral DNA synthesis. Due to increased GI absorption, plasma levels are higher than acyclovir. Use for the treatment of herpes zoster (shingles) and recurrent genital herpes.	May cause headache, weakness, fatigue, nausea, vomiting, dyspepsia, abdominal pain, renal damage, or allergic reactions.
Valproic acid	Depacon	Possible augmentation of GABA neurotransmission. Used in the treatment of all seizure types.	Severe hepatotoxicity possible, thrombocytopenia, and hyperammonemia.
Vancomycin	Vancocin Vancoled	An antibiotic that interferes with cell membrane synthesis. Primarily for Gram-positive. Organisms include beta-hemolytic streptococci, staphylococci, pneumococci, enterococci, clostridia, and corynebacteria.	Is ototoxic and nephrotoxic. May cause anaphylaxis and hypersensitivity reactions, "red neck" syndrome with IV administration, thrombophlebitis, super-infections, and transient leucopenia and eosinophilia.
Vardenafil HCL	Levitra	Used in the management of erectile dysfunction in men. It acts as an enzyme blocker for phosphodiesterase type 5 (PDE-5), which results in increased blood flow to the penis.	May cause headache, facial flushing, indigestion, and nasal decongestion. Contraindicated for those with heart problems or HTN.
Vasopressin	Pitressin	An extracted animal hormone from the posterior pituitary that has primarily an antidiuretic effect (no oxytocin effect). Effect is primarily due to increasing tubular reabsorption of water, creating a concentrated urine. Used in the management of diabetes insipidus, for dissipation of gas shadows on abdominal films, or reducing abdominal distention postsurgically. Has also been used as intranasal spray for maintenance treatment of diabetes insipidus and sometimes for enuresis.	Small doses may cause angina or MI and aggravate other preexisting heart conditions. May cause headache, water intoxication, and anaphylaxis, among other common drug side effects.
Varenicline	Chantix	Used in the management of smoking cessation. It is a partial agonist for alpha-1, beta-2 nicotinic acetylcholine receptors.	Is ototoxic and nephrotoxic. May cause anaphylaxis and hypersensitivity reactions, "red neck" syndrome with IV administration, thrombophlebitis, super-infections, and transient leucopenia and eosinophilia.
Verapamil HCL	Calan Covera Isoptin Verelan	A calcium channel blocker that decreases vasoconstriction (especially coronaries) and slow conduction at SA and AV nodes. Used in the management of Prinzmetal (variant) angina and various arrhythmias.	May cause headache, AV block, hypotension, constipation, elevated liver enzymes, or syncope.
Warfarin	Coumadin Panwarfin Warfilone	An anticoagulant that decreases the synthesis of vitamin K-dependent coagulation factors. Similar to heparin but actions are accumulative and prolonged. Used prophylactically for embolic and thromboembolic conditions such as deep vein thrombosis, transient ischemic attacks, prosthetic valves, pulmonary embolism, and atrial fibrillation with embolization.	May cause bleeding at any site. Caution when adjusting patients on Warfarin due to subarachnoid bleeds, bruising of skin, and other potential bleeding sites. May also cause anorexia, abdominal cramps, diarrhea, and may increase liver enzymes.

(continues)

Table B–8 Some Common Medications (Listed by Generic Name) (continued)

Name	Examples	Mechanism/Use	Some Side Effects/Concerns
Zafirlukast	Accolate	An oral leukotriene receptor antagonist. Leukotrienes are pro-inflammatory chemicals derived from arachidonic acid. Blocks the binding of leukotriene types D4 (LTD4) and E4 (LTE4). Used in the treatment of asthma, decreasing the inflammatory aspect of asthma.	May cause headache, GI distress, and an increase in respiratory infection in older patients.
Zidovudine	Retrovir (AZT)	When entering the host cell it is converted to triphosphate by thymidine kinase. It is then incorporated into DNA chains by reverse transcriptase, disrupting cell replication. Used in the treatment of HIV infections.	Causes many GI complaints, headache, fever, malaise, myalgia, dizziness, cough and wheezing, and bone marrow suppression.
Zoledronic Acid	Zometa	Used for hypercalcemia associated with metastasis, multiple myeloma, and Paget's. Blocks osteoclastic resorption of bone and release of calcium.	May cause fever, nausea, vomiting, abdominal or chest pain, leg edema, hypos (calcium, potassium, sodium), or pancytopenia.
Zolpidem	Ambien	A nonbenzodiazepine hypnotic medication with no muscle relaxation or anticonvulsant effects used in the short-term management of insomnia.	May cause headache upon waking, lethargy, fatigue, depression, anxiety, irritability, or dizziness. With doses greater than 10 mg, may report antegrade amnesia or memory impairment.

Table B–9 Alphabetical Listing by Product Name for Medications in Table B–8

Drug Name	Located on Page	Drug Name	Located on Page	Drug Name	Located on Page
A.S.A.	1254	Aristocort	1280	C.E.S.	1262
A/T/S/E-Mycin	1261	Aristospan	1280	Calan	1281
Abatacept	1251	Articulose	1280	Canesten	1258
Abelcet	1253	Aspergum	1254	Captopril	1255
Absorbocarpine	1273	AsthmaHaler	1261	Carafate	1277
Accolate	1282	AsthmaNefrin	1261	Carbatrol	1255
Achromycin	1279	Atarax	1265	Catapres	1257
Actonel	1276	Ativan	1268	Celebrex	1256
Acycloguanosine	1252	Atolone	1280	Celexa	1257
Adalat	1271	Aventyl	1271	Cenestins	1262
Adapin	1260	Avonex	1266	Cenocort	1280
Adipex-P	1273	Axura	1269	Chibroxin	1271
Aeroseb-Dex	1259	Azulfidine	1278	Chlorofair	1256
Akne-Mycin	1261	Bactrim	1280	Chloromycetin	1256
Alba-Dex	1259	Balminil	1259	Chlorpromanine	1256
Aldactone	1277	Banophen	1260	Cholestabyl	1258
Aldomet	1269	Barbital	1273	Cialis	1278
Alesse	1262	Bayer	1254	Cibalith-S	1268
Alestacon	1269	Baygam	1266	Cipro	1257

Table B–9 Alphabetical Listing by Product Name for Medications in Table B–8 (continued)

Drug Name	Located on Page	Drug Name	Located on Page	Drug Name	Located on Page
Aleve	1270	Belix	1260	Claritin	1268
Alka-Seltzer	1254	Benadryl	1260	Claritin RediTab	1268
Allerdryl	1260	Benahist	1260	Clinoril	1278
Alloprin	1252	Ben-Allergin	1260	Clonazepam	1257
Alupent	1270	Benemid	1274	Clopidogrel	1258
Ambien	1282	Benuryl	1274	Cognex	1278
Amcil	1253	Benylin	1259	Colace	1260
Amlodipine/Atorvastatin	1253	Benzylpenicillin	1272	Colestid	1258
Amoxil	1253	Betaseron	1266	Compazine	1274
Amphocin	1253	Bevacizumab	1254	Corgard	1270
Amphotec	1253	Bicillin	1272	Cosprin	1254
Anaprox	1270	Bio-Tropin	1277	Co-Trimoxazole	1280
Anexsia	1256	Bisacolax	1254	Coumadin	1281
Antegren	1271	Black Draught	1276	Covera	1281
Antilirium	1273	Blocadren	1279	Crinone Gel	1274
Antivert	1269	Bonamine	1269	Cryptocillin	1272
Atrazine	1269	Botulinum Toxin Type A	1255	Cuprimine	1272
Apo-Bisacodyl	1254	Bretylate	1255	Cyclamen	1259
Apo-Erythro Base	1261	Bretylol	1255	Cyclosporine	1258
Apo-Flurazepam	1264	Bromitin Mist	1261	Cycloflex	1258
Apo-Naproxen	1270	Bronkaid Mist	1261	Cylert	1272
Aricept	1260	Bronkodyl	1279	Cytomel	1268
Aripiprazole	1253	Dutasteride	1261	Dalalone	1259
Danocrine	1259	Dyrenium	1280	Dalmane	1264
Darvon	1275	Easprin	1254	Fumide	1264
Decaderm	1259	Ecotrin	1254	Fungizone	1253
Decadron	1259	Elavil	1253	Fungoid	1270
Decaspray	1259	Eldepryl	1276	Furomide	1264
Deficol	1254	Elixophyllin	1279	Gamimune	1266
Delsym	1259	Eltroxin	1267	Gammagard	1266
Demerol	1269	Enbrel	1262	Gammar P	1266
Demulen	1262	Empirin	1254	Gantrisin	1278
Depacon	1281	Enalapril	1261	Garamycin	1264
Depen	1272	Endep	1253	Gastrocrom	1258
Deronil	1259	Enlon	1261	Gengraf	1258
Desenex	1270	Entrophen	1254	Genoptic	1264
Desogen	1262	Epi E-Z Pen	1261	Genotropin	1277
Desyrel	1280	Epinephrine	1261	Gentlax	1276
Dethasone	1274	Epitrate	1261	Gesterol	1274
Detrol	1279	Epogen	1261	Glucophage	1269
Detrol A	1279	Eprex	1261	Glucophage XR	1269

(continues)

Table B–9 Alphabetical Listing by Product Name for Medications in Table B–8 (continued)

Drug Name	Located on Page	Drug Name	Located on Page	Drug Name	Located on Page
Dexasone	1259	Eryderm	1261	Glucotrol	1264
Dexedrine	1259	Ery-Tab	1261	Glucotrol XL	1264
Dexone	1259	Erythrocin	1261	Glynase	1264
DiaBeta	1264	Erythromid	1261	Gyne-Lotrimin	1258
Dichlor	1256	Eskalith	1268	Halcyon	1280
Diahist	1260	Estratab	1262	Haldol	1265
Dialose	1260	Eszopiclone	1262	H-BIG	1265
Diazepam	1259	Euglucon	1264	Hepalean	1265
Didronel	1263	Evista	1275	Heparin	1265
Dilantin	1273	Exelon	1276	Hep-B-Gammagee	1265
Dilaudid	1265	Ezetimibe and Simvastatin	1263	Hep-Lock	1265
Dilaudid-HP	1265	Ezetimibe	1263	Hexadrol	1259
Dilocaine	1268	Fastin	1273	Humalog (RCA)	1266
Diphenatol	1259	Femizole	1270	Humatrope	1277
Disodium cromoglycate	1258	Fenicol	1256	Humira	1252
Dispose-a-Med	1267	Fexofenadine	1263	Humulin	1266
Ditropan	1272	Fivent	1258	Hydrin	1279
Ditropan XL	1272	Flagyl	1270	Hydrocil	1275
Diuril	1256	Fleet	1254	Hyoscine	1276
Dizmiss	1270	Flexeril	1258	HyperHEP	1265
Dopar	1267	Flonase	1264	Ibandronate	1265
Drospirenone and Estradiol	1260	Fluticasone	1264	Iletin II	1266
Dulcolax	1254	Fluticasone Propionate with Salmeterol	1264	Illocyin	1262
Duloxetine	1260	Fosamax	1252	Imipramine	1265
Durapam	1264	L-Caine	1268	Medrol	1274
Imitrex	1278	Lestid	1258	Megacillin	1272
Imodium	1268	Levitra	1281	Menest	1262
Indameth	1266	Levlite	1262	Menrium	1262
Inderal	1274	Levora	1262	Mestinon	1275
Indocid	1266	Levothroid	1267	Metamucil	1275
Indocin	1266	Levoxyl	1267	Methylmorphine	1258
Indocin SR	1266	Libritabs	1256	Methylphenidate	1269
Infergen	1266	Librium	1256	Metizol	1270
INH	1266	Lidopen	1268	Metro-Gel	1270
Instant	1275	Lipo-Hepin	1265	Mevacor	1268
Intal	1258	Lipitor	1254	Micatin	1270
Invinex	1276	Liquaemin	1265	Micronase	1264
Ionamin	1273	Liquid Pred	1274	Midamor	1253
Isoptin	1281	Lithane	1268	Minims Pilocarpine	1273
Isopto Carpine	1273	Lithobid	1268	Minipress	1274
Isotamine	1266	Lithonate	1268	Miocarpine	1273

Table B–9 Alphabetical Listing by Product Name for Medications in Table B–8 (continued)

Drug Name	Located on Page	Drug Name	Located on Page	Drug Name	Located on Page
Isuprel	1267	Lo-CHOLEST	1257	Modane Bulk	1275
Iveegam	1266	Lodosyn	1255	Monistat (Derm, 3, 7)	1270
Jenest	1262	Loestrin	1262	Montelukast	1270
Kabikinase	1277	Lofene	1259	Murocoll	1276
Kaopectate	1267	Lomanate	1259	Mycelex	1258
Kaospan	1267	Lomotil	1259	Mycostatin	1271
Karasil	1275	Lomox	1259	Mymethasone	1259
Kariva	1262	Lopid	1264	Myochrysine	1265
Keflex	1256	Lopressor	1270	M-Zole	1270
Keftabs	1256	Lopurin	1252	Nadostine	1271
Kenacort	1280	Lorcet	1265	Namenda	1269
Kenalog-E	1280	Lorcet Plus	1265	Naprolen	1270
Kestrone	1262	Losec	1272	Naprosyn	1270
Kaolin w/Pectin	1267	Lotrimin	1258	Nardil	1273
Konsyl	1275	Lotronex	1252	NasalCrom	1258
Lamisil	1279	Low-Quel	1259	Necon	1262
Lamisil DermGel	1279	Luminal	1273	Neo-Estrone	1262
Lamictal	1267	Luramide	1264	Neoral	1258
Laniazid	1266	Maalox Antidiarrheal	1268	Nervocaine	1268
Lanoxicaps	1259	Marcaine	1255	Neurontin	1264
Lanoxin	1259	Marezine	1258	Nexium	1261
Lantus (RCA)	1266	Marzine	1258	NiAc	1271
Largactil	1256	Medilium	1256	Nicobid	1271
Larodopa	1267	Mediquell	1259	Nicolar	1271
Larotid	1253	Paraflex	1257	Nilstat	1271
Lasix	1264	Parafon-Forte	1257	Promapar	1256
Laxit	1254	Parlodel	1255	Promaz	1256
Nizoral	1267	Parnate	1280	Prometrium	1274
Nolvadex	1278	Paveral	1258	Pronestyl	1274
Norco	1265	Paxil	1272	Propecia	1263
Nordene	1262	Pediapred Oral Liquid	1274	Propyl-Thyracil	1275
Norditropin	1277	Penbritin	1253	Proscar	1263
Nordryl	1260	Pentids	1272	Prostigmin	1271
Noritate	1270	Pepcid	1263	Protostat	1270
Nor-Mil	1259	Pepto-Bismol	1255	Proventil	1252
Normodyne	1267	Pepto Diarrhea Control	1268	Prozac	1264
Noroxin	1271	Peptol	1257	Pulmophylline	1279
Novocain	1274	Percolone	1272	Questran	1257
Nolvadex-D	1278	Per Diem Plain	1275	Rebif	1266
NovoLog (RCA)	1266	Peridol	1265	Reginol	1257
Novasen	1254	Permapen	1272	Regulax	1260
Novochloroscap	1256	Pertussin	1259	Reguloid	1275

(continues)

Table B–9 Alphabetical Listing by Product Name for Medications in Table B–8 (continued)

Drug Name	Located on Page	Drug Name	Located on Page	Drug Name	Located on Page
Novo-Cimetine	1257	Pethadol	1269	Remicade	1266
Novocolchine	1258	Pethidine HCL	1269	Resectisol	1269
Novoflupam	1264	Pfizerpen	1272	Retrovir (AZT)	1282
Novo-Niacin	1271	Pilocar	1273	Reversol	1261
Novo-Poxide	1257	Pitressin	1281	Rheumatrex	1269
Novopropoxyn	1275	Platinol	1257	Ritalin	1269
Novopurinol	1252	Plavix	1258	Robimycin	1261
Novo-Rythro	1261	PMS Docusate	1260	Romalar	1259
Novospiroton	1277	Polymox	1253	Ropinirole	1276
Novolin	1266	Pravachol	1274	Rosiglitazone Maleate	1276
Nutropin	1277	Prednisolone	1274	Roxicodone	1272
Nyaderm	1271	Pregabalin	1274	Ru-Vert	1269
Nydrazid	1266	Premarin	1262	Rynacrom	1258
Nystex	1271	Prevalite	1257	S.A.S.-500	1278
Nytol with DPM	1260	Prilosec	1272	Salazopyrin	1278
Obenix	1273	Primacor	1270	Saizen	1277
Oby-Trim	1273	Primatene Mist	1261	Sandimmune	1258
Octocaine	1268	Probalan	1274	Sandoglobulin	1266
Ocusert	1273	Procan	1274	Sansert	1270
Ogestrel	1262	Procanbid	1274	Savacort-D	1259
Omnipen	1253	Procardia	1272	Senexon	1276
Ormazine	1256	Procrit	1261	Senokot	1276
Ortho-Cept	1262	Progens	1262	Senolax	1276
Osmitrol	1269	Progestaject	1274	Sensorcaine	1255
OxyContin	1272	Tegretol-XR	1255	Venoglobulin	1266
Oxyfast	1272	Tenormin	1254	Ventolin	1252
Pamelor	1271	Tensilon	1261	Varenicline	1281
Panwarfin	1281	Teriparatide	1279	Verelan	1281
Septra	1280	Tetterine	1270	Viagra	1277
Sereen	1256	Theodur	1279	Vibramycin	1260
Serevent	1276	Theospan	1279	Vicodin	1265
Serostim	1277	Theralax	1254	Vicodin ES	1265
Serpalan	1275	Therevac	1260	Vioxx	1276
Serutan	1275	Thorazine	1256	Vistacon	1265
Silybon	1275	Thor-Prom	1256	Vistacrom	1258
Sinemet	1255	Tiotropium	1279	Vistaject	1265
Sinequan	1269	Topamax	1280	Vistaril	1265
SK-Chlorothiazide	1256	Toprol XL	1270	V-Lax	1275
SK-Reserpine	1275	Totacillin	1253	Warfilone	1281
Slo-Bid	1279	Trandate	1267	Wellbutrin	1255
Slo-Phyllin	1279	Trastuzumab	1280	Wellbutrin SR	1255
Solifenacin	1277	Trexall	1269	Wellferon	1266

Table B–9 Alphabetical Listing by Product Name for Medications in Table B–8 (continued)

Drug Name	Located on Page	Drug Name	Located on Page	Drug Name	Located on Page
Solfoton	1273	Triadapin	1260	Wycillin	1272
Somazina	1256	Triam-Forte	1280	Xanax	1252
Somophyllin	1279	Triaphen-10	1254	Xenical	1272
St. Joseph's	1254	Trilone	1280	Xylocaine	1268
Staticin	1261	Trimox	1253	Xylocard	1268
Stemetil	1275	Triostat	1268	Zantac	1275
Strattera	1254	Triphasil	1262	Zarontin	1263
Streptase	1277	Triptone	1276	Zelnorm	1278
Streptomycin	1277	Tristoject	1280	Zestril	1268
Sulcrate	1277	Trivora	1262	Zithromax	1254
Sulfasalazine	1278	T-Stat	1261	Zocor	1263, 1277
Surfak	1260	Ultram	1280	Zoledronic Acid	1282
Syllac	1275	Uni-Dur	1279	Zoloft	1277
Symmetrel	1253	Unithroid	1267	Zolpidem Tartrate	1282
Synthroid	1267	Valacyclovir	1281	Zonalon	1260
Tadalafil	1278	Valdrene	1260	ZORprin	1254
Tagamet	1257	Valium	1259	Zovirax	1252
Talwin	1273	Vancocin	1281	Zyban	1255
Talwin NX	1273	Vancoled	1281	Zyloprim	1255
Tamofen	1278	Vasotec	1261		
Tamsulosin	1278				
Tapazole	1269				
Teebaconin	1266				
Tegretol	1255				

more extensive information on these and other medications. This table is intended to serve as a quick reference guide. Further information should be sought from more comprehensive sources available.

References

1. IMS Institute for Healthcare Informatics. The use of medicines in the United States: review of 2011. 2012.

2. Gu Q, Dillon CF, Burt VL. Prescription drug use continues to increase: U.S. prescription drug data for 2007-2008. *NCHS Data Brief*. Sep 2010(42):1–8.

3. Rodriguez-Fragoso L, Martinez-Arismendi JL, Orozco-Bustos D, Reyes-Esparza J, Torres E, Burchiel SW. Potential risks resulting from fruit/vegetable-drug interactions: effects on drug-metabolizing enzymes and drug transporters. *J Food Sci*. 2011;76(4):R112–124.

4. Manchikanti L, Helm S, 2nd, Fellows B, et al. Opioid epidemic in the United States. *Pain Physician*. 2012;15(3 Suppl):ES9–38.

5. McBride JT. The association of acetaminophen and asthma prevalence and severity. *Pediatrics*. 2011;128(6):1181–1185.

6. Watkins PB, Kaplowitz N, Slattery JT, et al. Aminotransferase elevations in healthy adults receiving 4 grams of acetaminophen daily: a randomized controlled trial. *JAMA*. 2006;296(1):87–93.

7. Curhan SG, Eavey R, Shargorodsky J, Curhan GC. Analgesic use and the risk of hearing loss in men. *Am J Med*. Mar 2010;123(3):231–237.

8. Curhan SG, Shargorodsky J, Eavey R, Curhan GC. Analgesic use and the risk of hearing loss in women. *Am J Epidemiol.* 2012;176(6):544–554.

9. Dagenais S, Haldeman S, eds. *Evidence-Based Management of Low Back Pain.* St. Louis, Elsevier; 2012:134.

10. Abrahamsen B, Vestergaard P. Proton pump inhibitor use and fracture risk—effect modification by histamine H1 receptor blockade. Observational case-control study using National Prescription Data. *Bone.* 2013;57(1):269–271.

11. Gill SK, O'Brien L, Einarson TR, Koren G. The safety of proton pump inhibitors (PPIs) in pregnancy: a meta-analysis. *Am J Gastroenterol.* 2009;104(6): 1541–1545; quiz 1540, 1546.

12. Canani RB, Cirillo P, Roggero P, et al. Therapy with gastric acidity inhibitors increases the risk of acute gastroenteritis and community-acquired pneumonia in children. *Pediatrics.* 2006;117(5):e817–820.

13. Black DM, Greenspan SL, Ensrud KE, et al. The effects of parathyroid hormone and alendronate alone or in combination in postmenopausal osteoporosis. *N Engl J Med.* 2003;349:1207–1215.

14. Finkelstein JS, Hayes A, Hunzelman JL, et al. Effects of parathyroid hormone, alendronate, or both in men with osteoporosis. *N Engl J Med.* 2003;349:1216–1226.

15. Neer RM, Arnaud CD, Zanchetta JR, et al. Effect of parathyroid hormone (I-34) on fracture and bone mineral density in postmenopausal women with osteoporosis. *N Engl J Med.* 2001;344:1434–1441.

16. LaCroix AZ, Cauley JA, Pettinger M, et al. Statin use, clinical fracture, and bone density in postmenopausal women: results from the Women's Initiative Observational Study. *Ann Int Med.* 2003;139:97–104.

INDEX

Note: Page numbers followed by *f* or *t* indicate material in figures or tables respectively. Page numbers in italics denote exhibits.